Carvers' Medical Imaging

Carvers' Medical Imaging

THIRD EDITION

Edited by

Elizabeth Carver, BSc(Hons), DCR(R), FAETC
Teaching Fellow,
Former Clinical Education Lead (Radiography),
Former Director of Student Experience for School of Health Sciences,
Bangor University,
Bangor, UK

Barry Carver, PgDipCT, PGCE, DCR(R)
Teaching Fellow,
Former Director of Radiography,
Bangor University,
Bangor, UK

Karen Knapp, BSc (Hons), PCAP, PgC, PhD, SFHEA
Associate Professor in Musculoskeletal Imaging,
Head of Medical Imaging,
Medical Imaging, University of Exeter,
Exeter, UK

Foreword by

Jonathan McNulty, BSc (Hons) Radiography, H.Dip. MRI, PhD
Associate Professor,
Associate Dean, School of Medicine,
Vice Principal for Teaching and Learning,
College of Health and Agricultural Sciences,
Fellow in Teaching and Academic Development,
University College Dublin,
Dublin, Ireland

ELSEVIER London New York Oxford Philadelphia St Louis Sydney 2021

First edition 2006
Second edition 2012
Third edition 2021

Notices

Practitioners and researchers must always rely on their own experience and knowledge in evaluating and using any information, methods, compounds or experiments described herein. Because of rapid advances in the medical sciences, in particular, independent verification of diagnoses and drug dosages should be made. To the fullest extent of the law, no responsibility is assumed by Elsevier, authors, editors or contributors for any injury and/or damage to persons or property as a matter of products liability, negligence or otherwise, or from any use or operation of any methods, products, instructions, or ideas contained in the material herein.

ISBN: 978-0-7020-6955-0

Content Strategist: Poppy Garraway/Trinity Hutton
Content Development Specialist: Veronika Watkins
Project Manager: Anne Collett
Design: Ryan Cook
Illustration Manager: Anitha Rajarathnam

Printed in the UK

Last digit is the print number: 9 8 7 6 5 4 3 2

Contents

Foreword

Carvers' Medical Imaging has established itself as a core or listed text for radiographic practice in institutions right around the world. This is testament to the efforts to enhance the text with each successive edition. Now retired from their leadership roles in radiography education, Elizabeth and Barry Carver, with renowned radiography educator and researcher Karen Knapp joining the editorial team, have once again managed to enhance what was already an essential textbook in this, the third edition. The editors have once again provided an opportunity for clinical radiographers, including many advanced practitioners, consultant radiographers, and academic radiographers, to contribute to a textbook for the first time. This approach helps ensure that fresh perspectives run throughout the chapters. It was for these reasons that I had no hesitation in agreeing to author this foreword for the third edition of *Carvers' Medical Imaging*.

One glance at the list of authors and the table of contents makes it immediately evident why this text will be a much used, and much relied on, resource for radiography students from the beginning of their studies, on to their graduation, and throughout their professional careers. The structure and content of this text also make it an accessible and useful resource for assistant practitioners, radiology trainees, medical students considering a future career in radiology, and medical physicists looking to gain a better insight into clinical applications and techniques.

The 30 chapters which comprise the third edition cover the essential topics of digital imaging, radiation dose, image quality, and preliminary clinical evaluation (PCE) before moving through all aspects of general radiography, including dedicated chapters on radiography in the emergency department, mobile and theatre radiography, and paediatric radiography. The text then moves on to the topic of contrast agents, specialist imaging of the gastrointestinal and genitourinary systems, vascular and interventional procedures, and breast imaging, concluding with chapters introducing computed tomography, magnetic resonance imaging, nuclear medicine, ultrasound, and DXA. In each of these chapters the expertise of the authors, and their passion and enthusiasm for their particular topic, is evident as one journeys throughout the text. All chapters are clearly well-researched and supported by extensive reference lists for those who wish to dive deeper into topics.

Of note is the incorporation of PCE in this edition, in Chapter 3, across the general radiography chapters, and for paediatric radiography. Illustrative PCE comments are provided throughout, and the impact of common errors on PCE comments or reports has now also been captured in the established 'common errors' tables in each chapter. This reflects the fact that PCE, and radiographer reporting, are now generally very well established across the UK, and will also be of interest to radiographers beyond the UK who are contributing to efforts to move beyond red dot and formally implement PCE and, potentially, full radiographer reporting.

Chapters 4 through 19 are much more than a simple '*how to examine the ..(insert body part)*' guide, with consideration throughout given to technique adaptations, problem-solving, and clinical decision-making. Chapters provide very clear descriptions of radiographic techniques and include excellent figures, photographs, radiographs, and diagrams to guide the reader. The layout within these chapters lends itself to quick reviews of key information when looking to refresh your mind or find solutions.

The paediatric radiography section is an excellent resource for radiographers with limited paediatric experience or those not working in a specialist paediatric centre. The gastrointestinal and genitourinary chapters are nicely presented and remain valuable resources, reminding us of the continued utility of these examinations alongside advanced imaging modalities. Again, the presentation within these chapters, together with the excellent figures and illustrations, make these chapters extremely practical for both students and clinicians alike.

Chapters 23 through 30 manage to provide us with the history of each modality, physical principles, technologies, safety considerations, clinical applications, and practical technique considerations. A new section on DXA is another excellent, and most welcome, addition to the third edition. This topic, often overlooked in medical imaging textbooks, has been authored by Karen Knapp and serves us all as a reminder of the important role DXA plays in evaluating bone health, and why this modality should not be neglected.

I have thoroughly enjoyed reading through this textbook where the editors, and authors, have done a fantastic job in making sure the third edition of *Carvers' Medical Imaging* remains a must have reference text for all educational institutions and for all clinical departments.

Dr. Jonathan McNulty
Dublin 2021

Preface

The developing role of the radiographer has meant that updating our book does not just apply to the techniques and procedures themselves. When our first edition was released, diagnostic radiographers had long been undertaking barium studies and administering intravenous contrast agents, but since then we have seen an explosion of role development in so many areas of our profession. A huge change has been how widespread the use of reporting radiographers has become, and in many Trusts radiographer reporting is now the norm; what a change from the dark ages when very knowledgeable radiographers weren't even allowed to say if an image was abnormal or normal! Then came 'red dot' systems and at last we were able to at least show that we had recognised a potential abnormality, followed by the first reporting radiographers some years later. We have no doubt that the hard work and success of reporting radiographers directly led to widespread implementation of preliminary clinical evaluation (PCE) as a regular part of clinical practice, and its inclusion in undergraduate courses; for this reason we realised that information on PCE was vital if this edition was to move forward and reflect current clinical practice.

It was clear from the beginning that there were excellent resources in terms of textbooks dedicated to image reporting, plus interactive courses (such as the Norwich Image Interpretation Course) and we didn't want to try to replace these, we just wanted to make sure there was a summary of examination-relevant checks in addition to those generic checks that relate to bone and cortical outlines, trabecular patterns, soft tissue outlines and recognition of normal versus abnormal anatomy. Since we now have a fabulous resource available to us in the form of reporting radiographers, it is the perfect time to press forward with including what we call 'PCE Comments' for the most commonly undertaken examinations. Indeed, the only areas that don't carry PCE comments are for rarely undertaken examinations, or those that are not normally commented upon by the radiographer undertaking the examination. For this edition we have welcomed (and thank most profusely) many reporting radiographers to our team, either as authors or advisors; for most, it is the first time they will see their name in a book. We hope that the text will become a well-used bench book in imaging departments, and that it will be used as reference and support by radiographers who are undertaking PCE as independent practitioners.

Another development of the text has been to add to the 'common errors' sections of each chapter, and include what impact each error has upon the accuracy of the report or PCE; again, we thank the reporting radiographers who contributed to this change. It's been our dream for a long time to include this as part of our message on image quality; we believe that it's a vital tool in emphasising why quality criteria must be adhered to wherever possible, and hope that the inclusion of this new aspect will help maintain high standards in image production.

Advanced and consultant radiographers have assisted with the general radiography sections of this edition for the first time; previous editions have used advanced and consultant practitioners for breast imaging, paediatrics, GI, CT, MRI, RNI and ultrasound, and for this edition we welcome new experts via our new inclusions: GI bariatric imaging, proctography, DXA scanning, and theatre and mobiles.

Writing about our new contributors brings to mind the authors who have worked on this book over the three editions: including ourselves, 50 people have written or advised on chapters since 2006 and of those 50, 38 are new authors who will have seen their name in a published book for the first time. Helping so many new authors to write and work through the publication process has been an amazing experience and such an honour for us; we hope our exacting editing demands haven't been too annoying!

For this edition we have been extremely pleased to welcome Karen Knapp on board as co-editor; her contribution to our profession was well known to us before we joined forces and we've had a fabulous time working with her, and her commitment, enthusiasm and excellent work ethic have been invaluable. We hope that she continues to work as editor in future editions. Thanks so much, Karen, it's been a blast!

Since the last edition we have been so saddened by the passing of a much-loved author and colleague, Darren Wood. Darren wrote several chapters in our first two editions and his knowledge of advanced practice in GI imaging was vital to the success of the first edition in particular. Darren's professional path crossed ours for over 30 years, from when he was a student, then as clinical supervisor and assessor of students, as author and later as colleague at Bangor University. He was always a dependable and supportive colleague, with a cheerful and often cheeky disposition; he will be very much missed.

We're so very proud to have been part of this fantastic profession and especially because of the way in which radiographers have not only seized the opportunity to take on new roles, but also because they have made such a success of them. At a recent international conference we attended it became clear, during end-of-session questions and discussion, that the rest of Europe has been long wishing to emulate the UK radiographer, simply because of our extended range of capabilities, opportunities and status as practitioners. We have also heard a visiting radiologist (based outside the UK) at a CT study day comment to UK radiologists: 'You have such high-quality radiographers to work with in the UK; you don't know how lucky you are.'

To close, we must give our appreciation for the unquestioning dedication of radiographers who have worked selflessly and, as a profession, almost anonymously to provide diagnostic imaging on every Covid-positive patient during the COVID-19 pandemic. And of course, you continued to provide an excellent service for all other patients.

– be proud, people, be proud.

Elizabeth and Barry Carver
Stoke on Trent, 2021

It's been an absolute pleasure to join Elizabeth and Barry editing the latest edition of *Carvers' Medical Imaging*. It was an honour to be invited to join their team and they have been wonderful mentors to me, introducing me to book editing and assisting me every step of the way. Their dedication and hard work in putting this book together cannot be underestimated and I am in awe of them.

I've felt that I've been able to bring a little bit of my areas of expertise into the book as well, with the addition of a new chapter on DXA and the introduction of Silver Trauma Pathways to the emergency medicine chapter, reflecting my research and practice in the osteoporosis field.

Like Elizabeth and Barry, I am proud to be a radiographer and to have the pleasure to educate the radiographers of the future. You will never know what an inspiration you all are to me, especially as I write this during the COVID-19 outbreak in the UK, when many of our third year students graduated early to start their careers sooner than anticipated, to support the response to the COVID-19 pandemic. I am lucky to work with an amazing team at the University of Exeter and with our clinical partners, some of whom have contributed to this book. Thank you for your time and effort and for humouring me in my requests. You have brought your clinical experience and expertise to updating chapters in our rapidly moving profession and I am very grateful.

Karen Knapp
Exeter, 2021

Acknowledgements

We are grateful to those who have provided or given permission for use of images for this or previous editions: Accuray Inc., Phillip Ballinger and Eugene Frank, Canon UK, Stephen Eustace, GE Medical, Christine Gunn, Professor P. Lauterbur, Linda Lee, Michelle McNicholas, Stephanie Ryan, Verdi Stickland, Robin Wilson, Andrew Evans, Professor Sir Peter Mansfield, Oncology Systems Ltd, Philips Medical Systems, Royal Stoke University Hospital, TomoTherapy, Toshiba Medical Systems, Xograph Medical Systems, Alexandra Unett Stow, Graeme Stow, James Unett Stow, Emilia (Mabel) Unett Stow, Ultrasound Now Ltd, Bracco UK, Eric Whaites.

For assistance with the MRI chapter, the author wishes to thank: Professor Sir Peter Mansfield for historical data and published papers; Professor Paul Lauterbur for his kind advice and help on the zeugmatography image; Philips Medical Systems for their commitment to furthering MRI education and their continuing support in providing images and advice.

For expert reviews of vascular and interventional chapters: Wendy Jones, Luke Popplestone, Danny Rhodes.

For advice on the contrast agents chapter: Christine Heales.

For advice on cervical spine imaging in trauma: Andy Appelboam.

For assistance with the paediatric chapter, the authors wish to thank Mary Smail, Clinical Scientist, University Hospitals Bristol and Weston NHS Foundation Trust.

We are grateful to those who provided us with information or support for our previous editions, valuable assistance that has underpinned information in this third edition: Neil Barker, Margaret Cliffe, Timothy Cox, Neil Deasy, Joanne Fairhurst, Chris Hale, Mark Hitchman, Mark Holmshaw, Lynn Gilman, Peter Groome, Julie Mead, Gillian Phillips, Graham Plant, Jack Reese, Meryl Rogers, Claire Shacklestone, Christine Smith, Mike Tatlow, undergraduate radiographers and physiotherapists at St Martins University, Carlisle.

We wish to thank those authors who originated or assisted with some of the chapters in the first and second editions and whose work was used as foundation material for this edition: Philip Cosson, Margot McBride, Jonathan McConnell, Michael Stocksley, Darren Wood, Andrew Layt, Patricia Fowler, Peter Hogg, David Wynn Jones, Julian McDonald, Mark McEntee, Sara Millington, Joanne Rudd, Rita Phillips.

At Elsevier we thank team members Anne Collett, Poppy Garraway, Trinity Hutton, Elaine Leek and Veronika Watkins.

The editors acknowledge the patience and commitment of the models who feature throughout the positioning sections of the text: Alexandra Unett Stow, Danny Rhodes, Deborah Walsh, Michael Gundry; and thanks to Paul Quinn, for photographs in Chapter 30.

For those who have loved or inspired us, for each other
-- and for 96 more.

EC and BC

To my family and friends who support me in everything I do.
Thank you for always being there.

KK

List of Contributors

The editors would like to acknowledge and offer grateful thanks for the input of all previous editions' contributors, without whom this new edition would not have been possible.

Saeed Alqahtani, BSc, MSc, PhD
Assistant Professor and Vice Dean,
Institute of Studies and Consulting Services,
Najran University,
Saudi Arabia

Lucy Banfield, BSc Diagnostic Radiography, MSc Clinical Reporting
Programme Lead, MSc Advanced Practice,
Senior Lecturer, Medical Imaging,
University of Exeter, College of Medicine and Health,
Exeter, UK

Rita Mary Borgen, MSc, DCR (R), FAETC
Consultant Radiographer,
East Lancashire Breast Screening Unit,
Burnley General Hospital,
Burnley, UK

Lisa Brown, PgDip CT colonography, DCR(R)
Advanced GI Practitioner,
Royal Stoke University Hospital,
University Hospitals of North Midlands,
Stoke-on-Trent, UK

Julie Burnage, DCR, DMU, FETC
Advanced Practitioner – human and small animal veterinary ultrasound,
Director, JB Imaging Solutions,
Bodfari, UK

Jeanette Carter, BSc Hons Diagnostic Radiography, MSc Radiography
Consultant Radiographer,
Royal Stoke University Hospital,
University Hospitals of North Midlands,
Stoke-on-Trent, UK

Barry Carver, PgDipCT, PGCE, DCR(R)
Teaching Fellow,
Former Director of Radiography,
Bangor University,
Bangor, UK

Elizabeth Carver, BSc(Hons), DCR(R), FAETC
Teaching Fellow,
Former Clinical Education Lead and Director of Student Experience,
School of Health Sciences,
Bangor University,
Bangor, UK

Mark Cowling, BSc, MB BS, MRCP, FRCR, MA(Med Ed)
Formerly Consultant Vascular Radiologist,
University Hospital of North Midlands NHS Trust,
Stoke-on-Trent, UK

Susan Cutler, MSc
Principal Lecturer,
Medical Imaging,
Teesside University,
Middlesbrough, UK

Donna Jane Dimond, MSc, PgCert(TLHE), BSc(Hons), DCR(R)
Senior Lecturer in Diagnostic Imaging,
Allied Health Professions,
University of the West of England,
Bristol, UK

Christine Eade, BSc, MSc, PGCE
Consultant Radiographer,
Royal Cornwall Hospital Trust,
Truro, UK

Patricia Fowler, MMEd, BSc(Hons), DCRR, CertCl, FHEA
Formerly Senior Lecturer,
Faculty of Health and Social Care,
London South Bank University,
London, UK

Robert Gordon, BSc (Hons) Biology PGDip Nuclear Medicine
Lead Technologist in Nuclear Medicine and PET-CT,
Royal Stoke University Hospital,
University Hospitals of North Midlands,
Stoke-on-Trent, UK

Rebekah Goulston, BSc (Hons) Diagnostic Radiography
Radiographer,
University Dental Hospital of Manchester,
Manchester University NHS Foundation Trust,
Manchester, UK

Hazel Harries-Jones, FCR DCRR PgC Clinical Reporting
Senior Lecturer in Medical Imaging,
University of Exeter,
Exeter, UK

Martine Harris, MSc, PGCert CT, BSc
Senior CT/Research Radiographer,
Radiology,
The Mid Yorkshire Hospitals NHS Trust,
Wakefield, UK

Delyth Hughes, DCR(R), FHEA
Professional Lead – Radiography,
Bangor University,
Wrexham, UK

James Hughes, BSc Diagnostic Radiography
Audit and Research Radiographer,
Radiology,
Mid Yorkshire NHS Trust,
Wakefield, UK

Judith Kelly, MSc, PgCert, DCR, Cert Mammography
Consultant Radiographer – Clinical Lead, Chester
Deputy Programme Director,
Wirral and Chester Breast Unit,
Honorary Senior Research Fellow,
University of Salford, UK

Karen Knapp, BSc (Hons), PCAP, PgC, PhD, SFHEA
Associate Professor in Musculoskeletal Imaging,
Head of Medical Imaging,
Medical Imaging, University of Exeter,
Exeter, UK

Andrew Layt, DCR(R)
Formerly Superintendent Radiographer, Neuroradiology,
King's College Hospital NHS Foundation Trust,
London, UK

Fiona MacGregor, MSc Diagnostic Radiography, MA History and Politics
Senior Lecturer Medical Imaging,
School of Health and Social Care,
Teesside University,
Middlesbrough, UK

Maria Manfredi, BSc Hons, PGCert, PGDip, FHEA
Reporting Radiographer, Lead for Clinical Education,
School of Health Sciences (Radiography),
Bangor University,
Wrexham, UK

Suzanne McLaughlan, BSc (Hons), PgD
General Superintendent/Reporting Radiographer,
Medical Imaging,
Royal Devon & Exeter NHS Foundation Trust,
Exeter, UK

Colin Monaghan, DCR(R), PgCert
Superintendent Radiographer,
Liverpool Heart and Chest Hospital,
NHS Foundation Trust,
Liverpool, UK

Kelley Ochiltree, DCR, PGCert
Royal Stoke University Hospital,
University Hospital of North Midlands NHS Trust,
Stoke-on-Trent, UK

Tim Palarm, MSc, BSc(Hons), DCR(R), FAETC
Regional Manager (Ultrasound sales), Canon Medical Systems Ltd (UK);
Formerly Senior Lecturer in Diagnostic Imaging and Postgraduate Programme Leader in Medical Ultrasound,
University of the West of England,
Bristol, UK

Sue Rimes, DCR(R), MbyRes(Medical Imaging)
Principal Radiographer,
Diagnostic Imaging Department,
Somerset NHS Foundation Trust,
Taunton, UK

Michael Smith, Hon PgDip Advanced Practice in Medical Imaging, SoR Accredited Consultant Practitioner
Imaging Department,
Royal Stoke University Hospital,
University Hospital of North Midlands,
Stoke-on-Trent, UK

Peter Sutton, DCR PGCert (adult chest reporting)
Royal Stoke University Hospital,
University Hospital of North Midlands,
Stoke-on-Trent, UK

John Talbot, MSc DCR(R) PGC(LT) FHEA
Senior Lecturer, Medical Imaging,
Director www.mrieducation.com

Linda Williams, MSc. Health Care Leadership (EGA), HDCR, IHSM(Cert), PgCert (teaching in HE),
Chief AHP and Radiology Manager,
Clatterbridge Cancer Centre,
Liverpool, UK

Georgia Willmott, BSc (Hons) Diagnostic Imaging
Advanced Clinical Practitioner, MRI,
University Hospitals Plymouth NHS Trust,
Plymouth, UK

Darren Wood†, DCR(R), PgCert, FHEA
Formerly Head of Radiography BSc Diagnostic Radiography and Imaging,
Bangor University,
Bangor, UK

Abbreviations

2D	two-dimensional
3D	three-dimensional
3VT	three-vessel and trachea view
3VV	three-vessel view
4D	four-dimensional
A-mode	amplitude mode (ultrasound)
AAA	abdominal aortic aneurysm
AC	abdominal circumference
ACR	American College of Radiology
ADC	analogue-to-digital conversion/converter
ADC	apparent diffusion coefficient
AEC	automatic exposure chamber
AED	automatic exposure device
AFM	after fatty meal
AFP	alpha-fetoprotein
AI	artificial intelligence
ALARP	as low as reasonably practicable
AO	anterior oblique
AP	anteroposterior
ARAS	atheromatous renal artery stenosis
ARSAC	Administration of Radioactive Substances Advisory Committee
aSe	amorphous selenium
aSi	amorphous silicon
ASIS	anterior superior iliac spine
ATLS	Advanced Trauma Life Support
AVM	arteriovenous malformation
AVN	avascular necrosis
B-mode	brightness modulated mode (ultrasound)
BaE	barium enema
BaFT	barium follow-through
BAT	brown adipose fat/tissue
BIR	British Institute of Radiology
BMD	bone mineral density
BMI	Body Mass Index
BMUS	British Medical Ultrasound Society
BPD	biparietal diameter
BPH	benign prostatic hyperplasia/hypertrophy
BPP	biophysical profile
Bq	Becquerel
CAD	computer-aided detection
CASE	Consortium for the Accreditation of Sonographic Education
CBCT	cone beam computed tomography
CBD	common bile duct
CBF	cerebral blood flow
CBV	cerebral blood volume
CC	craniocaudal
CCHR	Canadian CT Head Rule
CDH	congenital dislocation of the hip
CE	Conformité Européene
CEM	contrast-enhanced mammography
CEMRA	contrast-enhanced magnetic resonance imaging
CEUS	contrast-enhanced ultrasound
CFA	common femoral artery
CI-AKI	contrast-induced acute kidney injury
CIN	contrast-induced nephropathy
CLD	chronic liver disease
COPD	chronic obstructive pulmonary disease
COR	centre of rotation
CPD	continuing professional development
CPR	cardiopulmonary resuscitation
CR	computed radiography
CRL	crown–rump length
CRT	cathode ray tube
CSE	conventional spin echo
CSF	cerebrospinal fluid
CT	computed tomography
CT ratio	cardiothoracic ratio
CTA	computed tomography angiography
CTC	computed tomography colonography
CTDI	computed tomography dose index
CTLM	computed tomography laser mammography
CTPA	computed tomography pulmonary angiography
CVA	cerebral vascular accident
CVC	central venous catheter
CVP	central venous pressure
CVS	chorionic villus sampling
CW	continuous wave (Doppler)
CXR	chest X-ray
CZT	cadmium zinc telluride
DC	direct current
D&C	dilatation and curettage
DAP	dose–area product
DAS	data acquisition system
DCBE	double-contrast barium enema
DCE	dynamic contrast-enhanced
DCIS	ductal carcinoma in situ
DDF	direct digital fluoroscopy
DDH	developmental dysplasia of the hip
DDR	direct digital radiography
DGH	district general hospital
DI	deviation index
DLP	dose length product
DMIST	Digital Mammographic Imaging Screening Trial
DNA	deoxyribonucleic acid

DOBI	dynamic optical breast imaging
DP	dorsipalmar or dorsiplantar
DPO	dorsipalmar oblique or dorsiplantar oblique
DPT	dental panoramic tomography
DQE	detective quantum efficiency
DR	digital radiography
DRL	diagnostic reference level
DSA	digital subtraction angiography
DSI	digital spot image
DTPA	diethylenetriamine penta-acetic acid
DVT	deep vein thrombosis
DW	diffusion weighted
DWI	diffusion weighted imaging
DXA	dual energy X-ray absorptiometry
EAM	external auditory meatus
EBCT	electron beam computed tomography
ECG	electrocardiogram/electrocardiography
ED	Emergency Department
EDD	estimated date of delivery
EDE	effective dose equivalent
EFOV	extended field of view
eGFR	estimated glomerular filtration rate
EI	exposure index
EI_T	target exposure index
ELS	echocardiography in life support
EMA	European Medicines Agency
EOP	external occipital protuberance
EPI	echo-planar imaging
ERCP	endoscopic retrograde cholangiopancreatography
ESD	entrance surface dose or entrance skin dose
EUS	endoscopic ultrasound
ESWL	extracorporeal shockwave lithotripsy
FASP	Fetal Anomaly Screening Programme
FAST	Focused Abdominal Sonography for Trauma
FB	foreign body
FBP	filtered back projection
FDA	(US) Food and Drug Administration
FDG	fluorodeoxyglucose
FDP	fluorographic defecating proctography
FET	field effect transistor
FFD	focus–film distance
FISH	fluorescence in situ hybridisation
FL	femur/femoral length
FLAIR	fluid-attenuated inversion recovery
fMRI	functional MRI
FNA	fine needle aspiration
FNAC	fine needle aspiration cytology
FNST	fetal non-stress test
FO	fronto-occipital
FOD	focus object distance
FOOSH	fall onto outstretched hand
FOV	field of view
FRD	focus receptor distance
FSE	fast spin echo
FWHM	full-width half maximum
GCS	Glasgow Coma Scale
GE	gradient echo
GFR	glomerular filtration rate
GI	gastrointestinal
GOJ	gastro-oesophageal junction
GOR	gastro-oesophageal reflux
GSV	gestational sac volumes
GTD	gestational trophoblastic disease
Gy	Gray
HBL	horizontal beam lateral
HC	head circumference
HCA	healthcare assistant
hCG	human chorionic gonadotrophin
HCPC	Health and Care Professions Council
HDP	hydroxymethylene diphosphonate
HIDA	hepatobiliary iminodiacetic acid
HIV	human immunodeficiency virus
HLA	horizontal long axis
HMPAO	hexamethylpropylene amine oxime
HOCM	high osmolar contrast media
HRCT	high-resolution CT
HRT	hormone replacement therapy
HSG	hysterosalpingography
HU	Hounsfield unit
HyCoSy	hysterosalpingo-contrast sonography
IAM	internal auditory meatus
IARC	International Agency for Research on Cancer
ICH	intracranial haemorrhage
II	image intensifier
IOFB	intraocular foreign body
IR	image receptor
IR	iterative reconstruction
IR(ME)R	Ionising Radiation (Medical Exposure) Regulations
IUCD	intrauterine contraceptive device
IV	intravenous
IVC	intravenous cholangiogram *or* cholangiography
IVC	inferior vena cava
IVF	in vitro fertilisation
IVU	intravenous urogram/urography
keV	kilo electron volt
KUB	kidneys, ureters and bladder
kVp	kilovoltage peak
LAO	left anterior oblique
LBD	light beam diaphragm
LCD	liquid crystal display
LCR	low-contrast resolution
LCSF	lower cervical spine fracture
LEAP	low energy all purpose
LEHR	low energy high resolution
LFTs	liver function tests

LgM	log measurement
LMP	last menstrual period
LNT	linear no threshold
LOCM	low osmolar contrast media
LPO	left posterior oblique
lppm	line pairs per millimetre
LSJ	lumbosacral junction
LSO	lutetium oxyorthosilicate
LUQ	left upper quadrant
M-mode	motion mode (ultrasound)
MAA	macro-aggregated albumin
mAs	milliampere seconds
MCU	micturating cystourethrography
MDP	methylene diphosphonate
mGy	milliGray
MHRA	Medicines and Healthcare products Regulatory Agency
mHz	milliHertz
MI	mechanical index
mIBG	metaiodobenzylguanidine
MIP	maximum intensity projection
MIRD	medical internal radiation dose
MLO	mediolateral oblique
MML	meatomental line
MOI	mechanism of injury
MPI	myocardial perfusion imaging
mpMR	multi-parametric magnetic resonance
MR	magnetic resonance
MRA	magnetic resonance angiography
MRCP	magnetic resonance cholangiopancreatography
MRDP	magnetic resonance defecating proctography
MRI	magnetic resonance imaging
MRM	magnetic resonance mammography
MSD	mean sac diameter
MSK	musculoskeletal
MSP	median sagittal plane
MSS	maternal serum screening
mSv	milliSievert
mT	milliTesla
N	Newton
NAI	non-accidental injury
NBCSP	National Bowel Cancer Screening Programme
NCEPOD	National Confidential Enquiry into Perioperative Deaths
NEXUS	National Emergency X-radiography Utilisation Study
NHSBSP	National Health Service Breast Screening Programme
NICE	National Institute for Health and Care Excellence
NIPT	Non-Invasive Pre-Natal Testing
NM	nuclear medicine
NMR	nuclear magnetic resonance
NMV	net magnetic vector
NOF	neck of femur
NOGG	National Osteoporosis Guideline Group
NRPB	National Radiological Protection Board
NSF	nephrogenic systemic fibrosis
NST	non-stress test
NT	nuchal translucency
OA	osteoarthritis
OCD	osteochondral defect
ODS	obstructed defecation syndrome
OF	occipitofrontal
OFD	object–film distance
OGD	oesophagogastric duodenoscopy
OI	osteogenesis imperfecta
OM	occipitomental
OMBL	orbitomeatal baseline
OPG/OPT	orthopantomography
ORD	object receptor distance
PA	posteroanterior
PACS	picture archiving and communication system
PCA	phase contrast angiography
PCE	preliminary clinical evaluation
PCNL	percutaneous nephrolithotomy
PCOS	polycystic ovarian syndrome
PD	proton density
PE	pulmonary embolus/embolism
PET	positron emission tomography
PID	pelvic inflammatory disease
PGMI	perfect, good, moderate, inadequate (system)
PMT	photomultiplier tube
PoCUS	Point-of-Care Ultrasound
PPE	personal protective equipment
ppm	parts per million
PR	peri-rectal/per rectum
PSA	prostate-specific antigen
PSIS	posterior superior iliac spine
PSL	photostimulable luminescence
PSP	photostimulable phosphor
PTC	percutaneous transhepatic cholangiography
PW	perfusion weighted
PW	pulsed wave (Doppler)
QA	quality assurance
QDE	quantum detection efficiency
RA	rheumatoid arthritis
RCEM	Royal College of Emergency Medicine
RCR	Royal College of Radiologists
RF	radiofrequency
RNI	radionuclide imaging
RAO	right anterior oblique
ROI	region of interest
RPD	renal pelvic dilatation
RPO	right posterior oblique
RSD	reflex sympathetic dystrophy

RSNA	Radiological Society of North America
RUQ	right upper quadrant
SA	short axis
SAH	subarachnoid haemorrhage
SBE	small bowel enema
SC	sternoclavicular
SFA	superficial femoral artery
SFDM	small field digital mammography
SI	sacroiliac
SIGGAR	Special Interest Group in Gastrointestinal and Abdominal Radiology
SIJ	sacroiliac joint
SMV	submentovertical
SNR	signal-to-noise ratio
SCoR	Society and College of Radiographers
SOL	space-occupying lesion
SPA	suspected physical abuse
SPET	single photon emission tomography
SPECT	single photon emission computed tomography
SPR	scan projection radiograph
SSFSE	single-shot fast spin echo
STARR	stapled transanal resection of the rectum
STIR	short tau inversion recovery
SUFE	slipped upper femoral epiphysis
SUV	Standardised Uptake Value
Sv	Sievert
SVC	superior vena cava
SWE	shear wave elastography
SXR	skull X-ray
T	Tesla
TA	transabdominal
TAS	transabdominal scan
TB	tuberculosis
TE	time to echo
TFT	thin film transistor
TFTs	thyroid function tests
TGC	time gain compensation
TI	thermal index
TIA	transient ischaemic attack
TLD	thermo-luminescent dosimetry
TMJ	temporomandibular joint
TMT	tarsometatarsal
TNM	Tumour, Node, Metastasis
TOF	time-of-flight
TPN	total parenteral nutrition
TR	time to repetition
TS	transabdominal scan
TV	transvaginal
TVS	transvaginal scan
UAE	uterine artery embolisation
UCSF	upper cervical spine fracture
UE3	unconjugated oestriol
US	ultrasound
UTI	urinary tract infection
VA	vascular access
VACTERL	vertebral defects, anal atresia, cardiac defects, tracheo-esophageal fistula, renal anomalies and limb abnormalities
VDU	visual display unit
VFA	vertebral fracture assessment
VLA	vertical long axis
VENC	velocity encoding
V/Q	ventilation/perfusion
WRULD	work-related upper limb disorder
w/v	weight to volume

1 Digital Imaging

DELYTH HUGHES and BARRY CARVER

Since the early 1980s there has been an inexorable move towards digital imaging within radiography.[1] Digital radiography has a number of advantages over film screen radiography and the different types of digital imaging each have their own strengths and weaknesses.

Advantages of Digital Imaging

Manipulation: The digital image is formed by a matrix of pixels, each of which has a numerical value attached to it and it is this value that determines where on the grey scale that particular pixel will be. This means that the radiographer is able to manipulate the image to optimise it by altering the numerical value associated with the pixel and therefore altering where on the grey scale it will lie.

Transmission: As the image is comprised of a number of pixels all with their own numerical value which represents the attenuation of the X-ray beam, these images can be sent via a network anywhere, which enables remote diagnosis regardless of where the image was actually acquired.

Storage: Images can be easily archived due to their digital nature and furthermore can be compressed, enabling more efficient storage, and facilitating easier transmission.

Analysis/reconstruction: As the images consist of digital data it is possible to manipulate these data in ways that allow reconstruction, such as in 3D reconstruction in computed tomography (CT), which results in images very different to those normally displayed. Computer-aided diagnosis or artificial intelligence software in order to detect very small but potentially significant areas is available, as are packages for orthopaedic templating, which allows for better planning of surgical procedures.

There are currently two main types of system available: computed radiography (CR) and digital radiography (DR); DR is subdivided into two further types which can be described as direct digital radiography (DDR) and indirect digital radiography (IDR).

Computed Radiography

CR was first introduced in 1983[2] and its use is widespread in modern healthcare systems. It is a cassette-based system that uses photostimulable phosphors (PSPs) in combination with a receptor plate scanning system to produce a digital image, using alkaline–earth halides and alkaline halides as PSPs to record a latent image of any irradiated structure.

COMPONENTS OF A CR SYSTEM

There are four basic components to any CR system: the receptor plate, the CR cassette, the image reader and the image display device (image display is described separately later).

Receptor Plate

The structure of the receptor plate in CR is very similar to the structure of an intensifying screen in film/screen systems.

It consists of five layers:

1. A top layer, which is a thin protective layer and is electron beam cured to reduce the amount of laser beam reflection that occurs during the secondary excitation phase of image acquisition.
2. Directly beneath this protective layer is the PSP. The phosphor used is generally a barium fluorohalide with europium impurities, together known as europium-activated barium fluorohalide (BaFX:Eu). The most common of the halides used in storage phosphors are iodine and bromine (designated as X in the chemical formula above). The latent image is stored within this layer as higher levels of electron energy. The thickness of this PSP layer is typically between 0.1 and 0.3 mm; the thickness of this layer is related to the image quality.
3. The phosphor layer is attached to a dyed layer that is often described as the anti-halation layer. This layer stops or reduces the amount of laser light that is reflected back into the phosphor layer.
4. Underneath the anti-halation layer and part of the support polyurethane is a conductive layer which allows any static electricity to escape without causing damage to the image plate or stimulating the phosphor layer.
5. All the layers are supported by a polyurethane backing layer, which provides rigidity for the whole structure. The polyurethane is also attached to a layer of laminate, which provides further support, and the complete image plate is stored inside a tough cassette for further protection.

As the receptor plate is constructed of very small phosphor grains embedded in an organic binder coated onto the substrate material, the plate can scatter light. The amount of this light diffusion limits how thick the phosphor layer can be as internal diffusion of light in the phosphor layer will increase in proportion to an increase in thickness. There are other factors which also have an effect on the spatial resolution of the CR receptor, such as the readout time and the diameter of the laser used in the secondary excitation phase.

Theoretically, CR receptor plates can be reused many thousands of times if handled correctly but will eventually need replacing when the phosphor no longer reacts as efficiently, or due to any physical damage such as scratches.

CR Cassettes

CR cassettes will come in a variety of sizes and are commonly constructed of lightweight materials resistant to damage with a low attenuation coefficient. Polypropylene cassettes are warm to the touch, relatively inexpensive and have a good level of flexibility; however, they have a higher attenuation coefficient than carbon fibre cassettes. Carbon fibre cassettes are more expensive but attenuate less radiation, but they are also cold to the touch, which can be uncomfortable for patients, and they are relatively inflexible.

They require a lead backing of typically 150 μm to prevent backscatter which, as PSP are particularly sensitive to lower energy X-rays, is particularly important. An antistatic inner lining to prevent static and build up of dust and to reduce the risk of mechanical damage as they are put into the CR reader is also a necessity.

The biggest difference in CR cassettes as opposed to previous film screen cassettes is the omission of a patient ID window. When using CR the patient and examination details are 'attached' to the image digitally either through the use of an RF chip or a memory chip situated within the cassette.

Image Reader

In order for the image to be displayed, the cassette with the exposed receptor must be placed into a device that can read the information and convert the data into an image. The design of the image reader can have implications on the ergonomics and workflow of the department. There are two main designs of image reader:

Single Plate. As the name suggests, these readers can take one cassette at a time and the whole cycle of data processing must finish before a second cassette can be placed into it. This type of reader is best suited to areas where only one patient is being imaged at a time, e.g. single X-ray room or theatre. The radiographer must be present to remove the cassette from the reader once the processing image cycle is complete.

Multi Readers. These allow the loading of up to 10 cassettes at a time and incorporate an automatic loading system so that they can be left unattended. These readers are suitable to serve more than one room within departments and are usually located between two or more rooms.

CR IMAGE FORMATION

There are three distinct phases of CR image formation: primary excitation, secondary excitation and photomultiplication, and digitisation

Primary Excitation

The latent image is formed when X-ray photons incident on the imaging plate interact with the storage phosphor layer. The impurities in the PSP, typically europium, cause the formation of electron traps; it is the electrons in these traps that form the latent image. The number of trapped electrons is directly proportional to the number of photons incident on the storage phosphor plate. These trapped electrons are relatively stable but some may be prematurely released by receiving sufficient energy from sources such as background radiation or heating. Fading of the trapped signal will occur exponentially over time, consequently it is important to read the plate as soon as practicable after exposure.[3]

Secondary Excitation and Photo Multiplication

After exposure, the image reader will remove the receptor plate from within the cassette and transport it through the reader to the laser assembly. The plate can then be scanned in a raster pattern with a finely focused laser beam and a scanning mirror.

The laser stimulates the phosphor and gives the trapped electrons enough additional energy to release them. As the trapped electrons are released back to their resting state this drop in energy state of the phosphor releases electromagnetic energy in the form of light. This light released from the receptor plate is then directed to a photomultiplier tube which produces an electrical signal directly proportional to the light released from the receptor. This electrical signal is then amplified and sent to the digitiser, the image is built up pixel by pixel and line by line.

The imaging cycle is then completed by flooding the entire receptor plate with a high-intensity sodium discharge lamp that ensures any trapped electrons not released in the secondary excitation phase are returned back to their resting state and the receptor plate is prepared for its next use.

Digitisation

The electrical signal from the photo multiplier tube is digitised by an analogue to digital convertor by converting the continuously variable electrical signal into digital data in a two-step process – sampling and quantisation.

Sampling frequency is about deciding the matrix size and ensuring that there are enough samples per horizontal line to faithfully replicate the original analogue signal (the electrical signal from the photomultiplier tube). If a sampling frequency too low is used then you can get a phenomenon known as aliasing; aliasing can result not only in the loss of important high-spatial-frequency information but also in the introduction of false lower-frequency data.

Quantisation assigns a grey scale value to each pixel dependent on the intensity of the electrical signal formed within the photomultiplier tube.

Digital Radiography

Whilst CR is indeed a form of digital radiography, when talking about DR we are usually referring to a system that utilises a different process of X-ray detection and image production. DR usually refers to systems with an integrated readout system and was introduced at the end of the 1990s.

Whilst CR converts X-rays into an electrical signal through the use of photostimulable storage phosphors, DR converts them through the use of a thin film transistor (TFT) array. The TFT array can be mounted within a cassette and connected either wirelessly or tethered to the system or can be mounted within a fixed detector either within a table or a wall stand.

A simple description of the process is that each pixel of the TFT array is connected to switching controls in a way that allows all switches in a row of the array to be operated at the same time. During the exposure all the switches in the array are switched off; immediately following the exposure all the switches in the first row are turned on and the signal from each pixel is amplified and converted to digital data by the use of an analogue to digital convertor (ADC), then the switches in that first row are turned off and the ones in the second row turned on and so on, with all the rows being switched on, the signal being obtained, and then off again in a sequential manner.

The difference between direct conversion detectors and indirect conversion detectors is in the method used to record the amount of radiation reaching the detector. Direct conversion detectors use an X-ray sensitive photoconductor and a charge-collecting TFT array and indirect conversion uses a scintillator layer and a light-sensitive TFT array.

DIRECT CONVERSION SYSTEMS

A direct conversion system uses amorphous selenium (a-Se) within its receptor: selenium is a photoconductor, which can directly convert X-ray photo energy to signal without the use of a phosphor. Prior to exposure an electrical field is applied across the selenium layer of the detector. Following exposure the absorbed X-ray photons are converted into an electrical charge, the charge generated is proportional to the amount of radiation incident on the detector. These charges are then stored in the TFT charge collectors, are amplified and converted to a digital value for each pixel.

The a-Se is laid onto a predetermined matrix of TFTs, one for each pixel and each pixel area records its signal on a capacitor. Normally pixel pitch is 140 μm, but 70–85 μm pixels can be used for mammography.

The advantage to this system is the lack of any light scattering in a phosphor layer. The a-Se layer can be thick without the risk of increased noise, however, the thicker the layer the larger the voltage required across it to capture the electrons. A practical limit would be 1000 μm as this would require 10 000 volts. For lower photon energies, e.g. mammography, 200-μm thick detectors achieve 100% absorption with less than 5000 volts. However, the requirement for a high voltage system makes the detector relatively complex and bulky.

INDIRECT CONVERSION SYSTEMS

Indirect conversion systems use caesium iodide (CsI) or gadolinium oxysulphide (Gd_2O_2S) phosphors. The phosphors can be arranged in an unstructured or structured crystalline format: unstructured scintillators scatter a large amount of light which results in a reduction in their spatial resolution; structured scintillators use phosphor materials in a needle-like crystalline pattern which reduces lateral scatter and also increases the number of photon interactions.

In indirect conversion a thin layer of amorphous silicon (a-Si) is attached to the phosphor layer, the silicon is laid out in a fixed matrix of pixels, with each pixel behaving as a photodiode 'sensor'. When the phosphor layer is exposed to X-rays the energy from the incident beam is absorbed and converted into light; the amount of light produced is proportional to the number of X-ray photons incident on the phosphor layer. This light is then converted into an electrical charge by the amorphous silicon (a-Si) photodiode array.[4] This charge is converted to an electrical signal, the signal is read via the TFT, amplified and converted to a digital value, to be sent to the display.

The advantages to this system are the high sensitivity of CsI:Tl phosphor to X-rays and the relatively stable properties of amorphous silicon. CsI:Tl is also used in fluoroscopy systems, as it has a fast decay time, allowing for updated images at 30-plus frames per second without noticeable lag.

Detective Quantum Efficiency (DQE)

Indirect systems generally have a higher DQE than direct systems.

Defined as the ratio of the (image signal-to-noise ratio) squared to the number of incident X-ray photons, the DQE describes how efficiently a system translates incident X-ray photons into useful signal (relative to noise) within an image.

The DQE describes how efficiently a detector can produce an image: as DQE increases, the exposure needed to produce an image with the same signal to noise ratio decreases.

Detector Connections. Digital detectors can be fixed, tethered or use wireless technology; direct conversion detectors will be found in some fixed detector systems whilst indirect conversion can be fixed, tethered or wireless. The advantage of wireless detectors is that they can be utilised in X-ray rooms previously used for film screen or CR without the need to replace the X-ray set.

Image Display

Once all the data has been collected it needs to be converted into a form that can be viewed easily. Images are most commonly displayed on screens either on the CR reader, incorporated into the DR control panel, or on a high resolution reporting workstation. There are several types of display technology available but with the demise of cathode ray monitors, flat panel liquid crystal display (LCD) screens are the commonest in current use.

LCD DISPLAYS

LCD displays are primarily two sheets of polarised glass with a liquid crystal solution trapped between them. The liquid crystals used act as shutters that open or close to either stop light from transmitting or allow it. The liquid crystals used are known as nematic phase liquid crystals; their molecules are arranged in a definite pattern. The displays used for medical applications are active matrix backlit panels; backlit simply means that there is an external light source such as built-in microfluorescent tubes or LED-based backlighting placed above, besides and sometimes behind the LCD panel. A diffusion panel is used behind the LCD panel to scatter and direct light to ensure a uniform brightness across the display.

Display Resolution

Active matrix panels use TFT technology similar to that used in direct digital detectors. These panels have a set maximum resolution: resolution is typically expressed by identifying the number of pixels on the horizontal axis (rows) and the number on the vertical axis (columns). The Royal

College of Radiologists now recommends the use of 3Mp (2048×1536) for *'plain X-ray'*, and 2Mp (1600×1200) for other imaging modalities.[5] This matrix size is very important to resolution. Up to a point, the more squares on the matrix, the better the image will look and the more the image can be modified. In reality, the spatial resolution of a digital image is generally limited by the spatial resolution of the image detector rather than by the display system itself, consequently the requirement for a higher resolution screen for DI images as their native spatial resolution is greater than, for example, CT.

There is increasing use of colour displays in imaging. These are particularly used in functional scanning such as positron emission tomography (PET) scanning, radionuclide imaging, 3D CT reconstructions and Doppler ultrasound studies so more modern display screens are now colour monitors. To display colour on an LCD screen each pixel is divided into three sub pixels with red, green and blue filters within the pixel.

IMAGE STORAGE

Digital images can be stored as graphic files in a number of formats. Radiographs are generally stored as bitmap graphics; the common format used in medical imaging systems is DICOM, others are 'bmp' and 'jpeg'. Bitmapped graphics are stored as a series of numbers, rather than being described in terms of formulae as used in vector graphics (e.g. 'gif' files). Bitmaps are usually larger than vector graphics because areas of empty space must be recorded as well. Uncompressed they are the exact same size no matter what the image content.

A bitmap can be visualised by considering a chessboard pattern, each square ('pixel': picture element) is allocated a colour (in a bitmap this will be a numerical value to represent each shade) which best represents the contents of that square. The quality of the image produced will depend on the size of the 'chessboard', the number of squares (matrix) and the colours available (in radiography this will most often be shades of grey).

Changing the size of the image ('chessboard') will change the outer dimensions of the picture, but not add any detail to it, just make each square bigger. When the squares are big and noticeable the image is said to be 'pixelated'.

Increasing the number of pixels (squares on the chessboard) causes each to be smaller and therefore less noticeable, theory suggests that the smallest detail visible in any bitmap is twice the size of a pixel. A smaller pixel size also makes the selection of the allocated 'colour' easier as each pixel is representing a smaller area of the image. As there can only be one colour covering each pixel, the closest match to the average colour in that area of the image must be used. The smaller the area of the image and the more extensive the available colour selection (greyscale), the easier the choice and the more accurate the copy (stored image).

A standard chessboard has 8 rows and 8 columns of squares that form an 8×8 matrix, or array. The total number of pixels is 64. Each pixel is 50 mm square and is adjacent to its neighbour, therefore a pixel pitch of 50 mm. A computer represents the colour of a pixel by storing a number, called the pixel value. In computing, numbers are stored in binary form, i.e. a series of 0s and 1s. Each numerical value is termed a bit; the number of values the computer can use for each pixel (i.e. number of bits) is called the bit depth. For example if 6 bits were used, then binary values from 000000 to 111111 (0 to 63) would be available, that is 64 grey shades (pixel values). Computers generally group bits into units of 8 (8 bits = 1 byte), hence images are generally stored as 8, 16, 24, or 32 bit files.

Digital Image Manipulation

Perhaps the greatest advantage of digital imaging is the ability to duplicate, store, search and manipulate the acquired data. In acquisition and display, the emphasis is on fidelity. Recording the radiographic contrast emerging from the patient as faithfully as possible is paramount, which means displaying the pixel values and locations accurately and consistently. The number one benefit of all digital projection radiography systems is the ability to deal with changing radiographic exposure parameters, even incorrect ones! In this case we want to change the data coming in before displaying it because the pixel values are either too high (overexposed) or too low (underexposed). The computer achieves this adjustment by adding or subtracting an array from the stored bitmap before display.

The initial data acquired is stored in a file called the *raw data*. Any manipulation should be on a copy of this data, leaving the original intact. In some systems, after manipulation, only the new data is sent across the network to be viewed and stored; this can be with a reduced palette (e.g. 14 becomes 12 bit). Although this might be seen as a disadvantage, it does emphasise the radiographer's role in QA informed by clinical indications. Poor decisions at the QA station can cause loss of diagnostic information.

IMAGE PROCESSING

The process for processing the digital data in either CR, DR or any other digital imaging technique such as CT is broadly the same; each pixel is given a value dependent on the amount of light/charge produced at that point as discussed previously, and this value is then used by the processing software to form the image. Different manufacturers have different names for certain processes; they may carry out tasks in a different order and some have patented processes that are unavailable for scrutiny.

Histogram Analysis

Segmentation. Segmentation separates an image into distinct regions which contain pixels of similar value, these regions relate to specific features/areas of the image. Segmentation can either be non-contextual where no account of the spatial relationship of pixels is taken or contextual where pixels of similar grey scale level and in close proximity are grouped together. This segmentation analysis results in a histogram of the image produced

The Histogram. A histogram is a graphical representation of a series of numerical values: the x axis represents the amount of exposure, and the y axis the number of pixels for each exposure level. The computer software has histogram models for each anatomical region, each having a shape characteristic of the selected anatomic region and projection. These stored histogram models have values of interest (VOI), which determine what range of the histogram data set should be included in the displayed image. The range of values within the VOI area is what the software is 'expecting' to see.

Histogram analysis is used to maintain consistent image contrast despite overexposure or underexposure, known as automatic rescaling. The computer rescales the image based on the comparison of the histogram, which is actually a process of mapping the greyscale to the VOI to present a specific display of contrast and it will endeavour to match the actual values with those stored in the system histogram by rescaling the contrast.

Different manufacturers use different systems of histogram analysis assuming various ways in which radiographers are likely to use the system. These assumptions include:

- Area of interest is in the middle of the receptor (CR)
- Smallest size receptor used relative to the body part (CR)
- Field has not been split – i.e. only one exposure per receptor (CR)
- Collimation has been used.

If any of these is not true then this can result in an incorrect analysis which can impact on image quality.

Modern software is becoming increasingly sophisticated in being able to analyse deviations from the norm. One set of data they nearly all use is the selection of body part and projection, selected by the radiographer prior to making any exposure. If the incorrect body part is selected then the system will apply the algorithm pertinent to the body part selected not the actual body part, which can result in adverse effects on the image. Once analysis of the data is completed the imaging software will apply a body part-specific histogram to the data; digital imaging systems will attempt to match the pixel values in the raw data histogram to this desired optical density histogram. The optical density histogram for any given body part is within the software but can be altered either temporarily or permanently by the operator. Images which are under- or overexposed may appear as expected because of this ability of the software to match the raw data pixel values to the expected optical densities in the image. Similarly, if the radiographer selects the wrong body part then the image will be processed using the incorrect values and this can have a detrimental effect on image quality.

The image in Fig. 1.1(A) appears underexposed with a lack of density and contrast. This is due to the wrong body part being selected and consequently the wrong algorithm being applied. In Fig. 1.1(B) this has been rectified as a result of the correct algorithm being applied.

Exposure Control

In digital systems a figure for exposure control must be indicated somewhere in the system. Much has been made of the potential for over- and underexposure due to digital systems. Several systems aim for a value of 2.0 (antilog 2.0 is 100, i.e. 100% of the expected value). Radiographers who get a value of 2.3 seem within limits, but the antilog of 2.3 is 200, i.e. 200% (double) the expected value and this is a considerable overexposure.

With such a system, an audit of pelvic examinations showed that 28% of images accepted had exposure levels of 2.6–2.8, possibly indicating endemic 400%–600% overexposures.[6] Having said that, the exposure index or sensitivity is vital, but it may also be misleading. The value is unpredictable depending on collimation, positioning, time taken to develop the image and background scatter present before exposure. Lehning et al[7] showed a variation of up to a factor of 2 in sensitivity index values for the same exposure depending on conditions prior to and after exposure and prior to reading of the plate.

Exposure indices are further discussed in Chapter 2.

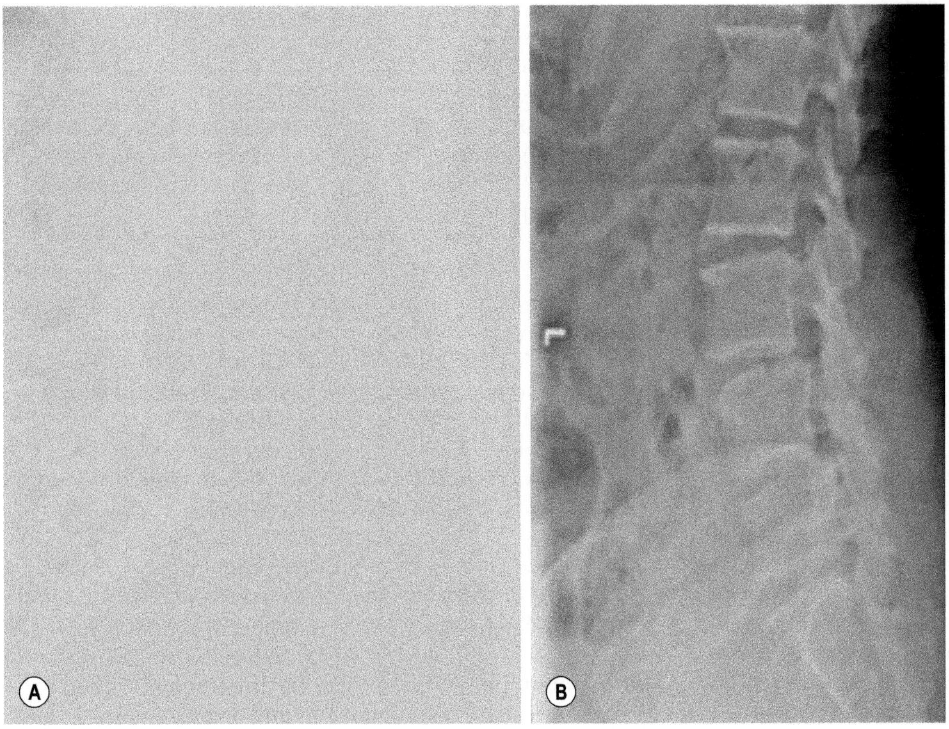

Fig. 1.1 Application of body part algorithm. (A) Incorrect body part chosen; (B) correct body part chosen, resulting in an acceptable image.

The Characteristic Curve and Inherent Response of CR and DR Systems

In film-based radiography, each film-screen system had a characteristic 'S-shaped' response curve, with which radiographers would be familiar. This representation of exposure response was seldom used by engineers or physicists, as any exposure response is energy-dependent and this was not represented on the graph. It is therefore difficult to find an exposure response graph in the literature for CR and DR systems. Most systems are said to have linear exposure response.

The film-screen type of response to radiation differs from a linear response in its poorer sensitivity to low energy radiation. Scattered radiation and extra focal radiation are both likely to be low energy and therefore are more likely to be detected by any CR/DR system. It is therefore vital that all collimated areas are screened with lead rubber or equivalent and that CR plates are erased daily and used in strict rotation.

Digital System Response and LUT

In the case of over- or underexposure of the imaging plate, the pixel value histogram will be shifted along the exposure axis; digital systems can create a new response curve with the aim of matching the pixel value histogram with the desired optical density histogram.

The algorithm employed uses a Look Up Table (LUT) specific to the body part; this in appearance is similar to the S shape film-screen response curve. The value of each pixel is translated to a grey scale value on the display using this LUT. When radiographers manipulate images by using the density and contrast controls what they are doing is temporarily changing the grey scale value assigned to any particular pixel value.

Multi-frequency Processing

Many systems now aim to reduce the complex content of the digital image into its constituent parts. Areas of mottle and noise are all very high frequency. Areas of clinically important detail, e.g. bony trabeculae, are said to be medium frequency. Areas of subtle shading over the whole image are said to be low frequency.

The low-frequency elements of the image can be digitally suppressed, as they are generally not felt to be helpful in image interpretation. This leads to an image with special properties that enhance fine details. Edge enhancement can be achieved through transforming the acquired data by applying a mathematical function to accentuate the difference between adjacent pixel values where one exists currently. This has the visual effect of enhancing any boundaries. These are high frequency structures: statistical variation, such as noise, is also high frequency so becomes much more apparent. The most unsatisfying digital images visually are those with low exposure and high edge enhancement. However, this is what is preferred in situations such as central venous pressure (CVP) line, long-line or chest drain location; it is possible using some equipment to have the set make an automatic copy of a chest image and apply edge enhancement processing to the copy resulting in two images from one exposure.

Algorithms that are applied to an image should suit the local requirements, and departments need to work with manufacturers to customise the standard algorithms to suit local preferences. There should also be specific algorithms for such examinations as foreign body demonstration and paediatric examinations and again these should be customised to suit local preferences.

Failure to ensure processing algorithms match the local needs results in a failure to maximise the potential digital imaging brings. Both DR and CR are digital modalities and as such should not be seen or treated as a simple replacement for film-screen imaging but rather should be configured to best suit the requirements of the local department.

COMMON ERRORS

Digital radiography is not an intelligent system. Some of the most common human errors found are not corrected by the digital radiography systems. For example:

- Digital radiography will not correctly rotate an AP image processed as a PA.
- The system will not correct misidentification of an image and incorrectly identified images once archived are difficult to retrieve unless the incorrect name placed on the image is known.
- The system will not correct processing errors. If the user puts a 'chest' through the processor as a 'cervical spine' the image will have the incorrect processing parameters applied to the image. Unless the raw data of the image has also been stored, the chances are high that the resultant image will not be diagnostic.
- The user must be aware that the diagnostic acceptability of an image must be judged on a monitor of diagnostic quality. The monitors provided with digital radiography systems for the initial appraisal of images are meant only as preview monitors for the assessment of gross positioning, inclusion of the region of interest, anatomical markers and identification.

Quality Assurance and Quality Control

In radiography we tend to use quality assurance as a blanket term that covers acceptance testing and ongoing monitoring of systems. There is, however, a subtle difference between quality assurance (QA) and quality control (QC); QA is primarily concerned with preventing defects and is process-driven whilst QC is about preventing problems by recognising deviations from the norm before they can cause issues and is more product-driven.

Both QA and QC help with quality improvement and are continuous activities to ensure optimal levels of performance in all systems. In the following paragraphs the term QA will be used to describe both processes as this is the norm in practice, but the routine 'QA' of systems is in fact technically quality control.

The first step in a programme of QA is acceptance testing of new equipment, including assessment by radiation protection advisors to ensure the system is operating safely. The purpose of acceptance testing is to ensure that the equipment is operating safely and within the specifications of the manufacturer. Ongoing QA tests are not always the same as acceptance testing but will use the data obtained

TABLE 1.1 QA for CR Equipment

Test	Frequency
Monitor and laser printer test	Acceptance testing and annually
Erasure efficiency	Acceptance testing and annually
Sensitivity index calibration and consistency	Acceptance testing and annually
Uniformity	Acceptance testing and annually
Scaling errors	Acceptance testing and annually
Blurring	Acceptance testing and annually
Limiting spatial resolution	Acceptance testing and annually
Threshold contrast detail detectability	Acceptance testing and annually
Dark noise	Acceptance testing and annually
Moiré patterns	Acceptance testing
General cassette condition check	3 monthly
Sensitivity index monitoring	3 monthly
Uniformity	3 monthly
Threshold contrast detail detectability	3 monthly
Limiting spatial resolution	3 monthly

Note: The processing parameters that should be used during quality control tests on a computed radiography system will vary between manufacturers, consequently there is the need to refer to their guidelines on processing parameters during quality control. In general little or no image processing will be used.

during acceptance testing as the baseline to track system performance over time and recognise any early indications of potential problems.

Tables 1.1 and 1.2 show typical examples of the type of tests that will be carried out. This list refers only to the QA of the receptors in CR or DR, and not the tube QA, which is a separate procedure.

TABLE 1.2 QA for DR Equipment

Test	Frequency
Monitor and laser printer set-up	Acceptance testing and annually
Image retention	Acceptance testing and annually
Sensitivity index consistency	Acceptance testing and annually
Uniformity	Acceptance testing and annually
Scaling errors	Acceptance testing and annually
Blurring and stitching artefacts	Acceptance testing and annually
Limiting spatial resolution	Acceptance testing and annually
Threshold contrast detail detectability	Acceptance testing and annually
Dark noise	Acceptance testing and annually
Moiré patterns	Acceptance testing
Detector calibration	6 monthly

References

1. Bansal GJ, Digital radiography. A comparison with modern conventional imaging. *Postgrad Med J.* 2006;82(969):425–428.
2. Sonoda M, Takano M, Miyahara J, Kato H. Computed radiography utilizing scanning laser stimulated luminescence. *Radiology.* 1983;148:833–838.
3. Mackenzie A. Effect of latent image decay on image quality in computed radiography. In: *Proceedings of UK Radiological Congress.* London: BIR; 2004:21.
4. Lanco. S Digital radiography – a technical overview: Part 1. *Radiography.* 2008;15:58–62.
5. Royal College of Radiologists. In: *PACS and Guidelines on Diagnostic Display Devices.* 3rd ed. London: RCR; 2019.
6. Field S, Blower C. *Moving to CR – impact on radiography practice. Proceedings of UK Radiological Congress.* London: BIR; 2004:41.
7. Lehning L, Günther-Kohfahl S, Maack I, et al. Exposure indicators in digital radiography: what is their relation to exposure? Proceedings of the European Congress of Radiology, Vienna, 2002. *Eur Radiol.* 2002;12(1 Suppl). C-0746.

2 Image Quality and Dose

BARRY CARVER and DELYTH HUGHES

Image Quality

For accurate diagnosis we require high-quality radiographic reproduction of the patient area being examined. What is a high-quality image? Signal to noise ratio can be used to define image quality, maximum signal with minimum noise could be said to produce the ideal image, but as increased signal in most cases in radiography equates to increased dose, these two factors need to be balanced in order to produce an *optimum* image.

Many factors need to be included in the assessment of an image to determine its quality: patient positioning and compliance will affect the resultant image, as will the image receptor and exposure used. Density and contrast are the photographic properties that affect image quality, commonly combined (inaccurately) to form 'exposure'. Although density and contrast are inextricably linked they can be differentiated on the image and the effects of each manipulated to optimise image quality. Unsharpness includes many aspects of image geometry which also contribute to the quality of the result. Taken together, these three factors may provide a means by which a radiographic image can be evaluated for 'technical quality'; other contributing factors, such as acceptability of positioning, will be discussed in the relevant chapters for each body part/technique.

DENSITY

Density may also be referred to as optical or radiographic density. Density in radiography is a measurable quantity: in its simplest sense it is the degree of 'blackening' seen on the image. For film/screen systems, when thought of in this way density was easy to evaluate and correct: is the film too dark (decrease exposure) or too light (increase exposure)?

Digital radiography systems do not make it this simple, consequently users need to be aware of the impact of over- and underexposure on the image. Underexposure of a digital radiographic image will not result in an image that has low density. In fact, the image will generally be manipulated by the system to be displayed with an adequate optical density of approximately 1.2 no matter how much or how little radiation the system receives.

Underexposure instead causes problems with the signal-to-noise ratio; insufficient exposure reduces acquired signal, and the image will appear grainy as a result of quantum mottle. The image must be closely examined to recognise this appearance, as from a distance the image may appear diagnostic. In most cases where fine detail is required for diagnosis, low signal-to-noise ratio in the image will result in the image being repeated.

Overexposure will also not result in an image of high densities. Again, the optical density of the overexposed image will be approximately 1.2, but in this case overexposures (high patient doses) result in high signal-to-noise ratios and image quality will be increased. The temptation, especially when using digital techniques, is to overexpose, as the safety net of image manipulation will prevent the need for a repeat examination, but this practice leads to each individual exposure being higher than necessary for the individual patient. Clearly this is a temptation to be avoided, and professional standards in the application of the 'as low as reasonably practicable' (ALARP) principle need to be maintained: give the right exposure for the individual patient.

Variation of applied mAs is often given as the controlling factor for density,[1] although the effect of variation of kVp on intensity, and therefore density, must also be considered. However, in general it is considered better to use a fixed kVp for each examination, using variations of mAs to control required changes in density.[2]

CONTRAST

Image contrast is a combination of subject contrast, which is the contrast produced due to the anatomical area under examination, and the receptor (radiographic) contrast, which is the contrast produced as a result of the image receptor being employed; and may be influenced by subjective contrast, which is the effect on contrast perception due to the observer or observing conditions.

The image itself is produced by means of differences in the attenuation of the X-ray beam within the patient. The differences thus produced in the transmitted beam are due to anatomical variations within the patient part under examination, in turn producing visible differences in density and contrast in the resultant image.

The contrast formed on the image in this way is termed 'subject contrast', due to the inherent 'contrast' which is the result of varying tissue types and densities of the body part under examination. Subject contrast can be influenced and manipulated by use of positive and negative contrast media, and the application of varying kVp techniques as described below.

Contrast can be shown to be inversely proportional to the applied kVp, hence in general at lower kVp values greater subject contrast is obtained, conversely at a high kVp a flatter more uniform image is produced.

There is again a dose trade-off, as use of low kVp may increase skin dose. Several studies support the use of high kVp as a means of dose reduction. Guidelines for paediatric radiography recommend the use of 55–60 kVp, even for extremity work,[3] but the increase in kVp will reduce subject contrast and hence image definition.[4] Commonly forgotten, in departments that have adapted this technique for adult use, is the requirement for additional copper filtration to optimise the useful spectrum. Failure to use this additional filtration results in a reduction in image quality without the full benefit of the dose reduction intended.

As digital systems manipulate the acquired image to produce a fixed image contrast, the direct relationship between kVp and subject contrast can be lost, however for intrinsically high contrast examinations such as the chest, the use of high kVp enables better visualisation of the structures of the lung despite the reduction in overall image contrast. This is because the 'flatter' image enables visualisation of structures with similar densities, which would not be differentiated in a high contrast 'more black and white' image. The 'flat' or grey appearance of such images does not suit all subjective tastes, and as such the technique is not universally accepted; however, this subjectivity is difficult to reconcile with accepted best practice, in terms of both image quality and dosimetry. Image readers need to educate themselves to accept these changes and embrace best practice,[3] the evidence for which is now long established.[5]

kVp is the exposure factor by which contrast can be manipulated. If an image has adequate density but lacks contrast, even after digital manipulation, then kVp should be reduced; however, as kVp reduction will also reduce the number of photons reaching the image receptor, decreasing the signal to noise ratio, an appropriate increase in mAs is required to maintain the final image quality.

Subject contrast will be affected both by pathological processes, which may change the appearance from the expected 'norm', and the effects of scatter, which are discussed below.

As mentioned above, subjectivity in image viewing can be an important factor when considering image contrast, and 'subjective contrast' requires some consideration.

Not to be confused with subject contrast as described above, subjective contrast is due to the observer rather than inherent in the image,[6] but is nonetheless important to consider. The observer needs to be considered: eye strain and fatigue can have an effect on perception and several short viewing (or reporting) sessions are preferable to a single extended session; aids to visual acuity should be used as required. Viewing conditions need to be optimal. Digital viewing stations should be of appropriate resolution and correctly adjusted, and viewed in appropriate ambient lighting.

As already stated, the amount of scatter reaching the image receptor will also affect image contrast. An increase in scatter reduces radiographic contrast by contributing a general increase in the overall acquired image density, but this is an effective increase in noise rather than signal.

Unfortunately, all examinations in the diagnostic range result in the production of scattered radiation, some of which inevitably reaches the image receptor. Consideration needs to be given to the most effective means by which scatter can be prevented from reaching the receptor in all circumstances. Scatter production can only be effectively limited by using appropriate collimation: minimising the irradiated volume minimises the scatter produced. Maximum use of appropriate collimation should be applied to *all* projections undertaken, as there are also clear dose implications.

Given that some scatter will be produced, lead rubber can be utilised to shield the unused part of the image receptor, which also assists in reduction of the amount of extra focal radiation reaching the receptor, as this may cause errors in histogram analysis. Use of lead rubber in this manner should not be confused with application of shielding in contact with the patient, which it is recommended should be discontinued in most circumstances, as discussed in Chapter 3.

For larger body parts where higher photon energies are used and more forward scatter is produced which is more likely to reach the IR, consideration should be given to the use of a grid. Placed between the patient and the image receptor, the grid will absorb scatter, but also – to a degree – primary radiation, leading to a requirement to increase exposure factors and consequently patient dose. Careful thought needs to be given as to whether the use of a grid is necessary to produce the image quality required: for example when undertaking fluoroscopy the use of a grid should not be automatic.[7] The use of virtual grids is becoming more common: no physical grid is used, instead post processing algorithms are used to remove the results of low energy photons which are likely to relate to scatter. This method aims to improve image quality without adverse effects on patient dose.

UNSHARPNESS

Having the 'correct' density and contrast on the resultant image is important, but if the image produced is unsharp then detail is lost and the diagnostic quality of the image reduced.

- Such unsharpness may be due to several causes, which include system geometry (penumbra, photographic) and lack of patient cooperation due to voluntary or involuntary movement.
- As the anode target produces a finite effective focal spot size rather than the ideal point source, there is inevitably some penumbral effect produced, as shown in Fig. 2.1.

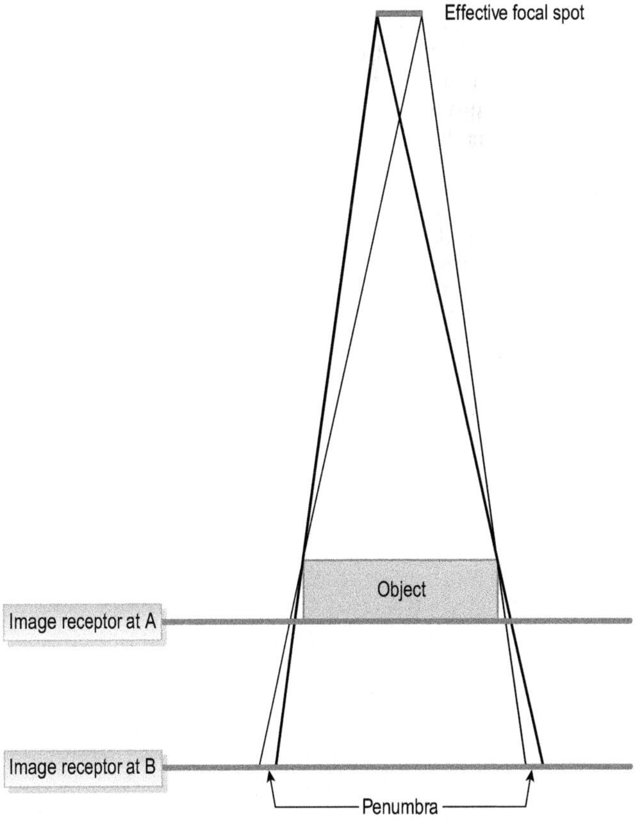

Fig. 2.1 Penumbral effect: as ORD is increased the size of the penumbra produced can be seen to increase.

- The penumbra causes geometric unsharpness within the resultant image. There are three ways in which this effect can be reduced:
  - Select the smallest useful focal spot size, which will minimise the size of the penumbra. Choice is limited in practice by tube loading considerations, but in general the smallest focal spot that enables the choice of the required exposure without compromise to tube life should be selected.
  - Minimise object receptor distance (ORD); as seen in Fig. 2.1, increasing ORD increases the size and therefore the effect of the penumbra.
  - If a broad focal spot is required and a large ORD cannot be avoided, e.g. when imaging a thick body part, consideration may be given to increasing focus receptor distance. Again this will lessen the penumbral effect due to the increase in focus object distance (FOD).
  - Unsharpness due to penumbral effects (geometric unsharpness) can be expressed as:

$$\text{Geometric Unsharpness} = \frac{\text{ORD} \times \text{Focal Spot Size}}{\text{FOD}}$$

Photographic unsharpness is inherent to the receptor system resolution; it depends on the size of the detector and detection technique. For modern digital systems this is as described in Chapter 1.

EXPOSURE FACTOR SELECTION

Digital systems generally have the advantage of offering wide exposure latitude in all situations. However, it should be noted that if a repeat is required, small increments of changes in exposure factors are to be avoided. This is because small incremental changes (the 1 or 2 kVp change by the supervisor which so infuriates students, and is anyway useless) have no effect on the resultant image. A wide latitude means that within that range of exposures a similar resultant image is produced.

Computed radiography (CR) systems and direct digital radiography (DDR) systems are not inherently dose reducing except for the reduction in repeats.[8] In low tube voltage examinations it has been shown that CR and amorphous selenium (a-Se) compare well with 200-class film/screen systems when exposed with equal mAs.[9] DDR amorphous silicon (a-Si) systems using CsI:Tl phosphors have been shown to have higher detective quantum efficiency (DQE) than film/screen, BaF(X) photostimulable phosphor (PSP) and a-Se systems. The thickness of these phosphors may allow lower than 400-class system exposure.[10] For all these systems, reducing exposure further will increase the appearance of noise and reduce image quality.

For digital imaging systems, the selection of kilovoltages has been debated by several authorities. Theoretically, any difference in the energy absorption spectra of CR and DDR detectors compared with film-screen systems could result in a different optimum kVp.

Data from Hubbell and Seltzer[11] and Nakano et al[12] for BaF(X)-based CR PSPs and a-Si/CsI:Tl indirect digital systems suggests broadly similar responses to those of film-screen. a-Se detectors, however, are highly kVp dependent and should always be used in the lower kVp range.

The ability to use signal processing techniques to amplify contrast can compensate for the reduced subject contrast available with high kVp techniques. This has led some authors to suggest increasing kVp to reduce patient dose. A thorough study of contrast detail detectability over the 60–120 kVp range concluded that BaF(X)-based CR PSPs performed slightly better than 400-class film-screen systems in demonstrating low contrast detectability, but only when receiving a 200-class exposure level. This study concluded that patient dose savings could be made, but only through the use of increased tube filtration, as previously mentioned.[13]

There are many situations, however, where high-quality images are not required, such as the examination of a total hip replacement, limb length measurement, or any other examination where only gross image detail is required. In these situations digital radiography can produce the required image quality at 80% less dose than film-screen radiography. The quantity of radiation required must therefore be considered on an examination-by-examination basis. A sensible way to approach dose reduction with digital radiography systems is to define the image criteria that must be visualised for a given examination and reduce the dose systematically until it is as low as is reasonably achievable while maintaining diagnostic efficacy.

Because digital systems adjust the optical density to correct for under- and overexposure, inappropriate exposure technique may be disguised. For example, if the operator overexposes a *film* the resultant image is too dark, and the next time the operator will use less radiation; this is called negative feedback. No such negative feedback exists with digital systems. Increasing the radiation reaching the storage phosphor will reduce the quantum mottle and associated noise factors in the image. When too little radiation reaches the storage phosphor the image will not be too light; however, there may be insufficient data in the image to allow an accurate diagnosis to be made and the image will have a noisy or grainy appearance (quantum mottle) due to decreased signal-to-noise ratio.

As a result, an indicator of the average exposure on the imaging plate is necessary to verify proper exposure selection and to provide a method of feedback to the radiographer, thus keeping patient dose to a minimum. Exposure indicators used in CR and DR indicate the dose reaching the image plate and provide no information as to the entrance surface dose received by the patient. For example, a patient of average size and body mass index will receive less radiation than a larger patient, even though the exposure indicator may be equal for both.

Exposure indicators are also affected by several other factors, including: radiation dose, kVp, mAs, focus receptor distance, patient position, patient size and composition, and equipment factors such as grid, table material and filtration. The initial choice of exposure factors significantly affects the resultant image because if they don't match the range set within the algorithm (body part) the image quality will be poor: if a low kV technique is employed for a chest examination but the pre-set kV range for image processing is high, this prevents optimisation of image quality because they do not match.

It is important not only to consider the exposure indicator but also the image quality when deciding whether to repeat or not.

EXPOSURE INDICATORS

Digital imaging technologies, either CR or DR, have the potential to reduce patient dose as the ability to manipulate images during post processing can reduce the number of repeats required, DR also can require lower exposure factors therefore reducing the dose even further.

When using digital imaging the software will endeavour to match the pixel values in the raw data histogram to the desired optical density histogram of the relevant body part and therefore a visual inspection of the image will not necessarily be a consistent indicator that the correct exposure factors have been selected. In order to assess the suitability of the selected exposure factors the radiographer must use the exposure indicator value. A complication to this is that different manufacturers use different methods to express this, although there has been a move towards a standardised measure.

Exposure indicator is *not* a measurement of the radiation dose received by the patient but it is a measure of the amount of radiation energy that has been captured by the detector and gives an indicator as to whether the image has been over- or underexposed. Exposure indicator value is affected by technical factors such as exposure factors selected, collimation, presence of metal artefacts such as joint replacements and scatter, amongst others, and should not be used to determine whether to repeat or reject an image.

Each manufacturer will have a recommended range of values which indicate that the exposure factors chosen were correct. The exposure indicator can be used to inform exposure factor choice, although the relationship between the exposure indicator and exposure factors is not always a linear one; it may be a logarithmic relationship, as described in Chapter 1 (Exposure Control).

System Sensitivity: S Number

Fuji CR systems use a system sensitivity number, which is the value sought by the computer during pre-processing in order to adjust the centre of the pre-processed histogram to the centre of the digital display range. The S number is calibrated in the factory settings and its relationship to dose is greatly influenced by beam energy. The digital system adjusts the sensitivity so that the mean optical density of the displayed image will always be 1.2. The sensitivity number is inversely related to the incident exposure.

As the S number is derived from exposure data recognition (EDR) processing it cannot be used as a direct exposure indicator, as the EDR depends on position and anatomy. However, if all things remain exactly the same, the S number will relatively reflect the exposure, i.e. double the dose, halve the S number.

Exposure Index (EI)

Carestream systems use an exposure index (EI), which provides a value directly proportional to an average exposure across the entire image plate. This is a relative measure of the number of X-rays that reach the receptor and form the relevant portion of the image. This does not include background scatter or collimated areas.

The EI is directly proportional to the average log incident exposure on the plate. Keeping all other factors the same, double the screen exposure results in an increase of 300 in the EI value. For example, in Fig. 2.2 the exposure index seemed to be low, however the image quality was adequate. The reason for this seeming anomaly is because exposure indicator, regardless of the unit of measurement, is an average of the exposure across the whole receptor. In this case the splitting of the receptor into two areas results in a lower exposure index.

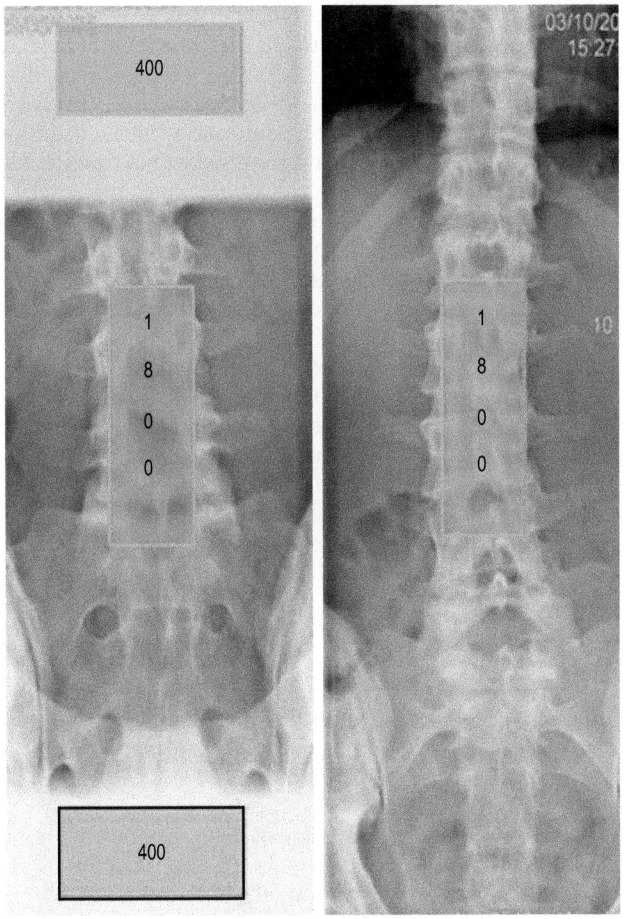

Fig. 2.2 Example of distribution of EI.

lgM

Agfa systems have a dose-monitoring tool that uses a relative exposure paradigm. The dose value is a log measurement (lgM) calculated for each scanned image and logged into a database. The database stores the lgM reading of the previous 100 exposures carried out for each specific radiographic examination. The mean is calculated and the current exposure compared against this value. The current exposure is determined as being overexposed (having an lgM greater than the average of the last 100 hundred exposures for that examination), underexposed or average.

When an image is presented to the radiographer a graphical indicator is displayed in the text fields indicating the statistical average mean exposure for the specific examination compared to the relative over- or underexposure level in the current image. If the exposure of the image plate exceeds the average of 100 exposures for the same examination the graph will indicate a red bar extending to the right; if the exposure is lower than the average the graph will indicate a blue bar extending to the left. The further the line extends to the left or to the right, the greater the deviation from the reference value.

Standardising the Exposure Indicator

In 2012 there was a proposal put forward to standardise and simplify the figure used in the exposure indicator. As different manufacturers use different calculations and many departments will have equipment from more than one manufacturer it could be a source of confusion.[14] The standard was developed in parallel with the International Electrotechnical Commission (IEC) standard and has established a common terminology to be used when discussing exposure indicators. This standardised exposure indicator uses the terms exposure index (EI) target exposure index (EI_T) and deviation index (DI).

The EI is determined by technical factors as already discussed, the EI_T is the ideal exposure, balancing image quality, patient dose and image noise. The DI measures how far the EI value differs from the EI_T and provides immediate feedback on how appropriate the selected exposure factors were. This value is determined by the formula:

$$DI = 10 \times \log 10\ (EI / EI_T)$$

Dosimetry

A full discussion on dosimetry is beyond the scope and intent of this text. There are many resources, particularly for students, that discuss the issues of dose measurement and radiation protection.[15–17] The commonest measures used are effective dose equivalent (EDE, quoted in milli-Sieverts, mSv), entrance surface dose (ESD, quoted in milli-Gray, mGy) and dose–area product (DAP, quoted in mGy/cm^2).

Optimisation of patient dose is a requirement of both European and international (ICRP) directives[18,19] and UK law,[20] each requiring doses to be kept 'as low as reasonably practicable'. IR(ME)R requires the setting of diagnostic reference levels; readings from DAP meters are often used to provide information for establishment of DRLs. ESD and EDE can also be used but require calculation from exposure factors or measurement with dose meters.

The current system for radiation protection uses the linear no threshold (LNT) model for assessment of the risk from medical exposures. This assumes a linear relationship between the exposure received and the risk of cancer induction. At high exposure levels (>200 mSv) there is evidence from epidemiological studies to show that this is the case; however, below this threshold there is little hard evidence. Current legislation, based on the LNT model, is a 'safe' approach assuming harmful effects from low doses in order to provide maximum protection to the public.[21]

It has been argued that individual molecular lesions may[22,23] or may not[24] induce cancer. There has been opinion in favour of radiation hormesis, the argument being that there may in fact be beneficial effects associated with low doses. Our bodies have very efficient repair mechanisms which cope with the ever-present effects of background radiation, as well as the more significant effects of deoxyribonucleic acid (DNA) damage from biological sources. Feinendegen argues that the stimulation of these processes at low doses may in fact be beneficial.[25]

Deterministic effects encountered in radiotherapy are also found in diagnostic imaging, e.g. erythema has been observed,[26] and lens opacities may be induced in children from doses of as little as 0.1 Gy[27] (a CT head scan can be 0.03–0.06 Gy in children).[28] These effects have now been taken into account, with dose limitation being included in IR(ME)R 2017.[21]

This is an extremely complex argument which is likely to continue for some time. Until proved otherwise, use of the LNT model as required by current legislation would seem to be a sensible approach. Research should continue – with an open mind: as Arthur Conan Doyle pointed out, *'premature assumption results in a tendency to interpret data to agree with the assumption'*.[24] An appropriate quotation for application by all researchers at whatever level.

References

1. Lampignano J, Kendrick L. *Bontrager's Textbook of Radiographic Positioning and Related Anatomy*. 9th ed. St Louis: Elsevier; 2018.
2. Dowd S, Tilson E. *Practical Radiation Protection and Applied Radiobiology*. 2nd ed. Philadelphia: Saunders; 1999.
3. Cook JV, Pettett A, Shah K. *Guidelines on Best Practice in the X-ray Imaging of Children*. Bristol: Ian Allan Printing; 1998.
4. Pizzutiello R, Cullinan J. *Introduction to Medical Radiographic Imaging*. Eastman Kodak; 1993.
5. European Commission. European Guidelines on Quality Criteria for Diagnostic Radiographic Images. *EUR 16260*. Luxembourg: Office for Official Publications of the European Communities; 1996.
6. Whitley AS, Sloane C, Hoadley G, et al. *Clark's Positioning in Radiography*. 12th ed. London: Hodder Arnold; 2005.
7. Lloyd P, Lowe D, Harty DS, et al. The secondary radiation grid; its effect on fluoroscopic dose-area product during barium enema examinations. *Br J Radiol*. 1998;71:303–306.
8. Field S, Blower C. Moving to CR – impact on radiography practice. In: *Proceedings of UK Radiological Congress*. London: BIR; 2004:41.
9. Zähringer M, Krug B, Kamm KF, et al. Detection of porcine bone lesions and fissures. *AJR Am J Roentgenol*. 2001;177:1397–1403.
10. Borasi G, Nitrosi A, Ferrari P, et al. On site evaluation of three flat panel detectors for digital radiography. *Med Phys*. 2003;30(7):1719–1731.
11. Hubbell J, Seltzer S. *Tables of X-ray Mass Attenuation Coefficients and Mass Energy-Absorption Coefficients*. Gaithersburg, MD: National Institute of Standards and Technology; 2004 (version 1.4) http://physics.nist.gov/xaamdi.
12. Nakano Y, Gido T, Honda S, et al. Improved computed radiography image quality from a BaFI:Eu photostimulable phosphor plate. *Med Phys*. 2002;29(4).
13. Lu Z, Nickoloff EL, So JC, et al. Comparison of computed radiography and film/screen combination using a contrast detail phantom. *J Appl Clin Med Phys*. 2003;4(1):91–98.
14. Whiting D, Apgar R. New exposure indicators for digital radiography simplified for radiologists and technicians. *AJR Am J Roentgenol*. 2012;199(6):1337–1341.
15. Allisy-Roberts P, Williams J. *Farr's Physics for Medical Imaging*. 2nd ed. London: Saunders; 2007.
16. Graham D, Cloke P, Vosper M. *Principles and Applications of Radiological Physics*. 6th ed. Edinburgh: Churchill Livingstone; 2012.
17. Bushong S. *Radiologic Science for Technologists*. 11th ed. St Louis: Elsevier; 2016.
18. European Commission Directorate-General for the Environment. *Radiation Protection 118: Referral Guidelines for Imaging*. Luxembourg: Office for Official Publications of the European Communities; 2000.
19. European Union. Council Directive 97/43 Euratom on health protection of individuals against the dangers of ionising radiation in relation to medical exposure. *Official Journal of the European Communities*. 1997:40.
20. *The Ionising Radiation (Medical Exposure) Regulations*. UK Statutory Instrument 2017 No. 1322; 2017. [IR(ME)R]. https://www.legislation.gov.uk/uksi/2017/1322/contents/made.
21. Martin C. UKRC 2004 debate: the LNT model provides the best approach for practical implementation of radiation protection. *Br J Radiol*. 2005;78:14–16.
22. Anoopkumar-Dukie S, McMahon A, Allshiree A, et al. Further evidence for biological effects resulting from ionising radiation doses in the diagnostic X-ray range. *Br J Radiol*. 2005;78:335–337.

23. Chadwick K, Leenhouts H. UKRC 2004 debate: radiation risk is linear with dose at low doses. *Br J Radiol.* 2005;78:8–10.
24. Cameron J. UKRC 2004 debate: Moderate dose rate ionising radiation increases longevity. *Br J Radiol.* 2005;78:11–13.
25. Feinendegen L. UKRC 2004 debate: evidence for beneficial low level radiation effects and radiation hormesis. *Br J Radiol.* 2005;78:3–7.
26. Mooney R, McKinstry CS, Kamel HA. Absorbed dose and deterministic effects to patients from interventional neuroradiology. *Br J Radiol.* 2000;73:745–751.
27. Wilde G, Sjöstrand J. A clinical study of radiation cataract formation in adult life following gamma irradiation of the lens in early childhood. *Br J Ophthalmol.* 1997;81:261–266.
28. Shrimpton P, Hillier MC, Meeson C, et al. *Doses from CT Examinations in the UK – 2011 Review.* Public Health England; 2014.

3 Introduction to General Radiography and Preliminary Clinical Evaluation

ELIZABETH CARVER and DELYTH HUGHES

What is covered in this chapter? To avoid repetition throughout the plain radiography (also known as projection radiography) chapters in this text, some safety, terminological and technical issues are addressed in this introductory chapter. Here we provide initial statements regarding projection names, patient preparation, selection and use of image recording media, dose reduction methods, image identification, anatomical markers and preliminary clinical evaluation.

Specific points to note when making preliminary clinical evaluation (PCE) comments on skeletal radiography will be included in Chapters 4–13; these will be under the heading 'PCE Comments'. Aspects of the image that can be assessed using generic points are included in this present chapter, again to avoid repetition. It should be assumed that these generic checks should be made in addition to the examination-specific points given in Chapters 4–13. Chest and abdominal radiography carry their own unique PCE considerations and these will be addressed within these anatomy-specific chapters.

Projection Names

Names of projections are always given as representations of the direction of beam, so that this gives the radiographer information on the initial patient position. This is in preference to a system that uses names for some projections that reflect the original describer of the projection (e.g. Towne's, Waters') but gives little or no information on the position. The UK system has for many years avoided overuse of named projections, and the use of position descriptors for projection titles is less confusing, making it unnecessary for the radiographer to learn eponymous titles. As a matter of interest, the editors of this text searched for all named projections in use, most popularly used in the United States; the total number found was 200 (projections for all body areas). Confusion caused by a lack of consistency in projection names/descriptors is further discussed in the facial bones section of Chapter 13, as it is a particularly relevant topic for that area.

In reality, a handful of eponymous titles are still considered mainstream and heard in use by radiographers in the clinical setting; when such a name is very commonly used in everyday practice, it will be given as an alternative in brackets.

Patient Preparation

For all examinations, patient preparation should always include:

- Appropriate and effective communication methods, which will ensure patient compliance or cooperation
- Removal of items of clothing or artefacts overlying the relevant examination area; in cases of severe trauma it may not be advisable or even possible to remove some items
- Accurate identification check
- Assessing justification for request
- Assessment of the possibility of pregnancy for examinations where this is required.[1]

Image Recording (CR Cassettes and Digital Plates)

With the current situation of image recording, where there can be a choice of computed radiography (CR), digital radiography (DR) and even film/screen systems for a few, it has been difficult to select a method of description that accurately embraces the use of all of these methods. It must be said that use of film/screen radiography is now almost obsolete in most countries but that it is still in use in some locations. As CR uses cassettes similar in appearance to conventional film/screen systems, there is little difference to film/screen methods for image receptor (IR) placement in relation to the body part; however, notable differences regarding DR exist. Since the second edition of this book, the term 'image receptor' has been used as an umbrella term. This is intended to include any of the recording systems that may be used by the radiographer. It should also be noted that use of lead rubber for masking is not advisable for CR and DR systems, although some of the positioning images do demonstrate this on a film/screen cassette.

In DR, wireless plates are now used extensively (Fig. 3.1), which further improves the flexibility and range of uses for digital plates, with some manufacturers producing DR support units that are flexible in their positioning rather than being fixed vertically or horizontally (Figs 3.2A and B). DR plates vary slightly in size and are usually square in shape, but generally do not come in the wider range of sizes found with film/screen or CR plates. They can be fixed under a stand or table surface, independent (wired or wireless), in a

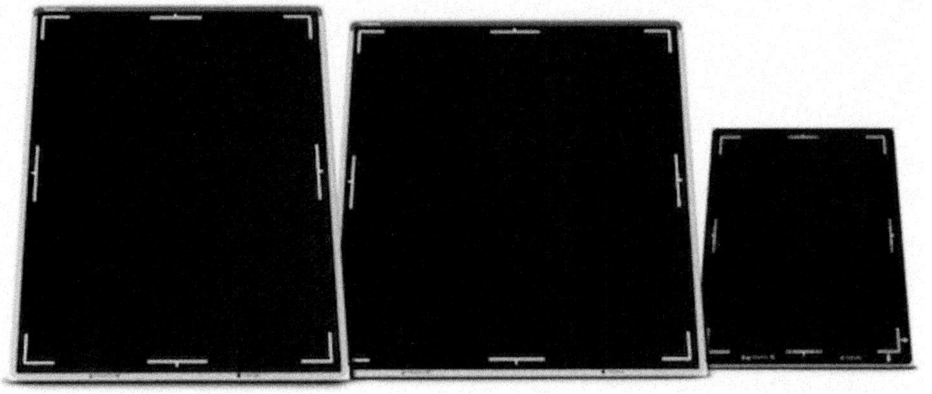

Fig. 3.1 Wireless image receptors. (Courtesy GE Medical.)

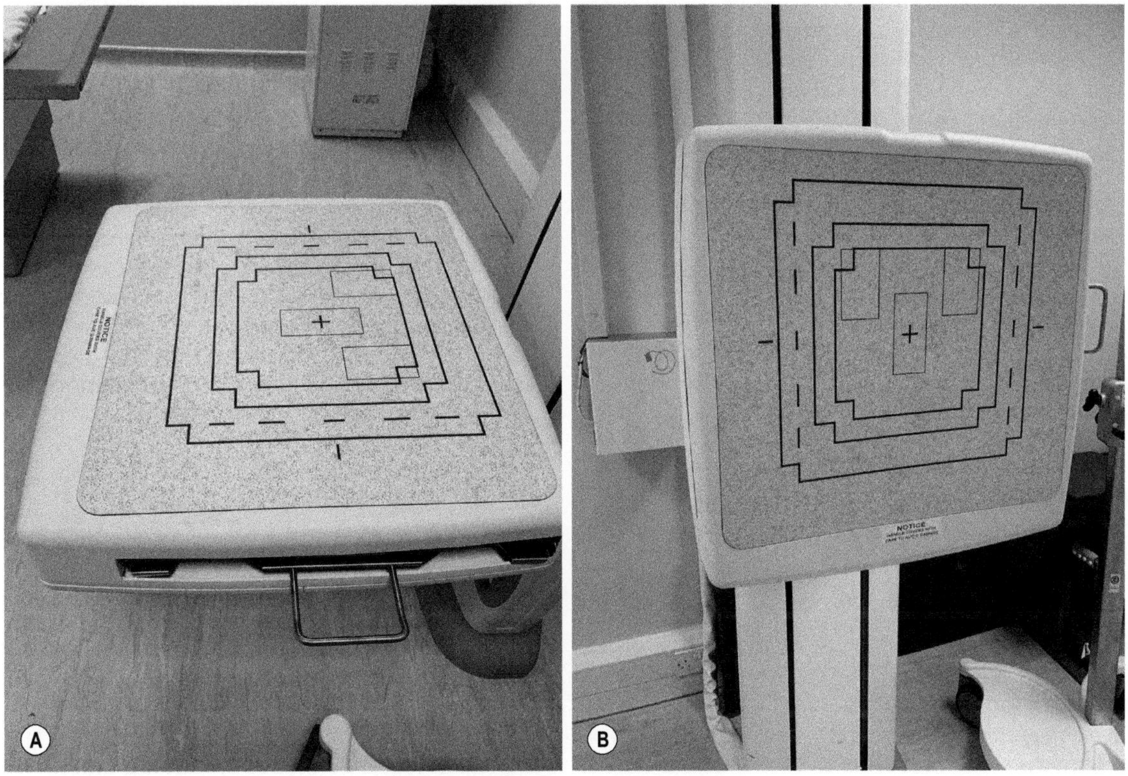

Fig. 3.2 Adjustable fixed plate detectors. (Courtesy GE Medical.)

tray used under the table-top or pulled from the side of the table-top for extremity work.

As a result of the range of possibilities for receptor arrangement, the IR positions are referred to as horizontal or vertical and no IR sizes will be given.

DR plates do not require the centre of the body part to be placed coincident with the middle, unlike CR cassette radiography. For this reason, the positioning descriptors provided in this book assume that the radiographer will always ensure that the body part lies within the IR, or within an unexposed section if the IR is used for more than one projection. At times it will be necessary to centre the body part to the middle of the DR plate, e.g. when that body part is large (as in chest or abdomen radiography), and this will be advised in descriptors for some sections, in order to ensure that the whole of the body part is included in the image. When using CR a general rule is that you should use the smallest possible receptor size for the body part under examination and that there should only be one exposure per cassette. This is because of the way the CR receptor is scanned during processing in order to produce the image (see Chapter 1, Digital Imaging). However, when imaging small body areas such as the fingers or scaphoid it is possible to make a maximum of two exposures and in this instance the use of lead rubber masking is acceptable. The exposures should be as close to the centre of the receptor as possible with no overlap of exposed areas and no unexposed area between the projections. Accuracy in positioning the lead rubber screening is of utmost importance; this is to ensure that no area of anatomy is obscured by scattered radiation, whilst at the same time ensuring that the areas under examination remain as close to the centre of the IR as possible. This should ensure that, during the secondary excitation phase (as described in Chapter 1) there is no unexposed area in the centre of the receptor which could lead to a reduction in image quality.

Another point to raise is the use of an antiscatter device (grid), which should be used in conjunction with the IR if scatter reduction is relevant. Their use will be indicated in descriptors when necessary.

Focus Receptor and Object Receptor Distance

With the disappearance of film/screen radiography it became necessary to reconsider these radiographic terms in order to ensure accuracy of reference. It has been noted that different terminologies have been introduced in recent years in an attempt to address this issue, and US texts initiated the use of the terms 'source image distance' and 'object image distance' as long ago as 2005[2] in an attempt to use more appropriate terms that did not include the word 'film'. However, we question the use of the word 'source': it is true that the tube target is a source of radiation but use of the word 'source' in a radiation environment does imply 'radioactive source', simply because 'source' is used more routinely when referring to radioactive materials (although it is not inaccurate to refer to electrically produced X-radiation as a source of radiation). In addition, use of the word 'image' can be considered inaccurate, as the image is latent until digitally processed and displayed. As a result, the terms *focus receptor distance* (FRD) and *object receptor distance* (ORD) have been used since 2012[3]; we feel that these are more appropriate, especially as the terms only include one changed word from old terminology, making them more easy to adopt.

In the following chapters a suggested FRD is given for each examination description; however in practice a range of FRDs (typically from 100 to 200 cm) may be used, dependent upon the examination to be performed, local protocol, and equipment used.

Anatomical Markers

It is assumed that anatomical markers will *always* be placed within the field of primary beam, clear of the essential area of interest before exposure. Most manufacturers include digital anatomical annotation in their post-processing software but they are not an acceptable substitute for the radiographer placing the correct anatomical marker within the field of the primary beam before making the exposure, which is the accepted gold standard of practice. Failure to place the correct anatomical marker within the primary beam prior to exposure could have serious medicolegal implications, including potential treatment of the body part on an incorrect side.[4,5] Additionally, it is important to comment on the dangers of applying anatomical markers over the required area of interest, and this includes soft tissue outlines as well as bony information. Instructions for placement of AP markers are not routinely included in projection descriptions because it should be assumed that this will always happen. Use of posteroanterior (PA) markers *will* be referred to but the authors do acknowledge that some imaging departments do not use PA markers. Anatomical markers do not always appear in positioning images as often they are too small to reproduce on a small photograph.

It will also be assumed that the radiographer will always check accuracy of anatomical markers on the resulting images as this is an important medicolegal requirement; therefore the image quality criteria will not refer specifically to this requirement.

Image Identification

Correct identification of the image is assumed to be an area that the radiographer should not need to be reminded of during image quality assessment, since this is a vital medicolegal requirement. This is therefore not included in the image evaluation lists in the text. It should be noted that correct image identification *must* include:

- correct patient name
- correct accession or examination number
- correct projection: it is important that the correct projection is selected in order that the correct *processing algorithm* is applied to the image and the accession number (a unique identifier used within PACS systems).

EXPOSURE FACTORS – EVALUATION OF IMAGES

The progression of digital radiography brought with it the possibility of image manipulation or post processing in order to optimise the image submitted for reporting but it is still important to state evaluation criteria for exposure factors, as in previous editions of this book. There are errors in exposure technique that should be addressed (Table 3.1) even if post processing of the image makes it possible to produce an image in line with required standards. The very nature of digital imaging means that an acceptable level of contrast density and noise should invariably be achieved, however this combined with the ability to manipulate the resultant images is no excuse for poor attention to the use of the optimal exposure factors for the area under examination. Particular attention should be paid to the exposure indicator which evidences if correct exposure factor selection has taken place, ensuring that the radiation dose to the patient is as low as reasonably practicable. Exposure indicators are discussed in more detail in Chapter 2 and are an important tool to be used in optimising exposure factors.

In all non-contrast radiography chapters (Chapters 4–16, 19 and 25), plus barium follow-through (Gastrointestinal Imaging, Chapter 21) and intravenous urography (Genitourinary Contrast Imaging, Chapter 22), image evaluation criteria include specifics for which structures should be seen clearly, and in contrast to other structures, for each examination. These should be used in conjunction with the generic assessment requirements for exposure factors provided in Table 3.1.

Dose Reduction Methods

Contact shielding has historically been used, and advocated in previous editions of this text, but recent guidelines recommend that shielding of this type is not generally required.[6] This relates to most diagnostic and interventional procedures, but devices such as gonad shields, (lead rubber) aprons or modified lead rubber shapes should be made *available*. They also recommend that each individual has the right to request (or indeed refuse) shielding.

TABLE 3.1 Exposure Factors Evaluation: Recognition of Common Faults

Exposure Indicator Reading	Image Appearance	Cause	Rectification
Within acceptable range	Too dark, with reduced contrast	Too much kV	Reprocess to improve contrast Reduce kV for subsequent examinations If using AEC, ensure body part is centred over chamber
Above acceptable range	Will appear to be of acceptable quality	Too much mAs	Reduce mAs for subsequent examinations
Above acceptable range	Image too dark, with reduced contrast and increased radiographic density	Too much kV and mAs	Reprocess to improve image Reduce both kV and mAs for subsequent examinations
Below acceptable range	Image quality *might* initially appear as acceptable quality but may have unsharpness and loss of detail	Too little mAs, which can lead to quantum mottle and loss of small detail such as bony trabeculae	Increase mAs in subsequent examinations
Below acceptable range	Image looks dark, with increased density	Too little mAs and too much kV	Reprocessing may not work as not enough data due to suboptimal exposure Increase mAs and reduce kV for subsequent examinations

Precautions such as avoidance of unnecessary irradiation of patient, fetus or personnel are of paramount importance; collimation is also a vital radiation dose limitation measure, specifically to:

- ensure that the required area of interest is definitely included on the image
- limit the radiation field to the area of interest as a dose limitation method
- reduce scatter in order to maintain image quality and reduce radiation dose.

Lead rubber protection will sometimes appear in positioning images in this text, as there is no valid reason to replace images, given that correct placement of contact shielding causes no risk to the patient.

Other recommendations for dose reduction are:

- The patient's head should be turned away from the primary beam and examination area during exposure, if possible in the position described, in order to minimise radiation dose to the radiosensitive lenses of the eyes and thyroid.
- Legs must never be placed under the table, to clear the femora and gonads from the primary beam, edge of collimation and scattered radiation.

Preliminary Clinical Evaluation (PCE) in X-ray Examination of the Skeleton

There are generic assessments that should be made, in order to provide PCE for referrers, and there are several commonly encountered pathological or injury types associated with the skeleton. Within chapters on body regions (skeletal system) there are specific comments that may relate to individual examinations but familiarity with common pathologies or fracture types is essential.

Generic assessments, in addition to normal medicolegal and quality checks, should always include the following:

- Assessment of the whole area, systematically avoiding the urge to focus only on immediately obvious abnormalities
- Examination of cortical outlines and trabecular patterns and including tracing bony outlines to assess for disruption
- Looking at the soft tissue (any change may indicate a subtle fracture)
- Checking any lines, zones and arcs that are relevant to the area of interest
- Referring back to any previous imaging if relevant

Radiographic examination of the human skeleton may identify a range of pathologies or appearances that identify traumatically induced changes. Many of the conditions listed below are found generally throughout the skeleton or its articulations, and for this reason are listed before chapters describing skeletal examination techniques (Chapters 4–13). Information related to specific areas of the skeleton will be included at the beginning of the appropriate chapter, or related to individual projections and PCE of the region if more appropriate. Not all conditions listed are necessarily justification for plain radiographic examination, nor is plain radiography necessarily the initial imaging method of choice for each condition. The pathologies given here are by no means exhaustive, but comprise those conditions most commonly encountered by the radiographer.

Commonly Encountered Pathologies that Affect the Skeleton and Its Articulations

Acromegaly

Overproduction of growth hormone due to a pituitary gland tumour may result in an increase in the size of the skeleton, even after full normal adult growth has been completed. The soft tissue of the heel outline shows an enlarged fat pad, whereas there is apparent increase in joint spaces, an increase in vertebral height, possible pituitary fossa enlargement and early arthritis.[7] Modern diagnostic methods have resulted in earlier detection of pituitary tumours, thereby significantly reducing the number of people suffering from increased growth. The radiographer will need to consider that patients with acromegaly often present with a larger skeleton than is considered average, and if CR plates are used an appropriate size relevant to the patient's size must be selected. If using DR systems the use of digital stitching of two or more images may be useful in some cases of acromegaly where the long bones have been affected by excessive growth hormone; it is essential to ensure that accuracy in implementation of this method is ensured to avoid false-positive or false-negative interpretation.[8]

Ankylosing Spondylitis

Most notably referred to as 'bamboo spine' in its advanced stages; inflammation of the fibro-osseous junctions leads to calcification of fibrous tissue. Eventually, vertebral bodies appear fused, with dense calcification that is wider than the bodies themselves. This gives the ridged appearance of the vertebral column, which is likened to a bamboo stick. Patients with ankylosing spondylitis are likely to have limited movement and may not be as able to cooperate with projectional requirements as easily as others.

Bone Age

Although not technically seen as skeletal pathology, epiphyseal appearance and fusions will determine bone age.[9] This type of assessment is requested when a child's physical development or size does not fall within the range considered to be normal. Among areas included in bone age surveys are hand and wrist, knee, elbow and iliac crests. Bones selected for the bone age survey vary according to the chronological age of the child.

Chondrosarcoma

This aggressive lesion is the third most common primary bone tumour and arises from cartilaginous tissue. There may be a soft tissue mass at the site, usually with cortical destruction. Slow-growing lesions will show cortical thickening.[10]

Enchondroma

Enchondroma consists of hyaline cartilage found as an island in bone. A noticeable lesion, with some sclerosis and containing small calcifications, may be accompanied by pathological fracture. There may be some soft tissue outline changes, especially if accompanied by a visible mass. Often the lesion is asymptomatic and findings may therefore be incidental.

Gout

Crystals of monosodium urate monohydrate are deposited in synovial fluid, which results in inflammation and erosion of cartilage and articular surfaces of bone. Radiologically there are likely to be narrowed joint spaces, a soft tissue outline indicative of swelling around the joint and small localised erosions over the bone surface.

Metastases

Metastases are malignant secondary tumours which spread to bone from a primary malignancy. They affect other tissue types in addition to the skeleton. In the skeleton lesions appear lytic, in some cases sclerotic (metastatic deposits from carcinoma breast and prostate); pathological fractures may be present.

Myeloma

This is a neoplastic condition arising from bone marrow. Lesions show as low-density lytic areas; they may appear as multiple lesions seen as clusters, which have a scalloped edge appearance.

Osteoarthritis

This wear-and-tear disease displays narrowed joint spaces which may show as asymmetry in weight-bearing joints; osteophytes; sclerosis and erosions. Bone density is likely to be preserved unless the patient is generally osteoporotic.[3,8,9] There may be increased bone density in the articulating parts of affected joints, and exposure factors should be modified to take this into account.

Osteochondritis

Osteochondritis is a condition affecting primary and secondary centres of ossification, leading to avascular necrosis of a portion of bone due to a cut in the blood supply. In children this is idiopathic; in adults it can be due to trauma or inflammation.[9,10] Appearances vary according to the locality of disease and include loose bodies apparent in joints, sclerosis of epiphyses, collapse of affected bone and soft tissue swelling.

Osteomalacia

This is low bone mineralisation causing low bone density, which may or may not be apparent radiologically. Vertebral bodies may collapse, causing a kyphosis seen on lateral spine radiographs. Small linear radiolucencies (Looser's zones) may appear and can develop into fractures that follow the same linear direction.

Osteomyelitis

Osteomyelitis is inflammation of the bone and bone marrow following soft tissue infection or, occasionally, injury. It most commonly, but not exclusively, affects children. In the acute stage radiological signs are not likely to appear for up to 10 days but, when present, will probably show as metaphyseal bone destruction and periosteal reaction. Radionuclide imaging is effective in early detection of the condition. More long-standing osteomyelitis can be very aggressive, leading to changes in the periosteum and even deformity of the bone.

Osteoporosis

Osteoporosis is bone demineralisation and mainly affects older women, but some older males may also suffer from the condition. The diagnostic route does not use plain radiography as the first choice as a significant percentage of demineralisation (approximately 30%) must occur before loss of bone density is shown on plain X-ray. Early diagnosis is made by osteoporosis screening methods (see Chapter 30). In addition to loss of bone density, plain images may reveal noticeable loss of cortical width and a wedge appearance of vertebral bodies. Patients with known osteoporosis will require a reduction of exposure factors for skeletal radiography, and possibly modification of technique if extreme kyphosis is present.

Osteosarcoma

Osteosarcoma is an aggressively malignant tumour which most often affects young patients. Soft tissue swelling and periosteal reaction (Codman triangle) are often seen on plain radiography.

Paget's Disease

Increased bone density, which is a result of this disease, is often referred to as having a 'cottonwool' appearance. The inexperienced can confuse the signs with the moth-eaten appearance of metastatic deposits in bone, but the mottled appearance of both can be distinguished thus: metastases erode (reducing the density of areas of bone compared to normal bone) whereas Paget's disease has areas of increased density compared to normal bone. Exposure factors for skeletal radiography must be increased to take into account the increase in bone density.

Perthes disease

This condition is categorised as an avascular necrosis of the head of femur and affects children. Radiologically there will be increased joint space at the hip, flattened femoral head, sclerotic appearance of the femoral epiphysis and areas of low density over the metaphysis.

Rheumatoid Arthritis

This is an inflammatory autoimmune disease which may affect any of the synovial joints, most commonly the hands and wrists. It results in synovial inflammation, joint articular destruction and deformity. Radiologically significant appearances include a soft tissue outline which indicates swelling at joints, osteoporosis, narrowing of joint spaces, joint deformity, subluxation and marginal erosions.[10–12] Reduction in bone density should be considered when selecting exposure factors for these patients.

Trauma

Most positive diagnoses involve fractures or dislocations, which are categorised as follows.

Avulsion Fractures. These fractures occur as a result of hyperflexion, hyperextension or unnaturally forced lateral movement of a joint; they are often seen in examinations of the fingers and thumb.

Comminuted Fracture. The fracture site consists of several fragments.

Compound Fracture. The fracture site is accompanied by an open wound on to the surface of the affected body part.

Complicated Fracture. Complications arise because of the involvement of the fracture with important functional sites of the body, usually a joint, vascular supply/drainage or nerves.

Dislocation. The articulating surfaces of bones are no longer normally aligned and within the normal joint capsule, showing as disruption of the normal radiographic appearance of the joint. This appearance varies according to joint type. Dislocation may occur at the site of any joint. Most commonly affected are the shoulder, hip and elbow. Incomplete dislocation is known as subluxation.

Depressed Fracture. The fracture is caused by an impact or forced pressure on the vault of the skull. The fragments are forced to lie under the normal position of the dome of the vault (calvarium). Fragments may overlap and appear as hyperdense areas at sites of overlap. There may be a stellate appearance of fracture lines radiating from a central point.[13]

Displaced Fracture. In this fracture fragments are separated, usually in more than one direction.

Epiphyseal Injuries. Fracture and/or separation of the epiphysis can occur, with varying severity which ranges from the most simple (Salter–Harris class I), involving fracture along the epiphyseal line, to Salter–Harris V, where the epiphysis is crushed[14] (Table 3.2).

Salter–Harris types VI–IX are extremely rare and include injuries to the periosteum, which affect membranous growth, and injury to perichondral structures and injuries that may affect endochondral ossification.

Greenstick Fracture. Greenstick fractures are almost exclusively found in the long bones of children and are frequently seen in the radius and ulna. This type of fracture does not traverse completely across the bone, which may appear bent rather than broken. A buckled appearance may be seen instead of an incomplete fracture, and this is known as a torus fracture. The torus fracture is most commonly found near the metaphysis of the bone, the most commonly affected bone being the radius.

Hairline Fracture. This is a fine fracture which has no displacement or separation of the fragments.

TABLE 3.2 Salter–Harris Fracture Types I–V

Salter–Harris type I	The fracture line passes along the epiphyseal line, or physis. If there is no displacement of the epiphysis, effusion may be the only indication
Salter–Harris type II	The fracture line runs along the physis and then obliquely, taking a triangular fragment of metaphysis (this is the most common Salter–Harris classification injury found)
Salter–Harris type III	The epiphysis is split in a vertical direction with a fragment displaced along the epiphyseal line
Salter–Harris type IV	The fracture extends through the metaphysis, the epiphyseal line and the epiphysis
Salter–Harris type V	This is compression or crush of the epiphyseal plate, which may not be noticed radiologically. Axial loading injury typically causes this type of fracture. It is rare in occurrence and causes interruption or cessation of normal growth at the site. It is often undetected and only investigated after growth disturbance becomes apparent. Prognosis is poor

Simple Fracture. A simple fracture is a fracture of the bone, usually into two fragments, with no involvement of other structures and no displacement.

Spiral Fracture. This is a fracture that travels along a bone shaft in a spiral direction. The fracture may be seen apparently travelling obliquely on each individual radiographic projection, rather than obviously demonstrated as a spiral in appearance.

Subluxation. Partial dislocation of a joint.

Torus Fracture. See section on greenstick fracture above.

References

1. *The Ionising Radiation (Medical Exposure) Regulations.* UK Statutory Instrument 2017 No. 1322; 2017. [IR(ME)R]. https://www.legislation.gov.uk/uksi/2017/1322/contents/made.
2. Bontrager K, Lampignano JP. *Textbook of Radiographic Positioning and Related Anatomy.* 6th ed. St Louis: Mosby; 2005.
3. Carver E, Carver B, eds. *Medical Imaging: Techniques, Reflection and Evaluation.* 2nd ed. Edinburgh: Churchill Livingstone; 2012.
4. Finnbogason T. Side markings of the neonatal chest: two legal cases of pneumothorax side mix up. *Eur Radiol.* 2002;12(4):938–941.
5. NHS England. Never Events list 2015/16. Online. Available at: https://www.england.nhs.uk/wp-content/uploads/2015/03/never-evnts-list-15-16.pdf.
6. British Institute of Radiology. *Guidance on Using Shielding on Patients for Diagnostic Radiology Applications.* London: BIR; 2020.
7. Burnett S, Taylor A, Watson M. *A–Z of Orthopaedic Radiology.* London: Saunders; 2000.
8. Faurie C, Williams N, Cundy PJ. A stitch in time: stitching errors in digital radiology. *Med J Aust.* 2017;207(5):224.
9. Ryan S, McNicholas M, Eustace S. *Anatomy of Diagnostic Imaging.* 3rd ed. London: Saunders; 2010.
10. Helms CA. *Fundamentals of Skeletal Radiology.* 5th ed. Philadelphia: Saunders; 2019.
11. Burgener F, Kormano M, Pudas T. *Bone and Joint Disorders.* 2nd ed. New York: Thieme; 2006.
12. Manaster BJ. *Handbook of Skeletal Radiology.* 2nd ed. St Louis: Mosby; 1997.
13. Heller M, Fink A, eds. *Radiology of Trauma.* Berlin: Springer; 2000.
14. Scally P. *Medical Imaging.* Oxford: Oxford University Press; 1999.

4 Fingers, Hand and Wrist

ELIZABETH CARVER and HAZEL HARRIES-JONES

Descriptions of projections of the upper limb in this chapter will refer to aspects of the arm in relation to the human body, in the anatomical position (i.e. with arms abducted and palms facing anteriorly). This means that the aspect of the limb that would normally be orientated outwards (laterally) in this position will be referred to as the lateral aspect, even when the hand is in pronation. The aspect of the arm which is normally nearest the trunk in the anatomical position (medial aspect) will always be referred to as the medial aspect, even for projections with the hand in pronation.

Throughout this chapter a suggested FRD is given for each examination description; however, in practice a range of FRDs (typically from 100 cm to 120 cm) may be used, dependent on local protocol.

PCE – GENERIC COMMENTS FOR FINGERS, HAND AND WRIST

Hand and wrist injuries account for 20% of injuries presenting to emergency departments.[1] These injuries can have a long-lasting or permanent detrimental effect on patients in terms of dexterity if mismanaged. There are patterns of likely injuries which tend to fall into groups defined by age.

Mechanism of injury (MOI) is also important to consider and knowledge of common fractures from each type of MOI is important. However, it is also important to recognise potential lack of accuracy in history of injury given by patients. Care should be taken not to be misled by this lack of accuracy, so carry out full systematic research on all images.

Common fractures are either extra-articular or intra-articular and treatment and outcomes for these fractures are different. This means it is important to distinguish between the two when commenting on the image.

Comment on angulation of the fracture site is also important for the management of patients, as is involvement of the soft tissues.

Thumb

PCE COMMENTS – THUMB

Fractures and/or fracture-dislocations of the first metacarpal are more common than fractures of the proximal phalanx of the thumb, and thumb series images will demonstrate these injuries well. The commonest of this type in the thumb is the *Bennett's fracture*, a fracture at the base of the first metacarpal, extending into the carpometacarpal joint. Bennett's fracture is almost always associated with subluxation or dislocation of the carpometacarpal joint. On thumb projections, assess the base of thumb for possible avulsed bone fragment caused by rupture of the ulnar collateral ligament.

Forced abduction of the thumb can rupture the ulnar collateral ligament and is often found among skiers, hence being known as skier's thumb, which is generally an acute injury. Years ago this type of injury was more associated with repetitive injury or strain, known as *gamekeeper's thumb*; repeated forced abduction (when wringing the neck of game) eventually caused rupture of the ligament. There may be a small avulsion fracture seen at the ulnar corner of the base of the proximal phalanx, or the carpometacarpal joint may appear widened at the ulnar side of the joint.[2]

ANTEROPOSTERIOR (AP) THUMB

Traditionally the AP thumb projection has been described with the patient seated,[3] but these positions create difficulties when trying to clear the hypothenar eminence from the field. Method 1 described here uses a position considered to be significantly more comfortable and achievable than others and may be at variance with other commonly performed methods (methods 2 and 3). The idea for method 1 was originally researched with the patient in an erect position,[4] with the later suggestion that immobilisation might be more effective if the patient is supine.[5]

It is clear that the patient's thyroid and the lenses of the eyes are close to the primary beam and edge of collimation in method 1, but if the head is turned away efficiently and the IR is placed as far away as possible from the trunk, risks can be minimised.

For all projections of the thumb the IR is placed horizontal unless otherwise specified.

Positioning

Method 1: Patient Supine (Fig. 4.1A,B).

- The patient is supine with the affected arm flexed at the elbow and the dorsum of the hand initially in contact with the IR
- The fingers are extended and separated from the thumb
- The anterior aspect of the thumb is placed in contact with the IR and adjusted until the long axis of the thumb is parallel to it; the hypothenar eminence is cleared from the thumb and thenar eminence
- As the dorsum of the hand is now not in contact with the IR, a radiolucent pad is used under the dorsum to aid immobilisation
- The head is turned away from the primary beam

Method 2: Patient Seated Alongside Table (Fig. 4.2).

- The patient is seated with the affected side next to the table

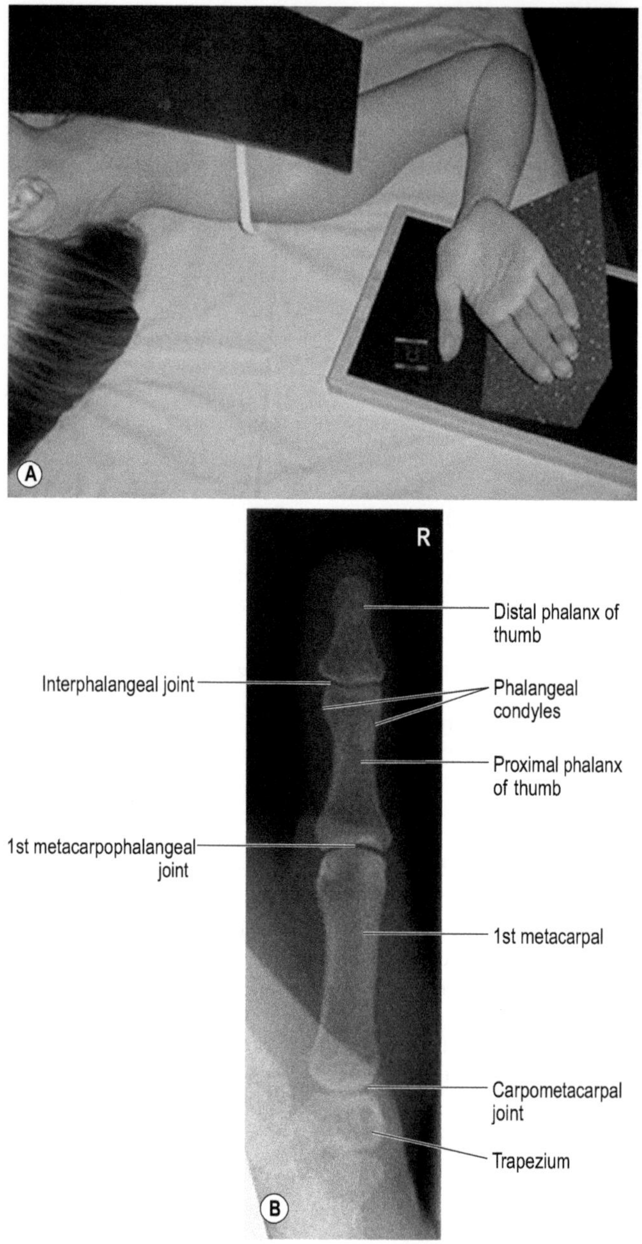

Fig. 4.1 (A) AP thumb with patient supine; (B) AP thumb.

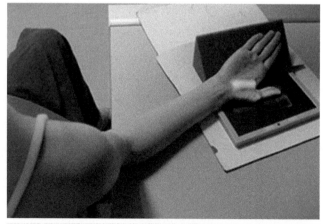

Fig. 4.2 AP thumb with patient seated next to the table.

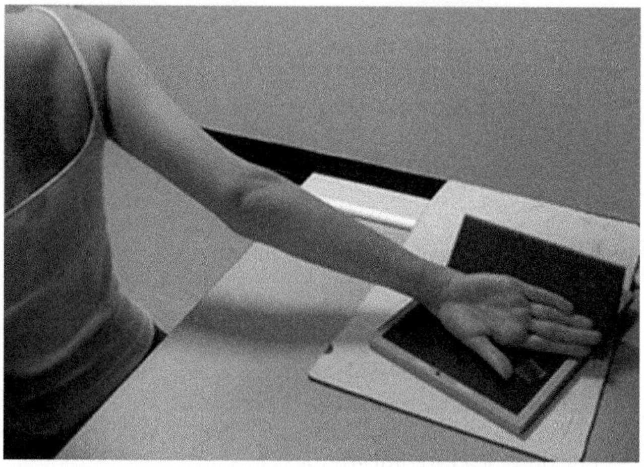

Fig. 4.3 AP thumb with patient's back to the table.

- The affected hand is externally rotated and the thumb cleared from the fingers
- The anterior aspect of the thumb is placed in contact with the IR; it may be necessary for the patient to lean towards the table in order to facilitate this
- A radiolucent pad is used under the dorsum of the hand to aid immobilisation
- Care must be taken to clear the hypothenar eminence from the first metacarpal
- The head is turned away from the primary beam

Method 3: Patient Seated with Back to Table (Fig. 4.3).

- The patient is seated with their back to the table
- The affected arm is abducted posteriorly and medially rotated
- The anterior aspect of the thumb is placed in contact with the IR; the hypothenar eminence is cleared from the thumb and thenar eminence
- A radiolucent pad is used under the dorsum of the hand to aid immobilisation
- Care must be taken to clear the hypothenar eminence from the first metacarpal

For patients who are unable to achieve any of these positions, the PA projection should be used. Principles of radiographic imaging indicate that there will be some magnification of the thumb with this projection, thereby increasing unsharpness. However, an increase in the focus receptor distance (FRD) will compensate for and reduce the effects of this. An increase in mAs will also be necessary to account for reduction in radiographic density due to the inverse square law. However, this is likely to be minimal and the balance of benefit versus risk should be considered.

Popular opinion would suggest that the creation of an air gap between the thumb and the IR also requires an increase in mAs, in order to effect further film blackening as compensation for the reduction in scatter. For denser body areas requiring higher exposure factors than the thumb, this would be a relevant consideration. However, as this projection is performed with the selection of a relatively low kVp, the dominant interaction process is one of absorption rather than production of scatter. Therefore this negates the requirement for an increase in mAs (see Chapter 2). Possible other disadvantages of using the PA projection are the possibility of poor maintenance of position and immobilisation; use of immobilisation aids therefore becomes of paramount importance.

POSTEROANTERIOR (PA) THUMB (FIG. 4.4)

Positioning

- The patient is seated with the affected side next to the table
- From a dorsipalmar (DP) position, the hand is externally rotated through 90° and the lateral border of the wrist placed in contact with the table
- The fingers are extended and superimposed vertically; the thumb is extended and cleared away from the fingers
- The long axis of the thumb is supported in a horizontal position by a radiolucent pad
- The thumb and thenar eminence are cleared from the hypothenar eminence and palm of the hand

Beam Direction and FRD (All AP Methods and PA Method)

Vertical, at 90° to the IR
100 cm FRD

Centring Point

Over the first metacarpophalangeal joint

Collimation

All phalanges, first metacarpal, trapezium, soft tissue outlines including that of the thenar eminence

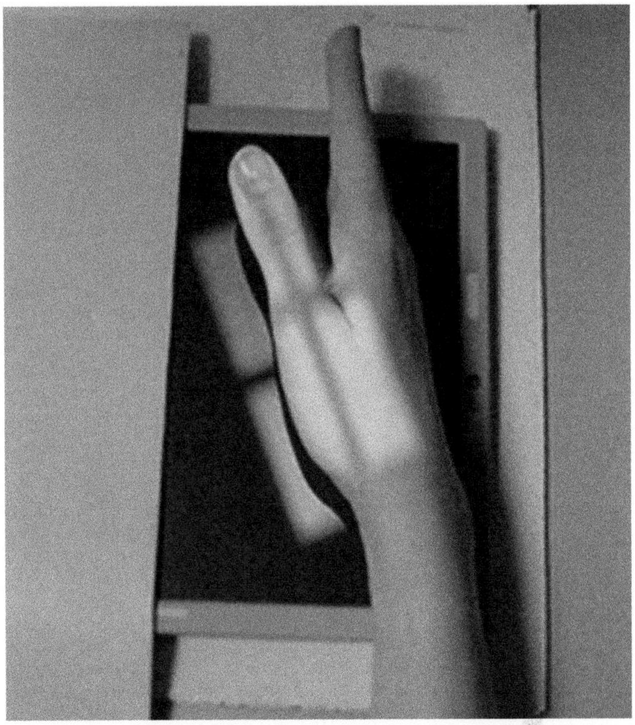

Fig. 4.4 PA thumb. The immobilisation pad is removed to show position more clearly.

Criteria for Assessing Image Quality: All AP Methods and PA Method

- All phalanges, first metacarpal, trapezium and soft tissue outline are demonstrated and clear of the hypothenar eminence
- Clear interphalangeal and metacarpophalangeal joint spaces; symmetry of the phalangeal condyles
- Sharp image demonstrating soft tissue margins of the thumb and thenar eminence, bony cortex and trabeculae; adequate penetration of thenar eminence to demonstrate first metacarpal and trapezium

Common Errors: PA Thumb

Common Errors	Possible Reasons	Potential Effects on PCE or Report
Interphalangeal joint space not clearly demonstrated	Long axis of thumb may not be parallel to IR	Intra-articular fractures may be missed Pathology may not be clearly visualised
Asymmetry of phalangeal condyles	Transverse axis of thumb may not be parallel to IR	Subtle pathology or fractures may be missed
AP METHODS 1–3		
Shadow of hypothenar eminence superimposed over first metacarpal and trapezium	Inadequate rotation of hand; rotate hand further to clear	Soft tissue shadows may obscure trabecular pattern and/or mimic a fracture site. Bearing in mind that a good proportion of thumb injuries affect the metacarpal, it is important that detail of this region is good
PA		
Shadow of thenar and hypothenar eminence superimposed over first metacarpal and trapezium	Thumb may be positioned too close to the rest of hand; clear thumb and first metacarpal from hand and fingers	Effects are the same as for errors in AP methods

LATERAL THUMB (FIG. 4.5A,B)

Positioning

- The patient is seated with the affected side next to the table
- In the DP position the thumb is cleared from the fingers and the hand is medially rotated until the thumb lies laterally, with its phalangeal condyles superimposed
- Because the medial aspect of the hand will be raised to achieve the correct position, a radiolucent pad is used under the palmar aspect of the hand to aid immobilisation
- An alternative method for immobilisation is to flex the fingers into the palm while maintaining separation of the thumb from the rest of the hand, using the fist to support the dorsum in the required position (Fig. 4.5B)

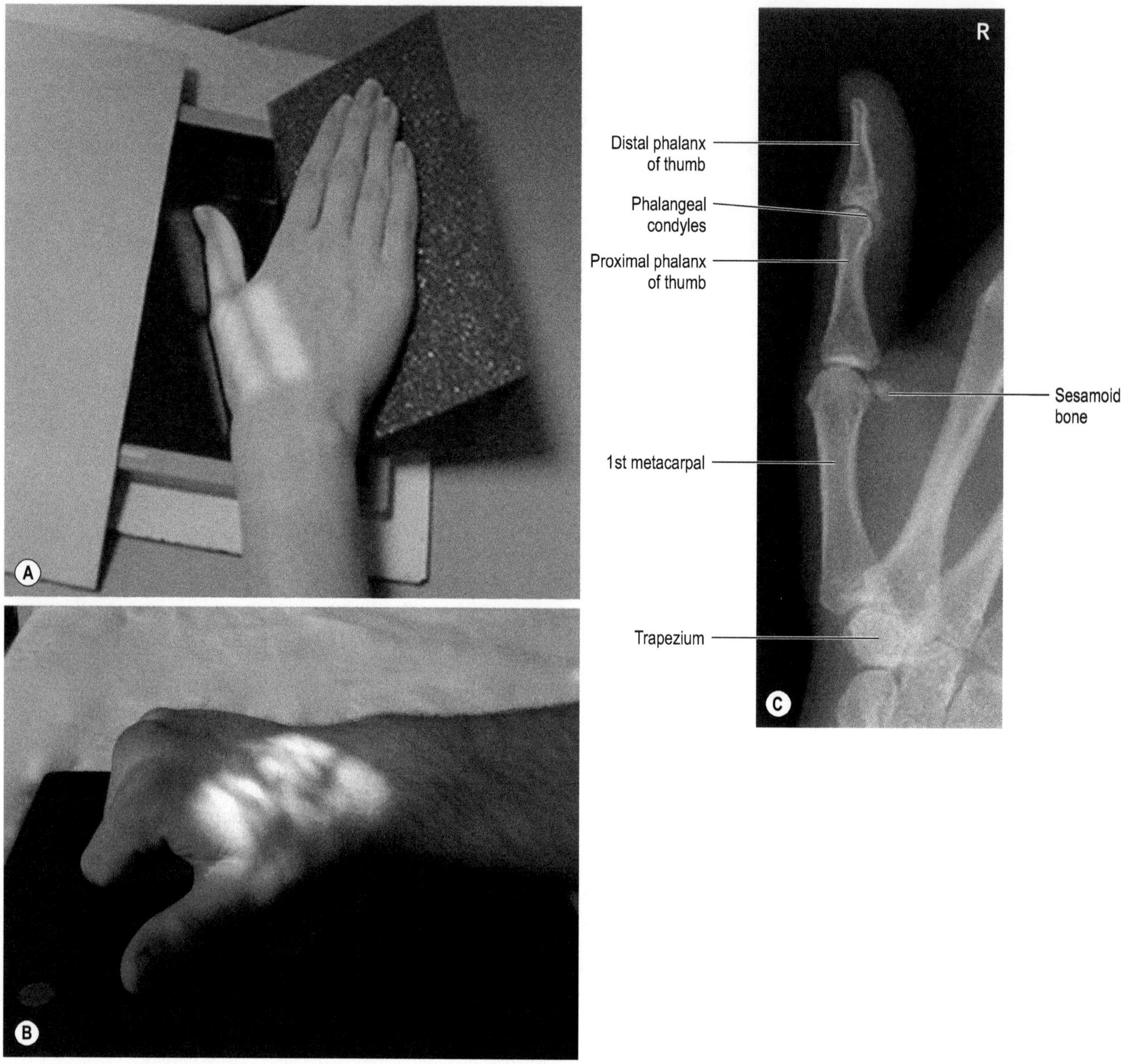

Fig. 4.5 (A,B) Lateral thumb positions; (C) lateral thumb.

Beam Direction and FRD

Vertical, at 90° to the IR
100 cm FRD

Centring Point

Over the first metacarpophalangeal joint

Collimation

All phalanges, the first metacarpal, trapezium, soft tissue outlines including that of the thenar eminence

Criteria for Assessing Image Quality

- All phalanges, first metacarpal, trapezium and soft tissue outlines are demonstrated
- The thumb, first metacarpal and trapezium are cleared from the fingers and hand
- Superimposition of phalangeal condyles to clear interphalangeal and metacarpophalangeal joint spaces
- Sharp image demonstrating the soft tissue margins of the thumb and thenar eminence, bony cortex and trabeculae. The thenar eminence should be penetrated to adequately demonstrate the first metacarpal and trapezium.

Common Errors: Lateral Thumb

Common Error	Possible Reason	Potential Effect on PCE or Report
Poor joint space visualisation and non-superimposition of phalangeal condyles	Hand has not been rotated accurately; medial or external rotation of the hand will facilitate superimposition of phalangeal condyles	Cortical margins and intra-articular fractures may be difficult to interpret

Fingers

The most frequent reason for imaging of the fingers is to demonstrate the results of trauma to the area. Avulsion fractures, such as those accompanying mallet finger, are often seen, as are dislocations, volar plate fractures from hyperextension injuries and foreign bodies.

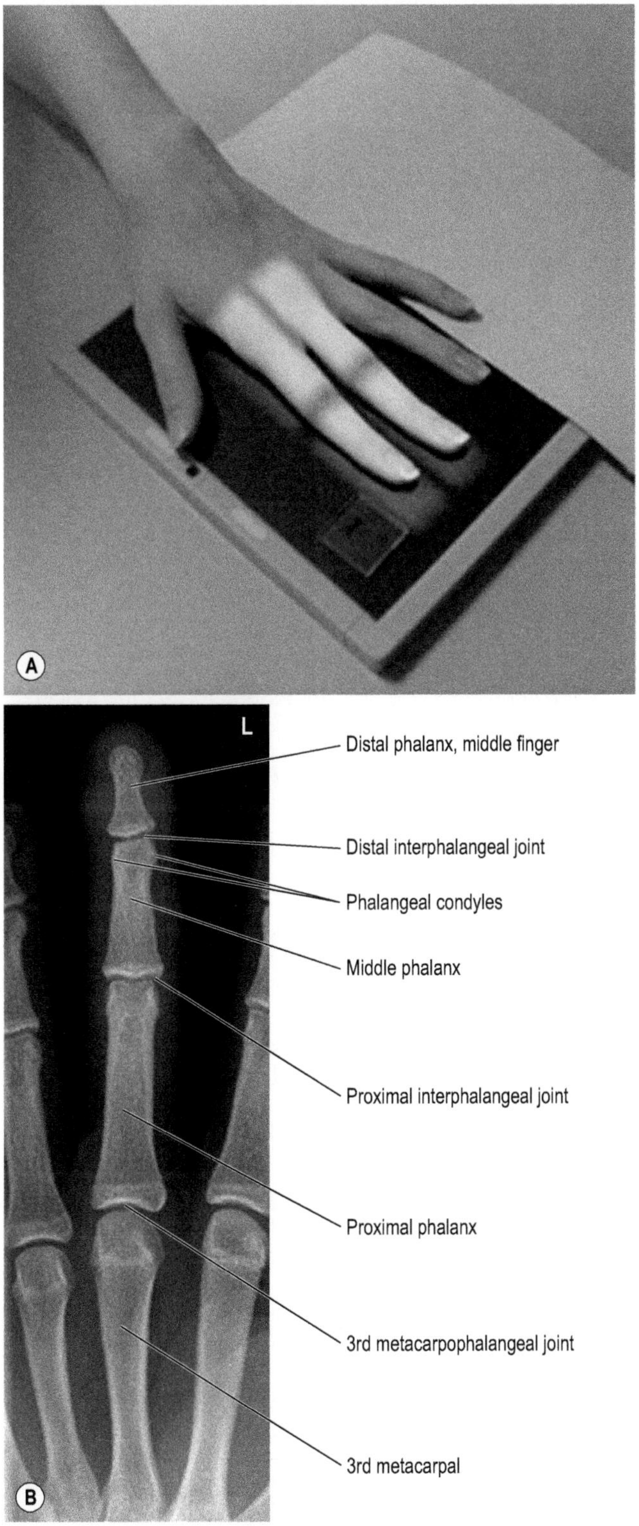

Fig. 4.6 (A) DP finger; (B) DP middle finger.

Opinions on centring points and the area for inclusion in the primary beam vary for finger examinations. The radiographer has a medicolegal responsibility to ensure that the correct digit has been examined and that there is evidence to support this.

One way to ensure this is to include the adjacent finger and nearest border of the hand in the field of collimation to ensure correct identification of the finger. Unfortunately this does involve irradiation of areas not required for examination and could theoretically be deemed to be in contravention of IR(ME)R 2017.[6] As a result, imaging department protocols should clearly identify the hospital's requirements for the radiographer, ensuring that there is uniformity of provision regarding finger images.

Centring points also vary, according to the area of interest required to be included in the field of radiation (see variation in descriptive section).

PCE COMMENTS – FINGERS

It is important not to miss small fractures of the fingers.

Forced flexion and extension injuries: these can result in avulsion fractures and knowledge of ligament insertions will guide accurate interpretation of fractures. Pay special attention to the volar plate area where avulsion fractures are common; they tend to be unstable and will require orthopaedic assessment. Mallet finger (fixed flexion deformity) can be associated with avulsion of a small fragment of bone from the dorsal aspect of the base of the phalanx. Volar plate fractures avulse from the palmar aspect involving the volar plate. These are best seen on the lateral projection.

Less commonly, there may be avulsion fractures on the lateral or medial margins originating from an avulsion of the collateral ligament.

Dislocations or subluxations of the interphalangeal joints: these are most commonly seen in the proximal interphalangeal joints and may be accompanied by a volar plate fracture. These dislocations should be described by mentioning direction of the dislocation relating to the displacement of distal phalanx (i.e. 'there is a dorsal dislocation of the proximal interphalangeal joint') and involvement of any avulsed fragment.

Articular surface: check to see if the articular surface is involved. Is the fragment small or a larger section of bone? (Treatment and follow up will vary according to fragment size; larger bone fragments may require surgical intervention.)

Spiral fractures: this type of fracture in the finger may be displaced but could involve the articular surface.

Paediatric cases: special attention should be paid to the metaphysis as this is the weakest part of the bone in a child. Look for steps in the cortex which can be subtle and can indicate a Salter–Harris type 2 fracture (see Chapter 3 for Salter–Harris fracture classifications). Other epiphyseal fractures are less common.

DORSIPALMAR (DP) FINGERS (FIG. 4.6A,B)

For all projections of the fingers the IR is horizontal.

Positioning

- The patient is seated with the affected side adjacent to the table

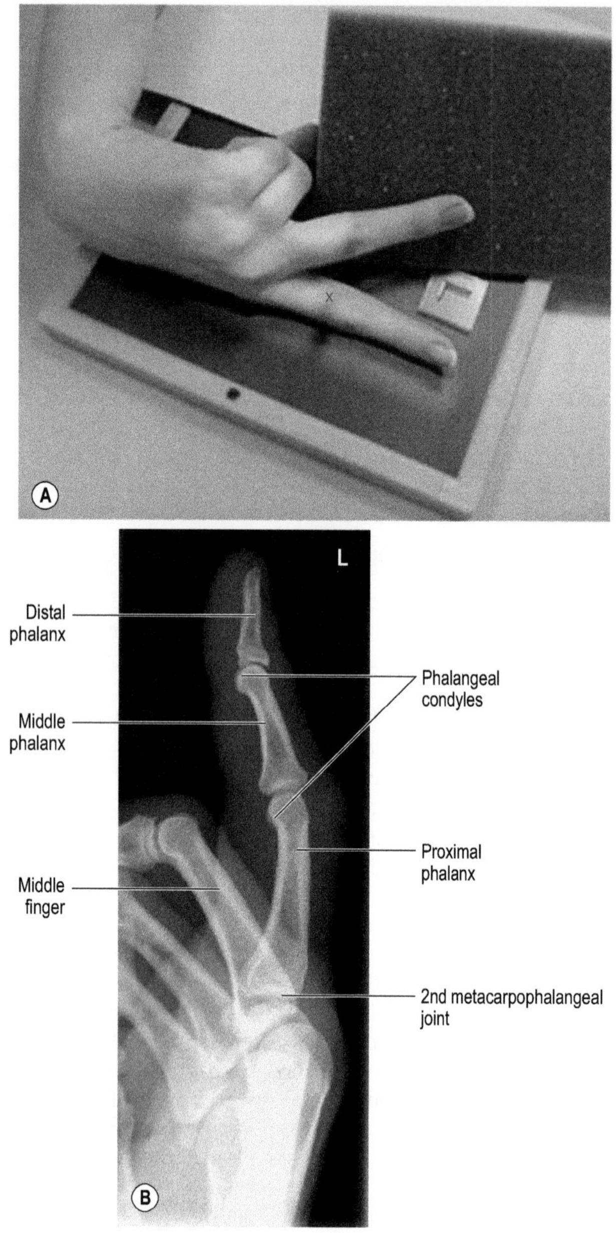

Fig. 4.7 Lateral index finger.

- The affected hand is pronated with the fingers extended, to facilitate visualisation of interphalangeal joint spaces, and slightly separated

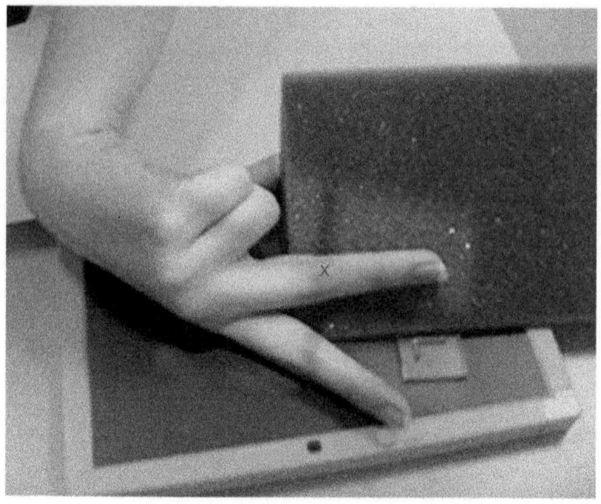

Fig. 4.8 Lateral middle finger.

Beam Direction and FRD

Vertical, at 90° to the IR
100 cm FRD

Centring Point

Method (a): Over the proximal interphalangeal joint or
Method (b): Metacarpophalangeal joint

Collimation

Centring method (a): All phalanges of the finger under examination; the metacarpophalangeal joint; adjacent finger/s to facilitate correct finger identification

Centring method (b): As above but to include associated metacarpal

Criteria for Assessing Image Quality

- *Centring method (a):* All phalanges and the metacarpophalangeal joint are demonstrated
- *Centring method (b)*: All phalanges, the metacarpophalangeal joint and the metacarpal are demonstrated
- Adjacent finger/s and soft tissue outline of the affected and adjacent fingers are demonstrated
- Symmetry of the phalangeal condyles
- The interphalangeal and metacarpophalangeal joint spaces are clearly visible and open
- Sharp image demonstrating the soft tissue margins of the finger, bony cortex and trabeculae

Common Errors: DP Fingers

Common Error	Possible Reason	Potential Effects on PCE or Report
Interphalangeal joint spaces not clearly demonstrated	Fingers may be flexed; extend to clear	Intra-articular fractures may be missed Important volar plate fractures may not be demonstrated

LATERAL FINGERS

Lateral projections of some fingers can prove difficult to achieve and maintain in position, especially when attempting to separate and immobilise middle, ring and little fingers. The injured or arthritic patient may be even less cooperative. Small wedge-shaped radiolucent pads are efficient aids in separating fingers for radiographic examination.

Positioning

Index (First) Finger (Fig. 4.7A,B).

- From the DP position the hand is internally rotated through 90° and the third and fourth fingers are flexed and held in position by the thumb
- The index finger is extended and positioned with its lateral aspect in contact with the IR

- The long axis of the index finger is separated from the palmar-flexed middle finger with a radiolucent pad

Middle Finger (Fig. 4.8).

- From the DP position, the hand is internally rotated 90° and positioned as for the lateral index finger projection
- The middle finger is extended and separated from the index finger with a radiolucent pad
- The middle finger is supported in a horizontal position by a radiolucent pad

Ring and Little Finger: Method 1 (Fig. 4.9).

- From the DP position the hand is externally rotated through 90°
- The index and middle fingers are flexed and held by the thumb; the little finger remains extended, as does the ring finger
- The medial aspect of the fifth metacarpal is in contact with the IR
- The ring finger is slightly dorsiflexed to clear it from the little finger
- If under examination, the ring finger is supported in a horizontal position; in any event it is separated from the little finger by a radiolucent pad

Ring and Little Finger: Method 2 (Fig. 4.10).

- From the DP position the hand is externally rotated through 90°
- The index finger is flexed and held by the thumb; the remaining fingers are slightly dorsiflexed and fanned out; their long axes remain horizontal
- If under examination, the ring finger is supported in a horizontal position; in any event it is separated from the other fingers by radiolucent pads

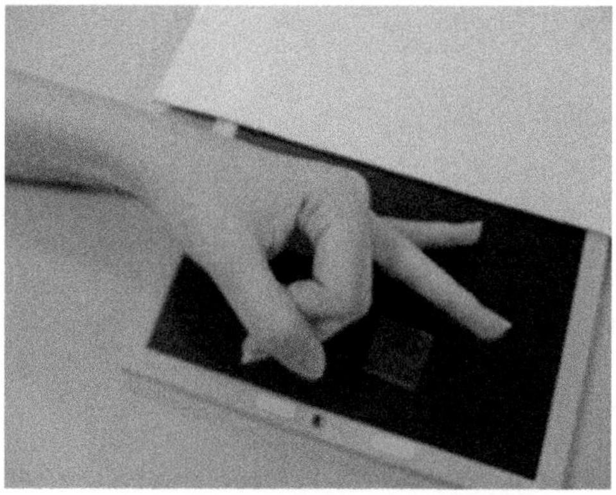

Fig. 4.9 Ring and little finger – method 1.

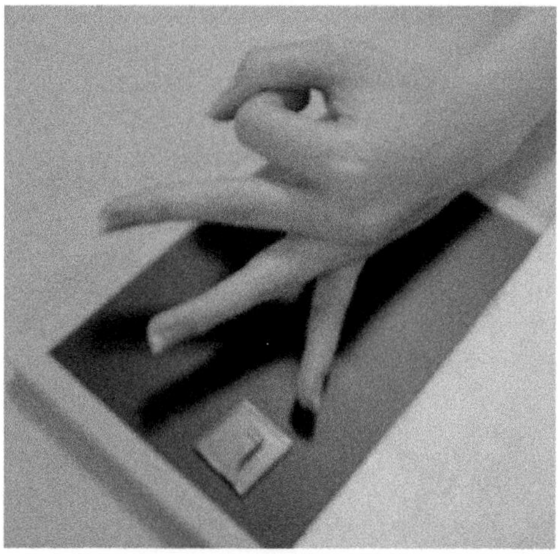

Fig. 4.10 Ring and little finger – method 2.

FOR ALL THE FINGERS AND POSITIONS

Beam Direction and FRD

Vertical, at 90° to the IR
100 cm FRD

Centring Point

Method (a): Over the proximal interphalangeal joint of the finger under examination or
Method (b): Metacarpophalangeal joint of the finger under examination

Collimation

Centring method (a): All phalanges, soft tissue outlines and the metacarpophalangeal joint. Evidence of the adjacent finger for confirmation of identification of the finger under examination

Centring method (b): All phalanges, soft tissue outlines and the associated metacarpal. Evidence of the adjacent finger for confirmation of identification of the finger under examination

Criteria for Assessing Image Quality

- *Centring method (a)*: All phalanges and the metacarpophalangeal joint are demonstrated, with the outline of adjacent finger/s
- *Centring method (b)*: All phalanges, the metacarpophalangeal joint and the metacarpal are demonstrated with the outline of adjacent finger/s
- Clear interphalangeal and metacarpophalangeal joints are demonstrated, with phalangeal condyles superimposed
- Sharp image demonstrating the soft tissue margins of the finger, bony cortex and trabeculae of phalanges under examination

Common Errors: Lateral – All Fingers and Positions

Common Error	Possible Reason	Potential Effect on PCE or Report
Poor joint space demonstration with non-superimposition of phalangeal condyles	Long axis of finger may not lie parallel to IR; reposition and support more effectively or angle beam to coincide with angle of interphalangeal joints if patient cannot comply	Intra-articular and volar plate fractures may not be visualised

Hand

PCE COMMENTS – HAND

Boxer's or *fighter's fractures*: these relatively common fractures occur at the neck of the fifth and sometimes the fourth metacarpal, resulting from the force of a punch. They are often clearly seen. Describe the position and degree of angulation of the fracture site as seen on the lateral projection.

Carpometacarpal dislocations: assess joint spaces for carpometacarpal dislocations or fractures; the lateral projection is best for this. Remember bones should not overlap in a normal radiograph. (Beware of projectional errors caused by poor positioning.)

Rheumatology patients: in rheumatology cases the ball catcher's projection will demonstrate subluxed joints and erosion of the articular surfaces. It is important to compare these views with previous imaging to assess disease progression. However, good management in the early stages of the disease has resulted in less advanced destructive disease being commonly seen.

Particular attention should be paid to the uniformity of *carpal joint spaces*. The proximal row of carpal bones articulate with the distal row. Any irregularity may indicate a fracture or ligament disruption. The carpal bones are each joined to the adjacent ones by intercarpal ligaments, and widening of any of these areas indicates disruption of the ligament. A good example of this is seen in scapholunate disruption, showing as widening in the joint space between the two bones and sometimes referred to as the Terry Thomas sign, David Letterman sign or even Madonna sign (so described because the widened gap between adjacent bones looks similar to the gapped front teeth displayed by all three people).[7]

Carpometacarpal joints should also be examined meticulously so as not to miss dislocations at this point. Lateral views of hand or wrist show this injury best.

Lunate or perilunate fracture/dislocations are the result of a high-impact injury. Pay particular attention to alignment of bones on the lateral projection and overlapping of carpal bones and joint spaces on the DP, AP or ballcatcher's projections.

Other important lunate/perilunate and trans-scaphoid perilunate injuries should be considered. These tend to result from high-impact trauma (often motorcycle accidents). Careful assessment should be made of the alignment of the radius, lunate and capitate on lateral views of hand and wrist. A key approach to assessing lunate, capitate and radius congruency is to use the apple/cup/saucer sign: the 'apple' (capitate) should sit in the 'cup' (lunate), which should sit in the 'saucer' (radius). If these are not aligned, then lunate or perilunate dislocation is indicated and the lateral image will help differentiate whether there is lunate or perilunate dislocation.[8,9]

Is there abnormal overlapping of the carpal bones on the PA projection? This may result in the lunate adopting a 'slice of pie'-shaped appearance (triangular appearance of lunate on the PA projection rather than the more usual trapezoid shape); this indicates lunate or perilunate dislocation. There will also be loss of uniformity of joint spaces.

Remember to look at the whole image. *Galeazzi* fracture dislocations of the forearm result in radioulnar joint disruption (also see PCE comments for forearm, Chapter 5). You may also see this on wrist images.

Scaphoid fractures often cannot be excluded on acute images, so advice over clinical correlation should be mentioned (also see PCE comments for the wrist).

The scaphoid fat pad sign can be used to supplement bony information, but the fat pad sign cannot be used as standalone evidence of injury.[10]

DORSIPALMAR (DP) HAND (FIG. 4.11A,B)

For all projections of the hand the IR is placed on the table-top.

Positioning

- The patient is seated with the affected side next to the table
- The hand is pronated and its palmar aspect placed in contact with the IR
- The fingers and thumb are extended and slightly separated

Beam Direction and FRD

Vertical, at 90° to the IR
100 cm FRD

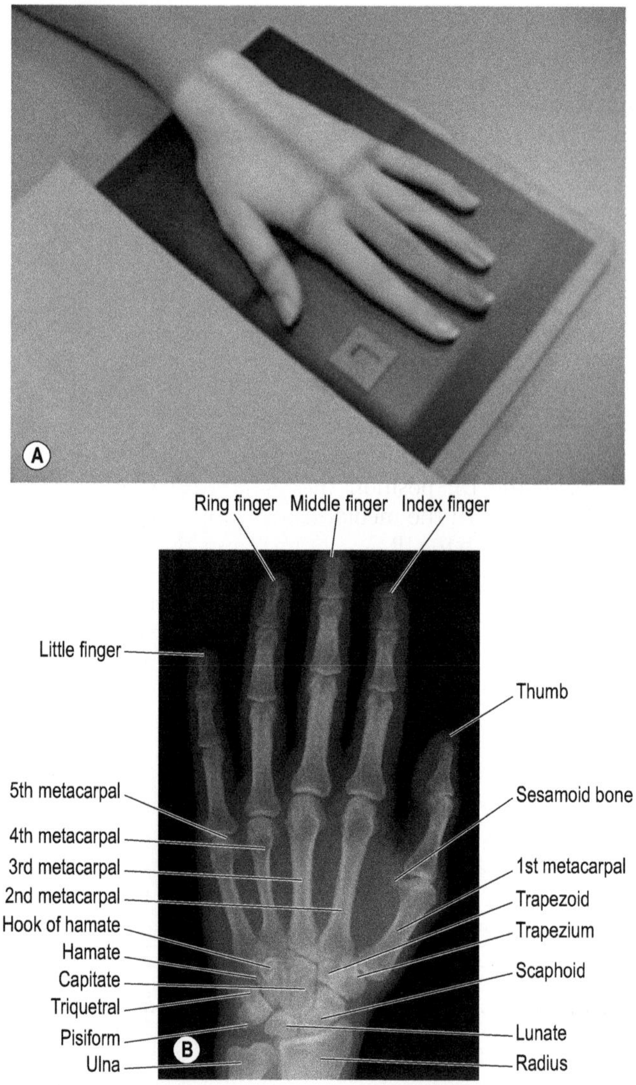

Fig. 4.11 DP hand.

Centring Point

Over the head of the third metacarpal

Collimation

All phalanges, soft tissue outline of the hand, wrist joint

Criteria for Assessing Image Quality

- All phalanges, the wrist joint and the soft tissue outline of the hand are demonstrated
- The fingers are separated, and the interphalangeal and metacarpophalangeal joints are clear
- Symmetrical appearance of the heads of metacarpals 2–4
- Obliquity of thumb and the heads of metacarpals 1 and 5
- Sharp image demonstrating the soft tissue margins of the hand, bony cortex and trabeculae
- Adequate penetration to demonstrate the hook of hamate whilst showing distal phalanges

Common Errors: DP Hand

Common Errors	Possible Reasons	Potential Effects on PCE or Report
Superimposition of soft tissue outlines of fingers	Fingers are not separated adequately	Soft tissue swelling or foreign bodies may not be visualised adequately Cortical outlines may be obscured
Poor demonstration of joint spaces	Fingers may not be extended; extend fingers or examine with hand in supination to use obliquity of rays around centre of beam, to 'open out' joints	Intra-articular fractures or dislocations may be missed on the DP projection Volar plate fractures may be missed

In this position it is to be noted that the fifth metacarpal and little finger are externally rotated into an oblique appearance. The concept of reducing this obliquity and the impact of this on the image has been discussed in the past,[11] yet it does not appear that there has been a widespread adoption of the measures suggested. Could this be because reporting radiographers and radiologists find that the projections of the fifth metacarpal provided by the DP and dorsipalmar oblique (DPO) positions are at sufficiently different angles? Or is familiarity with these more usual appearances enough to inspire confidence in outlining a report?

DORSIPALMAR OBLIQUE (DPO) HAND (FIG. 4.12A,B)

Positioning

- The patient is seated with the affected side next to the table
- From the DP position the hand is externally rotated through 45°; the medial aspect of the hand remains in contact with the IR
- A radiolucent pad is placed under the lateral aspect of the hand as immobilisation and to keep the fingers extended and horizontal. An alternative is to allow the fingers and thumb to dorsiflex gently and rest on the IR for support
- The fingers are separated

Beam Direction and FRD

Vertical, at 90° to the IR
100 cm FRD

Centring Point

Over the head of the third metacarpal

Collimation

All phalanges, soft tissue outline of the hand, wrist joint

Previous descriptions of the DPO hand have shown the selection of a range of centring methods.[3,5] Originally, in the UK, centring for this projection was stated as over

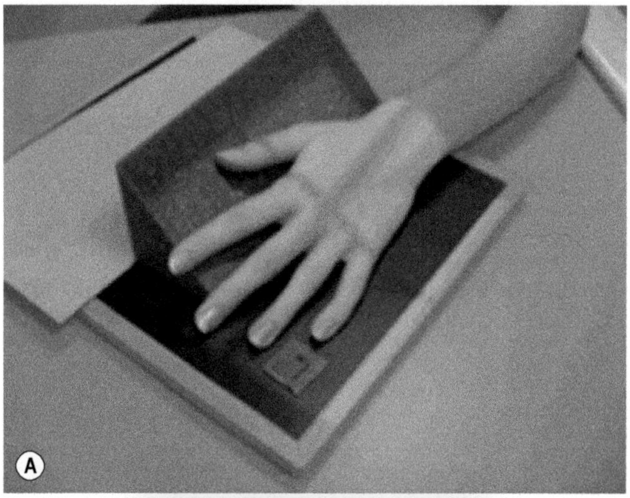

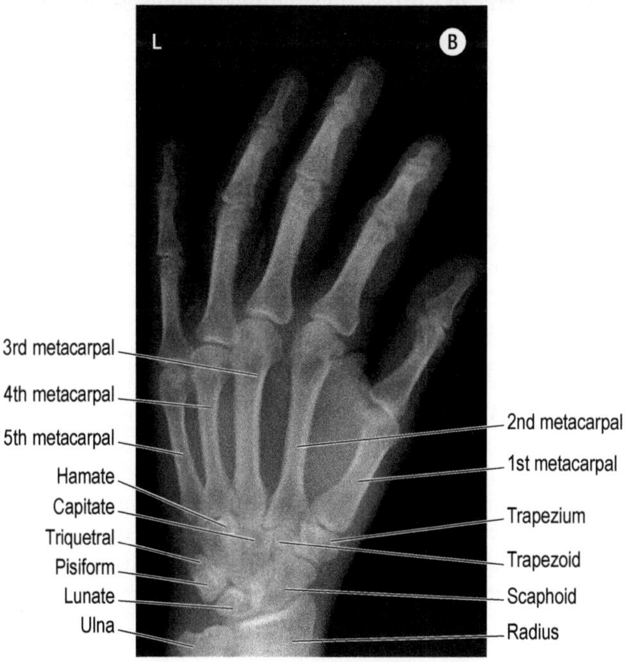

Fig. 4.12 DP oblique hand.

the head of the fifth metacarpal[12,13] in order to use the effect of the oblique rays which 'opened out' the spaces between the metacarpal heads. As the dose reduction culture gained influence in radiography, it became clear that this centring point required an unacceptably large field of radiation, almost half of which was not usefully employed. The result was to suggest that centring should remain the same, with the addition of angulation across the dorsum of the hand until the central ray lay over the head of the third metacarpal. This would allow closer collimation around the hand, yet maintain the effects of the oblique rays afforded in the original centring point.

In principle, of course, this sounds a logical amendment. However, questions have arisen regarding this method.[5] Because the FRD for this projection lies at 100 cm and the distance between the heads of the fifth and third metacarpals is generally around 3 cm, the oblique rays referred to will actually be around 2° and possibly even less. How useful would such a small angle be? Can the human eye detect differences in images taken with or without this angle?

Why even consider 'opening up' the spaces between metacarpal heads when they are well separated on the DP image? Different projections in radiography are always used to give a different view of what is essentially a two-dimensional image medium, and adding angle onto a DPO projection will only serve to reduce the usefulness of the obliquity. If it is really essential (and the authors question whether or not this would actually be the case, bearing in mind the previous sentence) then why not utilise 2° less obliquity on the rotation of the hand, although could 2° even be assessed accurately by the human eye?

For these reasons, in this book the centring is selected as the head of the third metacarpal with a vertical central ray.

Criteria for Assessing Image Quality

- All phalanges, wrist joint and soft tissue outline of the hand are demonstrated
- Separation of the shafts of the metacarpals but with some overlap of metacarpal heads 3–5
- Separation of the soft tissues of the fingers and intermediate phalanges and distal phalanges
- Joint spaces will not be demonstrated as clear
- Sharp image demonstrating the soft tissue margins of the hand, bony cortex and trabeculae

Common Errors: DPO Hand

Common Error	Possible Reason	Potential Effects on PCE or Report
Overlap of shafts of metacarpals	Excessive external rotation of the hand	Cortical outlines difficult to assess Trabecular patterns obscured, potentially causing a missed fracture

LATERAL HAND (FIG. 4.13A,B)

The lateral projection is most useful for demonstrating the direction of displacement in fractures of the metacarpals and is particularly useful to identify anterior displacement of distal bony fragments in the boxer's fracture. The fingers are superimposed and the adducted thumb overexposed, meaning that these structures are not well identified in this projection.

Positioning

- The patient is seated with the affected side next to the table
- From the DP position, the hand is externally rotated through 90°
- The fingers are extended and superimposed vertically, and the thumb is extended and abducted from the hand
- The thumb lies horizontally and supported on a radiolucent pad

Beam Direction and FRD

Vertical, at 90° to the IR
100 cm FRD

Centring Point

Over the medial aspect of the head of the second metacarpal

Collimation

All phalanges, soft tissue outline of the hand, wrist joint

Criteria for Assessing Image Quality

- All phalanges, the wrist joint and the soft tissue outline of the hand are demonstrated
- The fingers are superimposed, metacarpals 2–5 are superimposed and the thumb is cleared from other bones of the hand
- Sharp image demonstrating the soft tissue margins of the hand, bony cortex and trabeculae of the lunate. Outlines of superimposed bones are demonstrated but not showing trabecular detail. Penetration to demonstrate individual carpal bones

Common Errors: Lateral Hand

Common Error	Possible Reason	Potential Effects on PCE or Report
Poor superimposition of phalanges and poor superimposition of metacarpals	Over- or under-rotation of the hand; ensure dorsum of hand is at 90° to IR	Angulation of fracture site may be difficult to assess Carpometacarpal fractures may be overlooked

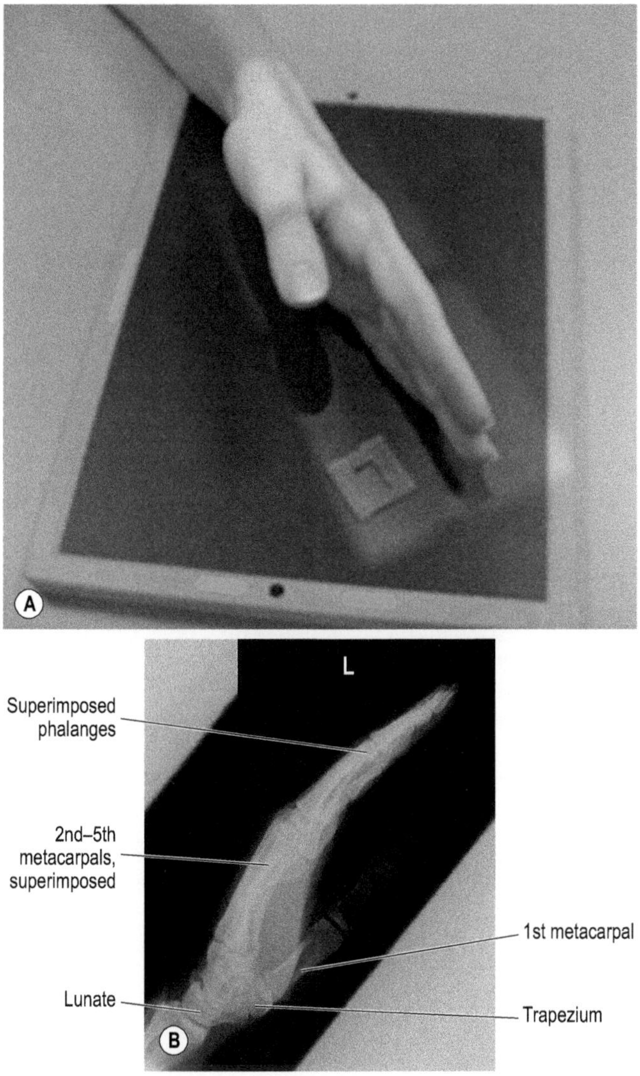

Fig. 4.13 Lateral hand.

PALMAR DORSAL OBLIQUE OF BOTH HANDS FOR RHEUMATOID ARTHRITIS ASSESSMENT (BALL CATCHER'S) (FIG. 4.14A,B)

Both hands are examined via the same single-exposure image. Hands are palm upwards with relaxed fingers and slight medial rotation. The hands appear as though the patient is poised ready to catch a ball, hence the alternative name *'ball catcher's projection'*.

Positioning

- The patient is seated alongside the table but it may be necessary to turn the trunk slightly towards the IR
- The arms are abducted forwards towards the IR and externally rotated to bring the region of the dorsum of the hands overlying the fifth metacarpal in contact with the IR
- The dorsum of the hands lie at 30° to the IR and the hands are supported in this position by radiolucent pads. The fingers are slightly relaxed

Beam Direction and FRD

Vertical, at 90° to the IR
100 cm FRD

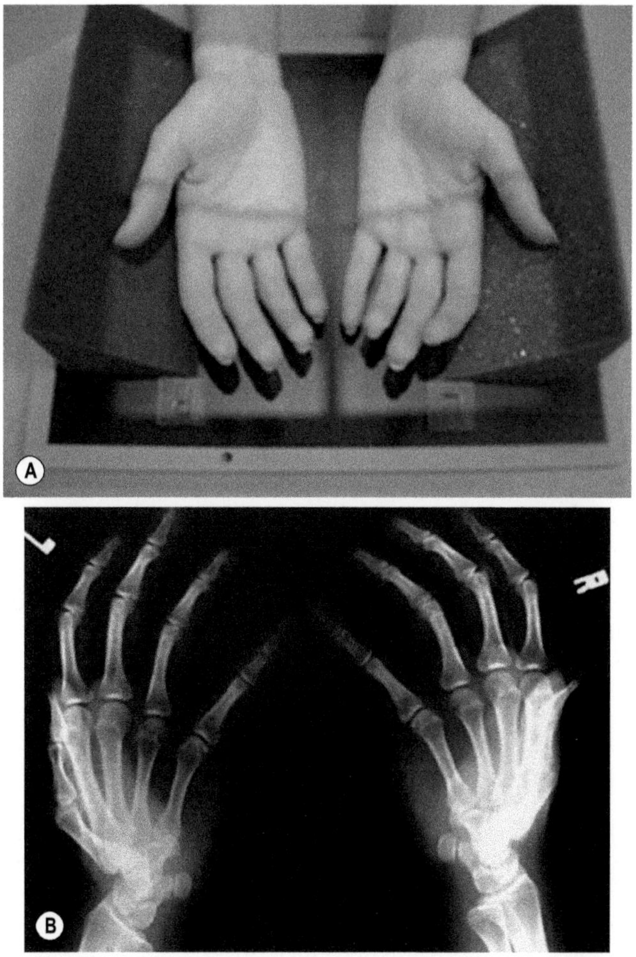

Fig. 4.14 Ball catcher's. (B, Reproduced with permission from Ballinger PW, Frank ED. *Merrill's Atlas of Radiographic Positioning and Radiologic Procedures.* 10th ed. St Louis: Mosby; 2003.)

Centring Point

Midway between the medial borders of the hand, level with the heads of the fifth metacarpals

Collimation

Both hands and wrist joints

Criteria for Assessing Image Quality

- Both hands and wrist joints are demonstrated
- Clear metacarpophalangeal joint spaces 2–5
- Sharp image demonstrating bony detail in contrast with the joint spaces

Wrist

It has been estimated that some 17% of fractures encountered in the Emergency Department involve the distal radius,[14] making radiological assessment of this area a fairly common occurrence.

Wrist examinations are often undertaken with the wrist in an immobilisation medium, which will have implications for selection of the exposure factor, according to density of the fracture immobiliser. If a dense medium is used, as in plaster of Paris, both kVp and mAs will need to be increased, although most immobilisers are less dense and require less or no increase in exposure factors. It should be noted that plaster of Paris is less frequently used than in the past. Any increase results in a higher radiation dose to the area.

PCE COMMENTS – WRIST

A fall onto outstretched hand (FOOSH) is a common presentation in the Emergency Department and can cause one of three groups of fractures; often the fracture types are age-relevant. Knowledge of these is useful in interpretation of these images. A rough guide is:

Children

Children tend to suffer from *greenstick fractures* that do not completely fracture across the bones due to the elasticity of the bones. They are mainly seen in the diaphysis and are most commonly seen in children under the age of 10. In some cases the bone may appear bowed, but with no apparent fracture.

A *torus fracture* appears as buckling of the cortex on the inner bend of the fractured bone; they show the convex surface as intact.

Epiphyseal fractures (found in the growth plate) are commonly encountered on images. It is very important not to overlook this as these fractures can result in long-term deformities.

Adults

Scaphoid fracture is often caused by falling onto an outstretched hand or by forced sudden hyperflexion (as in steering-wheel injuries). These fractures often are not obvious in the acute stage so mention of this and importance of clinical correlation is advised in PCE. Follow-up after 10–14 days will classically show callus along the healing fracture site as the indicator. A normal fat pad is seen best on PA and PA oblique wrist projections, and is seen as a radiolucent linear or triangular area of fat on the lateral, or ulnar, aspect of the scaphoid; an abnormal scaphoid may show a fat pad sign where the fat pad appears to be missing or laterally displaced. It is most commonly associated with scaphoid fracture but may indicate radial styloid fracture, or even a fracture of the first metacarpal. The fat pad sign alone cannot be considered unequivocal[10] and is not usually noted in patients under 12 years of age. Scaphoid fractures are more commonly found in patients aged 15–40 but can be seen in other adult age ranges. In addition to the scaphoid, other bones of the carpus should also be checked, as in comments given for PCE in hand projections.

Colles' fracture is a fracture of the distal radius with dorsal (posterior) angulation of the distal fragment, commonly found after fall onto an outstretched hand. In some cases the ulna may also be involved but this is much rarer in incidence. The Colles' fracture is most commonly found in patients over the age of 40. Ensure you describe the type of fracture, degree of angulation and involvement of the articular surface. Assess the palmar tilt of the radial articular surface to pick up subtle impacted fractures.

Smith's fracture is less commonly seen than the Colles' fracture, caused by impact on the dorsal forearm or falling onto the wrist in flexion. The fracture will be displaced in a palmar direction. Similarly, describe the direction of distal fragment, degree of angulation and if there is articular involvement.

Galeazzi fracture dislocations of the forearm result in radioulnar joint disruption (also see PCE comments for forearm, Chapter 5). You may also see this on hand images.

Don't forget to check for subtle fractures in all cases, following generic checks outlined in Chapter 3.

POSTEROANTERIOR (PA) WRIST (FIG. 4.15A,B)

For all projections of the wrist the IR is horizontal.

Positioning

- The patient is seated with the affected side next to the table
- The affected arm is flexed at the elbow and the wrist is internally rotated to pronate the hand
- The anterior aspect of the wrist is placed in contact with the IR; the fingers are relaxed to bring the forearm and wrist flat and in contact with the IR

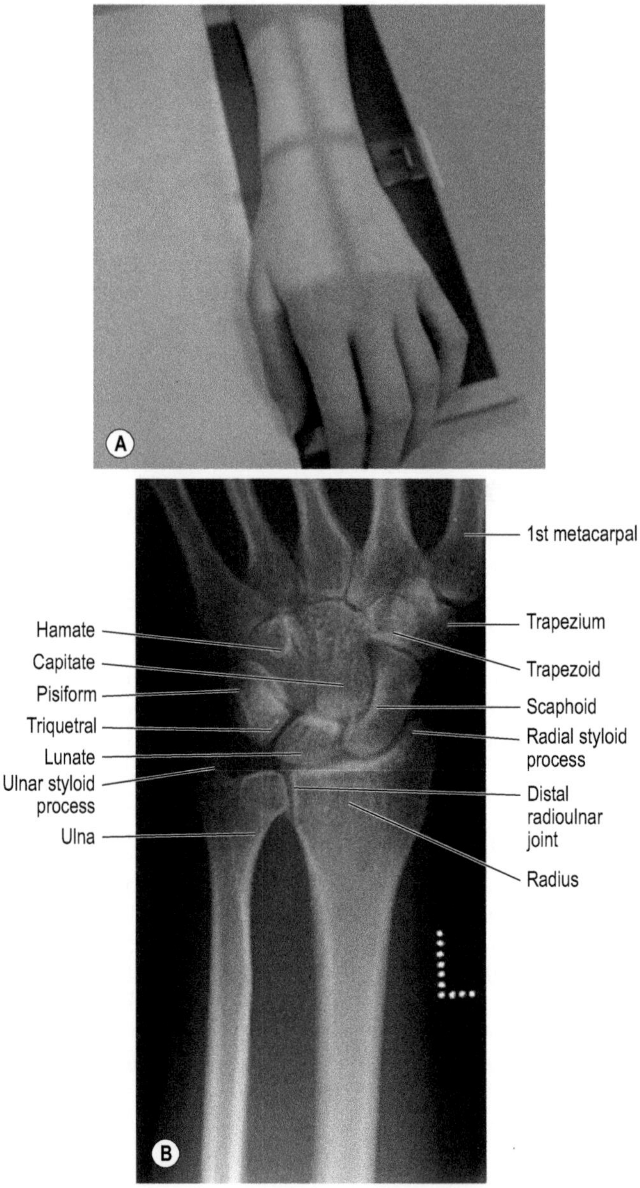

Fig. 4.15 PA wrist.

- The radial and ulnar styloid processes are equidistant from the IR

Beam Direction and FRD

Vertical, at 90° to the IR
100 cm FRD

Centring Point

Midway between the radial and ulnar styloid processes

Collimation

Proximal third of metacarpals, carpals, distal third of radius and ulna, soft tissue outlines of wrist

Criteria for Assessing Image Quality

- Proximal third of metacarpals, the carpals, distal third of radius and ulna, and soft tissue outlines of the wrist are demonstrated
- Clear demonstration of the distal radioulnar joint
- The radial and ulnar styloid processes seen on the lateral and medial margins of these bones
- Sharp image demonstrating the soft tissue margins of the area, bony cortex and trabeculae. Adequate penetration will demonstrate the hook of hamate clearly
- Good contrast is required over the soft tissue as there is evidence that changes the alignment and shape of the scaphoid fat pad

Common Errors: PA Wrist

Common Error	Possible Reason	Potential Effects on PCE or Report
Radial and ulnar styloid processes appear displaced from lateral and medial margins of these bones; superimposition of the radius and ulna over the distal radioulnar joint	Styloid processes are not equidistant from the IR	Intra-articular fractures are difficult to visualise Cortical outlines and symmetry of joint spaces may cause errors in interpretation Accurate assessment of angulation at fracture site may be compromised Forearm fractures causing dislocation of the distal radio ulna joint (Galeazzi fracture) may be overlooked

LATERAL WRIST (FIG. 4.16A,B)

Positioning

- The patient is seated with the affected side next to the table
- The wrist is externally rotated 90° from the PA position*
- The medial aspect of the wrist is placed in contact with the IR
- The wrist is externally rotated approximately 5° further, in order to superimpose the radial and ulnar styloid processes

*At this point it is important to discuss positioning for the lateral wrist, bearing in mind traditional approaches to this projection. Some texts have described the patient's position as with the arm abducted laterally, with a view to facilitate movement of the ulna to a position that is suggested to be at 90° to the PA,[5,10] and others described a position involving external rotation from the PA position only.[13,15] The first method is believed to ensure that the ulna lies at 90° to its position in the PA by moving the arm at the shoulder and putting the humerus in a lateral position; at this point it is important to discuss this further.

Study of the movement of the forearm, for both methods, demonstrates that the outline of the ulnar styloid process on the image does not change between projections, whatever technique is used. The only way that a difference of 90° can be achieved is with the hand in supination, as in an AP position, and with a lateral using any of the methods previously described[5,10,13–15] (Fig. 4.17A–F).

One can only wonder why wrist projections originated with two projections that provided images at 90° for only one of the bones required for demonstration, but a study of texts from the earlier days of radiography (over 70 years ago) show that the PA projection appears always to have been the projection of choice for this region.[16]

Beam Direction and FRD

Vertical, at 90° to the IR
100 cm FRD

Centring Point

Over the radial styloid process

Collimation

Proximal third of metacarpals, the carpals, distal third of radius and ulna, soft tissue outlines of wrist

Criteria for Assessing Image Quality

- Proximal third of metacarpals, carpals, distal third of radius and ulna, soft tissue outlines of the wrist are demonstrated
- Superimposition of the distal radius and ulna; the lunate should have a crescent-shaped appearance; distal scaphoid superimposed over pisiform;[17] long axes of radius and third metacarpal are aligned[18]
- Sharp image demonstrating the soft tissue margins of the wrist, bony cortex and trabeculae. Penetration of carpus to demonstrate individual carpal bones while demonstrating pronator fat stripe within soft tissue, anterior to radius

Inclusion of the anterior fat stripe in collimation is recognised as necessary as it may be the only (subtle) indication of injury.[17] The area of reduced radiographic density lies approximately 0.6 cm from the anterior aspect of the radial outline and curves very slightly, following the distal radial outline in a proximal direction. Positional criteria given are simple descriptors of recurrently recommended criteria,[13,17] but more complex requirements have been described as 'the palmar cortex of the pisiform bone should overlie the central third of the interval between the palmar cortices of the distal scaphoid pole and the capitate head'.[14] Needless to say, deformities caused by severe trauma to the wrist and carpus may render it impossible to ensure that such positional criteria can be achieved.

Common Errors: Lateral Wrist

Common Errors	Possible Reasons	Potential Effects on PCE or Report
Radius appears posteriorly in relation to ulna	Excessive external rotation	Angulation of fracture site and carpal bone position may be difficult to assess Subtle fractures and dislocations may be missed
Ulna appears posteriorly in relation to radius	Inadequate external rotation	Angulation of fracture site and carpal bone position may be difficult to assess Subtle fractures or dislocations may be missed

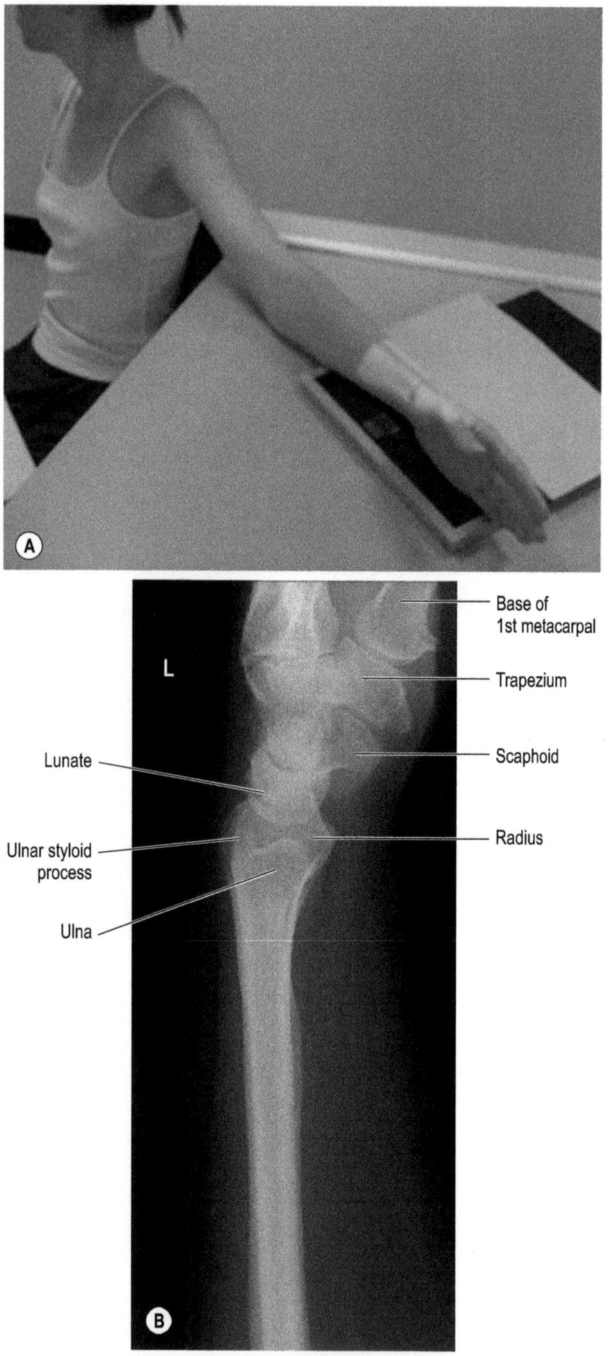

Fig. 4.16 Lateral wrist.

POSTEROANTERIOR (PA) OBLIQUE WRIST (FIG. 4.18A,B)

Positioning

- The patient is seated with the affected side next to the table
- From the PA position the wrist is externally rotated 45°
- The wrist is supported in this position with a radiolucent pad or by slight flexion of the fingers until their tips rest on the IR or table to support the obliquity; there should be no dorsiflexion or palmar flexion at the wrist

Beam Direction and FRD

Vertical, at 90° to the IR
100 cm FRD

Centring Point

Midway between the radial and ulnar styloid processes

Collimation

Proximal third of metacarpals, carpals, distal third of radius and ulna, and soft tissue outlines of wrist

Criteria for Assessing Image Quality

- Proximal third of metacarpals, carpals, distal third of radius and ulna, and the soft tissue outlines of the wrist demonstrated
- Overlap of the distal radioulnar joint
- Scaphoid and trapezium are clearly demonstrated
- Sharp image demonstrating the soft tissue margins of the wrist, bony cortex and trabeculae. Adequate penetration to demonstrate differentiation between overlapped carpal bones

Scaphoid

Scaphoid fractures are difficult to detect radiographically immediately after injury and are best demonstrated after 10–14 days, when callus formation can be seen as increased bone density on radiographs.

However, because fractures of the radius and ulna must also be excluded at the time of injury, wrist projections are undertaken initially. Disruption of the single blood supply to the proximal end of the scaphoid may result in bony necrosis and onset of bony degenerative changes if the fracture is not treated; as a result, even in the event of negative findings for radius and ulna at the initial stage, the wrist is treated conservatively, with the use of immobilisation. At the end of the 10–14-day callus formation period immobilisation is removed and well-collimated scaphoid projections are requested. It is possible that plain radiographic imaging may not provide useful information, and imaging may include use of MRI, radionuclide imaging or even ultrasound.[19]

Many projections that will demonstrate the scaphoid have been described and it is necessary to use the minimum that will provide the required information. Projections selected for description include ulnar deviation, to clear the scaphoid from adjacent carpal bones, and a 30° angle which has been shown to demonstrate fractures of the waist effectively. It may not be considered necessary to use all the projections described in one assessment of the scaphoid.

Descriptions include only those for the specifically centred, well-coned scaphoid assessment. In the PA wrist projection, where the centring point lies between the styloid processes, the scaphoid will be foreshortened owing to its orientation within the carpus. Centring over the scaphoid reduces this effect and the scaphoid is likely to be more clearly demonstrated, with minimum distortion. However, in an attempt to consider this concept realistically, it should be asked whether this improved visualisation would be detected by the human eye, since the obliquity of X-rays around the central ray at 100 cm FRD will only be approximately 2° through the fracture.

Initial assessment, which includes the wrist, should be positioned as described in the section on wrist examinations but with ulnar deviation applied. When using this medial flexion on the wrist, care should be taken not to flex the joint anteriorly or posteriorly as this can distort the image of the scaphoid itself.

In this book the term 'anatomical snuffbox' is used in centring point descriptions. The position of the scaphoid can be identified as lying under this 'snuffbox', a depression found on the lateral border of the carpus, between the base of the first metacarpal and the radius. It is particularly evident when the thumb is in lateral abduction.

For all projections of the scaphoid the IR is horizontal.

POSTEROANTERIOR (PA) WITH ULNAR DEVIATION (FIG. 4.19A,B)

Positioning

- The patient is positioned as for the PA projection of the wrist
- The 'snuffbox' is placed in the centre of the available space if an IR is used

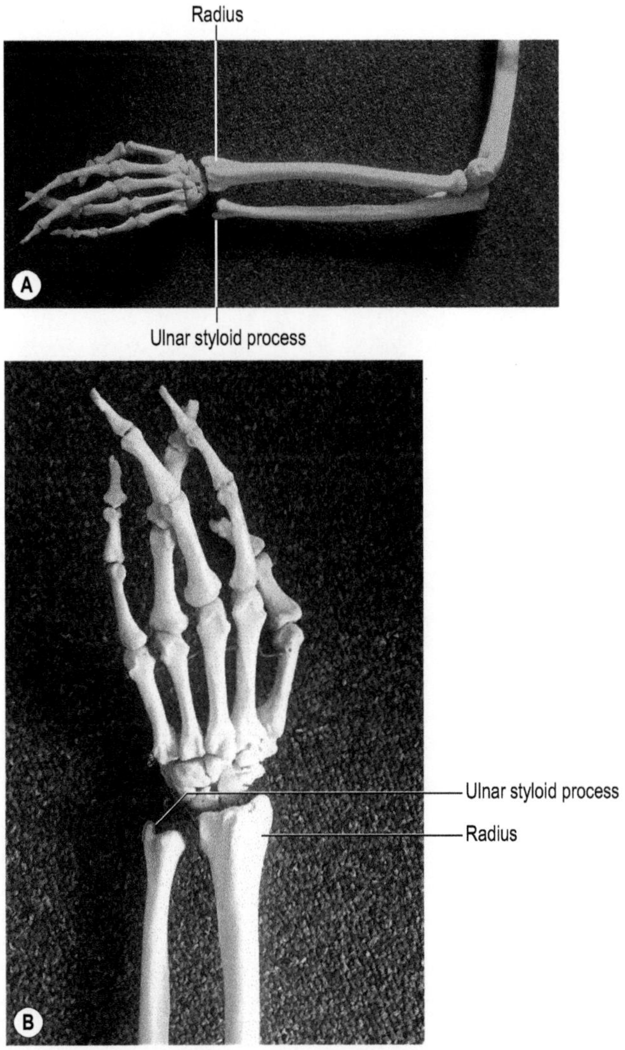

Fig. 4.17 Changing position of ulnar styloid process during forearm movements and rotation of the left wrist and forearm. (A,B) Ulnar styloid process position with the hand in pronation as in the PA wrist projection.

Continued

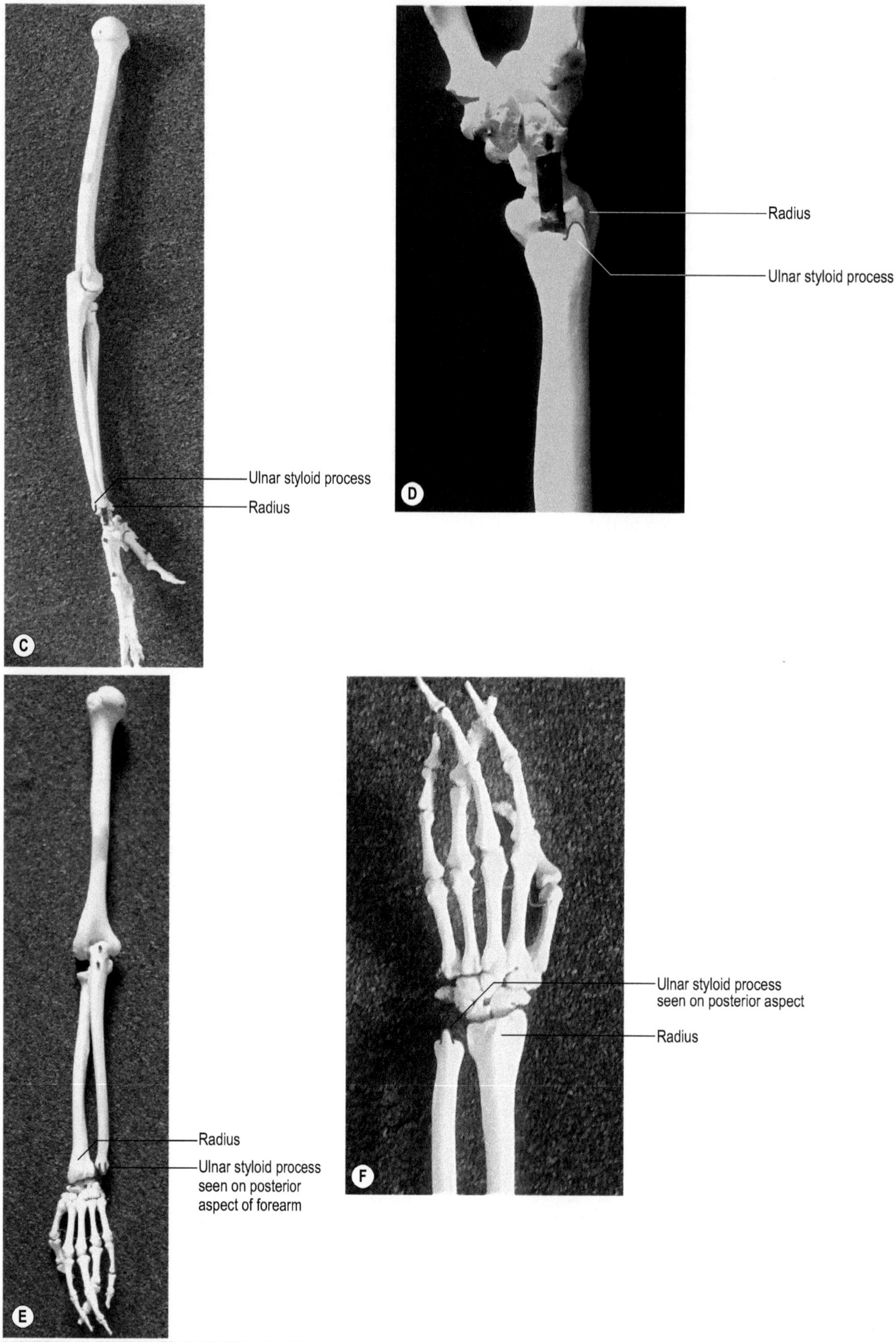

Fig. 4.17, Cont'd (C,D) Ulnar styloid process position with the arm in the lateral position (as seen from the medial aspect in order to show the distal ulna; to show it from the lateral aspect would superimpose the radius over the ulna) – note that it appears as a mirror image compared to the lateral radiograph in Fig. 4.16B because the bone is shown from its medial aspect; (E,F) ulnar styloid process position seen from the posterior aspect when the arm is in supination, showing the ulnar styloid process has shifted in position when compared to Fig. 4.17A–D. This is the only position that will show the styloid process at 90° to the lateral.

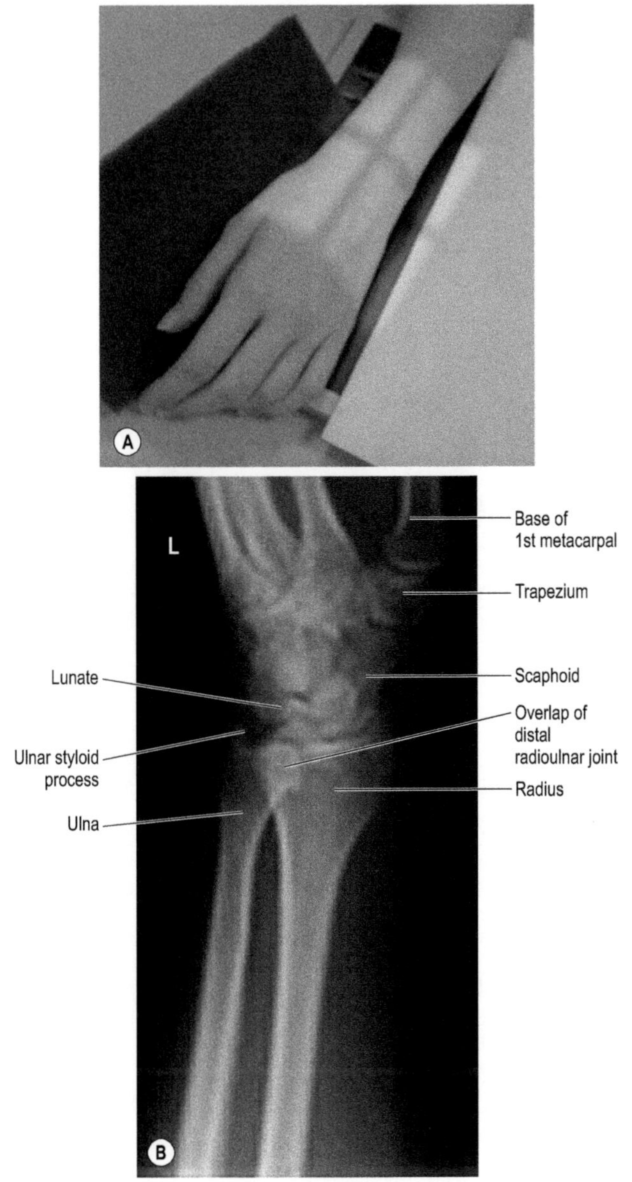

Fig. 4.18 PA oblique wrist.

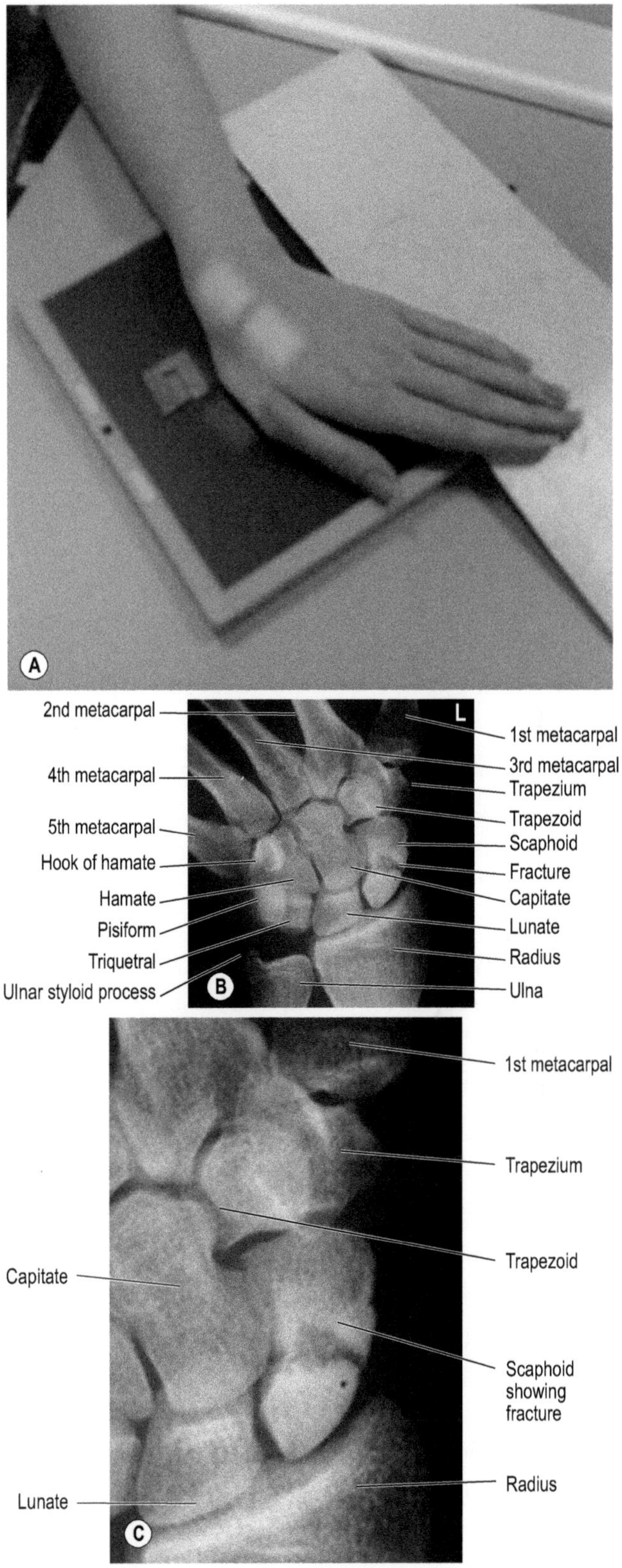

Fig. 4.19 Scaphoid PA with (A) ulnar deviation, (B) showing fracture, (C) demonstrating close collimation.

- The hand is adducted towards the ulna; there should be no other flexion of the wrist. The thumb is in contact with the lateral aspect of the second metacarpal

Beam Direction and FRD

Vertical, at 90° to the IR
100 cm FRD

Centring Point

Over the 'snuffbox'

Collimation

Scaphoid, trapezium, trapezoid, lunate, first carpometacarpal joint, radiocarpal joint

Criteria for Assessing Image Quality

- Demonstration of the scaphoid, trapezium, trapezoid, lunate, first carpometacarpal joint and radiocarpal joint
- Separation of the joint spaces around the scaphoid; adequate ulnar deviation will show the long axis of the first metacarpal following that of the radius (if included in the image)
- Sharp image demonstrating bony cortex and trabeculae. Optimum penetration to demonstrate overlap of carpal bones and contrast to allow for demonstration of the subtle scaphoid fat pad sign

Common Errors: PA Scaphoid with Ulnar Deviation

Common Error	Possible Reason	Potential Effect on PCE or Report
Poor separation of joint space around scaphoid	Inadequate ulnar deviation	Non-visualisation of cortical margins may cause fractures to be missed

POSTEROANTERIOR OBLIQUE (PAO) WITH ULNAR DEVIATION (FIG. 4.20A,B)

Positioning

- The patient is positioned as for the PAO projection of the wrist
- The 'snuffbox' is placed in the centre of the available space if an IR is used
- A radiolucent pad is used under the wrist to aid immobilisation
- The hand is adducted towards the ulna; there should be no flexion of the wrist

Beam Direction and FRD

Vertical, at 90° to the IR
100 cm FRD

Centring Point

Over the 'snuffbox'

Collimation

Scaphoid, trapezium, trapezoid, lunate, first carpometacarpal joint, radiocarpal joint

Please note that Fig. 4.20B shows less stringent collimation, to provide an example of the relationship of other carpal bones to the scaphoid.

Criteria for Assessing Image Quality

- Demonstration of the scaphoid, trapezium, trapezoid, lunate, first carpometacarpal joint and radiocarpal joint
- Separation of joint spaces around the scaphoid
- Sharp image demonstrating bony cortex and trabeculae. Adequate penetration to demonstrate differentiation between overlapped carpal bones

Common Errors: PAO Scaphoid with Ulnar Deviation

Common Error	Possible Reason	Potential Effect on PCE or Report
Poor separation of joint space around scaphoid	Inadequate ulnar deviation	Joint space symmetry and cortical outline appearances may be affected, potentially causing fractures to be missed

ANTEROPOSTERIOR OBLIQUE (APO) WITH ULNAR DEVIATION (FIG. 4.21A,B)

Positioning

- The patient is positioned initially as for the lateral projection of the wrist
- The wrist is externally rotated 45° and a radiolucent pad is placed under the wrist to aid immobilisation
- The 'snuffbox' should be in the centre of the available space if an IR is used
- The hand is adducted towards the ulna; there should be no flexion of the wrist

Beam Direction and FRD

Vertical, at 90° to the IR
100 cm FRD

Centring Point

Over the 'snuffbox'

Collimation

Scaphoid, trapezium, trapezoid, lunate, first carpometacarpal joint, radiocarpal joint

Please note that Fig. 4.21B shows less stringent collimation, to provide an example of the relationship of other carpal bones to the scaphoid.

Criteria for Assessing Image Quality

- Demonstration of the scaphoid, trapezium, trapezoid, lunate, first carpometacarpal joint and radiocarpal joint
- The scaphoid seen above the radius, partially overlapping the lunate but clear of the pisiform and triquetral
- Sharp image demonstrating bony cortex and trabeculae. Adequate penetration to demonstrate differentiation between overlapped carpal bones

LATERAL SCAPHOID (FIG. 4.22A,B)

Positioning

- The patient is positioned as for a lateral projection of the wrist
- The 'snuffbox' is placed in the centre of the available space if an IR is used

Beam Direction and FRD

Vertical, at 90° to the IR
100 cm FRD

Centring Point

Over the 'snuffbox'

Collimation

Scaphoid, trapezium, lunate, first carpometacarpal joint, radiocarpal joint, radial and ulnar styloid processes

Please note that Fig. 4.22B shows less stringent collimation, to provide an example of the relationship of other carpal bones to the scaphoid.

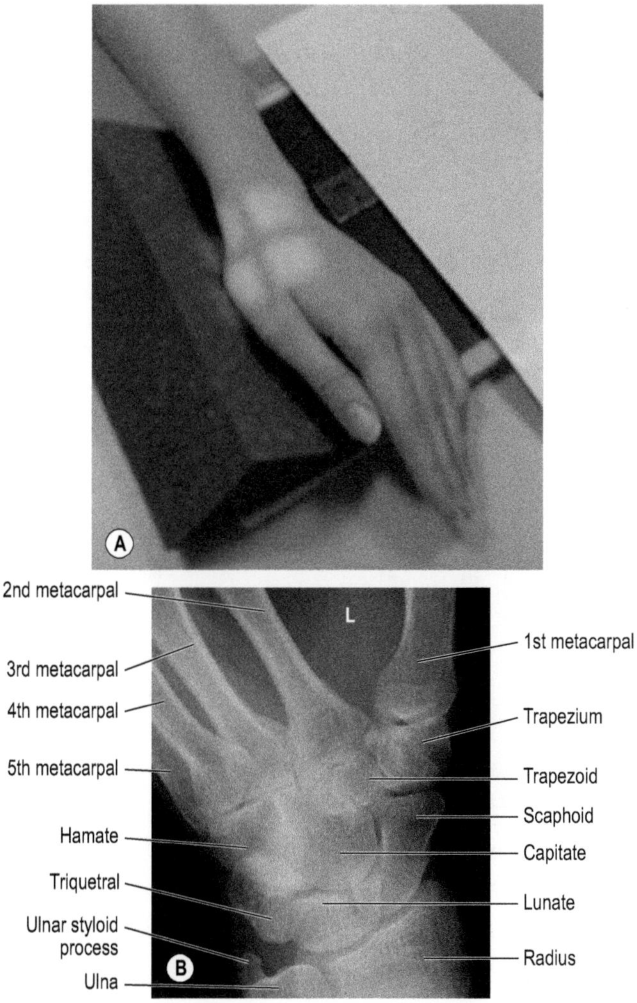

Fig. 4.20 (A) Scaphoid PA oblique; (B) showing fracture.

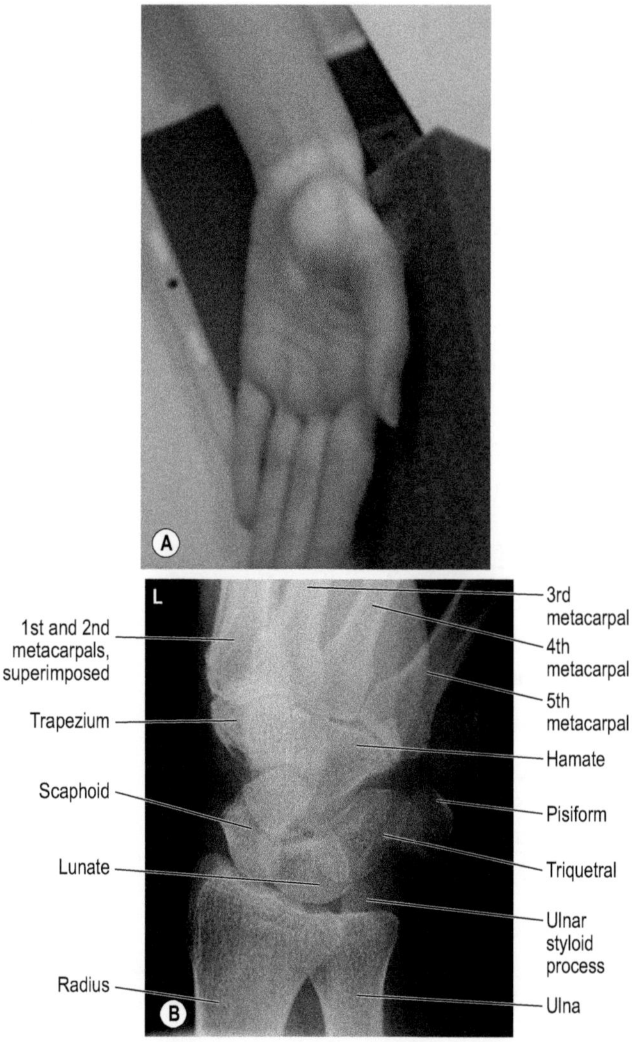

Fig. 4.21 AP oblique scaphoid.

Criteria for Assessing Image Quality

- Demonstration of the scaphoid, trapezium, lunate, first carpometacarpal joint, radiocarpal joint and radial and ulnar styloid processes
- The lunate projected as a crescent. The proximal end of the third metacarpal, capitate, lunate and distal radius should be in alignment. The waist of the scaphoid should be superimposed over the pisiform, with the tubercle of scaphoid clear of the pisiform anteriorly on the palmar aspect of the wrist
- Sharp image demonstrating bony cortex and trabeculae. Adequate penetration to demonstrate differentiation between overlapped carpal bones

POSTEROANTERIOR (PA) WITH 30° ANGULATION AND ULNAR DEVIATION

Positioning

Position is as for the PA scaphoid with ulnar deviation (Fig. 4.19A)

The 'snuffbox' is positioned coincident with the centre of the available space if an IR is used

Beam Direction and FRD

Initially vertical, then directed 30° towards the elbow
100 cm FRD

Centring Point

Over the trapezium at base of thumb

Collimation

Scaphoid and surrounding joints

This projection should be undertaken with the forearm positioned parallel to the median sagittal plain (MSP), so that the central ray is not directed towards the trunk when angled towards the elbow. To achieve this, the patient's chair should be placed next to the longer dimension of the table rather than at the end, to allow easy and accurate angulation of the X-ray tube in the correct plane.

There are three alternative projections which will also place the scaphoid into a position where it will lie at 30° to the central ray, thus negating the need for angulation.

WRIST IN DORSIFLEXION (FIG. 4.23)

Positioning

- An initial PA wrist position is modified by dorsiflexing the hand at the wrist until it makes an angle of 30° with the IR

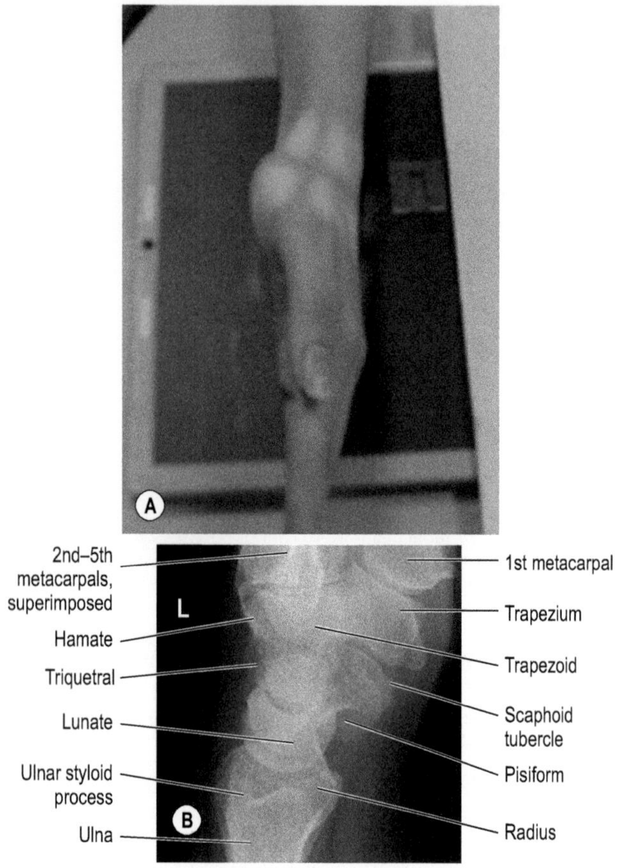

Fig. 4.22 Scaphoid lateral.

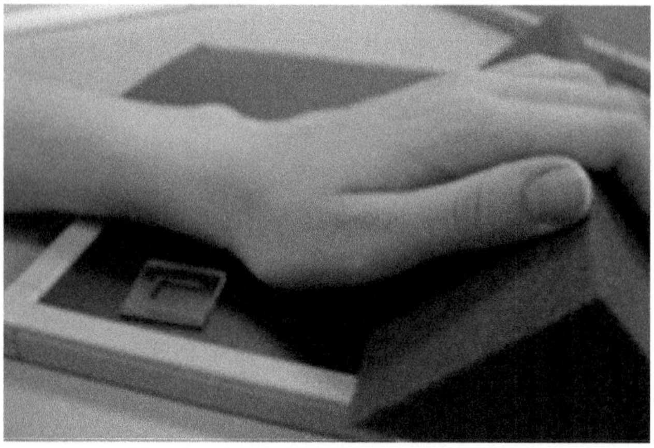

Fig. 4.23 Scaphoid with wrist in dorsiflexion.

- The hand is supported on a radiolucent pad and the wrist is placed in ulnar deviation. The anterior aspect of the wrist remains in contact with the IR

Beam Direction and FRD

Vertical, at 90° to the IR
100 cm FRD

Centring Point

Over the 'snuffbox'

Collimation

Scaphoid and surrounding joints

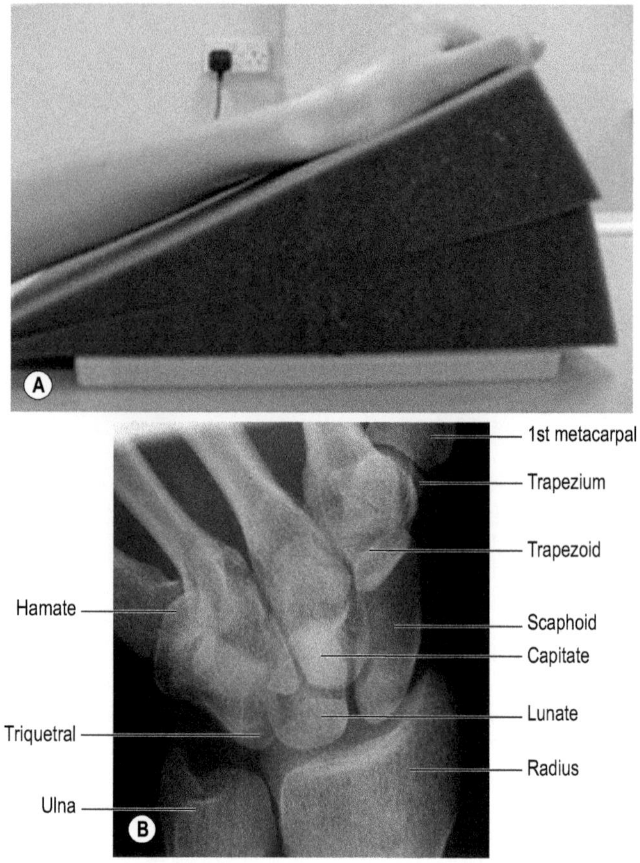

Fig. 4.24 (A) Scaphoid with forearm raised 30°; (B) scaphoid–PA 30° image.

FOREARM RAISED 30° (FIG. 4.24A,B)

Positioning

- With the wrist in pronation, the forearm is raised 30° at the elbow
- The elbow remains in contact with the table
- The forearm and hand are supported on a radiolucent pad and the wrist is placed in ulnar deviation; the hand and forearm remain in the same plane

Beam Direction and FRD

Vertical, at 90° to the IR
150 cm FRD, to reduce magnification caused by increased object receptor distance (ORD)

Centring Point

Over the 'snuffbox'

Collimation

Scaphoid and surrounding joints

This projection option with the forearm raised 30° will cause a significant amount of magnification unsharpness, but this can be counteracted by placing pads under the IR to raise it by 30°; the forearm is then placed directly on the IR, thereby reducing ORD, and a vertical central ray is used instead of 30° angulation

CLENCHED FIST WITH ULNAR DEVIATION

Positioning

- With the wrist in pronation, the fist is fully clenched to raise the dorsum of the hand through 30°, as for the lateral thumb position seen in Fig. 4.5B
- Ulnar deviation is applied to the wrist

Beam Direction and FRD

Vertical, at 90° to the IR
100 cm FRD

Centring Point

Over the 'snuffbox'

Collimation

Scaphoid and surrounding joints

Criteria for Assessing Image Quality: All 30° Projections

- The scaphoid and surrounding joints are demonstrated
- The scaphoid is cleared from other carpals due to ulnar deviation, with elongation due to 30° angle
- Sharp but elongated image demonstrating bony cortex and trabeculae of scaphoid (see Fig. 4.24B; please note that this image shows less stringent collimation, to provide an example of the relationship of other carpal bones to the scaphoid)

Common Errors: Clenched Fist with Ulnar Deviation

Common Error	Possible Reasons	Potential Effect on PCE or Report
Short appearance of scaphoid	Inadequate angle used or hand/forearm not raised enough	Trabecular pattern cannot be assessed and fracture line may be missed

Carpal Tunnel

Compression of the median nerve in the carpal tunnel on the anterior aspect of the wrist results in pain and paraesthesia of the fingers; the collection of these symptoms is known as carpal tunnel syndrome.[20] Whenever possible, MRI should be the imaging modality of choice for symptoms suggestive of this condition. However, bony spurs which emanate from the carpus, impinging on innervation at the wrist, can be detected using plain film radiography. In addition, when there are valid reasons contraindicating the use of MRI it may still be necessary to undertake plain radiographic examination of the carpal tunnel.

Several methods of producing images of this region are available and implications of dose to radiosensitive organs, projectional principles and patient condition or capability should be considered when selecting the most appropriate. Method 1 is given priority for description, as it is considered to show the least magnification unsharpness and, with the trunk turned away from the primary beam, is most effective in reducing dose to radiosensitive areas (thyroid, gonads, breast, eye lens). Unfortunately, carpal tunnel syndrome is highly likely to impair the patient's ability to forcibly dorsiflex the wrist, and in these cases method 3 should be selected.

No PCE comments are given for this region since it is not a commonly encountered examination in situations where PCE is required.

METHOD 1: SUPEROINFERIOR CARPAL TUNNEL – ERECT WITH PATIENT FACING AWAY FROM THE CENTRAL RAY (FIG. 4.25A,B)

An IR at the edge of a table is required for this projection, placed horizontal and with its edge aligned with the edge of the table.

Positioning

- The patient stands with their back to the table, which should be adjusted so that its height lies just below their waist
- The affected arm is internally rotated until the palm faces posteriorly, towards the table and IR
- The proximal half of the palm is placed in contact with the IR and the fingers are flexed around the edge of the receptor; the carpus should be as far away from the edge of the receptor as possible
- The patient effects dorsiflexion of the wrist in this position by leaning forward and exerting slight pressure on the forearm, which is extended at the elbow to allow maximum effect. The forearm is cleared from the wrist and carpus

METHOD 2: SUPEROINFERIOR CARPAL TUNNEL – ERECT WITH PATIENT FACING THE CENTRAL RAY (FIG. 4.26)

The IR is positioned as for method 1.

Positioning

- The patient stands facing the table, which should be adjusted so that its height lies just below their waist
- The affected arm is externally rotated until the palm is in supination, facing anteriorly towards the table and IR
- The proximal half of the palm is placed in contact with the IR and the fingers flexed around the edge of the receptor; the carpus should be as far from the edge of the receptor as possible
- The patient effects dorsiflexion of the wrist in this position by leaning back and exerting a slight pressure on the forearm, which is extended at the elbow to allow maximum effect. The forearm is cleared from the wrist and carpus

Beam Direction and FRD for Methods 1 and 2

Vertical, at 90° to the IR
100 cm FRD

Centring Point

Over the midpoint of the anterior part of the wrist, within the depression caused by the tunnel arrangement of the carpus

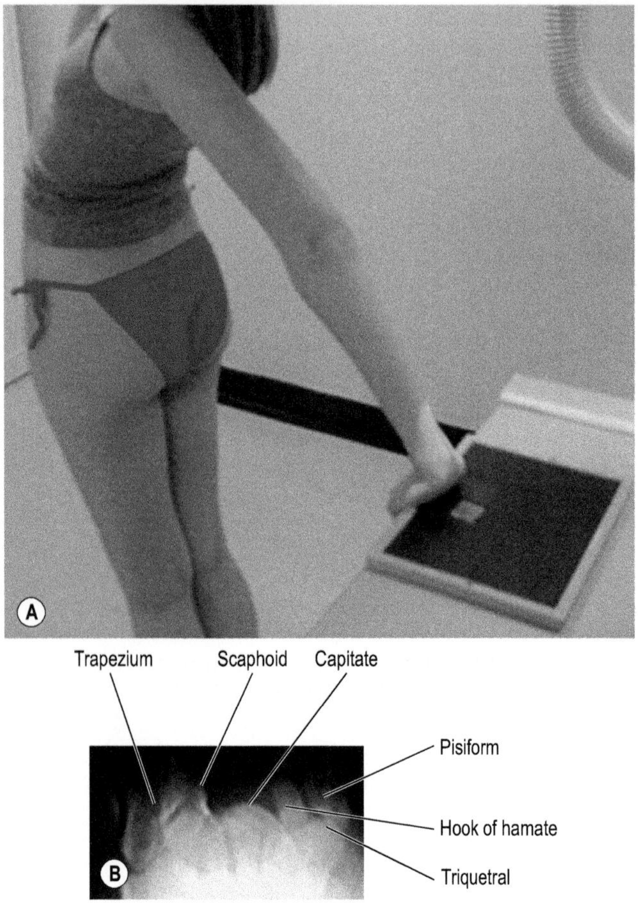

Fig. 4.25 Superoinferior carpal tunnel (method 1) with (A) patient's back to X-ray beam; (B) carpal tunnel.

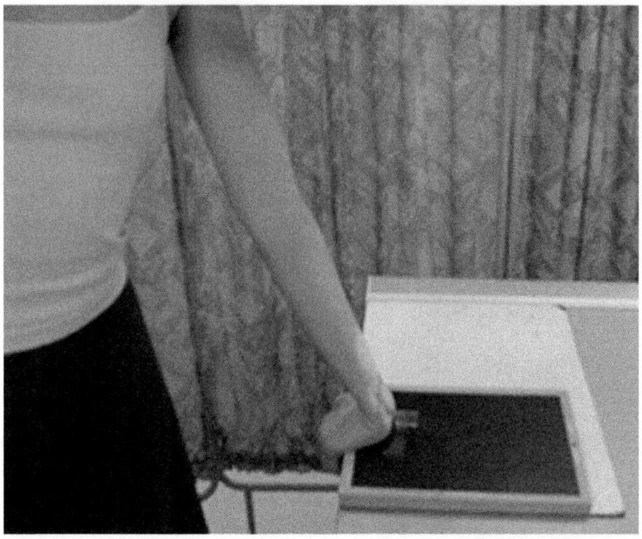

Fig. 4.26 Superoinferior carpal tunnel (method 2) with patient facing X-ray beam.

Collimation

Carpal bones, soft tissue of anterior aspect of wrist

METHOD 3: INFEROSUPERIOR CARPAL TUNNEL – PATIENT SEATED FACING THE TABLE (FIG. 4.27)

Positioning

- The IR is horizontal, 30–40 cm from the patient, and there must be enough table-top space for the patient to rest their elbow for immobilisation and positioning
- A 45° radiolucent pad is placed onto the IR
- The patient places the flexed elbow of the affected side onto the table
- Whilst maintaining some elbow flexion, the hand is pronated and the forearm rested on the pad
- The wrist should lie over, but not in contact with, the IR
- The hand is dorsiflexed at the wrist and a bandage passed around the fingers; pulling this bandage gently will facilitate the extent of dorsiflexion required to clear the forearm from the carpus
- The patient maintains the dorsiflexion by holding and pulling the ends of the bandage; the elbow remains in contact with the table-top
- The head is turned to the side, away from the primary beam

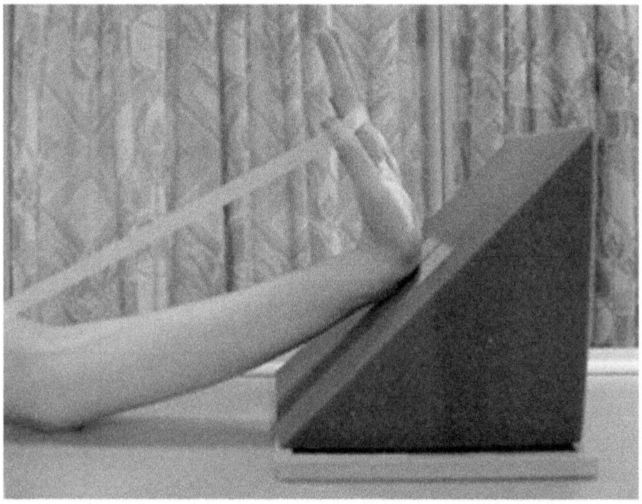

Fig. 4.27 Inferosuperior carpal tunnel (method 3) with patient seated.

Beam Direction and FRD for Method 3

Vertical, at 90° to the IR
150 cm FRD

Centring Point

Over the midpoint of the anterior part of the proximal portion of the hand, within the depression caused by the tunnel arrangement of the carpus

Collimation

Carpal bones, soft tissue of anterior portion of distal hand

Criteria for Assessing Image Quality: All Methods

- The carpal bones and soft tissue of the anterior portion of the wrist are demonstrated
- The carpal tunnel is seen as a curved, darker, soft tissue area anterior to the denser carpal bones
- The distal radius and ulna are cleared from the carpus to lie over the metacarpals

- The hook of hamate and pisiform are cleared from the rest of the carpus and on the medial aspect of the tunnel
- Sharp image demonstrating soft tissue of the carpal tunnel region, bony trabeculae of pisiform and the hook of hamate. Optimum penetration to demonstrate these bones, whilst maintaining contrast with required soft tissue. Superimposed carpals will not be fully penetrated

Common Errors: Carpal Tunnel

Common Errors	Possible Reasons	Potential Effects on PCE or Report
Image overall appears pale with no distinguishable bony features	1. Inadequate penetration and exposure	Dark soft tissue area defining carpal tunnel will not be seen Bony spurs will not be visualised
	2. Forearm may not have been cleared from carpus; improve dorsiflexion or consider examination using a method that may be more comfortable for the patient	The carpal tunnel cannot be assessed
Asymmetry of tunnel; fourth and fifth metacarpals are seen clear of forearm	Patient's arm is leaning towards radius; ensure forearm lies vertically over the hand and carpus	Correct assessment of tunnel, and detection of bony spurs not possible. Image is considered unacceptable
Asymmetry of tunnel; first and second metacarpals are seen clear of forearm	Patient's arm is leaning towards ulna; ensure forearm lies vertically over the hand and carpus	As above

References

1. British Society for Surgery of the Hand. Hand Surgery in the UK: a resource for those involved in organising, delivering and developing services for patients with conditions of the hand and wrist. In: *Report of a Working Party*. London: BSSH; 2017. https://tinyurl.com/yyy6ue4o.
2. Gaillard F, Dawes L, et al. Gamekeeper thumb. [online] Radiopaedia. https://radiopaedia.org/articles/gamekeeper-thumb/revisions?lang=gb (accessed 2019).
3. Whitley AS, Sloane C, Hoadley G, et al. *Clark's Positioning in Radiography*. 12th ed. London: Hodder Arnold; 2005.
4. Richmond B. A comparative study of two radiographic techniques for obtaining an AP projection of the thumb. *Radiogr Today*. 1995;61(696):11–15.
5. Unett EM, Royle AJ. *Radiographic Techniques and Image Evaluation*. London: Chapman and Hall; 1997.
6. The Ionising Radiation (Medical Exposure) Regulations 2017. UK Statutory Instrument 2017 No. 1322. https://www.legislation.gov.uk/uksi/2017/1322/contents/made.
7. Clark DL, von Schroeder HP. Scapholunate ligament injury: the natural history. *Can J Surg*. 2004;47(4):298–299.
8. Raby N, Berman L. *Accident and Emergency Radiology: A Survival Guide*. 3rd ed. Philadelphia: Saunders; 2014.
9. El-Feky M, Dixon AD. Piece of pie sign (wrist). [online] Radiopaedia. https://radiopaedia.org/articles/piece-of-pie-sign-wrist?lang=gb (accessed 2019).
10. Carver E, Carver B, eds. *Medical Imaging: Techniques, Reflection, Evaluation*. 2nd ed. Edinburgh: Churchill Livingstone; 2012.
11. Lewis S. New angles on radiographic examination of the hand. *Radiogr Today*. 1988;54(617):4–45 (618):20–30, (619):47–48.
12. Bell G, Finlay D. *Basic Radiographic Positioning and Anatomy*. London: Baillière Tindall; 1986.
13. Clark KC. *Clark's Positioning in Radiography*. London: Heinemann; 1939.
14. Goldfarb CA, Yin Y, Gilula LA, et al. Wrist fractures: what the clinician wants to know. *Radiology*. 2001;219:11–28.
15. Lampignano JP, Kendrick LE. *Bontrager's Textbook of Radiographic Positioning and Related Anatomy*. 9th ed. St Louis: Elsevier Mosby; 2018.
16. Sante LR. *Manual of Radiological Technique*. 2nd ed. Michigan: Edwards Brothers Inc; 1935.
17. McQuillen-Martenson K. *Radiographic Image Analysis*. 5th ed. St Louis: Elsevier; 2019.
18. Cooney W. *The Wrist: Diagnosis and Operative Treatment*. 2nd ed. Philadelphia: Lippincott Williams & Wilkins; 2010.
19. Machin E, Blackham J, Benger J. *Management of Suspected Scaphoid Fractures in the Emergency Department*. The College of Emergency Medicine. GEMNet; 2013. https://www.rcem.ac.uk/docs/College%20Guidelines/5z25.%20Suspected%20Scaphoid%20Fractures-%20(Flowchart)%20(Sept%202013).pdf.
20. Helms CA. *Fundamentals of Skeletal Radiology*. 5th ed. Philadelphia: Elsevier Saunders; 2019.

5 Forearm, Elbow, Humerus and Shoulder Girdle

ELIZABETH CARVER and JEANETTE CARTER

Forearm (Radius and Ulna)

This region of the upper limb most usually presents for imaging as a result of trauma. The Colles' fracture is the most usual finding after trauma to radius and ulna; this is outlined in Chapter 4 (Wrist).

PCE COMMENTS – FOREARM

Fractures in the forearm are mostly noted by using general steps for assessment that include cortical outlines, trabecular patterns and soft tissue outlines. Often fractures are seen in more than one location so look for secondary areas that display unusual appearances.

Assess both joints – if clinical concern of a specific joint, then designated imaging of this area may be warranted.

Specific to the forearm are complex fracture dislocations of the radius and ulna: the Galleazzi fracture is a fracture of the distal portion of the radius accompanied by subluxation or dislocation of the distal radioulnar joint. The Monteggia fracture, conversely, is a fracture of the ulna accompanied by dislocation of the radius proximally.

Throughout this chapter a suggested FRD is given for each examination description; however in practice a range of FRDs (typically from 100 cm to 120 cm) may be used, dependent on local protocol.

ANTEROPOSTERIOR (AP) FOREARM (FIG. 5.1A,B)

For all projections of the forearm the IR is placed horizontal unless otherwise specified.

Positioning

- The patient is seated with the affected side next to the table
- The arm is extended at the elbow, abducted away from the trunk and externally rotated until the hand lies in supination
- The posterior aspect of the forearm is placed in contact with the IR, to include elbow and wrist joints
- The joints must lie in the same plane
- The humeral epicondyles and radial and ulnar styloid processes are equidistant from the IR
- The head is turned away from the shoulder of the side under examination, aiming to reduce scattered radiation to the lenses of the eyes and thyroid

Beam Direction and FRD

Vertical, at 90° to the IR
100 cm FRD

Centring

Midway between the wrist and elbow joints

Collimation

Elbow, wrist, shafts of radius and ulna, soft tissue outlines of forearm

Criteria for Assessing Image Quality

- Wrist and elbow joints, radius, ulna and soft tissue outline of the forearm are demonstrated
- Partial superimposition of the radius and ulna at proximal and distal ends, with separation of the shafts. Radial tubercle should overlap the cortex of the ulnar shaft, but no further
- Humeral epicondyles equidistant from the coronoid and olecranon fossae
- Radial styloid process seen on the lateral aspects of this bone

Common Errors: AP Forearm

Common Error	Possible Reason	Potential Effects on PCE or Report
Radius cleared from ulna at the proximal end; radial head also shown clear	Externally rotated arm	May be difficult to assess: the olecranon within the olecranon fossa associated dislocations to any fractures of radius and ulna[1] alignment of displaced fractures at this site[2]
Radial tubercle superimposed over shaft of ulna	Internally rotated arm	May be difficult to assess: the distal and proximal radius – when looking for subtle fractures and displacement of fracture/s to the midshaft of the radius and ulna for alignment/surgical intervention associated dislocations in significantly displaced fractures[2]
Shafts of radius and ulna show adequate contrast and density but elbow is 'thin', under-penetrated and shows poor contrast or bony detail	Inadequate kVp selected	It is difficult to detect subtle breaks in the cortex and lucent lines, signs that indicate undisplaced fractures[1]
Elbow joint shows adequate contrast and density but shafts of radius and ulna are dark, showing poor contrast and bony detail	Selected kVp too high	Same effects as kVp too low Plus – difficult to assess soft tissue signs (such as elevated fat pads and soft tissue swelling) as often the soft tissues are also over-penetrated[1]

- Ulnar styloid process is shown in profile distally in the middle of the head of ulna
- Sharp image demonstrating soft tissue margins of the forearm, bony cortex and trabeculae. Adequate penetration to demonstrate overlap of the olecranon over the distal humerus while showing trabecular detail over the shafts of radius and ulna

LATERAL FOREARM (FIG. 5.2A,B)

Positioning

- The patient is seated with the affected side next to the table
- The arm is flexed at the elbow, abducted away from the trunk and internally rotated at the wrist
- The medial aspect of the forearm is placed in contact with the IR, to include elbow and wrist joints
- The shoulder, elbow and wrist joints must lie in the same plane
- The humeral epicondyles are superimposed, as are the radial and ulnar styloid processes. Ensuring the shoulder lies in the same plane as the wrist and elbow will help facilitate this
- The head is turned away from the shoulder of the side under examination, aiming to reduce scattered radiation to the lenses of the eyes and thyroid

Beam Direction and FRD

Vertical, at 90° to the IR
100 cm FRD

Centring

Midway between the wrist and elbow joints, on the medial aspect of the forearm

Collimation

Elbow, wrist, shafts of radius and ulna, soft tissue outlines of forearm

Criteria for Assessing Image Quality

- The wrist and elbow joints, radius, ulna and soft tissue outline of the forearm are demonstrated
- Superimposition of posterior portion of radial head over coronoid process of ulna; superimposition of distal radius and ulna
- Shaft of the radius is seen anterior to that of the ulna
- There will be some superimposition of trochlea and capitulum of humerus. However, it may be unrealistic to expect to see full superimposition of these structures as the obliquity of the beam at its periphery is likely to pass through the elbow at around 3–4°
- Sharp image demonstrating soft tissue margins of the forearm, bony cortex and trabeculae. Adequate penetration to demonstrate overlap of radial head over olecranon and distal radius over ulna, while showing trabecular detail over shafts of radius and ulna

Common Errors: Lateral Forearm

Common Error	Possible Reason	Potential Effects on PCE or Report
Distal radius seen anteriorly in relationship to ulna	Wrist is medially rotated	Difficult to assess: alignment for orthopaedic review subtle subluxations and fractures of the distal radius[2]
Distal radius seen posteriorly in relationship to ulna; shafts of radius and ulna superimposed along most of their length	Wrist and elbow are externally rotated; this usually only occurs when the humerus does not lie in the same plane as the forearm and the shoulder lies above the table-top	Same effects as for medial rotation (above)

Elbow

Degenerative change and trauma are both major indicators for plain radiographic imaging. Dislocations at the elbow can be demonstrated radiographically and the head of the radius is the most likely part to be subluxed.

The *supracondylar fracture* of the humerus has many implications for the future of the patient's arm. The vasculature of the arm can be damaged, or existing damage can be exacerbated, by forced extension of the elbow joint; this can cause an ischaemic state in the lower arm resulting in paralysis of the hand and forearm and, long term, in what is known as a *Volkmann's ischaemic contracture*. It is therefore essential that the radiographer undertakes modified projections of the elbow that cannot be extended; these are outlined in Chapter 17 on Emergency Department radiography.

PCE COMMENTS – ELBOW REGION

In addition to generic assessment of the area, there are other pertinent checks that should be made on elbow radiographs.

PCE COMMENTS – ELBOW REGION—Cont'd

Children: It is particularly relevant to check for supracondylar fracture and apophyseal fracture/avulsion of medial and lateral epicondyles.[3,4]

Adults: Radial head fracture, olecranon fracture.[5,6]

Radiocapitellar line (most usually found to be affected in injuries in children): On the AP projection, a line through the middle of the neck of radius should intersect the capitellum. If this line does not connect as described this indicates dislocation of the radial head, which is usually anterior in direction.[7]

Anterior humeral line: On the lateral projection, a line passing along the anterior humeral surface should pass through the middle third of the capitellum. If the line appears anteriorly or posteriorly to the mid third, this may indicate displacement of the capitellum, but it is possible that in some younger children the anterior humeral line does normally lie in the anterior third of capitellum. This highlights a need to inspect all aspects of the radiographic anatomy rather than focussing just on one aspect.[8]

If displacement of the capitellum is suspected, elbow effusion may be evident.

PCE COMMENTS – ELBOW REGION—Cont'd

Fat pads: These are seen anteriorly, and up to 45° angle from the long axis of humerus is to be considered normal. When significant trauma causes displacement of the pads there will be an appearance similar to a downturned rose thorn (seen as darker than the surrounding soft tissue) anterior and/or posterior to the distal humerus, just above the epicondyles. The normal positions of the fat pads are: supinator fat pad seen along the anterior aspect of the humerus; anterior fat pad seen anterior to the distal portion of the humerus just above the coronoid fossa; the posterior fat pad is positioned within the olecranon fossa posteriorly.[9] Flexion of the joint also affects fat pad appearance in the lateral elbow projection. Flexion <90° causes the olecranon to move towards the olecranon fossa, thereby displacing the posterior pad superiorly to a position that may be visible on the lateral radiograph. This may potentially mimic appearances suggestive of trauma and thus affect radiological comment.[2] It is important to remember that only fractures within the capsule cause elevation of the fat pads[1,10] and fractures outside the capsule will not cause elevated fat pads. Also, elevated fat pads can be caused by advanced arthropathy changes.[1]

ANTEROPOSTERIOR (AP) ELBOW (FIG. 5.3A,B)

For all projections of the elbow the IR is placed horizontal unless otherwise specified.

Positioning

- The patient is seated with the affected side next to the table
- The arm is extended at the elbow, abducted away from the trunk and externally rotated until the hand lies in supination
- The posterior aspect of the elbow is placed in contact with the IR
- The wrist, elbow and shoulder joints must lie in the same plane
- The humeral epicondyles are equidistant from the IR
- The head is turned away from the shoulder of the side under examination, aiming to reduce scattered radiation to the lenses of the eyes and thyroid

Beam Direction and FRD

Vertical, at 90° to the IR
100 cm FRD

Centring

Midway between the humeral epicondyles

Collimation

Proximal radius and ulna, elbow joint, distal shaft of humerus, soft tissue outlines surrounding elbow joint

Criteria for Assessing Image Quality

- The proximal radius and ulna, elbow joint, distal shaft of the humerus and soft tissue outlines surrounding the elbow joint demonstrated
- Partial superimposition of the radius and ulna at the proximal end (0.6 cm of radial head superimposed over ulna).[2] The radial tuberosity should overlap the cortex of the ulnar shaft, but no further
- Humeral epicondyles equidistant from the coronoid and olecranon fossae

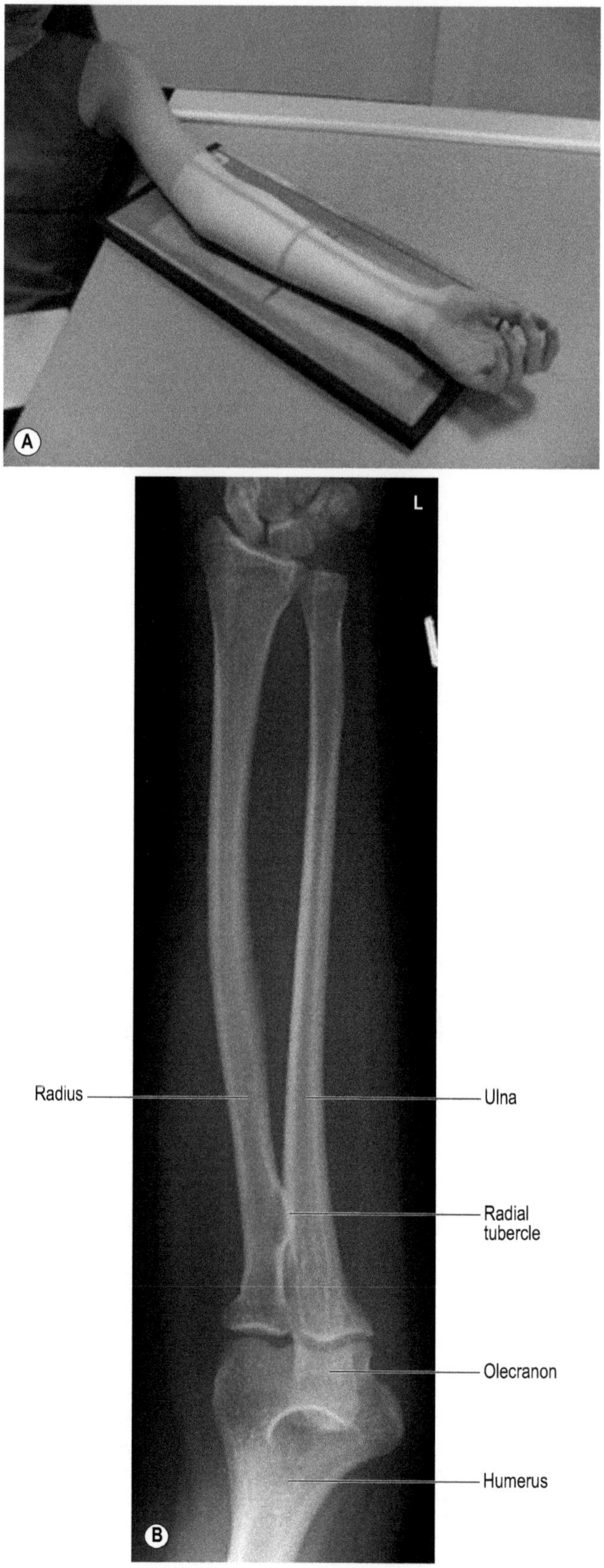

Fig. 5.1 AP forearm.

- Sharp image demonstrating soft tissue margins around the elbow, bony cortex and trabeculae. Adequate penetration to demonstrate overlap of olecranon over distal humerus

Common Errors: AP Elbow

Common Error	Possible Reason	Potential Effects on PCE or Report
Radius cleared from ulna; radial head also shown clear	Elbow is externally rotated	Difficult to assess: for supracondylar fractures, as the humeral head and proximal ulna appear oblique, (particularly difficult if subtle fracture) radiocapitellar line[11,12]
Radial head superimposed more than 0.6 cm over shaft of ulna	Internally rotated elbow	Difficult to assess: the radial head and therefore radial head fracture, which is the most common fracture of the adult elbow, occurring in approximately 20% of acute elbow injures severity of radial head fractures radiocapitellar line[12,13]
Radial head fully superimposed over ulna; distance between humeral epicondyles seems narrow	Hand may be in pronation rather than supination	Difficult to: visualise both angles of the radius and ulna detect subtle fractures due to overlapping visualise the joint space for pathology/dislocation[11–13]
Joint space between capitulum and radial head is closed; long axes of radius and ulna travel obliquely towards the lateral aspect of the arm away from the joint. Overlap of humerus with proximal radius and ulna	Arm not fully extended at the elbow	Difficult to: visualise the articular surfaces assess the radiocapitellar line[11–13]

LATERAL ELBOW (FIG. 5.4A,B)

Positioning

- The patient is seated with the affected side next to the table
- The arm is abducted from the trunk, internally rotated and flexed 90° at the elbow
- The wrist is externally rotated until the radial and ulnar styloid processes are superimposed
- The medial aspect of the elbow is placed in contact with the IR
- The shoulder, elbow and wrist joints must lie in the same plane
- The humeral epicondyles are superimposed. Ensuring the shoulder lies in the same plane as the wrist and elbow will help facilitate this more easily
- The head is turned away from the shoulder of the side under examination, aiming to reduce scattered radiation to the lenses of the eyes and thyroid

Beam Direction and FRD

Vertical, at 90° to the IR
100 cm FRD

Centring

Over the lateral humeral epicondyle

Collimation

Proximal radius and ulna, elbow joint, distal shaft of humerus, soft tissue outlines surrounding elbow joint

Criteria for Assessing Image Quality

- The proximal radius and ulna, elbow joint, distal shaft of the humerus and soft tissue outlines surrounding the elbow joint are demonstrated
- Superimposition of surfaces of trochlea and capitulum, with the posterior portion of the radial head shown over the coronoid process of the ulna. Evidence of joint space of the elbow seen
- Shaft of radius seen anterior to that of ulna
- Sharp image demonstrating soft tissue margins around the elbow, bony cortex and trabeculae. Adequate penetration to demonstrate overlap of radial head over olecranon and superimposed epicondyles. Exposure factors must ensure that the anterior and supinator fat pads are shown in contrast with the surrounding soft tissue (the posterior fat pad will only be demonstrated if there is bony injury, or sometimes in inflammatory joint disease such as rheumatoid arthritis)

The importance of optimum exposure factor selection cannot be emphasised enough, especially in the case of the elbow radiograph requested after trauma. Information on both bone and soft tissue becomes even more vital in trauma cases. This is because personnel assessing and/or reporting on the radiograph need to inspect the image for evidence of the fat pad sign.

The injured patient often finds it difficult or impossible to extend the elbow joint, making it impossible for the radiographer to undertake routine projections of the area. Techniques must be modified, especially if there is a risk of Volkmann's ischaemic contracture after supracondylar fracture. These modifications are covered in Chapter 17 on Emergency Department radiography.

Head of Radius

A significant proportion of the radial head is superimposed over the proximal ulna in both the AP and the lateral projections of the elbow joint. As a result, small fractures of the radial head may not be demonstrated by more routine projections. Modifications of these are recommended in order to provide the required information. These modified projections are undertaken in addition to AP and lateral projections.

OBLIQUE HEAD OF RADIUS: EXTERNAL ROTATION (FIG. 5.5A,B)

This projection will also demonstrate the proximal radioulnar joint.

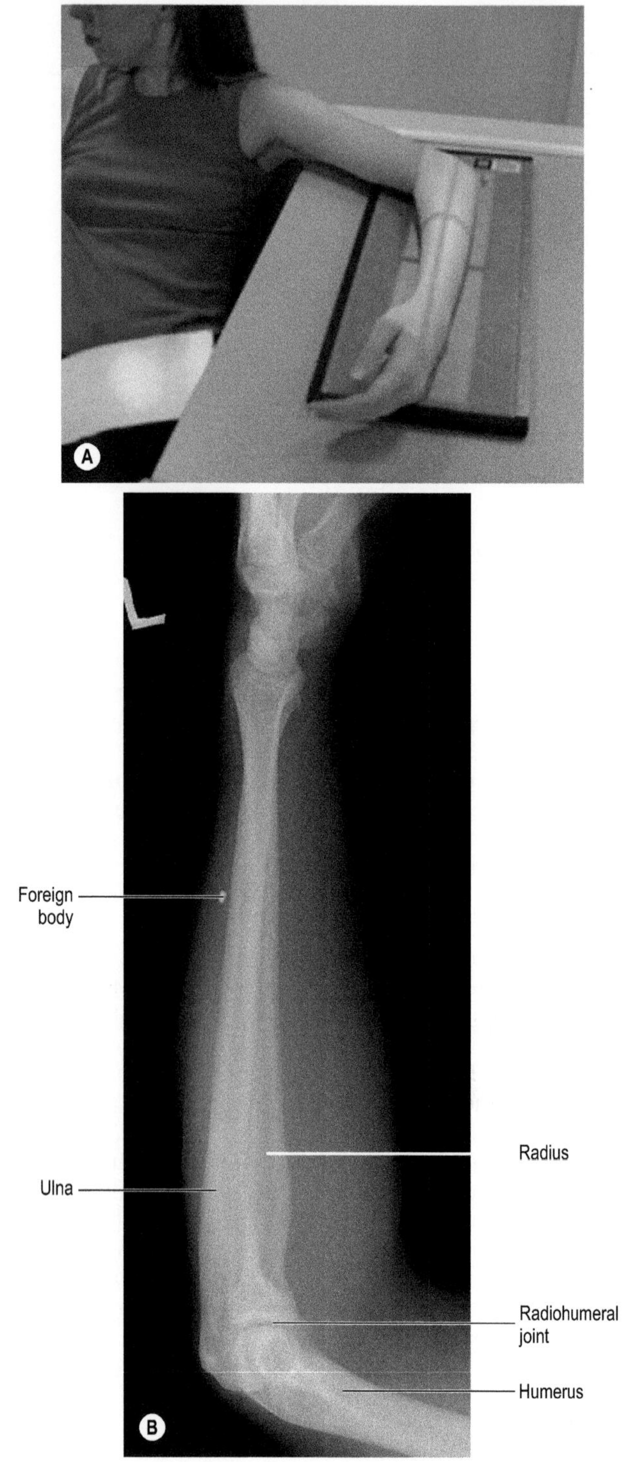

Fig. 5.2 Lateral forearm.

Positioning

- The patient is positioned initially as for the AP elbow projection
- The arm is externally rotated through approximately 20° to clear the radial head from the ulna. Asking the patient to lean sideways, towards the table and IR, will help facilitate this
- A radiolucent pad placed under the medial aspect of the forearm will aid immobilisation

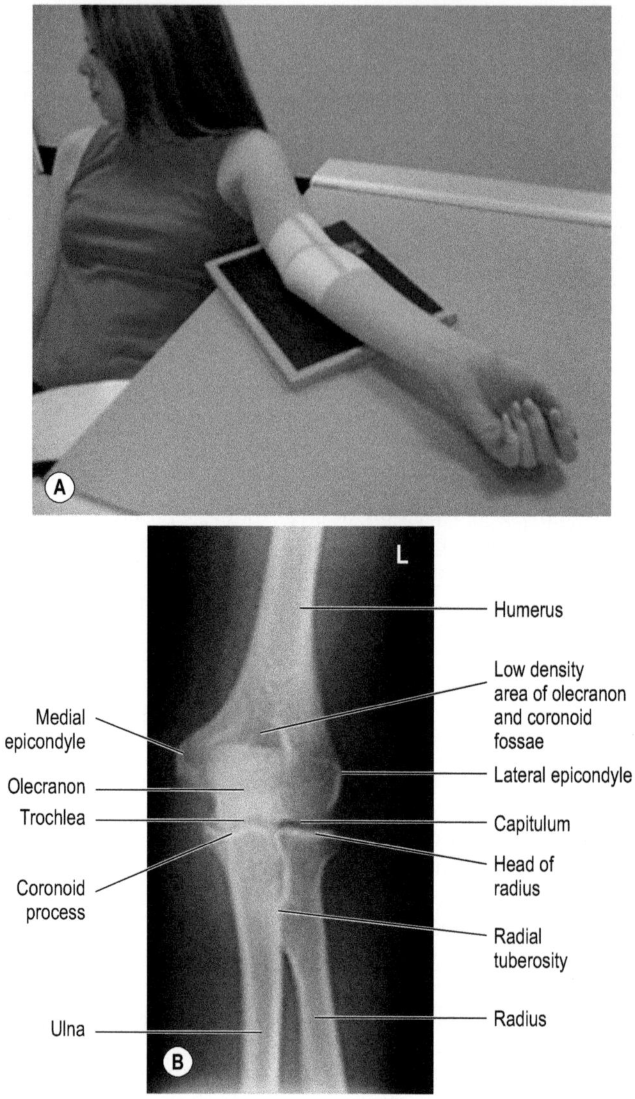

Fig. 5.3 AP elbow.

- The head is turned away from the shoulder of the side under examination, aiming to reduce scattered radiation to the lenses of the eyes and thyroid

Beam Direction and FRD

Vertical, at 90° to the IR
100 cm FRD

Centring

Over the middle of the crease of the elbow

Collimation

Proximal radius and ulna, elbow joint, distal shaft of humerus, soft tissue outlines surrounding elbow joint

Criteria for Assessing Image Quality

The proximal radius and ulna, elbow joint, distal shaft of the humerus and soft tissue outlines surrounding the elbow joint are demonstrated
Radial head is cleared from the ulna, and the proximal radioulnar joint is clear
Sharp image demonstrating soft tissue margins around the elbow, bony cortex and trabeculae

Common Errors: Oblique Head of Radius

Common Error	Possible Reason	Potential Effects on PCE or Report
Radial head not cleared from ulna	Inadequate external rotation	Difficult to assess the radial head for radial head fracture, which is one of the most common fractures to cause elevated fat pads[13]

Rotation as much as 45° has been suggested for demonstration of the radial head; this is significantly more than the 20° described here.[14] As 20° adequately demonstrates clearance of the head it seems excessive to expect the injured patient to aim for further rotation.

An alternative projection for clearance of the radial head from the ulna has been described as a *lateral with 45° lateromedial angulation of the primary beam.*[15] This projection is acknowledged to efficiently clear the radial head but will cause some significant distortion of the image (Fig. 5.5C). Angulation of the beam towards the trunk also has implications for a potential increase in radiation dose to more radiosensitive areas of the body. However, severe elbow trauma may render the patient incapable of adequate elbow extension for the oblique projection, and the lateral with 45° angle may be the only suitable alternative – clearly a situation when a risk–benefit assessment must be made by the radiographer.

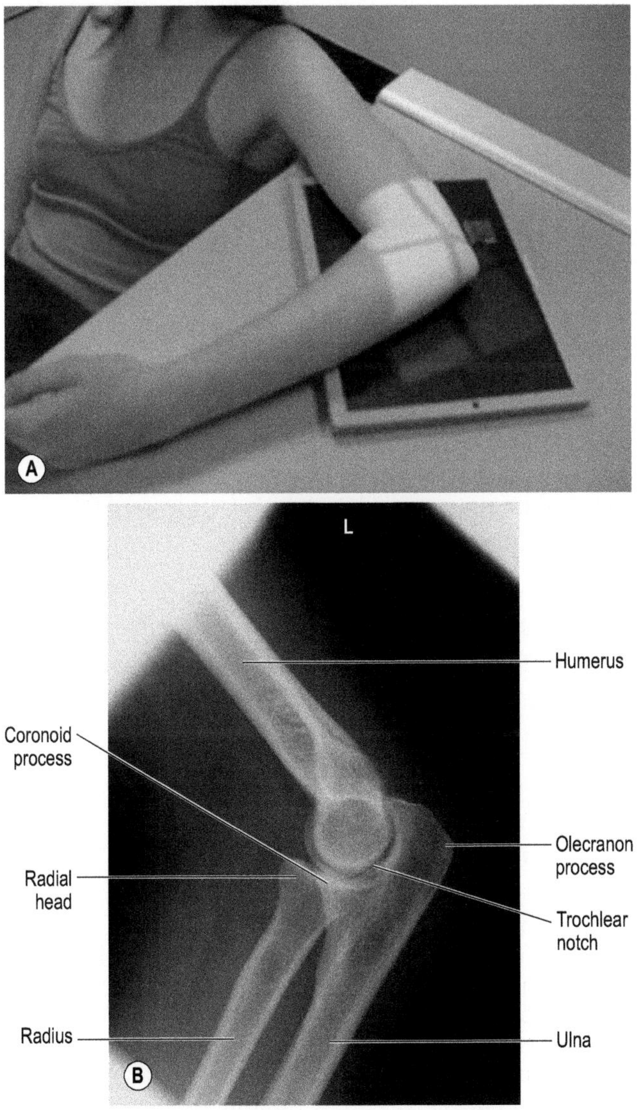

Fig. 5.4 Lateral elbow.

LATERAL HEAD OF RADIUS (FIGS 5.6A,B, 5.7A,B)

Although the externally rotated oblique projection for the radial head will clear it from the ulna to show more of its medial aspect, and its anterior aspect is seen on the lateral elbow projection, other aspects of the head will not have been well demonstrated on any of the routine elbow images.

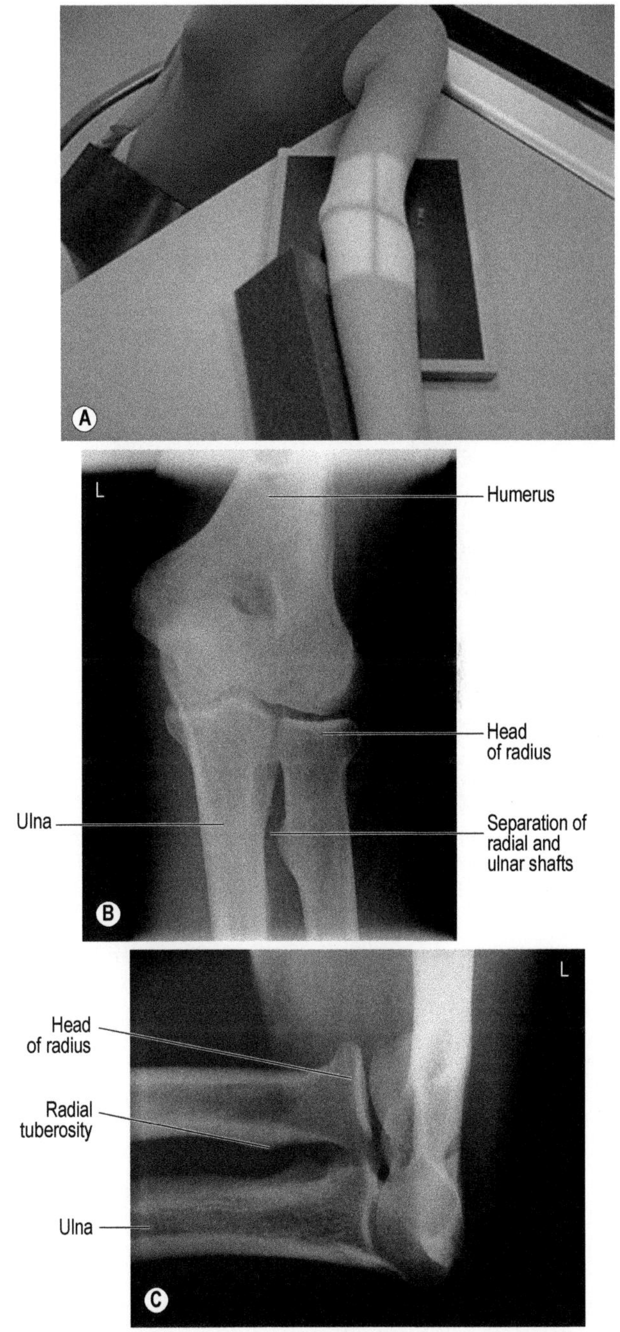

Fig. 5.5 (A,B) Head of radius – oblique; (C) head of radius – lateral elbow with 45° lateromedial angulation to clear radial head from ulna. (C, Reproduced with permission from Ballinger PW, Frank ED. *Merrill's Atlas of Radiographic Positioning and Radiologic Procedures.* 10th ed. St Louis: Mosby; 2003.)

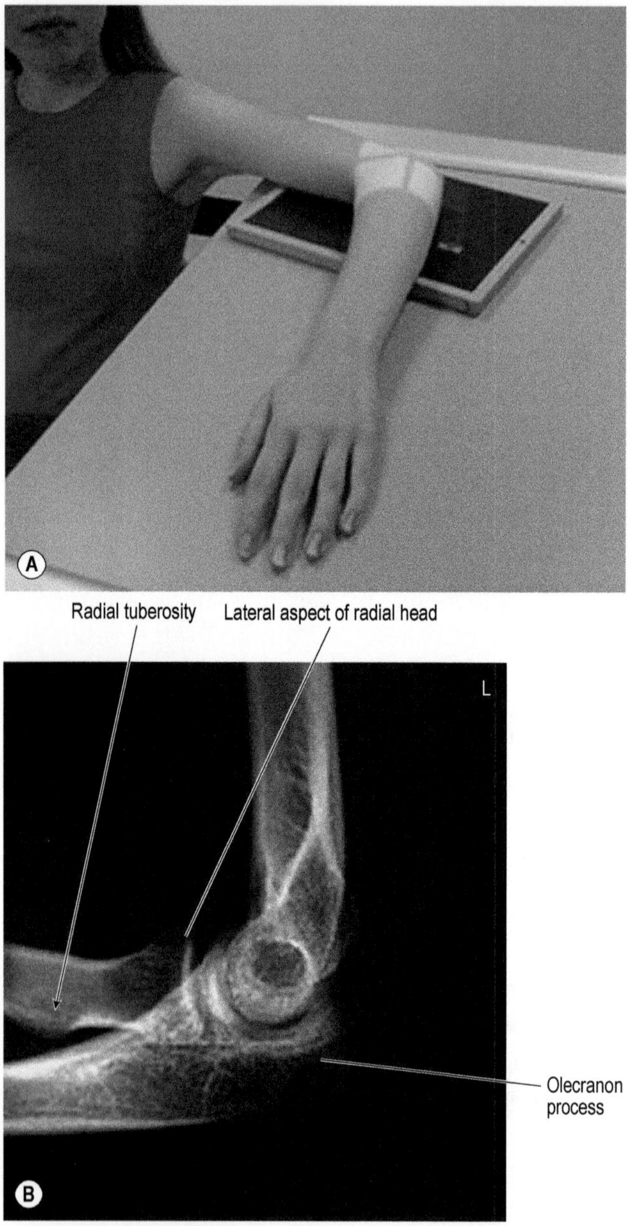

Fig. 5.6 **Lateral head of radius – hand pronated.** (B, Reproduced with permission from Ballinger PW, Frank ED. *Merrill's Atlas of Radiographic Positioning and Radiologic Procedures*. 10th ed. St Louis: Mosby; 2003.)

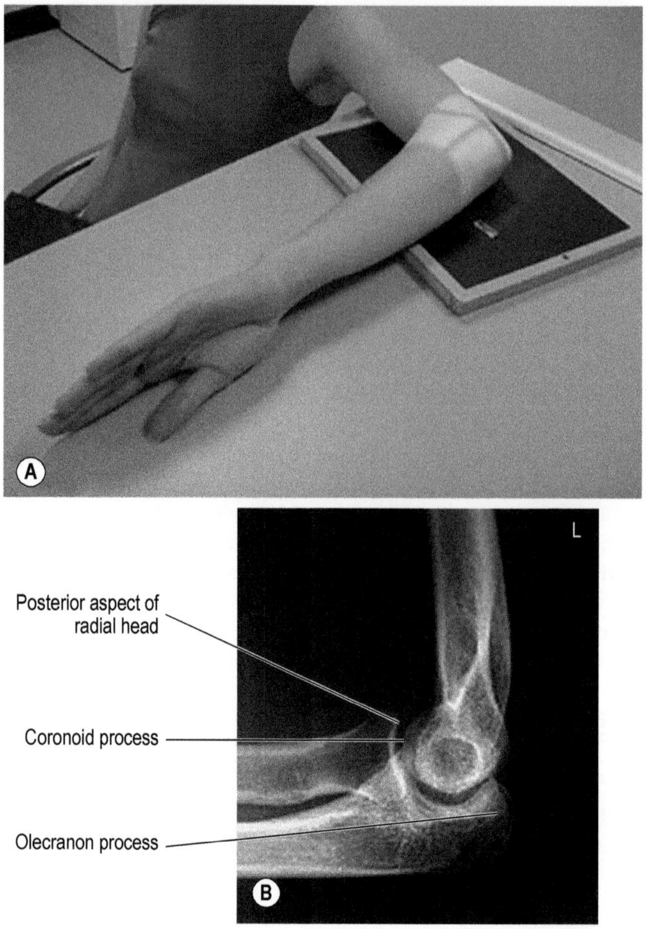

Fig. 5.7 **Lateral head of radius – hand medially rotated.** (B, Reproduced with permission from Ballinger PW, Frank ED. *Merrill's Atlas of Radiographic Positioning and Radiologic Procedures*. 10th ed. St Louis: Mosby; 2003.)

As a result it is necessary to provide profile projections of the radial head. These are achieved with the elbow in a lateral position and as described below.

Positioning

- The patient is positioned initially as for the lateral elbow projection
  (1) *To demonstrate the lateral aspect of the radial head*: Rotate the forearm internally until the hand is in pronation and in contact with the table-top
  (2) *To demonstrate the posterior aspect of the radial head*: From the position described in (1) above, the forearm is rotated further until its medial aspect is in contact with the IR and table-top
- A legend is applied to each image to identify the palm position used
- The head is turned away from the shoulder of the side under examination, aiming to reduce scattered radiation to the lenses of the eyes and thyroid

Beam Direction and FRD

Vertical, at 90° to the IR
100 cm FRD

Centring

Over the lateral humeral epicondyle (both forearm positions)

Collimation

Proximal radius and ulna, elbow joint, distal shaft of humerus, soft tissue outlines surrounding elbow joint

Criteria for Assessing Image Quality

- As for the lateral elbow, plus demonstration of change in position of the radial tubercle as it moves with rotation at the elbow. With the hand pronated (position 1) it should be seen as a slight prominence on the radius, projecting into the space between radius and ulna. With the hand further rotated medially (position 2) the tubercle appears more prominent and its outline will be nearer the outline of the ulna

OLECRANON AND CORONOID: AP OBLIQUE WITH INTERNAL ROTATION (FIG. 5.8A,B)

More detailed information of these areas on the ulna can be obtained by an internal oblique projection in cases where adequate AP and lateral projections cannot be undertaken because of the patient's condition.

Positioning

- The patient is positioned initially as for the AP elbow projection
- The forearm is pronated by rotation of the wrist, to effect crossover of the radius and ulna
- The whole arm is rotated medially through 45° at the shoulder
- A radiolucent pad placed under the lateral aspect of the forearm will aid immobilisation
- The head is turned away from the shoulder of the side under examination, aiming to reduce scattered radiation to the lenses of the eyes and thyroid

Beam Direction and FRD

Vertical, at 90° to the IR
100 cm FRD

Centring

Over the middle of the crease of the elbow

Collimation

Proximal radius and ulna, elbow joint, distal shaft of humerus, soft tissue outlines surrounding elbow joint

Criteria for Assessing Image Quality

- Proximal radius and ulna, elbow joint, distal shaft of the humerus and soft tissue outlines surrounding the elbow joint are demonstrated
- Proximal ulna appears as a 'spanner' with the olecranon process, trochlear notch and coronoid process shown in profile
- Olecranon process is superimposed over the olecranon fossa, the trochlear notch surrounds the outline of the trochlea and the coronoid process is shown clear of the radius
- Sharp image demonstrating soft tissue margins around the elbow, coronoid process in profile over soft tissue, bony cortex and trabeculae. Adequate penetration to demonstrate the olecranon process overlying the distal humerus

Common Errors: AP Oblique Olecranon and Coronoid

Common Error	Possible Reason	Potential Effect on PCE or Report
Coronoid process not cleared from radius	Inadequate medial rotation	Difficult to identify the coronoid clearly and, as such, trauma/pathology of the coronoid cannot be determined/excluded

Clearly this projection will not be possible in patients who cannot extend at the elbow joint, a common occurrence in cases of elbow trauma. An alternative has been suggested where the partially flexed elbow is positioned with the posterior aspect of the forearm in contact with the IR. A 45° central ray is then used and directed lateromedially, centred over the crease of the elbow. Appearance of the olecranon is similar to that in Fig. 5.8B, in that the olecranon is seen as spanner-shaped. This position can also be used to demonstrate the radial head, used in conjunction with a mediolateral central ray, which projects the radial head laterally from the ulna. For cases where supination is also not possible, the arm (which is flexed at the elbow with the hand in pronation) is abducted with the humerus at 45° from the trunk, the forearm is in contact with the table and the vertical central ray is centred over the lateral epicondyle[16,17]; this provides an image of the olecranon almost identical to that in Fig. 5.8B but with less distortion, as the central ray is not angled. The issue of benefit versus risk is certainly relevant regarding the projections described that have the hand in supination, as it appears that the patient's legs may come close to the primary beam and their trunk is leaning towards it.

ULNAR GROOVE

The ulnar groove lies between the medial humeral epicondyle and the trochlea. It acts as a channel along which the ulnar nerve passes, down to the forearm from the humerus. Ulnar nerve compression at this point can cause paraesthesia and neuralgia. Because of its excellent capacity for imaging soft tissue, MRI is most suited to investigation of possible ulnar nerve compression and should be the imaging method of choice wherever possible.

Positioning (Fig. 5.9A)

- The patient is seated with the affected side next to the table
- The arm is extended at the elbow, abducted away from the trunk and externally rotated until the hand lies in supination
- The posterior aspect of the elbow is placed in contact with the IR
- The elbow is fully flexed and the fist gently clenched. The wrist is also gently flexed, to bring the fingers and thumb in contact with the shoulder
- From a position when the humeral epicondyles are equidistant from the IR, the upper arm is externally rotated 45°. This is best achieved by asking the patient to lean over towards the affected side before effecting the external rotation. The fist remains in contact with the shoulder throughout

Beam Direction and FRD

Vertical, at 90° to the IR
100 cm FRD

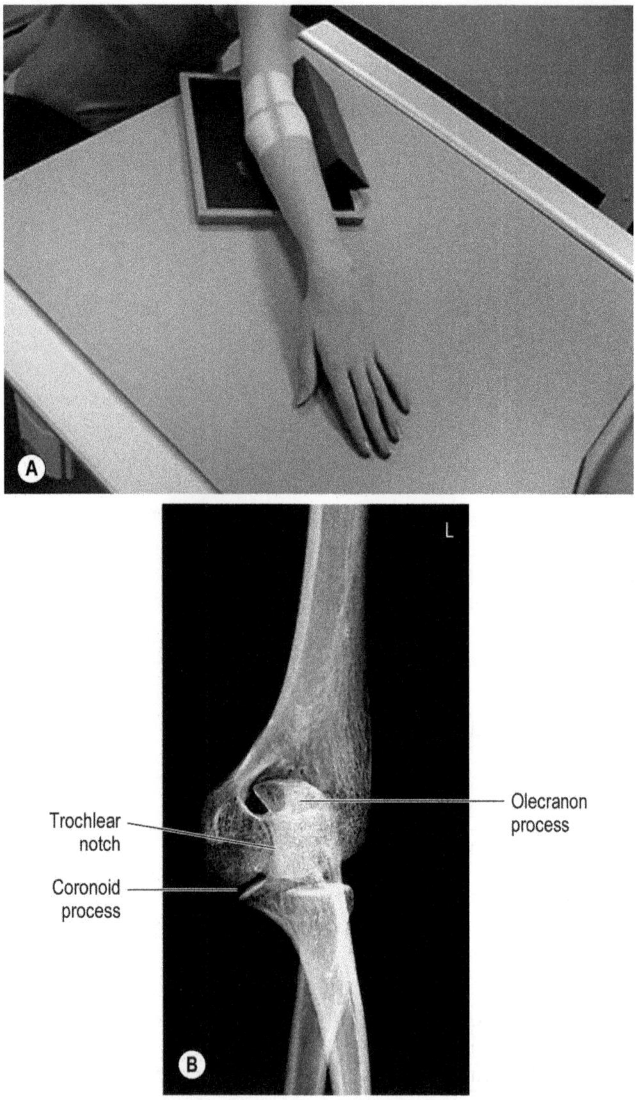

Fig. 5.8 Olecranon and coronoid – AP internally rotated oblique. (B, Reproduced with permission from Ballinger PW, Frank ED. *Merrill's Atlas of Radiographic Positioning and Radiologic Procedures.* 10th ed. St Louis: Mosby; 2003.)

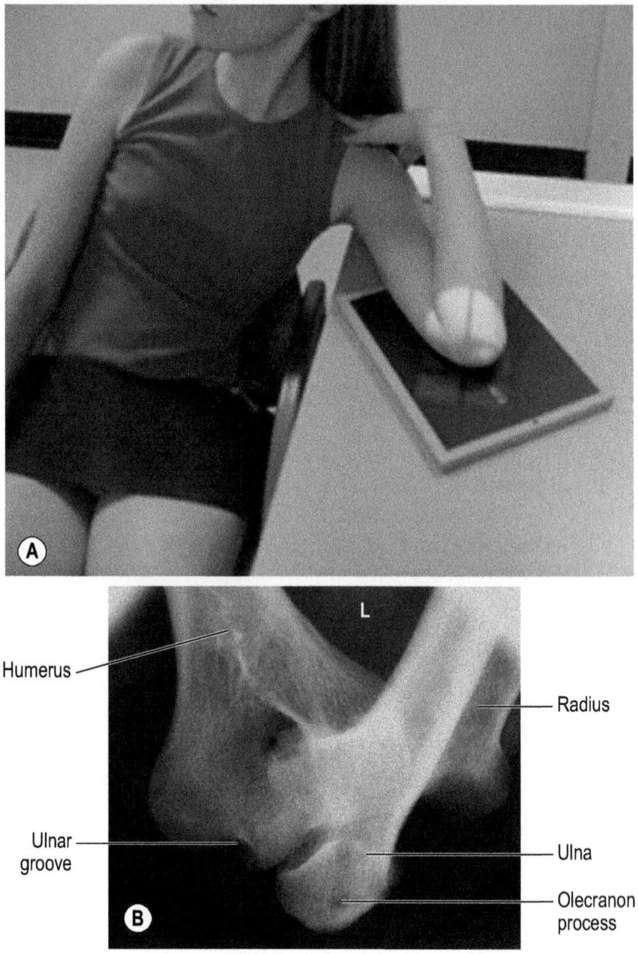

Fig. 5.9 Ulnar groove.

Centring

Over the medial epicondyle

Collimation

Olecranon process, distal humerus below shaft, soft tissue outlines around medial area of elbow

Criteria for Assessing Image Quality

- Olecranon process, distal humerus below the shaft and soft tissue outlines around the medial area of the elbow are demonstrated
- Forearm is shown superimposed over the lateral portion of the distal humerus and clear of the medial epicondyle
- Olecranon process is seen distally in relationship to the humerus
- Ulnar groove is seen as a notch between the medial epicondyle and the trochlea
- Sharp image demonstrating soft tissue margins around the medial aspect of the elbow, bony cortex and trabeculae of the non-superimposed portion of the humerus (see Fig. 5.9B)

Common Errors: Ulnar Groove

Common Error	Possible Reasons	Potential Effects on PCE or Report
Groove not seen as a distinct notch between trochlea and medial epicondyle	Inaccurate external rotation. If accompanied by superimposition of forearm over the midline of the humerus, this indicates inadequate external rotation. Superimposition of trochlea over the groove also indicates this If the medial epicondyle appears flattened, there is over-rotation of the arm	It will not be possible to assess the shape of the groove and potential compression of the ulnar nerve

Humerus

Referrals usually relate to trauma, suspected tumour, metastasis or cyst.

PCE COMMENTS – HUMERUS

Mid-shaft fractures are assessed by using generic assessment of bony outlines and trabecular pattern, with fractures in the adult being usually prominent. Fractures seen in children can be more subtle, especially spiral fractures.

Cysts: The proximal humerus is a common site for simple bone cysts (cyst = smooth and well-defined, lucent area, no periosteal reaction and may impinge on cortex without destroying it). Cysts can be an element of bone aneurysm (aneurysmal bone cyst), which may bulge within the bony outline without interrupting the cortex.

Sclerotic or *osteolytic* appearances should be noted.

Assessment of both joints: If there is clinical concern regarding a specific joint then designated imaging of this area may be warranted.

ANTEROPOSTERIOR (AP) HUMERUS (FIG. 5.10A,B)

For all projections of the humerus the IR is placed vertical. If a patient presents supine, as on a trolley in the Emergency Department, the IR can be used horizontally under the humerus, on the trolley-top, for the AP projection.

Positioning

- The IR is placed in the erect holder
- The patient stands erect facing the X-ray tube and the affected arm is extended and abducted from the trunk to avoid superimposition of the humerus and upper arm soft tissue over the soft tissue of the trunk
- The feet are slightly separated for stability
- The height of the IR is adjusted until its midpoint is coincident with the midshaft of the humerus
- Orientating the upper arm diagonally at 45° across the IR plate will maximise the available space for the area of interest which must include the shoulder and elbow joints on the image
- The palm faces forwards with the humeral epicondyles equidistant from the IR

Beam Direction and FRD

Horizontal, at 90° to the IR
100 cm FRD

Centring

To the middle of the humerus, on the anterior aspect of the arm

Collimation

Shoulder joint, shaft of humerus, elbow joint, soft tissues surrounding the area

Aligning the light beam diaphragm housing along the long axis of the humerus before collimating will allow more effective collimation around the area of interest.

Criteria for Assessing Image Quality

- Shoulder joint, shaft of humerus, elbow joint and soft tissues are demonstrated
- Humerus is clear of the soft tissue of the trunk
- Greater tuberosity of humerus is in profile laterally on the humeral head
- Humeral epicondyles are equidistant from coronoid and olecranon fossae
- Sharp image demonstrating soft tissue margins around the area of interest, bony cortex and trabeculae. Adequate penetration to demonstrate joints whilst maintaining trabecular detail over the humeral shaft

Common Errors: AP Humerus

Common Errors	Possible Reasons	Potential Effects on PCE or Report
Pale shadow overlying medial aspect of the humerus and soft tissue of upper arm	Arm not abducted adequately from the trunk	Difficult to assess: for fractures and soft tissues, as lines can mimic fracture/pathology; for subtle benign or malignant lesions
Humeral epicondyles not shown as equidistant around coronoid and olecranon fossae; greater tuberosity projected over the humeral head	Arm is rotated. This is most frequently medial rotation, as this is a more comfortable position for the patient than with the rotation required for a true AP position of the humerus	Difficult to assess any pathology of the greater tuberosity

LATERAL HUMERUS (FIG. 5.11A,B)

Positioning

- The IR is placed in the erect holder
- The patient stands erect facing the IR and the affected arm is extended and abducted from the trunk to avoid superimposition of the humerus and upper arm soft tissue over the soft tissue of the trunk
- The feet are slightly separated for stability
- The height of the IR is adjusted until its midpoint is coincident with the midshaft of the humerus
- Orientating the upper arm at 45° across the IR will maximise the available space for the area of interest, which must include the shoulder and elbow joints on the image
- The arm is medially rotated and the elbow flexed until the medial aspect of the hand comes into contact with the lower abdomen. The lateral aspect of the humerus is in contact with the IR. The humeral epicondyles are superimposed
- The head is turned away from the side under examination
- A PA anatomical marker is usually used for this projection

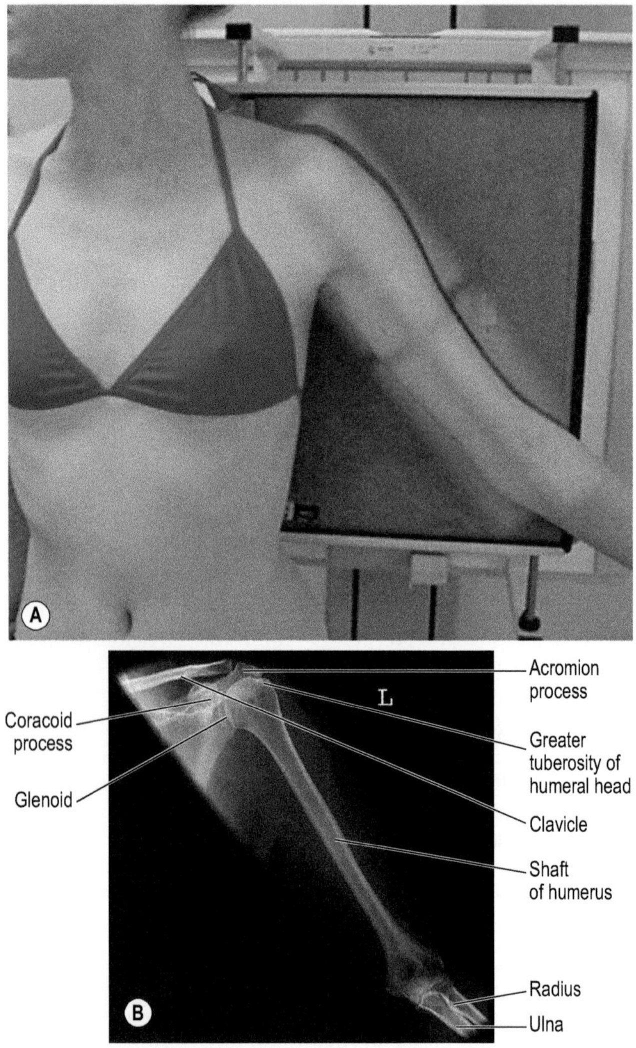

Fig. 5.10 AP humerus.

The lateral humerus projection can also be undertaken with the patient facing the X-ray tube, in an AP position, and this should be adapted for the trolley-bound patient who is supine, rather than attempting a PA approach.

For the AP projection the arm is flexed at the elbow and the limb medially rotated to bring the medial aspect of the humerus in contact with the IR. The hand is placed on the hip to immobilise the arm. Unfortunately this position is somewhat difficult, even for the uninjured patient, especially as the movement required at the shoulder results in the scapula being positioned almost perpendicular to the IR; this in itself is not disadvantageous, but the position of the scapula does push the posterior aspect of the upper humerus away from the IR, making lateral representation of the image of the bone less accurate. The action of the hand resting on the hip also makes superimposition of the humeral epicondyles difficult.

Beam Direction and FRD

Horizontal, at 90° to the IR
100 cm FRD

Centring

For patient in a PA position: to the middle of the humerus, on the medial aspect of the arm

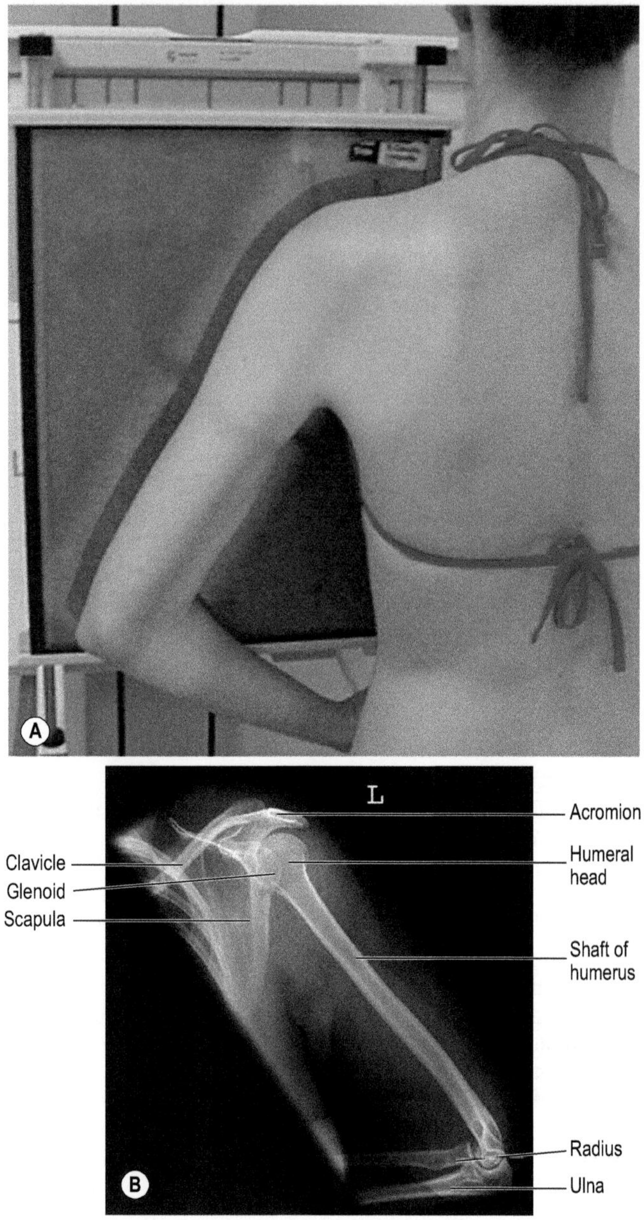

Fig. 5.11 Lateral humerus.

For patient in an AP position: to the middle of the humerus, on the lateral aspect of the arm

Collimation

Shoulder joint, shaft of humerus, elbow joint, soft tissues surrounding the area

Aligning the light beam diaphragm housing along the long axis of the humerus before collimating will allow more effective collimation around the area of interest.

Criteria for Assessing Image Quality

- Shoulder joint, shaft of humerus, elbow joint and soft tissues are demonstrated
- Humerus is clear of soft tissue of trunk and humeral head is cleared from the image of the scapula
- Greater tuberosity of humerus is seen over the middle of the humeral head

- Superimposition of the trochlea and capitulum is ideal, but it must be remembered that oblique rays around the central ray are likely to impinge upon this area at around 5–8°, varying with humeral length. This obliquity will almost certainly affect the superimposition of trochlea and capitulum. If this area of the humerus is of particular interest then elbow projections should be undertaken
- Sharp image demonstrating soft tissue margins around the area of interest, bony cortex and trabeculae. Adequate penetration to demonstrate joints whilst maintaining trabecular detail over the humeral shaft

Common Errors: Lateral Humerus

Common Errors	Possible Reasons	Potential Effects on PCE or Report
Pale shadow overlying the anterior aspect of the humerus (seen facing towards the thorax in this projection) and soft tissue of upper arm	Arm not abducted adequately from the trunk	Difficult as: soft tissues overlying bone make it possible to misread as a fracture or other pathology can miss subtle benign or malignant lesions
Greater tuberosity appears towards or over the lateral margin of the humeral head	Arm is externally rotated. This can be avoided by ensuring that the entire length of the lateral aspect of the humerus is in contact with the IR; this encourages the patient to maintain the lateral position	Difficult to assess subtle fractures of the greater tuberosity
Non-superimposition of trochlea and capitulum	Slight overlap, rather than full superimposition, can be explained by effects of obliquity of the beam around the central ray (see image quality criteria, above). However, when accompanied by incorrect appearance of the greater tuberosity (see point above) this may indicate external rotation of the humerus	Difficult to: visualise the elbow as it is not appearing on a true lateral angle detect any potential elevated fat pads

Intertuberous Sulcus (Bicipital Groove)

The intertuberous sulcus lies on the anterior aspect of the humeral head, between the greater and lesser tuberosities; insertion of the long head of biceps lies here. Its position makes it difficult to image because it travels vertically and cannot be seen on an AP projection of the humerus or shoulder.

The projection aims to demonstrate the groove in profile, which is only possible in the superoinferior or inferosuperior directions. There are many problems associated with either of these approaches, the most obvious being implementation of either position with the bulky light beam housings commonly found today. Other important considerations are dose implications when directing a beam caudally (for superoinferior projection), and immobilisation.

The option of the superoinferior method does cause serious concern for patient dose, as the caudal ray required would almost certainly irradiate anterior structures of the trunk in addition to the upper humerus, thereby raising questions as to its suitability.

Therefore, an inferosuperior approach may fit with the requirement for the radiographer to use a technique that reduces the risk of irradiating radiosensitive tissues. Older texts describe an inferosuperior method which involves the patient leaning over a tube head which is directed vertically but in a cranial direction.[18] Use of the old long cones, which were replaced by modern collimators, meant that the patient could use the cone as an aid to immobilisation. The IR was supported by a special holder. The method described in this book uses an adaptation of this, with the patient supine. In the absence of the long cone, the patient is immobilised by lying supine; a specialist receptor support is not always necessary but does prove useful.

INFEROSUPERIOR BICIPITAL GROOVE: METHOD 1 (FIG. 5.12)

Positioning

- The patient lies supine on the examination table
- The IR is supported vertically on the table with its tube side in contact with the superior aspect of the shoulder. Its centre is coincident with the humeral head

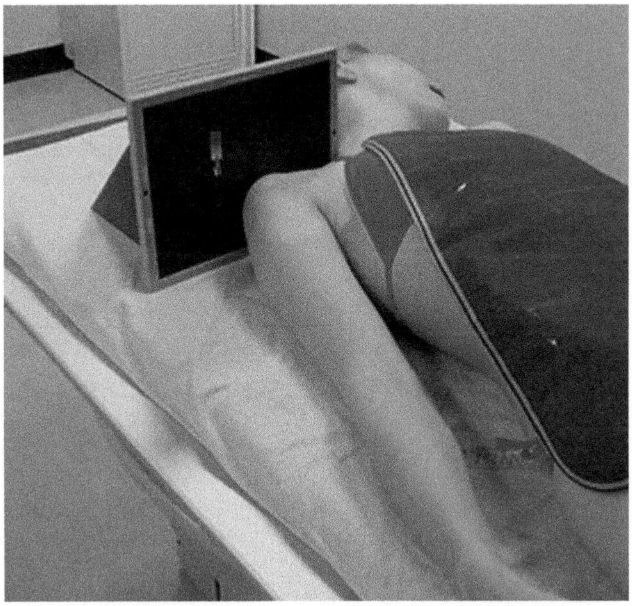

Fig. 5.12 Inferosuperior bicipital groove – method 1.

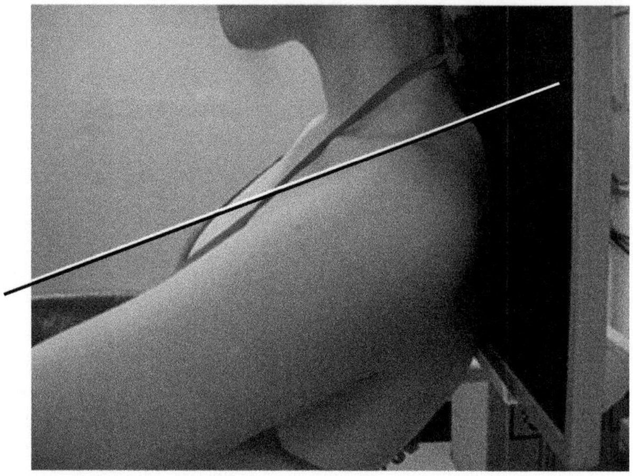

Fig. 5.13 Inferosuperior bicipital groove – method 2.

- The arm is abducted slightly from the trunk and externally rotated until the humeral epicondyles are approximately 45° to the table-top
- The greater and lesser tuberosities are palpated to ensure that the intertuberous sulcus is in profile superiorly
- The patient's head is turned away from the side under examination

Beam Direction and FRD

Initially horizontal, with a 5° caudal angle
FRD may vary according to the size of the tube mounting but should be no less than 100 cm

A slightly longer FRD may be beneficial, as there may be a relatively long object receptor distance (ORD) in patients who have a significant amount of adipose or muscle tissue over the shoulder joint.

INFEROSUPERIOR BICIPITAL GROOVE: METHOD 2 (FIG. 5.13)

The IR position is vertical.

Positioning

- The patient sits facing the X-ray tube, their back approximately 30 cm away from the IR
- The patient leans back, approximately 30° from vertical, until they lean against the IR
- The arm is abducted slightly from the trunk and externally rotated until the humeral epicondyles are approximately 45° to the median sagittal plane
- The arm is elevated slightly to bring the long axis of the humerus to make an angle of approximately 30° with the floor (60° to IR)
- The greater and lesser tuberosities are palpated to ensure that the intertuberous sulcus is in profile superiorly
- The patient's head is turned away from the side under examination

Beam Direction and FRD

Initially horizontal, with a 15–20° cranial angle
As for method 1, FRD may vary according to the size of the tube mounting but should be no less than 100 cm

Centring: Both Methods

Over the anterior aspect of the middle of the humeral head

Collimation

Anterior portion of humeral head, soft tissue overlying this area
Inclusion of the area within collimation can be ensured by checking that the outline shadow of the area lies within the light beam representation and the IR

Criteria for Assessing Image Quality

- Anterior portion of the humeral head and the soft tissue overlying it are demonstrated
- Bicipital groove is seen in profile as a notch superiorly over the outline of the anterior aspect of the humeral head, between the greater and lesser tuberosities
- Sharp image demonstrating soft tissue margins above the area of interest, bony cortex and its outline over the sulcus (Fig. 5.14)

Common Errors: Intertuberous Sulcus

Common Errors	Possible Reasons	Potential Effects on PCE or Report
Humeral head seen but sulcus not in profile	1. Sulcus projected medially or laterally due to inaccurate rotation of the limb *or* 2. Extreme obliquity of the arm positions the sulcus obliquely, rather than perpendicular to IR	It will not be possible to assess the shape of the sulcus and any impact its shape might have on long head of biceps
Dense soft tissue shadow overlying area of interest	Tube position too low; the soft tissues of the arm may be superimposed over the area of interest	Overlying soft tissues mimic pathology or hide subtle fractures or pathologies

The Shoulder Girdle

The use of plain imaging is still an essential starting point when investigating shoulder trauma, and plain radiography is indicated for fractures, dislocations and shoulder instability. Other imaging methods play an important part in assessment of the joint, with magnetic resonance imaging (MRI) and ultrasound useful for rotator cuff pain and injuries, and calcinic tendinitis.[19,20]

Computed tomography (CT) may be used in preoperative assessment of shoulder injuries, so that fractures are not underestimated (as can be the case in some instances with plain X-ray images) and 3D reconstruction can be used to fully demonstrate complex fractures and assist in surgical planning. Despite the obvious usefulness of MRI and ultrasound for demonstrating the shoulder joint, CT can be considered useful for preoperative planning in recurrent anterior shoulder instability, especially when there is a requirement to demonstrate glenoid defects.[21]

When imaging this region with plain radiography, radiation protection of the eyes and thyroid is an important consideration: the patient must always have their head turned away from the primary beam during exposure.

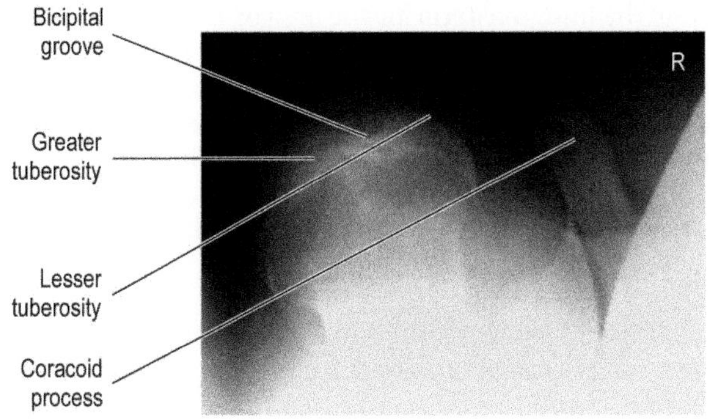

Fig. 5.14 Bicipital groove. (Reproduced with permission from Ballinger PW, Frank ED. *Merrill's Atlas of Radiographic Positioning and Radiologic Procedures*. 10th ed. St Louis: Mosby; 2003.)

This area of high subject contrast has implications for overexposure of some structures involved in the joint. This is especially true of the acromioclavicular (AC) joint, which is often lacking in detail due to overexposure, whereas details of denser structures of the region (e.g. the humeral head or glenoid) are adequately demonstrated. Repeat examinations are often required as a result, and can be avoided in the first instance by using a wedge filter placed between the IR and the upper shoulder. The most effective type of filter for this is rubberised and boomerang-shaped and can therefore sit comfortably and safely around and behind the upper shoulder. Use of a relatively high kVp and lower mAs can offer a solution in the absence of a filter, but the contrast of these images is somewhat reduced compared with those produced with a filter. Patients with very dense muscle (e.g. body builders and rugby players) will certainly need effective beam penetration. As long as the exposure index remains within the acceptable range, digital manipulation will also improve visualisation of the whole area.

INDICATIONS

Arthropathy

Erosions are a relatively late feature in patients with rheumatoid arthritis and the shoulder should only be examined by plain imaging if that joint is specifically affected. In patients with suspected osteoarthritis, X-ray is not indicated initially unless intervention is likely.

Common causes for pain in the shoulder which are indicative on radiographs include calcific tenditis where an area of dense calcification is noted within the shoulder joint, often from the supraspinatus tendon; further imaging with ultrasound is also recommended.[22] Rotator cuff arthropathies can often be indicative from a high riding humeral head and reduction in the subacromial space. This is often combined with slight sclerosis of the tendon attachments of the humeral head or inferior border of the acromion.[23] Ultrasound is often undertaken after the radiograph to further assess the joint.[24]

Fracture

This mostly affects the clavicle, humeral surgical neck, tuberosities of the humerus and scapula; fracture of the scapula is relatively uncommon, accounting for only 3–5% of shoulder injuries.

Fractures of the surgical neck of the humerus and the tuberosities have often been classified using Neer's method,[25] which considers the status and degree of displacement of the articular segment of the head of the humerus, the surgical neck of the humerus and the greater and lesser tuberosities. The reliability of such classification systems has been questioned and alternative classification methods suggested;[26] however, it must be mentioned that new methods, however reliable, need to be widely accepted so that they can be considered rigorous.

Dislocation

The shoulder joint is the most commonly dislocated joint in the human body,[27] with anterior dislocation most common; only up to 5% of dislocations occur posteriorly,[28] and an estimated 60–80% of these are missed on initial examination. As many as 50% of these uncommon dislocations can often be missed in the Emergency Department, highlighting the importance of an additional projection that can identify posterior dislocations.[29] Subluxation of the acromioclavicular joint can also occur.

PCE COMMENTS – SHOULDER

Plain X-ray imaging is most useful for demonstrating fractures and dislocations but calcifications seen in the region should be noted in a PCE report.

Remember not to focus on the obvious; the shoulder is not simply about the humerus and the glenohumeral joint. The clavicle, scapula, acromioclavicular joints and sternoclavicular joints must also be assessed.

Fractures: Proximal humeral fractures can be seen on the AP shoulder, and these are very common in elderly patients after trauma. Check that cortical outlines and the trabecular pattern of the humerus are not interrupted. Clavicular fractures are usually well demonstrated on the AP shoulder projection. For clavicle and scapular injuries, please see PCE comments noted in the section on the clavicle or scapula in this chapter.

If a dislocation is noted then there may be associated bony injury (see below).

Dislocations and subluxations: Anterior dislocation of the glenohumeral joint is the most common dislocation seen, with posterior dislocation comprising only up to 5%. The image should be also checked for: acromioclavicular joint subluxation or dislocation; glenohumeral joint trauma; widening of the AC joint space.

Posterior dislocation of the glenohumeral joint is seen in up to 5% of shoulder dislocations; presence of the light bulb sign of the humeral head, as opposed to the normal walking stick configuration, will alert the radiographer to this.

Inferior dislocations – the humeral head will be displaced directly below and a slightly medially to the glenoid fossa. These account for only around 1% of shoulder dislocations.[30]

Assessment of glenoid and humeral head is important, particularly in glenohumeral dislocations.

Bankart lesions are found in patients with anterior dislocation and affect the anteroinferior glenoid rim but are not easy to spot radiographically. They are commonly associated with a *Hill–Sachs lesion* which is a depressed fracture on the posterolateral aspect of the humeral head. If a Bankart lesion is in its most excessive form, there may be a fracture of the anteroinferior glenoid; this is termed *'bony Bankart'*. *Reverse Hill–Sachs lesions* are caused by posterior dislocation and are seen on the anteromedial humeral head (posterior dislocation).[30]

ANTEROPOSTERIOR (AP) SHOULDER (FIG. 5.15A,B)

This projection can be performed in the erect position, either standing or seated, depending on the patient's condition and ability. When examining a patient on a trolley, care should be taken to ensure either that the patient is in the fully erect position or the beam is accurately angled to compensate for any tilt on the trolley back rest; this will ensure that the central ray remains at 90° to the IR.

Positioning

- The patient sits or stands erect, with the posterior aspect of the shoulder under examination in contact with the vertical IR
- The arm is fully extended and slightly abducted with the palm of the hand facing forward to ensure the true anatomical position (with the greater tuberosity in profile on the lateral aspect of the humeral head)
- The patient's trunk is rotated approximately 20° towards the side under examination, to bring the scapula parallel to the IR
- The patient's head is turned away from the side under examination for radiation protection

Beam Direction and FRD

Horizontal at 90° to the IR
100 cm FRD

Centring Point

To the coracoid process of the scapula, palpable anteriorly just below the lateral third of the clavicle and medial to the middle of the humeral head

This centring point will bring the glenohumeral joint central to the IR but means that a large field of view is required to fulfil the image criteria for the area of interest. However, if the radiographic examination is for a general shoulder survey, the area of interest should be positioned to lie within the borders of the IR, with beam centring to the centre of the IR; this will ensure that the medial end of the clavicle, the whole of the scapula and the upper third of the humerus can be included in one image with the minimum field of radiation.

Collimation

The head and proximal third of humerus, scapula, clavicle, lateral soft tissues of proximal humerus

Criteria for Assessing Image Quality

- Head and proximal third of humerus, clavicle, acromioclavicular joint and the inferior end of the scapula are demonstrated
- Greater tuberosity is seen in profile on the lateral aspect of head of humerus
- Glenohumeral joint is obscured by head of humerus
- Acromion is demonstrated clear of the superior border of head of humerus
- Sharp image demonstrating the bony cortex and trabeculae of the head of the humerus in contrast with the shoulder joint and surrounding soft tissues; the acromioclavicular joint is seen clearly

The AP projection does not demonstrate the glenohumeral joint space clearly and orthopaedic departments may request either a 'True AP' or 'Grashey AP'[25] instead of, or to complement, the AP. This projection uses the same position and centring point as the AP described here but with an obliquity of the patient at 45° instead of 20°, to open the glenohumeral joint. The projection shows the glenohumeral joint tangentially, but published work has been varied in assessment of its effectiveness in demonstration of direction of dislocation.[31,32]

Common Errors: AP Shoulder

Common Errors	Possible Reasons	Potential Effects on PCE or Report
Inferior end of the scapula not included on the image	The IR is often positioned in the 'landscape' position; putting it in the 'portrait' position will usually prevent this	Difficult to identify fractures in this area
Foreshortening of the clavicle	The patient is rotated too much towards the side under examination	Difficult to assess as leads to distortion of the AC joint (causing potential of missing subtle Grade 1 AC joint dislocations). Can give a look of overriding of the clavicle upon itself, making even displaced fractures unable to be detected
The AC joint is over-penetrated	This is due to the difference in subject contrast in this area; the use of a wedge filter will prevent this	Difficult to assess: soft tissues (i.e. swelling) subtle cortical irregularities or break in cortex

AXILLARY/AXIAL PROJECTIONS OF THE SHOULDER

Evaluation of the shoulder joint, particularly for follow-up orthopaedic assessment, often requires an axillary projection to offer an image at 90° to the AP. Success of this projection will depend on the patient's condition and cooperation. Two methods are described here.

Method 1: Superoinferior Shoulder (Fig. 5.16A,B)

This method is often difficult to implement or inappropriate, particularly in trauma, owing to the extent to which the arm must be abducted.

IR is horizontal

Positioning

- The patient sits with the side under examination next to and slightly away from the table
- For radiation protection purposes the legs are placed so they are not under the table
- The arm is abducted fully and the patient leans laterally over the IR; the hand is internally rotated and pronated. The axilla is positioned over the IR in a position that will ensure inclusion of the relevant anatomy, and with the axilla as close to it as possible
- The patient's head and neck are abducted away from the shoulder under examination as far as possible to clear

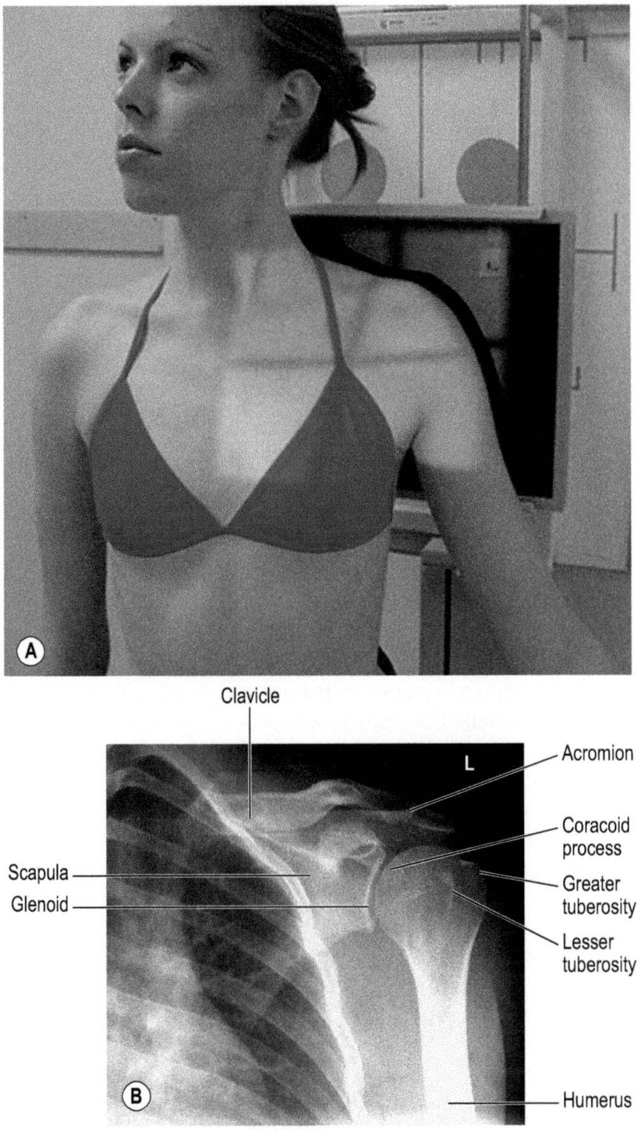

Fig. 5.15 AP shoulder.

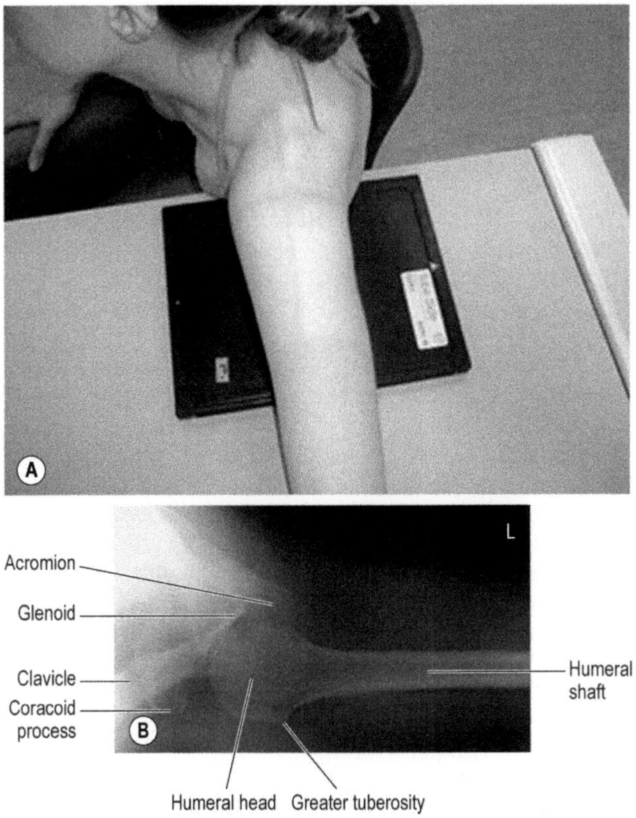

Fig. 5.16 Superoinferior shoulder.

them from the area of interest and reduce the radiation dose to these areas

Beam Direction and FRD

Vertical at 90° to the IR
100 cm FRD

Centring Point

To the superior aspect over the middle of the humeral head

Collimation

Head and proximal third of humerus, glenoid cavity, acromion, coracoid process, surrounding soft tissues

Criteria for Assessing Image Quality

- Head and proximal end of humerus, glenoid fossa, lateral end of clavicle, acromion and coracoid process are demonstrated
- Head of humerus appears above the glenoid 'like a golf ball on a tee'[29]
- Greater tuberosity should be seen in profile anteriorly
- Acromion and lateral end of clavicle are superimposed on the superoposterior aspect of head of humerus
- Coracoid process is demonstrated anterior to head of humerus
- Sharp image demonstrating the soft tissue margins, bony cortex and trabeculae of the humeral head with adequate image density to demonstrate the bony detail of the humerus in contrast to the glenohumeral joint, acromion and clavicle

Common Errors: Superoinferior Shoulder

Common Errors	Possible Reasons	Potential Effects on PCE or Report
The glenohumeral joint is not demonstrated within the boundaries of the IR	The patient may not be stretching across the IR sufficiently. If the patient is capable of leaning further, try lowering the table-top to enable the patient to flex more at the waist	Difficult to assess fractures if the whole area not demonstrated, therefore unable to assess for pathology/fracture/dislocation
Magnification and unsharpness of the resulting image, probably accompanied by foreshortening of humeral head	The axilla is not in close enough contact with IR and the humerus may not be fully abducted, causing its shaft to lie at an angle with the IR. Try using a pad to raise the IR or consider increasing the FRD to compensate for the large ORD	Distortion of the image can make pathology recognition difficult. Sometimes can cause false-positive result due to the distortion mimicking fracture lines

Method 2: Inferosuperior Shoulder (Fig. 5.17)

Method 2 is the method of choice for a patient with restricted movement of the humerus as there is more scope for adaptation to suit the patient's condition. Method 2 is sometimes referred to as the *Lawrence axillary projection.*[33]

Positioning

- The patient lies supine on the table
- A small radiolucent pad is placed beneath the shoulder to raise it slightly
- The head and neck are abducted as much as possible away from the side under examination to clear them from the area of interest and reduce radiation dose to these areas
- The IR is supported in the erect position, its tube side against the superior aspect of the head of the humerus and in contact with the neck
- The arm is abducted to 90° or as far as the patient's condition permits and the hand is supinated (although some internal rotation of the forearm is acceptable; supination acts mainly to help the patient maintain the correct relationship of the humerus to the IR)

Modern tube housings are usually too bulky to allow tube centring for this positioning. An alternative, *modified inferosuperior*, is suggested, as follows.

This technique can be achieved with as little as 30° arm abduction,[25] but the tube needs to be brought in as close to the patient's body as possible. By lying the patient in a slightly diagonal position across the length of the tabletop or trolley, access to the axilla is achievable (Fig. 5.18). Positioning the patient thus, diagonally across the tabletop, requires consideration for the safety of the patient; this is directly related to table width and should only be considered in the relatively cooperative patient.

Beam Direction and FRD (Inferosuperior and Modified Inferosuperior Projections)

Horizontal at 90° to the IR and coincident with the glenohumeral joint
100 cm FRD

The central ray must be at 90° to the IR and requires careful positioning to prevent a distorted image. To eliminate distortion, align the central ray with the patient first to ensure it is parallel to the glenohumeral joint, i.e. through the axilla, then position the IR until perpendicular to the central ray. This is suggested for both the inferosuperior and modified inferosuperior projections.

Centring Point

Through the axilla

Collimation

Head and proximal third of humerus, glenoid cavity, acromion, coracoid process, surrounding soft tissues

Criteria for Assessing Image Quality

- Head and proximal end of humerus, glenoid fossa, lateral end of clavicle, acromion and coracoid process should all be demonstrated
- Glenohumeral joint should be demonstrated
- Lesser tuberosity of humerus should be seen in profile
- Acromioclavicular joint will be superimposed on humerus
- Sharp image demonstrating the soft tissue margins, bony cortex and trabeculae of the humeral head with adequate image density to demonstrate the bony detail of the humerus in contrast to the glenohumeral joint

Common Errors: Inferosuperior Shoulder

Common Error	Possible Reason	Potential Effect on PCE or Report
The glenohumeral joint is not demonstrated within the boundaries of the IR	The head and neck may not be sufficiently abducted away from the side under examination to enable the IR to be positioned correctly. Always ensure the IR is closely tucked into the neck	If not demonstrated then unable to assess for pathology/fracture/dislocation

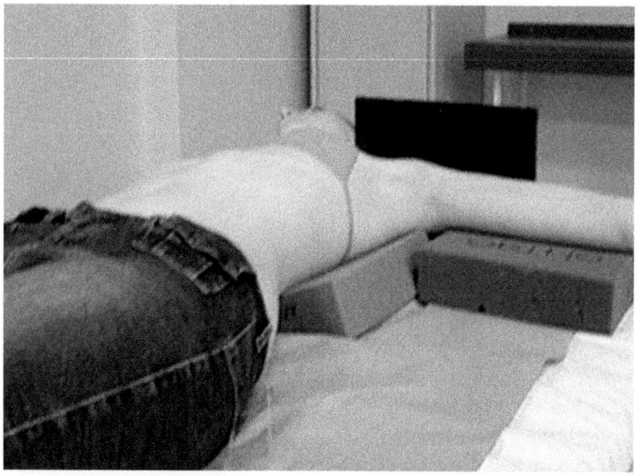

Fig. 5.17 Inferosuperior shoulder.

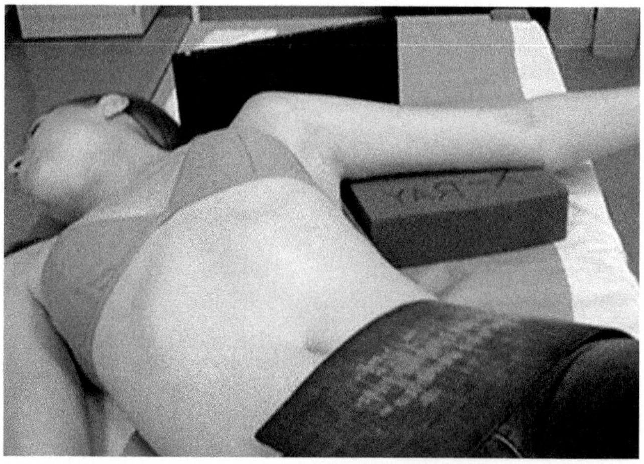

Fig. 5.18 Modified inferosuperior shoulder.

The inferosuperior projections can be adapted to demonstrate the classic Hill–Sachs compression fracture, seen in patients who have recurrent anterior dislocation of the shoulder. This adaptation involves maximum external rotation of the arm, with the patient aiming to press the thumb down towards the table- or trolley-top. Unfortunately, this manoeuvre can be difficult for patients to achieve and the AP shoulder with maximum internal rotation can also demonstrate this lesion adequately. In order to achieve the correct amount of rotation for this, the arm is medially rotated and flexed at the elbow; the dorsum of the hand is then rested on the waist. Yet another technique that can show Hill–Sachs lesions is the *Stryker notch projection*, where the palm of the hand is placed on top of the head with the fingers toward the back of the head and the long axis of the humerus parallel to the median sagittal plane (MSP); a 10° cranial angle is centred over the coracoid process for this projection.[34]

Bankart lesions are also recognised as an effect of recurrent anterior dislocation[35] and are best seen on the true superoinferior projection; clearly, superoinferior is recognised as difficult on the traumatised patient but feasible on patients with recovered range of shoulder movement following treatment.

30–45° MODIFIED SUPEROINFERIOR PROJECTION OF THE SHOULDER – 'APICAL OBLIQUE' (FIG. 5.19A,B)

This projection was described by Unett and Royle[33] and Raby et al,[27] and a similar projection was described by Long and Rafert[25] but with more obliquity of the patient (i.e. the patient is rotated 45° onto the side under examination as opposed to bringing the scapula parallel to the IR; this is known as the *Garth projection* or Garth apical oblique; see Fig. 17.16). Unett and Royle described this as 'modified Wallace and Hellier', but the resulting image achieved with the 30–45° modified projection is much less magnified and distorted, which makes it easier to interpret. It is therefore probably a misnomer to use the term 'modified Wallace and Hellier' for this projection, as the similarity is only the use of a caudal angle. The Wallace and Hellier projection (often called the 'Wallace' view) cannot be undertaken on the supine or semi-recumbent patient, as it requires the patient to sit with their back against the table, but uses a horizontal IR; the affected limb is 90° to the IR. The air gap between shoulder and IR will require some increase in exposure, thereby increasing radiation dose in the Wallace and Hellier projection. Another well-known alternative projection is the Velpeau projection; this is similar to the Wallace and Hellier in that the IR is placed horizontally but the patient leans back 30° over it. A vertical central ray is used, which creates less distortion, but there is still a rather long object receptor distance (ORD); clearly the imaging implications for this projection are more favourable than for Wallace and Hellier, but it still has negative points in comparison to the 30–45° projection.

It is easier to position the patient for the modified 30–45° projection, as the patient position is identical to that for the AP shoulder, with the angle of central ray directed 30–45° caudally. The patient can satisfactorily be positioned supine or on a trolley or in a chair, and this is therefore a very useful technique for trauma patients. Raby et al see the advantages of this method in terms of patient comfort and its ability to show small bony fragments easily; indeed, they state the only disadvantage as unfamiliarity due to its infrequency of use.[27] Despite the noticeable distortion caused by beam angulation, the humerus does still lie parallel to the IR, whereas in the Wallace and Hellier method the humerus lies at 90° to the IR and at 30° in Velpeau. In addition, Wallace and Hellier requires 45° caudal tube angulation; these combined factors cause more distortion than with the 30–45° AP shoulder.

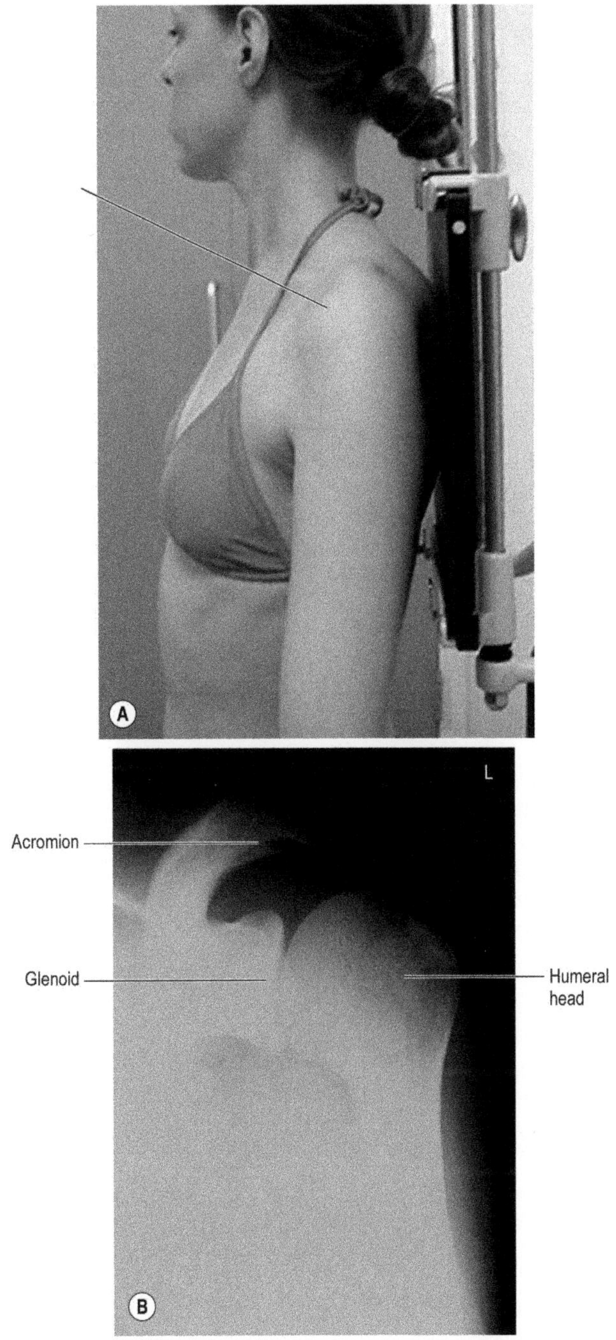

Fig. 5.19 30–45° modified superoinferior shoulder.

The 30–45° projection demonstrates the glenohumeral joint in coronal profile, and therefore an assessment of dislocation or intra-articular fractures can be made. The radiographer only needs to understand the basic radiographic principles involving effects of angulation on the image in order to assess direction of dislocation. Basically, the structure lying closest to the IR will be less obviously displaced than structures further from it; therefore, a posterior dislocation will show the humeral head superimposed over the acromion, and anterior dislocation will show the humeral head well below the acromion and low compared to the glenoid position. The Wallace and Hellier method does not appear to provide more useful information than the 30–45° modified projection and therefore its use should be questioned, considering that it appears to have more disadvantages than any other projection of its type.

Positioning (as for AP Shoulder)

- The IR is vertical or under/behind the patient's shoulder if supine or sitting on a trolley
- The patient can remain standing or be seated, with the posterior aspect of the shoulder in contact with the IR
- The arm is fully extended and slightly abducted with the palm of the hand facing forward to ensure the true anatomical position
- The patient is rotated approximately 20° onto the side under examination to bring the scapula parallel to the IR
- The patient's head is turned away from the side under examination for radiation protection

Beam Direction and FRD

Erect: Initially horizontal, directed caudally at 30–45° to the IR
Supine: Initially vertical, directed 30–45° caudally

If the patient is semirecumbent: The beam is initially positioned perpendicular to the IR and then directed a further 30–45° caudally from this angle
100 cm FRD

Centring Point

Above the coracoid process and slightly superior to the humeral head

Collimation

Head and proximal third of humerus, glenoid cavity, acromion process, surrounding soft tissues

Criteria for Assessing Image Quality

- Head and proximal shaft of humerus, glenoid fossa, lateral end of clavicle and acromion process should all be demonstrated
- Greater tuberosity is demonstrated on the lateral aspect of the humerus
- Elongation of head of humerus, the position of which will vary if the humeral head is dislocated
- The glenoid fossa and head of humerus are projected clear of the lateral margin of the rib cage
- Sharp image demonstrating the humeral head in contrast to the shoulder joint and surrounding soft tissues

'Y' VIEW/TRUE LATERAL (FIG. 5.20A,B)

This projection may be used in cases of suspected glenohumeral dislocation or fractures of the proximal humerus. It is similar to the basic lateral scapula projection but the humerus is not abducted in the same manner, to prevent it overlying the body of the scapula; in this case the humerus is adducted alongside the patient's trunk. It is relatively simple to position and requires little cooperation from the patient. The resulting image allows an assessment of fractures or glenohumeral dislocation, as the shoulder girdle is demonstrated in the true lateral position. Indeed, it has been claimed by some that the projection is superior to the axillary projection for the demonstration of dislocation.[36] If the patient is presented on a trolley the technique can be performed in the AP position with the patient rotating approximately 25° towards the uninjured side.

This technique is considered to be superior to the modified superoinferior or apical oblique (30–45° AP) described previously, as the modified axial can only help assess dislocations. This may then necessitate further radiographic examination. The 'Y' view is relatively simple to perform[35,36] and can

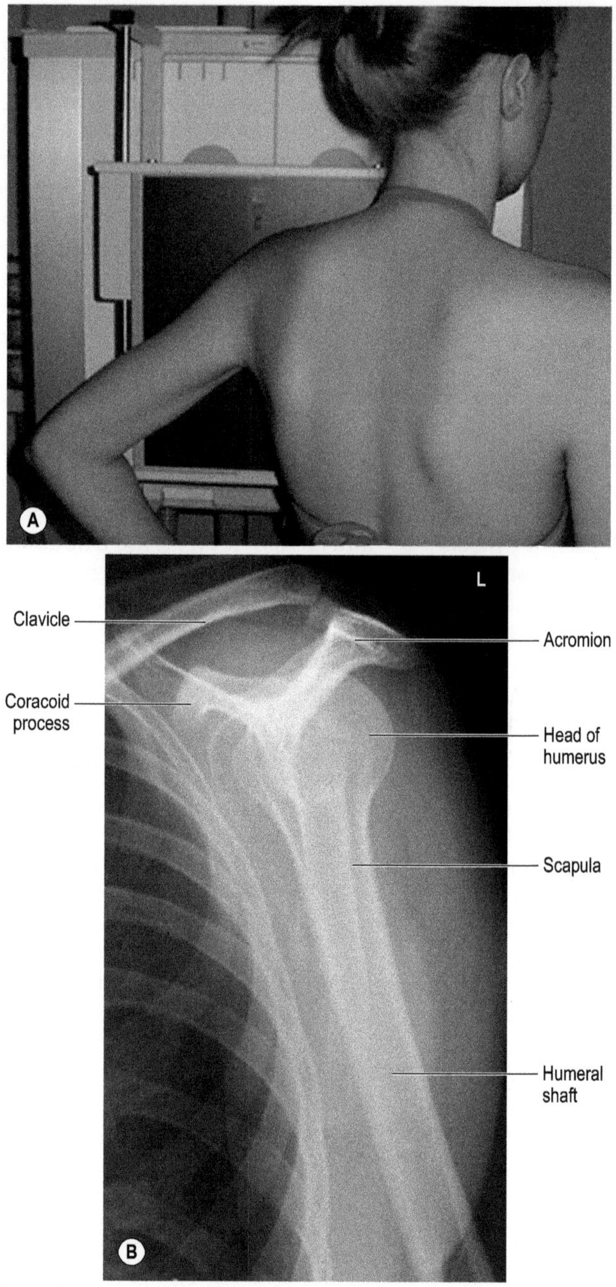

Fig. 5.20 Y view. Note that the arm position in (A) may not be achievable in injury and the arm may be adducted across the trunk as an alternative.

be achieved satisfactorily even if the patient presents supine on a trolley or in a chair, and it is therefore recommended for trauma patients.[37–39] It is believed that it will show fractures of the humeral head, scapula and coracoid process, plus dislocation of the humeral head and the direction of this,[40] but it can fail to demonstrate some intra-articular fractures well.[41]

In the normal shoulder the humeral head will be demonstrated superimposed on the glenoid process, as opposed to in the dislocated shoulder, where it will appear under the coracoid process in anterior dislocation and under the acromion in posterior dislocation.

Positioning

- The patient stands or sits erect, facing the IR with their back to the X-ray tube
- From an initial PA position, rotate the patient approximately 25° to bring the side under examination closer to, and bring the body of the scapula 90° to, the IR
- The arm on the side under examination is adducted from the trunk, with the elbow flexed and hand resting on the side of the waist. Alternatively, the elbow may be flexed with the forearm resting across the chest and the hand resting on the shoulder of the opposite side (this may be more comfortable for the injured patient)
- The scapula is palpated to check the lateral and medial borders are superimposed
- The patient's head is turned as far as possible towards the unaffected side

If the patient is *supine*, this projection can be achieved by rotating the trunk 25° away from the side under examination, placing radiolucent pads under the trunk for support. The scapula should still lie at 90° to the IR. Although this will cause some magnification and have implications for scattered radiation exposure to the thyroid, eye lenses and female breasts, it is an acceptable alternative when a PA position is unsafe owing to the patient's condition.

Beam Direction and FRD

Horizontal at 90° to the IR
100 cm FRD

Centring Point

To the upper end of the palpable medial border of the scapula to pass through the glenohumeral joint

Collimation

Scapula, the head and proximal third of humerus, surrounding soft tissues

Criteria for Assessing Image Quality

- Scapula and the head and proximal third of humerus are demonstrated
- Superimposition of the medial and lateral borders of the scapula
- Body of scapula is projected clear of the thorax
- Glenoid process is seen en face with the humeral head superimposed over it (in the normal shoulder)
- Sharp image demonstrating the bony cortex and trabeculae of the scapula and upper shaft of humerus in contrast with the surrounding soft tissue

The above technique can also be used with a *caudal angle of 10–15°* from the horizontal in cases of *suspected impingement syndrome.* The acromiohumeral space will appear more open than the true lateral scapula to show abnormalities of this area. The projection is sometimes referred to as the 'shoulder outlet'.[25]

Common Errors: 'Y' View/True Lateral Shoulder

Common Error	Possible Reason	Potential Effects on PCE or Report
Scapula not cleared from the ribs and thorax; not seen in profile	Inaccurate obliquity of position; there is often a temptation to turn the patient more than is required, as the correct trunk position does appear to be close to a PA projection	Difficult to assess for any malalignment of the glenohumeral joint as not a perfect 'Y' Difficult for satisfaction of search and detection of subtle fractures of humeral head

Clavicle

PCE COMMENTS – CLAVICLE

Midshaft fracture is the most commonly encountered bony injury (approximately 69% of total clavicular fractures but 90% of all child clavicular fractures), followed in frequency by distal fractures at 28% and proximal fractures comprising the remainder.[42] These figures show how important it is *not* to focus on just the common fracture locations, since it would be easy to miss the small proportion of fractures at the proximal end.

Checks should be made regarding the acromioclavicular joints and sternoclavicular joints and note if there is any associated dislocation. Acromioclavicular joint dislocation may be associated with avulsion fracture of the coracoid process. If fracture is noted, also check for pneumothorax in case severe displacement of bony fragments has caused penetration of the thorax.

PCE comments should include: fracture location in the shaft, any angulation and displacement, overlap.[43]

POSTEROANTERIOR (PA) CLAVICLE (FIG. 5.21A,B)

This projection is the method of choice, as opposed to an AP projection, because the object is in closer contact with the IR, thereby reducing magnification and distortion of the clavicle. However, if the patient is injured or in a sling then positioning for the AP clavicle may be more readily achievable and more comfortable.

IR is vertical

Positioning

- The patient sits or stands erect with the anterior aspect of the shoulder under examination in contact with the IR
- The arm is made comfortable and may remain in a sling if presented this way
- The patient is rotated slightly, until the long axis of the clavicle is parallel to and closer to the IR
- The patient's head is turned away from the side under examination for radiation protection

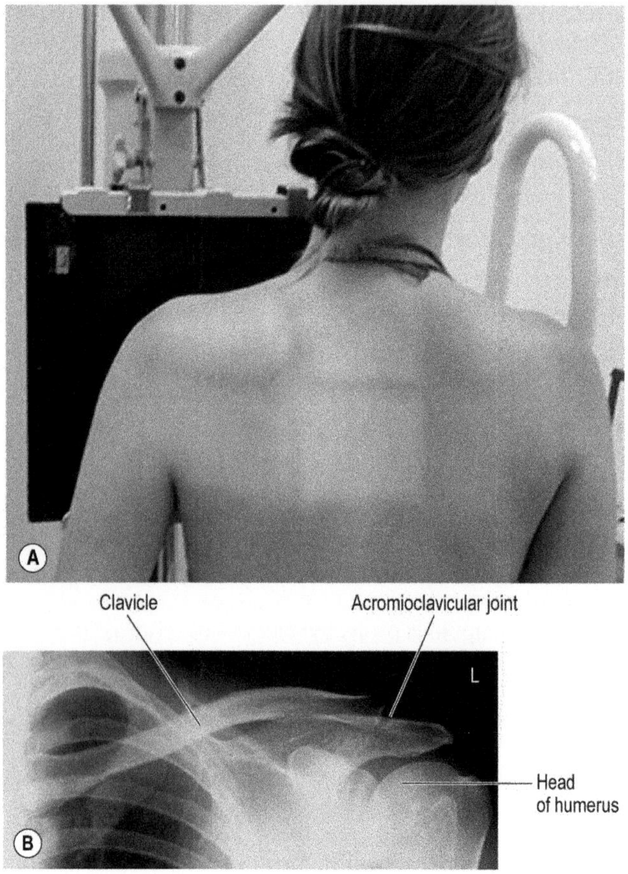

Fig. 5.21 PA clavicle.

Beam Direction and FRD

Horizontal at 90° to the IR
100 cm FRD

Centring Point

To the centre of the IR so that the central ray exits the mid shaft of the clavicle

Collimation

Clavicle, acromioclavicular joint, sternoclavicular joint

Criteria for Assessing Image Quality

See AP clavicle below.

ANTEROPOSTERIOR (AP) CLAVICLE (FIG. 5.22)

This can be undertaken if a patient's injuries prevent a PA approach.
IR is vertical

Positioning

- The patient sits or stands erect with the posterior aspect of the shoulder under examination in contact with the IR
- The arm is made comfortable and may remain in a sling if presented this way
- The patient stands with their MSP perpendicular to the IR or is rotated slightly towards the side under examination to bring the medial end of the clavicle away from the vertebral column
- The patient's head is turned away from the side under examination for radiation protection

Beam Direction and FRD

Horizontal at 90° to the IR
100 cm FRD

Centring Point

Over the mid point of the clavicle

Collimation

Clavicle, acromioclavicular joint, sternoclavicular joint

Criteria for Assessing Image Quality: AP and PA Projections

- Full length of the clavicle, including the acromioclavicular joints and sternoclavicular joints, is demonstrated
- No or minimal distortion along the length of the clavicle
- Acromioclavicular joint should be demonstrated
- Sharp image demonstrating the soft tissue margins, bony cortex and trabeculae of the clavicle. The clavicle should be demonstrated with even contrast along the length and without overexposing the medial and lateral ends

Common Errors: AP and PA Clavicle

Common Error	Possible Reason	Potential Effects on PCE or Report
High contrast on image which demonstrates the clavicle but the AC joint appears blackened	kVp insufficient to reduce the subject contrast	Soft tissues are difficult to be assessed for any swelling Bones can appear osteopenic when not and therefore subtle breaks in the cortex can be difficult to assess

INFEROSUPERIOR CLAVICLE

There are two methods described here to provide an inferosuperior projection of the clavicle. Method 1 is the easiest to achieve and is normally used to assess fracture union; method 2 can be used on the supine patient, e.g. when presented on a trolley, but only if a cassette-type IR is available. The AP projection is most frequently used alone, as fractures are rarely severely displaced; immobilisation with a sling is usually quite effective as treatment. Occasionally the clavicular fracture may be so displaced that the fragments do not unify, and these cases will almost certainly require an additional inferosuperior projection prior to a decision being made about surgical intervention to pin the bone.

Method 1 (Fig. 5.23A,B)

IR is vertical

Positioning

The patient is seated and then positioned as for the AP clavicle projection

The patient leans back by around 30°

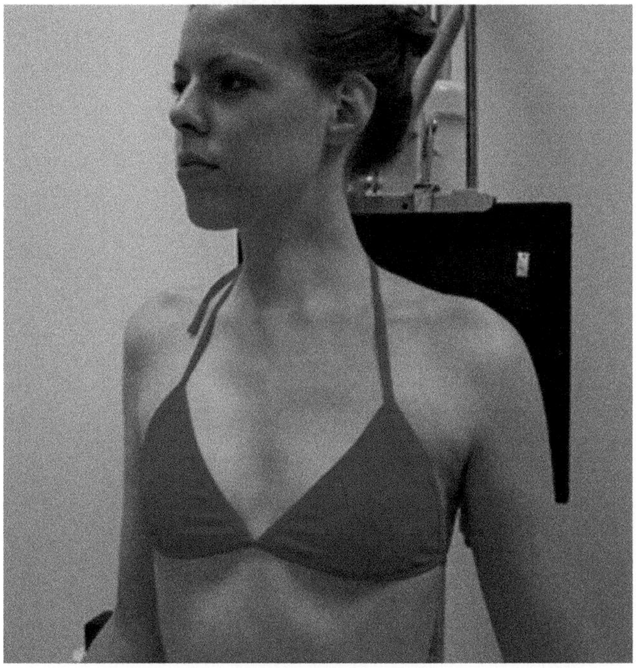

Fig. 5.22 AP clavicle.

Beam Direction and FRD

Initially horizontal, angled cranially 30–45°; the maximum angle achievable will be governed by equipment variables
100 cm FRD

Centring Point

Over the mid point of the clavicle

The image of the clavicle will be projected superiorly to the ribs and lung apices compared to the AP or PA clavicle (Fig. 5.23B), because of the cranial angle used. Therefore, the IR should be displaced cranially to compensate for this.

Collimation

Clavicle, acromioclavicular joint, sternoclavicular joint

Criteria for Assessing Image Quality

- The full length of the clavicle, including the acromioclavicular joint and the sternoclavicular joint, is demonstrated
- Clavicle is projected above the apex of the lung
- Acromioclavicular joint should be demonstrated
- Sharp image demonstrating the soft tissue, bony cortex and trabeculae of the clavicle. The clavicle should be demonstrated with even contrast along the length and without overexposing the medial and lateral ends

Method 2 (Fig. 5.24A)

IR is vertical

Positioning

- The patient lies supine with their arms resting at their side
- The IR is in contact with the superior aspect of the shoulder
- The head and neck are abducted for radiation protection of the eyes and thyroid

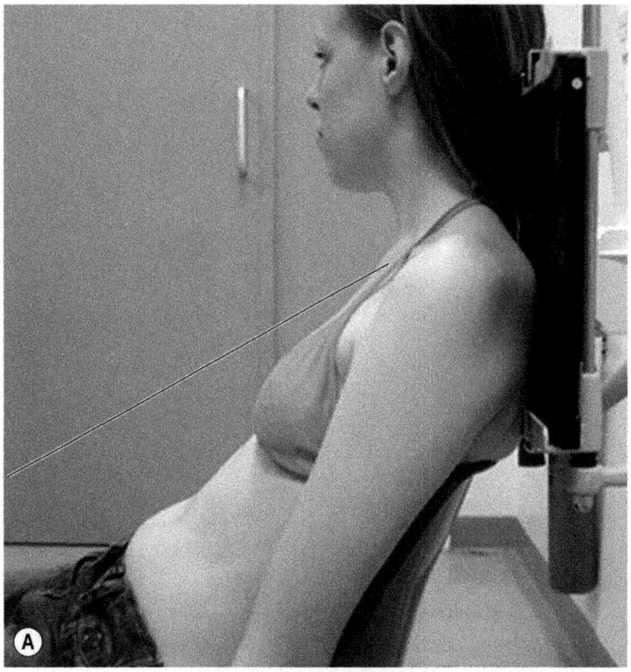

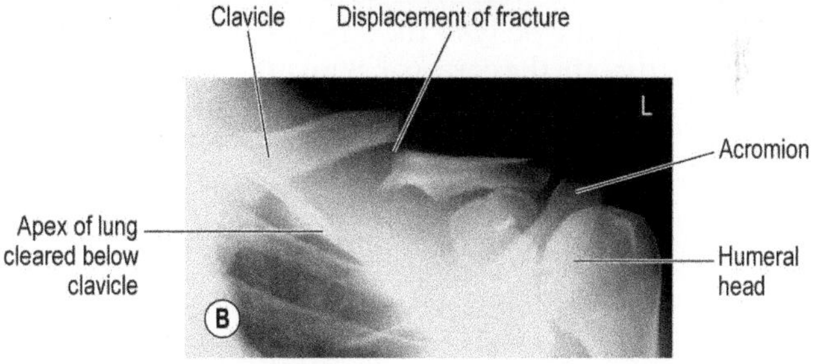

Fig. 5.23 (A) Inferosuperior clavicle – method 1; (B) inferosuperior clavicle.

Beam Direction and FRD

Initially vertical, angled at 45–60° towards the head, and 10–15° mediolaterally. *Again, the angle achieved will depend on equipment variables*
100 cm FRD

Centring Point

Over the mid point of the clavicle

For the supine inferosuperior projection, it is often not possible to position the X-ray tube low enough to achieve the required angulation (as is often the case with units that have large tube and light beam housing) and further modification may be necessary. The IR is placed in contact with the posterosuperior aspect of the shoulder and tilted backwards around 20° from vertical. The vertical central ray is then angled cranially until it is perpendicular to the IR, and an angle of approximately 10–15° mediolaterally away from the midline will clear the clavicle towards the centre of the IR. Centre over the middle of the clavicle (Fig. 5.24B).

Collimation

Clavicle, acromioclavicular joint, sternoclavicular joint

Criteria for Assessing Image Quality

- Full length of the clavicle, including the acromioclavicular joint and the sternoclavicular joint, is demonstrated

- Clavicle is projected above the apex of the lung
- Acromioclavicular joint should be demonstrated
- Tubercle of the clavicle is visible on its under-surface at the junction of the middle and lateral portions
- Medial end of the clavicle is slightly superior to the lateral end
- Sharp image demonstrating the soft tissue, bony cortex and trabeculae of the clavicle. The clavicle should be demonstrated with even contrast along the length and without overexposing the medial and lateral ends

Common Errors: Inferosuperior Clavicle

Common Errors	Possible Reasons	Potential Effects on PCE or Report
Clavicle not cleared from lung apices	Inadequate cranial angle used (both methods) *or* Patient not leaning back enough (method 1)	Overlying lung markings make assessment of the clavicle for subtle fractures/pathology difficult
Pale, soft tissue shadow overlying some or all of the area of interest	Thorax or abdomen lying in the path of the primary beam; this may be due to a large abdomen, large female breasts or too much angulation (method 1)	Difficult as: can be mistaken by soft tissue lesion/ pathology/swelling can make subtle breaks in the cortex difficult to visualise[33]

Scapula

PCE COMMENTS – SCAPULA

Injuries can be subtle – assess the full body of scapula in both AP and lateral.

Focussing on the body of the scapula only can result in missing fractures of the coracoid; Bankart lesions can be difficult to visualise (also see PCE comments for the shoulder).

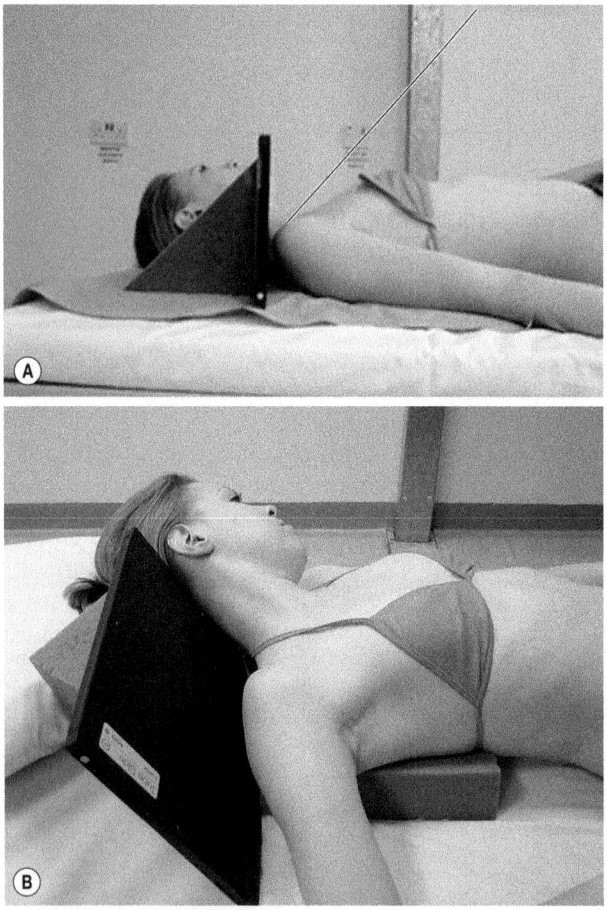

Fig. 5.24 (A) Inferosuperior clavicle – method 2; (B) alternative method for supine inferosuperior clavicle.

ANTEROPOSTERIOR (AP) SCAPULA (FIG. 5.25A,B)

IR is vertical

Positioning

- The patient sits or stands erect with the posterior aspect of the shoulder under examination in contact with the IR
- The arm is fully extended and slightly abducted with the palm of the hand facing forward to lie in the true anatomical position
- The patient is rotated approximately 20° towards the side under examination, to bring the scapula parallel to the IR
- The arm is flexed at the elbow and internally rotated, resting the dorsum of the hand on the patient's hip; this will move the scapula laterally away from the rib cage
- The patient's head is turned away from the side under examination for radiation protection

Beam Direction and FRD

Horizontal at 90° to the IR
100 cm FRD

Centring Point

To a point over the anterior chest (approximately 5 cm below the palpable coracoid process), to emerge over the mid-scapular area

Collimation

Scapula, the head and proximal third of humerus, the surrounding soft tissues

Criteria for Assessing Image Quality

- Head of humerus, the acromioclavicular joint and the superior and inferior angles of scapula are demonstrated
- Glenohumeral joint is obscured by the humeral head
- Scapula projected laterally, clearing as much of the rib cage from the medial border of the body as possible
- Acromion is demonstrated clear of the superior border of the humeral head
- Sharp image demonstrating the bony cortex and trabeculae of the scapula through the air-filled thorax. The bony detail of the scapula should be seen in contrast to the lungs, axilla and other soft tissue structures

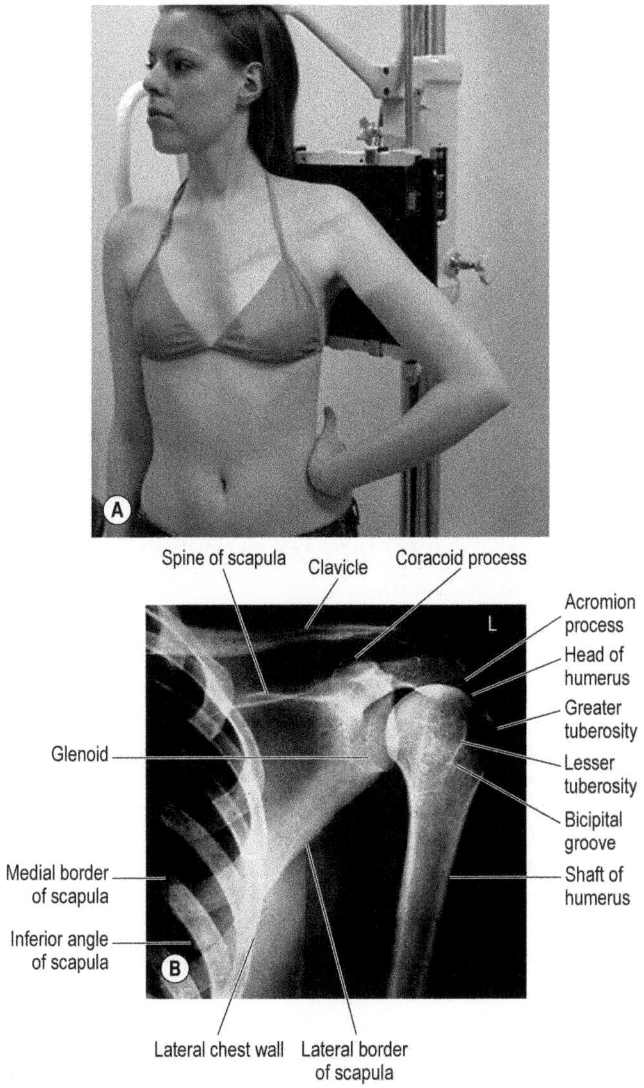

Fig. 5.25 AP scapula. (B, Reproduced with permission from Ballinger PW, Frank ED. *Merrill's Atlas of Radiographic Positioning and Radiologic Procedures*. 10th ed. St Louis: Mosby; 2003.)

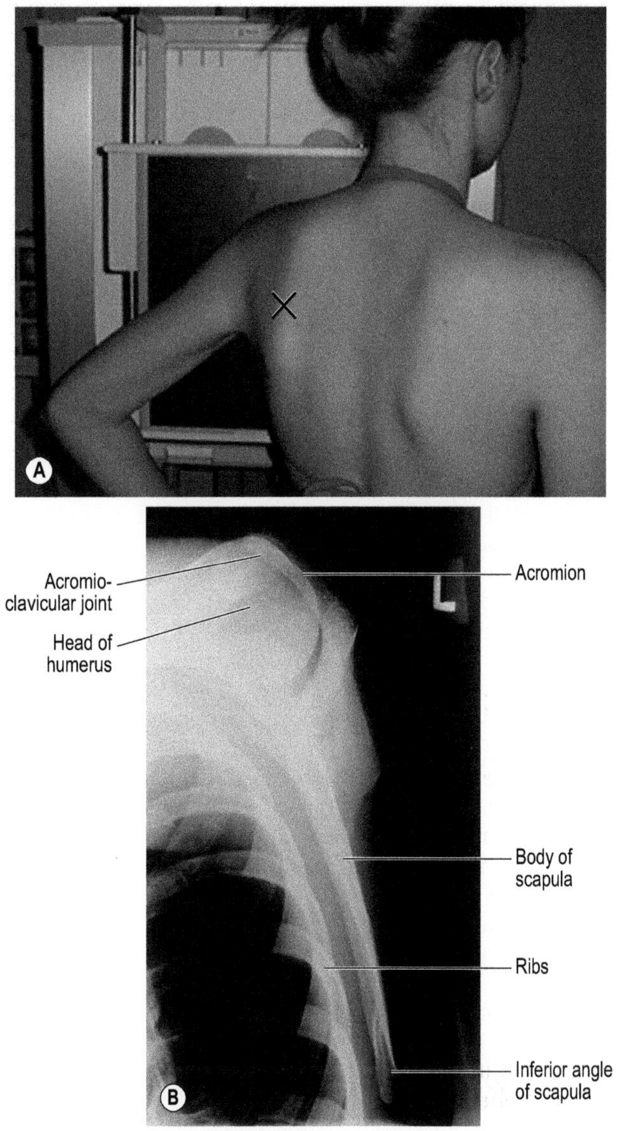

Fig. 5.26 Lateral scapula.

LATERAL SCAPULA (FIG. 5.26A,B)

IR is vertical

Positioning

- The patient stands or sits erect, facing the IR with their back to the X-ray tube
- From an initial PA position, rotate the patient approximately 25° to bring the side under examination closer to, and bring the body of the scapula 90° to, the IR
- The arm on the side under examination is flexed at the elbow, slightly abducted and the dorsum of the hand is placed on the hip; alternatively, the arm may rest across the chest with the hand resting on the shoulder of the opposite side (this may be more comfortable for the injured patient)
- The scapula is palpated to check the lateral and medial borders are superimposed

Beam Direction and FRD

Horizontal at 90° to the IR
100 cm FRD

Centring Point

To the middle of the palpable medial border of the scapula

Collimation

Scapula, the head and proximal third of humerus, the surrounding soft tissues

Criteria for Assessing Image Quality

- Scapula, the head and proximal third of humerus are demonstrated
- Superimposition of the medial and lateral borders of the scapula
- Shaft of humerus should not overlie the body of the scapula
- The body of the scapula is projected clear of the thorax
- Sharp image demonstrating the bony cortex and trabeculae of the scapula in contrast with the surrounding soft tissue

Common Errors: Lateral Scapula

Common Errors	Possible Reasons	Potential Effects on PCE or Report
Scapula not cleared from ribs and thorax; not seen in profile	Inaccurate obliquity of position; there is often a temptation to turn the patient more than is required, since the correct trunk position does appear to be close to a PA projection. Do not forget that the scapula will be moved into a position towards the lateral aspect of the thorax when the arm is placed in one of the required positions	Overlying bony or thorax outline can mimic fracture lines and can hide potential subtle fractures
Upper shaft of humerus superimposed over scapula	Arm not abducted *or* adducted sufficiently to clear the humerus from the body of scapula	Similar to above, the overlying humerus means that full evaluation of the scapula cannot be undertaken

Acromioclavicular Joints

These joints are normally examined to investigate subluxation of the joint following trauma. The radiographic examination should be requested following an orthopaedic assessment and not done routinely from Emergency Department referrals, as clinical examination of the joint by an experienced orthopaedic surgeon often proves to be diagnostically accurate, as severe disruption of the joint is palpable,[44] thereby rendering radiographic examination unnecessary. Weightbearing projections may be performed to assess the degree of subluxation, although initial shoulder radiographs should be examined first to exclude fracture, and because subluxation may be apparent without weights being given. However, research indicates that the weightbearing examination offers little in the diagnosis of subluxation[45–47] and therefore the technique is not described in this book. A fourth article[48] supports this research yet suggests a rather extensive series of radiographs for acromioclavicular joints, including:

- AP projection with arm in internal rotation
- AP with 10–15° cranial central ray (Zanca projection)[49]
- Axillary lateral (or lateral scapula or Wallace and Hellier projection if the axillary is unobtainable)

The full list of projections suggested by this article should not be routinely performed, particularly, as stated previously, as clinical examination frequently offers sufficient diagnostic information and the axillary lateral shoulder is only helpful when assessing a possible posterior dislocation. Comparative projections of both acromioclavicular joints should not be undertaken lightly, particularly in light of the requirements of the IR(ME)R 2017,[50] and this practice should be discouraged.

PCE COMMENTS – AC JOINTS

Sprains will likely show no anomaly radiographically. Comment on elevation of the clavicle superiorly away from the acromion. Detailed evaluation should be provided via a full imaging report rather than PCE.

Further information on appearances to suggest extent of ligament or tendinous injuries can be found in the Rockwood Classification.[51]

ANTEROPOSTERIOR (AP) ACROMIOCLAVICULAR JOINT (FIG. 5.27A,B)

IR is vertical

Positioning

- The patient sits or stands erect with the posterior aspect of the shoulder under examination in contact with the IR
- The arm is made comfortable and may remain in a sling if presented this way
- The patient is rotated approximately 10° towards the side under examination to bring the plane of the acromioclavicular joint perpendicular to the IR
- The patient's head is turned away from the side under examination for radiation protection

Beam Direction and FRD

Horizontal at 90° to the IR
100 cm FRD

Centring Point

Over the acromioclavicular joint

Collimation

Acromioclavicular joint, acromion process, surrounding soft tissues

Criteria for Assessing Image Quality

- Acromioclavicular joint, lateral end of the clavicle and soft tissue outlines are demonstrated
- If both joints are examined the images should be comparable in appearance
- Sharp image to demonstrate the bony trabeculae within the acromion and in contrast with the acromioclavicular joint and surrounding soft tissues

Common Errors: AP Acromioclavicular Joint

Common Error	Possible Reason	Potential Effects on PCE or Report
Dark image of joint with poor contrast between the joint and bones of the acromion and clavicle	Most obviously, exposure factors set too high but poor collimation will allow scatter to overblacken the image or reduce contrast	Due to overexposure the bones look osteopenic in appearance, masking subtle cortical abnormalities Acromion sometimes not visible at all, so any pathology is difficult to detect Soft tissues are also difficult to visualise

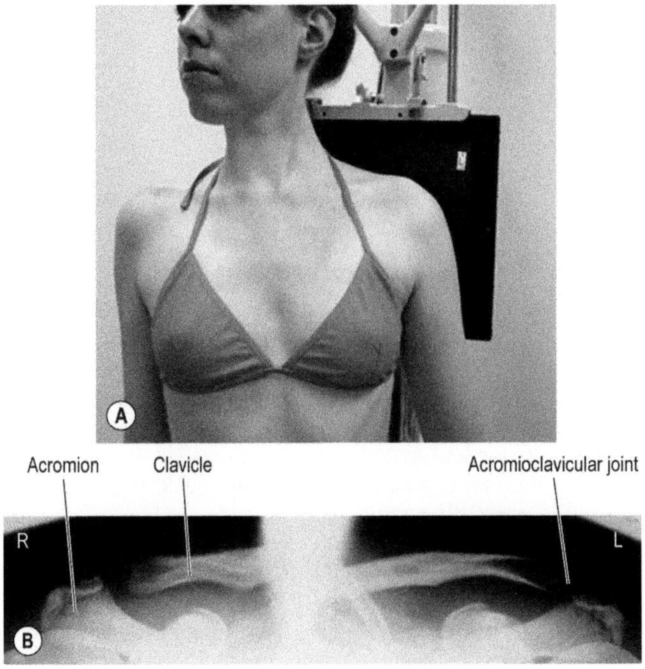

Fig. 5.27 AP acromioclavicular joint.

References

1. Goswami GK. Fat pad sign. *Radiology*. 2002;222:2. Available at: http://pubs.rsna.org/doi/full/10.1148/radiol.2222000365.
2. McQuillen-Martenson K. *Radiographic Image Analysis*. 5th ed. St Louis: Elsevier; 2019.
3. American Academy of Orthopedic Surgeons. *Elbow Fractures in Children*; 2019. Available at: https://orthoinfo.aaos.org/en/diseases-conditions/elbow-fractures-in-children/.
4. Elbow O. *Injuries in Children – Introduction*; 2011. Available at: http://www.orthoteers.org/(S(s2drpvwglit1rgx5x1p3qmsn))/mainpage.aspx?section=13&article=108.
5. American Academy of Orthopedic Surgeons. Radial head fractures of the elbow. 2014. https://orthoinfo.aaos.org/en/diseases--conditions/radial-head-fractures-of-the-elbow/.
6. Orthoteers. *Adult Elbow Injuries*; 2011. Available at: http://www.orthoteers.org/(S(s2drpvwglit1rgx5x1p3qmsn))/mainpage.aspx?section=13&article=107.
7. Bell JD, Jones J, et al. Radiocapitellar line. [online] Radiopedia. https://radiopaedia.org/articles/radiocapitellar-line?lang=gb (accessed 2017).
8. Knipe H, Jones J, et al. Anterior humeral line. [online] Radiopaedia. https://radiopaedia.org/articles/anterior-humeral-line?lang=gb (accessed 2017).
9. Scally P. *Medical Imaging*. Oxford: Oxford University Press; 1999.
10. Smithius R. *Elbow Fractures in Children*; 2008. https://radiologyassistant.nl/musculoskeletal/elbow-fractures-in-children.
11. Sheehan SE, et al. Traumatic elbow injuries: what the orthopedic surgeon wants to know. *Radiographics*. 2013;33:3. https://pubs.rsna.org/doi/10.1148/rg.333125176.
12. Nunn H. *The Elbow: Norwich Image Interpretation Course*; 2008. http://www.imageinterpretation.co.uk/elbow.php.
13. American Academy of Orthopedic Surgeons. *Radial Head Fractures for Elbow*; 2014. http://orthoinfo.aaos.org/topic.cfm?topic=A00073.
14. Lampignano JP, Kendrick LE. *Bontrager's Textbook of Radiographic Positioning and Related Anatomy*. 9th ed. St Louis: Elsevier Mosby; 2018.
15. Greenspan A, Norman A. The radial head capitellum view; a useful technique in elbow trauma. *Am J Radiol*. 1982;138:1186–1188.
16. Tomás FJ, Proubasta IR. Modified radial head-capitellum projection in elbow trauma. *Br J Radiol*. 1998;71:74–75.
17. Tomás FJ. Alternative radiographic projections of the ulnar coronoid process. *Br J Radiol*. 2001;74:756–758.
18. Clark KC. *Clark's Positioning in Radiography*. London: Heinemann; 1939.
19. Saraya S, El Bakry R. Ultrasound: can it replace MRI in the evaluation of rotator cuff tears? *Egypt. J Radiol Nucl Med*. 2016;47:1193–1201.
20. Tuite MJ, Small KM. Imaging evaluation of nonacute shoulder pain. *AJR Am J Roentgenol*. 2017;209:525–533.
21. Moroder P, Resch H, Schnaitmann S, et al. The importance of CT for the pre-operative surgical planning in recurrent anterior shoulder instability. *Arch Orthop Trauma Surg*. 2013;133(2):219–226.
22. Le Goff B, Berthelot JM, Guillot P, et al. Assessment of calcific tendonitis of rotator cuff by ultrasonography: comparison between symptomatic and asymptomatic shoulders. *Joint Bone Spine*. 2010;773:258–263.
23. Feeley B, Gallo RA, Craig EV. Cuff tear arthropathy: current trends in diagnosis and surgical management. *J Shoulder Elbow*. 2009;183:484–494.
24. American Academy of Orthopedic Surgeons. *Arthritis of Shoulder*; 2013. http://orthoinfo.aaos.org/topic.cfm?topic=a00222.
25. Long BW, Rafert JA. *Orthopedic Radiography*. Philadelphia: Saunders; 1995.
26. Mora Guix JM, Pédros JS, Castano Serrano A, et al. Updated classification system for proximal humeral fractures. *Clin Med Res*. 2009;7(1–2):32–44.
27. Raby N, Berman L, Lacey G. *Accident & Emergency Radiology: A Survival Guide*. 3rd ed. Philadelphia: Elsevier Saunders; 2014.
28. Sanders T, Jersey S. Conventional radiography of the shoulder. *Semin Roentgenol*. 2005;40(3):207–222.
29. Wilkinson K. Alternate trauma shoulder projection. *Radiol Technol J*. 2006;78:11–12.
30. Abrams R, Akbarnia H. *Shoulder Dislocations Overview*; 2019. StatPearls [Internet] https://www.ncbi.nlm.nih.gov/books/NBK459125/.
31. Schwartz D, Reisdorff E. *Emergency Radiology*. New York: McGraw–Hill; 2000.
32. Vear V. Routine projections for the trauma shoulder. *Radiographer J*. 1999;46:36–40.
33. Unett EM, Royle AJ. *Radiographic Techniques and Image Evaluation*. London: Nelson Thornes; 1997.
34. Ip D. *Orthopedic Traumatology: A Resident's Guide*. 2nd ed. Berlin: Springer; 2008.
35. Magee D. *Orthopedic Physical Assessment*. 5th ed. Philadelphia: Saunders; 2007.
36. Wilkie W. Back to basics: trauma shoulder. *Synergy J*. 2001;4:4–8.
37. Ianotti JP, Williams Jr GR. *Shoulder Diagnosis and Management*. 3rd ed. Philadelphia: Lippincott Williams & Wilkins; 2013.
38. Silfverskiold JP, Straehley DJ, Jones WW. Roentgenograph evaluation of suspected shoulder dislocation, a prospective study comparing the axillary and scapular Y view. *Orthopaedics*. 1990;13(1):63–69.
39. Wilson FC, Lin PP. *General Orthopedics*. New York: McGraw–Hill; 1997.
40. Grainger RG, Allison D. *Diagnostic Radiology*. 3rd ed. Edinburgh: Churchill Livingstone; 1997.
41. Edwards R, Jones H. Reporting on shoulder trauma. *Synergy J*. 2007;8:14–20.
42. Bentley TP, Journey JD. *Clavicle Fractures*; 2019. StatPearls [Internet] https://www.ncbi.nlm.nih.gov/books/NBK507892/.
43. Foster T, et al. Clavicular fracture. [online] Radiopaedia. https://radiopaedia.org/articles/clavicular-fracture?lang=gb.
44. Beim GM, Warner JJP. Clinical and radiographic evaluation of the acromioclavicular joint. *Operative Techn Sports Med*. 1997;5(2):65–71.
45. Varnarthos WJ, Ekman EF, Bohrer SP. Radiographic diagnosis of acromioclavicular joint separation without weight bearing, importance of internal rotation of the arm. *AJR Am J Roentgenol*. 1994;162:120–122.
46. Bossart PJ, Joyce SM, Manaster BJ, et al. Lack of efficacy of weighted radiographs in diagnosing acute acromioclavicular separation. *Ann Emerg Med*. 1998;17(1):20–24.
47. Yap JJL, Curl LA, Kvitne RS, et al. The value of weighted views of the acromioclavicular joint. *Am J Sports Med*. 1999;27(6):806–809.
48. Reeves PJ. Radiography of the acromioclavicular joint: a review. *Radiography*. 2003;9:1–4.
49. Zanca P. Shoulder pain: involvement of the acromioclavicular joint (analysis of 1000 cases). *AJR Am J Roentgenol*. 1971;112(3):493–506.
50. *The Ionising Radiation (Medical Exposure) Regulations*. UK Statutory Instrument 2017 No. 1322; 2017. [IR(ME)R]. https://www.legislation.gov.uk/uksi/2017/1322/contents/made.
51. Kiel J, Kaiser K. *Acromioclavicular Joint Injury*; 2020. StatPearls [Internet] https://www.ncbi.nlm.nih.gov/books/NBK493188/.

6 Foot, Toes, Ankle, Tibia and Fibula

SUZANNE MCLAUGHLAN, MARIA MANFREDI and LINDA WILLIAMS

Imaging of the foot and ankle requires removal of all artefacts, including socks, stockings and bandages. Extra care must be taken in cases of trauma and with those who have complications related to diabetes. Throughout this chapter a suggested FRD is given for each examination description; however, in practice a range of FRDs (typically from 100 cm to 120 cm) may be used, dependent on local protocol.

Foot and Toes

INDICATIONS

Examination of the foot for trauma should only be performed if there is true bony tenderness. The demonstration of a fracture in the toes rarely influences management, as the majority of phalangeal fractures are managed with immobilisation through buddy strapping.[1] Examination of the foot for hallux valgus is not indicated unless it is for preoperative assessment, in which case it must be performed weightbearing in order to assess the degree of valgus deformity.[2]

Other clinical indications for non-trauma imaging of the feet include: osteomyelitis, Charcot neuroathropathy, gangrene and arthropathies, including rheumatoid and osteoarthritis. It is important to differentiate between osteomyelitis and Charcot, as these conditions are associated with high morbidity rates and the therapeutic interventions vary considerably.[3] Whilst osteomyelitis is an infection of the bone, this can be located in any anatomical region, whilst Charcot neuropathy is typically an articular disease which is mainly located within the midfoot.[3]

March Fracture

March fractures, also known as fatigue or stress fractures, of the metatarsals are due to repetitive impact to this region[4]; it is common for some new periosteal bone formation to be demonstrated on the images, although this can often only become evident on plain film 2–3 weeks after injury.[5,6] Although stress fractures are most common in physically active people, underlying conditions, for example osteoporosis or other conditions that weaken the structure of the bones, may result in stress fractures during routine, everyday physical activity.[7]

Lisfranc Injuries

These are traumatic subluxations or dislocations at the base of the metatarsals at the tarsometatarsal (TMT) joints, with or without fracture. This injury may involve some or all of the joints. The mechanism of injury tends to involve rotational forces and can result from several events, such as the foot hitting the floor of a car in a road traffic accident, or missing a step or a kerb.[8,9]

A subtle cortical avulsion fracture can also occur at the Lisfranc ligament, resulting in a small 'fleck' sign; this site should be carefully evaluated.[9]

Jones' Fracture

This is a transverse fracture of the proximal third of the fifth metatarsal, usually as a result of an inversion injury to the foot, the same mechanism that causes an ankle sprain.[1]

PCE COMMENTS – FOOT

When undertaking the preliminary clinical evaluation, it is recommended to quickly assess the bony cortex, to ensure congruity and assess for any undisplaced fractures, cortical or osteochondral defects (see Fig. 6.8) or periosteal reactions that may be evident and then to assess the overlying soft tissues.

Hind Foot

It is recommended to closely inspect the anterior horn of the calcaneum on any oblique or lateral foot/ankle images, as it is not uncommon for fractures to be seen here during an inversion injury, but it is commonly missed in practice. Measuring Bohler's angle can assist with identifying fractures of the calcaneum (see Fig. 6.15), where the angle between the two lines (measured posteriorly) should be 30° or greater.

Review for avascular necrosis (Köhlers 'disease') in the navicular, with appearances of fragmentation and sclerosis.

Midfoot

Traumatic dislocations and subluxations should be carefully assessed through a review the alignment of the bones. Injury to the Lisfranc joint can be demonstrated by loss of the normal alignment at the base of the metatarsal. Review the image for bone fragments from the bases of the medial four metatarsals. If these are present, a tarsometatarsal subluxation should be suspected.[10]

Base of the Fifth Metatarsal

Remember the apophysis lies parallel to the metatarsal and it may appear displaced or even multifragmented. The base of the fifth metatarsal is a common site for an avulsion fracture at the insertion of the peroneus brevis tendon.[10]

Stress Fractures (March Fractures)

Stress fractures may be visualised in the metatarsal shafts, most commonly the second and third. Look for periostitis, especially in the diaphysis of the metatarsals.

DORSIPLANTAR (DP) FOOT (FIG. 6.1A,B)

For all projections of the foot and toes, the IR is horizontal (table-top) unless otherwise specified.

In both the dorsiplantar (DP) and DP oblique (DPO) positions, to enable the joint spaces between the tarsal bones to be demonstrated more clearly, a cranial angle may be used. The degree of the height of the medial arch of the foot will determine the angle required, which is typically between 10 and 15°.[11,12]

When using this projection the tarsometatarsal articulations are demonstrated without as much bony overlap as when a perpendicular central ray is used. The same image can be produced by using a 15° foam wedge directly under the foot, the thickest end being placed at the toe end; this removes the necessity for of the central ray directly towards the gonads. However, the image of the metatarsals and phalanges will be magnified if used in this way, as the object receptor distance will vary along the length of the foot. An alternative is to position the pad under the IR, which does remove the problem of magnification.

Exposure for a foot requires the toes and the tarsal bones to be demonstrated on the one image and a suitable kVp should be selected, which is high enough to reduce subject contrast without over-penetrating the thinner end of the area. The use of a slim wedge filter, the thickest part of the filter being placed at the toes, will have the effect of reducing subject contrast. The wedge can be used under the foot, but some magnification of the metatarsals and phalanges will occur in a similar way to that mentioned above.

Positioning – Non-weightbearing

- The patient is seated on the table with their legs extended and their hands are used to support themselves
- The patient's knee on the side under examination is flexed and the plantar aspect of the foot is placed in contact with the IR
- The opposite leg is abducted

Positioning – Weightbearing

- The IR is positioned on the floor, the patient places the affected foot on the IR putting their weight evenly through both feet

Beam Direction and FRD

- Vertical central ray, at 90° to the IR or a 10–15° cranial angle may be used
- 100 cm FRD

Centring Point

Over the base of the second metatarsal

Collimation

All phalanges, metatarsals, tarsals, soft tissues

Criteria for Assessing Image Quality

- Demonstration of the phalanges, metatarsals, navicular, cuboid and cuneiform bones and soft tissue shadowing of the outline of the foot
- Adjacent phalanges should be demonstrated separately with exception of the bases of metatarsals 2–5, which will be slightly overlapped. Toes of patients with toe deformities are unlikely to all be separated

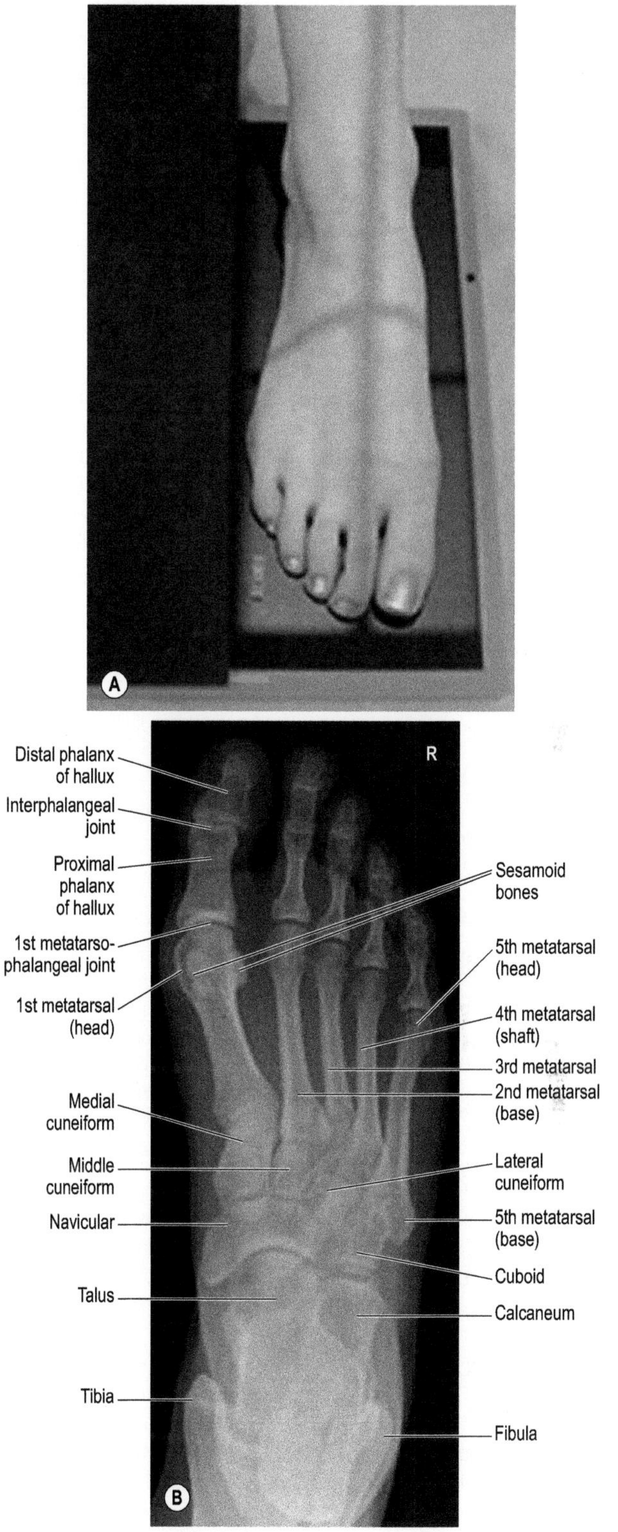

Fig. 6.1 DP foot.

- Shafts of the metatarsals separated
- Tarsal bones should appear overlapped
- Talus and calcaneum should be superimposed over the tibia and fibula
- Sharp image demonstrating the soft tissue margins, bony cortex and trabeculae of the phalanges, metatarsals and tarsus. The proximal calcaneum and talus will not be penetrated sufficiently to be demonstrated

Common Errors: DP Foot

Common Errors	Possible Reasons	Potential Effects on PCE or Report
Superimposition of the lower leg over the tarsal bones	Knee may be too flexed, encouraging too much ankle flexion	If tarsal bones are not clearly identified, subtle injury may not be excluded
TMT and navicular cuneiform joint spaces are not open	Knee is not flexed adequately; flex knee until foot is at a 90° angle to the lower leg or as close as possible	Lisfranc injury or subtle fracture may be missed if joints not clearly visualised

DORSIPLANTAR OBLIQUE (DPO) FOOT (FIG. 6.2A,B)

Positioning

- The plantar aspect of the foot is placed in contact with the IR
- From the DP position the patient's foot is internally rotated to bring the plane of the dorsum of the foot parallel to the IR
- A radiolucent 45° sponge pad is placed under the lateral plantar aspect of the foot for immobilisation
- The opposite leg is abducted

Beam Direction and FRD

Vertical central ray, at 90° to the IR or with a 10–15° cranial angle
100 cm FRD

Centring Point

Over the base of the third metatarsal

Collimation

All phalanges, metatarsals and tarsal bones, surrounding soft tissues

Criteria for Assessing Image Quality

- Demonstration of the phalanges, metatarsals, navicular, cuboid and cuneiform bones, the calcaneum and soft tissue shadowing of the outline of the foot
- Adjacent phalanges are not likely to all be separated, due to obliquity, especially in the case of patients with toe deformities (i.e. 'hammer toe')
- Shafts of metatarsals 2–4 separated
- Overlap of the bases of the first and second metatarsals
- Separation of the tarsal bones, although the medial and middle cuneiforms will appear superimposed, with some overlap of middle and lateral cuneiforms
- Talus and calcaneum are clear of the tibia and fibula
- Sharp image demonstrating the soft tissue margins of the foot, bony cortex and trabeculae of the phalanges, metatarsals and tarsus

Common Errors: DPO Foot

Common Errors	Possible Reasons	Potential Effects on PCE or Report
Superimposition of the lower leg over the tarsal bones	Knee may be too flexed, or the foot may be under-rotated	If tarsal bones are not clearly identified, subtle injury may not be excluded
Overlapping of metatarsals Longitudinal running foot joint, cuneiform-cuboid, navicular-cuboid and the 2nd–5th intermetatarsal joint spaces are closed	Over-rotation of foot	Lisfranc injury or subtle fracture may be missed if joints not clearly visualised
4th metatarsal tubercle is demonstrated without superimposition of the 5th metatarsal tubercle	Under-rotation of foot	Subtle fractures may be missed

Fractures to look out for that may commonly be missed are at the anterior horn of the calcaneum.

LATERAL FOOT (FIG. 6.3A,B)

Positioning

- With the leg extended, it is externally rotated until the lateral aspect of the foot is in contact with the IR and the patella is parallel to the table-top. This may be more comfortable if the knee is slightly relaxed and not fully extended. The plantar aspect of the foot is 90° to the IR
- Radiolucent foam pads may be placed under the lower leg and foot for support in this position

Beam Direction and FRD

Vertical central ray at 90° to the IR, however, a 10–15° cranial angle may be required to obtain superimposition of the talar dome
100 cm FRD

Centring Point

Over the navicular cuneiform region

Collimation

All phalanges, metatarsals, tarsals, soft tissues

WEIGHTBEARING LATERAL FOOT (FIG. 6.4A,B)

This projection is usually performed as part of an orthopaedic assessment. It is important to include the whole length of foot on the image, as the relationship between the joints of the tarsal bones and the metatarsals is an important indication of the degree of surgical intervention required following trauma, hallux valgus deformity or in the case of severe arthropathy. This is particularly important in Lisfranc injuries, where fracture dislocations are

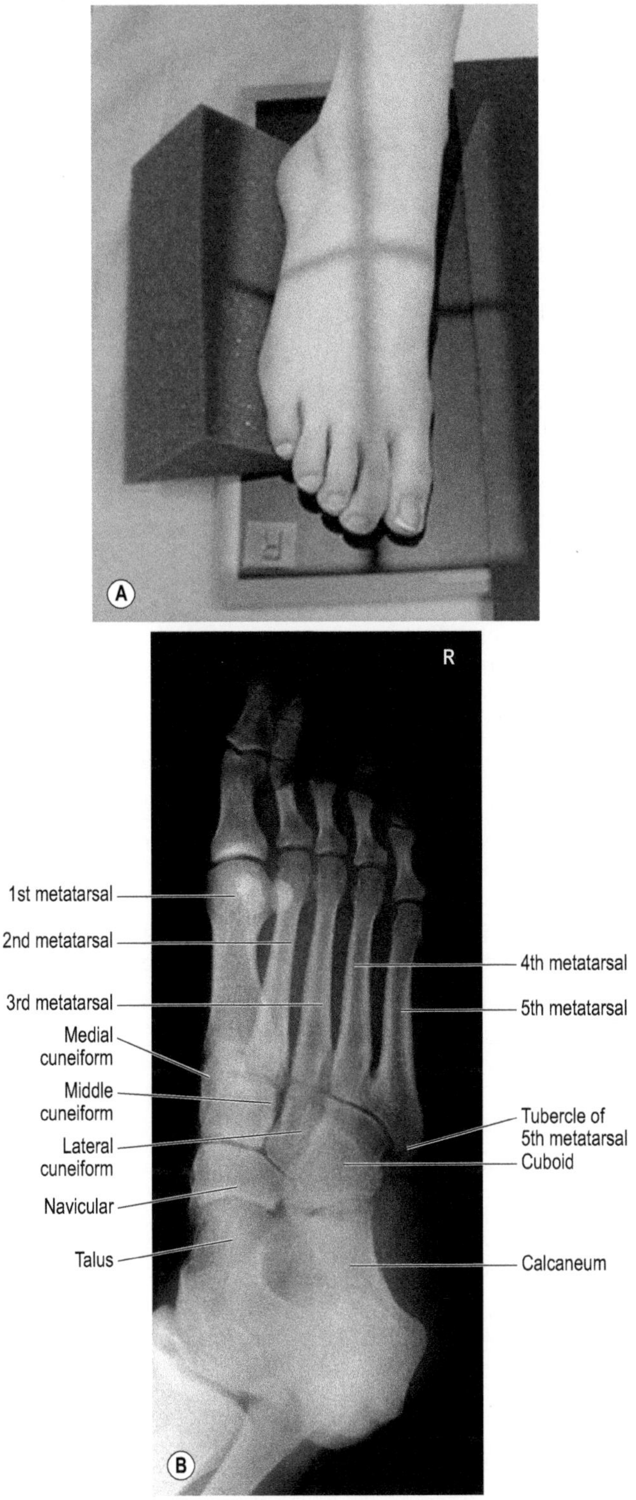

Fig. 6.2 DPO foot.

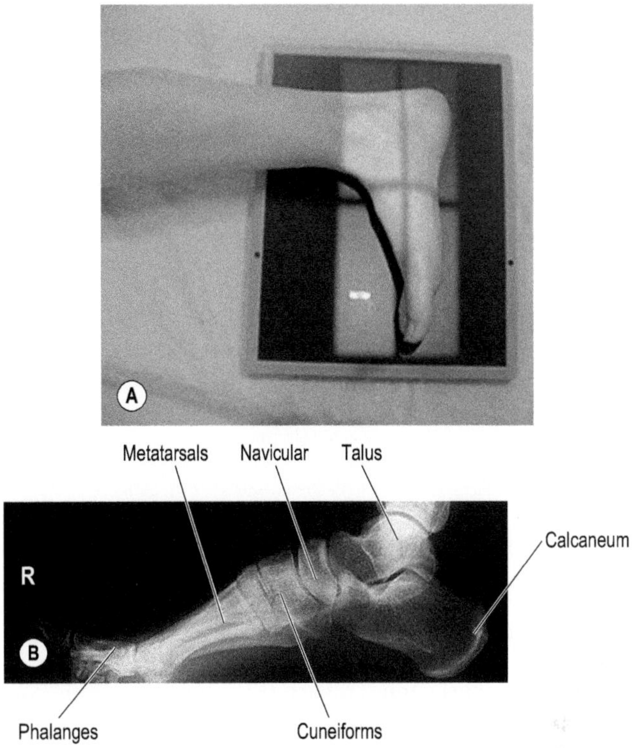

Fig. 6.3 Lateral foot.

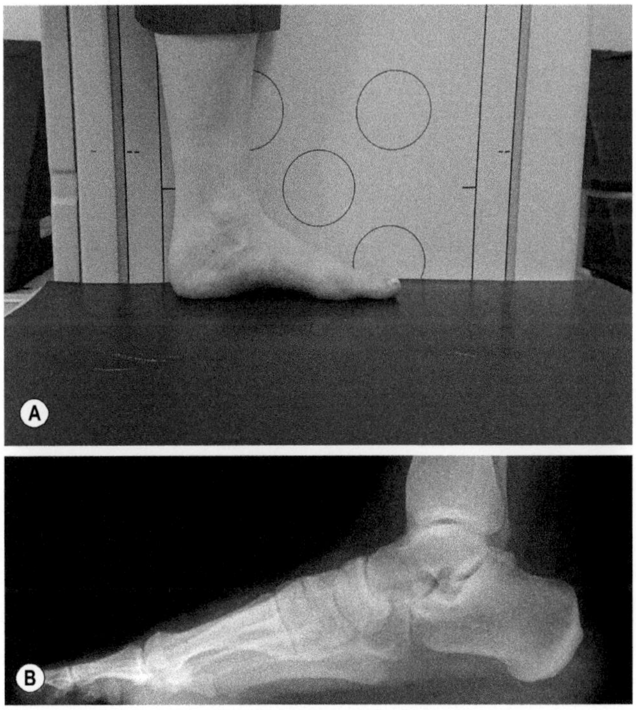

Fig. 6.4 Weightbearing lateral foot.

involved and a complete radiographic evaluation of the foot is required.[9]

A suitably designed platform or a stable step with handles for patient support is required for good radiography of this area. The platform or step should be made of radiolucent material that can be positioned against an erect IR or have a groove in the centre for positioning a flat plate IR vertically and to allow the IR to be placed at a level below the soft tissues of the plantar aspect of the foot to enable the soft tissues to be included on the image. The platform should be of a dimension to allow both feet to be placed comfortably on either side of the groove (Fig. 6.5) or for

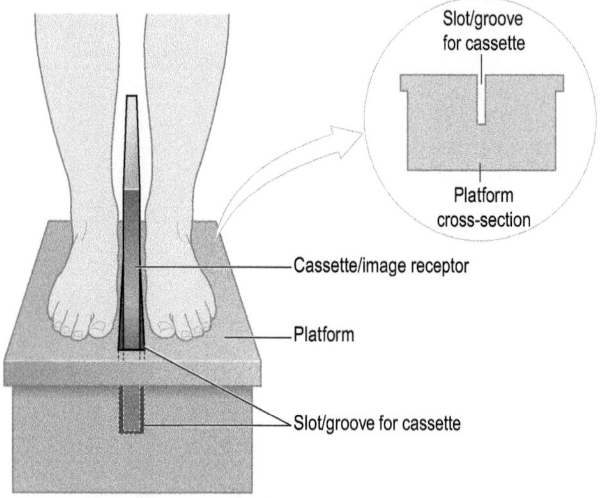

Fig. 6.5 Platform used for weightbearing lateral foot.

one foot to be positioned out of the primary beam. Most frequently, these platforms are made as a bespoke design in hospital workshops, rather than obtained from commercial sources.

The IR is placed vertical, in the groove of the support. This technique is only suitable when using a cassette/flat plate type IR.

Positioning

- Stand the patient on the specially designed platform
- Ensure the patient is stable and suitable support is provided to allow even distribution of the weight of both feet
- Support the IR in the erect, transverse position in the groove of the platform on the medial aspect of the foot
- Use a sheet of lead or lead rubber between the back of the IR and the foot that is not under examination for radiation protection
- The long axis of the foot should be parallel to the long axis of the IR

Collimation

The phalanges, metatarsals, tarsal bones, surrounding soft tissues

Beam Direction and FRD

Horizontal central ray, at 90° to the IR
100 cm FRD

Centring Point

Over the tubercle of the fifth metatarsal

Criteria for Assessing Image Quality

- Demonstration of the phalanges, metatarsals, navicular, cuboid, cuneiform bones, calcaneum and soft tissue shadowing of the outline of the foot
- Demonstration of the tibio-talar joint
- Superimposition of the talar dome
- Phalanges should be superimposed; the distal phalanges of the longest toe (hallux or second toe) will lie clear
- Metatarsals should be overlapped, with the first metatarsal lying most superiorly and the fifth inferiorly
- Sharp image demonstrating the superimposition of the phalanges and metatarsals and the bony trabeculae of the tarsal bones, navicular, talus and calcaneum

Toes

DP AND DPO TOES

In the case of trauma, guidelines discourage the imaging of the second to fifth toe, as patient management is not affected unless there is a clinical suspicion of an intra-articular fracture or dislocation. However, imaging of the toes is still considered in cases of localised infection (osteomyelitis) or in patients with diabetes where Charcot neuroarthropathy is suspected.

Positioning – DP

- The patient is seated on the table with their legs extended and their hands are used to support themselves
- The patient's knee on the side under examination is flexed and the plantar aspect of the toes is placed in contact with the IR
- The opposite leg is abducted

Positioning – DPO

- The plantar aspect of the foot is placed in contact with the IR
- From the DP position the patient's foot is internally rotated by approximately 40–45° to bring the plane of the dorsum of the foot parallel to the IR
- A radiolucent 45° sponge pad is placed under the lateral plantar aspect of the foot for immobilisation
- The opposite leg is abducted

Beam Direction and FRD

Vertical central ray, at 90° to the IR
100 cm FRD

Centring Point

To the metatarsophalangeal joint of the toe under examination to include the adjacent toe

Criteria for Assessing Image Quality

- All the phalanges and the distal half of the metatarsals should be included
- Symmetry of the phalangeal condyles
- Joint spaces of the interphalangeal joint spaces are demonstrated clearly. Separation of the toe or toes from the adjacent toes. Neither of these may be possible with patients with toe deformity
- Sharp image demonstrating the soft tissue margins of the toe/toes, bony cortex and trabeculae of the phalange/s

DP GREAT TOE/HALLUX (FIG. 6.6A,B)

Positioning

- The patient is seated on the table with their legs extended and their hands are used to support themselves
- The patient's knee on the side under examination is flexed and the plantar aspect of the toes is placed in contact with the IR
- The opposite leg is abducted

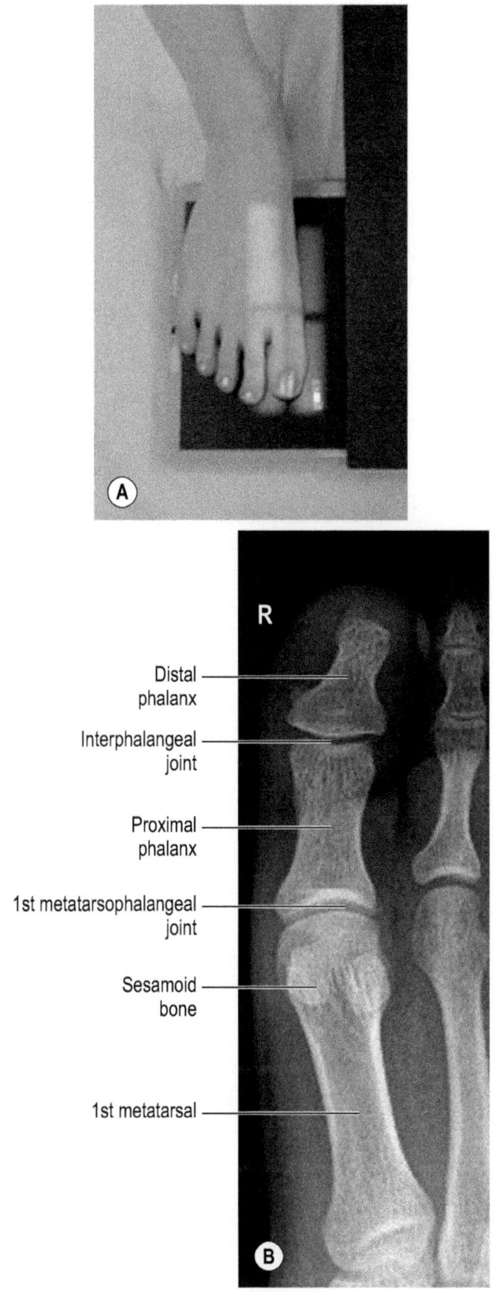

Fig. 6.6 DP individual toe – hallux.

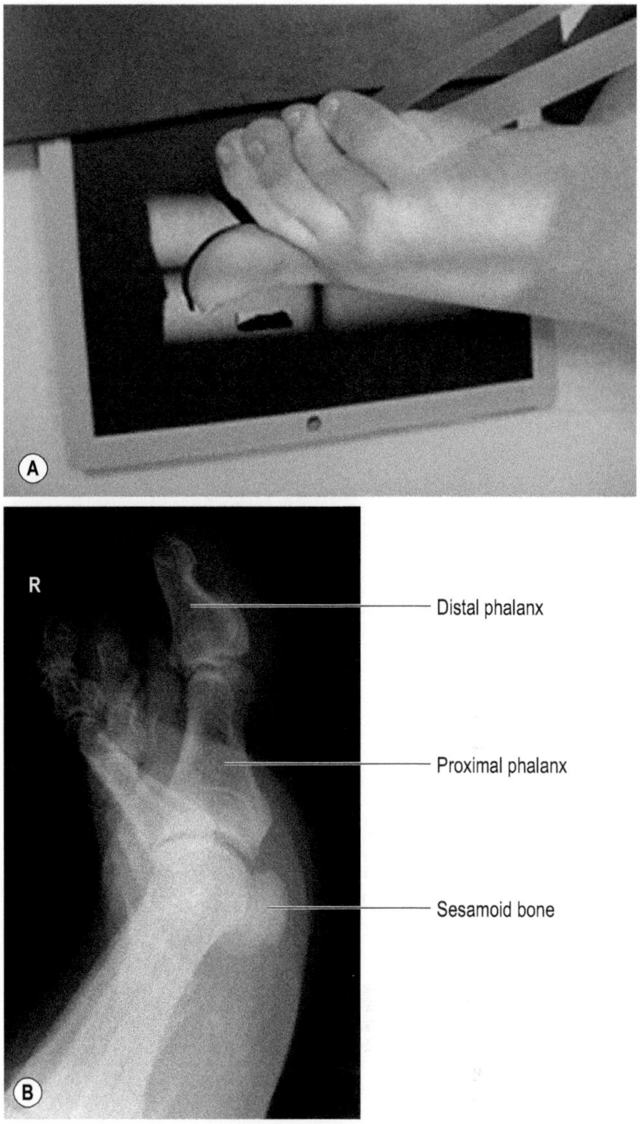

Fig. 6.7 Lateral hallux

Beam Direction and FRD

Vertical central ray, at 90° to the IR
100 cm FRD

Centring Point

To the great toe metatarsophalangeal joint (Fig. 6.6A)

Collimation

Distal half of metatarsal and phalanx of the relevant and also the adjacent toe

Criteria for Assessing Image Quality

- All the phalanges and the distal half of the metatarsals should be included
- Symmetry of the phalangeal condyles
- Joint spaces of the interphalangeal joint spaces are demonstrated clearly. Separation of the toe or toes from the adjacent toes. Neither of these may be possible with patients with toe deformity
- Sharp image demonstrating the soft tissue margins of the toe/toes, bony cortex and trabeculae of the phalange/s

LATERAL GREAT TOE/HALLUX (FIG. 6.7A,B)

Positioning

- The patient is seated on the table with their legs extended and their hands used to support themselves
- The plantar aspect of the toes are placed on the IR
- From the DP position the patient's leg is internally rotated so that the medial aspect comes in contact with the table
- The patient is asked to assist with use of a radiolucent band to pull the toes that are not being examined away from the toe under examination in either (1) a plantar direction (Fig. 6.7A) or (2) a dorsal direction (Fig. 6.7B), depending on the patient and how their

toes flex most easily. Bandages and gauze should be avoided as they can cause image artifacts when using digital imaging technologies. In the instance where a patient is unable to extend the great toe, the central ray may be angled proximally towards the calcaneus until it is perpendicular to the joint space of interest. This will cause magnification and distortion but may, however, give pertinent information in a trauma situation

- The opposite leg is abducted

Beam Direction and FRD

Vertical central ray, at 90° to the IR
100 cm FRD

Centring Point

To the metatarsal phalangeal joint

Collimation

Distal half of metatarsal and phalanges of the relevant toe

Criteria for Assessing Image Quality

- Relevant phalanges and the metatarsophalangeal joint demonstrated on the image
- Clear interphalangeal and metatarsophalangeal joints demonstrated, with the phalangeal condyles superimposed
- Sharp image demonstrating the soft tissue margins of the toe and the bony cortex and trabeculae of the phalanges

Common Errors: Toes

Common Errors	Possible Reasons	Potential Effects on PCE or Report
Poor joint spaces with non-superimposition of the phalangeal condyles	Long axis of the toe may not lie parallel to the IR, or the leg may not be rotated sufficiently medially	Subtle fractures at the plantar aspects of the phalangeal bases may be missed Early indicators of infective processes may be missed
Bony and/or soft tissue overlap	Utilisation of immobilisation to separate the structures, or utilise the method described using an oblique central ray	Subtle fractures at the plantar aspects of the phalangeal bases may be missed Early indicators of infective processes may be missed Displacement of fractures or degree of dislocation at the joints may be obscured

Ankle

Most ankle fractures involve one or both malleoli, and occasionally may include the third, posterior malleolus. However, osteochondral defects (Fig. 6.8) are also a common injury due to the mechanism of injury.[13] The particular fracture(s) and ligamentous damage is determined by the direction of the applied force.[11] A forced inversion injury, for example, may cause an avulsion fracture of the lateral malleolus.

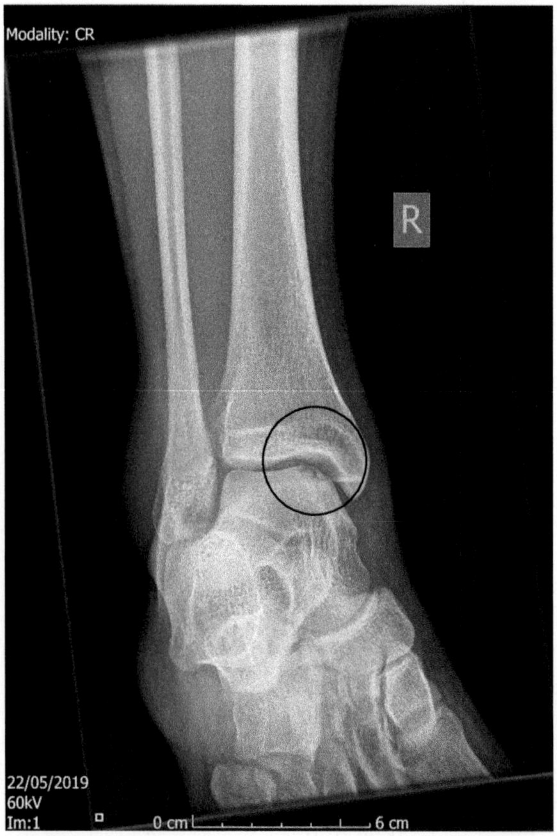

Fig. 6.8 Osteochondral defect.

Many injuries will be ligamentous, but will still require medical intervention. Indications of a ligament injury on a radiograph include widening at the fibula notch (interosseous membrane), soft tissue swelling at the medial and lateral malleoli which may result in the elevation of the anterior pre-talar fat pad or obliteration of the pre-Achilles triangle. This is not necessarily indicative of fracture and only indicates a joint effusion.[14] Figure 6.9 demonstrates soft tissue signs in the ankle.

Fractured ankles can be complex and many attempts have been made to classify them according to the degree of injury. There is also an increasing element of dislocation with each degree of fracture. Pott's fractures are one such method of classification; there are others available such as Webber. For the purposes of this chapter, the Potts classification system is outlined below:

Pott's Classifications

Abduction, External Rotation Type

Pott's I	A fracture of the lateral malleolus of the fibula
Pott's II	The fibular fracture, with also a transverse fracture of the medial malleolus and lateral subluxation of the talus
Pott's III	In addition to the fibular fracture, the posterior part of the medial malleolus is displaced upwards and the talus subluxed backwards

The above descriptions of the Pott's classifications are those most commonly found, but several more classifications are described for the more unusual adduction injury.

Adduction Type

Pott's I	Vertical fracture of the medial malleolus
Pott's II	The fractured medial malleolus is accompanied by a transverse fracture of the lateral malleolus and medial subluxation of the talus
Pott's III	The talus is dislocated backwards. There is a fracture of the posterior part of the medial malleolus and a transverse fracture of the lateral malleolus

Ankle Trauma in Children and Adolescents

It is much more likely for a child to suffer from an epiphyseal injury than a fracture or ligament tear because the ligaments in children are stronger than the physis.[15] The distal tibial epiphysis is only second to the radius in the number of bony injuries occurring in children over the entire skeleton. Salter–Harris classifications are used to describe these injuries; these are explained in the introductory section for skeletal radiography in Chapter 3.

The ankle joint may be examined for demonstration of the joint alone but is often examined for suspected fracture, and therefore the image usually requires inclusion of the lower third of tibia and fibula. If an isolated medial malleolus fracture is demonstrated on an ankle X-ray and the patient has bony tenderness over the head of the fibula then it may be necessary to undertake supplementary knee or tibia/fibula projections to rule out proximal fractures within the bony ring,[16] also known as a Maisonneuve fracture.

PCE COMMENTS – ANKLE

There are various soft tissue signs (see Fig. 6.9) that can be seen even when a fracture is not obvious, such as a joint effusion within the ankle joint, marked overlying soft tissue swelling or air trapped within the subcutaneous tissues, indicative of an open injury which may later be susceptible to infection.

In foot and ankle inversion injuries, pay attention to the malleoli as well as the base of fifth metatarsal, as these injuries can be seen in unison or separately. The talus should also be carefully reviewed in inversion injuries. These can result in impaction fractures, which are more commonly seen on the medial or lateral aspect of the talar dome. These may present as an irregularity of the cortex or a bone fragment.[10]

Be mindful of accessory ossicles in the ankle and don't diagnose these as a fracture.

The ankle forms part of a ring structure with the tibia, fibula and talus. If there is one fracture in the ring, it is important to look for a second. This may require further imaging of the proximal tibia and fibula to exclude a Maisonneuve fracture, which involves a medial malleolar fracture, medial collateral ligament rupture and a proximal fibular fracture along with distal tibiofibular syndesmosis disruption.[17]

In the absence of an ankle fracture, significant soft tissue swelling should be noted; this can be indicative of ligamentous injury, which may require clinical follow-up.

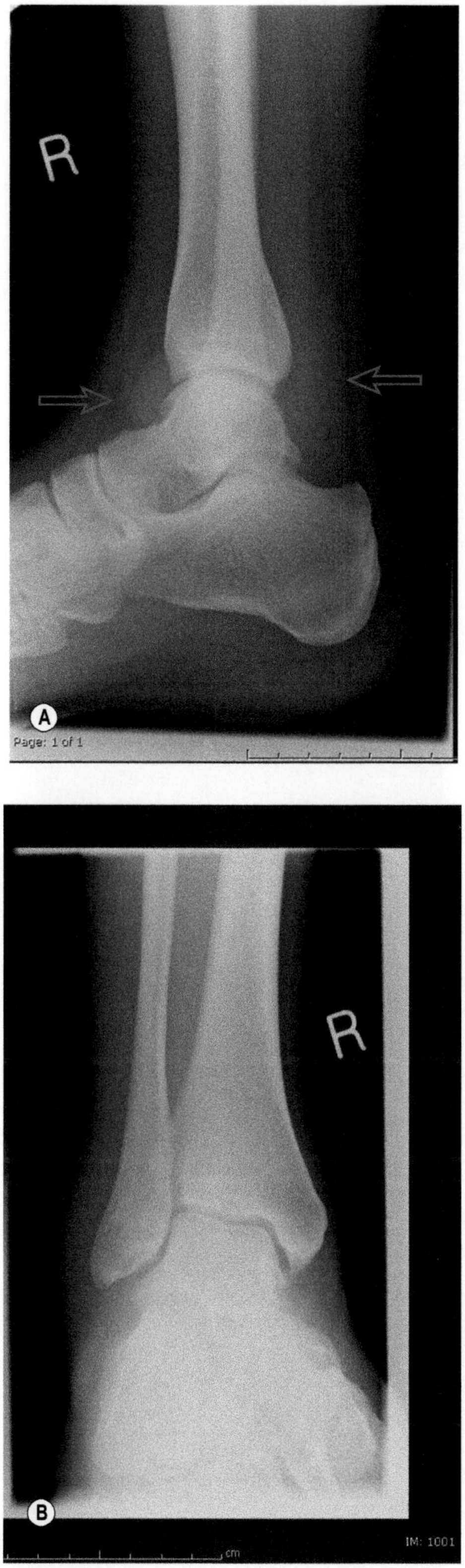

Fig. 6.9 Soft tissue signs in the ankle

ANTEROPOSTERIOR (AP) ANKLE (FIG. 6.10A,B)

The AP ankle is described in this book with the malleoli being equidistant from the IR. When the ankle is positioned in this way the distal tibia will be superimposed over the fibula and the distal tibiofibular joint will be obscured. The lateral aspect of the mortice, i.e. the

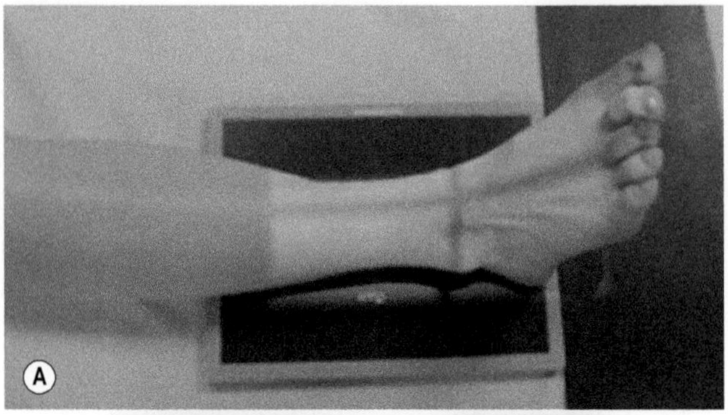

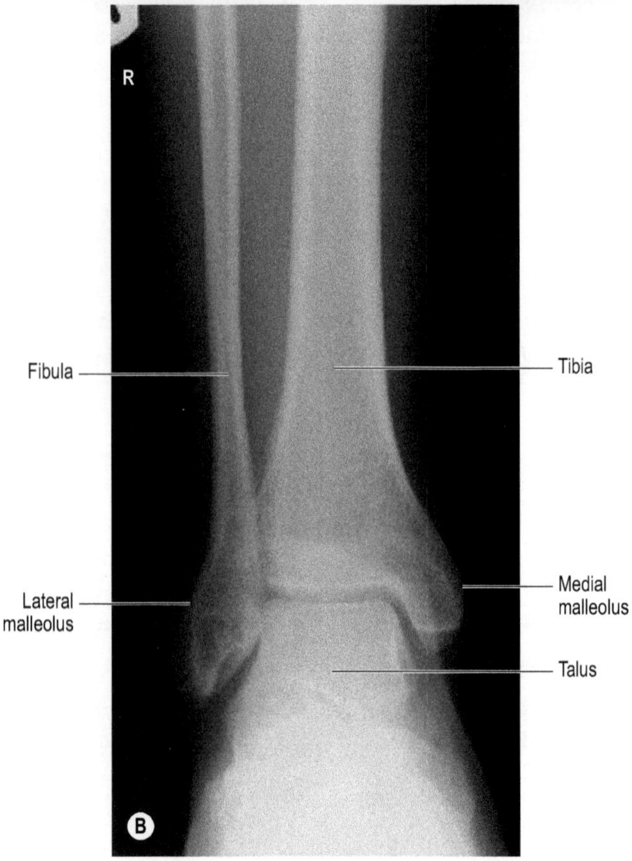

Fig. 6.10 AP ankle.

fibiotalar joint, will be demonstrated ('mortice' refers to the appearance of the joint space around the upper talus, in the AP ankle projection, as it fits between the distal tibia and both malleoli; this is likened to the mortice joint used in carpentry). Some texts[18,19] describe this position as an oblique ankle and suggest that, for the true AP, the intermalleoli line forms an angle of approximately 15–20° with the IR (with the lateral malleolus being closer to the IR than the medial malleolus). However, this positioning will obscure the most distal portion of the lateral mortice and demonstration of the distal fibula will be incomplete. Other texts[12,20,21] agree that, as described in this book, the malleoli should be equidistant from the IR and, as such, the mortice view, which is the routine projection, is commonly referred to as an AP.

Positioning

- The patient is seated on the table with their legs extended
- The leg under examination is adducted away from the opposite leg to offer protection from the main beam
- The posterior aspect of the lower leg is placed in contact with the IR
- The ankle joint is flexed to 90° (this is achieved by asking the patient to pull their toes towards their knee)
- The ankle is internally rotated to bring the medial and lateral malleoli equidistant from the IR

Beam Direction and FRD

- Vertical central ray, at 90° to the IR
- 100 cm FRD

Centring Point

Midway between the malleoli

Collimation

Lower third of tibia and fibula, ankle joint, lateral and medial malleoli, talus, surrounding soft tissues

Criteria for Assessing Image Quality

- Demonstration of the lower third of tibia and fibula, lateral and medial malleoli with soft tissue outlines
- Tibiotalar joint is well demonstrated, with equal space surrounding the superior aspect of the talus
- Talus and its articulation with the malleoli should be clearly demonstrated and free of superimposition
- Distal tibiofibular joint will be obscured
- Sharp image demonstrating the soft tissue margins, bony cortex and trabeculae of the distal tibia and fibula with the cortical margins of the superior aspect of the talus demonstrated

Common Errors: AP Ankle

Common Errors	Possible Reasons	Potential Effects on PCE or Report
Joint space not demonstrated between the talus and fibula	The leg is not sufficiently internally rotated; make sure the malleoli are equidistant from the table-top	Assessment for subtle avulsion fractures of the lateral malleolus or of the lateral aspect of the talar dome will not be possible
The tibiotalar joint is not clearly demonstrated	There is insufficient dorsiflexion of the foot	Assessment for subtle avulsion fractures of the medial malleolus will not be possible
Tibia superimposes less than half of the fibula	Too much internal rotation	The joint space between the lateral malleolus and the talus will not be visualised

LATERAL ANKLE (FIG. 6.11A,B)

To most easily achieve the best position for a lateral ankle, ask the patient to keep their leg extended and dorsiflexed at the ankle, and then roll over onto the side under examination; however, to ensure a true lateral, there should be a small degree of internal rotation, to allow for the superimposition of the malleoli. A common problem when performing the lateral ankle projection is that the patient tends to invert the foot, and it is difficult to rectify this once in the lateral position.

Positioning

- From the AP position the leg is externally rotated onto the side under examination until the malleoli are superimposed vertically
- The foot is dorsiflexed to bring the foot and tibia into an angle of 90°
- A small 15° foam pad can be placed under the lateral border of the forefoot to support the patient in this position, as the lateral aspect of the forefoot will not be in contact with the table-top when the malleoli are superimposed

Beam Direction and FRD

Vertical central ray at 90° to the IR, a 10–15° cranial angle may be required to support superimposition of the talar dome
100 cm FRD

Centring Point

Over the medial malleolus

Collimation

Lower third of tibia and fibula, talus, calcaneum, navicular, base of the fifth metatarsal, surrounding soft tissues

Criteria for Assessing Image Quality

- Lower third of tibia and fibula, talus, calcaneum, navicular, base of fifth metatarsal and the surrounding soft tissues are demonstrated
- Talar dome is superimposed to give a clear joint space
- Extreme distal aspect of the fibula is superimposed centrally over the distal tibia, although the shaft becomes more posterior proximally
- Single line representing superior articulatory surface of the talus, with clear tibiotalar joint space
- Sharp image demonstrating the soft tissue, bony cortex and trabeculae of tibia, fibula and talus

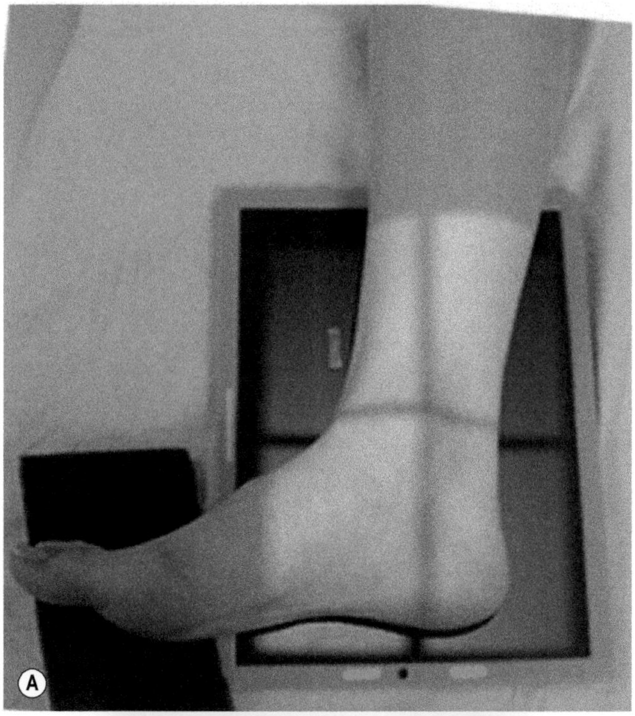

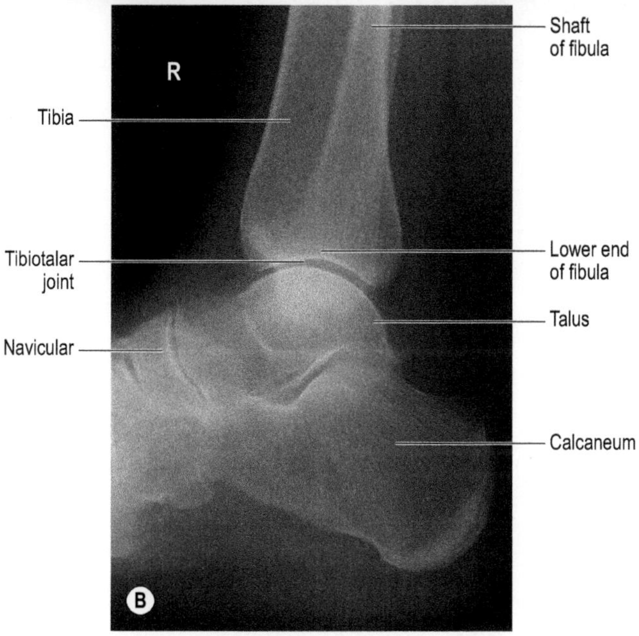

Fig. 6.11 Lateral ankle.

Common Errors: Lateral Ankle

Common Errors	Possible Reasons	Potential Effects on PCE or Report
Distal fibula projected posterior to the tibia	The leg is over-rotated laterally; make sure the malleoli are superimposed, using a small 15° wedge pad may assist with the correct positioning	Degree of displacement of fractures may be obscured
Shaft of the fibula projected over the tibia	The leg is under-rotated	Degree of displacement of fractures may be obscured
Loss of joint space and/or double edge to line representing superior articulatory surface of talus	Over- or under-rotation of the leg and/or inversion of the foot; poor flexion of the ankle	Subtle osteochondral defects may not be clearly visualised
Base of 5th metatarsal not included within the area of interest	Collimation too tight	Base 5th metatarsal fracture, which occurs from the same mechanism of injury, may be missed

ANKLE OBLIQUES

Obliques can be performed to further clarify or demonstrate any disruption to the joint, or to help in diagnosing a fractured malleolus. (a) Lateral/external and (b) medial/internal obliques with 45° rotation are usually required. In order to assess the distal tibiofibular joint, distal fibula, talus and its articulation with the lateral malleolus and tibia, the medial oblique has a reduced rotation of 30° (c). As previously described in the AP ankle section, the routine 'AP' projection is the mortice view, and as such is technically an oblique image.

It must be mentioned, however, that magnetic resonance imaging (MRI) is viewed by some as the method of choice when provision of a visual account of the biomechanics of the ankle joint is required due to its sensitivity when looking at soft tissue injuries, although it is noted that some imaging centres advocate ultrasound as the imaging method of choice.[22]

Positioning

(a) 45° Lateral/External Oblique (Fig. 6.12A,B)
- From the AP position the ankle is rotated 45° externally and a radiolucent foam pad is used to support the ankle in this position

(b) 45° Medial/Internal Oblique (Fig. 6.13A,B)
- From the AP position the ankle is rotated 45° internally and a radiolucent foam pad is used to support the ankle in this position

(c) 30° Medial/Internal Oblique (Fig. 6.14A,B)
- From the AP position the ankle is rotated 30° internally and a radiolucent foam pad is used to support the ankle in this position

Beam Direction and FRD

Vertical central ray at 90° to the IR, although a 15° cranial angle will clear the distal fibula more efficiently
100 cm FRD

Centring Point

For all projections, midway between the malleoli

Collimation

Medial and lateral malleoli, distal tibia and fibula, talus, surrounding soft tissues

Criteria for Assessing Image Quality

(a) 45° external rotation: The malleoli should be superimposed on the talus. The lower end of fibula should be obscured by the anterior aspect of the distal tibia
(b) 45° internal rotation: The lateral malleolus, lateral aspect of mortice and distal tibiofibular articulation should be well demonstrated. The medial aspect of the mortice will appear closed
(c) 30° internal rotation projection: The tibiotalar joint should be well visualised and the medial and lateral aspects of the mortice should be open. The medial and lateral malleoli should be well demonstrated

Subtalar Joint/Talocalcaneal Joints

The following projections are described here for completeness; however, it is now unusual to find them requested, as

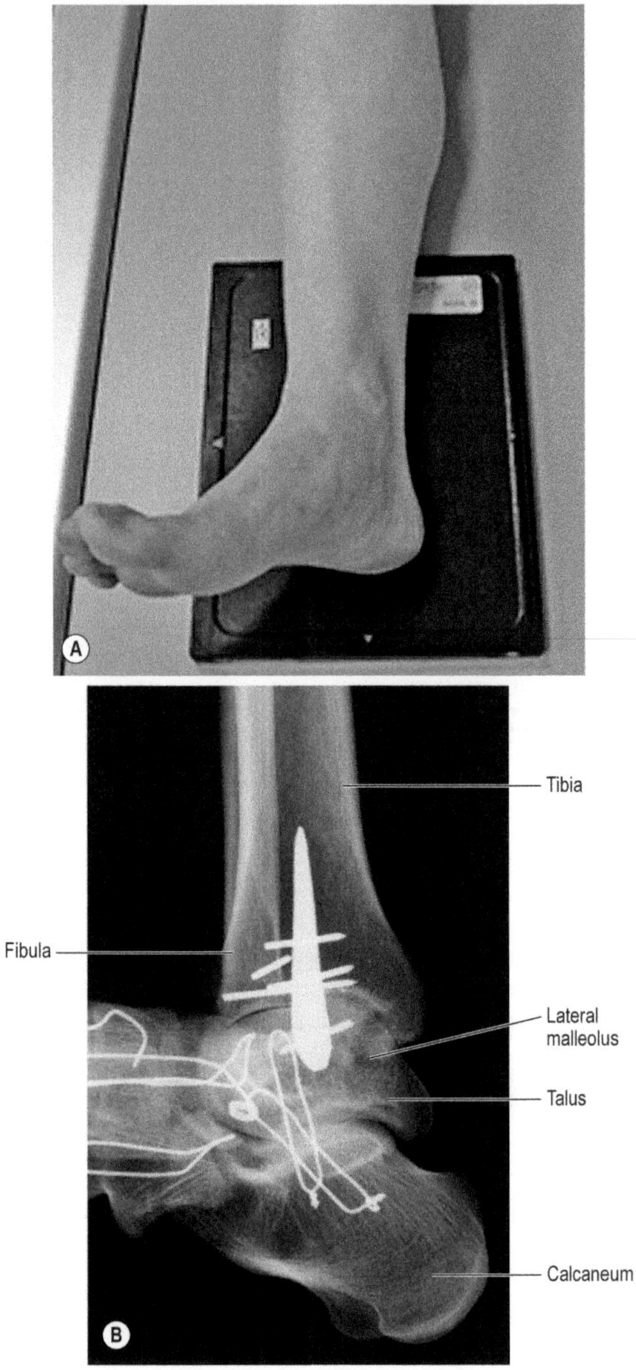

Fig. 6.12 45° external oblique ankle.

MRI will provide high contrast sensitivity and has multiplanar capabilities. It therefore facilitates superior demonstration of these articular surfaces.

MEDIAL OBLIQUE SUBTALAR JOINT

Positioning

As for 45° medial oblique (Fig. 6.13A)

Beam Direction and FRD

(1) *40° cranial angle* to show the anterior portion of the posterior talocalcaneal articulation

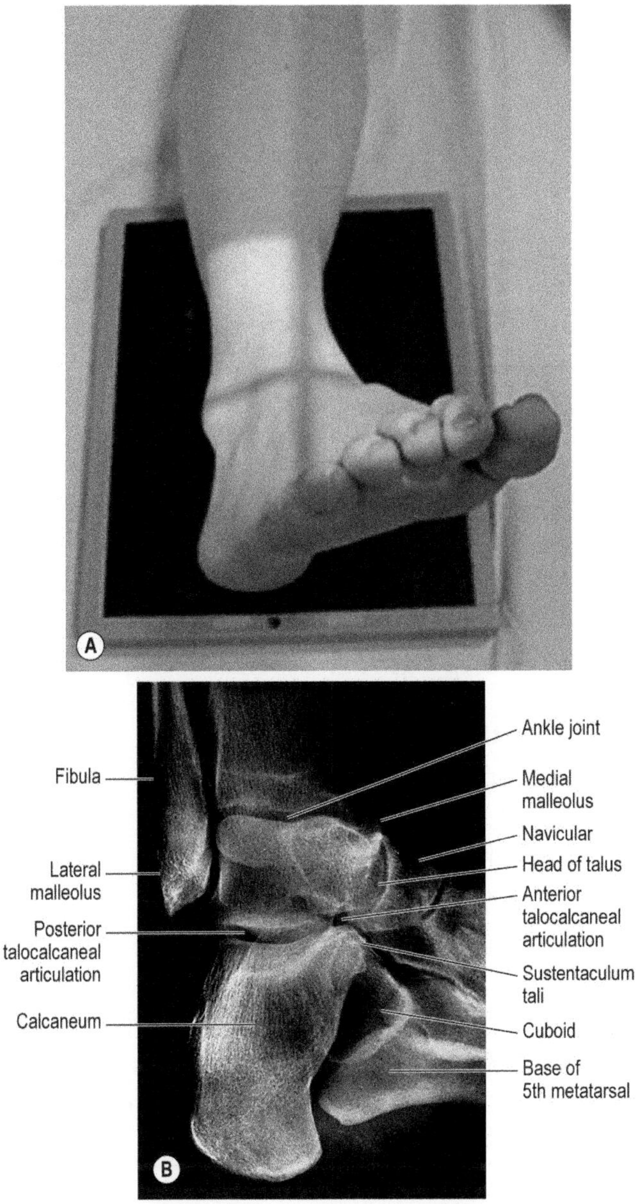

Fig. 6.13 **45° internal oblique ankle.** (B, Reproduced with permission from Bryan GJ. *Skeletal Anatomy*. 3rd ed. Edinburgh: Churchill Livingstone; 1996.)

(2) *30° cranial angle* to show the articulation between the talus and sustentaculum
(3) *10° cranial angle* to show the posterior portion of the posterior talocalcaneal articulation
100 cm FRD

Centring Point

All angulations – to a point beneath the lateral malleolus

Collimation

Distal end of the tibia and fibula, calcaneum, tarsal bones

Criteria for Assessing Image Quality

- Distal end of tibia and fibula, calcaneum and tarsal bones are demonstrated

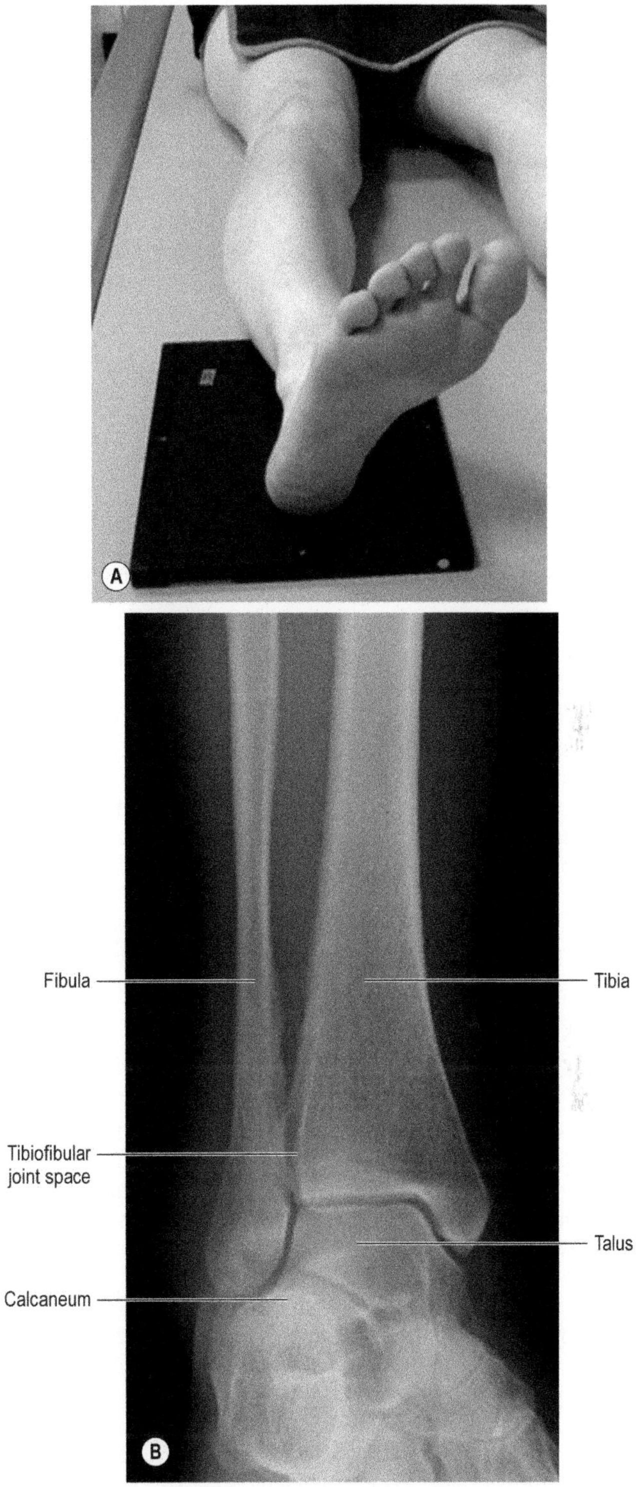

Fig. 6.14 30° internal oblique ankle.

(1) should demonstrate the anterior part of the posterior talocalcaneal articulation
(2) should demonstrate the articulation between the talus and sustenaculum
(3) should demonstrate the posterior part of the posterior talocalcaneal articulation. The sinus tarsi should be demonstrated as open on this projection

- Sharp image with adequate penetration to demonstrate the subtalar joint with visualisation of the bony cortex and trabeculae of the talus in contrast to the surrounding soft tissue margins

LATERAL OBLIQUE SUBTALAR JOINT

This demonstrates the posterior subtalar joint and will also confirm a fracture involving the joint surface[23] and disclose DP compression.

Positioning

- As for 45° external oblique projection (Fig. 6.12A)

Beam Direction and FRD

15° cranial angle
100 cm FRD

Centring Point

To a point just below and anterior to the medial malleolus

Collimation

Distal end of tibia and fibula, calcaneum, tarsal bones

Criteria for Assessing Image Quality

- Distal end of tibia and fibula, calcaneum and tarsal bones are demonstrated
- Posterior subtalar joint should be well demonstrated, with the middle and anterior subtalar joint obscured by the inferior aspects of the talar neck and head
- Sharp image with adequate penetration to demonstrate the posterior subtalar joint with visualisation of the bony cortex and trabeculae of the talus in contrast to the surrounding soft tissue margins

Calcaneum

The calcaneum is often examined when a patient presents after falling feet-first from height, but fractures of this area can result from a twisting injury. Some fractures will only become apparent when the Bohler's angle[16] is assessed; this angle is normally found to be between 30° and 40° and is reduced to below 30° when a fracture is present (Fig. 6.15). CT is useful for assessing the extent and involvement of fragments in the fractured calcaneum.

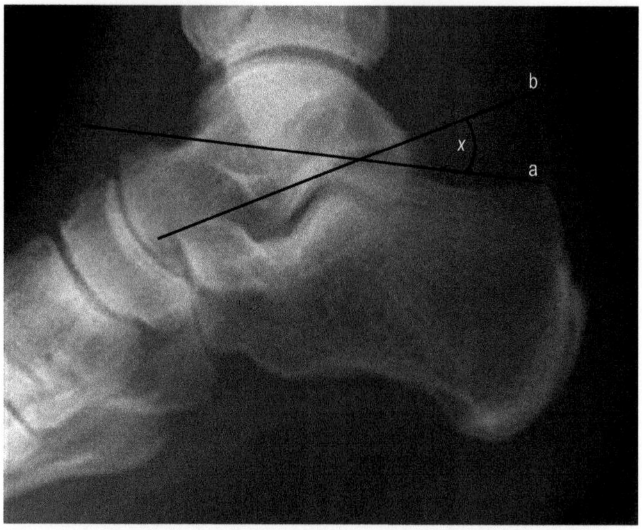

Fig. 6.15 Bohler's angle. Bohler's angle is assessed by drawing two intersecting lines (*a*) from the highest point on the posterior aspect of the calcaneum to its highest midpoint and (*b*) from the highest midpoint to the highest anterior point. The lines are extended here to demonstrate the angle more accurately. If the angle *x* is less than 30° this suggests a calcaneal fracture with compression.

LATERAL CALCANEUM (FIG. 6.16A,B)

Assessment of calcaneal spur is no longer routinely undertaken and therefore is not justified. However, it is still considered routine practice to perform imaging for plantar fasciitis and calcific tendonitis, which may both be associated with a calcaneal spur.[24]

Positioning

- The patient is seated on the table, and the ankle of the side under examination is rotated externally
- The lateral aspect of the foot is brought into contact with the IR
- The ankle is dorsiflexed to 90° and the rotation of the leg adjusted until the malleoli are superimposed

Beam Direction and FRD

Vertical central ray, at 90° to the IR
100 cm FRD

Centring Point

To the middle of the calcaneum below the medial malleolus

Collimation

Calcaneum, ankle joint, navicular, surrounding soft tissues

Criteria for Assessing Image Quality

- Calcaneum, talocalcaneal and cubocalcaneal joints and soft tissue outlines are demonstrated
- Distal fibula should be superimposed over the tibial malleolus
- Sharp image demonstrating the soft tissue margins, bony cortex and trabeculae of the calcaneum

AXIAL CALCANEUM

This projection can be achieved by several methods. It is commonly described with the patient seated on the table and the central ray directed 40° cranially towards the extended leg (method 4), but this has the X-ray beam directed towards the trunk and should be used only if the other methods described cannot be achieved due to the patient's condition.

Method 1 is easily achieved by the ambulant patient and methods 2 and 3 can be achieved in the less ambulant patient and most trolley patients. Methods 1–3 position the long axis of the calcaneum parallel to the IR, producing an image with minimal distortion. Method 4 positions the long axis of the calcaneum at 90° to the IR and produces maximum distortion to the image. All four techniques can be used to examine both calcanei simultaneously, with the X-ray beam centred between the heels, at the levels stated for the individual calcaneum. This will cause a degree of image distortion but will reduce the

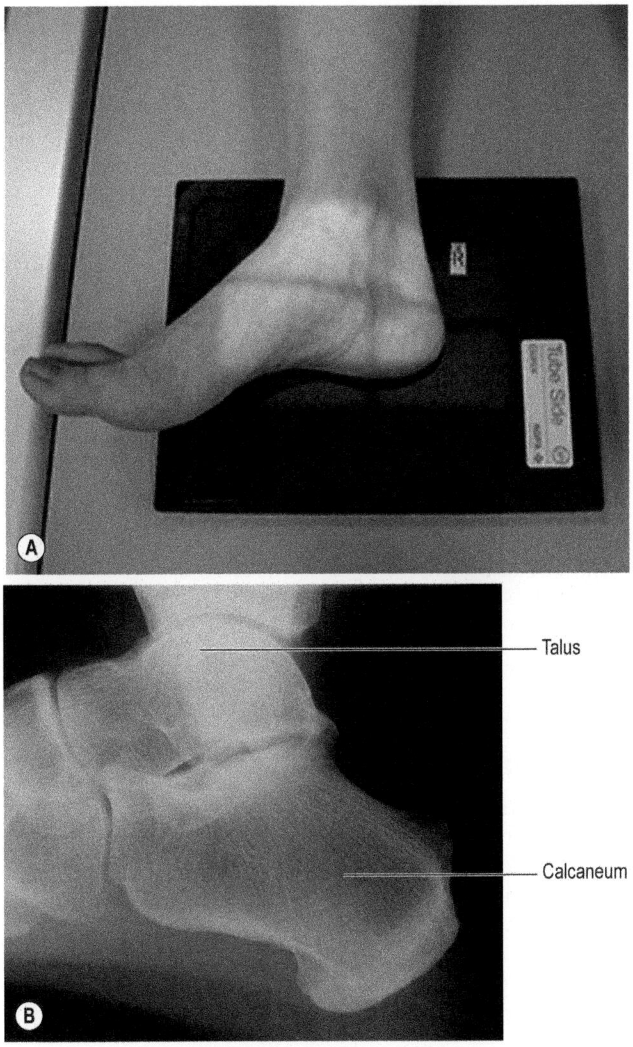

Fig. 6.16 Lateral calcaneum.

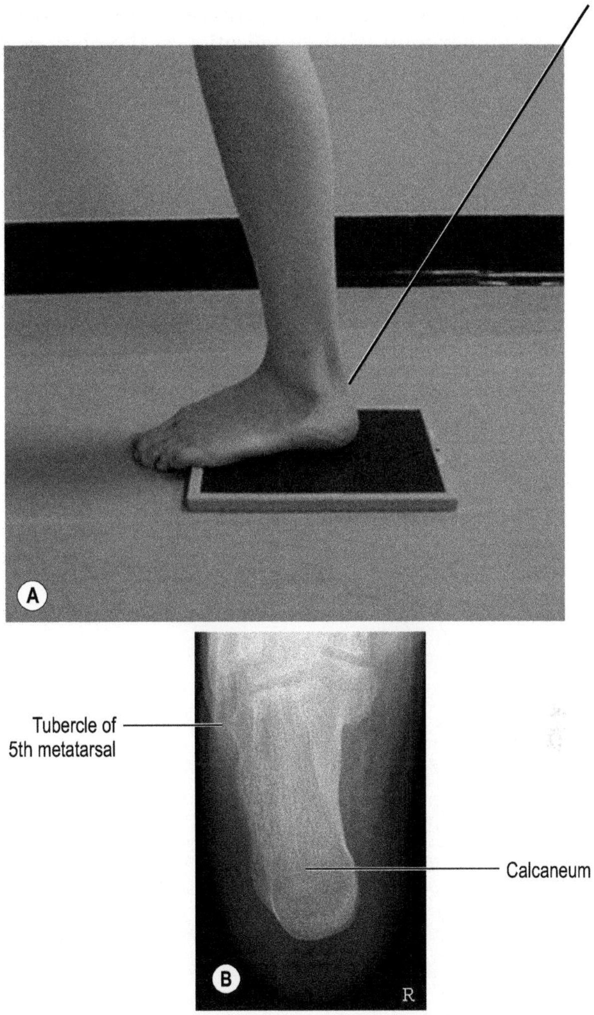

Fig. 6.17 (A) Erect axial calcaneum; (B) axial calcaneum.

number of exposures made to one; two separate exposures will increase the radiation dose but will provide less distortion due to accurate centring over each heel in turn. Methods 1 and 2 are not suitable for use with a fixed plate detector.

Method 1: Patient Erect (Fig. 6.17A,B)

Positioning

- The patient stands in the erect position with their back to the X-ray tube and the plantar aspect of the heel under examination is placed directly on the IR (consideration should be given to the weight limit of the receptor being used)
- The other leg is abducted to clear it from the radiation field
- With the patient's knees slightly flexed, the hands can be placed onto a fixed surface (i.e. table) in front for support
- The malleoli are checked until equidistant from the IR

Beam Direction and FRD

Initially vertical, the beam is directed 30° towards the toes, i.e. 60° to the IR
100 cm FRD

Method 2: Patient Prone (Fig. 6.18)

A vertical IR is required for this method. This method can be used with wireless receptors and where a fixed vertical receptor has a floor track which enables this patient position to be achieved.

Positioning

- The patient lies prone on the table with the toes projecting over the end of the table
- The IR is placed at the end of the table with the tube side of the IR facing the plantar aspect of the patient's feet
- Both legs are extended and the unaffected leg is abducted to clear it from the radiation field
- The plantar aspect of the foot under examination is placed in contact with the IR
- The malleoli are equidistant from the IR

Beam Direction and FRD

Initially horizontal, the X-ray tube is directed caudally towards the toes at approximately 30°, to create an angle of 60° with the IR
100 cm FRD

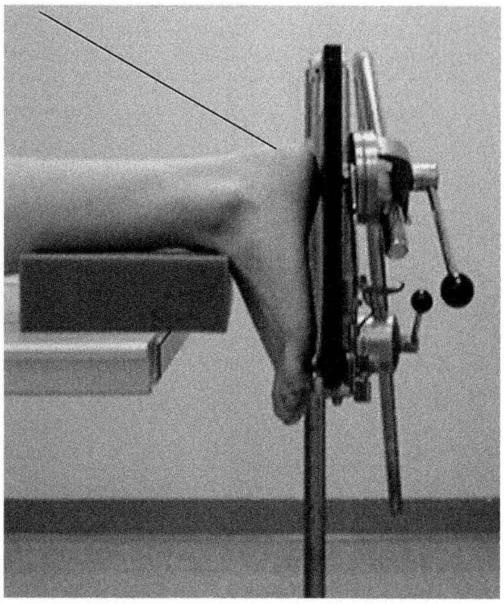

Fig. 6.18 Prone axial calcaneum.

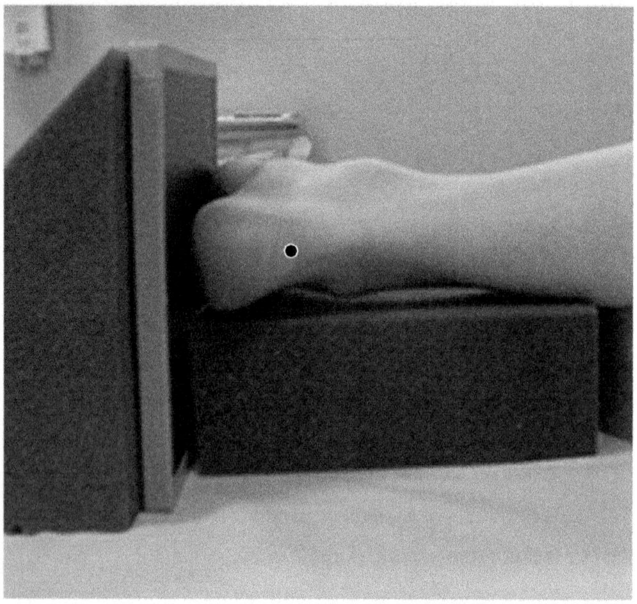

Fig. 6.19 Axial calcaneum with patient on their side.

Method 3: Patient Lying on Side (Fig. 6.19)

Positioning

- The patient lies in the lateral position on the side under examination
- The unaffected leg is abducted posteriorly and placed behind the side under examination
- The leg of the side under examination is supported above the table-top using foam pads and the IR is supported vertically, its tube side in contact with the plantar aspect of the heel
- The malleoli are equidistant from the IR

Beam Direction and FRD

Initially the beam is horizontal, directed towards the posterior aspect of the heel and coincident with the long axis of the calcaneum, *and then*

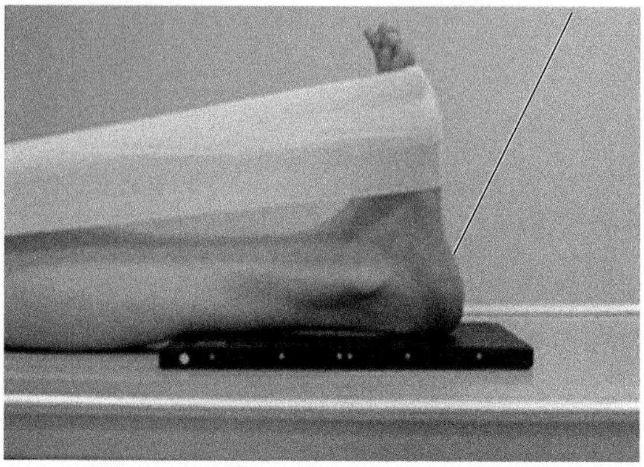

Fig. 6.20 Axial calcaneum with patient seated.

The angle is approximately 30° caudally towards the toes to form an angle of 60° with the IR
100 cm FRD

Centring Point Methods 1, 2 and 3

At the level of the malleoli, in the middle of the posterior aspect of the heel

Method 4: Patient Seated (Fig. 6.20)

Positioning

- The patient is seated on the table with their legs extended and separated
- The posterior aspect of the heel under examination is placed on the IR with the inferior border of the heel pad at the lower edge
- The foot is dorsiflexed; this position can be assisted and maintained by providing the patient with a bandage looped around the forefoot and pulled on towards the trunk. This is held by the patient
- The malleoli are equidistant from the IR

Beam Direction and FRD

A vertical central ray is directed 40° cranially
100 cm FRD

Centring Point

At a point midway on the plantar aspect of the heel, to pass through the malleoli

Collimation: All Methods

Calcaneum, talocalcaneal and cubocalcaneal joints, the soft tissue outline

Criteria for Assessing Image Quality: All Methods

- Calcaneum, talocalcaneal and cubocalcaneal joints and the soft tissue outlines demonstrated
- Cubocalcaneal joint space clearly visualised without the metatarsals superimposed
- Lateral malleolus demonstrated on the lateral aspect of the calcaneum
- Calcaneum demonstrated without rotation and distortion
- Sharp image demonstrating the soft tissue margins and bony cortex and trabeculae of the calcaneum, cubocalcaneal joint shown adequately without over-penetration of the distal aspect of calcaneum

Common Errors: Axial Calcaneum – All Methods

Common Errors	Possible Reasons	Potential Effects on PCE or Report
Elongated long axis of the calcaneum	Over-angulation of X-ray beam	Inadequate assessment of the body of the calcaneum can obscure subtle fractures
Foreshortening of long axis of the calcaneum	Not enough angulation on X-ray beam	Inadequate assessment of the body of the calcaneum can obscure subtle fractures
Cubocalcaneal joint not demonstrated	Not enough dorsiflexion of the foot	Intra-articular fractures may be obscured Bohler's angle may not be readily assessed if whole area of interest is not included on imaging

Tibia and Fibula

When examining the tibia and fibula both the knee and the ankle joint must be demonstrated. This is particularly important in the case of gross injuries in order to show general alignment and to be certain that a contracoup injury has not occurred. The fibula acts as a support for the tibia, and a fracture at one end of one bone often results in a fracture at the opposite end of the other. The ankle joint is often described as a bony ring, and this ring may be considered to extend into the knee. An external rotation injury of the ankle joint, resulting in a seemingly isolated fracture of the medial malleolus, may result in a fracture of the proximal fibula; this is called a Maisonneuve fracture.[16] In the case of spiral fracture the full length of the fracture may not be demonstrated if the full lengths of the tibia and fibula are not shown.

To ensure that the full lengths of the tibia and fibula are included it may be necessary to use two IRs per projection. However, most digital IRs are now 43 or 45 cm^2 or even 35×47 cm, and it may be possible to include the full length on one image for most patients if the IR is positioned diagonally under the patient.

PCE COMMENTS – TIBIA AND FIBULA

When undertaking the preliminary clinical evaluation, it is recommended to quickly assess the bony cortex, to ensure congruity and assess for any undisplaced fractures, cortical or osteochondral defects or periosteal reactions that may be evident and then to assess the overlying soft tissues. Check the medullary cavity for any obvious bony lesions, which may appear either sclerotic or radiolucent. The joints included within the image should also be checked as described for the ankle joint in this chapter and for the knee in Chapter 7, remembering that the centring point and divergent beam makes this a sub-optimal projection for joint assessment.

ANTEROPOSTERIOR (AP) TIBIA AND FIBULA (FIG. 6.21A,B)

Positioning

- The patient is seated on the table and may support themselves by leaning on their hands
- Both legs are extended and the leg that is not under examination is abducted to clear it from the radiation field
- The leg under examination is placed with its posterior aspect in contact with the IR

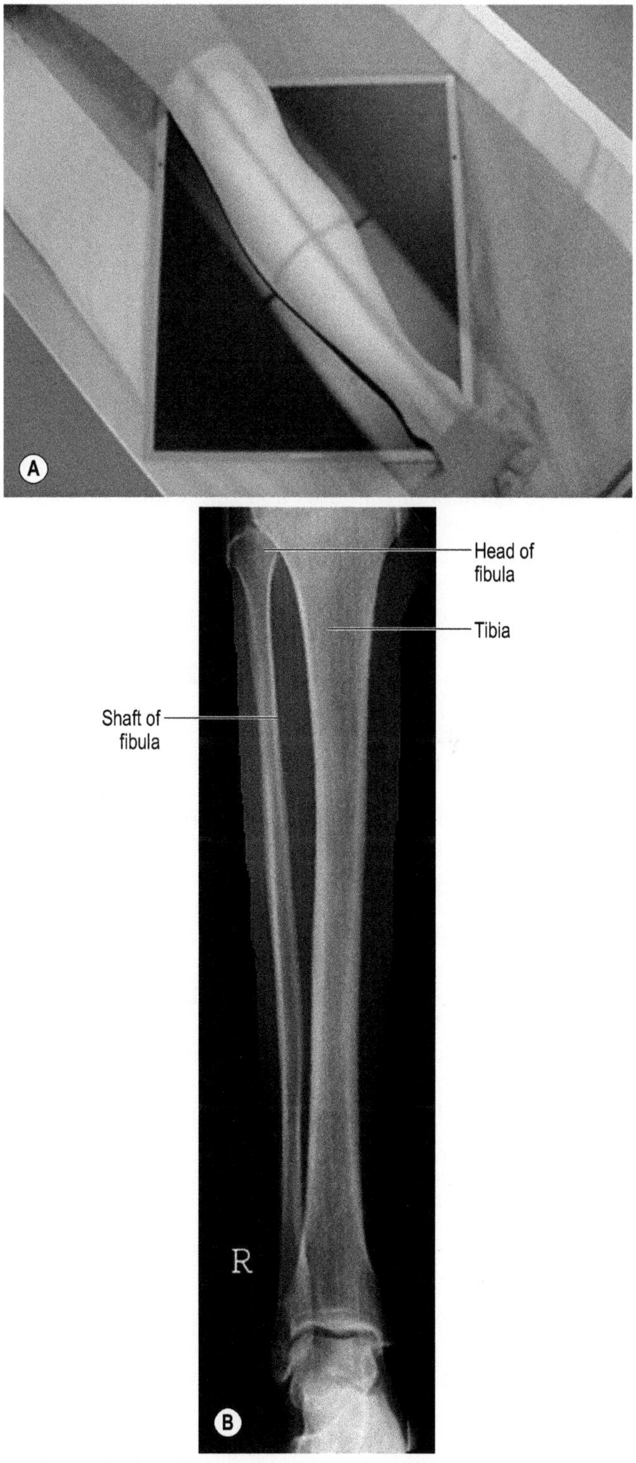

Fig. 6.21 AP tibia and fibula.

- The malleoli are positioned equidistant from the IR and the ankle is dorsiflexed; this position may be supported with use of a radiolucent pad and sandbag at the plantar aspect of the foot

Beam Direction and FRD

A vertical central ray, at 90° to the IR
100 cm FRD

Centring Point

Midway between the ankle and knee joint on the anterior aspect of the lower leg or, if both joints cannot be included on one image, in the middle of the area being exposed

Collimation

Tibia and fibula, ankle and knee joints, surrounding soft tissues

Criteria for Assessing Image Quality

- Tibia and fibula, ankle and knee joints and surrounding soft tissues are demonstrated
- Separation of the tibial and fibular shafts
- Proximal tibiofibular joint should show slight superimposition of fibula head behind the tibia
- The distal tibiofibular joint should have slight superimposition of tibia and fibula
- Demonstration of the joint space between the medial and lateral borders of the talus and the medial and lateral malleoli, respectively
- Sharp image demonstrating the soft tissue margins, bony cortex and trabeculae of tibia and fibula with adequate penetration to demonstrate both the ankle joint and knee joint

LATERAL TIBIA AND FIBULA (FIG. 6.22A,B)

Positioning

- From the AP position the leg is externally rotated onto the side under examination, however, in cases of trauma, a horizontal beam lateral should be performed to allow for assessment of effusions within the knee joint
- The opposite leg is abducted to clear from the main beam
- The lateral aspect of the leg is in contact with the IR, which is positioned to include the ankle and knee joint
- The long axis of the tibia and fibula should be parallel to the surface of the IR
- The ankle is flexed and the malleoli are superimposed
- A small 15° foam pad can be placed under the lateral border of the forefoot to support the patient in this position

Beam Direction and FRD

Vertical central ray at 90° to the IR
100 cm FRD

Centring Point

Midway between the ankle and knee joint on the medial aspect of the lower leg or, if both joints cannot be included on one image, in the middle of the area being exposed

Collimation

Tibia and fibula, ankle and knee joints, soft tissues

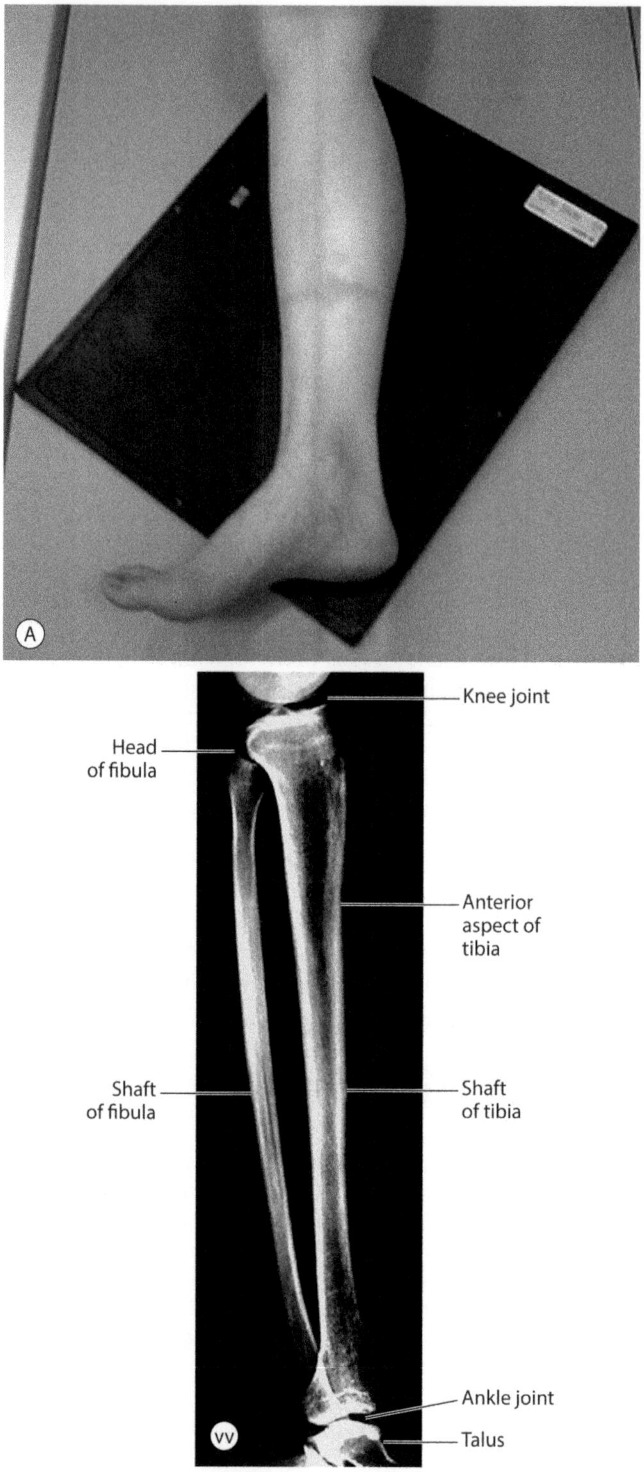

Fig. 6.22 Lateral tibia and fibula. (B, Reproduced with permission from Bryan GJ. *Skeletal Anatomy*. 3rd ed. Edinburgh: Churchill Livingstone; 1996 and Gunn C. *Bones and Joints*. 4th ed. Edinburgh: Churchill Livingstone; 2002.)

Criteria for Assessing Image Quality

- Ankle, knee joints and soft tissue demonstrated
- Mid-shaft of fibula should project slightly posterior to tibia
- Proximal end of fibula should be slightly posterior to tibia with partial superimposition

- The distal end of fibula should be superimposed over the middle of the distal tibia
- Sharp image demonstrating the soft tissue margins, bony cortex and trabeculae of tibia and fibula with adequate penetration to visualise the ankle and knee joints. The kVp should be sufficient to reduce the high subject contrast along the length of the tibia and fibula

Common Errors: Tibia and Fibula – All Methods

Common Errors	Possible Reasons	Potential Effects on PCE or Report
Condyles of the femur are not superimposed anteriorly and posteriorly and the patellofemoral joint space is not clear	Incorrect rotation: 1. If the head of the fibula is excessively or completely superimposed over the tibia then there is insufficient rotation – further external rotation is required 2. If the proximal tibiofibular joint is shown clearly then there is excessive rotation – less rotation is therefore required	1. Assessment of the fibula neck will not be possible. Assessment for condylar fractures or osteochondral defects will be difficult 2. Assessment for condylar fractures or osteochondral defects will be difficult
Condyles of the femur do not appear superimposed at the articulation with the tibial plateau	The leg is not parallel to the IR 1. If performing a turned lateral, the ankle joint must be positioned at the same level as the knee joint, a small (15°) wedge pad may be required under the ankle or a 10–15° cranial angle to achieve this 2. If performing a horizontal beam lateral (HBL) the leg must be positioned parallel to the IR and the tube or a 10–15° cranial angle to achieve this	Assessment for condylar fractures or osteochondral defects will be difficult

References

1. Murray J, Holmes E, Misra R. *A–Z of Musculoskeletal and Trauma Radiology*. Cambridge: Cambridge University Press; 2008:341–344.
2. Smith D. Lower-extremity radiographs: weight-bearing, please. *BC Med J*. 2018;60(7):365–367.
3. Schoots I, Maas M, Smithuis R. Diabetic Foot–MRI Examination. https://radiologyassistant.nl/musculoskeletal/diabetic-foot-mri-examination.
4. Murray J, Holmes E, Misra R. *A–Z of Musculoskeletal and Trauma Radiology*. Cambridge: Cambridge University Press; 2008:321–322.
5. Patel D, Roth M, Kapil N. Stress fractures: diagnosis, treatment and prevention. *Am Fam Phys*. 2011;83(1):39–46.
6. Manaster B. Metatarsal fractures. In: Jeffrey R, et al., ed. *Diagnostic Imaging: Emergency*. Salt Lake City, UT: Amirsys; 2007:182–185. Part 1, section 4.
7. Welck MJ, Hayes T, Pastides P, et al. Stress fractures of the foot and ankle. *Injury*. 2017;48(8):1722–1726.
8. Manaster B. Metatarsal fractures. In: Jeffrey R, et al., ed. *Diagnostic Imaging: Emergency*. Salt Lake City, UT: Amirsys; 2007:178–181. Part 1, section 4.
9. Llopis E, Carrascoso J, Iriarte I, et al. Lisfranc injury imaging and surgical management. *Semin Muscoskel Radiol*. 2016;20(02):139–153.
10. Raby N, Berman L, de Lacey G. *Accident and Emergency Radiography: A Survival Guide*. 2nd ed. Philadelphia: Saunders; 2005:216–245.
11. Lampridis V, Gougoulias N, Sakellariou A. Stability in ankle fractures: diagnosis and treatment. *EFORT Open Rev*. 2018;3(5):294–303.
12. Whitley AS, Sloane C, Hoadley G, et al. *Clark's Positioning in Radiography*. 12th ed. London: Hodder Arnold; 2005.
13. Zengerink M, Szerb I, László H, et al. Current concepts: treatment of osteochondral ankle defects. *Foot Ankle Clin*. 2006;11(2):331–359.
14. Porter DA, Jaggers RR, Barnes AF, et al. Optimal management of ankle syndesmosis injuries. *Open Access J Sports Med*. 2014;5:173–182.
15. Benton C. Physeal fractures, pediatric. In: Jeffrey R, et al., ed. *Diagnostic Imaging: Emergency*. Salt Lake City, UT: Amirsys; 2007:186–189. Part 1, section 4.
16. Pastides P, Gulati P, Peena S. Maisonneuve injury: beware of the 'isolated' medial malleolus or proximal fibula fracture. *Hong Kong J Emerg Med*. 2011;18(5):343–346.
17. Osamah AAA, Hartley L, et al. Ankle Radiograph (An Approach). [online] Radiopedia https://radiopaedia.org/articles/ankle-radiograph-an-approach?lang=gb.
18. Bontrager KL. *Textbook of Radiographic Positioning and Related Anatomy*. 6th ed. St Louis: Mosby; 2018.
19. Eisenberg RL, et al. *Radiographic Positioning*. 2nd ed. Boston: Little Brown and Company; 1995.
20. Unett EM, Royle AJ. *Radiographic Techniques and Image Evaluation*. London: Nelson Thornes; 1997.
21. Bell GA, Finlay DBL. *Basic Radiographic Positioning*. Eastbourne: Baillière Tindall; 1986.
22. Mulligan M. *Imaging in Ankle Fractures*; 2017. [online] https://emedicine.medscape.com/article/398578.
23. McQuillen-Martenson K. *Radiographic Image Analysis*. 3rd ed. Philadelphia: Saunders; 2010.
24. Royal College of Radiologists. *iRefer: Making the Best Use of Clinical Radiology*. 8th ed. London: RCR; 2017. https://www.rcr.ac.uk/clinical-radiology/being-consultant/rcr-referral-guidelines/about-irefer.

7 Knee and Femur

SUZANNE MCLAUGHLAN and LINDA WILLIAMS

Introduction

The knee has a complex arrangement of ligaments, tendons and muscles which together provide stability to the joint. Because of the anatomical location and the complex biomechanics of the knee, it is susceptible to a variety of injuries.[1] The knee and femur are often investigated in the event of trauma; however, this should only be the case if there is a suspected fracture, as ligamentous and meniscal injuries may appear normal on projection radiographs.[2] The knee should not be investigated for knee pain unless there is locking and restricted movement or a suspected loose body. Osteoarthritic changes are commonly found in the knee, and radiographic examination should only be undertaken if surgery is being considered.[3]

Projection radiography of the knee is complemented by magnetic resonance imaging (MRI), which is the method of choice for imaging the joint structures (Chapter 27). This is because of its high contrast sensitivity and multiplanar imaging capabilities. It is particularly effective in investigating the effects of trauma to the anterior and posterior cruciate ligaments and menisci.[4] The images of non-bony parts of the joint obtained by MRI are far superior to, and carry more information than, projection radiographs, and diagnosis and appropriate management of this complex joint is established with greater confidence after MRI examination.[3]

Ultrasound is also used as a method of imaging some lesions of the knee joint, e.g. Baker's cyst; these can show as a vague mass behind the knee on projection radiographs, but ultrasound will give a clear account of the full extent of the cyst.[4]

There is, however, still an important role for projection radiography of the knee for initial diagnosis in trauma follow-up orthopaedic assessment and assessment of osteoarthritic and degenerative changes.

Throughout this chapter a suggested FRD is given for each examination description; however in practice a range of FRDs (typically from 100cm to 120cm), may be used, dependent on local protocol.

PCE comments for the region are given at the end of the chapter.

FRACTURES AND INJURIES AFFECTING THE REGION OF KNEE AND FEMUR

Fractured Shaft of Femur

The shaft is usually fractured as a result of considerable force to the femur, commonly in road traffic accidents, fall from heights or a crush injury.

Supracondylar Fracture

These are fractures superior to the femoral condyles; the gastrocnemius muscle may pull the distal fragments posteriorly. These fractures usually occur following high-energy trauma, however, it may also be seen in the elderly after a low-energy trauma.[5]

Tibial Plateau Fracture

These fractures are often associated with considerable damage to the medial collateral or cruciate ligaments. The most common finding is depressed lateral tibial plateau[6] caused by a car bumper injury; this is seen in 80% of tibial plateau cases.[1,7]

Patella Fractures

Patellar comminuted fractures are usually the result of a direct blow.[6] Muscle spasm (quadriceps), if severe enough, can cause transverse fractures.[6] The bipartite patella (unfused secondary ossification centre) can be confused with a fracture, but these have well-defined, corticated margins and are usually seen at the superolateral aspect.[8] The patella may also be *dislocated* medially or laterally, and can be recurrent due to a shallow intercondylar groove. Dislocations usually occur following a twisting force, typically in sports injuries.

Knee

ANTEROPOSTERIOR (AP) KNEE (FIG. 7.1A–C)

In cases of trauma, this should always be performed with the IR horizontal and the patient positioned on the table or trolley.

Positioning

- The patient is seated on the table with their legs extended
- The posterior aspect of the knee under examination is placed over the IR
- The unaffected leg is abducted from the leg under examination to clear it from the field of radiation
- The leg is rotated to bring the tibial condyles equidistant to the IR. The patella may appear centralised but this is not consistent for all patients

Orthopaedic requests very often require this projection to be undertaken with the patient erect, weightbearing. This allows for assessment of joint space narrowing and alignment of the joint during weightbearing, prior to surgery.[1] Its use is now more widespread in that published evidence suggests that a weightbearing technique has advantages over the conventional sitting method, and that a posteroanterior (PA) rather than an AP approach may be even better.[9] Positioning for the erect AP remains the same as for the seated version, but with the patient standing with the back of their knee against the IR and still facing the X-ray tube. The stability of the patient should also be considered in the erect position and there should be a support for them to hold. The patient must be asked to distribute their weight evenly on both feet.

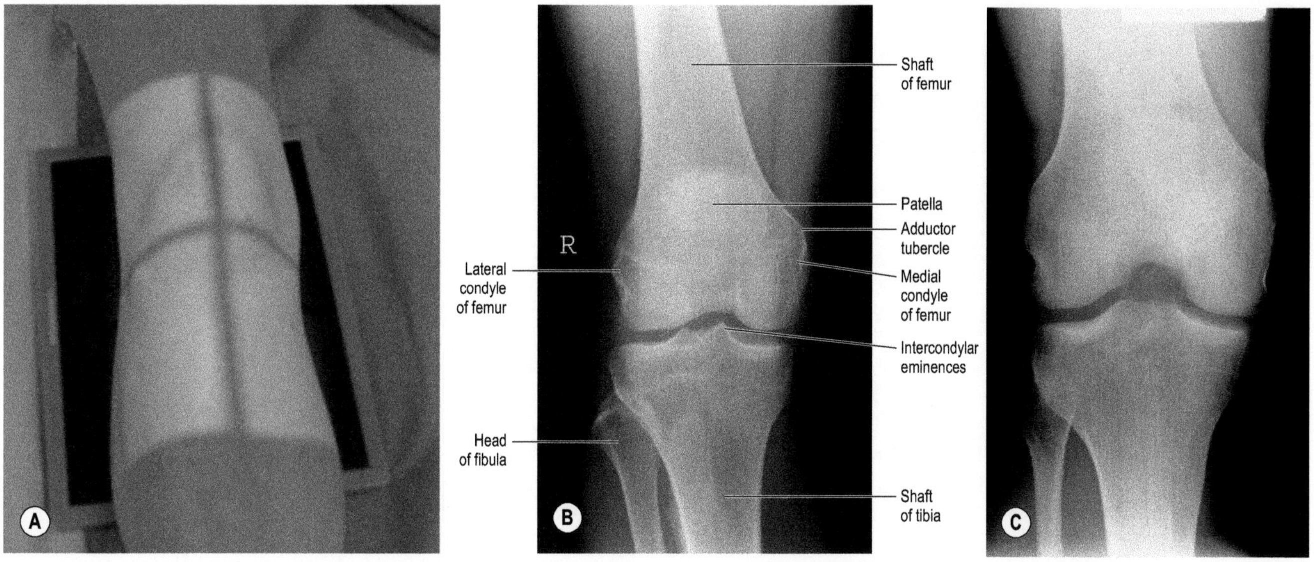

Fig. 7.1 (A,B) AP knee; (C) patella not centralised but joint space shown adequately.

Similarly, erect PA will require the patient to distribute their weight evenly, but with the patella in contact with the IR.

Beam Direction and FRD

Patient seated: Vertical central beam, at 90° to the IR *or* 90° to the long axis of the tibia (which will improve joint space demonstration if the patient cannot fully extend the knee)
Patient erect: Horizontal beam, at 90° to the IR *or* long axis of the tibia
100 cm FRD

Centring Point

AP: On the anterior aspect of the knee in the middle of the joint space, midway between the tibial condyles
PA: On the posterior aspect of the knee in the middle of the joint space, midway between the tibial condyles

A point 2.5 cm below the apex of the patella is often cited as the centring point for AP of this joint, but this specific measurement does not allow for variations in patient build.

Collimation

Lower third of femur, knee joint, proximal third of tibia, head of fibula, surrounding soft tissues

Criteria for Assessing Image Quality

- Distal third of femur, proximal third of tibia, head of fibula, patella and soft tissue outlines are demonstrated
- Medial and lateral epicondyles of the femur are demonstrated in profile
- Head of fibula should appear partially obscured by the tibia
- Shafts of tibia and fibula should be separated
- Joint space should appear clear and the upper margin of the tibial plateau should be shown in profile
- Sharp image demonstrating the soft tissue margins, bony cortex and trabeculae of tibia, fibula, femur and patella, with sufficient penetration to visualise the bony trabeculae and cortical outline of the patella over the femur
- Demonstration of the knee joint space in contrast to bony areas

Common Errors: AP Knee

Common Errors	Possible Reasons	Potential Effects on PCE or Report
The patella appears medially in relation to the femur and the proximal tibiofibular joint is demonstrated. The joint space may appear narrowed or obscured, unilaterally or bilaterally. Part, or all, of the tibial plateau does not appear to be seen in profile	The leg is excessively internally rotated; ensure the tibial condyles are equidistant from the IR and the patella is centralised. However, take care to note whether the patient has a naturally medially positioned patella or knock knees before attempting repeat projection. If the tibiofibular joint appears to be demonstrated correctly, and joint space shown clear, then it is likely that the patient's patella does not naturally lie centrally positioned; an example of this is shown in Fig. 7.1C	Incorrectly rotated images will prevent accurate assessment of potential bony injury, patellar dislocation or degenerative changes in the case of orthopaedic assessment
The patella is projected laterally in relation to the femur and the proximal tibiofibular joint is obscured by the tibia. The joint space may appear narrowed or obscured, unilaterally or bilaterally. Part or all of the tibial plateau does not appear to be seen in profile	There is excessive external rotation of the leg. Patellae are less likely to naturally lie on the more lateral aspect over the femur than medially, as above, but note should still be made to check if this is the case	Incorrectly rotated images will prevent accurate assessment of potential bony injury, patellar dislocation or degenerative changes in the case of orthopaedic assessment
There is no bony detail of the patella demonstrated – pale image of patella but femur may show trabecular detail outside the periphery of the patella	The radiograph is under-penetrated; increase kVp	Under-penetrated images prevent accurate assessment of patellar fractures or bony abnormality

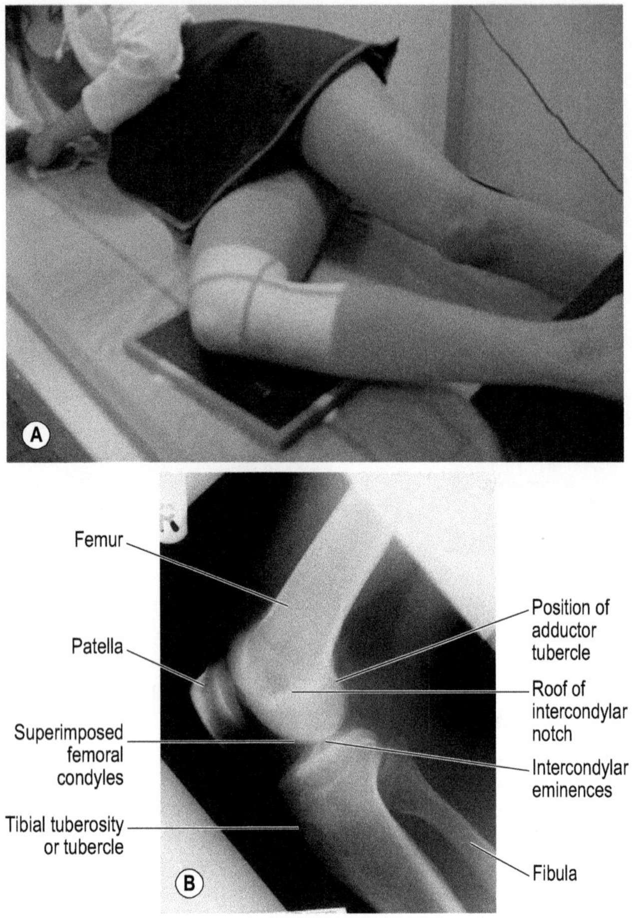

Fig. 7.2 Lateral knee.

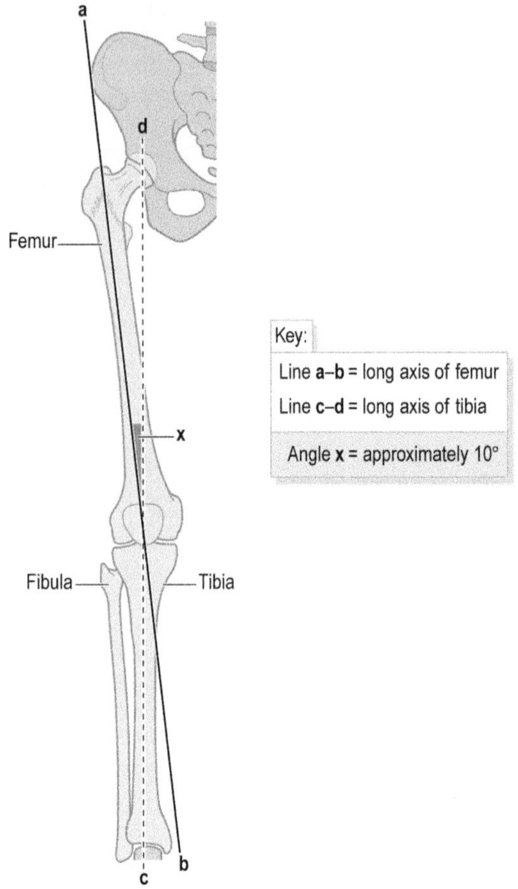

Fig. 7.3 Alignment of shafts of femur and tibia.

LATERAL KNEE (FIG. 7.2A,B)

In cases of trauma horizontal beam laterals (HBL) must be performed; this method will demonstrate any joint effusion displacing the suprapatellar bursa, which may contain fat released from the bone marrow following fracture.[2] A fat–blood effusion may be seen within the suprapatellar bursa (lipohaemarthrosis, see PCE Comments and Fig. 7.13), indicating a fracture even if not seen on the resulting radiograph. Use of a horizontal beam will also ensure that the unstable joint is not disrupted further, or fracture fragments further displaced. This is especially a risk in the case of transverse patellar fracture or fractures of the femoral shaft.

Positioning – HBL

- The patient is seated on the table with their legs extended, with the affected leg being parallel to the IR
- The IR is vertical, to the medial aspect of the affected knee
- The condyles of the femur are superimposed; this may be achieved by using a small external rotation of the affected leg

Note on Superimposing the Femoral Condyles. Criteria for assessing the lateral knee radiograph require the knee joint to be demonstrated with the condyles of the femur superimposed. However, there is often difficulty in producing this as the femur and tibia do not follow a straight line. The femoral shaft angles medially through approximately 10° from hip to knee, yet the plane of the articular surface of the knee joint is at right-angles to the long axis of the tibia (Fig. 7.3); this means that there is an angle of approximately 170° between femur and tibia at the lateral aspect of the knee joint. To correct this, a 5–10° cranial angle may be required.[10,11]

Beam Direction and FRD

Horizontal at 90° to the IR and coincident with the transverse axis of the joint
100 cm FRD

Centring Point

Over the middle of the medial tibial condyle, through the middle of the knee joint
2.5 cm below and behind the apex of the patella has been described for the centring point for this projection but, as discussed in the AP knee projection description, this does not allow for variation in patient build.

Collimation

Lower third of femur, knee joint, proximal third of tibia, head of fibula, surrounding soft tissues

Criteria for Assessing Image Quality

- Distal third of femur, proximal third of tibia, head of fibula and soft tissues should all be demonstrated

- Knee joint is demonstrated as clear, with the condyles of femur superimposed
- Patellofemoral joint space is demonstrated. However, if the patella is not naturally positioned centrally over the femur, the patellofemoral space will not be seen despite good superimposition of the femoral condyles. This is seen in Fig. 7.2B
- Head of fibula is partly superimposed over tibia (approximately one-third to half of the head should be overlapped)
- Head of fibula is seen posteriorly in relation to tibia
- Sharp image demonstrating the soft tissue margins, bony cortex and trabeculae of femur, tibia, fibula and patella. Joint space is shown in contrast to denser bone

Common Errors: Lateral Knee

Common Errors	Possible Reasons	Potential Effects on PCE or Report
The condyles of the femur are not superimposed anteriorly and posteriorly and the patellofemoral joint space is not clear	Incorrect rotation, but is the leg over-rotated or under-rotated? The head of fibula is a good indication of the direction to correct rotation: 1. If the head of fibula is excessively or completely superimposed over the tibia then there is insufficient rotation – further external rotation is required 2. If the proximal tibiofibular joint is shown clearly then there is excessive rotation – less rotation is therefore required	Assessment of the fibula head/neck will not be possible. Assessment for condylar fractures or osteochondral defects (OCDs) will be difficult Assessment for condylar fractures or OCDs will be difficult
	The *adductor tubercle*, found on the posterior upper aspect of the medial femoral condyle, can also be used as an indicator when assessing knee rotation. In the correct position the tubercle is hardly discernible but in cases of incorrect rotation it becomes more apparent and can be used as follows: 1. If the tubercle lies anteriorly in relationship to the other condyle, the knee is over-rotated 2. If the tubercle lies posteriorly, the knee is under-rotated	Assessment for condylar fractures or OCDs will be difficult Assessment of the fibula head/neck will not be possible.
	The *patellofemoral* joint space will clear once the rotation is corrected but it must be remembered that the patella may not be centralised naturally and this may result in unavoidable loss of joint space. If the condyles are superimposed and the patellofemoral space is not evident, this may be due to a naturally occurring non-centralised patella (this will also have been apparent when positioning for the AP projection) or may also be due to degenerative change within the patellofemoral joint resulting in narrowed joint space	Assessment of OCDs or subtle avulsion fractures may be affected
	Another method for assessing direction of rotation is to estimate the relative *size of each condyle*; it is assumed that the outline of the apparently larger condyle will be that most remote from the IR (the medial condyle) since it will be more magnified than the lateral condyle on a turned lateral. Unfortunately it is difficult to make this assessment when only part of the condyle lies clear of the other. Some patients also have one slightly flattened condyle (usually on its anterior aspect), which will never appear superimposed over the other, more normally curved, condyle	Full assessment of condyles and the joint space may be obscured
Femoral condyles not superimposed along the knee joint surface, i.e. nearest the upper surface of the tibial plateau	The tibia is not parallel to the table-top; usually this is due to a lack of attention to adequate padding of the lower leg. It is more difficult to assess correction requirements in this situation but estimation of size of condyles (as described above) may help. It is more likely that the lower leg is inadequately raised rather than excessively raised	Full assessment of the joint space may not be achieved and subtle fractures or osteochondral defects may be missed

Intercondylar Notch

Projections for this area are sometimes referred to as 'tunnel' projections, as the appearances are similar to that of a railway tunnel. It is commonly performed to investigate knee pain if there is locking, restricted movement and a suspected loose body. These requests are usually only made by orthopaedic teams and are used to examine the tibial plateau and femoral intercondylar spaces.[12] Three methods will be described here to achieve this projection: methods 1 and 2 are the methods of choice as the primary beam is not directly pointing towards the gonads. Method 3 will also provide a more distorted, magnified image; the third method should only be attempted in patients who are unable to achieve the positions required for methods 1 or 2.

METHOD 1 (FIG. 7.4A–C)

IR is horizontal

Positioning

- The patient kneels on the table with the knee of the leg under examination on the IR, their hands placed on the table for support
- The unaffected leg is separated from that under examination to clear it from the radiation field
- The angle between the tibia and femur should be 120°
- The femoral condyles should be equidistant to the table-top and the patella centralised between them

Beam Direction and FRD

1. Vertical central beam, at 90° to the long axis of the tibia.
   This will demonstrate the posterior aspect of the notch.

This is the only projection necessary to demonstrate loose bodies, as the whole of the notch can be visualised, with the exception of its anterior aspect.

2. Cranial angle at 70° to the tibia
   This will demonstrate the anterior aspect of the notch.

100 cm FRD

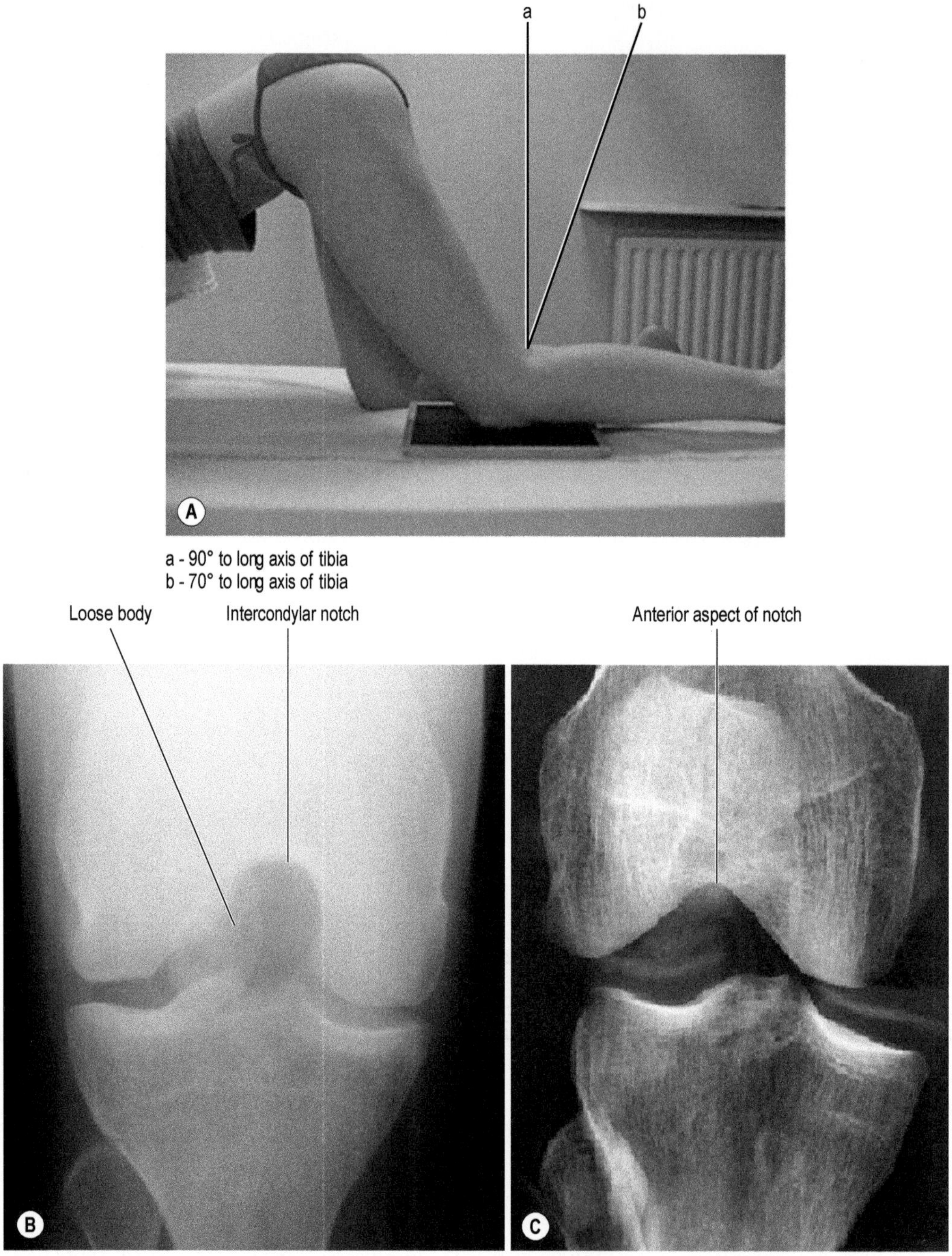

Fig. 7.4 (A) Intercondylar notch – method 1; (B) with beam 90° to tibia; (C) with beam 70° to tibia.

Centring Point

In the middle of the crease of the knee

METHOD 2 (FIG. 7.5)

IR is horizontal

Positioning

- The patient lies prone on the table with the knee under examination in contact with the IR
- The unaffected leg is separated from that under examination to clear it from the radiation field
- The knee is flexed until the tibia is at an angle of 45° to the table-top and is supported in this position
- The femoral condyles are adjusted to centralise the patella

Beam Direction and FRD

1. Caudal central beam at 45° to the IR and femur. This will demonstrate the whole of the notch, with the exception of the anterior aspect
2. Caudal angle at 65° to the femur. This will demonstrate the anterior aspect of the notch
100 cm FRD

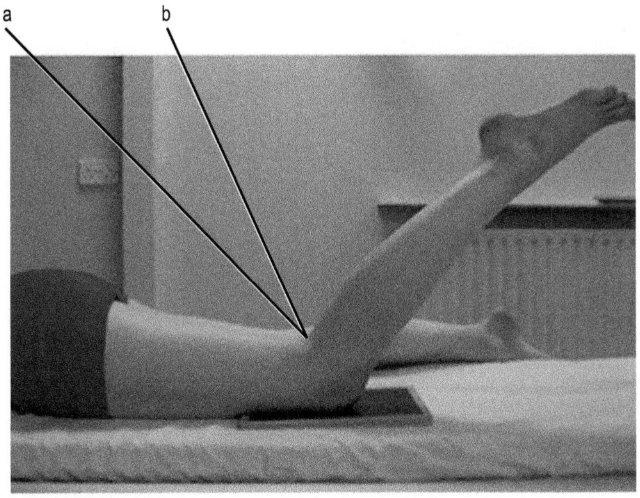

Fig. 7.5 Intercondylar notch – method 2.

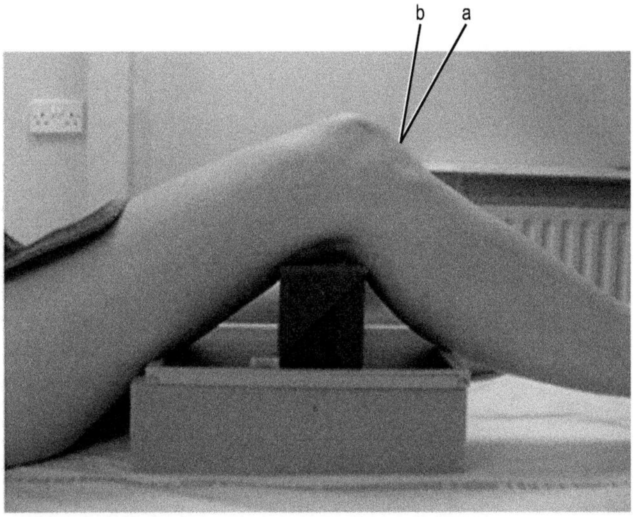

Fig. 7.6 Intercondylar notch – method 3.

Centring Point

In the middle of the crease of the knee

METHOD 3 (FIG. 7.6)

Positioning

- The patient is seated on the table with the leg under examination flexed through 60° until the angle between the tibia and femur is 120°
- The unaffected leg is separated from that under examination to clear it from the radiation field
- The IR is supported on a pad under the flexed knee so that it is elevated high enough to ensure the upper and lower leg are in contact with it
- The femoral condyles should be equidistant to the IR to centralise the patella

Beam Direction and FRD

1. Initially vertical, the central beam is angled cranially until at 90° to the long axis of tibia. This will demonstrate the whole of the notch, with the exception of the anterior aspect
2. Initially vertical, the central beam is angled until at 110° to the long axis of the tibia. This will demonstrate the anterior aspect of the notch

100 cm FRD

Angulation can be estimated accurately by initially positioning the tube housing or light beam housing parallel to the long axis of the tibia, then checking the angulation indicator on the unit before adding the required angulation to this reading.

Centring Point

Immediately below the apex of the patella

Collimation

Femoral and tibial condyles

Criteria for Assessing Image Quality

- Femoral and tibial condyles are included in the image
- Patella is cleared above the intercondylar notch and central between the femoral condyles
- Tubercles of the intercondylar eminences of tibia are visualised
- Tibiofemoral joint space should be clear
- *For the whole notch*: The notch should be seen as tunnel or 'n'-shaped, with almost vertical lateral margins and an arched roof
- *For the anterior aspect of the notch*: The notch is shallower than required for the full notch, rather like an inverted 'v' with sloped lateral margins and narrow roof
- Sharp image demonstrating the soft tissue in the notch in contrast to the adjacent bone, intercondylar eminences and any loose bodies

Common Error: Intercondylar Notch – All Methods

Common Error	Possible Reason	Potential Effect on PCE or Report
Patella superimposed over notch	Beam angle not correctly set in relation to tibia (too much cranial angle in PA projections, methods 1 and 2; not enough cranial angulation in method 3, AP projection). Incorrect flexion can also cause this	The intercondylar region cannot be fully assessed if the patella is superimposed

Patella

POSTEROANTERIOR (PA) PATELLA (FIG. 7.7A,B)

Although the PA is the preferred method for the patella projection, as it is in close contact with the IR, the patient may not be able to achieve the position because of injury or their general condition. In these cases a satisfactory image can be obtained by positioning the patient as for an AP knee projection, with a 10 kVp increase on exposure factors. Consideration must be given to increasing the FRD to compensate for the relatively large object receptor distance.

The IR is horizontal.

Positioning

- The patient lies prone on the table with their legs extended and the affected patella in contact with the IR
- The unaffected leg is separated from that under examination to clear it from the radiation field
- The leg is rotated to align the patella between the femoral condyles and a small pad is placed under the tibia to prevent rotation of the leg

Beam Direction and FRD

Vertical central beam, at 90° to the IR
100 cm FRD

Centring Point

In the middle of the crease of the knee

Collimation

Femoral and tibial condyles, knee joint, surrounding soft tissues

Criteria for Assessing Image Quality

- Distal third of femur, proximal third of tibia, head of fibula, patella and soft tissue outlines should all be demonstrated
- Patella is centralised over the femur
- Head of fibula should appear slightly obscured by tibia
- Shafts of tibia and fibula should be separated
- Sharp image demonstrating the bony cortex and trabeculae of patella in contrast to the femur

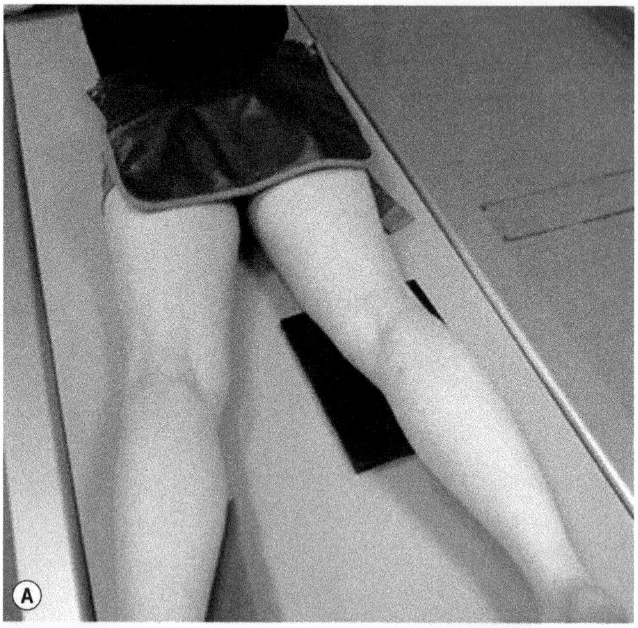

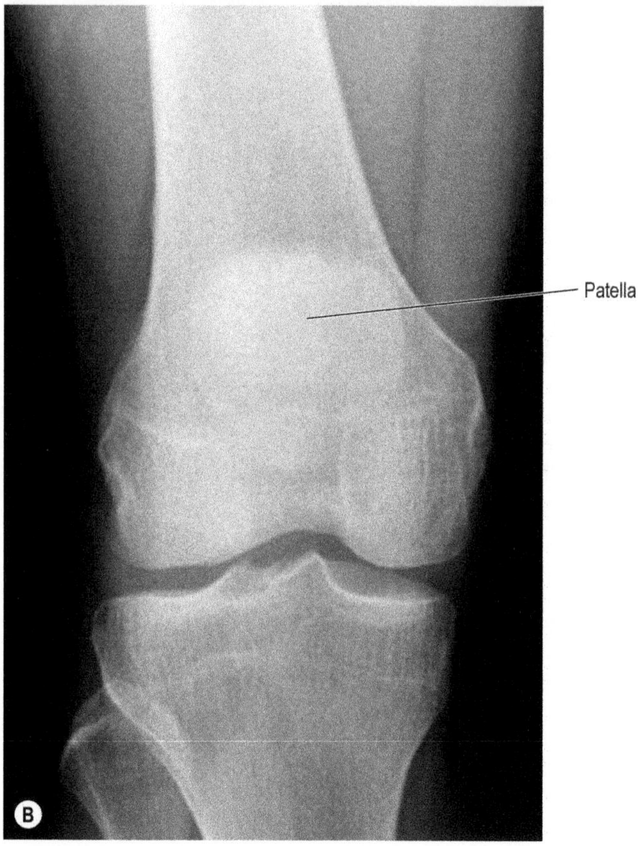

Fig. 7.7 PA patella.

INFEROSUPERIOR PATELLA (SKYLINE/SUNRISE PROJECTION)

This projection is often undertaken to evaluate the patellofemoral joint in an orthopaedic assessment before and after knee surgery. It must not be attempted if there is a suspected fracture of the patella, as in the case of a transverse fracture, because the fragments can be further separated and thus exacerbate the effects of injury. However, if the patient presents with some flexion of the knee, method 3 below may be considered.

There are several methods for achieving this projection and three will be described here. Method 1 is the preferred method as the central ray is not directed directly towards the gonads. In method 2, although the main beam is not directly towards the patient's abdomen, it is still aimed in the direction of the trunk. Method 3 is commonly described with the patient seated and supporting the IR themselves.[1,11,13,14] However, where the patient is supine[15] and the IR can be placed vertically, not only will greater radiation protection be achieved for the patient, i.e. the main beam will not be directed at the patient's torso and towards their fingers, but the risk of movement unsharpness from the patient holding the IR will be removed. Many digital radiography (DR) detectors are quite cumbersome and a computed radiography (CR) cassette may be preferable for this projection.

To demonstrate lateral movement of the patella if subluxation is suspected, the projection can be performed with the knee at varying angles of flexion, e.g. 30°, 60° and 90°.[16]

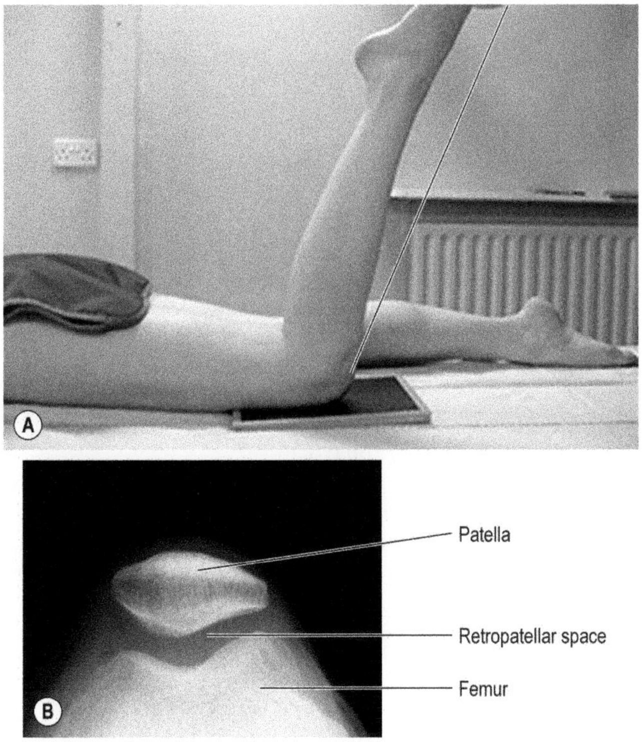

Fig. 7.8 (A) Inferosuperior patella – method 1; (B) inferosuperior patella.

Positioning

Method 1 (Fig. 7.8A,B)

- The IR is horizontal
- The patient lies in the prone position with the IR below the knee of the leg to be examined
- The unaffected leg is separated from the leg under examination to clear it from the radiation field
- The knee is flexed through 60° and immobilised with the use of a bandage around the ankle; this is held by the patient. Alternatively, radiolucent pads and sandbags may be placed under the lower leg for support (although a significant depth of pad would be required for this)
- The patella is centralised over the femur

Method 2 (Fig. 7.9)

- The IR is vertical
- The patient lies on the side under examination with knee flexed through approximately 75°
- The unaffected leg is cleared backwards, away from the leg under examination, to clear it from the radiation field
- The patient's arms are used as support
- The IR is positioned in the vertical position on the table, tube side in contact with the lower end of the femur and at 90° to the long axis of the patella, or support using pads and sandbags

Method 3 (Fig. 7.10)

- The patient lies supine on the table with the affected knee flexed through 60°
- The unaffected leg is separated from the leg under examination to clear it from the radiation field
- The IR is supported vertically, its lower edge in contact with the lower end of the femur and at 90° to the long axis of the patella (the tube side of the IR is towards the knee and feet)

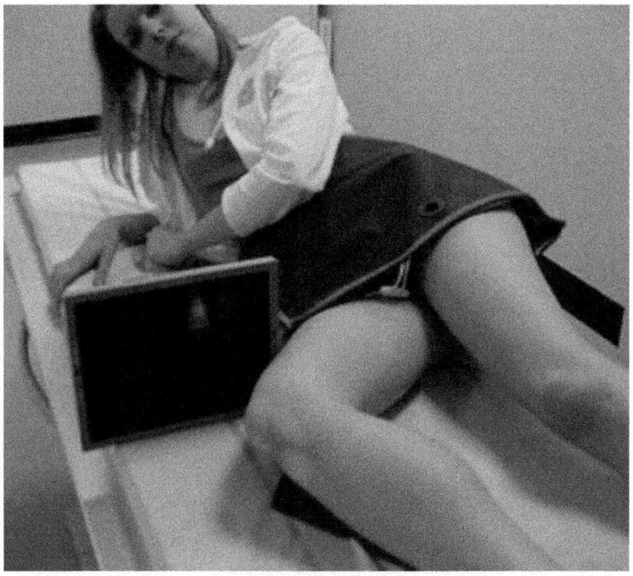

Fig. 7.9 Inferosuperior patella – method 2.

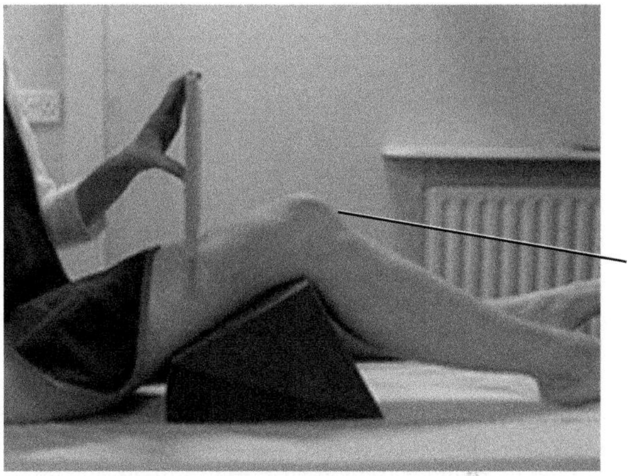

Fig. 7.10 Inferosuperior patella – method 3.

- If no holder is available the IR must be supported by the patient, but this leads to an increased radiation dose, especially to the trunk and hands. There is also increased potential for movement unsharpness and distortion of image if the patient does not maintain the correct relationship of the IR to the patella

Beam Direction and FRD

Method 1: Vertical, directed cranially (approximately 15°) to coincide with the long axis of the patella
100 cm FRD
Method 2: Horizontal, at 90° to the IR and to coincide with the long axis of the patella
Method 3: Horizontal, directed cranially up to approximately 15° and to coincide with the long axis of the patella

Centring Point: All Methods

Immediately below (behind) the apex of the patella

Collimation

Patellofemoral joint space, articular surfaces of the femur, anterior surface of the patella, surrounding soft tissues

Criteria for Assessing Image Quality

- Patella is projected clear from the femoral condyles for a clear view of the patellofemoral joint space
- Sharp image demonstrating the joint space and surrounding soft tissues, in contrast to the bony cortex and trabeculae of patella

Femur

The femoral shaft is mainly imaged after trauma, or when there is suspicion of metabolic bone disease or malignant deposits.[5]

The femur has a wide variation in subject contrast from the hip joint, through the shaft and down to the knee joint; to reduce this it is advisable to use a kVp of at least 75.

In the Western world in particular, people are getting taller,[17] but this has not been reflected in the availability of significantly larger IRs and, unfortunately, average limb length has been seen to have increased even more than trunk length. This has implications for radiographic examination of the femur, which ideally should have only one exposure per projection, with the entire femur from hip to knee included. In reality, limitations of IR space very often require the radiographer to provide images of the upper and lower femur on two overlapping images of the same projection.

CR cassettes remain at a maximum 35×43 cm in size, but most DR IRs have a maximum size of 43 or 45 cm^2 or 35×47 cm. There will be increased space for the femoral length on the larger receptor if it is positioned diagonally, compared to the space available across the diagonal of the 35×43 cm cassette. Simple mathematical calculation of the length of the diagonal in the 43 cm^2 receptor shows it to be 60.8 cm, compared to 55 cm in the case of the 35×43 cm cassette, although it must be noted that this only relates to the extreme measurement from corner to corner. The 35×47 cm IR will facilitate even more of the body area.

If the femur really is too long for inclusion on one image, the leg should remain in the same position for both images used for the same projection, to assess the rotation of any fracture, and there should be overlap of the mid shaft of the femur on each image. Follow-up images taken for orthopaedic assessment only require demonstration of the fracture site and associated or nearest joint (unless there is a surgical prosthesis or pin present), thereby reducing the radiation exposure for these assessments to one projection. It is possible to use a radiopaque ruler positioned at the side of the patient to demonstrate that there is true overlap of the images.

Radiation protection is an essential consideration and the 28-day rule should be applied when the whole femur is to be demonstrated.

ANTEROPOSTERIOR (AP) FEMUR (FIG. 7.11A–C)

IR is horizontal

Positioning

- The patient lies supine on the table or trolley with their legs extended
- The posterior aspect of the femur under examination is placed in contact with the IR and positioned to include the hip and knee joint if possible. If this is not possible, ensure that the knee is included if the lower two-thirds of the femur is required (Fig. 7.11A). If the upper third is required, the hip joint should be included. Where a single image is not possible, the IR should be used in conjunction with a grid for the hip exposure, either within the table bucky or under the trolley.
- The unaffected leg is separated from the leg under examination to clear it from the radiation field
- The leg is internally rotated approximately 15° to bring the femur into the true AP position and the neck of the femur parallel to the IR

Beam Direction and FRD

Vertical at 90° to the IR
100 cm FRD

Centring Point

Mid shaft, on the anterior aspect of the femur*

Collimation

Knee and hip joints, surrounding soft tissues*

*Note that the asterisked sections will require consideration for amendment if two images of the projection are required, when femoral length dictates this. Realistically, the *central ray* can be considered to be in the middle of the area covered by the IR space.

Criteria for Assessing Image Quality

- Knee and hip joints, patella and all the soft tissue outlines should be demonstrated (or the area intended for inclusion if the whole femur cannot be included on the IR)
- Greater trochanter should be seen in profile on the lateral aspect of the upper femur and cleared from the neck
- Lesser trochanter, if included, should be seen on the medial aspect of the femur
- Sharp image demonstrating the soft tissue margins, bony cortex and trabeculae of femur; care should be taken in kVp selection to reduce the inherent contrast in the femur

Common Errors: AP Femur

Common Errors	Possible Reasons	Potential Effects on PCE or Report
Both joints not demonstrated	Inaccurate assessment of adequacy of receptor size *or* IR not positioned accurately Patient simply may have long legs	Accuracy of overlap cannot be assessed if a marker or ruler is not used
Greater trochanter overlaps neck of femur	Inadequate internal rotation of leg	Potential neck of femur fractures or proximal femoral fractures or bony lesions may not be accurately assessed

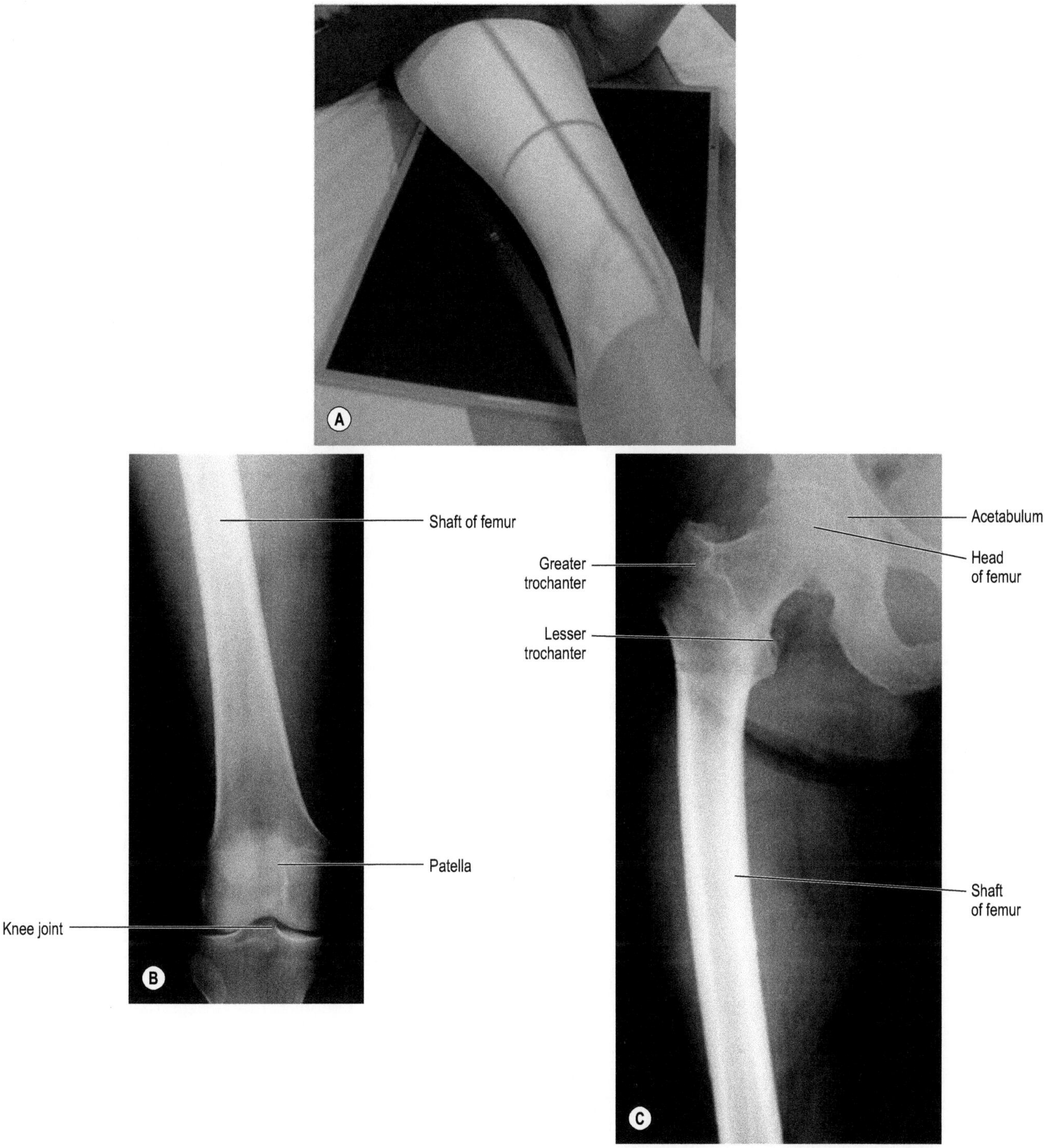

Fig. 7.11 **(A) AP lower femur; (B) AP lower femur; (C) AP upper femur.** (B,C, Reproduced with permission from Bryan GJ. *Skeletal Anatomy*. 3rd ed. Edinburgh: Churchill Livingstone; 1996 and Gunn C. *Bones and Joints*. 4th ed. Edinburgh: Churchill Livingstone; 2002.)

LATERAL FEMUR (FIG. 7.12A–C)

IR is horizontal

Positioning – Non-trauma

- From the AP position the patient is rotated onto the side under examination with the opposite leg placed behind them, on the table-top
- With the knee and hip slightly flexed, the femur is positioned to include the hip and knee joint if possible. If this is not possible, ensure that the knee is included if the lower two-thirds of the femur is required (Fig. 7.12A). If the upper third is required, the hip joint should be included
- The femoral condyles are superimposed and a sandbag or small wedge pad is placed under the ankle joint to help facilitate this. The more the hip is flexed, the easier it becomes to rotate the patient into a lateral position

Beam Direction and FRD

Vertical at 90° to the IR

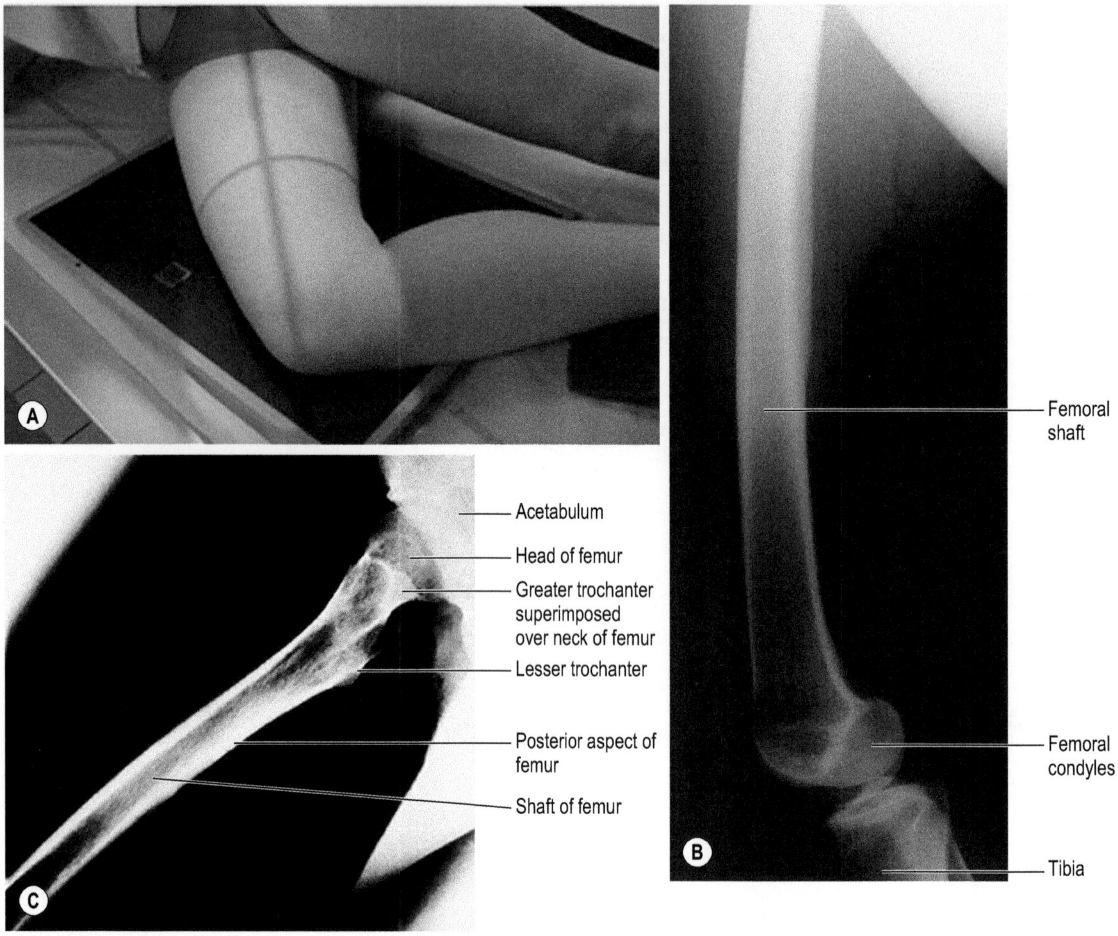

Fig. 7.12 **(A) Lateral femur; (B) lateral lower femur; (C) lateral upper femur.** (C, Reproduced with permission from Bryan GJ. *Skeletal Anatomy*. 3rd ed. Edinburgh: Churchill Livingstone; 1996 and Gunn C. *Bones and Joints*. Edinburgh: Churchill Livingstone; 2002.)

100 cm FRD

Centring Point

Mid shaft, on the medial aspect of femur*

Collimation

Hip and knee joints, surrounding soft tissues*

*As for the AP femur, these will vary according to the amount of femur that can be included on the image receptor.

Following *trauma* or *surgery*, horizontal beam laterals (HBLs) should be performed. In either of these cases consider undertaking a horizontal beam lateral neck of the femur as described in Chapter 8, and horizontal beam lateral of the knee and lower two-thirds of the femur. To take this mediolateral approach, the opposite leg must be uninjured so that it can be raised. If this is not possible, a lateromedial approach should be used for the lower two-thirds of the femur, with appropriate protection for the other leg, and a mediolateral oblique used as for the femoral neck lateral.

Criteria for Assessing Image Quality

- Hip, knee joint, patella and surrounding soft tissues are demonstrated, or the area intended for inclusion if the whole of the femur cannot be included on the image receptor
- Patellofemoral joint space is visualised (unless the patella is not naturally centralised on the individual patient)
- Greater trochanter is superimposed on the shaft of femur
- Lesser trochanter is seen in profile on the posterior aspect of the femur
- Sharp image demonstrating the soft tissue margins, bony cortex and trabeculae of femur; care should be taken in kVp selection to reduce the inherent contrast in the femur

PCE COMMENTS – KNEE AND FEMUR

The Knee

There are various soft issue signs that can be seen even when a fracture is not obvious, such as a joint effusion within the ankle or knee joints, marked overlying soft tissue swelling or air trapped within the subcutaneous tissues, which is indicative of an open injury which may later be susceptible to infection.

The Patella

Rupture of the patellar tendon can be identified when a high position of the patella is visualised. In the normal patient the distance from the tibial tubercle to the lower pole of the patella should not exceed the length of the patella by more the 20%.[18]

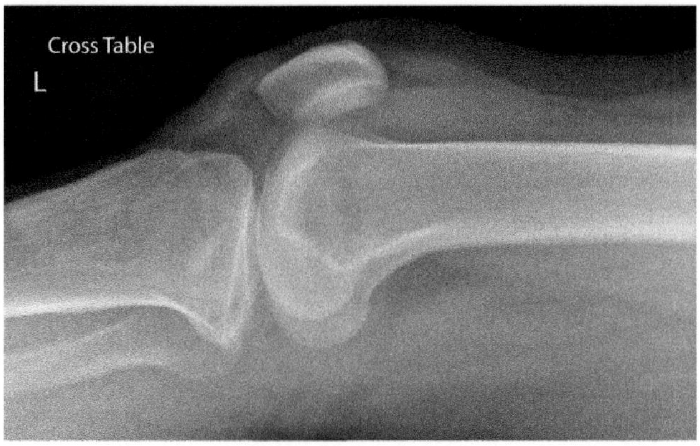

Fig. 7.13 Lipohaemarthrosis.

Patella fractures may be visualised on the AP and lateral projections; they can be vertical, horizontal or comminuted. Osteochondral fractures of the articular surface may be more subtle and may require an inferosuperior (skyline) projection. Fat–fluid levels in the suprapatellar bursa indicate an intra-articular fracture, even if one cannot be visualised.

A bipartite or tripartite patella may be present and this should not be confused with a fracture – they will have a well-defined corticated edge.[18]

Fractures of the Knee

Many fractures of the knee are relatively easy to detect, but some are more subtle. However, in some fractures, the only indication of an intra-articular fracture will be the presence of a lipohaemarthrosis, where a fat–fluid level is demonstrated on a horizontal beam lateral knee radiograph (Fig. 7.13).

Tibial plateau fractures may be difficult to see – check for sclerotic areas due to bone compression. The lateral margin may be displaced and this can be identified by the following rule:

a perpendicular line drawn at the most lateral margin of the femur should not have more than 5 mm of the adjacent margin of the tibia beyond it.[18]

Review the neck of the fibula for fractures. These fractures can be associated with ligament damage.[19]

Avulsion Fractures

The knee is a complex joint with multiple ligament insertions. A fracture of the intercondylar eminence commonly results from an avulsion of the anterior cruciate ligament. This is rare in adults, but may be seen in adolescents. A small avulsion of the lateral tibial plateau, called a Segond fracture, is associated with disruption of the anterior cruciate ligament in 75% of cases.[20]

The Femur

Fractures of the femur will be generally relatively easy to identify. However, there is one fracture type which is important not to miss, and which may be overlooked. Patients on bisphosphonate treatments for osteoporosis or cancer are at risk of atypical femoral fractures due to over-suppression of bone turnover (Fig. 7.14).

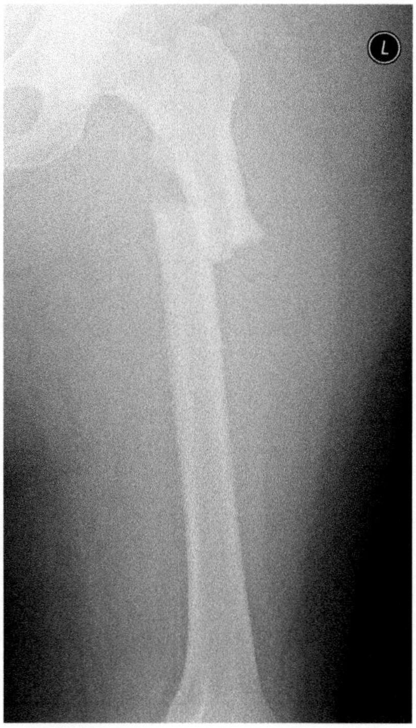

Fig. 7.14 Atypical femoral fracture.

Atypical femoral fractures may be complete, as in Fig. 7.14, in which case they are difficult to miss. However, it is important to detect incomplete atypical femoral fractures, since these will often require prophylactic surgical intervention. The lateral cortex of the femur should be examined for localised periosteal reactions resulting in thickening of the cortex, also referred to as 'beaking'. There may be a lucent line visualised within the thickened cortex. Many atypical femoral fractures are bilateral, so there should be consideration of imaging the contralateral side.

The American Society for Bone and Mineral Research have developed the following as characteristics of an atypical femoral fracture:

Major features

- Located anywhere along the femur from just distal to the lesser trochanter to just proximal to the supracondylar flare
- Associated with no trauma or minimal trauma, as in a fall from a standing height or less
- Transverse or short oblique configuration
- Non-comminuted
- Complete fractures extend through both cortices and may be associated with a medial spike; incomplete fractures involve only the lateral cortex

Minor features

- Localised periosteal reaction of the lateral cortex
- Generalised increase in cortical thickness of the diaphysis
- Prodromal symptoms such as dull or aching pain in the groin or thigh
- Bilateral fractures and symptoms
- Delayed healing
- Comorbid conditions (e.g., vitamin D deficiency, rheumatoid arthritis, hypophosphatasia)
- Use of pharmaceutical agents (e.g., bisphosphonates, glucocorticoids, proton pump inhibitors)[21]

Interpretation of fractures of the hip will be covered in Chapter 8.

References

1. Long BW, Rafert JA. *Orthopedic Radiography*. Philadelphia: Saunders; 1995.
2. Raby N, Berman L, de Lacey G. *Accident and Emergency Radiography: A Survival Guide*. 2nd ed. Philadelphia: Saunders; 2005.
3. European Commission Directorate-General for the Environment. *Radiation Protection 118: Referral Guidelines for Imaging*. Luxembourg: Office for Official Publications of the European Communities; 2000.
4. Burnett S, Taylor A, Watson M. *A–Z of Orthopaedic Radiology*. London: Saunders; 2000.
5. Murray J, Holmes E, Misra R. *A–Z of Musculoskeletal and Trauma Radiology*. Cambridge: Cambridge University Press; 2008:307–311.
6. Murray J, Holmes E, Misra R. *A–Z of Musculoskeletal and Trauma Radiology*. Cambridge: Cambridge University Press; 2008:326–331.
7. Manaster B. Tibial plateau fracture. In: Jeffrey R, et al., ed. *Diagnostic Imaging: Emergency*. Salt Lake City, UT: Amirsys; 2007:154–157. Part 1, section 4.
8. Chapin R. Patellar fracture. In: Jeffrey R, et al., *Diagnostic Imaging: Emergency*. Salt Lake City, UT: Amirsys; 2007:146–149. Part 1, section 4.
9. Vince AS, Singhania AK. What knee X-rays do we need? A survey of orthopaedic surgeons in the United Kingdom. *Knee*. 2000;7(2):101–104.
10. McQuillen-Martensen K. *Radiographic Image Analysis*. 3rd ed. Philadelphia: Saunders; 2010.
11. Eisenberg RL, et al. *Radiographic Positioning*. 2nd ed. Boston: Little Brown and Company; 1995.
12. Knipe H, et al. Knee (Beclere method intercondylar view). [online] Radiopaedia. https://radiopaedia.org/articles/knee-beclere-method-intercondylar-view).
13. Whitley AS, Sloane C, Hoadley G, et al. *Clark's Positioning in Radiography*. 12th ed. London: Hodder Arnold; 2005.
14. Bontrager KL. *Textbook of Radiographic Positioning and Related Anatomy*. 5th ed. St Louis: Mosby; 2001.
15. Bontrager KL, Lampignano JP. *Textbook of Radiographic Positioning and Related Anatomy*. 7th ed. St Louis: Mosby; 2010.
16. Unett EM, Royle AJ. *Radiographic Techniques and Image Evaluation*. London: Nelson Thornes; 1997.
17. Cole TJ. Secular trends in growth. *Nutr Sociol*. 2000;59(2):317–324.
18. Raby N, Berman L, de Lacey G. *Accident and Emergency Radiography: A Survival Guide*. 2nd ed. Philadelphia: Saunders; 2005:216–245.
19. El-Khoury GY, Daniel WW, Kathol MH. Acute and chronic avulsive injuries. *Radiol Clin North Am*. 1997;35:747–766.
20. Ling Y, Gaillard F. Segond fracture. [online] Radiopedia. https://radiopaedia.org/articles/segond-fracture.
21. Shane E, Burr D, Abrahamsen B, et al. Atypical subtrochanteric and diaphyseal femoral fractures: Second Report of a Task force of the American Society for bone and Mineral Research. *J Bone Miner Res*. 2014;29:1–23.

8 Pelvis and Hips

ELIZABETH CARVER, JEANETTE CARTER and MARIA MANFREDI

The pelvis and hips may be examined for assessment of trauma or pathology, and most commonly osteolytic or sclerotic lesions, degenerative change or congenital abnormality. In osteoarthritis, radiographic examination should only be performed if the patient is likely to require hip replacement.

Throughout this chapter a suggested FRD is given for each examination description; however, in practice a range of FRDs (typically from 100 cm to 120 cm) may be used, dependent on local protocol.

PCE COMMENTS – PELVIS AND HIPS

Note: it is important to assess the request, or even have a conversation with the referrer, regarding red flag areas. However, there is always a chance something unexpected will appear.

Trauma

The whole region should be assessed, so avoid the temptation to focus on obvious fractures; don't forget that the area is a bony ring and more than one region may be affected by trauma. Don't forget that the sacrum also forms part of the pelvic ring.

Assess *bony symmetry*, as asymmetry may be an indicator of open book fracture.

Follow the *sacroiliac joints*: disruption and asymmetry in these are significant and should be commented upon. These appearances can be missed as they can be subtle, or may be obscured by abdominal contents such as faecal matter or bowel gas.

Sacral fractures are under-diagnosed – take care to assess the sacral arcuate lines or 'sacral eyebrows' (Fig. 8.1), which should be contiguous (arched and smooth).[1] Loss of continuity of the arch is an indicator of fracture; classic appearance of a fracture is that the sacral eyebrow looks more like a tent than an arch.

Pelvic ring fractures may show as subtle steps or loss of alignment of the iliopectineal and ilioischeal lines (Fig. 8.1).

Iliopectineal and ilioischeal lines also assist in assessment of the acetabular ring, where fractures are often subtle: a lucent line leading from the acetabulum through to the iliopectineal and ilioischeal lines indicates acetabular fracture. This type of fracture may not even show displacement yet it carries severe implications if undetected.

Avulsion fractures may show as asymmetry in pelvic structures. Avulsion fractures of the ischial tuberosity and the anterior inferior iliac spine (AIIS) can present as a result of relatively low impact trauma or even as a result of sporting injury such as hamstring or rectus femoris injury. Hamstring attachment is at the ischial tuberosity and rectus femoris at AIIS, so it is important to check for small detail over these aspects of the pelvis. The commonest incidence of avulsion fractures in the pelvis is in children.

Neck of femur (NOF) fractures: Shenton's line (Fig. 8.1) shows NOF integrity or displacement. It follows the curve of the upper border of the obturator foramen and continues to travel inferiorly down the medial border of the femoral neck. This line can be used as a guide to compare the two sides when checking for injury, as a disruption in the normally smooth, curved line indicates subluxation, dislocation or change in femoral neck position as a result of fracture. The primary function of the line is to assess for NOF fracture: check for loss of alignment of the line in the neck and linear bands of sclerosis or lucent lines seen across the line, as these appearances are considered significant. Lucency across the line indicates fractured NOF and a sclerotic line may indicate an impacted fracture. A line drawn along the middle of the long axis of the femoral neck should bisect the femoral head (Fig. 8.1).

Intertrochanteric fractures are usually easily spotted and this highlights the importance of including all trochanters on the image, *and* in the correct projection *if* patient presentation permits. Although a forgone conclusion, it must be stressed that fractures of the femoral neck and/or trochanters must be brought to the attention of the referrer quickly, to ensure correct patient management begins as soon as possible.

Slipped upper femoral epiphysis (SUFE): the epiphysis is displaced, usually posteriorly and medially, and the patient often presents with spontaneous groin pain. Age groups to look out for are 8–15 (girls) and 10–17 (boys). Check if there is an increase in density over the proximal metaphysis (due to the capital epiphysis being superimposed over NOF) and also the line of Klein (a line along the *lateral* femoral neck which should intersect the *lateral* epiphysis);[2] if the line does not intersect the lateral section of the epiphysis, then this is suspicious. Also look for metaphyseal displacement.

Hip dysplasias: most commonly seen in children. Use Shenton's line to check alignment of the same structures as used in assessment of the adult pelvis. Abnormalities often show with accompanying shallow acetabular ring.

Perthes' disease: this childhood disease of the upper femoral epiphysis manifests as osteonecrosis of the capital femoral epiphysis[3] where the growing epiphysis shows ischaemic changes and abnormal growth. It presents most commonly in children aged 4–9 years, and boys are four times more likely to be affected than girls.[4] Perthes shows with the femoral head epiphysis as sclerotic, small and irregular in outline. The head can appear flattened and should be compared with the other femoral head but, uncommonly, Perthes can be bilateral. Frog lateral is required for accurate assessment of Perthes (see Chapter 19).

Degenerative Disease

Osteoarthritis: check for acetabular narrowing and sclerosis of the acetabulum and osteophytic lipping.

Avascular necrosis of the hip (AVN): initially presents on X-ray as a linear 'crescent sign' (subarticular lucency in the

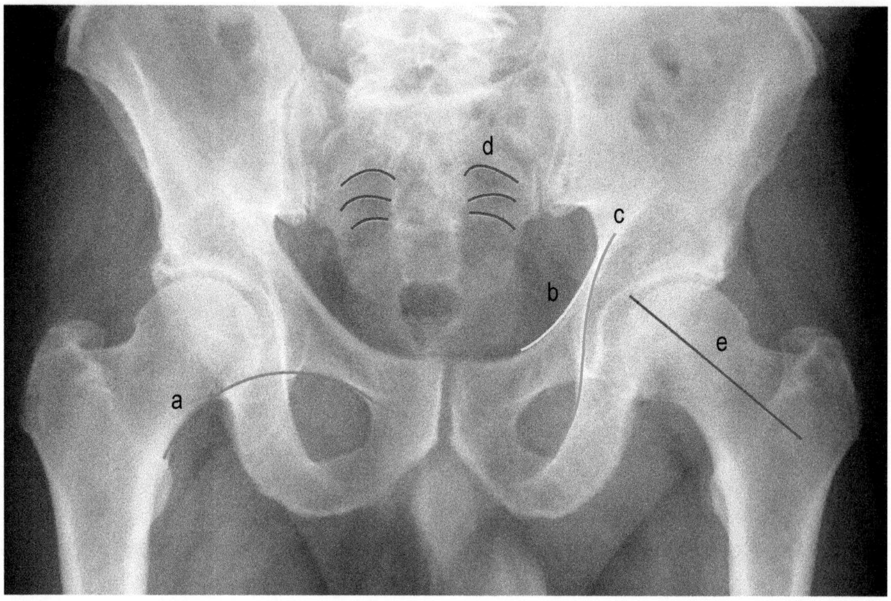

Fig. 8.1 Assessment lines: *a*, Shenton's line; *b*, iliopectineal line; *c*, ilioischial line; *d*, sacral arcuate lines; line *e* should bisect the femoral head if this region is uninjured.

femoral head running parallel to the superior femoral head). This can show on AP and/or a lateral projection. AVN progresses to flattening of the femoral head. It is important to differentiate between AVN and OA when making a clinical diagnosis, so it is important to comment as accurately as possible. AVN is more speedy in progression than OA but treatment is the same (hip prosthesis).

Metastatic and Malignant Disease

Look for lucent or sclerotic lesions which can appear anywhere in the pelvis and hip region. Myeloma will show osteolytic lesions.

Paget's Disease

There will be sclerotic (very dense) and misshapen bone caused by bone resorption, formation and remodelling. Classically this is described as a cotton wool appearance. It is easy to focus on an immediately obvious area affected by Paget's disease and therefore important to check all of the pelvis and upper femora for other suspicious appearances.

Other Diseases of the Hip and Femoral Head

Hip dysplasias: most commonly seen in children. Use Shenton's line to check alignment of the same structures as used in assessment of the adult pelvis. Abnormalities often show with accompanying shallow acetabular ring.

Perthes' disease: this childhood disease of the upper femoral epiphysis manifests as osteonecrosis of the capital femoral epiphysis[3] where the growing epiphysis shows ischaemic changes and abnormal growth. It presents most commonly in children aged 4–9 years, and boys are four times more likely to be affected than girls.[4] Perthes shows with the femoral head epiphysis as sclerotic, small and irregular in outline. The head can appear flattened and should be compared with the other femoral head but, uncommonly, Perthes can be bilateral. Frog lateral is required for accurate assessment of Perthes (see Chapter 19).

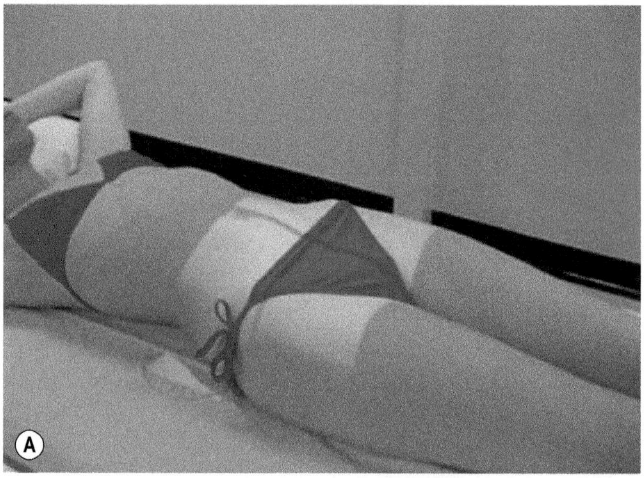

Fig. 8.2 (A) Supine AP pelvis and hips.

ANTEROPOSTERIOR (AP) PELVIS AND HIPS (FIG. 8.2A–C)

The AP pelvis has traditionally been undertaken supine[5–7] but there has been more recent suggestion that a weight-bearing approach may be more appropriate in some cases.[8] In any case, requirements for the examination may indicate that either the whole pelvis and both hips should be included on the image, or the region of hips only. The 'hips only' projection is usually requested for follow-up after hip replacement surgery and may be referred to as a 'low centred' pelvis. However, it is a valid and recognised projection, having been described in texts for many years.[6,7,9] Radiographers should not, therefore, assume that this is simply a 'mis-centred pelvis' and consider it to be a suboptimal procedure. Field size is as for the pelvis and hips AP, as it is often necessary to include a longer section of the femur to ensure the whole length of hip prosthesis is demonstrated (if relevant).

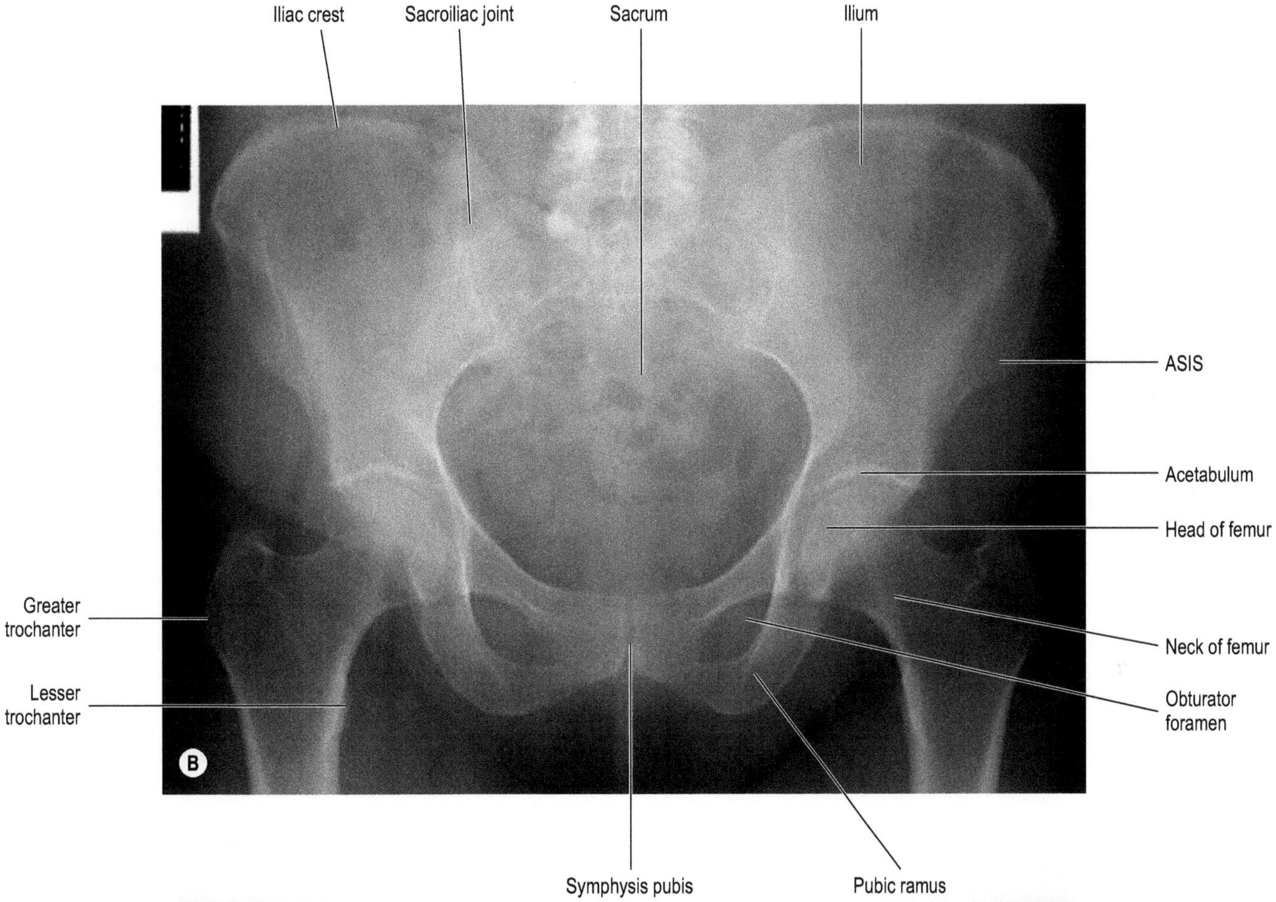

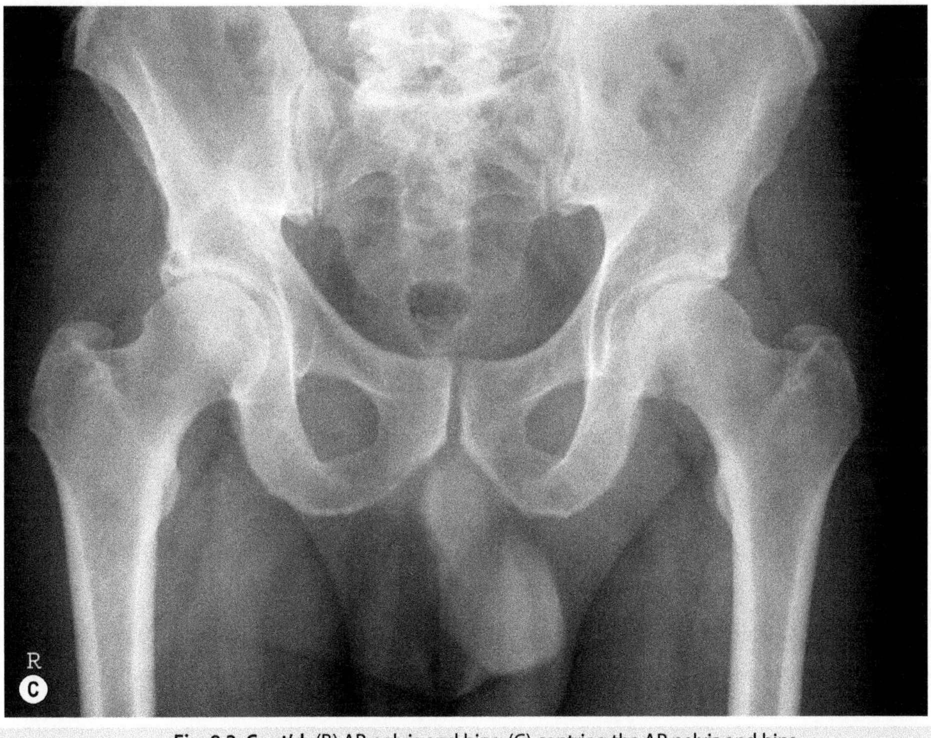

Fig. 8.2, Cont'd (B) AP pelvis and hips; (C) centring the AP pelvis and hips.

Regarding use of an erect weightbearing technique, standardisation for positioning should be ensured by using a hand support to ensure stability and an adjustable footprint indicator to provide the correct degree of internal rotation required to bring the femoral necks parallel to the IR.[8]

The IR is horizontal for the supine technique, or vertical for the erect technique. An antiscatter grid is employed (for adults and older children).

The 28-day rule should always be used in women of reproductive capacity when examining this area.

Positioning – Supine Technique

- The patient lies supine on the table with their legs extended and their head resting on a pillow (Fig. 8.2A)
- The median sagittal plane (MSP) is at 90° to the table-top and the anterior superior iliac spines (ASISs) should be equal distance from the table-top; this ensures minimal rotation
- The arms are raised onto the pillow
- The legs are slightly internally rotated to bring the necks of femora parallel to the table-top

Positioning – Erect Technique

- The patient stands with their back to the IR and separates their feet until at the required internally rotated position, holding a hand support to ensure immobilisation
- The MSP is at 90° to the IR and the ASISs should be equal distance from it
- The legs are slightly internally rotated to bring the necks of femora parallel to the table-top

For both methods the feet are internally rotated slightly during positioning to bring them into the true anatomical position and allow the NOF to lie parallel to the IR.[7] This facilitates demonstration of the femoral neck with minimal foreshortening, and also clears the greater trochanter from the femoral neck, the lesser trochanter appearing in profile medially. As the femoral neck has normal anteversion of between 10 to 15°, the patient's legs should be internally rotated 10–15° at the hip joint.

In the case of trauma, the supine approach is always used and the patient's foot position can provide an indication of a fractured NOF, when they will present with the affected leg in noticeable external rotation, often with the lateral aspect of the foot in contact with the trolley-top; there is usually apparent shortening of the leg. No attempt must be made to move or internally rotate this leg.[3]

Overexposure of the greater trochanters can be a problem in this projection, particularly in thin patients who have little soft tissue in this region. This can be resolved by careful consideration of exposure factors: a reduction in mAs will reduce the degree of image blackening, and to cater for this a kVp of at least 70 will reduce the level of subject contrast.[7] It is suggested that a minimum of 70 kVp be used in all AP pelvis examinations.

Some patients will present with a body shape that is relatively slim over the legs and hip joint but larger over the pelvis and abdomen. This shape appears to occur most frequently in elderly women and can pose a problem in producing an image with a useful range of densities. The use of a kVp even higher than 70 may be useful in these cases, as the central region of the pelvis may appear underexposed when the hips appear correctly exposed (and vice versa) on the image when insufficient kVp is used. Use of an automatic exposure device can create problems in patients with this type of build: use of the outer chambers will result in termination of exposure related to thinner body tissue areas, therefore the central pelvic area will be of low radiographic density; use of the central chamber may mean that the area over the hips is over-blackened.

Beam Direction and FRD

Supine AP: vertical at 90° to the IR
Erect AP: horizontal at 90° to the IR
115–120 cm FRD

Note that the focus receptor distance (FRD) suggested is longer than the 100 cm used for the majority of radiographic projections. The buttocks elevate the pelvis, which is a relatively large structure, thereby increasing object receptor distance (ORD) and magnification of the pelvis. The larger pelvis will potentially be less likely to be included within the perimeter of the IR; to overcome this, increasing the FRD reduces this magnification and improves on image sharpness.

Those patients with a noticeably larger amount of adipose tissue will, in effect, find their pelvis raised even higher above the IR than slimmer patients. Therefore, FRD of 120 cm is recommended in these patients.

Centring Point

For pelvis and hips: in the midline, midway between the ASIS and the upper border of the symphysis pubis

While centring, it is wise to check that the tops of the iliac crests lie within the upper border of the IR; this will ensure that the maximum amount of anatomy distal to the iliac crests is demonstrated on the image.

For hips: in the midline, 2.5 cm above the superior border of the symphysis pubis (the upper border of the symphysis pubis is located level with the greater trochanters)

Collimation

For pelvis and hips: iliac crests, proximal portion of femora, greater and lesser trochanters

The IR may be aligned with the X-ray beam before examining the patient[7] and collimation can be adjusted at this. This avoids the temptation to open the collimators wider than necessary when X-raying a larger than average patient.

For hips: acetabulae, greater and lesser trochanters, upper third of femur or full length of the prosthesis (if present)

If previous images are available it is recommended that they be viewed to establish the length of any surgical device that may be present in the hip/s to ensure that the IR is positioned correctly for their inclusion.

Criteria for Assessing Image Quality

- Iliac crests and greater and lesser trochanters are demonstrated for full pelvis, acetabulae, trochanters and appropriate amount of femur for the hips only
- Iliac bones, heads and necks of femora and the greater and lesser trochanters and obturator foramina should be symmetrical
- Sharp image demonstrating the range of densities of the bony cortex and trabeculae of the pelvis and its soft tissues, hips and trochanters

Common Errors: AP Pelvis and Hips

Common Errors	Possible Reasons	Potential Effects on PCE or Report
Asymmetry of structures	MSP not 90° to table-top (rotated patient). This could be due to muscular atrophy or simply the patient lying awkwardly. Use of radiolucent pads may help correct this in the case of muscular atrophy. The notable features in the pelvis are the obturator foraminae and iliac bones; study of a rotated pelvis image will show a larger obtutator foramen (compared with the other obturator foramen) and narrowed ilium on the side that is *raised* from the table	Symmetry of the pelvis is identified as important in the PCE Comments of this chapter. As a result, asymmetry will compromise assessment of the following: open book fracture; sacroiliac joint fractures and dislocations; avulsion fractures; pubic rami fractures; NOF to check for fractures; SUFE; Perthes'; AVN
Greater trochanters obscured and overlying the NOF	Feet are not internally rotated (but this is unavoidable in patients with fractured NOF)	Not possible to exclude subtle fracture of NOF, as the neck will seem artificially foreshortened
Overexposed image (see section after Positioning, for overexposure of the greater trochanters and uneven exposure of hips and pelvis)	If an automatic exposure device (AED) has been used for a patient with hip prostheses the exposure will continue for longer than necessary to try to expose the hips correctly. An AED device should not be utilised if a patient has a hip prosthesis There are other problems associated with AED use (see comments after the Positioning section for the pelvis). Setting a manual exposure is a suitable solution in both events described there. Digital manipulation can help, especially if within acceptable range on indicator	Affects appearance of sacrum, sacral eyebrows and sacroiliac joints in particular (see PCE Comments). Disruption and symmetry in these are significant and may be missed if exposure factors are inappropriate Subtle fractures may be missed (all areas) Subtle lucency indicative of AVN may be missed Small lesions indicative of metastatic disease may be missed

ANTEROPOSTERIOR (AP) SINGLE HIP (FIG. 8.3A,B)

This projection is most likely to be undertaken as a post-operative check after hip replacement surgery.

IR is horizontal, an antiscatter grid is employed

Positioning

- Initial positioning is as for AP pelvis
- The leg of the side under examination is slightly internally rotated
- The unaffected leg is abducted to clear it from the radiation field

Beam Direction and FRD

Vertical at 90° to IR

100 cm FRD

Centring Point

Over the femoral pulse

The femoral pulse (and therefore the centre of the head of femur) is located thus: draw an imaginary line from the ASIS to the upper border of the symphysis pubis; bisect this line perpendicularly and then locate a point 2.5 cm distally along this bisecting line (Fig. 8.4).

Collimation

ASIS, greater and lesser trochanters, proximal third of femur; full length of prosthesis if relevant

Criteria for Assessing Image Quality

- ASIS, proximal third of the femur and trochanters are demonstrated
- Greater trochanter is seen cleared from and laterally to the NOF, and slightly in profile
- Lesser trochanter is visible on the medial aspect of the femur
- Obturator foramen is seen 'open' and not obscured by the ischium
- Sharp image demonstrating the soft tissue margins, bony cortex and trabeculae of the distal ilium, ischium and proximal femora while demonstrating the greater trochanter

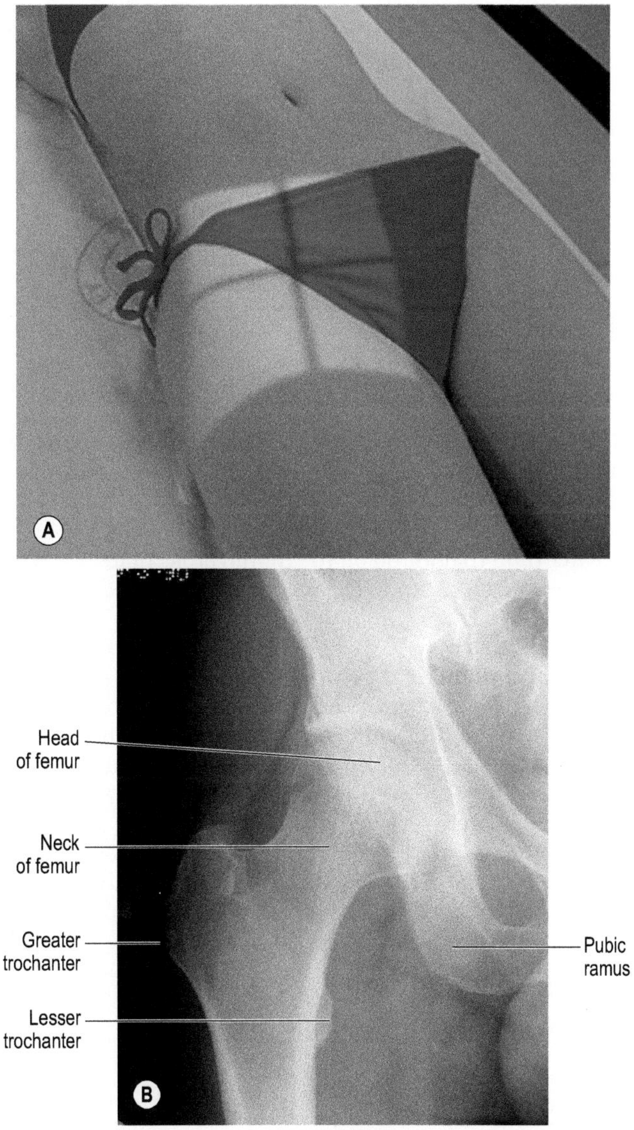

Fig. 8.3 AP single hip.

Common Errors: AP Single Hip		
Common Errors	**Possible Reasons**	**Potential Effects on PCE or Report**
Length of hip prosthesis not fully demonstrated	Inaccurate centring or presence of prosthesis not known or considered. Ensure previous images are available to view and if necessary, use a larger IR or field	If the complete section that includes cement and ball bearing is not seen, fracture or damage through the cement may be missed
Greater trochanter obscured and overlying the NOF	Lack of internal rotation	As for AP pelvis
Overexposed image	See discussion section under AP pelvis above, for overexposure of the greater trochanters and use of automatic exposure device (AED) for patients with hip replacement	Subtle fractures may be missed

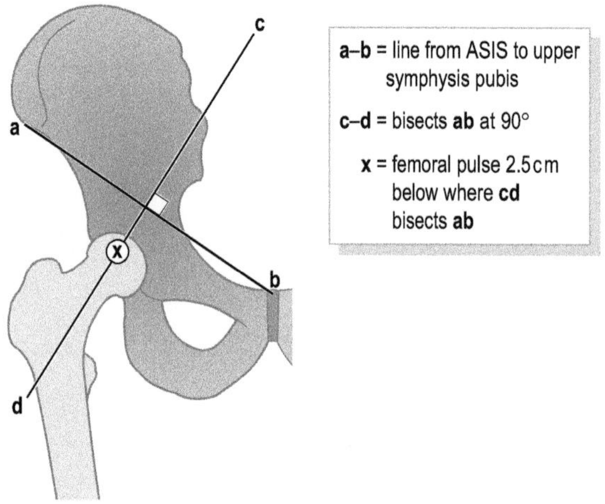

Fig. 8.4 Location of femoral pulse.

LATERAL OBLIQUE SINGLE HIP (FIG. 8.5A,B)

This projection must not be used in the case of trauma and is usually performed to supplement an AP pelvis when examining patients with non-specific hip pain. However, its use is rarely justified, as information gained is not significantly greater than that found on the AP hip projection.

IR is horizontal, an antiscatter grid is employed

Positioning

- Initial positioning is as for AP pelvis
- The MSP is 90° to the table; from this position the patient is rotated laterally through 45° onto the side under examination and supported in this position with foam pads
- The knee and hip are flexed and externally rotated to bring the lateral aspect of the thigh in contact with the table-top; the more flexion at the knee, the easier the patient finds it to achieve and maintain this position
- The arms are rested on the pillow

Beam Direction and FRD

Vertical at 90° to the IR

100 cm FRD

Centring Point

Over the femoral pulse (see Centring Point for AP single hip)

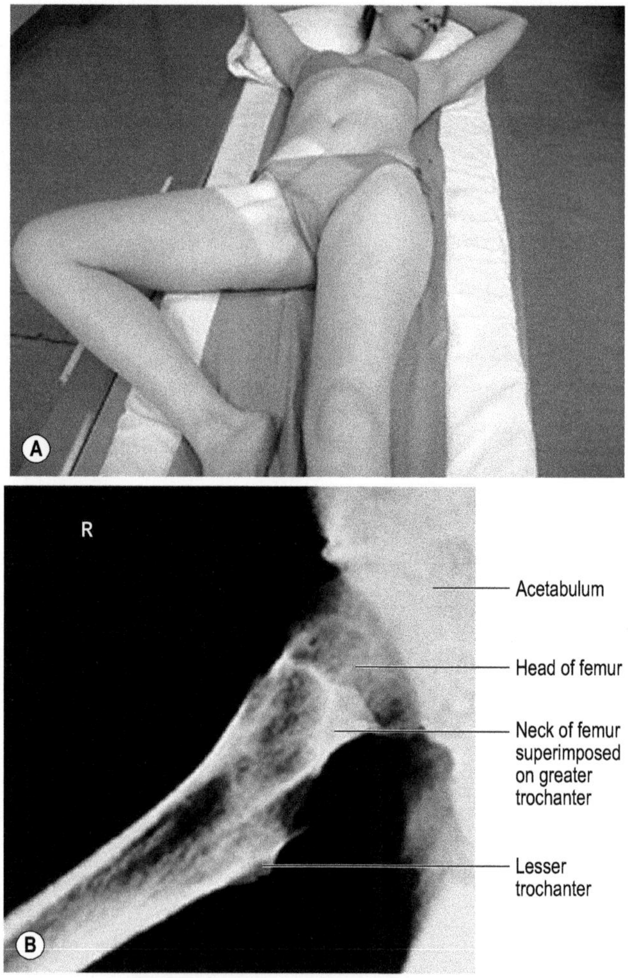

Fig. 8.5 (A) Lateral oblique single hip. (B) Lateral oblique. (B, Reproduced with permission from Bryan GJ. *Skeletal Anatomy*. 3rd ed. Edinburgh: Churchill Livingstone; 1996 and Gunn C. *Bones and Joints*. 4th ed. Edinburgh: Churchill Livingstone; 2002.)

Collimation

ASIS, greater and lesser trochanters, anterior and posterior soft tissue outline of the femur

If, after positioning, the long axis of the femur lies obliquely across the table-top, rotate the light beam diaphragm to coincide with the long axis of the femur, to enable closer collimation.

Criteria for Assessing Image Quality

- Acetabulum and proximal third of femur are demonstrated
- Greater trochanter is superimposed over the NOF
- Lesser trochanter is seen in profile on the medial aspect of the upper femur
- Ischium and pubic ramus will be superimposed
- Sharp image demonstrating the bony cortex and trabeculae of the proximal femora with sufficient penetration to demonstrate the acetabulum

Common Error: Lateral Oblique Single Hip

Common Error	Possible Reason	Potential Effect on PCE or Reporting
Hyperdense area over the hip, increasing distally over the femoral shaft. Foreshortened femoral neck; the greater trochanter not superimposed over the NOF	Inadequate external rotation of the leg can cause these errors. The cause is usually inadequate flexion of the knee and insufficient rotation of the patient towards the side under examination; good knee flexion facilitates more comfortable and correct external rotation until the thigh is in contact with the table	The full extent and position of any prosthesis may not be shown adequately

HORIZONTAL BEAM LATERAL FOR NECK OF FEMUR (FIG. 8.6A,B)

Two initial approaches to positioning are given here, one to allow for tube angulation and the other to oblique the trolley as an alternative; both result in the same projection.

This projection must always be used if a lateral is required in cases of hip or pelvic trauma, and following surgery to the hip. In these cases it is inadvisable to move the patient, but a projection at 90° to the AP projection is still often required. It is the most frequent lateral performed on the hip, despite being described in most texts as an adaptation to technique. Despite this extensive use, discussion suggests that it need not be employed routinely in all cases of hip injury, and that an AP alone may be sufficient.[10]

The NOF lies at 45° to the MSP and correct positioning of the IR, at 45° to the MSP and parallel to the NOF, will produce an image of the femoral neck at 90° to the AP hip image. The IR is best positioned using a 45° radiolucent pad placed next to the patient's thigh (see Positioning section).

As the projection requires the use of a medial approach to the hip, with horizontal beam, the unaffected leg must be cleared from the primary beam. This is achieved by the use of a leg support; this support must be radiolucent and with a comfortable lower leg and foot rest. One example of this is the 'Poole' leg support (Fig. 8.7). Great consideration for the maintenance of patient dignity and comfort is essential when positioning the leg on the support, as the position can be difficult to achieve, revealing what is considered a very private area (patients are often in a hospital gown after removal of clothing for clinical assessment). Maintenance of patient dignity and comfort at all times is paramount.

Care should be taken when selecting exposure factors, as the inherent contrast of this area is high, from the dense hip joint down to the shaft of femur; the use of a compensating filter should therefore be considered.[11]

Positioning

Method 1 – Tube Angulation (Fig. 8.8A)

- A grid is usually employed with method 1 to reduce scatter in image production
- The patient is supine on the emergency trolley, with the MSP perpendicular to the trolley-top. The long axis of the trolley should be parallel to the ceiling track of the X-ray tube
- The MSP should also be coincident with the long axis of the trolley *or parallel to the ceiling track of the X-ray tube if the patient is lying obliquely on the trolley*

Method 2 (Fig. 8.8B)

- The X-ray tube is positioned next to the unaffected side, its light beam housing directed horizontally and 90° towards the patient
- The trolley is then rotated to bring the leg on the patient's unaffected side nearer to the X-ray tube, until the patient's MSP is at 45° to the beam

Both Methods

- The IR is placed vertically. The upper edge of the IR is adjacent to, and gently pushed into, the soft tissues immediately above the iliac crest on the affected side; it is then positioned at 45° to the MSP and parallel with the NOF (this must be done with great care to avoid discomfort to the patient)
- The use of a 45° foam pad between the patient and IR aids in correct assessment of receptor angle for this positioning
- The holder is then adjusted to ensure that the IR and grid are pressed firmly down onto the mattress; this prevents the ischial tuberosity being omitted from the image
- A leg support (see Fig. 8.7) is placed on the table-top and the unaffected leg is flexed at the knee and hip to bring the anterior aspect of the femur as close to the trunk as possible (and at least into the vertical position to prevent superimposition of the thigh on the image). Vertical position of the thigh is vital to clearance of soft tissue from the head of femme and acetabulum
- The ankle and foot are placed on the leg support. The greater the knee flexion, the more effective the clearance of the thigh from the hip under examination. If the patient's condition permits slight external rotation of the uninjured limb, this will clear the soft tissues of this thigh even more efficiently

Studies have shown that a viable option is to use an air gap of approximately 60 cm between the IR and the patient when using method 2 for the trolley position, and with an increased FRD to counteract image magnification. The IR can be supported in an erect stand for this method. The method is advocated as a radiation dose-reducing technique,[12] reducing dose by negating the use of a grid. FRD should be a minimum of 3 metres.[13]

Note that, if using an air gap, the IR will *not* be in contact with the patient, and it is important to ensure the area of interest will lie within the IR boundaries at this increased FRD.

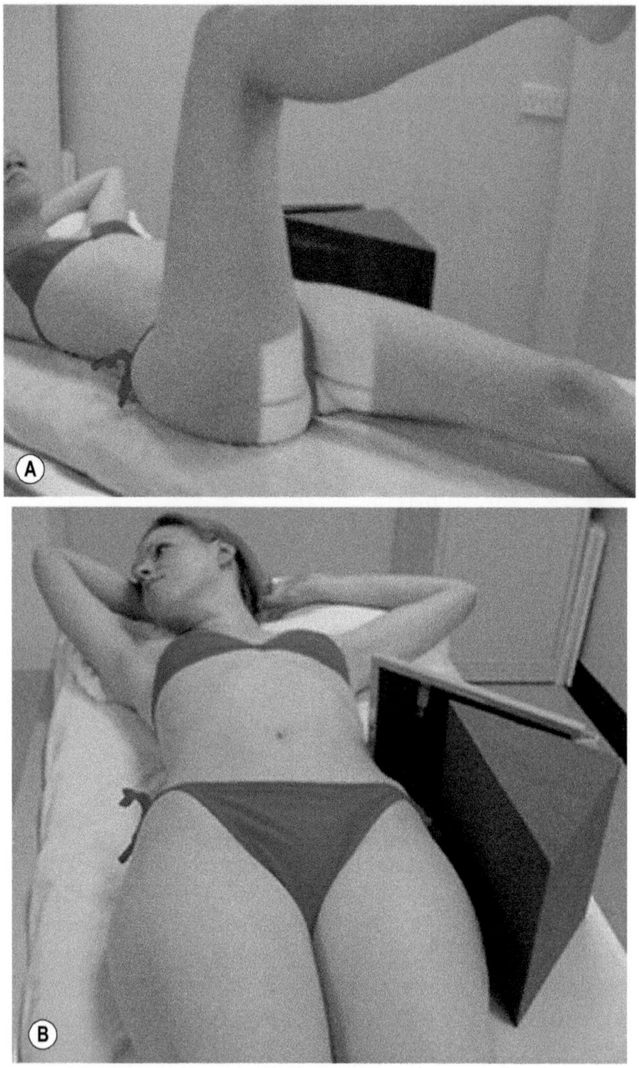

Fig. 8.6 (A) Horizontal beam lateral for NOF – method 1. (B) Cassette position for horizontal beam lateral hip, positioned before the thigh is raised.

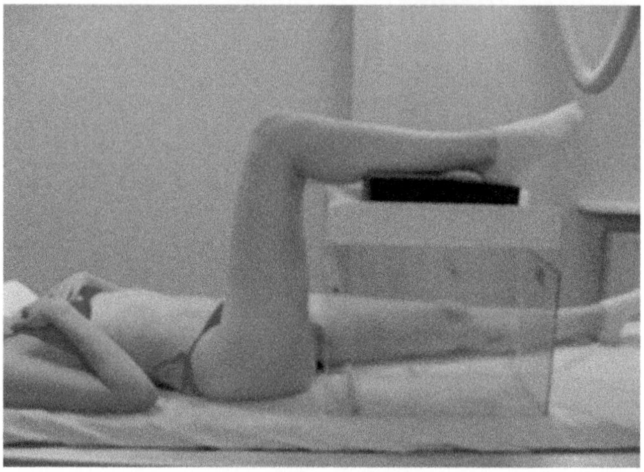

Fig. 8.7 'Poole' leg support.

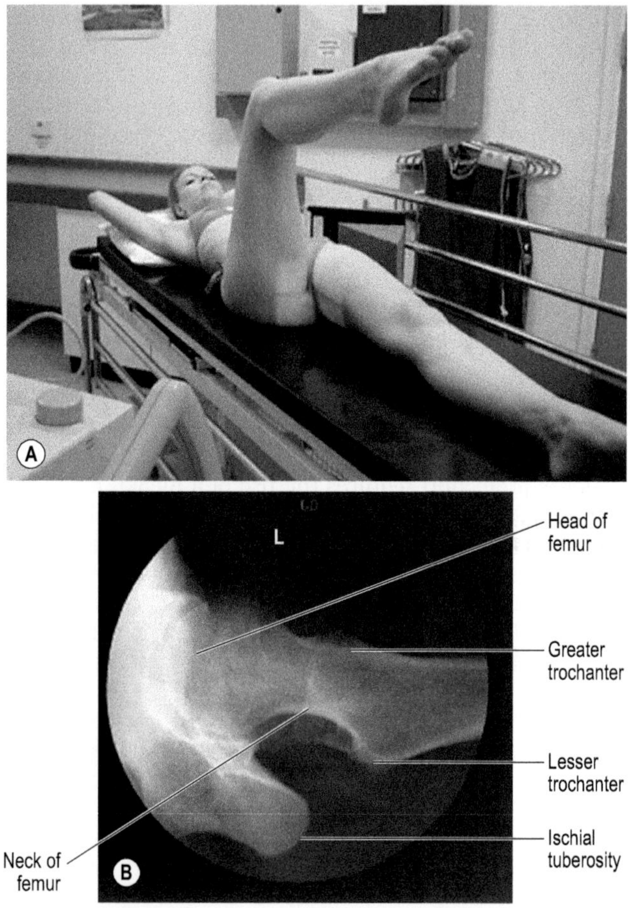

Fig. 8.8 (A) Horizontal beam lateral for NOF – method 2. (B) Horizontal beam lateral. (B, Reproduced with permission from Ballinger P, Frank E. *Pocket Guide to Radiography*. 5th ed. St Louis: Mosby; 2003.)

Beam Direction and FRD

Horizontal at 90° to the IR (the tube will require 45° rotational adjustment to achieve this in method 1, but not method 2 where the trolley has been rotated 45°)

100 cm FRD; 3 m FRD for air gap technique

Centring Point

To the middle of crease of the internal and medial aspect of the groin of the affected leg

Collimation

Acetabulum, proximal femur, trochanters, anterior and posterior soft tissue outlines

Criteria for Assessing Image Quality

- Head of femur and acetabulum clearly demonstrated
- Greater trochanter superimposed on NOF
- Lesser trochanter superimposed inferiorly on greater trochanter
- Soft tissue shadowing of raised thigh cleared from head and neck of femur
- Ischial tuberosity demonstrated posteriorly
- Sharp image demonstrating the soft tissue margins of the thigh, bony cortex and trabeculae of the head neck and proximal femur. The kVp chosen should be sufficient to demonstrate the acetabulum and head of femur, but the femoral neck should not be over-penetrated

Common Errors: HBL Neck of Femur

Common Errors	Possible Reasons	Potential Effects on PCE or Report
The acetabulum and joint space not clearly demonstrated (dense soft tissue shadow overlying area)	The soft tissues of the opposite leg have obscured the area of interest and the exposure factors used were insufficient to penetrate them. Flex the knee and hip of the opposite leg to a greater degree	Fractures and dislocations of the region may be missed, especially if subtle
Part of the image has grid cut off (if a grid is used)	The grid is either not in a vertical position or the central ray is not at 90° to the grid	Affects contrast that is vital for assessment of fractures and dislocations
The acetabulum and joint space are clearly demonstrated but the NOF is overexposed	Incorrect exposure factors may have been chosen, check that the exposure index is within acceptable range and post process image to improve quality. Consider the use of a filter	Affects contrast that is vital for assessment of fractures
The image appears very grey and it is difficult to distinguish features	The benefit of effective collimation cannot be underestimated. Insufficient collimation results in too much scattered radiation reaching the receptor. Collimate more closely and consider the use of a lead rubber sheet over the anterior aspect of the patient's thigh on the side under examination	Affects report or PCE as in all comments above

Acetabulum

Acetabular fractures carry significant clinical sequelae but are difficult to assess in some cases, for example when the femoral head has pushed through the acetabulum but sprung back by the time the radiograph is taken, leaving only subtle soft tissue signs. Correct recognition and classification of acetabular fracture is essential and this is best achieved by obtaining CT data that can be used in 3D reconstruction.[14]

The techniques described here are sometimes referred to as Judet obliques, first described by the brothers Judet in 1964;[3] the two obliques can be distinguished from each other by using the terms 'acetabulum en face' and 'profile'[7] which are quite meaningful terms when considering the aspect of the acetabulum demonstrated by each projection. The projections, if taken in conjunction with an AP pelvis, allow for a more complete assessment of the acetabulum. Both obliques are necessary for a complete examination.

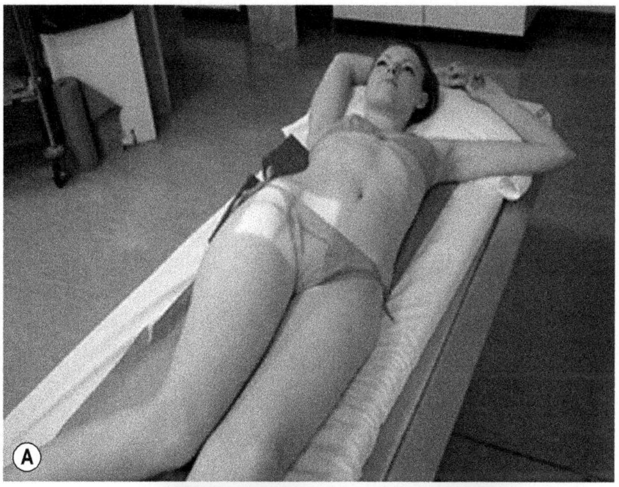

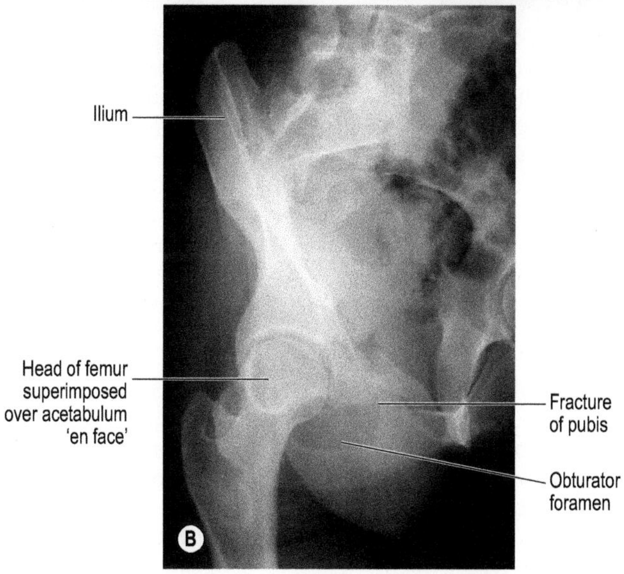

Fig. 8.9 Acetabulum posterior rim/obturator oblique.

ACETABULUM POSTERIOR RIM/EN FACE/ OBTURATOR OBLIQUE (FIG. 8.9A,B)

IR is horizontal, an antiscatter grid is employed

Positioning

- The patient lies supine on the table with their legs extended and their head resting on a pillow
- Initially the MSP is 90° to the table; from this position the patient's trunk is rotated through 45°, *away* from the side under examination
- The raised side is supported in this position with radiolucent pads

ACETABULUM ANTERIOR RIM/PROFILE/ILIAC OBLIQUE (FIG. 8.10A,B)

IR is horizontal, an antiscatter grid is employed

Positioning

- The patient lies supine on the table with their legs extended and their head resting on a pillow
- Initially the MSP is 90° to the table; from this position the patient's trunk is rotated through 45° *towards* the side under examination
- The raised side is supported in this position with radiolucent pads

Beam Direction and FRD

Vertical at 90° to the IR
100 cm FRD

Centring Point

Over the femoral pulse (see Fig. 8.4)

Collimation

ASIS, ischium, pubic ramus

The obliques described should be undertaken when a complete orthopaedic assessment of the patient's pelvis has been carried out and it has been established that the pelvis is stable enough for movement. If not, and it is possible to lower the unaffected side of the pelvis, the projection for acetabulum en face can be undertaken as normal. For acetabulum in profile the patient remains in this position and the IR is supported vertically behind the raised side, using a horizontal central ray. Centre over the raised hip.

If injury to both acetabulae is suspected it is possible to examine one acetabulum in the en face position while the opposite one is in the lateral position, and vice versa, with wider collimation to include both sides on one image. This will cut the number of exposures from four to two but, by centring in the midline, the accuracy of the resulting radiograph of each acetabulum will not be as assured as when performing separate well-centred projections. The central portion of the pelvis will also be irradiated, when it is likely that this area would not be irradiated if four well-collimated exposures were made.

If there is access to a fluoroscopy suite with transverse C-arm rotational function, the injured patient can be moved across onto the table, using a suitable patient handling aid, and be examined using this equipment. The C-arm is rotated through 45° towards either side and this will achieve the same images as described above. This technique could potentially be used with an ordinary X-ray tube and table, but problems with cross-gridding arise unless the bucky can be adjusted to bring the grid slats 90° to the long axis of the table-top. Using a stationary grid can allow the grid slats to be placed in the correct direction, but this method does require placement of the IR in a holder under the table or trolley, and will depend on the type of imaging system available. Equipment which employs a virtual grid rather than a physical grid may mitigate these problems.

Criteria for Assessing Image Quality

Acetabulum Posterior Rim/En Face/Obturator Oblique

- The head and neck of femur are demonstrated with the acetabular rim outlined as a circle ('en face')
- The posterior rim of the acetabulum is particularly well demonstrated
- The ilium is demonstrated in profile with the obturator foramen seen open
- Sharp image demonstrating the bony cortex and trabeculae of the head of femur and cortical outline of the acetabular rim

Acetabulum Anterior Rim/Profile/Iliac Oblique

- The anterior acetabular rim is superimposed across the head of femur
- The iliac wing is seen 'en-face' and without foreshortening
- The ischial spine is demonstrated in profile medial to the acetabulum
- Sharp image demonstrating the bony cortex and trabeculae of the head of femur and cortical outline of the acetabular rim

LATERAL ILIUM AND ANTEROPOSTERIOR (AP) ILIUM

IR and Positioning

Lateral ilium: As for the acetabulum posterior rim/obturator oblique position (see Fig. 8.9A)

AP ilium: As for the acetabulum anterior rim/iliac oblique position (see Fig. 8.10A)

Beam Direction and FRD for Both Projections

Vertical at 90° to the IR
100 cm FRD

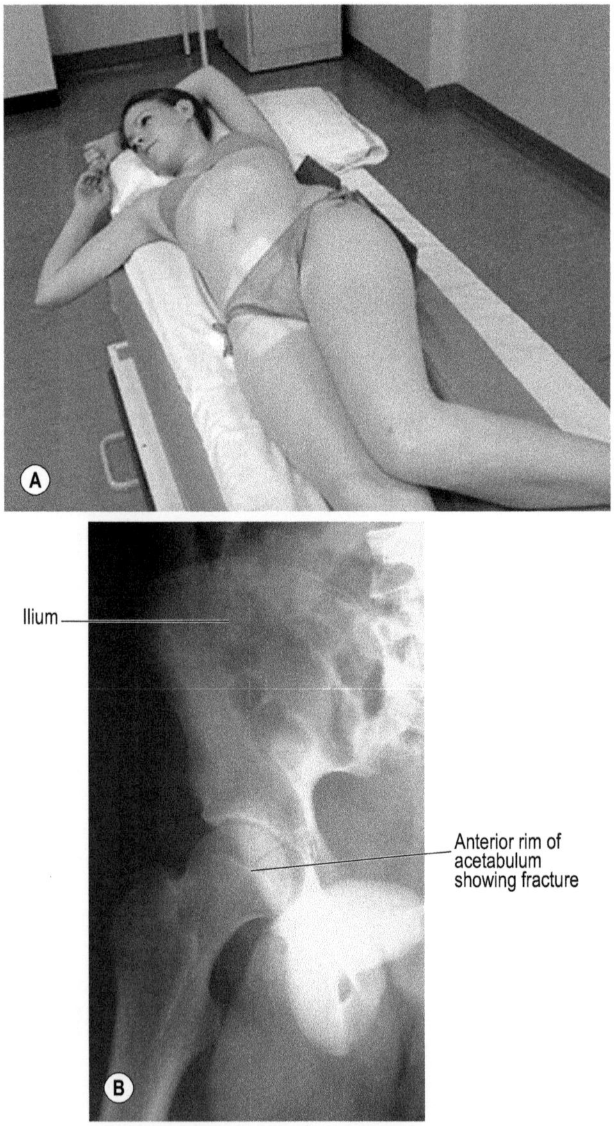

Fig. 8.10 Acetabulum anterior rim/iliac oblique position.

Centring Point

Lateral ilium: Over the ASIS of the raised side

AP ilium: Midway between the midline and the ASIS of the raised side

Collimation

Sacroiliac joint, iliac crest, ischium, pubic ramus

Criteria for Assessing Image Quality

Lateral Ilium

- Iliac crest, symphysis pubis, sacroiliac joint and ASIS are demonstrated
- Ilium is demonstrated in profile
- Opening of the obturator foramen as compared to the AP pelvis
- Sharp image demonstrating the bony cortex and trabecular patterns of the ilium, pubis, acetabulum and femoral head

AP Ilium

- Iliac crest, symphysis pubis, sacroiliac joints and ASIS are demonstrated
- Ilium demonstrated 'en face' with the iliac fossa seen without foreshortening
- Obturator foramen will appear closed
- Sharp image demonstrating the bony cortex and trabecular patterns of the ilium, acetabulum and femoral head

Pelvimetry

The imaging examination of the maternal pelvis is known as pelvimetry. In circumstances when obstetricians need to decide whether a caesarean section is required, accurate measurements of the pelvic inlet and outlet are taken and compared with the biparietal diameter of the baby's skull, which has been measured during ultrasound examination. Any cephalopelvic disproportion can then be established. The examination is usually performed around the 38th week of pregnancy when the radiation risk to the viable fetus has been reduced. In some circumstances the examination is taken after a caesarean section to establish the mother's measurements for future pregnancy and delivery.

In the last decade of the 20th century, accurate CT became the method of choice for this assessment, superseding the traditional method of plain film pelvimetry. Although CT is seen as a high-dose examination, CT pelvimetry involves a relatively low-dose yet accurate technique compared to plain X-ray pelvimetry.[15] One method uses AP and lateral scanogram/scout scans to identify the fovea over the femoral heads and a single axial CT slice to take the pelvimetric measurement. Alternatively, a single lateral scanogram from iliac crests down to include symphysis pubis may be used. MRI is also known be an excellent choice for this assessment.[16–18] Use of transperineal ultrasound in assessment for labour dystocia has also been described.[19]

It is clear that plain radiographic pelvimetry need not and should not be undertaken unless other methods are not available. Indeed, descriptions of plain film pelvimetry have long been deliberately discontinued by some authors.[20]

References

1. Rodrigues-Pinto R, Kurd MF, Schroeder GD, et al. Sacral fractures and associated injuries. *Global Spine J*. 2017;7(7):609–616.
2. Setia R, Gaillard A, et al. Line of Klein. [online] Radiopaedia. https://radiopaedia.org/articles/line-of-klein/revisions?lang=gb.
3. Long BW, Rafert JA. *Orthopaedic Radiography*. Philadelphia: WB Saunders; 1995.
4. Burnett S, Taylor A, Watson M. *A–Z of Orthopaedic Radiology*. London: Saunders; 2000.
5. Lampignano JP, Kendrick LE. *Bontrager's Textbook of Radiographic Positioning and Related Anatomy*. 9th ed. St Louis: Elsevier Mosby; 2018.
6. Whitley AS, Sloane C, Hoadley G, et al. *Clark's Positioning in Radiography*. 12th ed. London: Hodder Arnold; 2005.
7. Carver E, Carver B, eds. *Medical Imaging: Techniques, Reflection, Evaluation*. 2nd ed. Edinburgh: Churchill Livingstone; 2012.
8. Alzyoud K, Hogg P, Snaith B, et al. Video rasterstereography of the spine and pelvis in eight erect positions: a reliability study. *Radiography*. ePub June 27, doi: https://doi.org/10.1016/j.radi.2019.06.002.
9. Kreel L, Paris A. *Clark's Positioning in Radiography*. 10th ed. London: Heinemann Medical; 1979.
10. Almazedi B, Smith CD, Morgan D, et al. Another fractured neck of femur: do we need a lateral X-ray? *Br J Radiol*. 2011;84:413–417.
11. Long BW, Hall Rollins J, Smith BJ. *Merrill's Atlas of Radiographic Positioning and Procedures*. 13th ed. St Louis: Mosby; 2015.
12. Barrall T. Lateral hip air gap technique. *Synergy: Imaging in Therapy and Practice*. 2004. January:20–23.
13. Martin C. Optimisation in general radiography. *Biomed Imaging Interv J*. 2007;3(2):e18.
14. Scheinfeld MH, Dym AA, Spektor M, et al. Acetabular fractures: what radiologists should know and how 3D CT can aid classification. *Radiographics*. 2015;35(2):555–577.
15. Gilstrap L, Corton MM, Vandorsten P. *Operative Obstetrics*. 2nd ed. New York: McGraw–Hill; 2002.
16. Al-Ahwani S, Assem M, al-Mahallawi N, et al. Magnetic resonance imaging of the female bony pelvis: MRI pelvimetry. *J Belge Radiol*. 1991;74(1):15–18.
17. Kurjak A, Chervenak FA. *Donald School Textbook of Ultrasound in Obstetrics and Gynaecology*. Delhi: Jaypee Brothers; 2008.
18. Zaretsky MV, Alexander JM, McIntire DD, et al. Magnetic resonance imaging pelvimetry and the prediction of labor dystocia. *Obstet Gynecol*. 2005;106(5 Pt1):919–926.
19. Yeo L, Romero R. Sonographic evaluation in the second stage of labor to improve the assessment of labor progress and its outcome. *Ultrasound Obstet Gynecol*. 2009;33(3):253–258.
20. Bontrager KL. *Textbook of Radiographic Positioning and Related Anatomy*. 5th ed. St Louis: Mosby; 2001.

9 Cervical and Thoracic Spine

BARRY CARVER, LUCY BANFIELD, ELIZABETH CARVER AND LINDA WILLIAMS

Cervical Spine

INDICATIONS FOR THE CERVICAL REGION

Trauma

Cervical spine injury is relatively common and is typically seen in association with road traffic accidents, falls from a height and sporting injuries. Most neck injuries are caused by transmission of force to the neck from force applied to the head. Consequently, evidence of head or facial trauma, particularly in patients with poor neurological response, requires 'clearance of the cervical spine'.[1] The overriding concern is of damage to the spinal cord, as this may result in varying degrees of paralysis or even death.

Positive yield of plain X-ray examination is extremely low, as injuries to the cervical spine have been found to occur in between 2% and 6.6% of patients suffering blunt trauma. Much work was done as long ago as the late 1990s and onwards, particularly in Canada and the United States (National Emergency X Radiography Utilization Study – NEXUS), to establish criteria that will ensure suitable imaging referral.[2–8] Today it is commonly accepted that there is reduced value in use of plain radiography in the traumatised patient and guidelines reflect this.[9] Application of these clinical criteria has been reported to have the potential to reduce requests for cervical spine radiography by up to 25%.[10] Significant savings could be made in staff and patient time, leading to financial savings as well as reductions in radiation dose to the patient.

A small but significant number of all victims of blunt head trauma suffer injury to the spinal column, many of whom are young adults under the age of 40 years and it is acknowledged that this is an essential consideration when assessing the injured patient.[11–13] Damage to the spinal cord, secondary to spinal trauma and due to squeezing or shearing forces caused by displaced bone, herniated disc material or buckling of ligaments, is an important consideration in this group of patients. Despite the fact that at least three times as many spinal column injuries occur without neurological deficit compared to those with neurological deficit, care must be taken and the cervical spine immobilised until the need for it is eliminated.[14] This caution must be observed, as spinal cord injury without radiographic abnormality is a well-known phenomenon; it is most commonly described in children.[15] In addition, hyperextension injuries of the cervical spine may injure the spinal cord without apparent damage to the spine seen on radiographs.

Another cause of spinal cord injury is the 'whiplash' injury, which involves extremes of flexion and extension of the neck. This is most frequently the result of a road traffic accident. As the occupant of a vehicle who is restrained by a seatbelt, the patient's head can often be whipped backwards if the vehicle is struck from behind. Alternatively, the vehicle may stop abruptly, causing sudden forward flexion of the neck followed by forced extension. Most commonly muscular injury is seen, but in extreme circumstances quadriplegia may result from a violent whiplash injury.[14]

As stated above, all patients whose mechanism of injury is such that injury to the spinal column is suspected should be immobilised by the application of a spinal collar or similar device until such time as the presence or absence of such injury is proven. Initial imaging must be obtained with minimal patient movement to avoid aggravating potentially unstable injuries.

Mechanism of injury is an important consideration, as symptoms of spinal injury may be masked by other distracting injuries,[16] or are difficult to determine because of cranial or facial trauma.[17,18] Reliance on the mechanism of injury for referral criteria is controversial,[19] but there are specific mechanisms associated with high risk of injury.[20,21]

Spinal clearance should, however, be achieved as promptly as possible, as there is significant morbidity associated with the prolonged use of spinal immobilisation in those who have undergone significant trauma.[22]

Neck Pain

Radiographic examination of the cervical spine is not recommended for the routine investigation of neck pain. However, cervical spine radiography may be useful where there is a history of trauma, or worsening/unresolved neurological symptoms, and in children where such pain is uncommon without a cause.[23]

Torticollis

This causes the neck to lie in abnormal lateral flexion with the head and neck rotated to the same side. This is usually caused following trauma, due to spasm in the sternocleidomastoid and trapezius muscles, and in isolation is not an indication for radiographic examination.

Degenerative Disease Processes

Symptoms of degenerative disease are commonly due to disc or ligamentous changes not demonstrated by plain X radiography.[23]

Rheumatoid Arthritis. This can cause instability of the atlantoaxial joint. Subluxation may be demonstrated by a lateral projection in flexion.[23]

Osteoarthritis. Osteoarthritis is not normally an indicator for radiography unless osteophytic impingement requires demonstration.

Neoplasia

See section in Chapter 3 on commonly encountered pathologies that affect the skeleton.

Congenital Processes

Klippel–Feil Syndrome. Short neck and fused cervical vertebrae. This is not an indicator for cervical spine radiography and is seen as an incidental finding.

Cervical Rib. This is an extra rib arising from C7. Cervical ribs vary in size and shape and clinical symptoms may bear little relationship to size. Its position relative to adjacent anatomy is the determining factor for severity of symptoms. It may cause compression of the subclavian artery or the brachial plexus.

RECOMMENDED PROJECTIONS FOR THE CERVICAL REGION

Imaging of the cervical spine, particularly in cases of trauma, has been the ongoing subject of worldwide debate for some considerable time. Although the cervical spine radiograph was long the routine method for imaging this anatomical region, imaging department protocols varied widely as to the required 'routine' series to be undertaken. More recently, computed tomography (CT) has been used as an essential examination for equivocal findings, but the growing body of evidence that suggested that CT should be used as the first-line investigation has resulted in significant direction towards CT in investigation of the cervical spine in tra uma,[2,9,19,24–26.] The increased capabilities of multidetector CT allow for better image detail and thereby enable the detection of injuries not seen on plain X-ray images.

UK guidance issued by the National Institute for Health and Care Excellence (NICE) recommends that computed tomography (CT) is performed in adults over the age of 16 years if imaging is indicated by the Canadian C-spine rule. In practice, CT is usually the first line investigation for all patients 65 years and over with suspected cervical spine injury as patients in this age range are considered high risk.[27] Regarding the elderly, it has been noted that there is a potential correlation between low-impact injuries and occurrence of upper cervical spine fractures (UCSF) in the oldest patients, with higher-impact injuries causing more lower cervical spine fractures (LCSF).[28]

The NEXUS study[4] looked at its appropriateness for imaging and has proposed that there is no risk of cervical spine injury if 'low risk' criteria are met on patient examination. These criteria are:

No posterior midline tenderness
Not intoxicated
Normal level of alertness
No focal neurological deficit
No painful distracting injuries

Regarding suggestion for a routine projectional series, there has never been an apparent consensus in the literature as to what should be used. Harris et al.[29] reported that whereas 81% of Orthopaedic Trauma Association members responding to their survey used a three-view series, only 31% of the National Association of Spinal Surgeons respondents did so.

Studies such as that performed by West et al[30] compared single-view to three-view screening, finding an increase in sensitivity from 81.8% to 83.3%, respectively, in a comparatively small sample. A similar study in paediatrics by Baker et al[31] found that a lateral projection had a sensitivity of 79% for cervical spine injury, compared to 94% for a three-view series. MacDonald et al[32] had similar findings to West and concluded that even a three-view series was not always sufficient for adequate diagnosis.

There are other suggestions in the literature. Holliman et al[33] suggested that the AP C3–C7 projection adds little to the diagnostic ability of the series; Turetsky et al[34] suggested its replacement by 30° trauma obliques. Doris and Wilson[35] advocated the use of obliques in a routine five-view series.

A problem with including oblique views as a five-view series is the question of 'which obliques?': 30° as above, 60° as advocated by Abel,[36] or something in between, such as 45° as is a familiar suggestion in radiographic positioning texts?[37]

Daffner[38] goes further and discusses a routine six-view series: the five-view series as discussed above (but again with no mention as to the angle of obliquity) with the addition of a swimmer's projection. It is interesting, from the perspective of a UK radiographer, to look at Daffner's results for plain X-radiography: examinations taking up to 46 minutes, with 13 radiographs being taken in one case, and 77% of patients requiring at least one repeat radiograph – standards related to radiation dose and patient care that has long been unacceptable in the UK. If this multiprojectional approach were to be used *in addition* to CT the radiation burden would certainly be high enough to question the benefit–risk ratio.

Following performance and evaluation of the lateral and such accessory views as may be required, the 'cervical spine series', including anteroposterior (AP), open mouth and oblique views, can be completed if no significant instability has been previously demonstrated.[39]

Some studies advocate the inclusion of flexion and extension radiographs[40] in the 'routine cervical spine series' (seven-view?), but care must be taken depending on the degree of suspicion of instability. Where a small subluxation is demonstrated, significant ligamentous injuries may be revealed by flexion and extension views. However, Pollack et al[41] found that flexion and extension images failed to demonstrate any injuries not already demonstrated by other images; hence their usefulness is to be questioned.

The cost and clinical efficacy of such protocols was called into question many years ago, by Mirvis et al.[42] They queried the use of 'routine' CT for clarifying areas of uncertainty, or non-visualised areas in asymptomatic patients, finding a less than 1% positive yield, and that finding was said to be a clinically unimportant injury. Careful clinical assessment of the was is held to be more effective.

Also, information gained from the initial lateral image can be readily, if not necessarily fully, interpreted by the attending emergency doctor with assistance from radiographers who use a system of preliminary clinical evaluation (PCE). In fact, UK guidelines state that X-ray report by a clinician trained in interpretation should be available within 1 hour of the examination and this 'hot reporting' facility is available in many UK Trusts, where this hot reporting is frequently performed by radiographers. This is less likely with CT examination, which requires radiological interpretation, or at the very least a 'provisional' report within an hour of the scan.[27] CT has, however, been shown to be a more cost-effective option for imaging medium- to high-risk patients.[25]

Nunez et al[43] found that 35% of fractures detected by CT were not seen on initial plain radiography in the most seriously ill group of patients, and that a third of these fractures were unstable, located mostly at C1/2 or C7/T1, again stressing the importance of adequate visualisation of C7. Suboptimal examinations were often found to be due to patient condition, and the suggestion is that CT must be included for this most seriously injured patient group.

Throughout this chapter a suggested FRD is given for each examination description; however, in practice a range of FRDs may be used, dependent on local protocol.

PCE COMMENTS – CERVICAL SPINE

Lateral

Importance of prevertebral soft tissue appearances: In the cervical spine lateral radiograph, a careful evaluation of the soft tissues may provide significant information about the location and extent of an injury. Even this can be the subject of debate. In adult patients it is said that the normal distance between the posterior aspect of the pharyngeal air column and the anterior vertebral margin measured at the body of C3 should be less than 7 mm[44]; however, in their study Herr et al[45] quote less than 4–5 mm. The distance from the posterior aspect of the trachea to the anterior vertebral margin measured at the inferior aspect of C6 is more uniformly referred to as 21 mm or less.[44,46] In any case, an increase in these measurements is strongly indicative of the presence of a haematoma. More recently, published work has declared that assessment of the prevertebral soft tissues may be of less value than commonly thought,[47] but it should be said that the methodology included a relatively small sample size that may affect the reliability of the suggestion. Considering the overall information on evaluation of soft tissues, it is clear that inclusion of soft tissue is essential in the lateral projection.

Such prevertebral soft tissue haematomas are common in patients with injury to the anterior spinal column, commonly avulsion fracture or hyperextension injury.[45] Ligament damage can occur without fracture; visualisation of the prevertebral haematoma will help demonstrate the presence of such an injury, but is insensitive as a predictor of fracture or injury site.

Revisiting the importance of checking the prevertebral soft tissue shadow: An abnormal prevertebral soft tissue shadow may be an indicator of injury but it is worth remembering that other reasons for this appearance may exist, infection for example. A normal prevertebral shadow does not, however, exclude an injury. To summarise results after discussion on prevertebral soft tissue measurements, the following soft tissue measurements are considered normal:

1. C1–C4: 30% vertebral body width (approx. 7 mm or less)
2. C5–C7: 100% vertebral body width (approx. 21 mm or less)[44]

Vertebral alignment: This can be demonstrated on the lateral cervical spine radiograph and is commonly assessed using examination of continuous convex lines as described below and shown in Fig. 9.1:

Lines 1 and 2: The anterior and posterior *spinal lines* join the respective portions of the vertebral bodies.

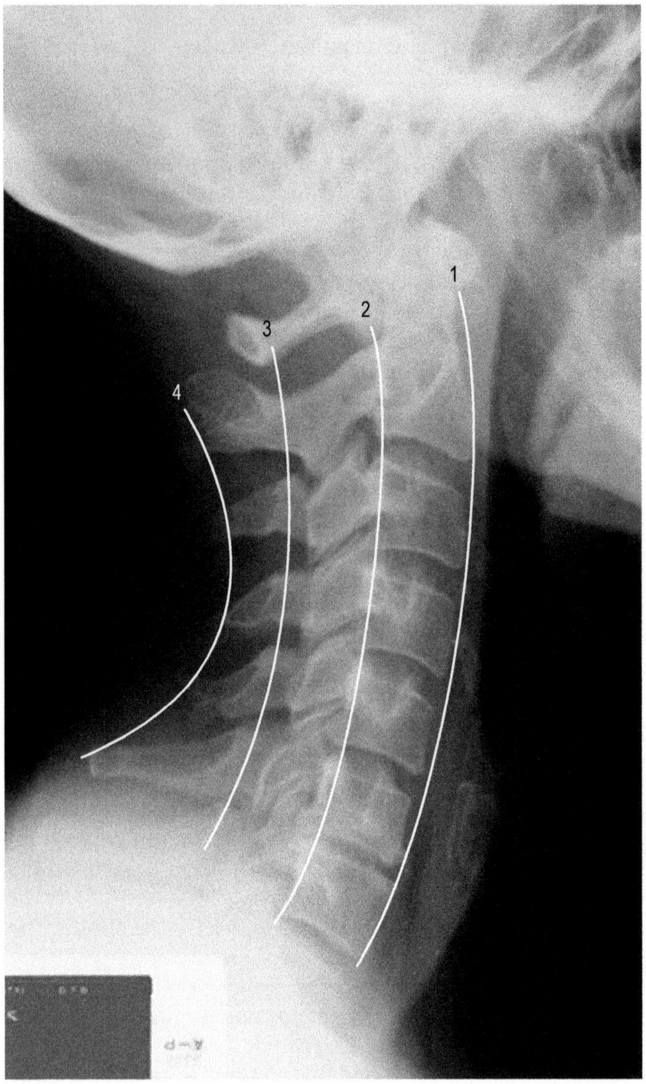

Fig. 9.1 Assessing alignment of cervical vertebrae.

Line 3: The *spinolaminar* line joins the anterior margins of the junctions of the laminae and spinous processes.

Line 4: The fourth line joins the tips of the spinous processes.

Disruption of one or more of these lines can be indicative of injury. For example, if an upper vertebral body is anterior to the one below, this may be an indication of disruption of the posterior ligaments.

The cervical spine is normally lordotic in curvature; loss of lordosis has been said to be an indication of severe muscular spasm and is taken as a sign of cervical spine injury,[14] commonly seen in 'whiplash' type injuries. However, such loss of lordosis can be accentuated by neck position and may be a normal finding if a 'stiff neck' is held in a slightly flexed position during imaging. Hence it is not a reliable sign of definite injury. To ensure this is not considered caused by position, the radiographer should ensure that the mandible is clear of the vertebral bodies (if safe to do so).

So, it is important to check alignment using the four spinal lines as previously mentioned (Fig. 9.1):

1. The anterior vertebral line
2. The posterior vertebral line
3. The spinolaminar line
4. Tips of the spinous processes

Predental space (atlantodens) should not measure more than 3 mm in adults and 5 mm in children. If the space is increased then a fracture of the odontoid process or disruption of the transverse ligament is a potential cause.

Pseudosubluxation versus traumatic subluxation: It is helpful to be aware of physiological or pseudosubluxation when reviewing the lateral projection. This is the normal mobility of C2 on C3 (and sometimes C3 on C4) in flexion that can be mistaken for traumatic subluxation and is a feature that is sometimes seen in young children. It is believed to be due to increased ligamentous laxity seen in children and due to the more horizontal nature of the facet joints.[48] In normal circumstances, this anterior displacement only occurs in flexion, and should not occur in extension.

Uniformity and normal anatomy: In addition to vertebral alignment and the soft tissues, it is also important to examine the vertebral bodies, posterior elements (facets, spinous processes etc.) and the disc spaces for uniformity. Unusual widening of disc spaces and interspinous distances can indicate soft tissue trauma.

Anteroposterior

When interpreting the AP projection there are some important points to consider:

- The height of each vertebral body should be approximately equal
- The spinous processes should be in a straight line and central within the vertebral body
- The intervertebral disc spaces should be equal, as should the space between spinous processes

It is worth remembering that the spinous processes in the cervical spine can often be bifid, particularly at the C4 and C5 levels.

Open Mouth Projection of C1/2

For this projection, commonly known as the open mouth or peg view, there are two main areas to consider for interpretation: alignment of C1 relative to C2, and the integrity of the peg itself.

Alignment: Can be assessed by examining whether the lateral masses of C1 align with the lateral borders of C2, and whether the distance between the dens and the lateral masses of C1 are equal. If the patient is rotated then the latter can appear asymmetrical, therefore evaluation of the head position is an important feature to keep in mind when interpreting this projection.

Joint spaces should also be assessed for symmetry of the articular spaces between the lateral masses of C1 and body of C2 (C1/2 joint spaces either side of the odontoid process), highlighting the importance of ensuring the articular spaces are not obscured by teeth, mandible or overzealous collimation.

Odontoid process: This should be scrutinised for any signs of fracture, such as lucent lines or breaks in the bony cortices. Superimposition of the teeth or the occiput over the peg should not be confused for a fracture line.

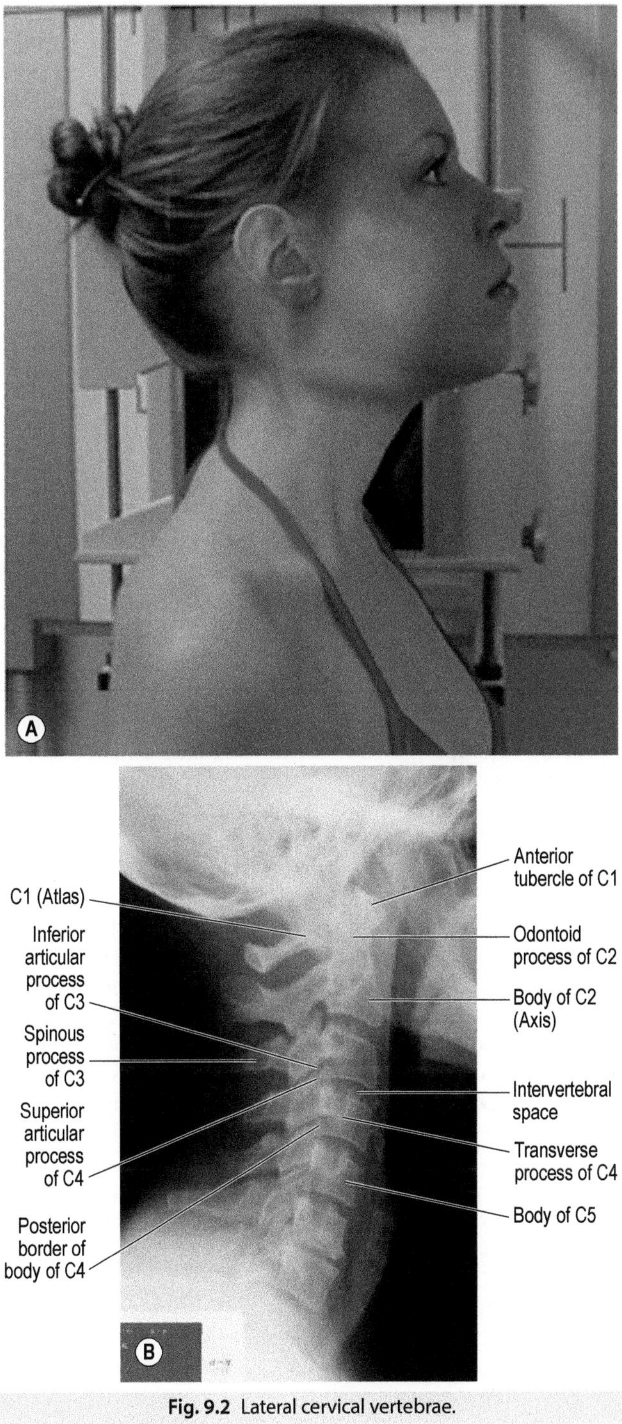

Fig. 9.2 Lateral cervical vertebrae.

Lateral Projections

LATERAL CERVICAL SPINE

IR is vertical

Positioning

Method 1: Patient Standing/Sitting Erect (Fig. 9.2A,B)

- The patient is seated/standing with the lateral aspect of their shoulder resting against the IR
- The median sagittal plane (MSP) is parallel to the IR, with the neck extended to raise the jaw and prevent the angles of the mandible being superimposed over the vertebral bodies

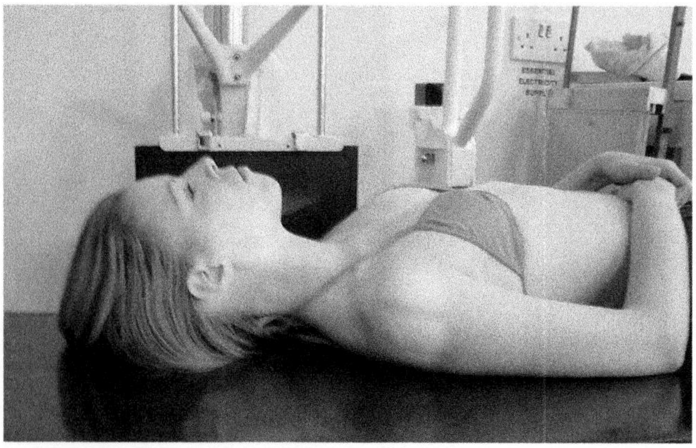

Fig. 9.3 Lateral cervical vertebrae – supine (trauma) position.

- The shoulders should be relaxed and depressed as much as possible as they may obscure the lower cervical vertebrae and the cervicothoracic junction. It has been suggested that patients with broad muscular shoulders should be given a weight to hold in each hand to help project the shoulder masses below the level of C7.[37] However, this is often counterproductive, as patients frequently hunch their shoulders in an attempt to hold the weights firmly while keeping still. This is especially likely if what is being attempted is not carefully explained to the patient. Exposing the radiograph on arrested expiration may help.

Method 2: Patient Supine (Fig. 9.3)

This is a modification of method 1 to account for the change in patient position. This position is typically used in trauma, therefore movement of the patient for the performance of this projection is contraindicated. Before attempting the examination, it is always worth checking for necklaces beneath cervical collars that should have been, but often are not, removed at initial examination of the patient.

Superimposition of the shoulders can be more problematic in this position and methods of applying shoulder traction (when safe to do so) may be used.[49] The key to success is, again, careful explanation to the patient to achieve their cooperation; traction should be applied above the elbow joints, and slowly to prevent the patient working against the application of traction.

- The IR must be positioned to ensure that its inferior border is low enough to include the spinous processes of the cervical vertebrae
- The trolley is positioned to ensure that the long axis of the cervical vertebrae is parallel to the wall or ceiling track of the X-ray tube
- 200 cm FRD is selected and the tube is centred approximately to the middle of the lateral aspect of the neck; approximate collimation to the neck should also take place at this point
- The IR is placed vertically at the side of the neck remote from the tube, its long axis parallel to the patient's MSP. Support for the IR may be via independent support designed for emergency department examinations, erect holder/detector or sponge pads and sandbags

Beam Direction and FRD: Both Methods

Horizontal, at 90° to the IR and the MSP

200 cm FRD – to minimise magnification caused by object receptor distance (ORD), which does, however, provide an air gap that reduces scatter reaching the IR

Centring Point

Below the mastoid process, at the level of the thyroid eminence

Traditionally a range of centring points have been described for this examination. Fixed centring points, such as 2.5 cm posterior and inferior to the angle of mandible,[50] take no account of patient size or shape and in a larger than average person would lead to the beam being centred at soft tissues anterior to C2/3 rather than in the centre of the cervical column at level of C4.

Collimation

Atlanto-occipital articulations, body of T1, cervical spinous processes, soft tissue structures of the pharynx

Soft tissues must be included, particularly in cases of trauma, where, as previously discussed, changes in appearance of the soft tissues can be a strong indicator of the presence of bony injury.[22,45]

Criteria for Assessing Image Quality

- Atlanto-occipital articulations, body of T1, cervical spinous processes and soft tissue structures of the pharynx are included on the image
- Mandible should be cleared from the vertebral bodies, and the angles of the mandible in close approximation
- Left and right posterior borders of the vertebral bodies are superimposed to show no rotation
- There should be clear intervertebral joint spaces with no overlap of superior and inferior borders of vertebral bodies, to show no tilt of the cervical column
- Sharp image demonstrating soft tissue structures of the pharynx in contrast to bone and air in the trachea, detail of the bony cortex and trabeculae, the joint space between C7 and T1 and spinous processes of the cervical vertebrae

Common Errors: Lateral Cervical Spine

Common Errors	Possible Reasons	Potential Effects on PCE or Report
Posterior borders of the vertebral bodies not superimposed	Rotation of neck; MSP not parallel to IR (accuracy in positioning may be affected if the patient is supine and immobilised)	Difficult to assess: posterior vertebral line for alignment presence of posterior marginal osteophytes
Superior borders of the vertebral bodies not superimposed; joint spaces may be obscured	Tilt of the neck in relationship to IR; MSP not parallel (accuracy in positioning may be affected if patient is supine and immobilised)	Difficult to assess: adequacy of disc spaces evidence of intervertebral disc disease potential for muscle spasm facet joints for congruity

Common Errors: Lateral Cervical Spine—cont'd

Common Errors	Possible Reasons	Potential Effects on PCE or Report
Superimposition of the mandible over vertebral bodies	Failure to raise the chin adequately – again may be difficult in the immobilised patient	Difficult to assess: anterior vertebral line anterior vertebral bodies of upper C-spine (usually C1 and C2) prevertebral soft tissues cannot assess normal lordotic curve accurately
Failure to demonstrate the body of T1	Usually due to superimposition of the shoulders over the field *or* insufficient kVp may have been used	Unable to exclude a fracture and/or dislocation of the cervicothoracic junction

Bony injury can manifest in many ways; fractures of the vertebrae may be obvious or very subtle, a typical example being the 'fat C2' sign, where the body of C2 appears wider than the body of C3 on a lateral radiograph.[51] This suggests the possibility of an oblique fracture of the body of C2, which may or may not be readily apparent on the lateral radiograph.

It has been estimated that, in acute cervical spine injury, up to 33% of fractures and dislocations have been missed,[14] hence the requirement for high-quality appropriate imaging. Given this figure, it is not surprising that there has been a culture of ordering radiography on all possibly neck-injured patients but widespread adherence to recommendations[27] should ensure that this is not the case.

In the 2018 guidelines issued by the American College of Radiology it is considered that CT scanning for patients admitted after major blunt trauma is appropriate, and that plain radiography of the region may also be appropriate.[19] However, where CT is not initially available it is clear that a three-view series should be used, in order to give required information of the whole region. In any case when plain radiography is performed, a three series examination should be undertaken: AP, lateral, and a view of C1 and C2. Regarding lateral cervical radiographs of C1–C7, inclusion of C7 and its junction with T1 is vital, although not always easy! Unfortunately, the incidence of injuries at this level has been reported as up to 30% of patients with cervical spine injury, but C7 is not demonstrated in some studies in up to 40% of cases where horizontal beam lateral ('cross table'`) technique is used.[14]

MODIFIED PROJECTIONS TO SUPPLEMENT THE LATERAL

As previously mentioned, the cervicothoracic junction is often inadequately demonstrated on lateral projections of the cervical spine owing to superimposition of the shoulders. Where it is suspected that this may be the case, traction should be applied whenever possible (and if safe) to help prevent superimposition; failure to do so inevitably results in a substandard and useless/unnecessary radiograph.

Should the body of T1 still not be demonstrated, alternatives such as the use of beam shaping filters or CT of the area should be considered. If neither is available the *swimmer's view* may be considered as a last resort. Despite the apparent popularity of this projection,[52,53] there are concerns regarding its utility in terms of image quality and dose, with up to 45% of swimmer's views failing to add to the patient's diagnosis.[54] CT is the best alternative; if unavailable, trauma oblique projections should be considered.

Swimmer's View of C7/T1 Junction (Fig. 9.4A–C)

Consideration should be given to the suitability of this projection for trauma patients because of the movements required. Visualisation of the required anatomy is poor due to the overlying structures; this is exacerbated in larger patients owing to the significant increase in exposure factors required by the projection and their size. Scatter is also considerable. CT should now be the first option; if not available, alternatives such as obliques,[34–36,55] or methods for moving the shoulders down and clear from the C7/T1 junction[55,56] should be considered.

Positioning

IR is vertical, an antiscatter device is employed

The patient should be seated/standing, or may be supine, with the lateral aspect of the shoulder resting against the IR; MSP is parallel to it

The centre of the IR is level with the heads of the humeri

Without altering the relationship of the MSP to the IR, the arm nearest the X-ray tube is raised and flexed at the elbow with the forearm resting across the top of the head

The shoulder nearest the IR is lowered as far as possible

Beam Direction and FRD

Horizontal at 90° to the IR

100 cm FRD

Centring Point

Over the superior aspect of the head of humerus on the side nearest the tube (note that the superior aspect will lie inferiorly to the shaft when the arm is in the correct position)

Collimation

C6, T2, the anterior aspect of the vertebral bodies, the spinous processes

Criteria for Assessing Image Quality

- C6–T2, the vertebral bodies and spinous processes are included on the image
- Right and left posterior, superior and inferior borders of the vertebral bodies are superimposed to show no rotation or tilt
- There should be vertical separation of the right and left shoulder masses enabling visualisation of the cervicothoracic junction
- Sharp image demonstrating detail of the bony cortex and trabeculae within the vertebral bodies of C6–T2, joint space between C7 and T1 and spinous process of seventh cervical vertebra

Common Errors: Swimmer's View

Common Errors	Possible Reasons	Potential Effects on PCE or Report
Failure to demonstrate the cervicothoracic junction – due to under-/overexposed image	Exposure factors and their effect on image detail are the main problems in producing diagnostic radiographs of the cervicothoracic junction. This may be overcome with the use of an automatic exposure device with the centre chamber selected. Good collimation must be used to ensure correct exposure	Unable to exclude a fracture and/or dislocation of the cervicothoracic junction
Failure to demonstrate cervicothoracic junction – due to the humeri overlying vertebrae	The shoulders not adequately displaced: if due to patient condition consider other investigations to demonstrate the area (CT recommended)	As above
Low-contrast 'grey' image	Strict collimation will significantly improve the quality of the image through a reduction in scatter	Whilst the gross alignment may be visible, bony detail will be suboptimal, and therefore excluding a fracture involving the cervicothoracic junction would not be possible

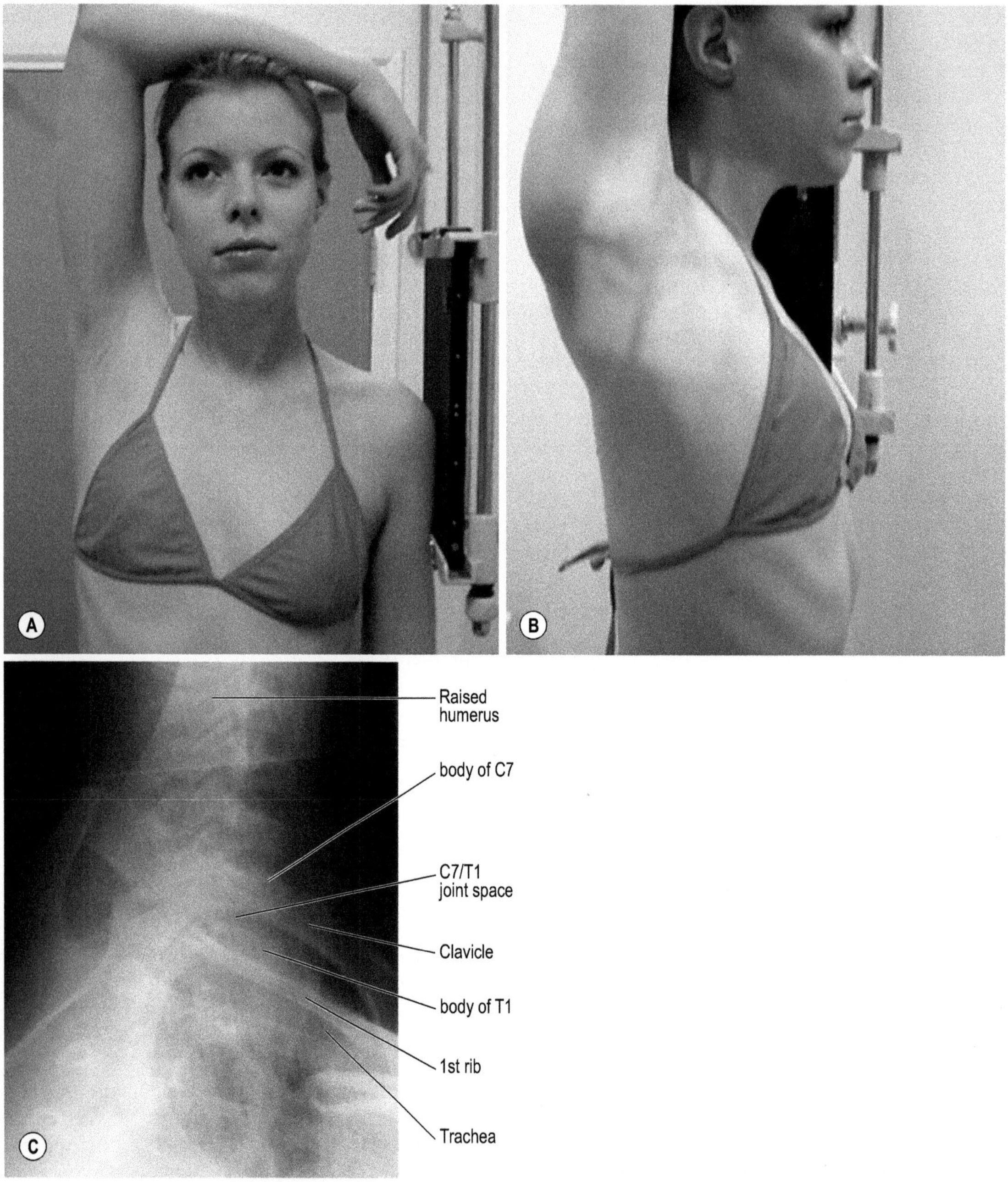

Fig. 9.4 (A) Swimmer's projection of C7/T1; (B) centring and collimation for swimmer's view; (C) swimmer's view.

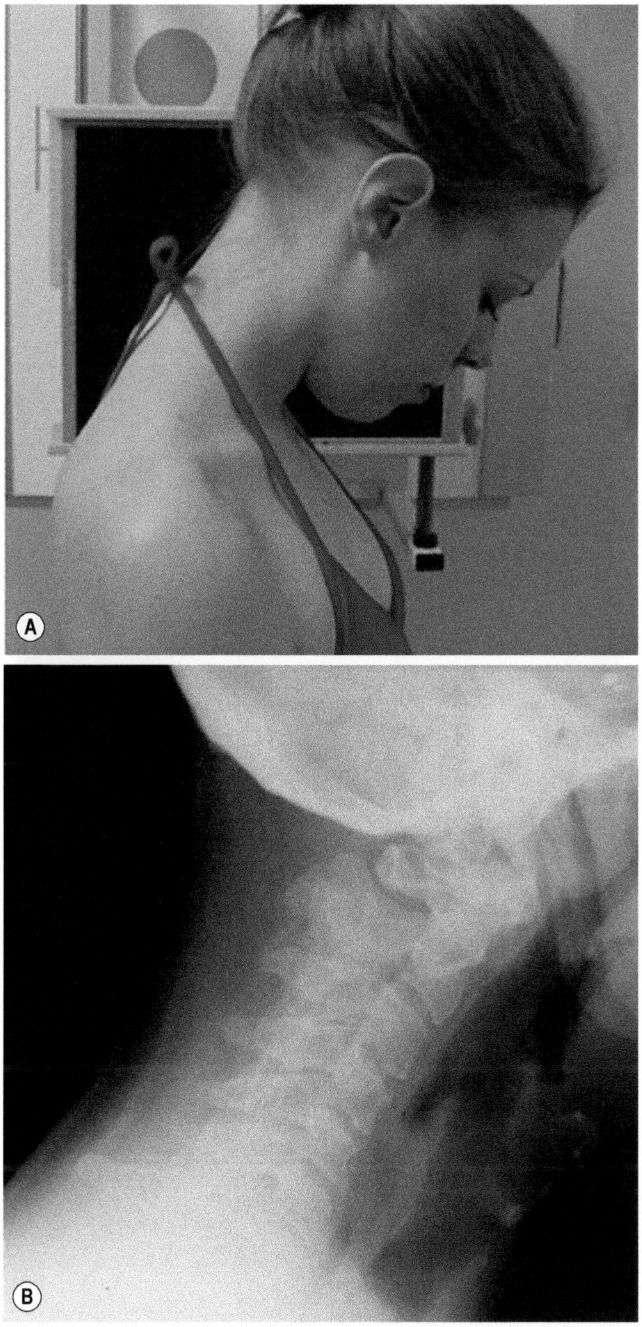

Fig. 9.5 (A) Neck in flexion; (B) C-spine in flexion.

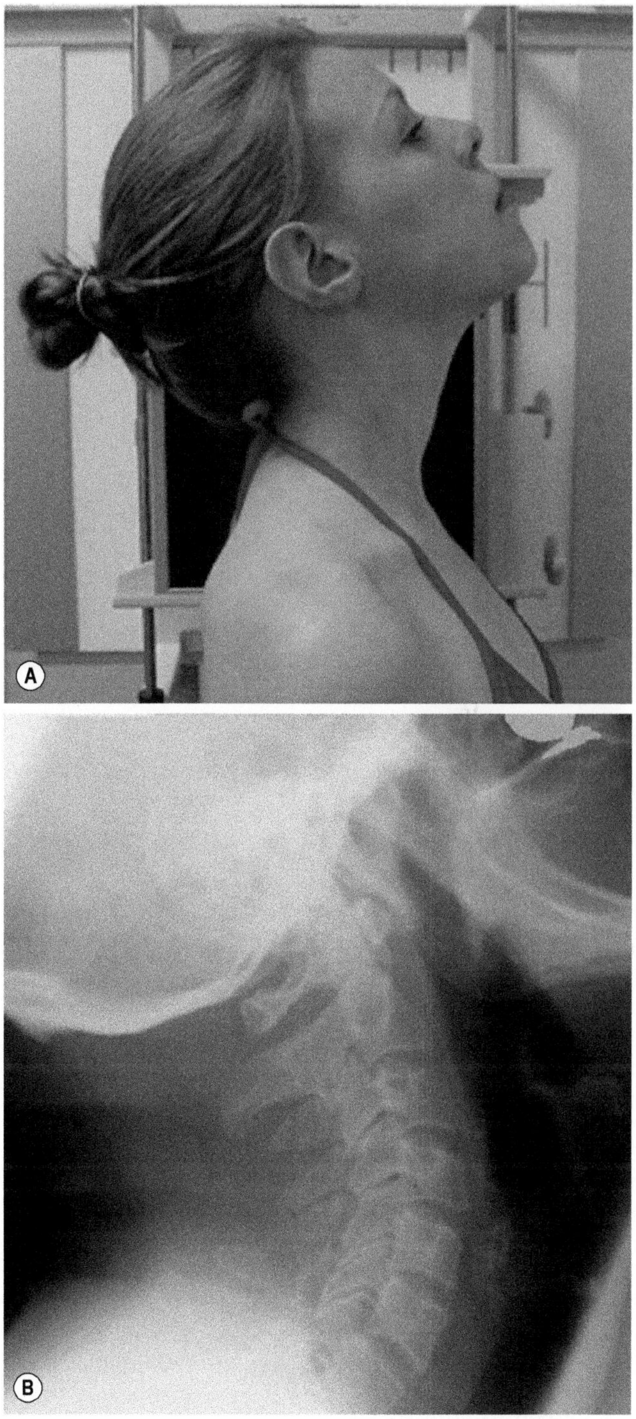

Fig. 9.6 (A) Neck in extension; (B) C-spine in extension.

LATERAL IN FLEXION AND EXTENSION (FIGS 9.5A,B, 9.6A,B)

This projection is used to demonstrate abnormal movements or deformities such as atlantoaxial instability, and in cases of suspected ligamentous injury when the initial radiographic examination is normal; careful use of fluoroscopy has been advocated as an alternative to the projections described below.[23]

Positioning

The principles of the technique are the same as described for the lateral projection above. The centre of the IR is coincident with the middle of the neck, with the long axis of the IR parallel to the long axis of the neck. For flexion the IR is most suitably placed in a landscape orientation in the holder, and for extension, with a portrait orientation.

Two exposures are made, one with the neck in full flexion and one in full extension; the degree of movement will be determined by patient condition and clinical indications, and should take place under medical supervision as required. The movements should not be forced and will be limited by the patient. This may be uncomfortable for the patient, so the position should be maintained for as short a time as possible.

Beam Direction and FRD

Horizontal, at 90° to the IR
200 cm FRD

Centring Point

To the middle of the neck at the level of the thyroid eminence; use of the mastoid protuberance as a vertical location point may not be appropriate for flexion and extension views

Collimation

Atlanto-occipital articulations, the body of T1, the anterior and posterior soft tissues

Criteria for Assessing Image Quality

- Atlanto-occipital articulations, body of T1, anterior soft tissue structures of neck and spinous processes demonstrated
- Superimposition of right and left posterior, superior and inferior borders of vertebral bodies
- Sharp image demonstrating soft tissue structures of the pharynx in contrast to bone and air in the trachea, detail of bony cortex and trabeculae, joint space between C7 and T1 and spinous processes of cervical vertebrae

Anteroposterior (AP) Projections

AP CERVICAL SPINE: C3–C7

IR is vertical, an antiscatter device is not required unless the patient is very large

Positioning

Method 1: Patient Standing or Sitting Erect (Fig. 9.7A,B)

- The patient is sitting or standing with the back of their neck resting on the IR
- The MSP is 90° to the IR
- The chin is slightly raised to superimpose the symphysis menti and the base of occiput and therefore provide clear visualisation of C3

Method 2: Patient Supine (Fig. 9.8A,B)

- This, as for the lateral cervical spine method 1, is usual for trauma, when the patient typically presents on a trolley
- The IR is placed beneath the neck or supported beneath the trolley on a tray. If placed beneath the neck then the lateral projection *must* have been inspected prior to patient movement. If supported beneath the trolley in a tray, effects of the increased ORD must be taken into account
- The MSP should be perpendicular to the IR wherever safely possible
- Superimposition of the symphysis menti and occiput is as for method 1, but this may not be possible with an immobilised patient

Beam Direction and FRD: Both Methods

90° to the IR; cranial angulation, which is often used 'routinely', is not necessary if symphysis menti and occiput are superimposed
100 cm FRD

Consider the effect of increased ORD if the patient is supine; a grid is not usually required but consideration needs to be given to patient size: a large patient may necessitate the use of a grid.

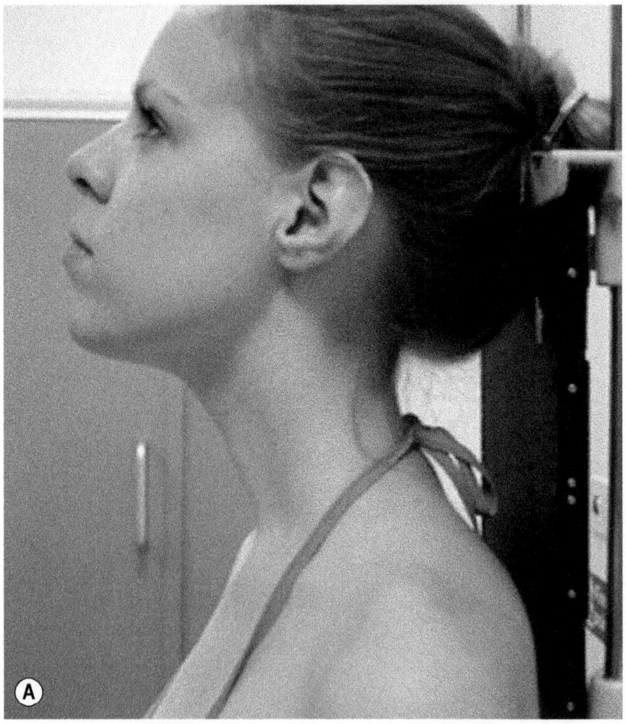

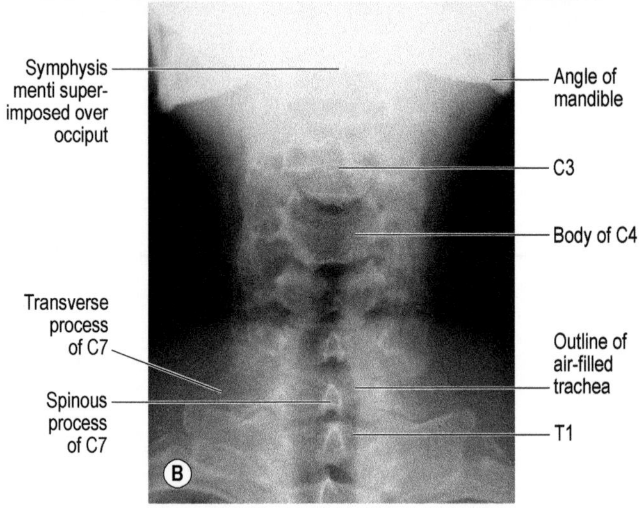

Fig. 9.7 (A) AP C3–C7 with patient erect; (B) AP C3–C7.

If the patient has undergone trauma and/or is in a cervical collar, or even has neck stiffness, it may not be possible to raise the chin, in which case a cranial angle should be applied to the X-ray beam; this should be sufficient to superimpose the lower mandible over the base of the occiput. The angle selected should equate to the line joining the symphysis menti to the occiput. Some neck immobilisation collars actually keep the chin elevated and superimpose the occiput over C3; in these cases a *caudal* angle should be employed. If angulation is used, it may be necessary to displace the IR to ensure the image falls within its boundaries.

Centring Point

Over the MSP at the level of the thyroid eminence

Collimation

C2/3, T1, the transverse processes of all vertebrae included on the image

Criteria for Assessing Image Quality

- C2/3 joint space, T1, and transverse processes are demonstrated
- Lower border of the mandible is superimposed on the base of occiput
- There is no rotation; the spinous processes are equidistant to the pedicles on each side
- Sharp image demonstrating air in the pharynx/trachea in contrast to the detail of the bony cortex and trabeculae; intervertebral disc spaces seen

Common Errors: AP Cervical Spine

Common Errors	Possible Reasons	Potential Effects on PCE or Report
Failure to visualise C3 – obscured by the mandible	Chin not raised sufficiently to superimpose the mandible over the base of occiput If a cranial angle has been used, angle applied has been insufficient	Difficult to adequately assess C3 and therefore difficult to exclude injury or pathology
Failure to visualise C3 – obscured by the occiput	Chin raised too much If a cranial angle has been used, too much angle has been applied	As above

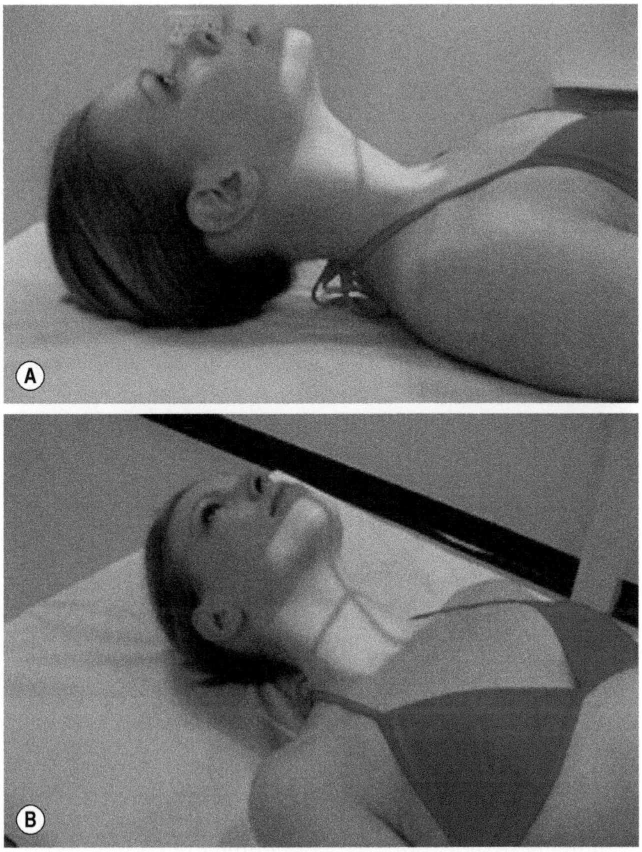

Fig. 9.8 (A) AP C3–C7 with patient supine; (B) AP C3–C7 showing centring.

CERVICAL RIB AND THE AP PROJECTION

If it is suspected that a patient has a cervical rib, the AP cervical spine projection is modified as follows: the patient position is as described above but the central ray is directed over the sternal notch and collimation includes C3–T5 and the lateral soft tissues of the neck.

AP PROJECTION FOR C1/C2 – 'OPEN MOUTH' (FIG. 9.9A,B)

IR is vertical, an antiscatter device is not necessary

Positioning

The patient initially is positioned as for the basic AP cervical spine position, erect or supine

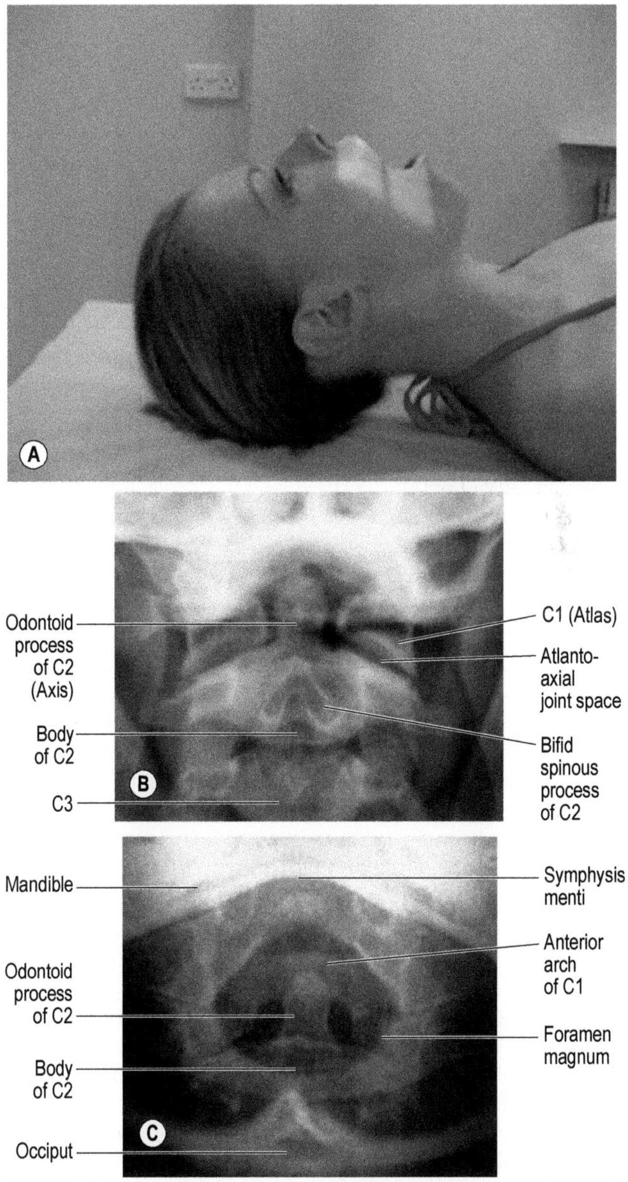

Fig. 9.9 (A) AP C1–C2 (odontoid process); (B) AP C1–C2; (C) axial odontoid process. (C, Reproduced with permission from Ballinger PW, Frank ED. *Merrill's Atlas of Radiographic Positions and Radiologic Procedures*. St Louis: Mosby; 2003.)

The patient opens their mouth as much as possible; if moving the head is an option it should be adjusted to bring the hard palate perpendicular to the IR. This can be achieved using the alatragal line (see Chapter 14, Fig. 14.3), which lies parallel to the hard palate, as a guide. Positioning of the hard palate in this way superimposes the lower border of the upper incisors over the base of the occiput, thus clearing these structures from the odontoid process and C1/C2 joints

The mouth is checked to ensure it is open far enough to adequately clear the teeth and mandible from the C2/C3 joint spaces

Beam Direction and FRD

Parallel to the alatragal line; this is especially useful as a guide for beam angulation in trauma cases where head movement is contraindicated
100 cm FRD

Centring Point

Through the open mouth at the level of the lower border of the upper incisors

Collimation

Atlanto-occipital joints, C2/C3 joint space, the transverse processes on each side

Criteria for Assessing Image Quality

- Odontoid process, atlas, axis and atlantoaxial articulations are demonstrated and visualised symmetrically
- Upper incisors and base of the skull are superimposed
- Lower incisors are superimposed over the body of C3 but cleared from the C2/C3 joint space
- No rotation; the spinous processes are demonstrated centrally to the vertebral bodies
- Sharp image demonstrating the bony cortex and trabeculae, in contrast to adjacent soft tissues

Common Errors: AP for C1/C2 – 'Open Mouth'

Common Errors	Possible Reasons	Potential Effects on PCE or Report
Odontoid process obscured by upper incisors	Chin not raised sufficiently *or* a caudal beam angle is too great	Obscures the odontoid process and does not allow for adequate visualisation in order to exclude fracture Superimposition of the teeth can give false appearance of a fracture line over the odontoid process
Odontoid process obscured by the occiput	Chin raised too much *or* a cranial beam angle is too great	As above – superimposition of the occiput can give false appearance of C2/odontoid process fracture
C1 and C2 not symmetrical *and/or* the lower teeth on one side obscure the C2/C3 joint space on one side	Rotation of the head	Difficult to assess atlanto-axial joint space Can give false impression of joint incongruency Teeth can obscure lateral margins making accurate evaluation of position of lateral masses challenging
Lower teeth obscuring C2/C3 joint space bilaterally	Mouth not open sufficiently	Unable to confirm that lateral margins of lateral masses are in alignment therefore unable to exclude fracture of C1

The difficulty of obtaining the AP C1/C2 projection in unconscious patients is no longer an issue since CT is recommended for these patients, but clearly there may be instances when CT is not available (most especially related to areas that are remote from CT facilities). For other (non-trauma) patients, for whom it is difficult to obtain an image of the odontoid process, and when the C2/C3 joint space has been adequately demonstrated, an axial odontoid peg projection can be undertaken. It is easier to undertake supine, as the chin is raised as much as possible and requires the patient to maintain a position that is more difficult to hold than the routine open mouth approach. The central ray is angled 25° cranially and directed midway between the angles of the mandible. The image produced shows the odontoid process through the foramen magnum (Fig. 9.9C).

Oblique Projections

For neurological referrals the usefulness of magnetic resonance imaging (MRI) examination of the neck far outweighs the effectiveness of oblique projections of the cervical spine, which were used in the past to demonstrate the shape of the intervertebral foramina. The main use for obliques is for cervical spine in the case of trauma, although, as discussed earlier in this chapter, CT is now the imaging modality of choice (unless this facility is unavailable). Trauma obliques are a modification of 'routine' erect obliques and are described at the end of the section on obliques.

It should be noted that a wide variety of oblique projections have been described, the main variation being the tube angulation applied.[34,36,37,57] Which of the alternatives is selected should be dependent on the pathology to be demonstrated, but those used are all too often selected from habit or protocol. For the sake of clarity and uniformity of approach, 45° neck obliquity (or 45° lateromedial tube angulation to produce appearances equivalent to 45° neck obliquity in the injured patient) is used throughout the following section, but this does not mean that it is necessarily the 'recommended technique'; reference must be made to the individual circumstances and the texts mentioned above before selecting the appropriate obliquity.

Whatever obliquity is ultimately selected, the technique is broadly the same; to change from one to another simply insert the number of degrees required (not forgetting to displace the IR appropriately if using lateromedial angulation!).

Where practicable, PA obliques should be used in preference to AP obliques because of the potentially lower absorbed dose to the thyroid in this position.

ANTERIOR OBLIQUES OF THE CERVICAL SPINE (FIG. 9.10A,B)

Don't forget that anterior obliques have the anterior aspect of the patient facing the IR
The *right anterior oblique* demonstrates the *right* intervertebral foramina

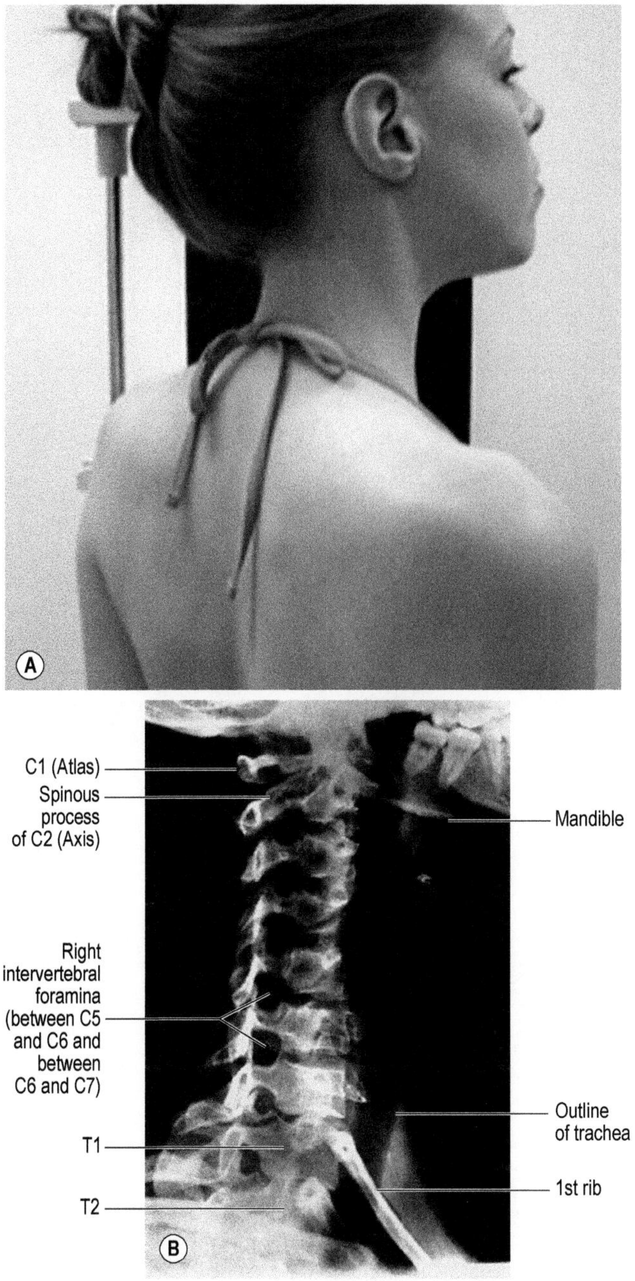

Fig. 9.10 Anterior oblique cervical vertebrae.

The *left anterior oblique* demonstrates the *left* intervertebral foramina
IR is vertical

Positioning

The patient is erect, facing the IR
The patient is rotated *away* from the side under examination, until the MSP is at 45° to the IR. The head is turned a further 45° until the MSP of the head is parallel to the IR
The chin is raised sufficiently to clear the mandibular rami from the upper vertebrae

Beam Direction and FRD

Horizontal central ray
200 cm FRD

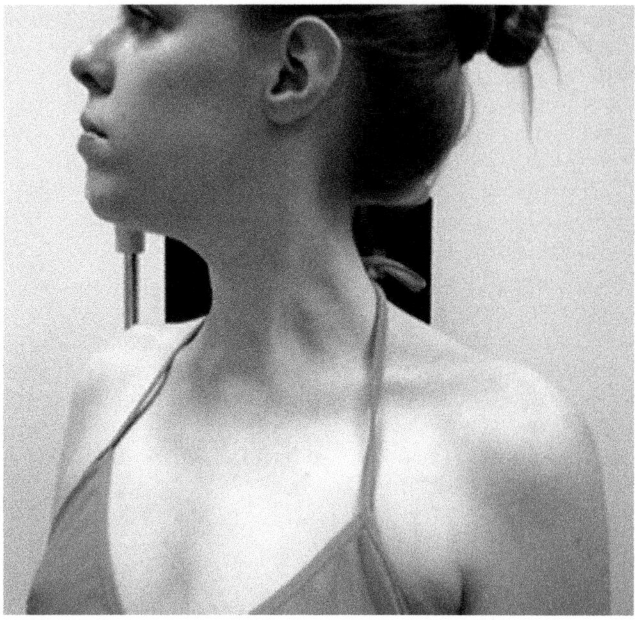

Fig. 9.11 Posterior oblique cervical vertebrae.

A 15° caudal angulation may be applied to better demonstrate the intervertebral foramina.

Centring Point

To a point in the middle of the neck, at the level of the thyroid eminence

Collimation

Atlanto-occipital joints, T1, lateral soft tissue outlines

Criteria for Assessing Image Quality

- Base of the occiput, the body of T1 and soft tissue outlines of the neck are demonstrated
- Mandible is cleared from the upper vertebrae
- Intervertebral foramina is demonstrated on the opposite side of the spine to the mandible; should be symmetrical ovoids
- Pedicles of the opposite side are projected centrally at the superior border of the vertebral bodies
- Spinous processes are demonstrated posterior to the intervertebral foramina
- Soft tissue structures of the neck are demonstrated anterior to the vertebral bodies
- Sharp image demonstrating detail of the bony cortex and trabeculae in contrast to the intervertebral foramina and adjacent soft tissue structures

POSTERIOR OBLIQUES OF THE CERVICAL SPINE (FIG. 9.11)

This projection may be used as an alternative to the anterior oblique; however, it should be noted that this position will lead to increased absorbed dose in the thyroid gland since the patient faces the X-ray tube.

This projection may be achieved in trauma cases with the patient supine, but the modified technique for trauma must be used, not the routine projection, as this requires patient movement, which is contraindicated for the trauma setting.

The *right posterior oblique* (RPO) demonstrates the *left* intervertebral foramina
The *left posterior oblique* (LPO) demonstrates the *right* intervertebral foramina
IR is vertical

Positioning

- The patient is erect, facing the X-ray tube and with their back against the IR
- The upper border of the IR is placed level with the top of the pinna of the ear
- The patient is rotated *away* from the side under examination, until the MSP is at 45° to the IR. The head is turned a further 45° until the MSP of the head is parallel to the IR
- The chin is raised sufficiently to clear the mandibular rami from the upper vertebrae

Beam Direction and FRD

Horizontal central ray
200 cm FRD

A 15° cranial angulation may be applied to better demonstrate the intervertebral foramina.

Centring Point

To a point in the middle of the neck at the level of the thyroid eminence

Collimation

Atlanto-occipital joints, T1, lateral soft tissue outlines

Criteria for Assessing Image Quality

These are the same as for the anterior obliques.

MODIFIED TECHNIQUE FOR TRAUMA (FIG. 9.12A,B)

Oblique projections of the cervical spine may be required as a supplementary examination in trauma cases where there is concern over the integrity of the facet joints.

AP oblique projections can be undertaken without moving the patient, using lateromedial angulation to provide an apparently oblique neck image.

The *RPO* demonstrates the *left* facet joints and intervertebral foramina
The *LPO* demonstrates the *right* facet joints and intervertebral foramina
IR is horizontal

Positioning

- The patient is supine and the IR is supported beneath the trolley-top
- The patient position is as close as possible to that for the AP cervical spine projection

Beam Direction and FRD

The beam is angled 45° lateromedially across the patient from either side in turn. The IR should be displaced from the centre (horizontally) sufficiently to ensure that its centre is coincident with the central ray, allowing for the applied beam angulation 100 cm FRD, which may need to be increased if there is a long ORD (such as when an IR tray is used).

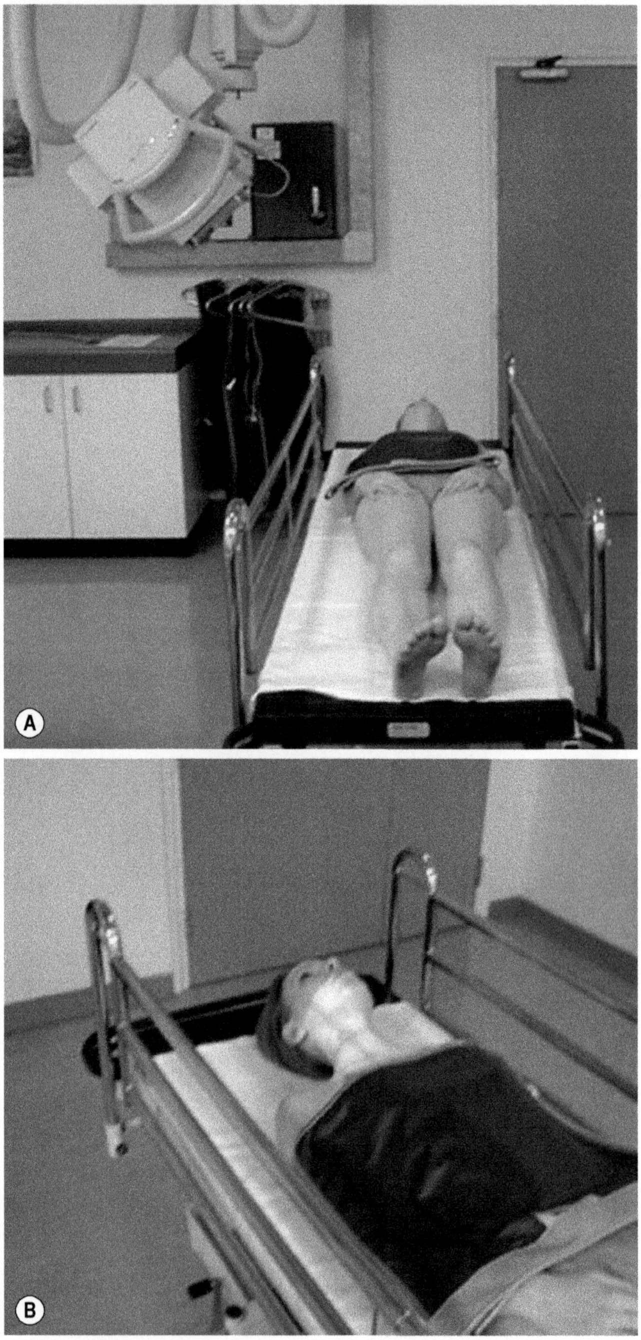

Fig. 9.12 (A) Trauma cervical oblique; (B) trauma oblique showing collimation.

If a 15° cranial angulation is required, this may be obtained by rotating the X-ray tube 15° around its horizontal axis after the initial lateromedial angulation.

Centring Point

To a point in the middle of the neck, at the level of the thyroid eminence, on the side nearest the X-ray tube

Collimation

Atlanto-occipital joints, T1, lateral soft tissue outlines

Criteria for Assessing Image Quality

These are the same as for the erect obliques.

Common Errors: Oblique Projections for Trauma

Common Errors	Possible Reasons	Potential Effects on PCE or Report
Narrowed foramina	Under-rotation of the neck	Unable to identify potential sites of nerve compression Sternoclavicular joint will be superimposed over lower vertebrae
Foreshortening of the pedicles	Over-rotation of the neck	May falsely imply congenitally short or hypoplastic pedicles
The foramina distorted/disc space not demonstrated	Insufficient cranial/caudal tube angulation	Unable to fully assess: alignment of posterior elements disc spaces sites of potential impingement

Note that if lateromedial angulation is used, as for modified projections in trauma, this will cause more image distortion than projections using neck rotation

Other Imaging Modalities and the Cervical Spine

Even though CT provides the most detailed evaluation of bony injuries, MRI has some clear advantages, being the most sensitive modality for the detection of intrinsic spinal cord pathology, and also providing the most detailed evaluation of the soft tissues. An added advantage is that there is no loss of resolution in areas such as the lower cervical spine, where the shoulders may interfere with visualisation, even with the use of CT.

It would be fantastic if MRI were available in the Emergency Department setting at all times, as readily and routinely available as plain X-ray imaging; however, even MRI is not without its disadvantages, particularly with the group of patients under consideration. Artefact can be a problem, from either the posterior fat pad in adults or the pulsatile flow of cerebrospinal fluid in children.[58] Studies have shown the effectiveness of using MRI in addition to CT,[2,59] particularly for diagnosis of ligamentous injury and cord impingement; however, it is unnecessary for diagnosis of unstable fractures,[60] as CT has been shown to have 100% sensitivity for this group of patients.[61]

There are other suggestions as to how imaging may be used in this group of patients. Brookes and Willett, researching in Oxford, proposed a protocol for spinal clearance involving dynamic screening of the cervical spine in unconscious trauma patients to enable rapid, safe discontinuation of spinal precautions.[22]

As with all debates in the field of medical imaging, it is not practicable to provide a concrete 'once and for all answer' to the question as to which of the above imaging methods is 'best'; the practice of medical imaging changed dramatically in the later decades of the 20th century and into the 21st, with a constant stream of new technologies that shows no sign of slowing down. For example, CT has become unrecognisable from the slice-by-slice technology of the late 20th century, with the introduction and development of wide multidetector and dual energy systems, and the readily available 3D reconstructions that were once but a dream for the future.

Thoracic Spine

INDICATIONS

Trauma

Useful advice is provided by NICE guidelines on spinal trauma, where the following is given in relation to the thoracic spine:

- X-ray as first-line investigation for suspected spinal column injury minus abnormal neurological signs or symptoms in thoracic or lumbosacral regions T1 to L3.
- CT if abnormality noted on X-ray, or if there are clinical signs or symptoms of spinal injury.
- If a new spinal column fracture is confirmed, image the rest of the spinal column.
- The clinical significance of wedge fractures should not be overlooked, as occasionally there may be fragments displaced within the spinal canal that could cause spinal cord compression.[62]

Fractures of the upper and middle sections of the thoracic spine do not occur as frequently as those of the cervical vertebrae and thoracolumbar region. However, with thoracic spine fractures there is a higher incidence of spinal cord injury.[63]

Multiple Myeloma

The thoracic spine may be examined as part of a skeletal survey to stage the condition and assess which lesions may benefit from radiotherapy. However, guidelines published by NICE indicate that MRI or CT should be first-line investigations when myeloma is suspected, and used in disease monitoring (unless contraindicated, or declined by the patient).[64]

Osteomyelitis

MRI is the modality of choice for the evaluation of vertebral osteomyelitis,[65] however when the patient is contraindicated for MRI, or MRI is not available, a two- to three-phase skeletal scintinogram is more sensitive than an X-ray examination and therefore a good alternative imaging modality. Plain X-ray imaging is not routinely indicated, however in the later stages of the disease an area of porosis may be seen; the diagnosis at this stage can usually be made by blood cultures.[66]

Pain

The thoracic spine should not be routinely examined by radiography for pain without trauma, unless in the elderly when osteoporosis may cause sudden collapse of vertebrae. MRI may be indicated if localised pain persists.

The 28-day rule should be applied when examining the thoracic spine in patients of reproductive capacity, as the inclusion of the lower thoracic vertebrae will also irradiate the medial portion of the upper abdomen.

PCE COMMENTS – THORACIC SPINE

Anteroposterior

Bone density and quality: It is important to assess and evaluate bone density and bone quality. Bony outlines should be sharp and fine and the intervertebral disc spaces should be uniform. The pedicles should be positively identified; absence of a pedicle may indicate the presence of a neoplastic process.

The paraspinal line is produced by the interface between the paravertebral soft tissues and the adjacent lung. It runs parallel to the lateral margin of the thoracic vertebral bodies on the left side only. A bulge or displacement in the paraspinal line may indicate:

- Haemorrhage
- Tumour
- Infection/inflammation

It should not be confused with the normal appearance of the aorta, which may begin to demonstrate unfolding with age.

Adjacent structures: Lastly, don't forget to examine the periphery of the image to ensure that no rib fractures or pneumothoraces are missed.

Lateral

Assess for gross abnormality and obvious sclerotic or lucent lesions; review the vertebral alignment. Smooth curves with a mild mid-thoracic kyphosis should be appreciated.

Anterior and posterior longitudinal lines – check for normal alignment.

Height of each vertebral body should be approximately equal to its neighbours, however, the bodies do increase in size as the anatomy progresses towards the lumbar spine.

Distance between spinous process should be relatively equal.

Trace the posterior elements: pedicles, laminae and spinous processes.

It helps to ask the following questions:

- Have all the vertebrae been included?
- Is a further projection required for the upper thoracic spine?
- Has the thoracolumbar junction been included adequately?

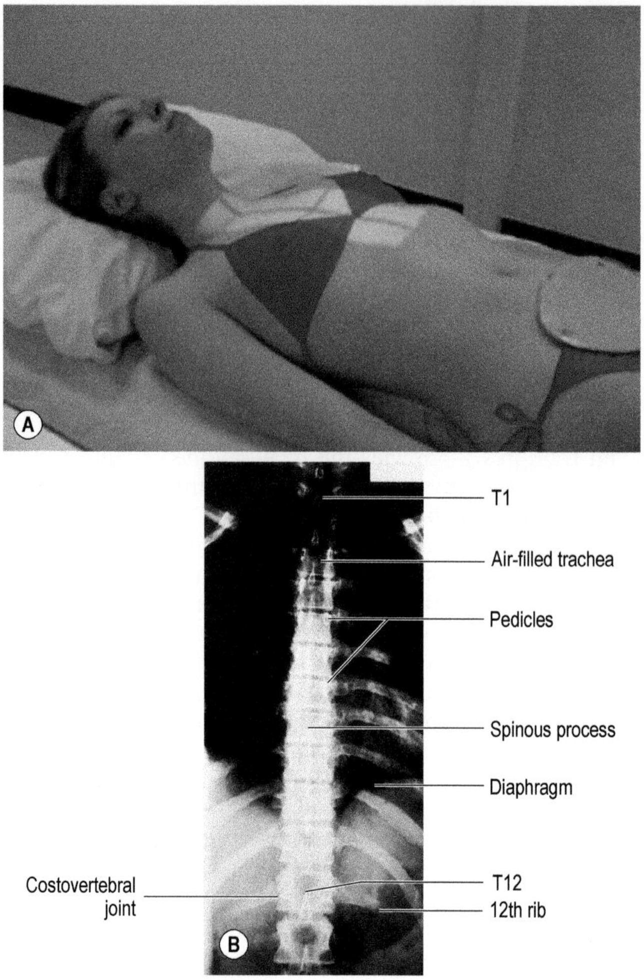

Fig. 9.13 AP thoracic spine. (B, Reproduced with permission from Bryan GJ. *Skeletal Anatomy*. 3rd ed. Edinburgh: Churchill Livingstone; 1996 and Gunn C. *Bones and Joints*. 4th ed. Edinburgh: Churchill Livingstone, 2002.)

ANTEROPOSTERIOR (AP) THORACIC SPINE (FIG. 9.13A,B)

Much research has been undertaken on the advantages and disadvantages of the PA versus the AP projection of the *lumbar* spine, particularly in relation to dose reduction. Brennan and Madigan,[67] in their article analysing the PA projection of the lumbar spine, recommend the use of this procedure to facilitate dose reduction without loss of image quality. However, it must be remembered that, owing to the natural kyphotic curvature of the thoracic spine, oblique rays from the X-ray beam will be angled in the opposite direction to the intervertebral joint spaces. The resulting PA image is therefore not likely to demonstrate the intervertebral joint spaces as adequately as the AP projection. This is somewhat unfortunate, as the PA projection may reduce radiation dose to the breast, eyes and thyroid, all radiosensitive areas. However, breast shields may be used, and with good collimation this can significantly reduce the dose. Levy et al studied the use of the PA projection in examining the whole spine for scoliosis in adolescents.[68] Their work suggested that a PA study of the spine will effect a reduction in dose to the patient without any loss of image quality; although assessment for scoliosis using plain radiography has reduced significantly with increased use of other imaging methods, their work indicates that PA thoracic spine examination may be a possibility in some cases.

A consideration when examining the thoracic spine is the variation in densities along the length of this section of the vertebral column, the upper end having the air-filled trachea superimposed and vertebrae 5–12 having the heart and great vessels superimposed. Abdominal contents are usually superimposed over T11 and T12 and the size of individual vertebrae increases gradually, with T1 being significantly smaller than T12.

Clearly this range of densities has implications for the choice of exposure factors to provide adequate contrast and density along the entire length of the region under examination. To achieve even density certain techniques may be employed, as follows:

1. A high enough kVp can be used to reduce the subject contrast along the length of the spine.
2. A wedge filter can be used with the thicker end at the upper region of the thoracic spine.
3. A flour filter can be used, consisting of flour inside a radiolucent bag (usually plastic, which is covered by a cotton bag that can be washed). The contents of the bag can be shaken to distribute the flour into a thicker layer at one end; this thicker end of the bag is then placed over the upper end of the sternum and the flour is patted by the radiographer until the thickness decreases towards the lower end of the thoracic vertebrae. The filter is therefore adaptable to any patient size, unlike set-size aluminium filters. The filter can be made extremely cheaply and requires no specialist attachment feature on the light beam mounting, although manufacture of such a filter should only be attempted after consultation with health and safety and cross-infection specialists from the hospital where the filter is to be used.

Some texts suggest the use of the anode heel effect to help reduce the subject contrast along the length of the spine.[69] However, it must be suggested that this is a somewhat outdated approach: anode targets in modern X-ray tubes are set at such an angle that this effect will have little or no difference on the resultant image.

The use of digital receptors clearly assists in overcoming the issues raised here, regarding variation in tissue thickness, but radiographers must always ensure that exposure factors are within optimum ranges.

When using an automatic exposure device (AED) for the thoracic spine, accurate centring and good collimation are essential. If the beam is not collimated sufficiently then the AED will end the exposure before the required radiographic density of the image is achieved. This is due to the effect of additional scatter from the excess irradiated tissue lateral to the spine.

The AP thoracic spine is exposed on arrested inspiration to ensure the diaphragm is lowered and a maximum number of thoracic vertebrae are demonstrated. However, it has also been suggested that the use of arrested expiration to reduce the amount of air in the thorax will provide a more uniform density over the thoracic spine, by helping to reduce the subject contrast of the air-filled lungs against the mediastinum and spine.[52,70] This is a questionable suggestion in that there will always be air in the lung fields, even in expiration.

IR is horizontal, an antiscatter grid is employed

Positioning

- The patient is supine with their arms at their sides and legs extended
- A low radiolucent pillow or pad may be used to support the head, and the knees may be supported slightly with a pad for comfort
- The median sagittal plane (MSP) is at 90° to the table-top and the coronal plane is parallel to the table-top
- Note that this technique may be performed erect, either standing or seated; the positioning is the same for each but a vertical IR is used. The direction of the central ray is adjusted accordingly.

Beam Direction and FRD

Vertical central ray, at 90° to the IR
100 cm FRD

Centring Point

In the midline approximately two-thirds of the distance between the sternal angle and the xiphisternum, nearest the xiphoid end

Some texts have quoted the centring point for this projection as midway between the sternal notch and the xiphisternum.[71,72] This point locates the central ray over T6, i.e. numerically at the middle of the thoracic vertebrae, and seems a logical selection; yet vertebrae T1–T6 are shorter than T7–T12 and a centring point over T6 will therefore not lie over the midpoint of the thoracic section of the vertebral column. Indeed, it will be in a relatively high position in relation to the actual midpoint of the area. Other texts quote a centring point as either between the sternal angle and the xiphisternum, or 3–5 cm below the sternal angle to a point over T7[73]; is this low enough to coincide with the actual midpoint of the thoracic vertebrae? In the first edition of this book it was thought necessary to reassess the situation and consider AP thoracic spine radiographs in an attempt to see whether there was a standard midpoint; in other words, which references suggested the most accurate midpoint of the thoracic spine? Several images were studied by the authors and it was noted that the actual halfway point between T1 and T12 lies, in fact, approximately over T7/8 disc space. As anterior surface markings need to be used for assessing this point, it has been identified, from skeletons and radiographs, that T7/8 junction lies two-thirds of the way down the sternum itself (including xiphisternum) – hence the centring point chosen (Fig. 9.14).

Collimation

C7–L1, all transverse processes

Expose on arrested respiration

Criteria for Assessing Image Quality

- C7 down to L1 and all their transverse processes are demonstrated
- The thoracic vertebrae are in the centre of the collimated area
- Spinous processes are centralised over the midline of the vertebral bodies
- Paraspinal line[62] should be clearly demonstrated
- Intervertebral joint spaces are demonstrated
- Sharp image demonstrating the bony cortex and trabeculae of the vertebral bodies of C7 down to L1, adequately penetrated through the denser mediastinal and upper abdominal structures without over-blackening of the upper vertebrae

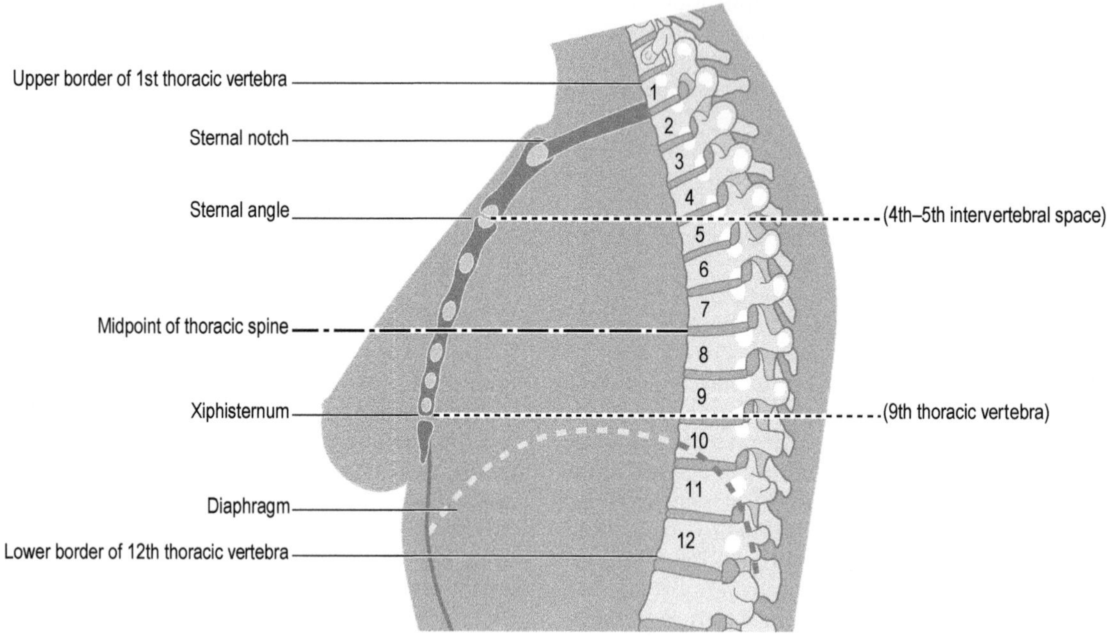

Fig. 9.14 Level of midpoint of thoracic spine.

Common Errors: AP Thoracic Spine

Common Errors	Possible Reasons	Potential Effects on PCE or Report
Overexposure of the upper region or underexposure of the lower region	Failure to employ any of the techniques described above for even image density throughout	Unable to adequately demonstrate vertebral bodies to assess for trauma Pedicles would not be adequately visualised
Superimposition of portions of the vertebral bodies vertically	The long axis of the spine is not near parallel to the table-top. Reducing the size of the head support and giving the patient a small pad beneath the knees for support can rectify this. (However, severely kyphotic patients may require two exposures with beam angled in each direction of the kyphosis)	Unable to gain true picture of vertebral body and intervertebral disc heights

LATERAL THORACIC SPINE (FIG. 9.15A,B)

As in the case of the AP projection, there also exists a range of densities along the area covered by the lateral thoracic spine projection. The more dense area in this case is the upper end of the thoracic region, as the average person is wider and denser at the shoulders than they are lower down the thoracic region. The use of the filter described earlier in this chapter is used with the thicker end orientated in the opposite direction to that used for the AP, i.e. the thinner end at the shoulder end. This will even out the densities encountered along the length of the spine. Comment on improved visualisation of the region by using digital image receptors and associated manipulation is clearly valid here, but selection of optimum exposure factors is again vital.

Use of the breathing technique, using a low mA and long exposure time (2 seconds plus) to provide the required mAs will blur rib shadows and lung markings that lie over the vertebrae, thereby enabling the viewer to see the vertebral bodies more clearly.[70,71,73] However, it is also suggested that, as the ribs are actually attached to the vertebrae, when using the breathing technique the rib shadow cannot be blurred without blurring the vertebrae too; in other words, what is actually happening is that, during breathing, the vertebral bodies are moving but to a lesser extent than the ribs. This gives the vertebral bodies an apparent sharpness owing to the differential sharpness between the ribs and the bodies themselves.

There is sometimes difficulty in demonstrating the intervertebral joint space of all the thoracic vertebrae on one image and this can be overcome by the use of a longer focus receptor distance (FRD) (150 cm). This relatively long distance means there is less divergence of the beam around the central ray when it reaches the thoracic spine, and more chance of the joint spaces being demonstrated on the image, especially those at the extreme ends of the thoracic spine. Although this method has been used by many radiographers for many years it was not until 2003 that a study by Thomas provided evidence to support the practice, also showing that magnification and unsharpness are reduced.[74] This technique would require adjustment of exposure factors, with due attention to the inverse square law, if an AED is not used.

A lead rubber sheet placed behind the patient, next to the skin surface, will absorb some of the scattered radiation

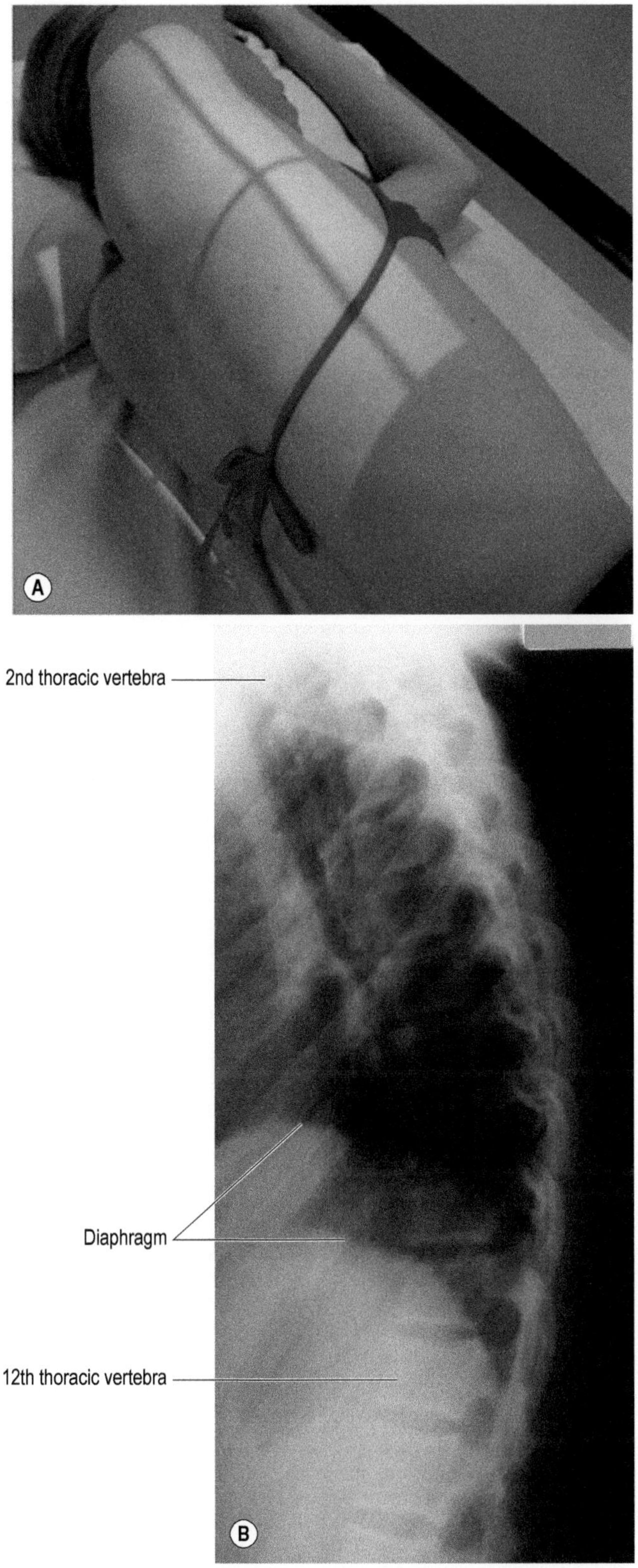

Fig. 9.15 Lateral thoracic spine.

produced during exposure and enhance the image. Some research disputed the necessity of placing lead rubber behind the patient for the lateral spine projection, arguing that the resulting radiograph is not enhanced by this practice. It also claimed that it is not necessary with the use of the accurate collimators available today which prevent any scatter reaching the IR. However, Thomas's 2003 study actually supports the use of lead rubber in this way, claiming that the resulting radiographic contrast is improved as a result of less scatter reaching the receptor.[74]

IR is horizontal, an antiscatter grid is employed

Positioning

- From the AP position the patient is turned 90° onto their side to bring the coronal plane 90° to the table-top and the MSP parallel to it, with their back to the radiographer for ease of positioning
- The patient's head is rested on a low radiolucent pad or pillow and the knees and hips are flexed for stability
- The patient's upper arm is placed stretched above their head to help bring the spine parallel to the table-top and clear the humerus and soft tissue of the arm from the field. The lower arm is raised onto the pad or pillow to clear it from the field
- The spinous processes are palpated and assessed to ensure that the long axis of the spine and the MSP are parallel to the table-top; this may require the use of a firm radiolucent pad under the lowered end of the thoracic spine if not parallel, but comments after the beam angulation section for this projection should also be noted before considering this. If the spine has a lateral curvature when the patient is lying on their side, with the curve appearing as a slight 'u' shape, it is usually not necessary to make adjustments to the central ray or to use pads. This is because the oblique rays around the central ray are likely to correspond with the obliquity of the intervertebral joint spaces. If a curvature appears as a slight 'n' shape, it will be more advantageous to turn the patient onto their opposite side for this projection. In any case, lateral curvature is often best assessed by viewing the AP projection before attempting the lateral position. If the vertebral column is straight, but not parallel to the IR, angulation will be required to ensure the central ray is perpendicular to the long axis of the spine (see Beam Direction below).

Beam Direction and FRD

Vertical at 90° to the long axis of the thoracic spine

Reference has already been made to the use of radiolucent pads to help the spine lie parallel to the IR, but it must be remembered that the effectiveness of this will vary according to the weight of the patient (heavier patients will squash the pad more than slimmer patients, thereby reducing the effect of the pad). Variations in the anatomy of individual patients will require varying compensation to allow the thoracic column to lie parallel to the IR. Insertion of pads can also be somewhat difficult when a patient is elderly, obese, or suffering from back pain and lying in the lateral position. Angulation of the beam in a direction that will ensure the central ray strikes the long axis of the thoracic vertebrae at 90° can also be used as an alternative strategy. It is easier to use this, rather than the pad method, and beam angulation will more accurately facilitate the correct 90° beam–vertebral column relationship. Most frequently patients with broad shoulders present with the elevated end of the thoracic spine at their shoulder level, requiring cranial angle.

115–150 cm FRD

Note the range of FRDs offered; this is after consideration of the comments made in the introductory notes for this projection.

Centring Point

At the level of T8 approximately 2–3 cm behind the mid-axillary line, and 7–9 cm anterior to the spinous process of T7.

Note that the spinous process of T7 lies level with the body of T8. T8 can also be located from the posterior aspect of the patient by palpating the inferior angle of the scapula, which lies level with T8, even when the arm is raised. Approximations in given measurements are due to the vast differences in patient shapes and sizes.

Collimation

C7 to L1, anterior vertebral bodies, spinous processes

Criteria for Assessing Image Quality

- T2 should be demonstrated and not obscured by the upper arms and shoulders; the body of L1 should be included inferiorly (it is not usually possible to demonstrate T1 on the lateral projection because of the shoulder thickness; it may be necessary to take a supplementary projection of this area if the clinical history indicates a need for this)
- All anterior bodies and spinous processes are demonstrated
- There is superimposition of the posterior ribs and superimposition of the anterior and posterior borders of the vertebral bodies
- Superimposition of the inferior and superior borders of the vertebral bodies and intervertebral disc spaces is demonstrated
- There is blurring of the ribs and lung markings if the breathing technique is used
- Correct image density to demonstrate the bony cortex and trabeculae of all the vertebrae with sufficient penetration of the shoulder region to visualise the upper vertebrae, without over-blackening of the lower vertebrae

Common Errors: Lateral Thoracic Spine

Common Errors	Possible Reasons	Potential Effects on PCE or Report
Collimation may result in some of the vertebral column being excluded from the image	Apart from poor centring and collimation, this may be caused by a kyphosis; this should be obvious on visual inspection of the patient and collimation must take the effects of kyphosis into consideration	If there are parts of the vertebral column missing from the image then it would be impossible to confidently exclude bony trauma or pathology
The anterior and posterior borders of the bodies are not superimposed	The patient is either rotated too far forward or too far back; ensure the coronal plane is 90° to the table-top	Anterior and posterior alignment of the vertebral bodies would be more difficult to interpret. Osteoporotic collapse may be more difficult to determine
The intervertebral joint spaces are not demonstrated; upper and lower borders of the vertebral bodies are not superimposed	The long axis of the spine is not parallel to the table-top. Care should be taken to ensure the spinous processes are all parallel to the table-top, with use of radiolucent pads if necessary, or the beam should be angled to strike the spine at 90° to its long axis	More subtle pathology or trauma would be less readily apparent Anterior dislocation or subluxation, although uncommon in this area, could be misinterpreted

References

1. Anderson P, et al. Clearing the cervical spine in the blunt trauma patient. *J Am Acad Orthop Surg.* 2010;18:149–159.
2. Menaker J, et al. Computed tomography alone for cervical spine clearance in the unreliable patient. Are we there yet? *J Trauma Injury Infect Crit Care.* 2008;64:898–904.
3. Hoffman JR, et al. Selective cervical spine radiography in blunt trauma. *Ann Emerg Med.* 1998;32(4):461–469.
4. Mower WR, et al. Selective cervical spine radiography of blunt trauma victims. *Acad Emerg Med.* 1999;6(5):451.
5. Stiell IG, et al. Obtaining consensus for a definition of 'clinically important cervical spine injury' in the CCC study. *Acad Emerg Med.* 1999;6(5):435.
6. Stolberg HO. The development of radiology guidelines in Canada. *Canad Assoc Radiol J.* 1999;50(83–8):152–155.
7. Stiell IG, et al. The Canadian C-spine rule for radiography in alert and stable trauma patients. *J Am Med Assoc.* 2001;286(15):1841–1848.
8. Stiell IG, et al. Application of the NEXUS low-risk criteria for cervical spine radiography in Canadian Emergency Departments. *Acad Emerg Med.* 2000;7(5):566.
9. National Institute for Health and Care Excellence (NICE). Pathway for C-spine imaging of neck with head injury. Overview; 2019. https://pathways.nice.org.uk/pathways/head-injury.
10. Kerr D, et al. Implementation of the Canadian C-spine rule reduces cervical spine X-ray rate for alert patients with potential neck injury. *J Emerg Med.* 2005;28:127–131.
11. Hills MW, Dean SA. Head injury and facial injury: is there an increased risk of cervical spine injury? *J Trauma.* 1993;34:549–554.
12. Paiva S, et al. Spinal cord injury and its association with blunt head trauma. *Int J Gen Med.* 2011;4:613–615.
13. NICE (National Institute for Health and Care Excellence). Take head injuries seriously. Clinical guideline [CG176]; 2019. https://www.nice.org.uk/guidance/cg176/documents/take-head-injuries-seriously-says-nice-.
14. Melville GE, Taveras JM. Traumatic injuries of the spinal cord and nerve roots. In: Taveras J, Ferrucci J, eds. *Radiology on CD-ROM.* Philadelphia: Lippincott; 2001.
15. Pang D, Pollack I. Spinal cord injury without radiographic abnormality in children – the SCIWORA syndrome. *J Trauma.* 1989;29:654–663.
16. Ullrich A, et al. Distracting painful injuries associated with cervical spinal injuries in blunt trauma. *Acad Emerg Med.* 2001;8(1):25–29.
17. Link TM, et al. Substantial head trauma: value of routine CT examination of the cervicocranium. *Radiology.* 1995;196:741–745.
18. Hackl W, et al. Prevalence of cervical spine injuries in patients with facial trauma. *Oral Surg Oral Med Oral Pathol Oral Radiol Endodont.* 2001;92(4):370–376.

19. American College of Radiology. ACR appropriateness Criteria® suspected spine trauma. https://acsearch.acr.org/docs/69359/Narrative/; 2018.
20. Thompson W, et al. Association of injury mechanism with the risk of cervical spine fractures. *Canad J Emerg Med Care.* 2009;11(1):14–22.
21. Stiell IG, et al. How important is mechanism of injury in predicting the risk of cervical spine injury? *Am Emerg Med.* 2001;8(5):456–457.
22. Brookes RA, Willett KM. Evaluation of the Oxford protocol for total spinal clearance in the unconscious trauma patient. *J Trauma.* 2001;50(5):862–867.
23. European Commission. *Radiation Protection 118: Referral Guidelines for Imaging.* Luxembourg: European Commission Directorate-General for the Environment; 2000.
24. Gonzalez-Beicos A, Nunez D. Role of multidetector computed tomography in the assessment of cervical spine trauma. *Semin Ultrasound CT MRI.* 2009;30(3):159–167.
25. Grogan E, et al. Cervical spine evaluation in urban trauma centers: lowering institutional costs and complications through helical CT scan. *J Am Coll Surg.* 2005;200(2):160–165.
26. Harris T, et al. Clearing the cervical spine in obtunded patients. *Spine.* 2008;33(14):1547–1553.
27. NICE (National Institute for Health and Care Excellence). Spinal injury: assessment and initial management. NICE guideline [NG41]; 2016. https://www.nice.org.uk/guidance/ng41.
28. Fuller N, et al. Cervical spine fractures in the elderly: are there missed opportunities for prevention? Open research Exeter. https://ore.exeter.ac.uk/repository/bitstream/handle/10871/35658/NOS%20poster%20FINAL.pdf?sequence=1.
29. Harris MB, et al. Evaluation of the cervical spine in the polytrauma patient. *Spine.* 2000;15(22):2884–2891. 25.
30. West OC, et al. Acute cervical spine trauma: diagnostic performance of single view versus three view radiographic screening. *Radiology.* 1997;204:819–823.
31. Baker C, et al. Evaluation of paediatric cervical spine injuries. *Am J Emerg Med.* 1999;17:230–234.
32. MacDonald RL, et al. Diagnosis of cervical spine injury in motor vehicle crash victims: how many x-rays are enough? *J Trauma.* 1990;30(4):392–397.
33. Holliman CJ, et al. Is the anteroposterior cervical spine radiograph necessary in initial trauma screening? *Am J Emerg Med.* 1991;9(5):421–425.
34. Turetsky DB, et al. Technique and use of supine oblique views in acute cervical spine trauma. *Ann Emerg Med.* 1993;22(4):685–689.
35. Doris PE, Wilson RA. The next logical step in the emergency radiographic evaluation of cervical spine trauma: the five view trauma series. *J Emerg Med.* 1985;3:371–375.
36. Abel MS. The exaggerated supine oblique view of the cervical spine. *Skelet Radiol.* 1982;8:213–219.
37. Unett EM, Royle AJ. *Radiographic Techniques and Image Evaluation.* London: Chapman and Hall; 1997.
38. Daffner RH. Cervical radiography for trauma patients: a time-effective technique? *Am J Roentgenol.* 2000;175:1309–1311.
39. American College of Radiology. ACR standard for the performance of radiography of the cervical spine in children and adults. [online]; 1999. http://www.acr.org/departments/stand_accred/standards/dl_list.html.
40. Platzer P, et al. Delayed or missed diagnosis of cervical spine injuries. *J Trauma-Injury Infect Crit Care.* 2006;61(1):150–155.
41. Pollack CV, et al. The utility of flexion-extension radiographs of the cervical spine in blunt trauma. *Acad Emerg Med.* 2001;8(5):488.
42. Mirvis SE, et al. Protocol-driven radiologic evaluation of suspected cervical spine injury: efficacy study. *Radiology.* 1989;170:831–834.
43. Nunez DB, et al. Cervical spine trauma: how much do we learn by routinely using helical CT? *Radiographics.* 1996;16:1307–1318.
44. Matar LD, Doyle AJ. Prevertebral soft-tissue measurements in cervical spine injury. *Australas Radiol.* 1997;41:229–237.
45. Herr CH, et al. Sensitivity of prevertebral soft tissue measurement of C3 for detection of cervical spine fractures and dislocations. *Am J Emerg Med.* 1998;16(40):346–349.
46. Deng F, et al. Perivertebral space. [online] Radiopaedia. https://radiopaedia.org/articles/perivertebral-space.
47. Patel MS. Are soft tissue measurements on lateral cervical spine X rays reliable in the assessment of traumatic injuries? *Eur J Trauma Emerg Surg.* 2013;39(6):613–618.
48. Ghanem I, et al. Pediatric cervical spine instability. *J Child Orthop.* 2008;2(2):71–84.
49. Carver BJ, Roche D. An alternative technique for visualisation of the C7/T1 junction in trauma. *Br J Radiol.* 2000;73:73.
50. Swallow R, et al. *Clark's Positioning in Radiography.* 11th ed. London: Heinemann; 1986.
51. Pellei DD. The fat C2 sign. *Radiology.* 2000;217:359–360.
52. Fell M. Cervical spine trauma radiographs: swimmers and supine obliques; an exploration of current practice. *Radiography.* 2011;17(1):33–38.
53. Lampignano JP. *Bontrager's Textbook of Radiographic Positioning and Related Anatomy.* 9th ed. St Louis: Mosby; 2018.
54. Rethnam U, et al. The swimmer's view: does it really show what it is supposed to show? A retrospective study. *BMC Med Imag.* 2008;8(2).
55. Kaneriya PP, et al. The cost-effectiveness of oblique radiography in the exclusion of C7–T1 injury in trauma patients. *AJR Am J Roentgenol.* 1998;171:959–962.
56. Carver E, Carver B. *Medical Imaging: Techniques, Reflection, Evaluation.* 2nd ed. Edinburgh: Churchill Livingstone; 2012.
57. Woodford MJ. Radiography of the acute cervical spine. *Radiography.* 1987;53(607):3–8.
58. Westbrook C. *Handbook of MRI Technique.* 3rd ed. Oxford: Blackwell Science; 2008.
59. Schoenfeld A, et al. Computed tomography alone versus computed tomography and magnetic resonance imaging in the identification of occult injuries to the cervical spine: a meta-analysis. *J Trauma Injury Infect Crit Care.* 2010;68(1):109–114.
60. Tomycz N, et al. MRI Is unnecessary to clear the cervical spine in obtunded/comatose trauma patients: the four-year experience of a level I trauma center. *J Trauma Injury Infect Crit Care.* 2008;64(5):1258–1263.
61. Hogan G, et al. Exclusion of unstable cervical spine injury in obtunded patients with blunt trauma: is MR imaging needed when multi-detector row CT findings are normal? *Radiology.* 2005;237:106–113.
62. Raby N, et al. *Accident and Emergency Radiology: A Survival Guide.* 3rd ed. London: Saunders; 2014.
63. Long BW, Rafert JA. *Orthopaedic Radiography.* Philadelphia: Saunders; 1995.
64. NICE (National Institute for Health and Care Excellence). Myeloma: diagnosis and management. NICE guideline [NG35]; 2018. https://www.nice.org.uk/guidance/ng35.
65. Graeber A, Cecava ND. Vertebral osteomyelitis. StatPearls [Internet]. https://www.ncbi.nlm.nih.gov/books/NBK532256/.
66. Duckworth T. *Lecture Notes on Orthopaedics and Fractures.* Oxford: Blackwell Science; 1995.
67. Brennan PC, Madigan E. Lumbar spine radiology; analysis of the posteroanterior projection. *Eur Radiol.* 2000;10:1197–1201.
68. Levy AR, et al. Reducing the lifetime risks of cancer from spinal radiographs amongst people with adolescent idiopathic scoliosis. *Spine.* 1996;21(13):1500–1507.
69. Eisenberg RL, et al. *Radiographic Positioning.* 2nd ed. Boston: Little Brown and Company; 1995.
70. McQuillen-Martensen K. *Radiographic Critique.* 3rd ed. Philadelphia: Saunders; 2010.
71. Unett EM, Royle AJ. *Radiographic Techniques and Image Evaluation.* London: Nelson Thornes; 1997.
72. Bell GA, Finlay DBL. *Basic Radiographic Positioning.* Eastbourne: Baillière Tindall; 1986.
73. Ballinger PW, Frank ED. *Merrill's Atlas of Radiographic Positioning and Radiologic Procedures.* 10th ed. St Louis: Mosby; 2003.
74. Thomas A. Imaging the lateral thoracic spine. *Synergy.* 2003. April:10–13.

10 Lumbar Spine, Sacrum and Coccyx

ELIZABETH CARVER, BARRY CARVER and JEANETTE CARTER

Referrals for plain radiography of the lumbar region have been dwindling since the early 1990s, with magnetic resonance imaging (MRI) being recognised as superior for diagnosis of a range of conditions affecting the spine and its associated anatomy. Computed tomography (CT) is also recognised as having a key role in spinal imaging, especially in diagnosis and assessment of fractures.[1]

Back pain, whether acute or chronic, is not itself an indicator for plain radiography; however, back pain may be associated with more serious features, in which case MRI is the investigation of choice.

Studies have shown that only a very small percentage of requests for plain radiography change patient management[2] and so they are not cost-effective.[3] The high radiation dose associated with lumbar spine radiography should not be used to provide patient reassurance, or indeed reassurance for the referrer.[4]

MRI is generally recognised as the most appropriate modality for lumbar spine imaging in many circumstances.[1,3] Cost and availability are factors that will still predispose some global regions to the continued use of plain radiography; the significant radiation dose burden must, however, always be considered for justification of this procedure.[5]

CT has been advocated for demonstration of pars interarticularis abnormalities which lead to spondylolisthesis,[6] but its role in imaging the intervertebral disc should be limited to patients unable to undergo MRI. CT also has a role in significant trauma where modern multislice scanners can use multiplanar and 3D bony reconstruction techniques.

CT is best for assessing osseous integrity in metastatic disease but MRI is superior for assessment of soft tissue involvement. Positron emission tomography (PET) and PET/CT are also useful for assessment in metastatic disease.[7]

Please note that, although a recommended FRD is given for each projection in this chapter, local protocols and equipment-specific guidance may differ.

PCE COMMENTS – LUMBAR REGION

Check alignment of vertebral bodies on both AP and lateral in the lumbar region. Often pathologies are well demonstrated by assessing alignment. It is important to assess posterior vertebral body alignment on laterals, which will show anterolisthesis and retrolisthesis.

Note if there is loss of intervertebral joint space (which may indicate lumbar disc prolapse).

Look on the lateral for evidence of lordosis or kyphosis, and on the AP note any scoliosis.

On the AP – are spinous processes in line? This may indicate facet joint dislocations if not in line.

Fracture and dislocation: These can cause misalignment of the vertebral column. Also check for loss of vertebral body height on both AP and lateral – wedge, compression and burst fractures are most commonly seen; wedge fractures can occur when the anterior border of a vertebral body is crushed due to flexion or vertical pressure, i.e. a high fall landing on the feet or head.

Transverse process fractures and spinous process fractures should also be commented on in both projections.

Pars interarticularis fractures are best identified with MRI or CT imaging, but can be seen on oblique lumbar spine projections (which are rarely undertaken when MRI or CT is readily available). Fractures of the pars can occasionally be seen on the lateral radiograph.

Spondylolisthesis (forward slippage of one vertebra in relation to the vertebra below) is seen on lateral radiographs, although plain radiography may not be the most appropriate investigative method. L5 slippage on the first sacral segment (S1) is most frequently found. These are often incidental findings on images and are not usually directly related to specific traumatic incidents. Presence of spondylolisthesis should be commented upon, giving information on vertebrae involved, and identifying which vertebra has slipped forward.

Metastatic disease is characterised by secondary deposits seen as lytic, and in some cases sclerotic, lesions; pathological fractures may be present. Note if there is a winking owl[8] (or winking eye) on the AP. On a normal AP the pedicles appear rounded, as in owl's eyes; when one eye (pedicle) is missing, or 'winking', this is a sign of malignancy or infection. There needs to be 50% bone destruction before the sign can be seen, but it can often be the first red flag. Nuclear medicine imaging or MRI are generally the most appropriate examinations for early detection.

Note if there is *spondylosis*, seen as bony outgrowths (osteophytes) on superior and inferior vertebral bodies (AP and lateral projections). Is there any evidence of advanced spondylitic disease, such as ankylosis spondylitis?

Check the sacroiliac joints for alignment and for *sacroiliitis*. Sacroiliitis appears as a roughly triangular area of increased density over the sacroiliac joint.

Spina bifida occulta may be seen on an AP radiograph; the defect does not involve the meninges or spinal cord and is usually an incidental finding on an AP radiograph of the area.

Challenges of the Lumbar Spine Examination

There are a number of challenges the radiographer will encounter when positioning a patient, not only due to the patient's physical shape and size but in judging the radiographic planes of the body in relation to the patient and X-ray table. The following tips may be helpful in overcoming difficulties that may be encountered.

Positioning Tips

When initially studying a patient's X-ray request form, prior knowledge of their clinical history assists in the problem-solving and decision-making processes crucial for the optimum choice of positioning technique required, in order to achieve a high-quality diagnostic image. Initial clinical evaluation of the shape of the spine will assist in any positioning adjustment requirements if the patient is placed on the X-ray couch for the examination. This is particularly important for patients with abnormal configurations of the spine.

The patient should be made to feel comfortable and relaxed; tension can cause difficulty when attempting to move a patient into position. The examination gown should be adjusted if necessary to ensure that no folds will interfere with their movement into the required position and that the anatomical landmarks can be easily palpated. If the gown design includes a split, this must be at the back of the patient, to allow for visualisation of the spinal column while palpating its surface markings.

Palpation of the prime anatomical landmarks is important when adjusting the patient into the correct position for each projection. Clinical palpation is a skill which, if practised with reservations, can lead to mistakes. Physical contact involving the lower trunk, as required for lumbar spine examination, requires a degree of tact and diplomacy while using precision and gentleness but firmness.

A key requisite for accurate positioning of the lateral lumbar projections is to assess the position of the long axis of the vertebral column in relation to the image receptor (IR). The column should be palpated *and* visually assessed along the lumbar section, with the *eyes at the level of the lumbar vertebrae.* Radiographers often assess visually from a point that is higher than the spine; this does not give a true impression of the vertebral position. Palpation of the spinous processes is also essential and must be implemented in addition to visual assessment, as the muscles on the posterior aspect of the patient can sag (especially in the middle-aged and elderly), giving an inaccurate impression if visual assessment only is used.

For lumbar spine X-ray examinations the anatomical landmarks chosen during positioning set-up techniques are considered reasonably standard, although their position relative to the surrounding anatomical structures can vary due to osteological changes. Excessive fatty tissue can also cause difficulty in palpation techniques and there is a large variation in total body fat in individuals of varying age and between populations. Therefore, standardisation of the anatomical sites used for positioning and palpation is important.

AP and Lateral Projections

ANTEROPOSTERIOR (AP) LUMBAR SPINE (FIG. 10.1A,B)

The projection may be undertaken erect or supine. If using an erect technique, ensure the patient is able to stand safely. The images shown are for the supine approach.

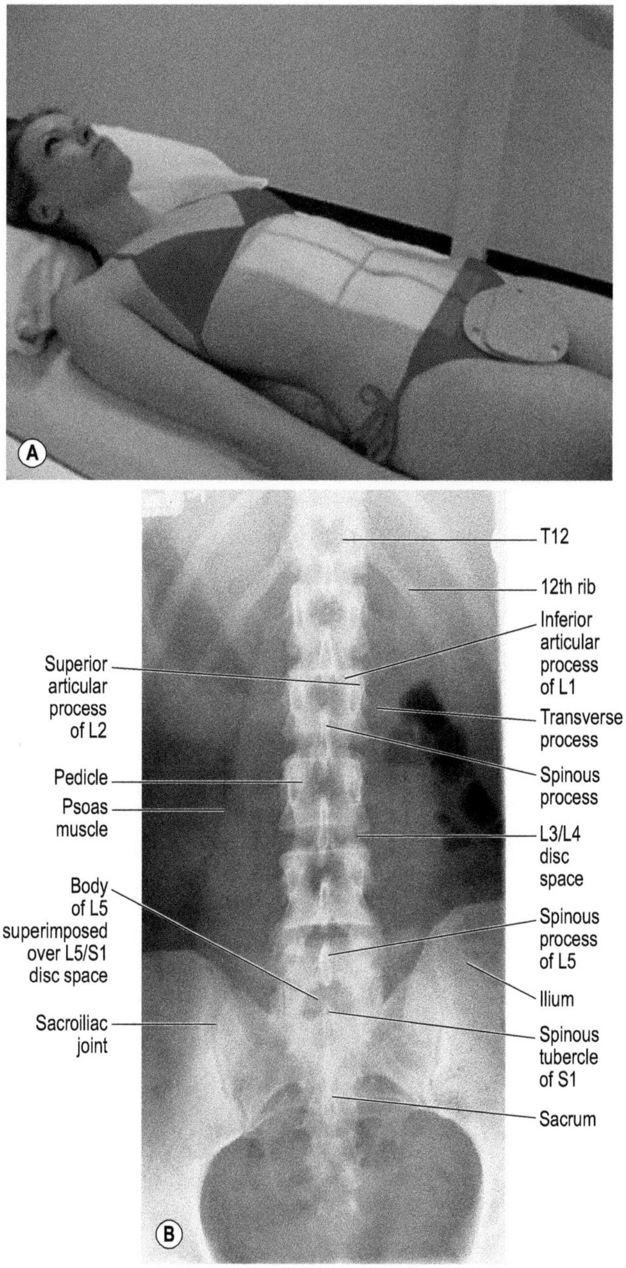

Fig. 10.1 AP lumbar spine.

IR is horizontal for a supine patient, or vertical for an erect approach

An antiscatter grid is employed

Positioning

- The patient is supine or erect, with their arms placed on the pillow when supine or abducted from their trunk if erect. In the erect position weight should be distributed evenly, so slight separation of the feet is recommended (this will also improve stability)
- In the supine patient the knees may be supported with a pad for patient comfort; to reduce the lumbar lordosis and enable better visualisation of the intervertebral joint spaces, the legs should be supported with the femora at 45° or more to the table-top. For the erect approach the patient may require a secondary

aid to hold while standing; it is important to make sure that the patient uses the immobilisation aid in such a way that their weight is evenly distributed and their spine position remains as required for the projection

- The mid-sagittal plane (MSP) is 90° to the IR and the coronal plane is parallel to it

Beam Direction and FRD

90° to the IR
100 cm FRD

Centring

In the midline, at the level of the lower costal margin (level of L3)

Collimation

Psoas muscles, transverse processes of LV1–LV5, T12/L1 joint space, sacroiliac joints

Criteria for Assessing Image Quality

- Psoas muscles, transverse processes of LV1–LV5, T12/L1 joint space, sacroiliac joints are demonstrated
- Spinous processes are in the centre of vertebral bodies, demonstrating no rotation
- L2/L3 and L3/L4 joint spaces are demonstrated; other intervertebral spaces will be projected obliquely due to lumbar curvature
- Sharp image demonstrating soft tissue of abdominal viscera in contrast to bone and air in the gastrointestinal tract; detail of bony cortex and trabeculae; spinous processes visualised through vertebral bodies

Notes on Exposing on Arrested Respiration for the AP Projection

Exposure is made on arrested respiration, to prevent blurring of abdominal contents. The respiratory phase is unimportant as the diaphragm will not move over the body of L1 in either phase. It is likely, though, that selection of exposure factors will be affected by opposite phases of respiration, as extreme inspiration will increase the volume and density of abdominal tissue overlying the lumbar area. This will be likely to necessitate an increase in exposure factors, which will result in an increase in radiation dose to the patient and a decrease in image contrast due to increased scatter from the greater tissue volume and density.

An alternative to demonstrate the transverse processes free from overlying gas shadows is to use a long exposure with the patient gently panting, using the effect of autotomography to prevent the gas obscuring bony detail.

Common Errors: AP Lumbar Spine

Common Errors	Possible Reasons	Potential Effects on PCE or Report
Spinous processes not in the midline of vertebral bodies	1. Rotation of the spine – MSP not perpendicular to the IR. Adjust the patient position so that the pelvis and shoulders are not rotated	Makes assessment of pedicles difficult; rotation will mean the pedicles are not clearly demonstrated. Therefore the chance of possible malignancy/metastases being missed is increased (winking owl sign can be missed)
	2. Scoliosis may cause this appearance and may not be improved upon. This is distinguishable from rotation due to position error by the distinct lateral curve of the column and potential variation of rotation down its length[9]	Scoliosis assessment is difficult, including identification of potential rotational issues
No intervertebral discs clearly demonstrated	Excessive lordosis – the direction of the primary beam can be adjusted so that the beam is directed through the required joint spaces *(see comments below)*	Vertebral body heights cannot be accurately assessed; this will mean that potentially fractured vertebral bodies can be missed or over-called. Disc space height cannot be accurately assessed; there will be risk of both under-/over-calling loss of disc space height
Lateral collimation too close, and psoas muscles are not seen in their entirety		The sacroiliac jojnts cannot be considered fully demonstrated. It will not be possible to check for loss of alignment, degenerative changes, RA changes or sacroiliitis (which is usually seen on the iliac aspect of the SIJ)
T12 omitted from the image		In trauma cases this is a common injury site, especially after whiplash injury. Omission of this vertebra clearly compromises injury identification

It has commonly been believed that the curvature of the lumbar spine can be reduced by an angled pad being placed under the knees, if the AP projection is undertaken supine, enabling better visualisation of the intervertebral joint spaces by associated flattening of the lumbar lordotic curve. The effectiveness of knee flexion is traditionally claimed to be felt by a simple experiment: if one lies supine with the legs extended a flat hand will slide easily under the arch made by the lumbar curve. When the knees and hips are flexed, the hand feels the lumbar area press down onto its dorsal aspect, suggesting a reduction in lumbar curve. The more the hips and knees are flexed, the more the curve appears to reduce. But is the movement felt by the hand merely muscular movement rather than reduction of lordosis? Would an increase in knee/hip flexion actually show a more significant lumbar curve reduction?

The effect was disputed by Murrie et al,[10] but this research was undertaken on a very small sample of seven examinations and this raises questions on the validity of the research. It is also noted that Murrie et al flexed the knees over a pad, which may not offer adequate *hip* flexion to reduce the lumbar curve.

Further research on this topic was performed on a larger sample of 60 volunteers by Downing,[11] who found that the lumbar curve was effectively reduced by up to 64% by hip and knee flexion, but in order that flexion is effective the femora should be at 45° to the table-top, as described in the technique description in this chapter. Note that the key is the angle between the femora and the table-top, *not* the angle of flexion of the knees.

However, the question must be asked 'Do we require all joint spaces to be visualised on an AP?': information regarding intervertebral disc spaces is more readily available on the lateral view, and on MRI, which after all is the investigation of choice for most lumbar pathologies. Indeed, given the erect AP is often undertaken, this issue becomes redundant if using this approach.

PA or AP?

Owing to the anterior curvature of the lumbar spine it would seem reasonable that the posteroanterior (PA) projection could be preferable to the anteroposterior, as in this position the diverging X-ray beam coincides more closely with the intervertebral joint spaces, enabling better demonstration.

This is not, however, a commonly adopted practice, reasons being the magnification and consequent unsharpness due to increased object receptor distance (ORD). This could be compensated for by an increase in focus receptor distance (FRD) and exposure factors.

Colleran[12] showed that the magnification produced does not cause a significant reduction in image quality and indeed recommends its adoption because of the superior demonstration of the sacrum, sacroiliac joints and intervertebral joint spaces. Her work resulted in the adoption of the PA projection in a small number of imaging departments, and is used extensively in the chiropractic community.

LATERAL LUMBAR SPINE (FIG. 10.2A,B)

The projection may be undertaken erect or on the table. As for the erect AP, ensure that the patient can stand safely for the erect lateral position.

Images shown are for the table-top approach
IR is horizontal for a supine patient, or vertical for an erect approach
An antiscatter grid is employed

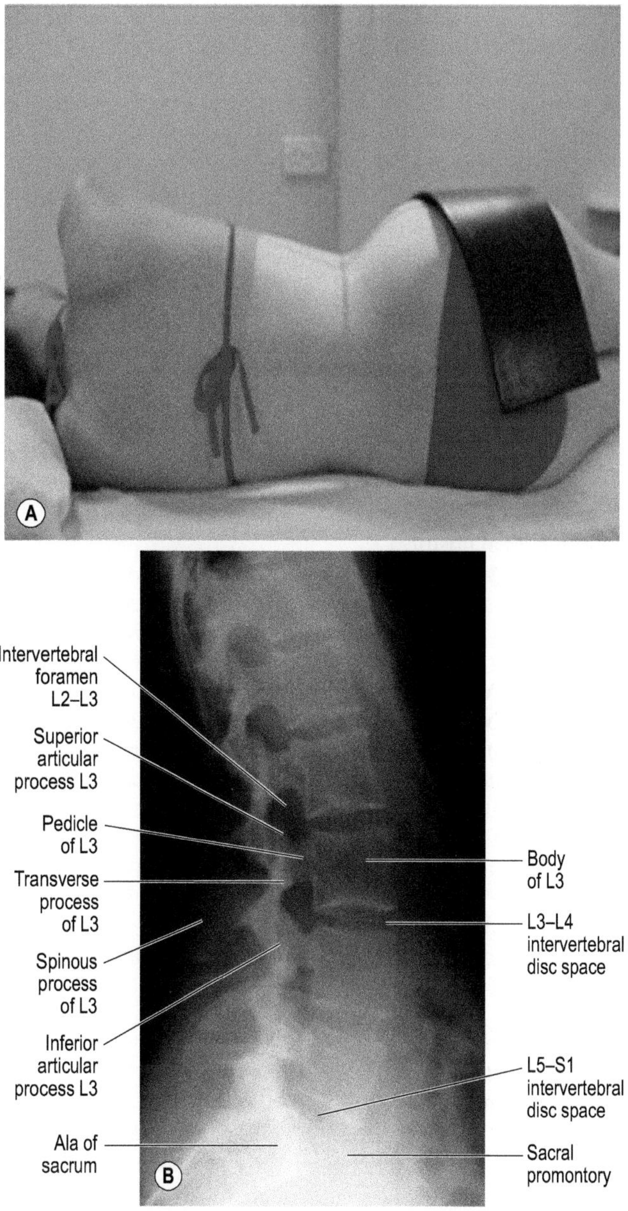

Fig. 10.2 Lateral lumbar spine.

Positioning

- From the AP position the patient is turned 90° towards their *left* side to bring the coronal plane 90° to the IR and the MSP parallel to it, with their back to the radiographer for ease of positioning
- For table-top examinations the knees and hips are flexed for stability and comfort and the arms are rested on the pillow in front of the patient's head; this clears the patient's arms from the required area. A pad may be inserted between the knees to aid positioning, patient comfort and stability. Note that the choice of size is important: it should be of a size that ensures that the raised knee does not affect the parallel position of the MSP in relationship to the couch
- For erect lateral the patient should slightly separate their legs for stability and cross their arms across their chest if they can stand unaided. It may be necessary to offer something to the patient to help keep their balance, and this should be assessed when admitting the patient to the examination room; it is important to make sure that the patient uses the immobilisation aid in such a way that their weight is evenly distributed and their spine position remains as required for the projection
- The spinous processes are palpated and assessed to ensure that the long axis of the spine and the MSP are parallel to the IR; if not, it will be necessary to angle the beam in a direction that will ensure the central ray strikes the long axis of the lumbar vertebrae at 90°. Very often, even in erect techniques, the female pelvis causes the spine to tilt upwards (or outwards if erect) towards the pelvic end of the vertebral column, whereas the male shoulders can cause the opposite effect (although this has more effect on the lateral thoracic spine projection). Radiolucent pads, placed between the lateral aspect of the upper end of the tilted vertebral column, can be used to address this problem. However, the accuracy and effectiveness of this is in question and beam angulation is likely to be more effective (see Chapter 9 regarding the lateral thoracic spine). The alignment of the spinous processes must be assessed with the eyes level with the spine to ensure accuracy. Palpation of the posterior superior iliac spines

(PSISs) to check their superimposition will assure accurate lateral positioning of the pelvic end of the lumbar vertebrae. The shoulder end of the column should also be assessed so that the posterior aspect of the patient's shoulders is 90 degrees to the IR; too frequently patients will rotate the upper shoulder region and this must be avoided

- Table-top examination: if the spine has a lateral curvature when the patient is lying on their side, with L1 and L5 higher than the middle vertebrae, it is not usually necessary to make adjustments in the central ray or to use pads. This is because the oblique rays around the central ray are likely to correspond with the obliquity of the intervertebral joint spaces. If a slight curvature appears with L1 and L5 lower than the middle vertebrae (not commonly encountered), it will be more advantageous to turn the patient onto their opposite side for this projection. In any case, lateral curvature is often best assessed by viewing the AP projection before attempting the lateral position
- If the patient has scoliosis, it is recommended that the side to which the largest curvature is more prominently demonstrated is placed nearest the IR. The central ray is then directed towards the lowest point of the convex shape of the curvature. This ensures that the oblique rays that penetrate each of the vertebral bodies produce an image that assists in reducing the superimposition of the vertebral bodies over intervertebral joint spaces, demonstrating the joint spaces as efficiently as is possible under the circumstances
- Unless otherwise indicated, e.g. by scoliosis, the left lateral should be routinely performed as this results in up to 38% less effective patient dose.[5,13] However, there is some evidence that the right lateral may be preferable in paediatric patients owing to the greater radiosensitivity of the liver in children.[14,15]

Beam Direction and FRD

Vertical central ray 90° to the long axis of the lumbar spine
100–150 cm FRD

Consider using the longer FRD (e.g. 150 cm) to compensate for long ORD. This will also enable better visualisation of the intervertebral joint spaces, as shown in Fig. 10.3A,B.

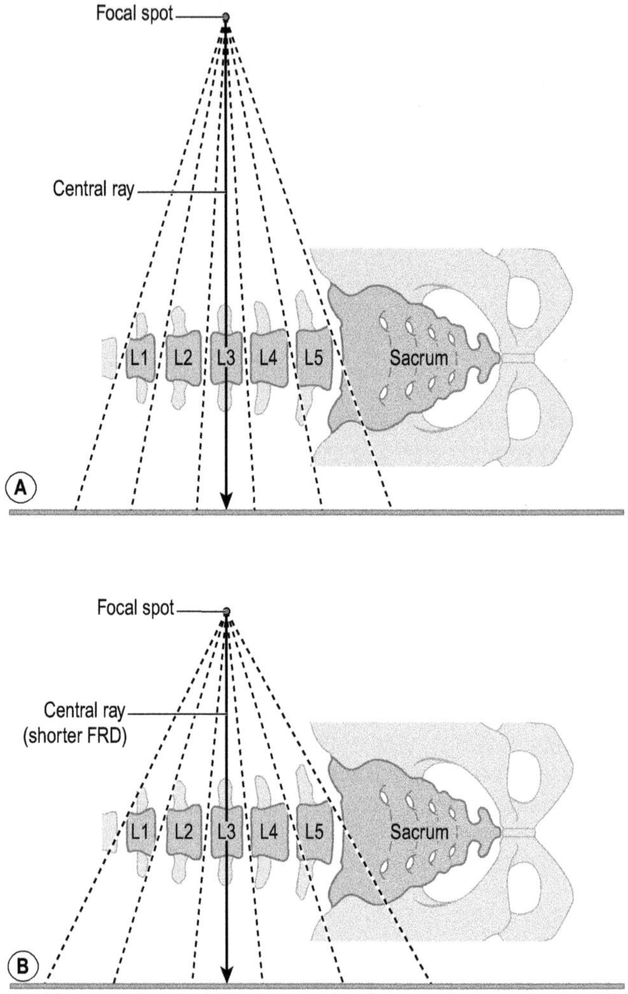

Fig. 10.3 Effects of varying FRDs on joint space demonstration. This is a diagrammatic representation of the lumbar vertebrae in the lateral position. (A) shows the position, which uses a longer FRD than in (B). Notice how the obliquity of the rays at the periphery (L5/S1 and T12/L1) increases with the shorter FRD and increases the chances of vertebral overlap on the image. L3 is unaffected as it lies below the central ray.

Centring Point

At the level of the lower costal margin, which is coincident with L3

The beam is required to be directed through the vertebral body of L3; this can be located 7.5–10 cm anterior to the spinous process of L3, the distance varying with patient build.

Collimation

T12 to S1, anterior aspects of the vertebral bodies, spinous processes

It may be useful to include the aorta anteriorly in patients in whom calcification may indicate the presence of atheromatous degeneration in the aorta. Localised deviation (apparent bulge) of the calcified outline of the aorta is indicative of abdominal aortic aneurysm.

Expose on arrested respiration

The exposure is made on expiration, to ensure the posterolateral aspects of the diaphragms do not overlie L1.

Exposure Factors

A kVp high enough to allow penetration and visualisation of the L5/S1 joint space, as well as to demonstrate the lumbar vertebrae, should be used. EU guidelines suggest 80–95 kVp.[16]

Criteria for Assessing Image Quality

- T12 to S1, spinous processes and soft tissues anterior to vertebral bodies are demonstrated on the image
- Posterior, superior and inferior borders of each vertebral body should be superimposed
- Posterior ribs and superior surfaces of the sacral alae should be superimposed
- Joint spaces between each vertebra should be clearly demonstrated
- Sharp image demonstrating soft tissue structures anterior to the vertebral bodies in contrast to detail of bony cortex and trabeculae; bone seen in contrast with intervertebral joint spaces between T12 and L1 down to L5/S1. Spinous processes of lumbar vertebrae visualised

Common Errors: Lateral Lumbar Spine

Common Errors	Possible Reasons	Potential Effects on PCE or Report
The posterior condyles of the vertebral bodies are not superimposed	Rotation of the patient – MSP not parallel to the table-top. Adjust the hips and/or shoulders so that they are superimposed	Makes assessment of the posterior alignment difficult. This would mean an over- or under-call of loss of alignment of the vertebral bodies. In trauma this can be a significant finding Also if there is a fracture of one of the vertebral bodies it can mean that assessment of the inclusion of the posterior column can be difficult. This again is a vital assessment as it will establish if the fracture is stable, or not
Disc spaces are not clearly demonstrated – the superior and inferior surfaces of the vertebral bodies are not superimposed	The long axis of the vertebral column is not parallel to the table-top (tilt). See notes in positioning section for methods that may be used to correct or compensate	Cannot assess disc space height or cortical irregularities. Subtle wedge fractures and compression fractures may be missed as a result
	Is there a degree of scoliosis which may be affecting joint space demonstration?	
Pale (low density) over L5/S1 region, rest of lumbar spine well demonstrated	Inadequate kVp selected	Limits vertebral body assessment
T12 omitted from the projection		In trauma cases this is a common injury site, especially after whiplash injury. Omission of this vertebra clearly compromises injury identification

Modification of Technique for Trauma

Clearly it is important not to move the patient if trauma is indicated; consequently, it is necessary for the lateral view to be obtained using a horizontal beam with the patient supine.

LATERAL LUMBOSACRAL JUNCTION (LSJ) (FIGS 10.4A,B, 10.5A,B)

The LSJ or L5/S1 projection is normally only required if the joint space is not adequately demonstrated on the lateral projection (i.e. if there is overlap of the vertebral body of L5 onto S1, or if there is insufficient penetration to demonstrate the joint space or bony detail of S1), to enable assessment of the intervertebral height. Under no circumstances should this projection be undertaken 'routinely', without first having assessed the lateral projection for suitability.

It is unnecessary for the joint space to be 'perfectly' demonstrated: some superimposition of the superior surfaces of S1 and the inferior surfaces of L5 is acceptable. A clear disc space with no superimposition of the vertebral bodies is the ideal result and is what we should be looking to achieve; however, the radiation dose burden of this examination needs to be considered. In order to avoid undertaking a lateral L5/S1 projection in addition to the lateral lumbar, assessment of disc space height can often be made on a less than perfect image, as shown in Fig. 10.4B, which shows the lower end of the lumbar vertebrae as they might appear on a lateral lumbar spine image. As long as the four surface edges can be identified then an assessment of joint space is possible, and an additional view of the LSJ is *not* required. These measurements can only be made when the lateral lumbar spine image shows adequate penetration and exposure that provides good detail of the bony trabeculae of the first sacral segment.

The projection may be undertaken erect or on the table. Immobilisation considerations apply as for the AP and lateral if an erect technique is used.

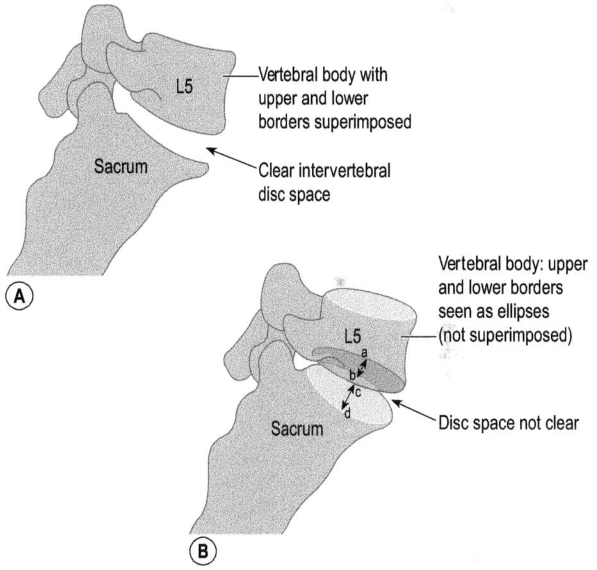

Fig. 10.4 'Tilted' lateral lumbar image: assessment of joint space. (A) 'Perfect' – L5/S1 showing disc space as seen in (B); (B) acceptable – because disc height can be assessed as indicated, by measuring *a–b* and *c–d*.

Images shown are for the table-top approach
IR is horizontal for a table-top examination, or vertical for an erect approach
An antiscatter grid is employed

Positioning

- The patient is positioned as for the lateral projection, with their MSP parallel to the IR
- An imaginary line adjoining the PSISs will demonstrate the plane of the L5/S1 joint space. If not superimposed, the beam should be angled to coincide with this line

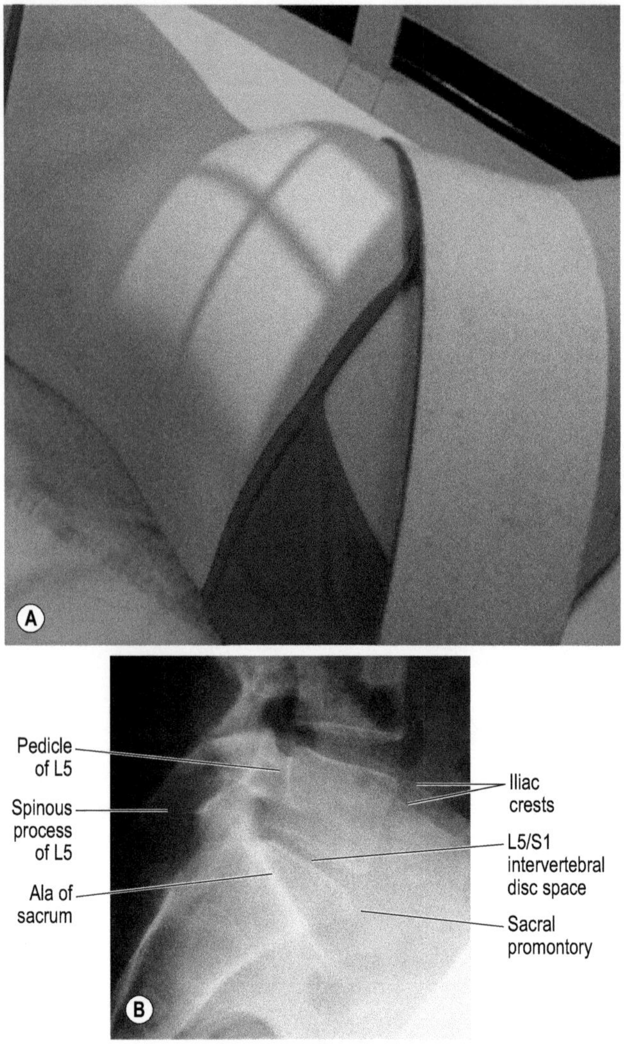

Fig. 10.5 Lateral lumbosacral junction.

Beam Direction and FRD

A central ray coincident with the L5/S1 joint space (alignment of PSISs) should be used. Beam angulation may be required to ensure the central ray is directed through the joint space, which should be assessed by viewing:

1. The AP projection to see if there is a lateral tilt of the lower lumbar spine and/or the joint space at the LSJ. The AP projection *must* be available for assessment before attempting the lateral L5/S1 projection
2. The position of the PSISs when in the lateral position. They should be aligned in order to justify use of a perpendicular central ray. Deviation from this position will mean that the central ray must be angled to coincide with the angle made by the PSISs
3. The lateral lumbar spine image. The radiographer *may* have used a vertical, caudally or cranially angled central ray for the lateral lumbar projection and the appearance of the lateral L5/S1 area on the lateral lumbar spine can be used as a reference point for assessment of the central ray. Modification of the central ray for this projection can be summarised thus:
   If the lateral lumbar image undertaken with a perpendicular central ray shows a good L5/S1 joint space (but is underexposed or under-penetrated), angle approximately 5–7° caudally when the beam is centred over the LSJ
   If the lateral lumbar image undertaken with a caudally angled central ray shows a good L5/S1 joint space (but is underexposed or under-penetrated), add more caudal angulation before centring the beam over the LSJ
   If the lateral lumbar image undertaken with a cranially angled central ray shows a good L5/S1 joint space (but is underexposed or under-penetrated), use a vertical beam centred over the LSJ
   If the lateral lumbar image undertaken with a perpendicular central ray shows a poor L5/S1 joint space it is most likely that a perpendicular central ray will actually be required for the lateral L5/S1 projection unless the AP projection and the PSISs show the opposite is required

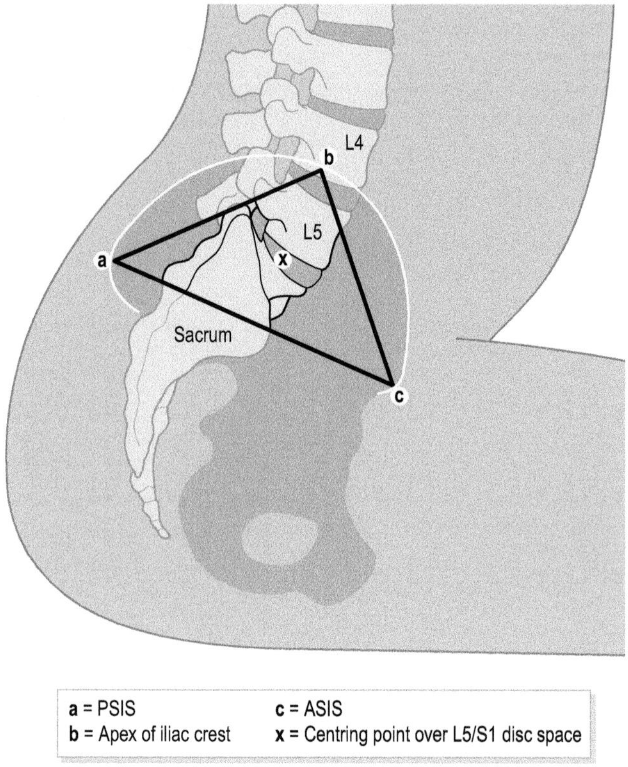

Fig. 10.6 Location of centring point for lateral L5/S1 projection. *a, b* and *c* show the landmarks which make the triangle around the centring point. The triangle is not necessarily equilateral or isosceles, but this is still an effective way to centre accurately.

100–150 cm FRD

Again, consider using the longer FRD to compensate for long ORD.

Centring Point

Through the lumbosacral junction, which lies anterior to the spinous process of L5

This is most readily located as shown in Fig. 10.6. An imaginary triangle is drawn between the readily palpable anterior superior iliac spine (ASIS), PSIS and apex of the iliac crest. The L5/S1 junction lies in the centre of this triangle.

Collimation

Body of L5, first sacral segment, spinous processes

Criteria for Assessing Image Quality

- Bodies of L5 and S1, spinous processes and soft tissues anterior to vertebral bodies are demonstrated on the image
- Posterior, superior and inferior borders of L5 and S1 should be superimposed
- L5/S1 joint space should be clearly demonstrated (but see Fig. 10.4)
- Ala of sacrum superimposed (see *)
- Sharp image demonstrating soft tissue structures anterior to the vertebral bodies in contrast to detail of bony cortex and trabeculae, joint space and spinous process of L5

* Use of the term 'ala' refers to the oblique white lines noted on the lateral projection, which have previously been described as the iliopectineal lines or basis ossis sacri.[17] The lines, whatever their correct name, do lie coincident with the sloped and expanding ala of the sacrum as they join with the pelvis at the sacroiliac joints but experimentation designed to accurately identify the structures proved equivocal; in this case the authors suggested that the lines are simply referred to as 'pelvic lines'.[17] Since the lines have origins associated with the ala the use of the term 'ala' relates to associated anatomy in the projection, as we feel it is simple and less confusing.[18]

Common Errors: Lateral Lumbosacral Junction

Common Errors	Possible Reasons	Potential Effects on PCE or Report
Both sides of ala of sacrum not superimposed; posterior parts of L5 do not appear superimposed	Rotation of the patient. MSP not parallel to the table-top (rotated) – adjust the hips and shoulders so that they are superimposed	Same points as in lateral lumbar are also relevant here
Disc spaces are not clearly demonstrated – the superior and inferior surfaces of the vertebral bodies are not superimposed	Incorrect choice of beam angulation *or* the long axis of the vertebral column is not parallel to the table-top	

ANTEROPOSTERIOR (AP) L5/S1 JUNCTION (FIG. 10.7A,B)

Because of the orientation of the lumbar curve, L5 tilts in opposition to the oblique rays of the X-ray beam; thus the L5/S1 joint space is not well demonstrated on the standard AP projection. The AP L5/S1 projection is rarely used but may be employed for additional evaluation in relevant clinical circumstances,[19] which is most commonly requested for specialist orthopaedic assessment.
IR is horizontal, an antiscatter grid is employed

Positioning

The patient is positioned as for an AP supine lumbar spine projection

Beam Direction and FRD

Initially vertical, with a cranial angle of 10–20°, according to the patient's lumbar lordosis, which tends to be more extreme in the female adult.[20] The lateral projection should be viewed before assessing the angulation required

Centring Point

In the midline, level with the ASISs; this may vary slightly according to cranial angle used

Collimation

L4/L5 junction, L5, transverse processes, L5/S1 junction

Criteria for Assessing Image Quality

- L4/L5 junction, L5, transverse processes, and L5/S1 junction are demonstrated
- L4/L5 and L5/S1 joint space shown clearly
- Spinous process of L5 centralised over vertebral body
- Sharp image showing contrast between bony trabeculae of vertebral bodies and the joint spaces between

Common Error: AP L5/S1 Junction

Common Error	Possible Reason	Potential Effects on PCE or Report
Poor joint space visualisation	Inaccurate angle selection	Joint space cannot be assessed

Oblique Projections

Oblique projections are rarely undertaken in the 21st century, given that CT imaging provides information that is superior to plain X-radiography. If obliques are undertaken, they are carried out as supine obliques, or posterior obliques. Oblique projections demonstrate the apophyseal joints, laminae, pedicles and pars interarticularis. They are used in particular to demonstrate defects in the pars interarticularis which may result in spondylolisthesis. Both obliques are undertaken, for comparison.

POSTERIOR OBLIQUES (FIG. 10.8A,B)

IR is horizontal, an antiscatter grid is employed

Positioning

- The patient lies supine, their MSP coincident with and perpendicular to the midline of the table

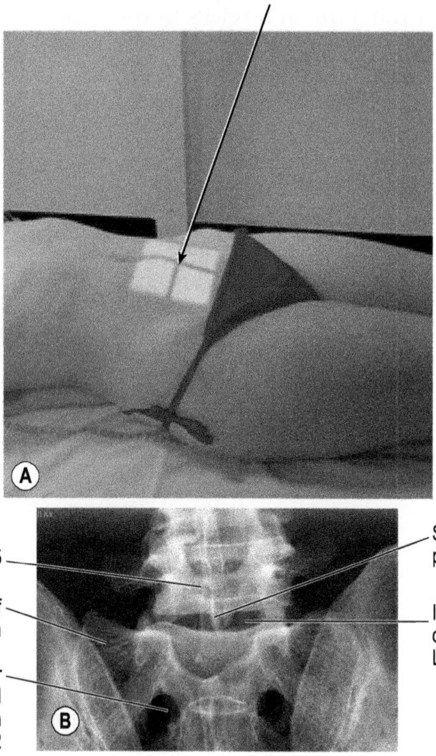

Fig. 10.7 (A) AP LSJ. (B) Notice how the appearances of L5 and its spinous process and L5/S1 joint space change from the AP lumbar spine image (Fig. 10.1B) to this, the AP L5/S1 image. This is because (1) the oblique rays in the AP lumbar image are caudal and the lumbar curve tilts the body of L5 forwards over the joint space; (2) the beam is angled opposite to this (cranially) for the AP L5/S1 projection, coinciding with the disc space.

- The arm on the side under examination is raised onto the pillow, for comfort and ease of positioning
- The patient is rotated 45° *towards* the side under examination
- Radiolucent pads are placed under the trunk and raised shoulder for support. The arm on the unaffected side must be clear of the area under examination

Beam Direction and FRD

Vertical *or*
For lordotic patients the beam is angled with a cranial or caudal tilt of between 10° and 15°. The degree of angle used is dependent upon the degree of lordosis and the direction of angle relates to which vertebrae are under examination (e.g. caudal angle for L1 and L2, cranial for L4 and L5)
100 cm FRD

Centring Point

Over the raised side of the trunk at the level of the lower costal margin (level of L3), in the midclavicular line

Collimation

T12/L1 junction, L5/S1 junction, bodies and transverse processes of lumbar vertebrae

Criteria for Assessing Image Quality

- T12/L1 junction, L5/S1 junction, bodies and transverse processes of lumbar vertebrae are demonstrated

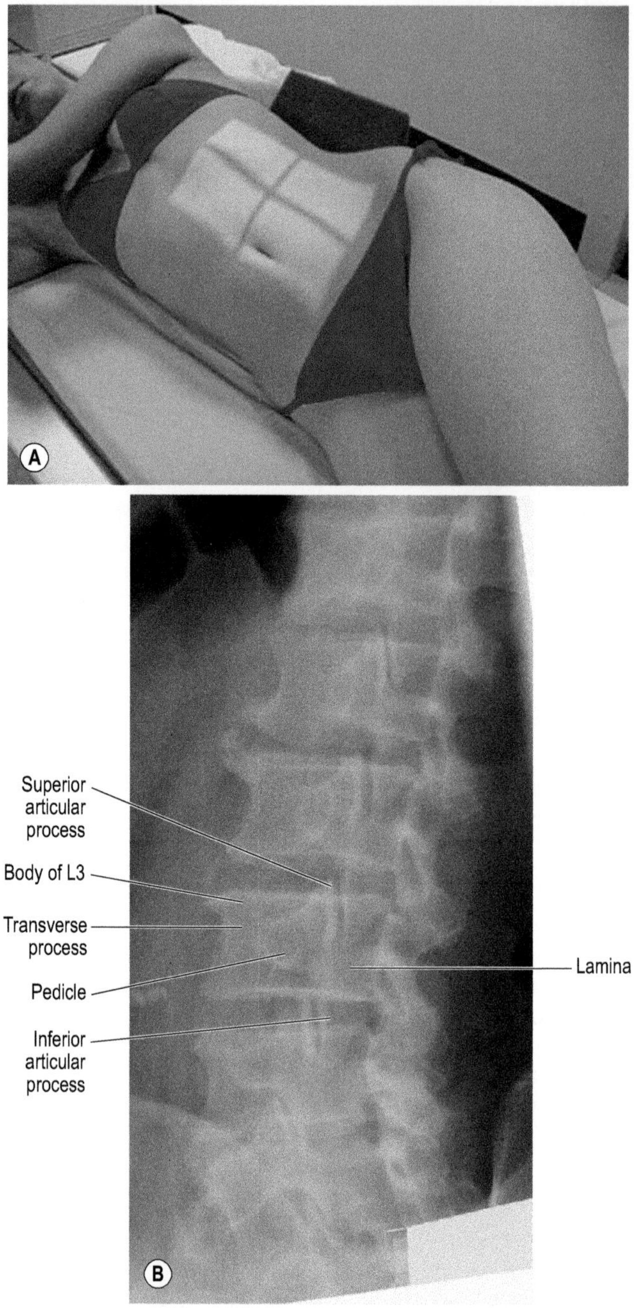

Fig. 10.8 Posterior oblique lumbar spine.

- 'Scottie dog' appearance seen within the associated vertebral body, with a dog's nose seen touching the edge of the vertebral body and the back of the dog's front leg coincident with the middle of the vertebral body. Structures correspond to the dog as follows:
  Nose = transverse process
  Eye = pedicle
  Ear = superior articular process
  Body = lamina
  Neck = pars interarticularis
  Front leg = inferior articular process

Please note that the position of the dog in relationship to its associated vertebral body will vary slightly in a longitudinal direction, according to the relationship of the vertebral body and its distance from the central ray. It is suggested that L3 is used to assess positional accuracy, as it lies most perpendicular to the central ray.

- Sharp image showing soft tissue in contrast with bone and 'Scottie dog' in contrast with the bony trabeculae of the associated vertebral body

Common Errors: Posterior Obliques

Common Errors	Possible Reasons	Potential Effects on PCE or Report
Dog's nose is elongated and most of it lies outside the vertebral body outline	Inadequate rotation	Distortion will make appearances of the pedicle difficult to assess. Fracture through the pars may not be seen
Dog's nose squashed and lies well within vertebral body outline	Excessive rotation	Overlying structures will make subtle pathologies difficult to spot. Fracture through the pars may not be seen

POSTERIOR OBLIQUE L5 (FIG. 10.9A,B)

For this projection positioning is as for the posterior oblique lumbar vertebrae, with the following adjustments because of the position of the vertebral body and its extreme tilt at the end of the lumbar lordosis. Anterior obliques may also be considered, with the direction of beam angulation in opposition to that used for posterior obliques and the centring point adapted to lie over the PSIS of the raised side.

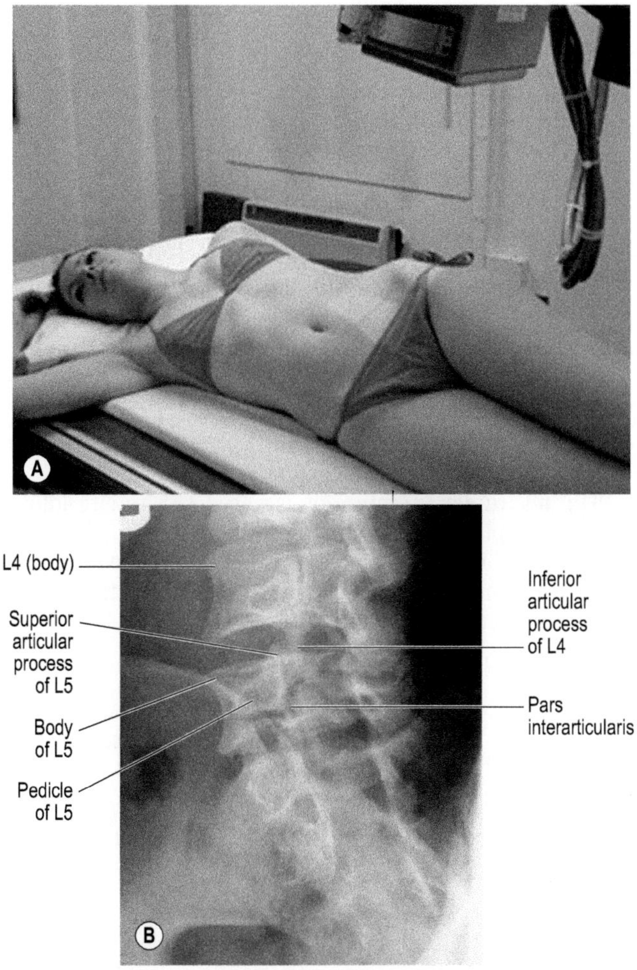

Fig. 10.9 Posterior oblique L5. Compare the pars interarticularis on this image to that of L3 on Fig. 10.8B. The neck of the 'Scottie dog' in Fig. 10.8B is intact, whereas here there appears to be a dark line or collar, which is suggestive of spondylolisthesis.

Beam Direction and FRD

Initially vertical, angled 10–20° cranially. The IR is displaced until coincident with the primary beam
100 cm FRD

Centring Point

Level with the ASIS in the midclavicular line

Collimation

L4/L5 junction, L5, S1

Criteria for Assessing Image Quality

- L4/L5 junction, L5 and S1 are demonstrated
- 'Scottie dog' appearance seen within L5 as explained for oblique lumbar vertebrae
- Clear joint space between L4 and 5, and L5 and S1
- Sharp image showing soft tissue in contrast with bone and 'Scottie dog' in contrast with the bony trabeculae of L5. Bone seen in contrast with joint spaces

Erect Laterals in Flexion and Extension

Flexion and extension views may be used to demonstrate the range of movement within the lumbar spine. With the development of erect scanning, it is possible to perform this examination using MRI.[21]
IR is vertical, an antiscatter grid is employed

Positioning

- The patient is in the erect lateral position, either seated or standing. The MSP is parallel to the erect bucky, usually with the left side in contact with it
- For the flexion projection the patient bends forward, flexing the spine as far forward as possible, arms extended forward, holding a fixed support or their legs to aid immobilisation
- For the extension projection the patient leans backwards, extending the spine as far as possible; again, immobilisation devices can be provided

Central Ray, FRD, Centring Point

Central ray horizontal, at 90° to the long axis of the spine. The rest of the technique is as for the lateral projection

Sacroiliac Joints

The sacroiliac joints (SIJs) are difficult to assess on AP projections of the lumbar spine or pelvis, owing to the oblique nature of the joints. The sacral angle, which lies in opposition to the oblique rays at the periphery of the X-ray beam, causes foreshortening of the joints on the AP lumbar projection. On the AP pelvis projection, the sacral and sacroiliac joint angle is far greater than the obliquity of X-rays around the central ray. The joints travel from the back of the sacrum and pelvis in an anterolateral direction (approximately 15°), again crossing the oblique rays in any AP position, rather than lying coincidentally with them. Therefore it is necessary to use a technique that considers the effects normal anatomy has on the demonstration of these joints.

Many years ago it was believed that the joints were demonstrated with a prone patient position and very short FRD; the short FRD was suggested in order to provide maximum angulation of oblique rays around the central ray and pass more accurately through the joints. This was combined with the prone position, which placed the sacral angle in a more suitable orientation. Unfortunately, although a prone position is often recommended to reduce the dose to the gonads, this method significantly increases the skin dose and is not likely to provide noticeable improvement of joint visualisation; it has been estimated that an unobtainable and unfeasible FRD of 18 cm would be required in order to provide obliquity of rays that will coincide with the 15° angles of the joints.[22] A prone projection at 100 cm FRD, with the caudal angle selected to pass through the sacral angle at 90°, is therefore recommended if a single projection is required. Alternatively, individual posterior oblique projections of each joint will demonstrate the joints most effectively, but will require the patient to be exposed to ionising radiation twice (although close collimation will reduce the associated risks of exposure to ionising radiation).

PRONE SACROILIAC JOINTS (SIJs) (FIG. 10.10A,B)

IR is horizontal, an antiscatter grid is employed

Positioning

- The patient lies prone, arms placed on the pillow and head turned to the side for comfort
- The MSP is perpendicular to the table-top and positioned to lie coincident with the long axis of the table

Beam Direction and FRD

A vertical central ray is angled caudally until at 90° to the long axis of the sacrum
100 cm FRD

Centring

Midway between the PSISs

Collimation

SIJs, L5/S1 joint

Criteria for Assessing Image Quality

- SIJs and L5/S1 joint are demonstrated
- Symmetry of sacrum and SIJs

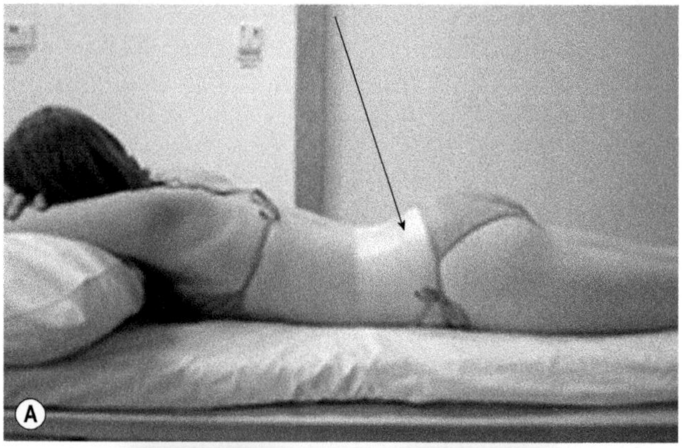

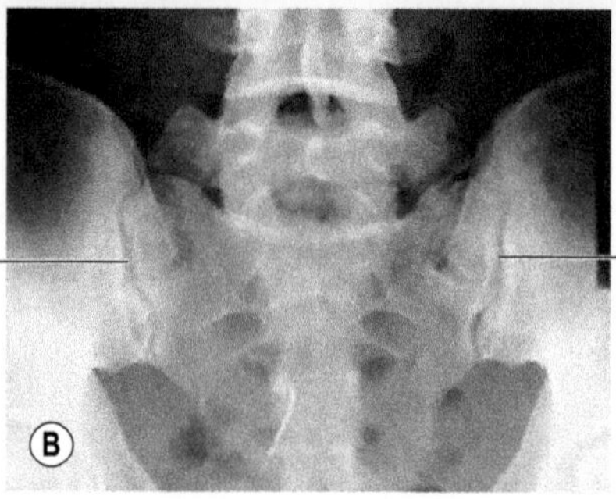

Fig. 10.10 Prone SIJs.

- Sharp image demonstrating the trabecular pattern of sacrum and ilium and lower density of the SIJs in contrast with the sacrum and ilium

POSTERIOR OBLIQUE SACROILIAC JOINTS (SIJs) (FIG. 10.11A,B)

Both joints are examined for comparison
IR is horizontal, an antiscatter grid is employed

Positioning

- The patient lies supine, with the MSP initially coincident with the long axis of the table
- The side under examination is raised 15° and a radiolucent pad placed under the raised side for immobilisation
- The arm on the lowered side is placed on the pillow for comfort and the leg on the same side flexed at the knee to aid stability

Beam Direction and FRD

1. Vertical *or*
2. Angled 10–15° cranially, to compensate for the sacral angle

The second option can, in some cases, project the image of the ischium over the inferior aspect of the SIJ. This is more likely in males, due to the shallower pelvis.
100 cm FRD.

Centring

1. 2.5 cm medial to the ASIS on the raised side
2. 2.5 cm medial to and below the ASIS on the raised side

Collimation

SIJ on the raised side

Criteria for Assessing Image Quality

- SIJ is demonstrated
- SIJ is shown clear of iliac crest and ASIS
- Joint space seen clearly
- Sharp image showing bony trabeculae of sacrum and ilium and the lower density joint in contrast with sacrum and ilium

Common Errors: Posterior Oblique Sacroiliac Joints

Common Errors	Possible Reasons	Potential Effects on PCE or Report
Joint space overlaps	Because the joint surfaces are not flat, some irregularity of the joint will be noted. Total loss of joint space is due to inaccurate obliquity. There may be indistinct or lost joint space in cases of degenerative diseases, such as ankylosing spondylitis	May not be possible to assess alignment of the joint
Ilium superimposed over joint	Too much obliquity	As above

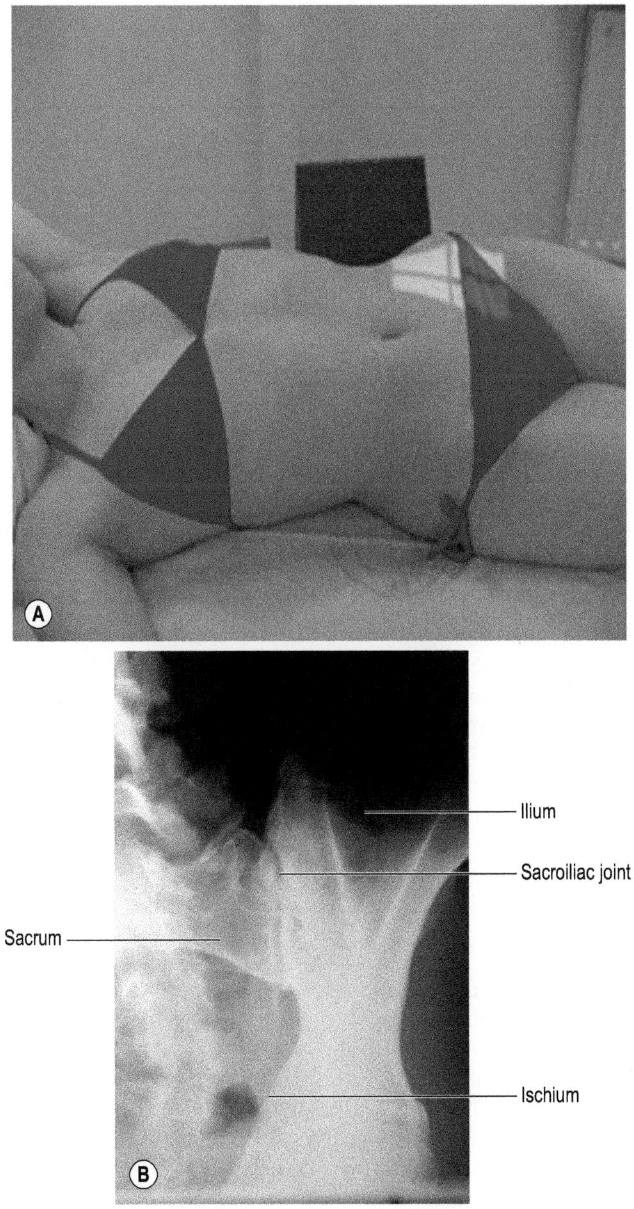

Fig. 10.11 Posterior oblique SIJs.

Sacrum

Trauma relating to the sacrum may well be associated with other injury to the pelvic ring and imaging of the pelvis is likely to be required in addition to examination of the sacrum. In cases of severe trauma it is inadvisable to undertake a lateral projection of the sacral area in the position described in this section; a horizontal beam approach would be the method of choice. However, as serious pelvis trauma will probably be assessed by initial pelvis images which will be supplemented by CT examination, a lateral sacrum image is unlikely to be required.

The sacrum may be a site for metastatic spread of malignancy and plain images of the region would demonstrate such lesions if the secondary tumour has eroded at least 40% of the bone. MRI is most appropriate for assessing bone metastases. Today it is rare to find radiography requested for assessment of this area, and there is no longer specific reference to assessment of the sacrum in UK guidelines for referrals.[23]

The lumbar curve varies with each individual patient and causes variation in the angles created between the sacrum and lumbar vertebrae. As a result it is suggested that the cranial angulation required to strike the sacrum at 90° in the AP position will vary from 10° to 25°, according to the individual patient's build. The most efficient strategy for making a decision on appropriate angulation is to undertake the lateral projection first and use it to assess the required angle before proceeding with the AP projection. This also applies to the coccyx.

If the examination request outlines that information on the coccyx is required, the lateral projection of the coccyx can be included on the lateral sacrum projection, to reduce the number of exposures. For this reason, the coccyx is also referred to in the description of the lateral projection.

For all projections of the sacrum and coccyx, the image receptor (IR) is horizontal and an antiscatter grid is employed.

PCE COMMENTS – SACRUM

Since injury to the sacral area usually necessitates assessment of the pelvic ring, assessment of the sacrum can often be made during study of pelvic X-ray imaging. If a separate sacral X-ray examination is undertaken, the sacral arcuate lines ('eyebrows') should be studied on the AP projection, as described in Chapter 8 (Pelvis and Hips).

LATERAL SACRUM (FIG. 10.12A,B)

Positioning

- The patient lies on their side, with hips and knees flexed to maintain stability and the feet placed together to prevent the patient from rolling forwards or backwards. The arms are flexed at the elbow and raised to rest on the pillows for comfort and to clear them from the area of interest
- The palm of the radiographer's hand is used to palpate the posterior aspect of the sacrum and ensure that its transverse axis is perpendicular to the table-top
- The long axis of the sacrum is parallel to the table-top; this should be checked with the area at the radiographer's eye level for accuracy. If patient build affects the relationship of the sacrum to the table-top a compensating cranial or caudal central ray can be used (see Beam Direction, below)

Beam Direction and FRD

Vertical, directed at 90° to the long axis of the sacrum once this has been assessed
100 cm FRD

Centring

Midway between the PSISs and sacrococcygeal junction

As the coccyx is more difficult to palpate than the sacrum, the level of its first segment may be difficult to locate. An alternative method to palpation uses the relationship of sacrococcygeal junction, which lies approximately level with the midpoint of the upper border of the symphysis pubis; palpation of the symphysis pubis anteriorly will allow the radiographer to estimate the level of the first coccygeal segment posteriorly.

Collimation

Lumbosacral junction, sacral promontory, soft tissues overlying the sacrum posteriorly, coccyx

Criteria for Assessing Image Quality

- Lumbosacral junction, sacral promontory, soft tissues overlying the sacrum posteriorly and coccyx are demonstrated. Omission of the coccyx from the field may be acceptable if demonstration of the coccyx is not required specifically for the examination
- Joint space at the lumbosacral junction is demonstrated
- Ala of sacrum superimposed
- Sharp image demonstrating bony trabeculae. Adequate penetration to demonstrate detail of sacrum and less dense coccyx on the one image

Common Errors: Lateral Sacrum

Common Errors	Possible Reasons	Potential Effects on PCE or Report
Non-superimposition of ala	Rotation	Any misalignment in fractures of sacrum will be difficult to comment on accurately
Sacrum demonstrated but detail of coccyx less so, or not seen	1. kVp may not be correct to demonstrate the range of densities encountered over sacrum and coccyx 2. A combination of the higher exposure factors and increased scatter associated with larger patients may have affected image contrast and quality. This is not necessarily considered a radiographer error; close collimation will reduce scatter but will not eliminate it *If information relating to the coccyx is not required for the examination, repeat examination should not be attempted*	Lack of detail will render it difficult to establish injury

ANTEROPOSTERIOR (AP) SACRUM (FIG. 10.13A,B)

Positioning

- The patient is supine with arms abducted from the trunk
- The median sagittal plane (MSP) is coincident with the long axis of the table
- ASISs are equidistant from the table-top

Beam Direction and FRD

The lateral sacrum projection is examined to assess the angle of the sacrum

Initially, the central ray is vertical, angled 10–25° cranially until 90° to the long axis of the sacrum

Centring

In the midline, midway between the level of the ASISs and the upper border of symphysis pubis

The IR must coincide with the emerging central ray, and to ensure that the collimated area lies within it

Collimation

Lumbosacral joint space, sacrococcygeal junction, sacroiliac joints

Criteria for Assessing Image Quality

- Lumbosacral joint space, sacrococcygeal junction and sacroiliac joints are demonstrated
- Symphysis pubis is superimposed over coccyx
- Symmetry of sacral foraminae
- Sharp image demonstrating bony detail of spinous tubercles in contrast with the body of the sacrum and all bony detail of the sacrum in contrast with the soft tissues of the pelvic cavity

Common Errors: AP Sacrum

Common Errors	Possible Reasons	Potential Effects on PCE or Report
Asymmetry of sacral foramina	Rotation about the MSP	Difficult to assess for potential impact of bed sores on the sacral bone Difficult to clearly assess the sacrum for any smaller pathologies, in particular fractures or osteomyelitis
Symphysis pubis superimposed over lower sacral segments	Angle of beam is too great	As above
Foreshortened sacrum	Inadequate angle used	As above
Ala of sacrum seen but sacral segments 2–4 superimposed; fifth segment seen	Angle selected is in wrong direction (caudal)	As above

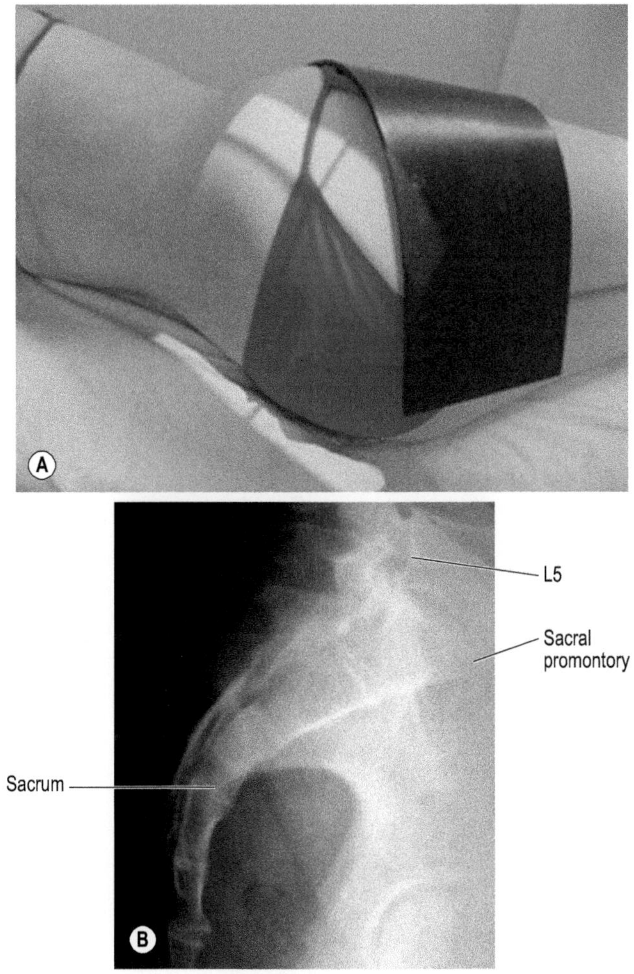

Fig. 10.12 Lateral sacrum.

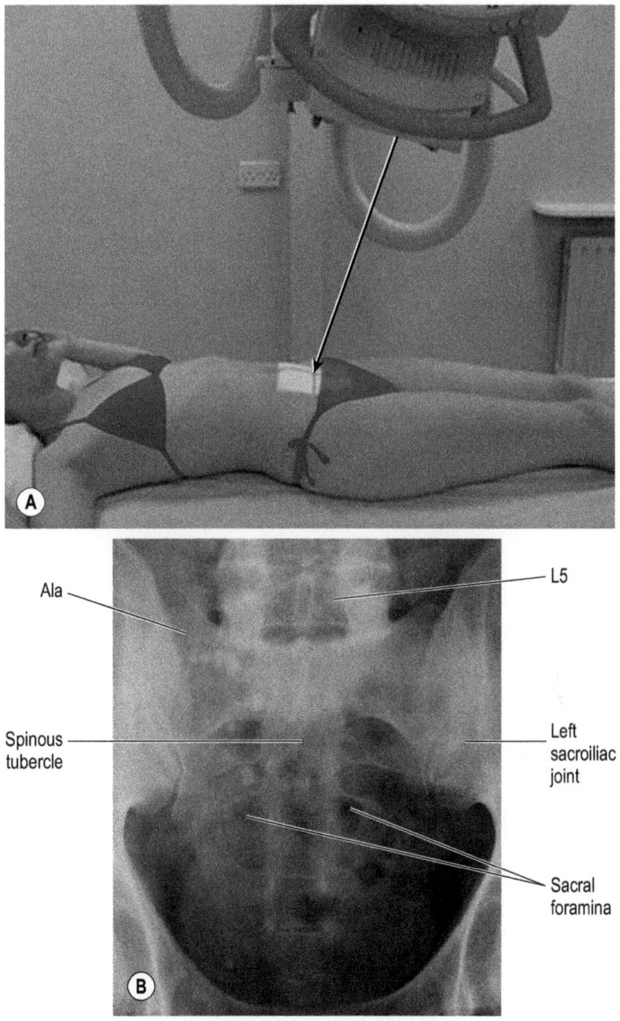

Fig. 10.13 AP sacrum.

Coccyx

Trauma to the coccyx and coccidynia are not routine indicators for radiographic examination of the coccyx, since confirmation of effects on the coccyx does not alter patient management. Variations in 'normal' appearances of the human coccyx can make radiological assessment difficult. However, although guidelines rule it out,[23] the most frequently encountered problems associated with the coccyx are extreme pain and trauma and these may necessitate radiographic examination.

For all projections of the coccyx, the IR is horizontal and an antiscatter grid is employed.

LATERAL COCCYX (FIG. 10.14A,B)

Positioning

- The patient lies on their side and is positioned as for the lateral sacrum and coccyx projection

Beam Direction and FRD

Vertical, directed at 90° to the long axis of the sacrum and coccyx
100 cm FRD

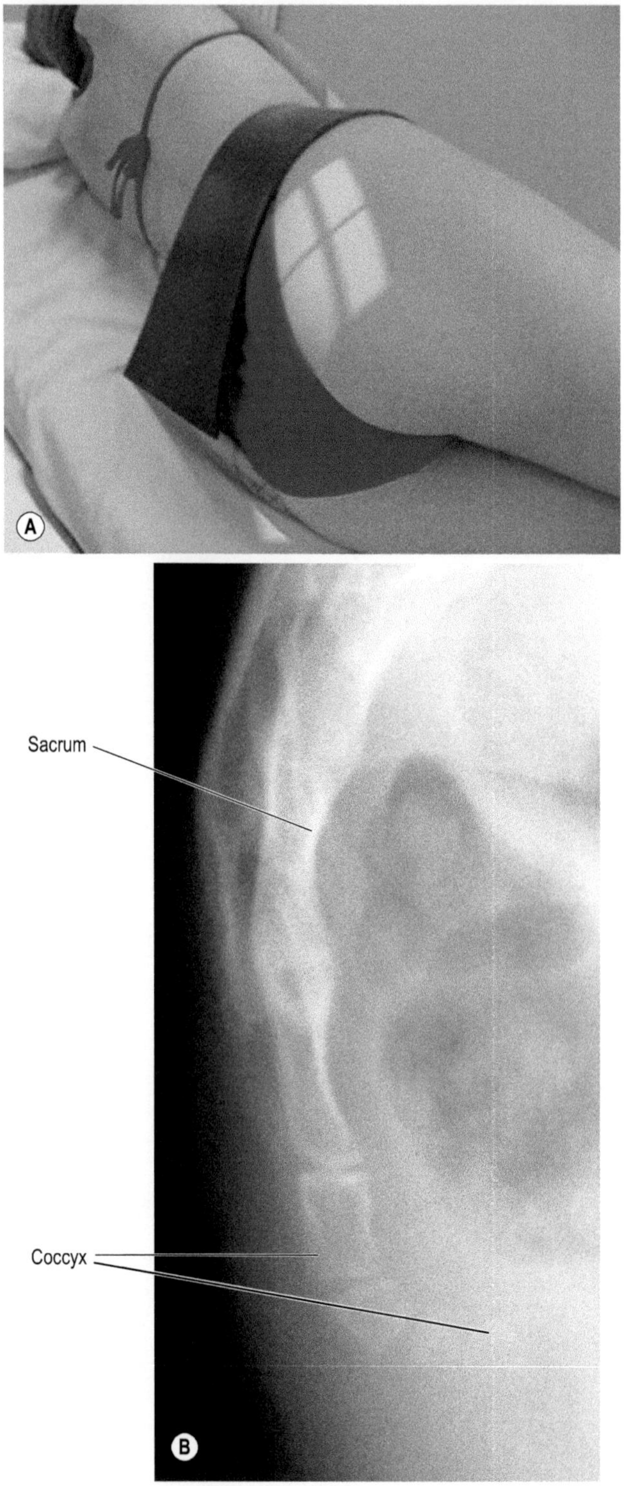

Fig. 10.14 Lateral coccyx.

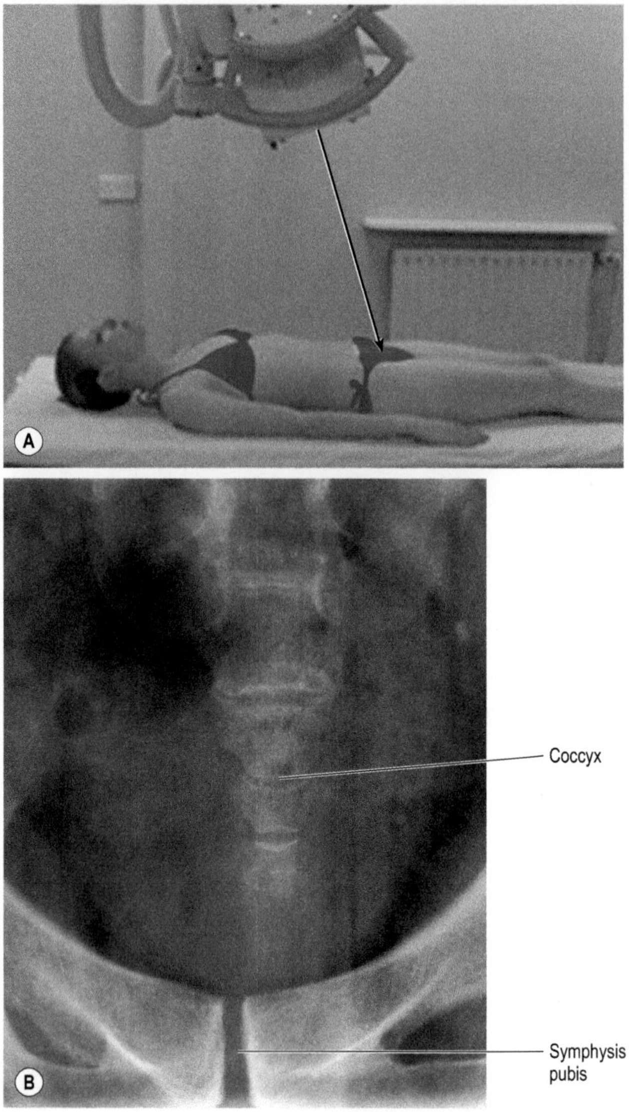

Fig. 10.15 AP coccyx.

Centring

At the base of the sacrum, level with the midpoint of the symphysis pubis

Collimation

Coccyx, sacrococcygeal junction

Criteria for Assessing Image Quality

- Coccyx and sacrococcygeal junction are demonstrated
- Sharp image demonstrating separate coccygeal segments in contrast to the surrounding soft tissues

Common Error: Lateral Coccyx

Common Error	Possible Reason	Potential Effect on PCE or Report
Inadequate contrast to distinctly demonstrate coccyx in contrast to soft tissues of buttocks	Usually due to patient build and implications of associated scatter (see errors section under AP coccyx)	Any displacement in cases of injury will not be shown

ANTEROPOSTERIOR (AP) COCCYX (FIG. 10.15A,B)

Positioning

The patient is supine as for the AP sacrum projection

Beam Direction and FRD

The lateral coccyx or sacrum and coccyx projection is examined to assess the angle of the coccyx
Initially the central ray is vertical, angled approximately 15–20° caudally until 90° to the long axis of the coccygeal segments
100 cm FRD

Centring

In the midline, midway between the level of the ASISs and the upper border of symphysis pubis

The IR must coincide with the emerging central ray, and to ensure that the collimated area lies within it

Collimation

Sacrococcygeal junction, all coccygeal segments

Criteria for Assessing Image Quality

- Sacrococcygeal junction and all coccygeal segments are demonstrated
- Symphysis pubis is cleared from the coccyx
- Foreshortened sacrum
- Sharp image demonstrating coccygeal segments in contrast with the soft tissues of the pelvic cavity

Common Errors: AP Coccyx

Common Errors	Possible Reasons	Potential Effects on PCE or Report
Poor contrast between coccyx and soft tissues or coccyx not demonstrated	1. Although the coccyx itself is not particularly dense, the pelvic area in the larger patient is an area of relatively large body thickness. Increased scatter associated with larger patients may thus have affected image contrast and quality. This is not necessarily considered a radiographer error and may be unavoidable in some cases 2. Faecal matter and bowel gas may also overlie the area and mask the low-density structure of the coccyx	Visualisation of any displacement in injury, or coccyx pathology may be difficult.
Coccygeal segments superimposed over the sacrum	Excessive angle used	Visualisation of any displacement in injury, or coccyx pathology may be difficult.
Sacrum not foreshortened; coccygeal segments foreshortened or superimposed	Angle selected is in wrong direction (cranial)	Visualisation of any displacement in injury, or coccyx pathology may be difficult.

References

1. Rao D, Scuderi G, Scuderi C, et al. The use of imaging in management of patients with low back pain. *J Clin Imaging Sci*. 2018;8:30.
2. Kendrick D, Fielding K, Bentley E, et al. Radiography of the lumbar spine in primary care patients with low back pain: randomised controlled trial. *Br Med J*. 2001;322:400–405.
3. Miller P, Kendrick D, Bentley E, et al. Cost-effectiveness of lumbar spine radiography in primary care patients with low back pain. *Spine*. 2002;27(20):2291–2297.
4. Editor's choice. Challenges to orthodoxy? *Br Med J*. 2001;322(7283):0.
5. Nicholson R, Thornton A, Sukumar VP. Awareness by radiology staff of the difference in radiation risk from two opposing lateral lumbar spine examinations. *Br J Radiol*. 1999;72:221.
6. Mayor P. Invited review: spondylolysis: current imaging and management. *Proceedings of UK Radiological Congress 2003. Br J Radiol*. 2003;76(Suppl):35.
7. Shah LM, Salzman KL. Imaging of spinal metastatic disease. *Int J Surg Oncol*. 2011. https://www.hindawi.com/journals/ijso/2011/769753/.
8. Bell DJ, et al. Winking owl sign (spine). [online] Radiopaedia. https://radiopaedia.org/articles/winking-owl-sign-spine/revisions?lang=gb 2018.
9. McQuillen-Martenson K. *Radiographic Image Analysis*. 5th ed. St Louis: Elsevier; 2019.
10. Murrie VL, Wilson H, Hollingworth W, et al. Supportive cushions produce no practical reduction in lumbar lordosis. *Br J Radiol*. 2002;75:536–538.
11. Downing N. Does flexion of the knees and hips reduce lumbar lordosis during AP lumbar spine examinations? *Proc UK Radiol Congr*. 2005;97.
12. Colleran C. PA lumbar spines; a future concept. *Radiogr Today*. 1994;60(681):17–20.
13. Hart D, Jones DG, Wall BF. *Estimation of Effective Dose in Radiology from Entrance Surface Dose and Dose Area Product Measurements*. Chilton: National Radiological Protection Board; 1994. NRPB 262.
14. Hart D, Jones DG, Wall BF. *Coefficients for Estimating Effective Doses from Paediatric X-ray Examinations*. Chilton: National Radiological Protection Board; 1996. NRPB 279.
15. Chapple C, et al. Awareness by radiology staff of the difference in radiation risk from two opposing lateral lumbar spine examinations. *Br J Radiol*. 2000;73:568.
16. European Commission Directorate-General for Research and Innovation. *European Guidelines on Quality Criteria for Diagnostic Radiographic Images. EUR 16260 Luxembourg: Office for Official Publications of the European Communities*; 1997.
17. Wong-Chung J, Jamsheer N, Nabar U, et al. Two parallel linear densities on lateral radiographs of the lumbosacral spine: neither iliopectineal lines nor basis ossis sacri. *Br J Radiol*. 1997;70:58–61.
18. Carver E, Carver B. *Medical Imaging: Techniques, Reflection, Evaluation*. 2nd ed. Edinburgh: Churchill Livingstone; 2012.
19. *ACR–ASSR–SPR–SSR Practice Parameter for the Performance of Spine Radiography*. ACR; 2017. https://www.acr.org/-/media/ACR/Files/Practice-Parameters/Rad-Spine.pdf.
20. Murrie VL, Dixon AK, Hollingworth W, et al. Lumbar lordosis measurement: a study in patients with and without low back pain. *Clin Anat*. 2001;14:298.
21. Jinkins J, Dworkin JS, Damadian RV. Upright, weight-bearing, dynamic-kinetic magnetic resonance imaging of the spine – review of the first clinical results. *J Hong Kong Coll Radiol*. 2003;6:55–74.
22. Unett EM, Royle AJ. *Radiographic Techniques and Image Evaluation*. London: Chapman and Hall; 1997.
23. Royal College of Radiologists. *iRefer: Making the Best Use of Clinical Radiology*. 8th ed. London: RCR; 2017. https://www.rcr.ac.uk/clinical-radiology/being-consultant/rcr-referral-guidelines/about-irefer.

11 Principles of Radiography of the Head

ELIZABETH CARVER

Introduction

Radiography of the head is commonly termed 'skull radiography' but, because the word 'skull' refers to the cranial vault and its bones, 'skull radiography' would technically exclude the facial bones, some paranasal sinuses, mandible and temporomandibular joints.

From the mid-1980s onwards there was a reduction in the number of requests for plain radiography of the head, as computed tomography (CT) and magnetic resonance imaging (MRI) provided more detailed and useful information (but plain radiography of the facial bones is still regularly requested). These imaging methods now provide information that is either unlikely to be provided by plain radiographic images or is only likely to be demonstrated by it in the later stages of disease processes. There came a reduction in the number of projections advocated per examination over the years, in order to reduce radiation dose to patients. Bearing in mind the superiority of MRI and CT, current guidelines do not recommend plain radiography of the cranial vault, even in cases of trauma, unless CT is not available at the time of examination; the exception to this is in cases of non-accidental injury in children.[1]

Despite the drop in numbers of requests and projections undertaken, chapters on the head will include a full range of descriptions of projections in order to provide information for regions where CT and MRI are not readily available. Where relevant, a discussion on the suitability of plain radiography versus specialised techniques will be presented throughout the section as each area is covered, but PCE comments are not offered as they can be found in area-specific descriptions (see Chapters 12 and 13).

A Logical Approach to Technique

Historically, texts on radiography presented radiographers and students with information that has included up to approximately 50 projections.[2,3] This proved daunting for radiographers in training, to say the least, and it is possible that the decline in frequency of use of plain radiography of the head likely exacerbates this.

However, if radiography of the head is approached logically it is realised that all projections are based upon a very few basic head positions, or projections, which require modification and variation by use of angulation and differing centring points. Collimation will also vary, according to the area of interest for each projection. With reference to centring points, it will appear that there are as many of these as there are projections. However, on examination of radiographs, it becomes clear that centring points used are logically selected as being in the middle of the area of interest; so it is recommended that, if in doubt, simply ensure the area of interest lies centrally in the collimated field. Realistically, the radiographer need only quote specific centring points when disseminating information to others.

Familiarity with the bony features of the skull and face, and their radiographic appearances, is vital when assessing radiographs for quality. The most important structures for recognition are:

- Orbits and the bones forming the orbits
- Bones of the vault and sutures
- Maxilla
- Sphenoid, including lesser and greater wings, sphenoid sinus, sella turcica and pterygoid processes/plates
- Petrous portion of temporal bone and its ridge
- Zygomae and arches
- Features of the mandible, temporomandibular joints
- Paranasal sinuses
- Nasal septum
- External and internal auditory meati
- Foramen magnum and atlanto-occipital joints

Description of basic projections relies heavily on the use of planes, baselines and surface markings, and the radiographer must be similarly familiar with these (Figs 11.1 and 11.2).

Surface Markings, Planes and Baselines

Glabella. The glabella is situated in the midline of the forehead just above the level of the superior orbital margins; it lies over the frontal sinuses.

External Occipital Protuberance (EOP). The EOP is palpable and situated in the midline, inferiorly, over the occiput.

External Auditory Meatus (EAM). The EAM is the hole surrounded by the pinna of the ear.

Nasion. The nasion is situated below the glabella, and is a depression between the orbits and above the nasal bone.

Coronal Plane. The coronal place is coincident with the coronal suture and separates the body into anterior and posterior halves.

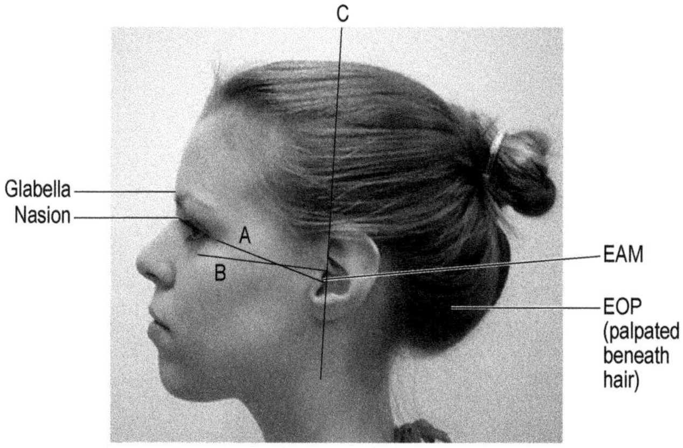

A. Orbitomeatal baseline (OMBL)
B. Anthropological baseline
C. Auricular line

Fig. 11.1 Surface markings, planes and baselines – 1.

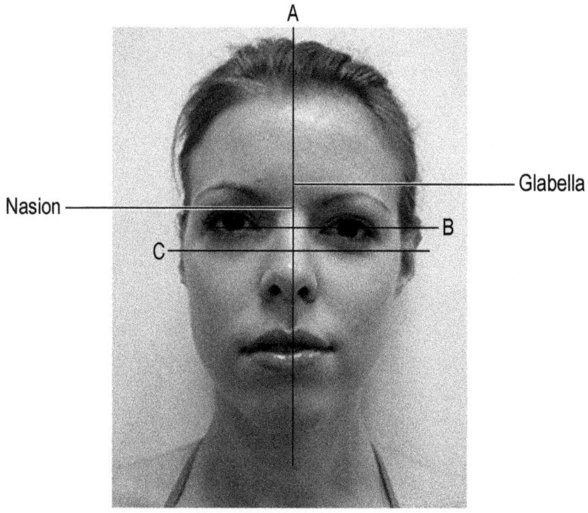

A. MSP
B. Interpupillary line
C. Infraorbital line

Fig. 11.2 Surface markings, planes and baselines – 2.

Infraorbital Line. The infraorbital line connects the inferior orbital margins and lies parallel to the interpupillary line.

Interpupillary Line. The interpupillary line is a horizontal line connecting the pupils of the eyes.

Median Sagittal Plane (MSP). The MSP is a vertical plane in the midline of the head, separating the left and right sides.

Orbitomeatal Baseline (OMBL). The OMBL is an imaginary line extending from the outer canthus of the eye to the middle of the EAM. It is used in conventional radiography techniques of the head.

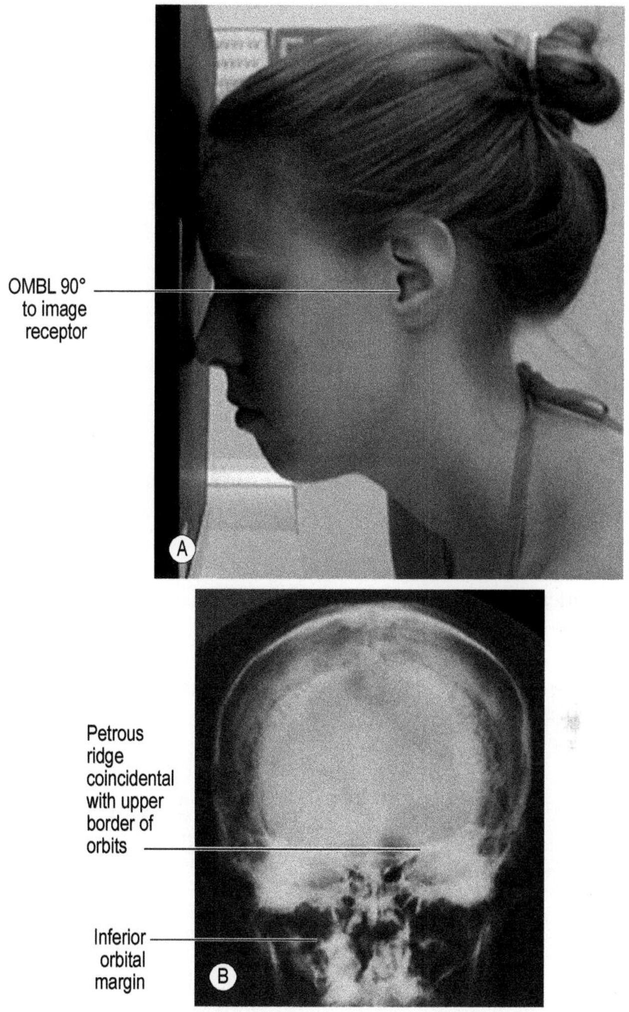

Fig. 11.3 (A) Basic OF position; (B) OF.

Basic Positions of the Head

In this book the names of projections are always given as a representation of the direction of the beam, so that this gives the radiographer information on the initial patient position. This is in preference to a system that uses names for some projections which reflect the original describer of the projection (for example Towne's, Waters') but gives little or no information on the position. When such a name is very commonly used in everyday practice, it will be given as an alternative in brackets.

OCCIPITOFRONTAL (OF) (FIG. 11.3A,B)

This is a posteroanterior (PA) position, with the forehead in contact with the image receptor (IR) and the OMBL at 90° to it. It is easiest to achieve with the patient seated erect. Traditionally it is referred to as a 'PA skull' position, but as the occipitomental (OM) position is also PA this does not describe the true position of the head for the OF.

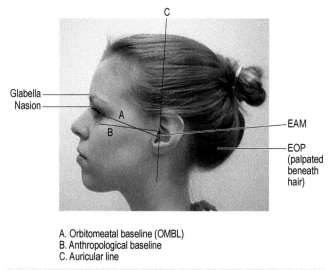

With an OF projection, beam angulation will affect the position of the ridge of the petrous portion of the temporal bone: caudal angulation lowering it in relation to the orbits and cranial angulation raising it. The effects of caudal angulation can be compared using Figs 11.4A–C. These positions rely on accurate positioning of the OMBL at 90° to the IR and accurate angle selection. The effects of errors on the appearance of the petrous ridge in the OF position are outlined below.

Common Errors: OF Projections

Common Errors	Possible Reasons
Petrous ridge appears higher within the orbits than required, or appears above superior orbital margins	OMBL not 90° to the IR, chin down too far. Caudal tube angle selected, if used, is less than required for projection. Direction of angle incorrect
Petrous ridge appears lower within the orbits than required, or appears below inferior orbital margins	OMBL not 90° to IR, chin raised slightly. Caudal tube angle selected, if used, is more than required for projection
Symmetry of the structures on either side of the head is a requirement of all AP or PA radiographs of the head. Rotation of the head, away from the position with the MSP perpendicular to the IR, will affect this symmetry. The most obvious identifiable appearance suggestive of rotation is increased distance of the lateral orbital border from the lateral outer table of the vault on one side compared to the other	

It has been noted that it is common practice for radiographers to initially ask the patient to place their nose and forehead in contact with the IR and that nose size will affect OMBL relationship if this method is used.[4] For this reason it is advocated that the patient is asked to place only their forehead against the IR, with the radiographer adjusting OMBL position as necessary.

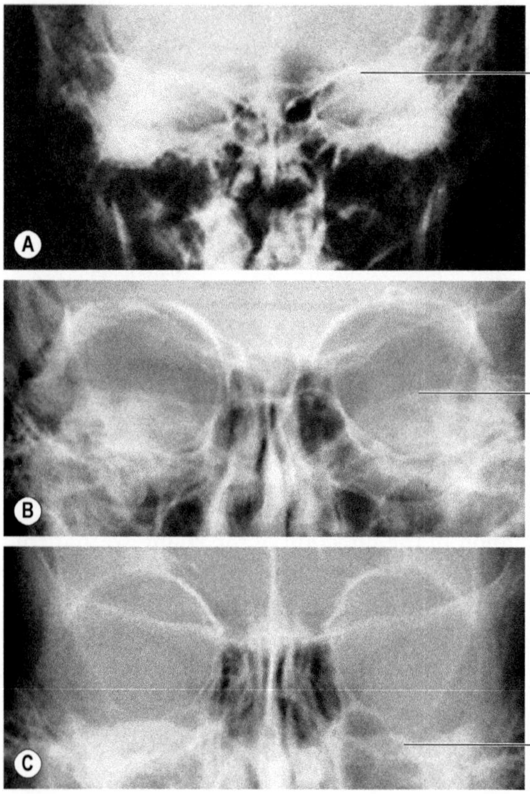

Fig. 11.4 Effects of caudal angulation on petrous ridge in the OF position: (A) no angle; (B) 10° angle; (C) 20° angle.

FRONTO-OCCIPITAL (FO) (FIG. 11.5)

This is an AP position, with the occiput in contact with the IR and OMBL at 90° to it. It can be undertaken erect or supine and is most often used in cases of trauma when patient condition is not suitable for an OF projection; if this is the case, any caudal angulation normally given in conjunction with the OF position is directed *cranially rather than caudally*. It is used when radiographers avoid PA projections of the head because of potential difficulty in achieving and maintaining the correct position. Caudal angulation may also be applied in the FO position routinely, as for the FO 30° half axial (Towne's) projection (see Chapter 12 on the cranial vault).

The appearance of the FO projection, with no tube angulation, should be identical to those for the OF, with the exception of relative orbital size. In the FO position the lateral orbital borders will appear very close to, or even superimposed over, the lateral outer table of the vault. The OF projection will show the lateral orbital borders well within the outer margins of the vault (Fig. 11.6A,B). Clearly this is due to the difference in magnification of the orbits, as they lie close to the IR in the OF position and further away in the FO position; the distance of the lateral aspects of the vault from the IR will be similar for both and magnification of the area will also be similar.

Errors in positioning have the same effects as those for the OF projection, OMBL position affecting the position of the petrous ridge and rotation affecting symmetry. A raised chin in the FO position will have the same effect as the same action in the OF position, which is that of lowering the

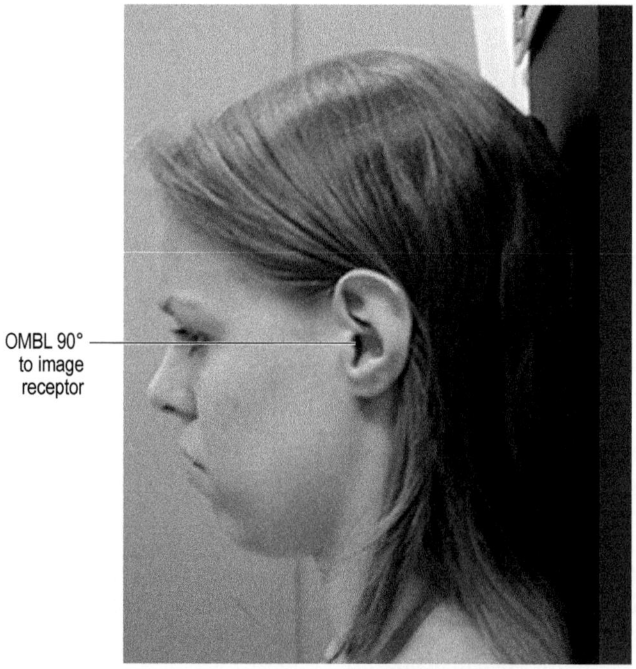

Fig. 11.5 Basic FO position.

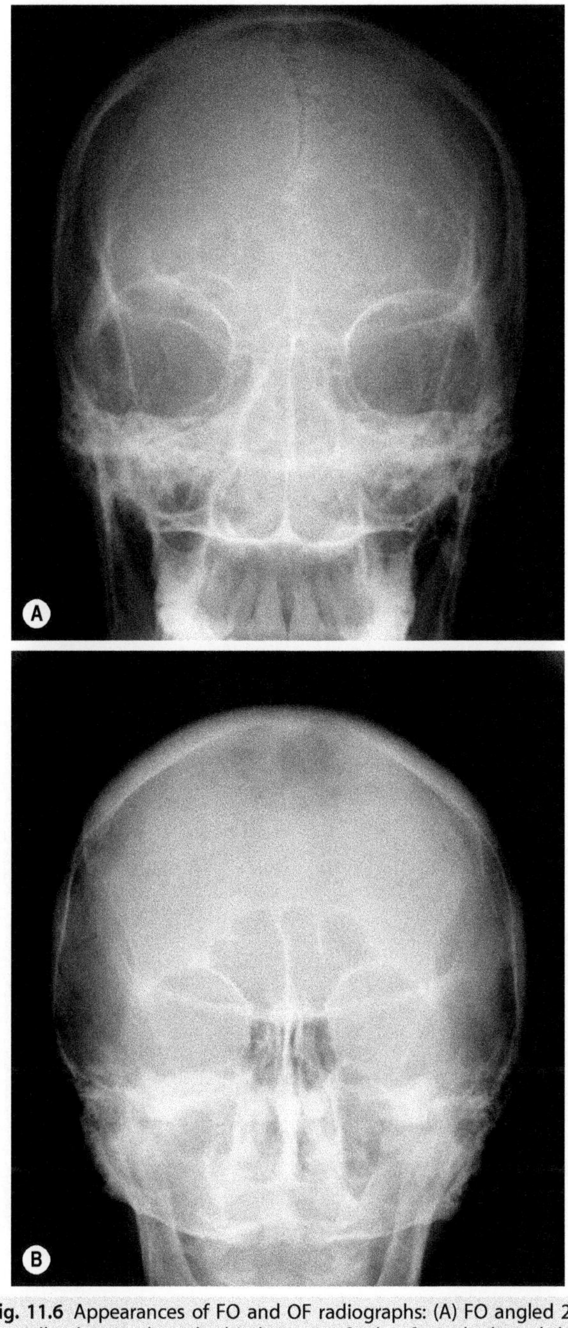

Fig. 11.6 Appearances of FO and OF radiographs: (A) FO angled 20° cranially, showing lateral orbital margins further from the lateral skull margins than in (B), OF angled 20° caudally.

petrous ridge, whereas a dropped chin will raise it. The FO with caudal angulation will show the petrous ridges rising above the orbital outlines, and becoming increasingly 'V' shaped as the angle increases. More specific guidelines on FO projectional errors are given in Chapter 12.

Positioning the OMBL at 90° to the IR can be difficult in this AP position, especially in the patient who is of stocky build or is kyphotic. If sitting erect, the patient will find it easier to press the occipital area against the IR, and achieve the correct relationship of OMBL to it, if the chair they use is placed slightly forward of the receptor unit. Leaning back towards the unit initially until their shoulders come into contact with it, they are then asked to push the back of their neck against the unit, flexing their neck until the occipital area is also in contact. It has been noted that this method is more effective than asking the patient to simply put the back of their head against the IR while dropping the chin, as the back of the head generally lies at the top of the occiput rather than in its centre.[4]

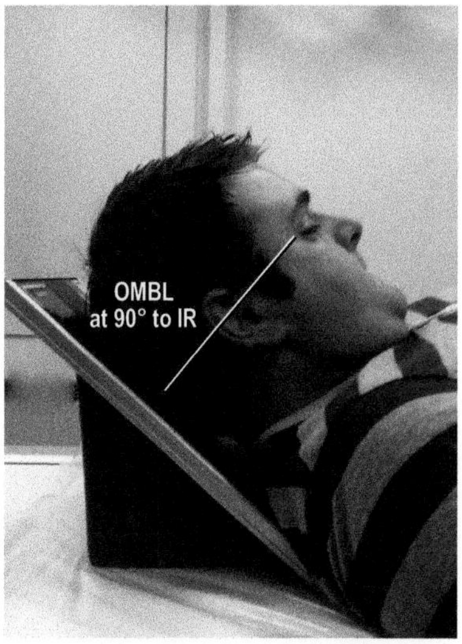

Fig. 11.7 Cassette supported for supine patient.

Positioning of the OMBL is more difficult for the supine patient, and it is worthy of note that most trauma patients requiring skull images will present supine on a trolley; use of a non-opaque pad under the head may help facilitate the position but is not considered ideal, as the increase in object receptor distance (ORD) causes magnification unsharpness which increases in severity towards the vertex of the skull. For the non-neck-injured patient it is preferable to use a support under an IR with stationary grid, positioned directly under the patient's head and at 90° to the OMBL (Fig. 11.7). Other solutions and suggestions will also be considered in Chapter 12 on the cranial vault.

OCCIPITOMENTAL (OM) (FIG. 11.8A,B)

This is a PA position, with the chin raised and in contact with the IR. The relationship of the OMBL to the IR varies and is usually between 30° and 45° from the perpendicular, according to the requirements of the examination. With the OMBL at 30° the nose is close to, or even in contact with, the IR, but this does vary according to shape of the nose; the chin is well elevated if a 45° relationship to the IR is required, and in this position the nose is very unlikely to be in contact with it. This projection is often called the Waters' view in the USA.

As for the OF and FO projections, the location of the petrous ridge on the image is also used to assess accuracy of positioning for the OM. The required level for most OM projections requires the petrous ridge to be seen at either the midpoint or the lower border of the maxillary sinuses. Caudal angulation will further lower the position of the petrous ridge on this projection.

With further reference to the assessment of projectional accuracy using the petrous ridge, as for the OF and FO positions: a higher position of the ridge than that required indicates that the chin is inadequately elevated; if the ridge is lower than required the chin is over-elevated. Again, evidence of rotation is assessed by symmetry of the facial structures, especially the distance of the lateral orbital margins and rami of the mandible from the lateral aspect of the vault.

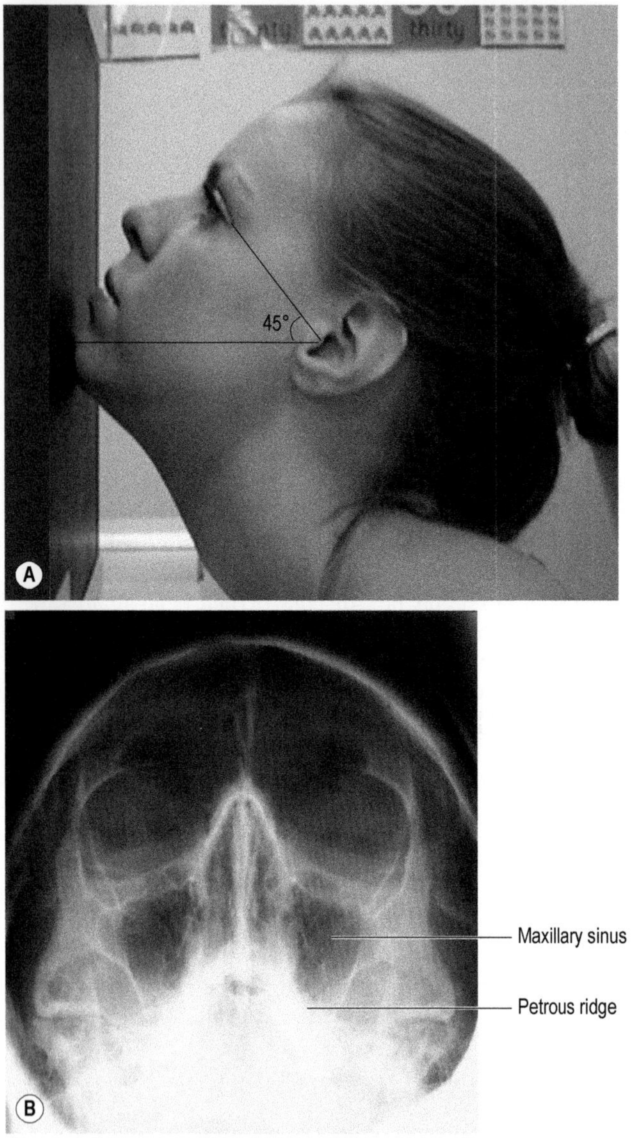

Fig. 11.8 (A) Basic OM position: chin raised 45°; (B) OM 45°.

LATERAL (FIG. 11.9A,B)

This is a familiar position, with the MSP parallel to the IR. Angulation can be used for some lateral oblique projections, such as those for mandible or temporomandibular joints. Both tilt and rotation of the head will affect the appearance of the lateral projection. This projection can be undertaken with the patient seated or prone but it can be difficult for them to achieve the required position; if undertaken erect, turning the patient's head into position while maintaining the MSP parallel to the IR may be more easily achieved with the chair placed very close to the IR and the patient's vertebral column vertically positioned. If a patient leans forward towards the unit there is more likelihood of tilt. Another solution lies in the use of a cassette-type IR with grid in an erect holder, or supported vertically against the side of the supine patient's head (which is elevated on a radiolucent pad), enabling the patient to be positioned with their whole MSP (head and body) parallel to the IR. This reduces the difficulty associated with turning the head and obtaining an accurate position.

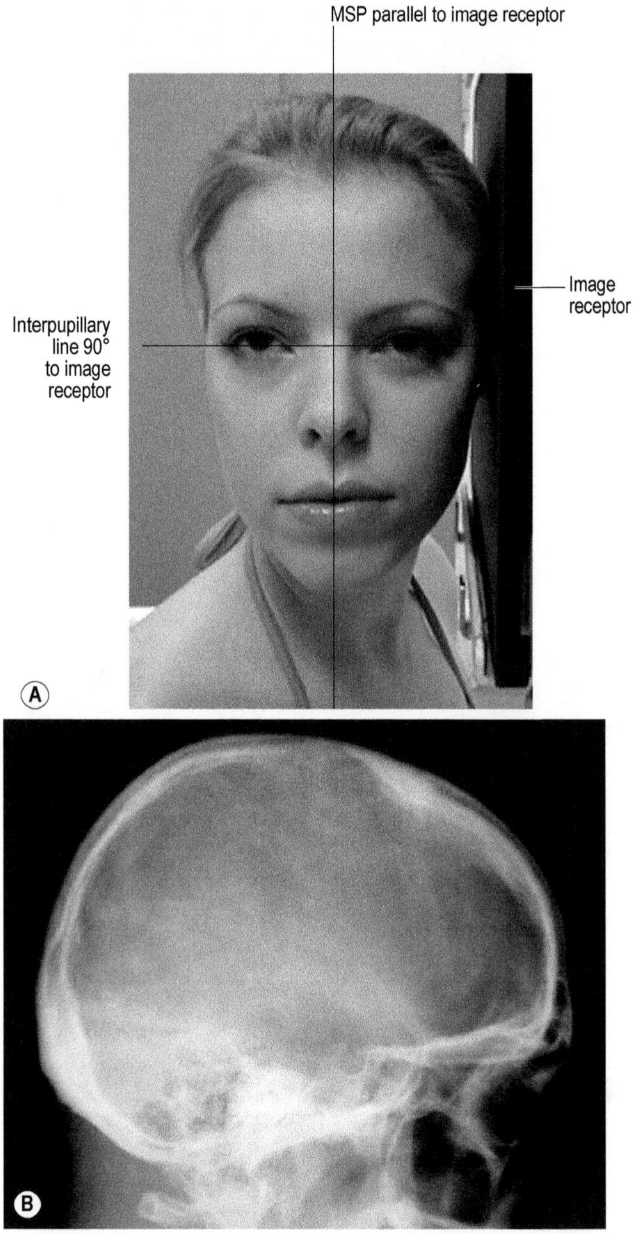

Fig. 11.9 (A) Basic lateral position; (B) lateral.

SUBMENTOVERTICAL (SMV) (FIG. 11.10A,B)

The vertex of the skull is placed in contact with the IR for this projection, facilitated by the patient initially sitting facing the X-ray tube and extending the neck and head backwards. The OMBL is parallel to the IR. The projection is not in common use as the information it provides is minimal and even inadequate compared to that given by CT and MRI. The projection can be quite difficult for some patients to achieve and maintain, especially as pressure on the vertex of the skull can be quite painful even when there is no superficial injury over the vertex.

Table-Top/Trolley or Erect Technique?

Although radiographic examination of the skull can be undertaken erect or supine, erect positioning is easier for the

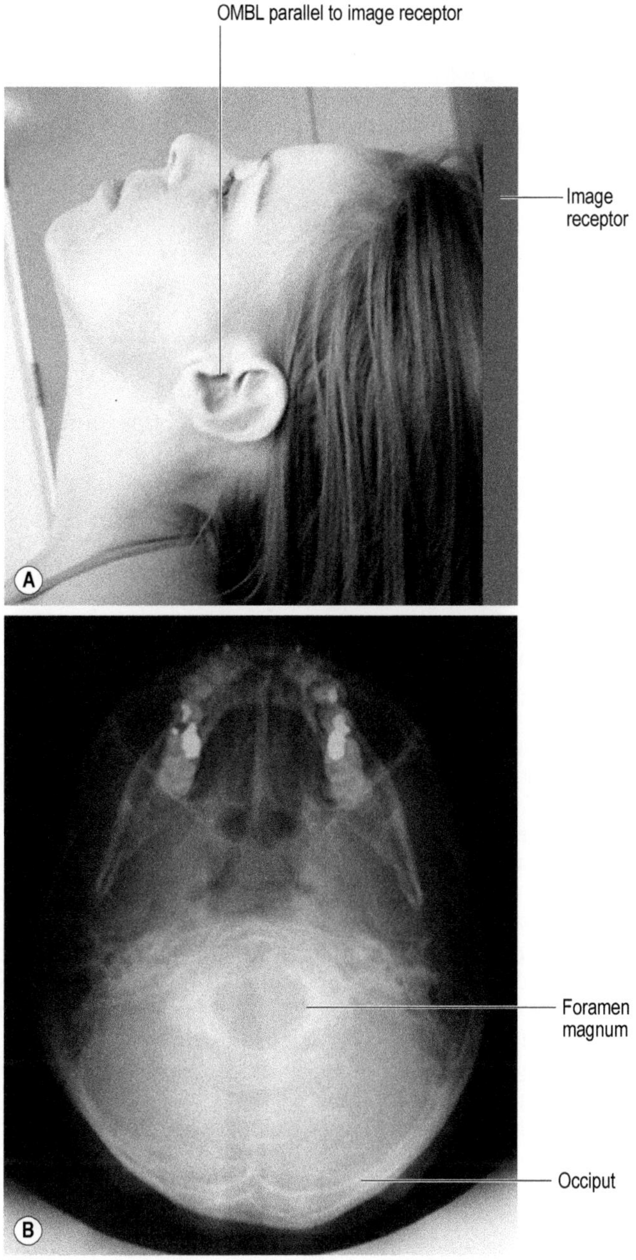

Fig. 11.10 (A) Basic SMV position; (B) SMV.

patient for most positions, especially PA positions. As already mentioned, lateral projections can be difficult to achieve when the patient is erect with their head turned, but a supine horizontal projection, with the whole of the body's MSP parallel to the IR, is easier for the patient. As this method usually uses a stationary grid, this could similarly be employed using an erect IR support with the patient seated. The patient's shoulder fits comfortably under the support, without the patient needing to turn their head. A lateral with the patient prone can be very difficult and, in any case, any prone position is out of the question for the injured patient. Achieving the perpendicular relationship of the OMBL for the FO projection is also quite difficult for the supine patient. Because of this, the method selected for descriptions of radiography of the head (conventional method) is the erect technique. Modifications for the supine patient can be found in Chapter 17.

Summary

There is a small range of basic projections (OF, FO, lateral, OM, SMV) upon which radiography of the head is based, and this range can be seen to be simplified when it is remembered that:

- the OF and FO projections are simply the reverse of each other
- the lateral projection is a familiar concept and therefore not a difficult one
- the SMV projection is little used
- erect positioning is often easier to achieve.

Chapters 12 and 13 give the relevant projections for specific areas of the head and these are described in more detail, showing use of these basic projections with modifications in angles used, centring points and collimation requirements.

References

1. Royal College of Radiologists. *iRefer: Making the Best Use of Clinical Radiology*. 8th ed. London: RCR; 2017. https://www.rcr.ac.uk/clinical-radiology/being-consultant/rcr-referral-guidelines/about-irefer.
2. Bontrager K, Lampignano JP. *Textbook of Radiographic Positioning and Related Anatomy*. 7th ed. St Louis: Mosby; 2010.
3. Whitley AS, Sloane C, Hoadley G, et al. *Clark's Positioning in Radiography*. 12th ed. London: Hodder Arnold; 2005.
4. Unett EM, Royle AJ. *Radiographic Techniques and Image Evaluation*. London: Chapman and Hall; 1997.

12 Cranial Vault and Specialised Projections of the Head

ELIZABETH CARVER, LUCY BANFIELD and BARRY CARVER

Skull radiography has been in decline for many years. It is still in limited use for the investigation of some metabolic and bone disorders, and as part of the skeletal survey protocol for cases of suspected physical abuse (SPA). In cases of trauma, even where still used, fewer projections have been recommended for a number of years – two rather than the 'traditional' three being advised.[1]

Why is this? The easy answer is minimisation of radiation dose, availability of superior imaging methods and not forgetting reduction in transition time and speedier treatment for the patient.

The story of the demise of plain X-ray examination of the skull began as long ago as the1970s: Eyes and Evans, in a study of 504 patients in two Liverpool teaching hospitals, found a very low yield of positive findings on plain skull radiographs, suggesting that they were of limited value in the management of patients with head injury.[2] Two other studies in the United States agreed with these findings, the yield of fractures varying but with a low of 2.7% in agreement with the above UK study.[3–5]

Head injuries are the cause of around 1.4 million hospital attendances each year in England and Wales, with approximately 700,000 of these being under the age of 15.[6] Imaging of the head injury patient is directed at detecting the nature of the underlying pathology; once this is accomplished the brain can be protected against greater damage. Optimal imaging is dependent on the nature of the injury, with evaluation of the brain normally being of paramount importance. Computed tomography (CT) has had a massive impact on the diagnosis and treatment of traumatic head injury, allowing rapid non-invasive identification of both diffuse injury and surgically treatable lesions.

It should be noted that cervical spine injury is relatively common in patients with head injury, hence it is important to exclude such an injury prior to mobilisation, the minimum examination being a high-quality lateral examination C1–C7.[7]

Elimination of unnecessary skull radiographs has long been on the agenda in the UK and measures to achieve this have been successful. Common practice is to adopt the Canadian CT head rule (CCHR)[8,9] to reduce or eliminate the need for radiography of the skull in trauma; the exception is where CT is unavailable, or in the case of SPA in children.

In the UK, guidance issued by the National Institute for Health and Care Excellence (NICE) directs implementation of imaging for head injury patients.[8] Application of CCHR has been shown to be effective in the management of patients with minor head trauma, significantly reducing the amount of scans required in this group. However, patients in the high- and medium-risk groups do require CT.[9]

Given its ability to demonstrate bony detail as well as much greater detail of the underlying soft tissues within the cranial vault, CT is the investigation of choice in many circumstances. Thus the use of skull radiography, particularly in trauma, has diminished greatly, but its use may not yet be obsolete in global regions where CT is not readily available in emergency situations: indeed, in some countries skull radiography remains in use. Consequently, it is still necessary for the radiographer to be competent in X-ray examination of the cranial vault.

Projections for the cranial vault may be undertaken erect, or with the patient supine or prone. The technique described here uses erect positioning, and the table-top or trolley technique must be modified by remembering that erect anteroposterior (AP) becomes supine, and erect posteroanterior (PA) becomes prone, etc. For the *injured patient*, no projections are undertaken prone, and occipitofrontal (OF) projections must be adjusted to become fronto-occipital (FO), with any cranial or caudal angulations directed in the opposite direction to those given for OF projection. For example, if an OF 20° with caudal angle is required, the FO uses a 20° cranial angle in order to reproduce the required appearances on the image.

As skull projections are still sometimes employed either for the identification of foreign bodies within the soft tissues of the scalp, or for the presence of metallic foreign bodies which may contraindicate magnetic resonance imaging (MRI), care should be taken to ensure that any hair bands or hair clips should be removed prior to imaging to avoid false-positive findings. Tightly braided or bunched hair can also potentially result in an artefact on the image which may result in a false-positive conclusion.

Throughout this chapter a suggested FRD is given for each examination description; however in practice a range of FRDs may be used (typically 100–120 cm), dependent on local protocol.

PCE COMMENTS – CRANIAL VAULT

As with all radiographic image interpretation, adequacy of the projection is the first consideration. The images obtained should be appropriate to address the clinical question raised by the referrer. This may involve specific projections when a query of craniosynostosis, for example, is raised and an appreciation as to the resultant anatomy demonstrated should be taken by the radiographer.

It is vital to be familiar with the normal appearances of the sutures and vascular markings.

Abnormalities can be seen in the form of changes to density, size and shape of the skull as well as any structural defects.

Vascular markings: May appear as grey lines with some evidence of branching and peripheral narrowing. Diploic, or venous lakes are seen as well-defined lytic areas within the skull vault, often with visible diploic vessels entering them.

Sutures: Tend to appear characteristically as serpentine with sclerotic edges. They, along with developmental fissures are usually bilateral, with exception of the sagittal and metopic sutures. Another anatomical consideration is the occipital bone as, during development, numerous fissures and sutures may appear, increasing the complexity of interpretation.

When viewing *paediatric* skull images it is important to be able to recognise the Mendosal suture, also known as the accessory occipital suture; this is commonly seen in neonates and should not be confused for fracture. The majority of these will close by 6 years of age.

Intracranial calcifications: Can be seen as age-related processes and unaccompanied by disease. For example, it is estimated that around two-thirds of the adult population will demonstrate calcification of the pineal gland.[10] The key is to recognise when the calcification is of an unusual size for the location or if it is seen in those patients under 9 years of age; these factors may raise suspicion of pathology.

General bony appearances: Examine for any breaks in the cortex and, when checking the skull vault, care should be given to the density of the bone. Although many skull fractures are linear, one must be aware of the potential for a depressed fracture and this might only be demonstrated by an increase in density as a consequence of the bone fragments overlapping.

Vascular markings can be differentiated from fractures as fracture lines appear more densely black due to the involvement of both inner and outer tables of the skull. In addition, fractures do not have branches that taper; they also lack sclerotic margins.

Pneumocephalus refers to free air within the skull vault; this appearance would be indicative of open fracture or of an injury involving the sinuses, so careful scrutiny should be made of the cortex and the sinuses themselves.

As plain radiography imaging of the skull in the context of trauma is not usually common practice, it is more likely that the skull vault is being imaged for pathology. In this case evaluation of the bony architecture is key, and any areas of sclerosis or lucency should be identified. The thickness of the skull vault might also need to be reviewed as certain pathological processes can increase the diploic space; Paget's disease is one such example.

OCCIPITOFRONTAL (OF) CRANIUM (FIG. 12.1A,B)

IR is vertical, an antiscatter grid is employed

Positioning

- The patient is seated facing the IR, their forehead in contact with it
- The orbitomeatal baseline (OMBL) and median sagittal plane (MSP) are perpendicular to the IR. The MSP position can be checked by ensuring that the distances between both external auditory meati (EAMs) and the IR are equidistant

Beam Direction and FRD

There are a range of beam directions used, which affect the position of the petrous ridge on the image produced (see Chapter 11, Fig.11.4); *20° caudal angulation* clears the ridge to the lowest border of the orbits and this angulation is probably that used most frequently, since it maximises the amount of vault shown above the maxilla

Centring

In the midline of the occiput, to emerge through the glabella

Owing to angulation, it is necessary to ensure that the collimated field lies within the IR boundaries.

Collimation

Vertex of vault, inferior border of occiput, lateral margins of vault

When a patient presents on a trolley, after a head injury, or when they cannot turn face-down for a table-top technique, the FO projection (described later) is used and adapted by using a 20° cranial angle. Centring is over the glabella.

Criteria for Assessing Image Quality

- Vertex of vault, inferior border of occiput, and the lateral margins of vault are demonstrated
- Superior border of petrous ridge shown level with superior orbital margins, if no angle is used. For techniques using beam angulation, the petrous ridge should appear halfway down the orbits for 10° caudal angle and at the bottom of the orbits for 20° angle
- Lateral borders of orbits equidistant from lateral borders of skull
- Sharp image showing the dense petrous ridge in contrast with the orbits and occiput, and frontal bone in contrast with the adjacent air-filled sinuses

Common Errors: OF Cranium

Common Errors	Possible Reasons	Potential Effect on PCE or Report
Petrous ridge is seen above required level in relationship to orbits	Inadequate angle selected or OMBL used is incorrectly positioned (chin down too far)	An insufficient amount of the skull vault will be demonstrated Frontal bone would be obscured by the facial skeleton
Petrous ridge is seen below required level in relationship to orbits	Angle selected is too great or OMBL used is incorrectly positioned (chin not down enough)	The frontal bone will be foreshortened and not adequately demonstrated
Distance between lateral orbital margins is not equal	Rotation of the head; the orbit demonstrating the shortest distance between its lateral border and the lateral aspect of the vault coincides with the side towards which the head is rotated	As with other anatomical structures, symmetry is useful when interpreting the image – rotation would not allow for adequate demonstration of the appropriate anatomy and reduce the potential to compare sides

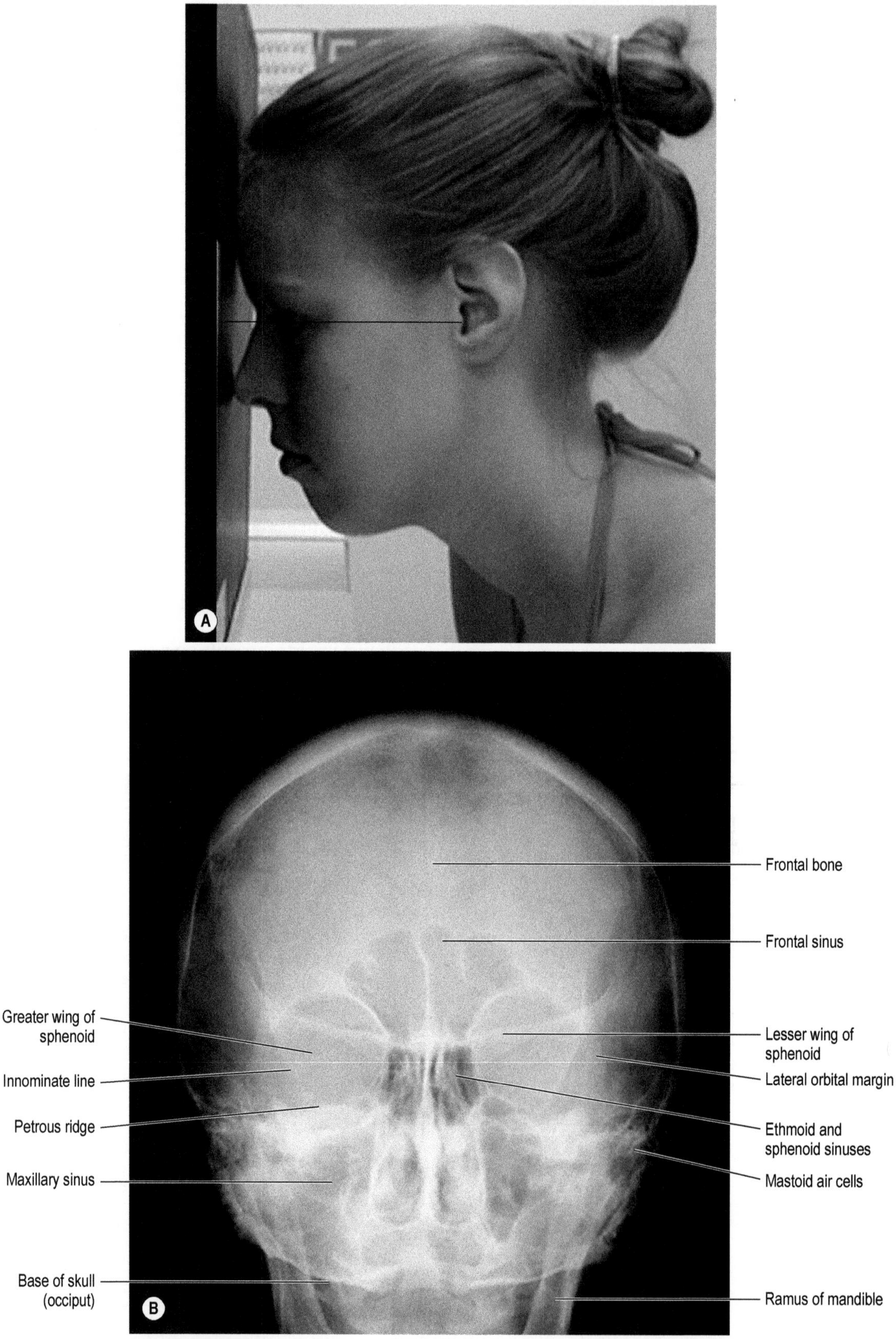

Fig. 12.1 (A) OF cranium; (B) OF 20° cranium. The OF 20° projection shows the petrous ridge level with the bottom of the orbits, thus projecting as much of the cranial vault as possible above the maxilla and petrous portion of temporal bone.

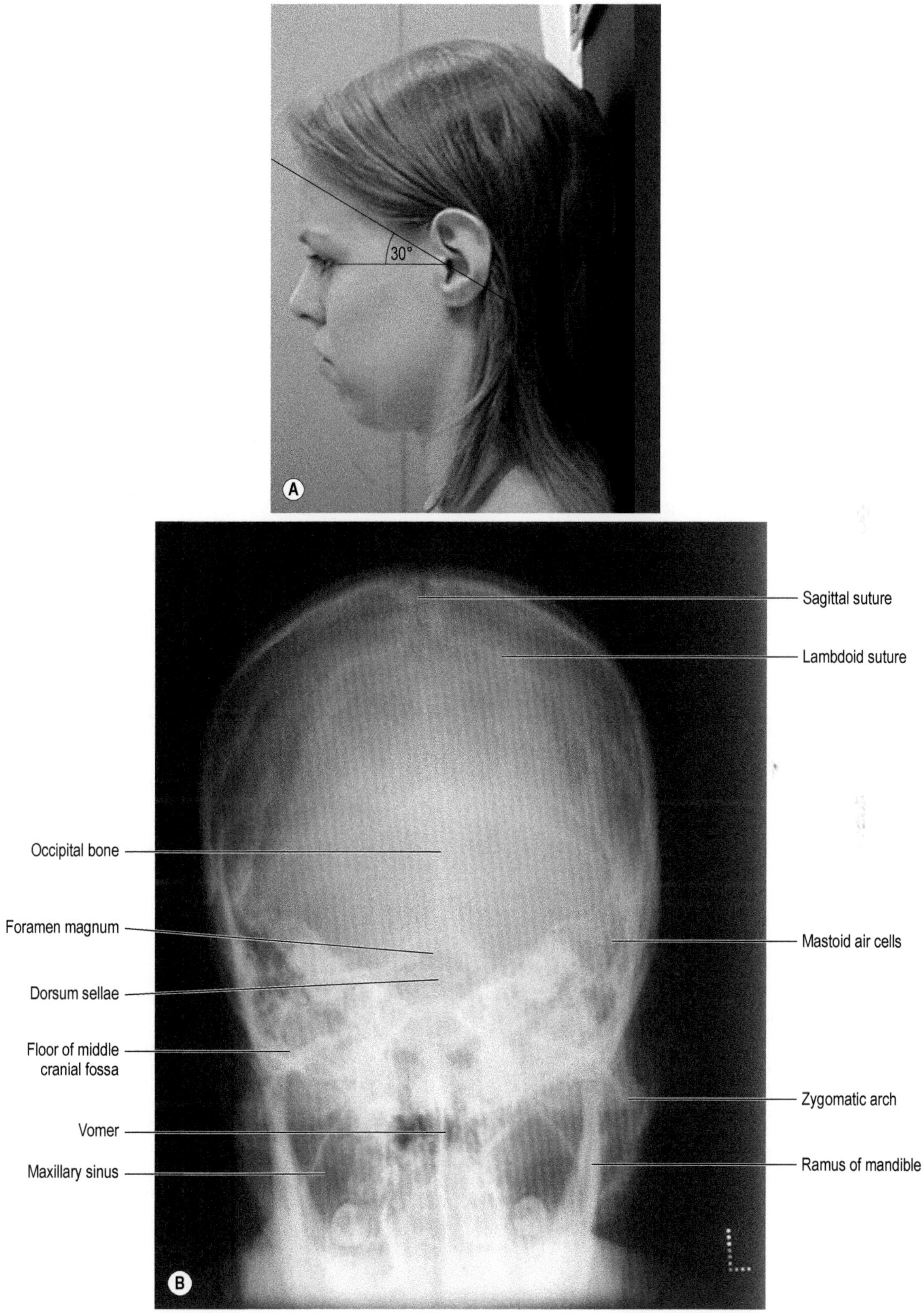
30°
A
Sagittal suture
Lambdoid suture
Occipital bone
Foramen magnum
Mastoid air cells
Dorsum sellae
Floor of middle cranial fossa
Zygomatic arch
Vomer
Maxillary sinus
Ramus of mandible
L
B

Fig. 12.2 FO 30°.

FRONTO-OCCIPITAL (FO) 30° CRANIUM (TOWNE'S) (FIG. 12.2A,B)

This projection may also be referred to as the *Towne's* or *half-axial* projection and may also be produced as an OF with a 30° cranial angle. The OF approach is seldom used in conventional skull techniques as the projection is mostly used to show the occiput, which is positioned closest to the IR in the FO position. However, the OF position is easier to achieve if the patient is seated erect, and the risks associated with radiation dose to the eye lens and thyroid are less severe. It would therefore be pertinent to stress that the FO approach should be used wherever possible.

IR is vertical, an antiscatter grid is employed

Positioning

- The patient sits erect facing the X-ray tube
- The OMBL and MSP are perpendicular to the IR. The MSP position can be checked by checking that the distances between the EAMs and the IR are equidistant. Avoid using facial structures such as eyebrows to assess symmetry of the position, as such soft tissue structures generally are not symmetrical in their position

For notes on how to overcome difficulties when positioning the OMBL for the FO in conventional technique, see Chapter 11.

Beam Direction and FRD

Initially horizontal, then angled 30° caudally

Centring

Traditional centring is often described as being approximately 5 cm above the glabella, but this has been mentioned to cause unnecessary irradiation of the neck and thyroid.[11] Radiographers may be familiar with the instruction to 'centre at the hairline', but unfortunately, not only do hairlines vary in their position, they are also non-existent in many patients. Alternatively, the central ray can be directed to a point above the glabella, ensuring that its path travels through the foramen magnum (found approximately midway between the EAM and mastoid process from the lateral perspective). Changing the centring point and central ray angle can have the effect of reducing dose to the thyroid.[12]

1. The horizontal beam is collimated to the size of the vault and angled 25° caudally

2. The beam is re-centred over the vault to include it in the collimated field; further longitudinal collimation may be possible at this point. It will be noted that the centring point is higher than when using the 30° angle

Collimation for Conventional FO 30° Projection

Occiput, parietal bones, foramen magnum, petrous temporal bone, lateral aspects of vault

Owing to angulation, it is necessary to ensure that the collimated field lies within the IR boundaries.

OCCIPITOFRONTAL (OF) WITH 30° CRANIAL ANGULATION (REVERSE TOWNE'S)

IR is vertical, an antiscatter grid is employed

Positioning

- The patient is seated facing the IR, their forehead in contact with it
- The OMBL is perpendicular to the IR as for other OF projections
- The MSP is perpendicular to the IR

Beam Direction and FRD

Initially horizontal, then angled 30° cranially
100 cm FRD

Centring

Below the external occipital protuberance (EOP) to emerge above the glabella. The beam should pass through the foramen magnum (found approximately midway between the EAM and mastoid process from the lateral perspective)

The IR will require cranial displacement to ensure its centre coincides with the central ray.

Collimation

Occiput, parietal bones, foramen magnum, petrous temporal bone, lateral aspects of vault

Criteria for Assessing Image Quality (OF and FO Methods)

- Occiput, parietal bones, foramen magnum, petrous temporal bone and lateral aspect of vault are shown
- Foramen magnum is demonstrated with dorsum sellae seen centrally within its borders
- Petrous ridge is seen as a shallow 'V' either side of the foramen magnum
- Sharp image showing dorsum sellae in contrast with the less dense foramen magnum; bones of the vault in contrast with the petrous portion of temporal bone

Common Errors: OF with 30° Cranial Angulation (Reverse Towne's)

Common Errors	Possible Reasons	Potential Effects on PCE or Report
Foramen magnum appears short or is not evident. Dorsum sellae may be visible above the portion of the foramen magnum that is seen	Angle selected is inadequate or OMBL is positioned incorrectly (chin not down enough)	Does not adequately demonstrate the occipital region and the foramen magnum May imply false-positive pathology regarding foramen magnum
Large foramen magnum seen but curve of the posterior arch of C1 is seen in its lower third, rather than the anvil-shaped dorsum sellae	Angle selected is too great or OMBL is not positioned correctly (chin down too far)	Foreshortens occipital region May imply false-positive pathology regarding foramen magnum
Dorsum sellae not seen centrally in foramen magnum and petrous portions of temporal bone are asymmetrical	Rotated head; direction of rotation coincides with the direction of shift of the sella within the foramen	May falsely indicate pathology associated with pituitary fossa

LATERAL CRANIUM (FIG. 12.3A,B)

IR is vertical, an antiscatter grid is employed

Positioning

- The patient is seated, facing the erect IR
- The head is turned through 90°, away from the side of interest, and the side of the head is placed in contact with the IR
- The MSP is parallel to the IR

Beam Direction and FRD

Horizontal, at 90° to the IR (must also be 90° to the MSP)
100 cm FRD

Centring

Midway between the glabella and EOP

Collimation

Vertex of skull, occiput, frontal bone

Criteria for Assessing Image Quality

- Vertex of skull, occiput and frontal bone are demonstrated
- There is superimposition of the floor of the anterior cranial fossa, superimposition of the outlines of the sphenoid and pituitary fossa; superimposition of the inner table of occiput; superimposition of the inner table of frontal bone; superimposition of the petrous portions of temporal bone
- Sharp image demonstrating bony detail of the vault in contrast with the less dense sutures, mastoid air cells and air-filled sphenoid sinus. The petrous portions of temporal should appear slightly underpenetrated in comparison to the temporal bones and the EAMs should be identified within the dense area of the petrous portions of temporal

Many structures are identified for superimposition in the lateral skull projection and not all are included in the list of image criteria above. Those not listed here include temporomandibular joints, angles of mandible and orbital outlines.

In the real world of clinical practice, experience has shown that these paired structures are almost never *all* superimposed on one lateral image. The main reason for this is the varying distance of these structures from the central ray, accompanied by the distance between the structures themselves; this serves to project the outline of the structure nearer the central ray away from the outline of the other structure in the pair.

For example, consider the lateral orbital outlines, which, on the average male adult, lie around 6 cm away from the centring point: at an FRD of 100 cm this would create obliquity of the ray passing through the lateral orbit. This obliquity can be assessed mathematically to be around 3.5°, which is enough to displace the image of the orbital outline furthest from the IR. Other structures, such as angle of mandible furthest from the IR, are even more remote from the central ray.

Common Errors: Lateral Cranium

Common Errors	Possible Reasons	Potential Effects of PCE or Report
Vertical aspects of structures not superimposed and appear *side by side*. These include: anterior clinoids, posterior clinoids, anterior aspect of sphenoid sinus, lateral orbital margins, temporomandibular joints, petrous ridges	MSP not perpendicular to the IR; rotation of the head	May falsely imply pathology involving the pituitary fossa Unlikely to demonstrate fluid level in the sphenoid sinus if present Potentially would not allow for accurate location of a foreign body
Horizontal aspects of structures not superimposed and appear *one above the other*. These include: floor of the anterior cranial fossa, anterior clinoids, posterior clinoids, floor of sphenoid sinus, floor of the pituitary fossa, orbital outlines, temporomandibular joints, petrous ridges	MSP not perpendicular to the IR; tilt of the head *Note that the image produced may demonstrate both tilt and rotation*	As above

Frequently the pituitary fossa is used as the main focus for assessment of position but it must be noted that a seriously tilted lateral may show a single pituitary fossa outline, suggesting good positioning. Severe tilt will displace one side of the fossa and lower its outline sufficiently so as to mask its outline with inferiorly positioned structures; this leaves one side of the fossa appearing to be a beautifully superimposed image of the full pituitary fossa. It is therefore recommended that the pituitary fossa is used only for position assessment in conjunction with at least one other pair of structures, for the lateral skull image.

SUBMENTOVERTICAL (SMV) CRANIUM (FIG. 12.4A,B)

IR is vertical, an antiscatter grid is employed

This projection is not possible as part of table-top technique unless equipment is available that can support the patient's trunk and legs above the table-top and allow extension of the neck to bring the vertex of the head in contact with the table-top.

Positioning

- A chair or stool is placed in front of the erect unit and pulled approximately 30 cm from it. If using a chair, its back should be perpendicular to the IR, rather than parallel with it. Brakes must be applied if the stool or chair has wheels
- The patient is seated with their back to the IR

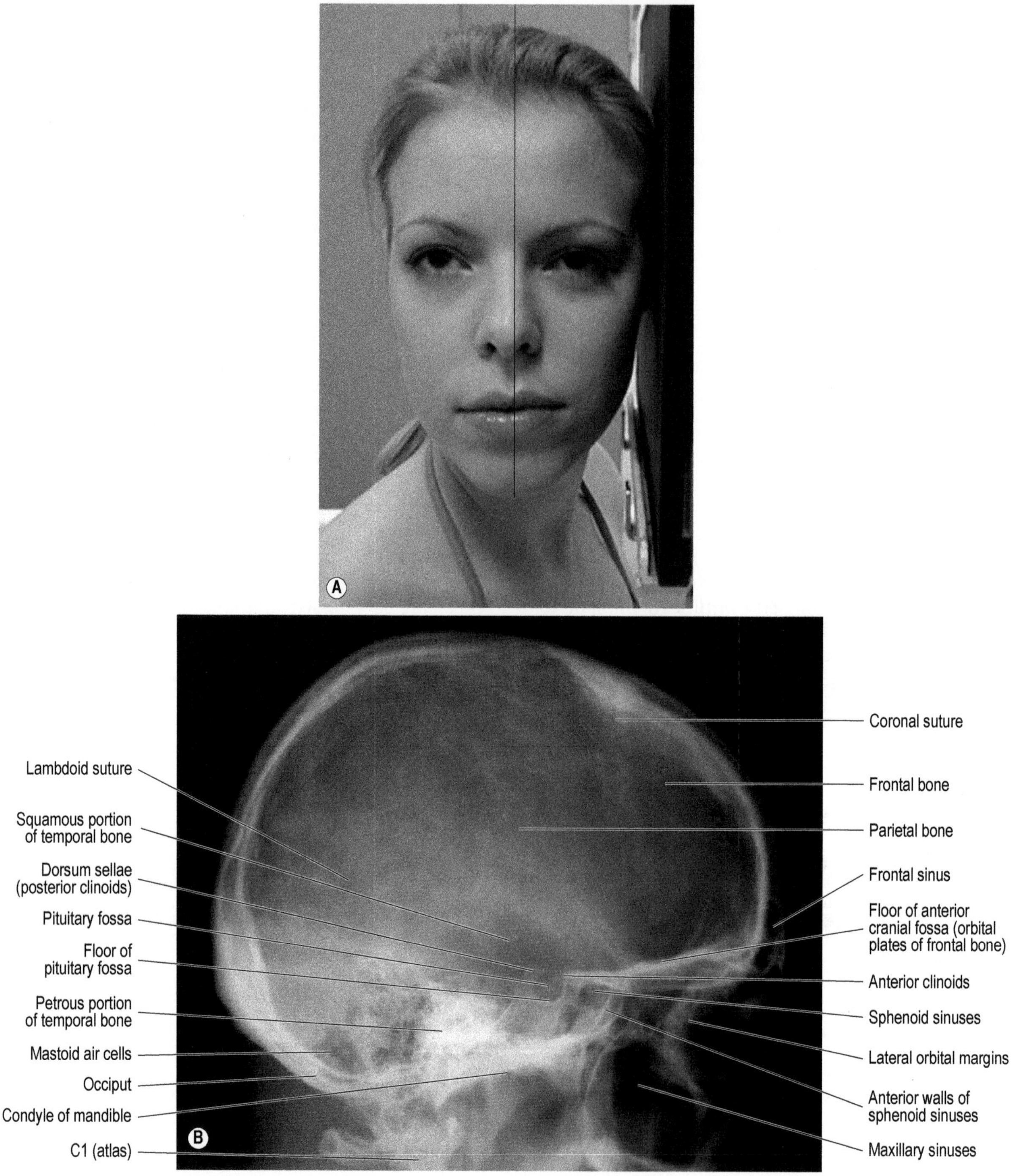

Fig. 12.3 Lateral cranium.

- The patient is asked to lean back and extend their neck; the radiographer should support their shoulders gently but should avoid taking the patient's full weight
- The patient is asked to place the vertex of their head in contact with the IR
- MSP of the head is perpendicular to the IR and the OMBL parallel to it

Beam Direction and FRD

Horizontal, then angled 5° cranially
100 cm FRD

Centring

Midway between the angles of the mandible

Collimation

Frontal bone, occiput, parietal bones

Maintenance of the required SMV position is very difficult for patients and their body weight is borne by the vertex of the skull; this is actually quite painful and can leave the patient feeling quite nauseous. The radiographer must position the patient confidently and efficiently, to ensure that their patient experiences minimum discomfort.

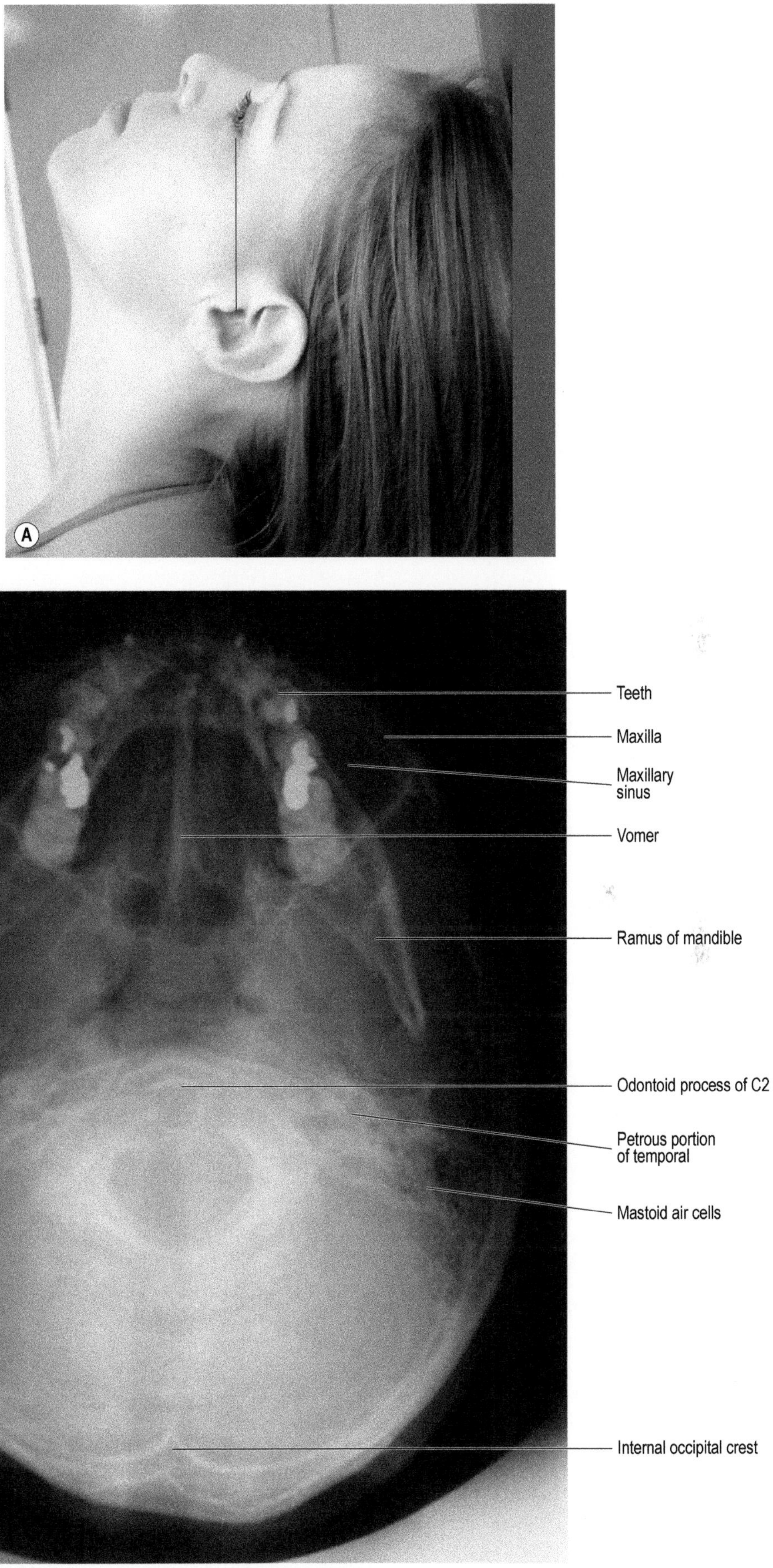

Fig. 12.4 SMV cranium.

Criteria for Assessing Image Quality

- Frontal bone, occiput and parietal bones are demonstrated
- Circular image of the odontoid process seen under the anterior rim of the foramen magnum
- Body of the mandible passes through the centre of the maxillary sinuses; symphysis menti is seen just inside the frontal bone
- Angles of the mandible are superimposed over corresponding temporomandibular joints
- Sagittal suture is seen centrally and bisects the foramen magnum; the cervical vertebrae are superimposed centrally down the MSP
- Symmetry of bilateral structures of the skull

Common Errors: SMV Cranium

Common Errors	Possible Reasons	Potential Effects on PCE or Report
Body of the mandible below maxillary sinuses; odontoid process seen more elongated, similar to its appearance on the AP C1–C2 projection; symphysis menti seen through the sphenoid or ethmoid sinuses; angles of the mandible below temporomandibular joints	OMBL not parallel to the IR; inadequate chin elevation	As this view is primarily aimed at assessing the base of the skull, poor positioning would mean that the mandible in particular will overlie key structures, making adequate assessment of this region difficult
Asymmetry of anatomical structures	MSP not perpendicular to the IR (tilt of the head)	Asymmetry will hinder evaluation and may confuse interpretation in an area that is anatomically complex

Specialised Projections of the Skull

In the 21st century, the majority of hospitals in the Western world have access to specialised imaging modalities. Of these, CT and MRI have largely replaced plain radiography in the diagnosis of diseases that were once only assessed with plain radiography. Unfortunately, plain radiography frequently only provides information when disease is very advanced; CT provides more detailed and high-quality information, and MRI has the advantage of providing information on neurological and other soft tissues (with no patient dose from ionising radiation) before any bony effects are seen. Recommended imaging methods are summarised in Table 12.1.

Information on plain radiography is still provided in this book, as support for radiographers working in areas with limited or no access to MRI and CT. PCE comments are not given since it is unlikely that there will be requirement for PCE at radiographer level in these situations.

SELLA TURCICA (PITUITARY FOSSA)

To clarify the use of terms in this chapter, the name 'pituitary fossa' refers to the depression within the sella turcica in which lies the pituitary gland. The sella turcica itself forms the top of the central portion of the sphenoid bone, lying over the sphenoid sinus in the midline.

An enlarged and eroded sella can be a sign of a pituitary tumour or raised intracranial pressure, but this appearance is an effect of long-term disease.

For all projections of the sella turcica the IR is vertical and an antiscatter grid is employed.

LATERAL SELLA TURCICA (FIG. 12.5A,B)

Positioning

- The patient is initially seated facing the IR
- The trunk is brought as close as possible to the receptor unit and the patient is asked to sit with their spine as erect as possible. This helps the patient turn their head more easily into the required lateral position
- The head is turned through 90° to bring the side of the head in contact with the IR
- The median sagittal plane (MSP) is parallel to the IR; there should be no tilt or rotation of the head. This can be assessed by checking the midline of the cranium over the top and symmetry of the frontal bone and orbits

Beam Direction and FRD

Horizontal, at 90° to the IR
100 cm FRD

Centring

Midway between the posterior tubercle of the first cervical vertebra and the glabella *or* 2.5 cm anterior to the external auditory meatus (EAM), along the OMBL, and 2.5 cm above this point

The second centring point will have variable efficacy due to variations in the skull size of the individual patient.

TABLE 12.1 Recommended Skull Imaging Modalities

Region	Recommendation
Pituitary	MRI[13]
Mastoids	CT[14]
IAMs and auditory nerves	MRI[15]
Optic foramina and optic nerve	MRI[16] with recognition of the use of CT for anatomic assessment of the optic canal[17]
Jugular foramina	For analysis of bony margins, CT; MRI for assessment of tumours and their size, characteristics, vascularisation and relationship to adjacent anatomy[18]

Collimation

Sphenoid bone from lesser wing (anterior clinoid processes) anteriorly and posterior clinoids posteriorly

Criteria for Assessing Image Quality

- Anterior and posterior clinoid processes, sella turcica, sphenoid sinus and dorsum sellae are demonstrated
- Superimposition of both sides of the floor of pituitary fossa and floor of the anterior cranial fossa
- Anterior clinoid processes are superimposed
- Posterior clinoid processes are superimposed
- Sharp image demonstrating outline of the clinoids and pituitary fossa in contrast with the temporal bones and sphenoid sinus

Common Errors: Lateral Sella Turcica

Common Errors	Possible Reasons	Potential Effects on PCE or Report
Both pairs of clinoid processes overlapped, seen one above the other	Tilted skull	Difficult to determine whether there is any enlargement of the pituitary fossa, which can occur with pathology such as adenoma or hypothyroidism
Both pairs of clinoid processes overlapped, seen side by side	Rotated skull	As above
'Double' floor of sella turcica; two lines over floor area	Tilted skull or floor is eroded on one side by tumour	As above

OCCIPITOFRONTAL (OF) SELLA TURCICA (FIG. 12.6A–C)

The OF 20° projection will demonstrate the floor of the sella turcica, seen as asymmetry of the floor if the floor is eroded on one side. The OF 30° projection has limited value, demonstrating the dorsum sellae through the foramen magnum; the dorsum will appear as low density if it is eroded. IR is erect

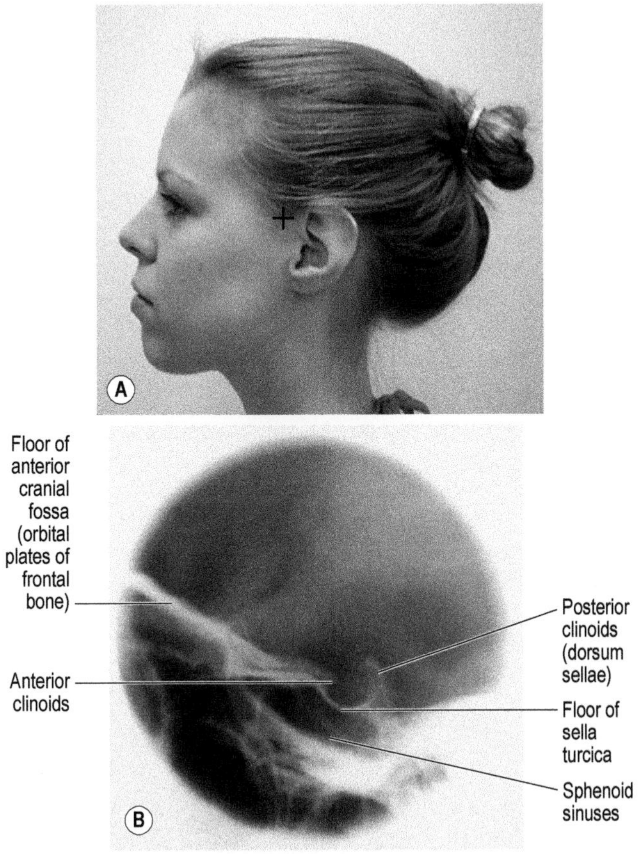

Fig. 12.5 Lateral sella turcica.

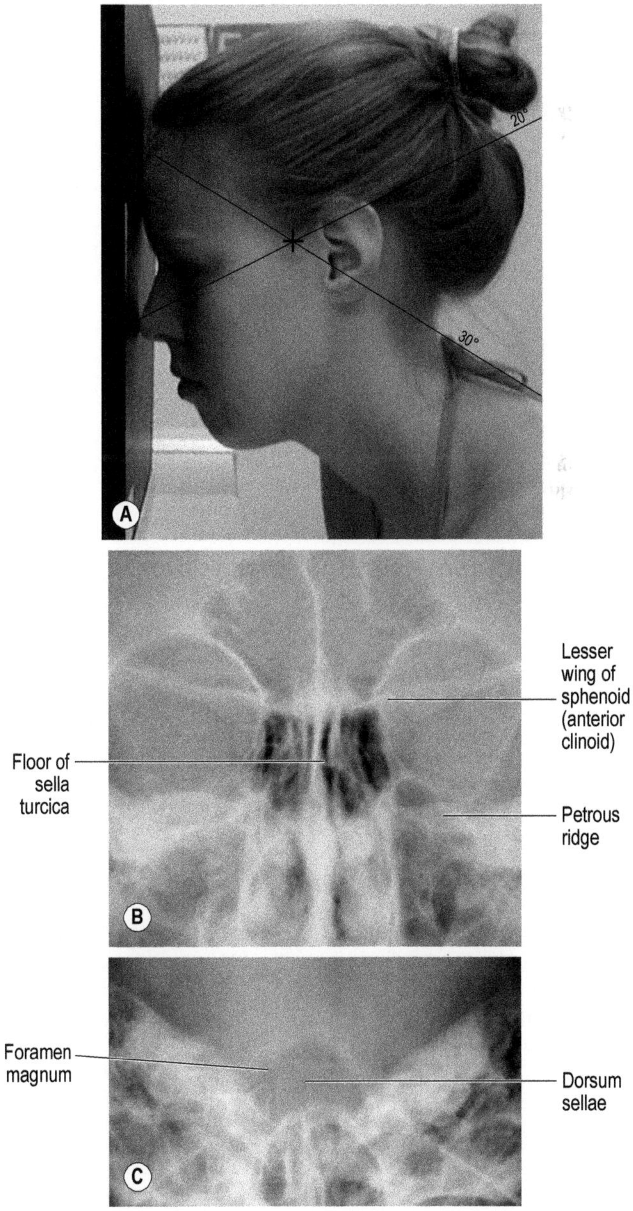

Fig. 12.6 (A) OF sella turcica; (B) OF 20° sella turcica; (C) OF 30° sella turcica.

Positioning

- The patient is seated facing the bucky, their forehead in contact with it
- The OMBL and MSP are perpendicular to the IR

Beam Direction and FRD

(a) Initially horizontal, a *20° caudal* angle will demonstrate the floor of the pituitary fossa through the ethmoid and sphenoid sinuses

(b) A *30° cranial* angle will demonstrate the dorsum sellae through the foramen magnum

100 cm FRD

Centring

(a) With *20° caudal* angle: above the EOP to emerge through the nasion

(b) With *30° cranial* angle: below the EOP, on the neck, to emerge through the glabella

Collimation

OF 20°: lesser wing of sphenoid, sphenoid and ethmoid sinuses

OF 30°: ethmoid sinus, foramen magnum

Criteria for Assessing Image Quality

OF 20°:

- Lesser wing of the sphenoid, sphenoid and ethmoid sinuses are demonstrated
- Medial aspects of the superior border of petrous ridge are shown superimposed on the inferior orbital margin
- Lesser wing of sphenoid seen medially and symmetrically across the upper portion of the orbits
- Medial borders of the orbits are equidistant from nasal septum
- Floor of pituitary fossa is seen as a horizontal line across the ethmoid sinuses. In cases of erosion of the floor of the fossa, this line may deviate from horizontal orientation
- Sharp image showing the fine line indicating the floor of the pituitary fossa in contrast with the air-filled ethmoid sinus

OF 30°:

- Foramen magnum is demonstrated
- Dorsum sellae is seen in the centre of the foramen magnum
- Sharp image showing dorsum sellae in contrast with the less dense foramen magnum

Common Errors: OF Sella Turcica

Common Errors	Possible Reasons	Potential Effects on PCE or Report
OF 20°		
Petrous ridge seen above the level of the inferior orbital margins	Inadequate angle selected *or* OMBL is incorrectly positioned (chin down too far)	The projection requires that structures should be visualised through the frontal bone. The floor of the pituitary fossa would be obscured by superimposed anatomy
Petrous ridge seen below the level of the inferior orbital margins	Angle selected is too great *or* OMBL is incorrectly positioned (chin not far enough down)	As above
OF 30°		
Foramen magnum appears short or is not evident. Dorsum sellae may be visible above the portion of the foramen magnum that is seen	Angle selected is inadequate *or* OMBL is positioned incorrectly (chin not far enough down)	If distortion of dorsum sellae occurs due to incorrect angulation, or there is superimposition of bony structures, then accurate measurement would not be possible and changes that may be associated with pathology such as adenoma would be missed. Symmetry of structures would potentially be difficult to determine
Large foramen magnum seen but curve of the posterior arch of C1 is seen in its lower third, rather than the anvil shape of dorsum sellae	Angle selected is too great *or* OMBL is not positioned correctly (chin too far down)	As above

Mastoids

LATERAL OBLIQUE MASTOIDS (FIG. 12.7A,B)

Positioning for this projection is identical to that for lateral oblique temporomandibular joints (TMJs), although the centring point differs. The pinna of the ear must also be cleared from the mastoid area. Both sides are examined for comparison.

IR is vertical, an antiscatter grid is employed

Positioning

- The patient is initially seated, facing the IR
- The trunk is brought as close as possible to the receptor unit and the patient is asked to sit with their spine as erect as possible. This helps the patient turn their head more easily into the required lateral position
- The head is turned through 90° to bring the mastoid on the side under examination over the IR. The location of this bone can be detected by palpating the mastoid process, which lies inferiorly and posteriorly to the EAM
- The pinna of the ear on the side nearest the IR is then gently pulled forward and the head rests against the IR to keep the pinna forward. This clears the image of the pinna from the area of interest
- The MSP is parallel to the IR; there should be no tilt or rotation of the head. This can be assessed by checking the midline of the cranium over the top, symmetry of the

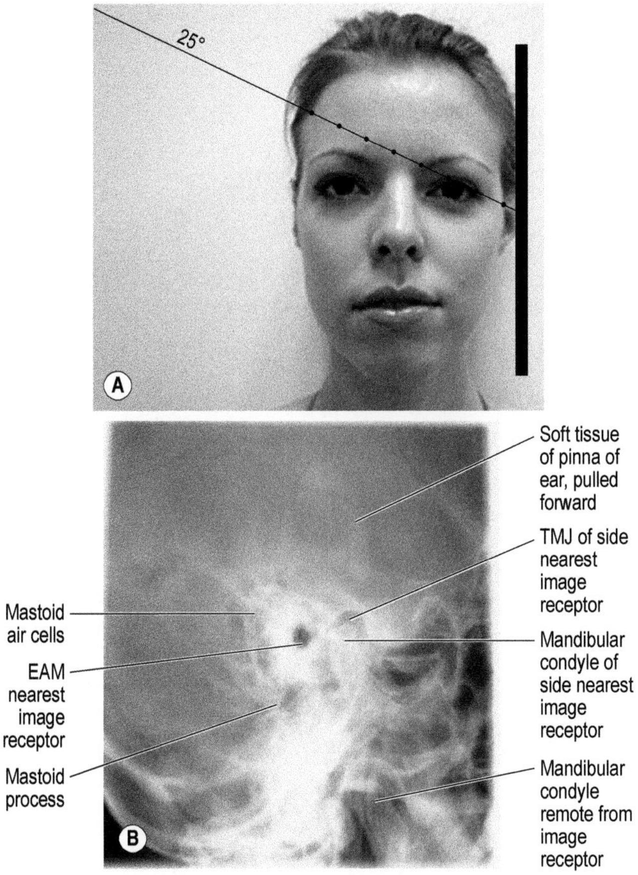

Fig. 12.7 Lateral oblique mastoids.

frontal bone and orbits and that the interpupillary line is perpendicular to the IR

- Asking the patient to close their eyes will assist in maintenance of the position; as the radiographer leaves the receptor unit, a patient will often follow this movement with their eyes and potentially affect the position of the head

Beam Direction and FRD

Initially horizontal, angled 25° caudally
100 cm FRD

Centring

Above the mastoid process on the side remote from the IR, to emerge over the mastoid process on the side nearest the IR

Collimation

EAM, mastoid process, air cells behind the pinna of the ear

Criteria for Assessing Image Quality

- EAM and air-filled mastoid are demonstrated posterior to the EAM
- Condyle of mandible and mastoid air cells of the opposite side are projected clear from those under examination
- Soft tissue of ear is seen as folded forward and cleared from the mastoid
- Air cells of the mastoids are seen in contrast to bone; bony detail of the mastoid bone is demonstrated

Common Errors: Lateral Oblique Mastoids

Common Errors	Possible Reasons	Potential Effects on PCE or Report
Mastoid closest to tube not cleared from mastoid under examination	1. Inadequate angle used *or* 2. Head is tilted with its vertex towards the IR, which effectively reduces the effects of angulation	Will be unable to determine which side was affected by pathology of the mastoids if they are not separated sufficiently
TMJ of opposite side not cleared from mastoid	Inadequate angle, or tilt as above *or* the head is rotated with the face away from the IR	Superimposition of the TMJ of the opposite side over the mastoid air cells under examination would potentially obscure any pathology

PROFILE OF MASTOID PROCESS (FIG. 12.8A,B)

Both sides are examined for comparison
IR is vertical

Positioning

- The patient is initially positioned as for an FO projection
- The head is rotated approximately 30° away from the side under examination, until the process is in profile and cleared from the ramus of the mandible

Beam Direction and FRD

Initially horizontal, angled 25° caudally
100 cm FRD

Centring

Over the mastoid process under examination (nearest the IR)

Collimation

Mastoid air cells, mastoid process

Criteria for Assessing Image Quality

- Mastoid and mastoid process are demonstrated
- Mastoid process is cleared from the mandible and zygoma
- Mastoid bone is seen in contrast to air-filled cells and soft tissues of the neck

Common Errors: Profile of Mastoid Process		
Common Errors	**Possible Reasons**	**Potential Effects on PCE or Report**
Mandible and/or zygoma overlying mastoid process	Inadequate obliquity	Anatomical structures will obscure the mastoids due to rotation and resultant superimposition
Occiput overlies mastoid process	Excessive obliquity	As above

OCCIPITOFRONTAL (OF) 30° MASTOIDS (FIG. 12.9 A,B)

IR is vertical, an antiscatter grid is employed

Positioning

- The patient is seated facing the bucky, their forehead in contact with it
- The OMBL and MSP are perpendicular to the IR

Beam Direction and FRD

Initially horizontal, angled 30° cranially
100 cm FRD

Centring

In the midline of the neck, to travel through the mastoid processes

It may be necessary to further displace the IR, to ensure the area of interest lies within its borders.

Collimation

Temporal bones, mastoid processes

Criteria for Assessing Image Quality

- Air-filled mastoid bones are demonstrated on the lateral portions of the temporal bones
- Dorsum sellae and posterior clinoid processes are projected through the centre of the foramen magnum
- Petrous temporals seen as a slight 'V' shape about the foramen magnum
- Symmetry of the petrous portions of the temporal around the midline
- Sharp image demonstrating the air-filled mastoids in contrast to the denser bones of the vault

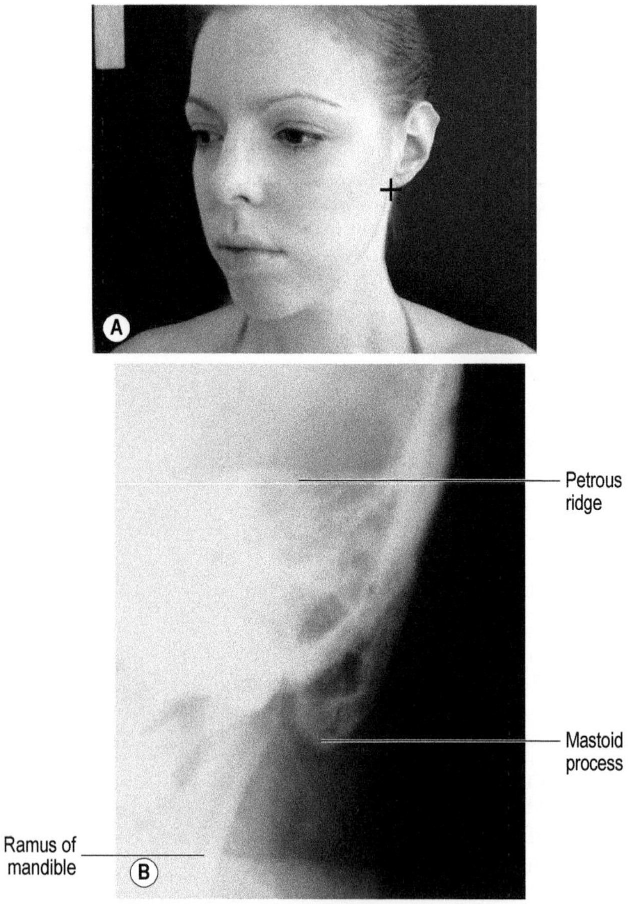

Fig. 12.8 Profile of mastoid process.

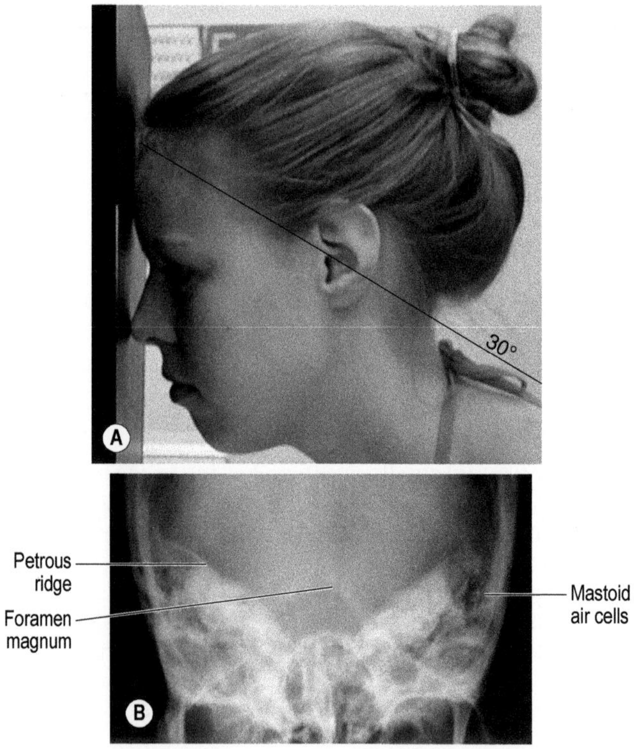

Fig. 12.9 OF 30° mastoids.

Common Errors: OF 30° Mastoids

Common Errors	Possible Reasons	Potential Effects on PCE or Report
Foramen magnum appears short or is not evident. Dorsum sellae may be visible above the portion of the foramen magnum that is seen	Angle selected is inadequate *or* OMBL is incorrectly positioned (chin not far enough down)	Will not adequately demonstrate mastoid air cells – subtle pathology or opacification of air cells could be missed
Large foramen magnum seen but curve of the posterior arch of C1 is seen in its lower third, rather than the anvil shape of dorsum sellae	Angle selected is too great *or* OMBL is incorrectly positioned (chin too far down)	As above

Temporal Bone: Petrous Portion for Internal Auditory Meati (IAMs)

OCCIPITOFRONTAL (OF) 5° IAMs (FIG. 12.10A,B)

IR is vertical, an antiscatter grid is employed

Positioning

- The patient is seated facing the bucky, their forehead in contact with it
- The OMBL and MSP are perpendicular to the IR
- The nasion is coincident with the middle of the IR

Beam Direction and FRD

Initially horizontal, angled 5° caudally
100 cm FRD

In older radiographic texts, central ray perpendicular to the IR was previously described[19] for this projection, but as the petrous ridge lies coincident with the upper border of the orbits, location of the IAMs can be difficult. Use of the 5° caudal angle brings the ridge just below the upper border of the orbits; this acts as a distinguishable landmark, below which lies the low-density channels for the IAMs (Fig. 12.10B).

Centring

Above the EOP to emerge through the nasion

Collimation

Superior orbits and base of skull (occiput)

Criteria for Assessing Image Quality

- Superior orbits and base of skull (occiput) are demonstrated
- Petrous ridge is seen just below the superior margins
- Symmetry of structures is seen through the orbits; semicircular canals seen at the outer limits of the IAMs can be assessed as to their equidistance from the lateral orbital outlines
- Sharp image demonstrating contrast of the petrous portions of temporal bones with the outline of the orbits and the less dense IAMs lying within the petrous portion

Common Errors: OF 5° Internal Auditory Meati

Common Errors	Possible Reasons	Potential Effects on PCE or Report
Petrous ridge seen above required level in orbits	Inadequate angle selected *or* OMBL is incorrectly positioned (chin too far down)	Will be unable to adequately identify IAMs due to possible superimposition of superior orbital margin
Petrous ridge seen below required level in orbits	Angle selected is too great *or* OMBL is incorrectly positioned (chin not far enough down)	Potential for superimposition of inferior orbital margins/facial bones over IAMs

ANTERIOR OBLIQUE (OF OBLIQUE) IAMs (STENVER'S) (FIG. 12.11A,B)

This projection is also known as *Stenver's projection.*[19] It aims to place the petrous portion of the temporal bone parallel to the IR while using a cranial angle to clear the image of the petrous bone above the zygomatic arch and over the flatter, less detailed image of the temporal and parietal bones. The obliquity of the petrous portion of the temporal bones for the Stenver's position is given as approximately 45° but variations according to head shape have been highlighted as ranging from 40° in the dolichocephalic head (long narrow vault as seen from above), through 47° in the mesocephalic ('average') and as much as 54° in the brachycephalic (short and broad vault when seen from above).[20]

IR is vertical, an antiscatter grid is employed

Positioning

- The patient is initially positioned in an OF position
- The head is rotated 45° away from the side under examination

Beam Direction and FRD

Initially horizontal, angled 12° cranially
100 cm FRD

Centring

Midway between the EOP and the EAM remote from the IR, to emerge midway between the EAM nearest the IR and outer canthus of the eye

It may be necessary to displace the IR to ensure the area of interest lies within its borders.

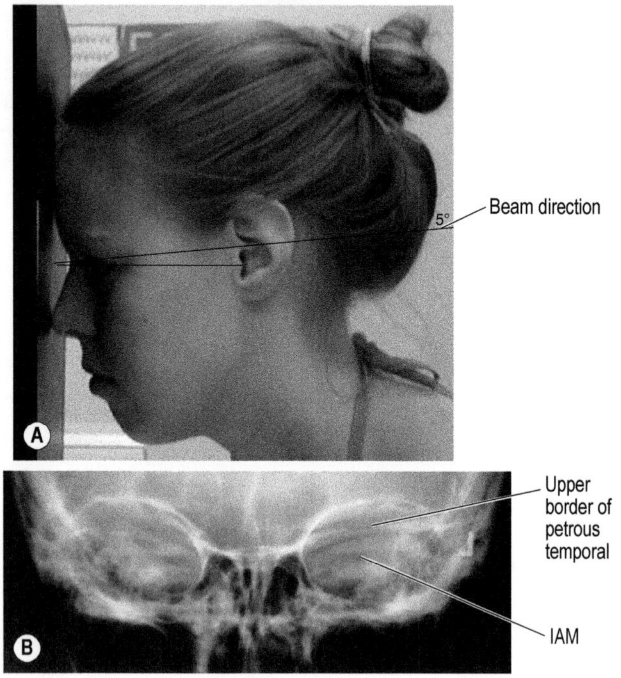

Fig. 12.10 OF 5° IAMs.

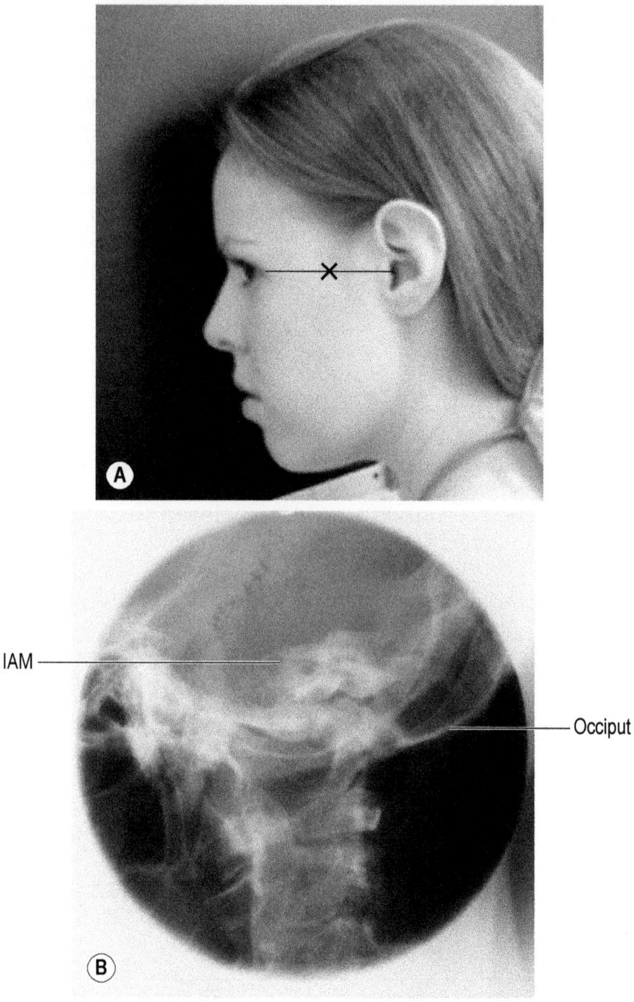

Fig. 12.11 AO (OF oblique) IAMs.

Collimation

Temporal bone under examination

Criteria for Assessing Image Quality

- Orbits, base of occiput and petrous portion of the temporal bone are demonstrated
- Mastoid air cells of the side under examination projected shown laterally in relation to semicircular canals
- Image of the curve of the occipital outline (of the side not under examination) travels through the mastoid air cells
- Lines representing the right and left sides of the base of the skull are horizontal and at the same level
- IAM, semicircular canals and vestibule of the ear are seen below the arcuate eminence, above the head of mandible
- Sharp image demonstrating the dense petrous portion of temporal bone in contrast to the IAM, semicircular canals and the vestibule

Common Errors: Anterior Oblique IAMs (Stenver's)

Common Error	Possible Reason	Potential Effect on PCE or Report
Short meatus	Incorrect rotation; this will show the internal occipital crest crossing the meatus or semicircular canals	Will not allow for complete and optimal appreciation of the structure under examination

OCCIPITOFRONTAL (OF) 30° PETROUS TEMPORAL (FIG. 12.12A,B)

IR is vertical, an antiscatter grid is employed

Positioning

The patient is seated facing the bucky, their forehead in contact with it

The OMBL and MSP are perpendicular to the IR

Beam Direction and FRD

Initially horizontal, angled 30° cranially

100 cm FRD

Centring

In the midline of the neck, to travel through the level of the EAMs

It may be necessary to displace the IR to ensure the area of interest lies within its borders.

Collimation

Temporal bones to include petrous portion

Criteria for Assessing Image Quality

- Temporal bones, including petrous portions, are demonstrated
- Dorsum sellae and posterior clinoid processes are projected through the centre of the foramen magnum
- Petrous temporals are seen as a slight 'V' shape about the foramen magnum
- Symmetry of petrous portions of temporal around the foramen magnum
- Sharp image with dense petrous portions of temporals seen in contrast to the less dense IAMs and the occiput

Common Errors: OF 30° Petrous Temporal

Common Errors	Possible Reasons	Potential Effects on PCE or Report
Foramen magnum appears short or is not evident. Dorsum sellae may be visible above the portion of the foramen magnum that is seen	Angle selected is inadequate *or* OMBL is incorrectly positioned (chin not far enough down)	Inadequate demonstration of the petrous ridge as it will not be cleared from other skull structures as required by the projection
Large foramen magnum seen but curve of the posterior arch of C1 is seen in its lower third, rather than the anvil shape of dorsum sellae	Angle selected is too great *or* OMBL is incorrectly positioned (chin too far down)	Petrous ridge will be distorted by incorrect angulation

Optic Foramen

OCCIPITOMENTAL (OM) OBLIQUE/ANTERIOR OBLIQUE (AO) OPTIC FORAMEN (FIG. 12.13A,B)

Both optic foramina are examined for comparison.
IR is vertical, an antiscatter grid is employed

Positioning

- The patient is seated, facing the IR
- The chin is placed in contact with the IR
- The chin position is adjusted until the OMBL has been raised 30°; the head is then rotated through 30°, away from the eye under examination

Beam Direction and FRD

Horizontal, at 90° to the IR
100 cm FRD

Centring

Behind and above the mastoid process nearest the X-ray tube, to emerge through the middle of the orbit under examination

Collimation

Bony outline of the orbit under examination

Criteria for Assessing Image Quality

- Outline of orbit is demonstrated in full
- Optic foramen seen as a low-density circle within the orbit, level with its midpoint and nearer the lateral margin of the orbit
- Sharp image demonstrating the low-density foramen in contrast to the bones forming the orbit and the overlying bones of the vault

Common Errors: OM Oblique/AO Optic Foramen

Common Errors	Possible Reasons	Potential Effects on PCE or Report
Lateral orbital margin obscuring part, or all, of the foramen	Head is rotated too far	Unable to visualise or assess shape and diameter of the optic canal
Inferior orbital margin obscuring part, or all, of the foramen	Chin is raised too far	As above
Foramen appears elliptical and is located nearer to the medial aspect of the orbit than is required	Inadequate rotation	May falsely imply narrowing or stenosis of the canal
Foramen appears to be cylindrical and is located in the upper half of the orbit	Inadequate raising of the chin	

Jugular Foramina

SUBMENTOVERTICAL (SMV) 20° JUGULAR FORAMINA (FIG. 12.14A,B)

IR is vertical, an antiscatter grid is employed

Positioning

- A seat is placed midway between the X-ray tube and the erect bucky; the patient sits on the stool, facing the X-ray tube
- The patient leans back gently onto the radiographer's arm and flexes their neck and back until the vertex of their head can be placed in contact with the bucky

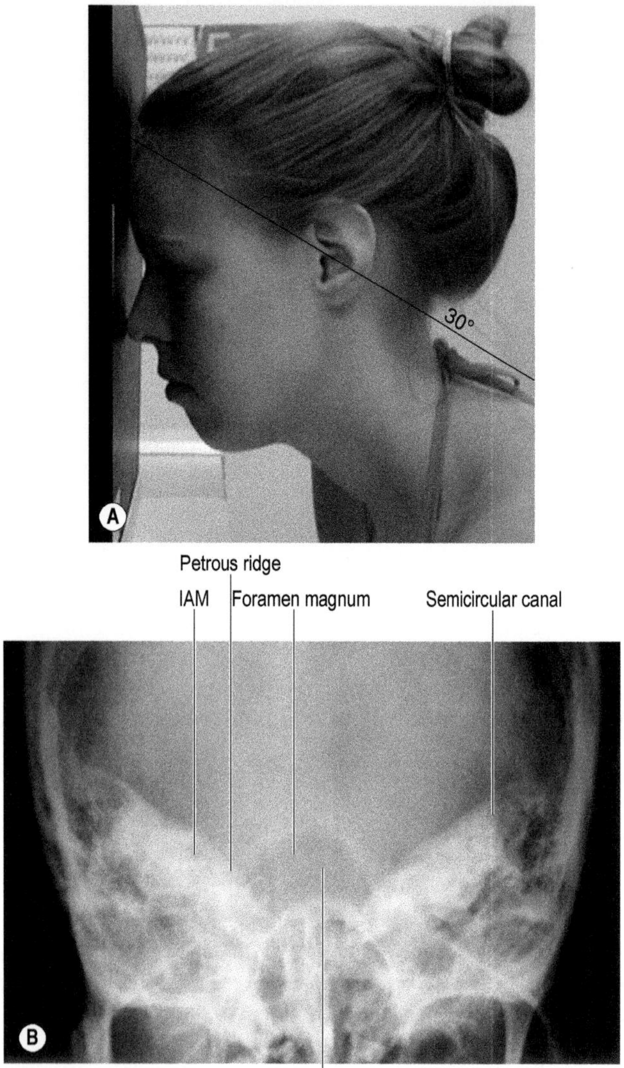

Fig. 12.12 OF 30° petrous temporal.

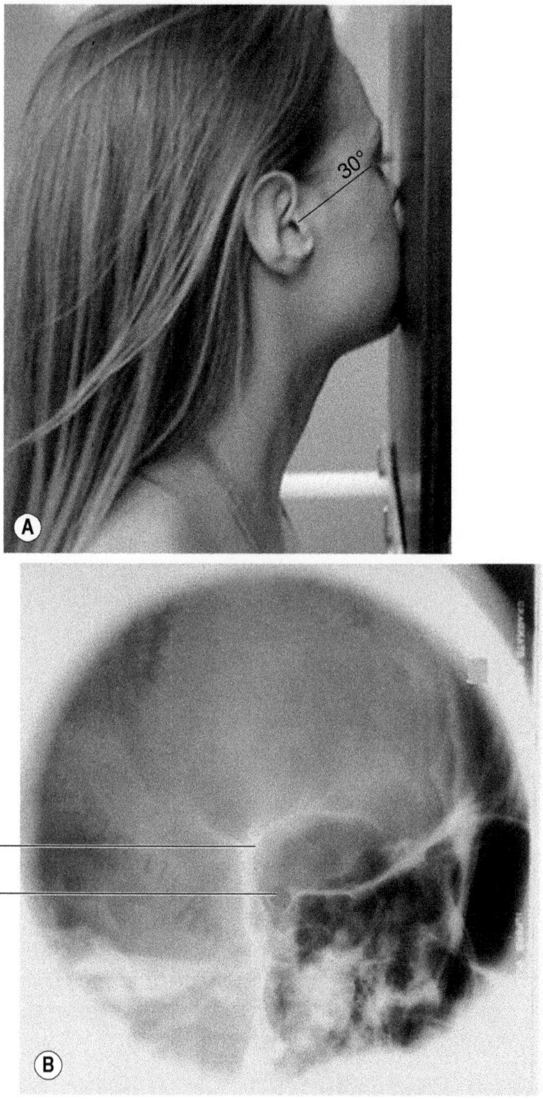

Fig. 12.13 AO optic foramen.

Beam Direction and FRD

20° cranially
100 cm FRD

It may be necessary to displace the IR to ensure the area of interest lies within its borders.

Centring

Midway between the angles of the mandible

Collimation

Angles of mandible, symphysis menti, foramen magnum

Criteria for Assessing Image Quality

- Angles of the mandible, symphysis menti and foramen magnum are demonstrated
- Odontoid process of C2 is demonstrated, through the upper half of the foramen magnum
- Mandible is raised clear of the jugular foramina and superimposed as an arch over the petrous temporal bones
- Both jugular foramina are demonstrated symmetrically on either side of the midline, midway between the edge of the foramen magnum and angle of mandible
- Sharp image demonstrating dense bone of the skull base, in contrast with the jugular foramina

The jugular foramina are variable in size and symmetry under normal circumstances, so in this instance loss of symmetry would not be a reliable indicator of pathology. However, the foramen should always appear well corticated, therefore it is the appearance of the bony margins that will act as a useful diagnostic tool in this instance.

Common Errors: SMV 20° Jugular Foramina

Common Errors	Possible Reasons	Potential Effects on PCE or Report
Mandible overlying foramina	Chin is not elevated enough	Foramina not visible – unable to evaluate
Mandible is clear but foramina not clear	Chin is elevated too much	As above

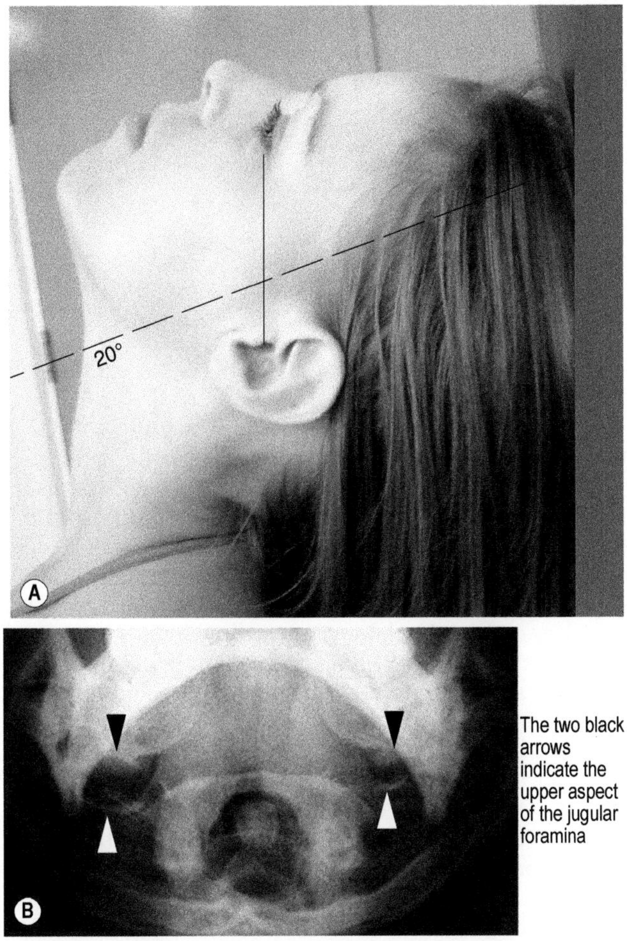
20°
A
B
The two black arrows indicate the upper aspect of the jugular foramina

Fig. 12.14 (A) SMV jugular foramina; (B) SMV 20° jugular foramina. (B, Reproduced with permission from Ballinger PW, Frank ED. *Merrill's Atlas of Radiographic Positioning and Radiologic Procedures.* 10th ed. St Louis: Mosby; 2003.)

References

1. McGlinchey I, Fleet MF, Eatock FC, et al. Comparison of two or three radiographic views in the diagnosis of skull fractures. *Clin Radiol.* 1998;53:215–217.
2. Eyes B, Evans A. Post-traumatic skull radiographs. Time for a reappraisal. *Lancet.* 1978;2(8080):85–86.
3. Balasubramaniam S, Kapadia T, Campbell J, et al. Efficacy of skull radiography. *Am J Surg.* 1981;142:366.
4. Strong I, MacMillan R, Jennett B. Head injuries in accident and emergency departments at Scottish hospitals. *Injury.* 1978;10:154.
5. St John EG. The role of the emergency skull roentgenogram in head trauma. *AJR Am J Roentgenol.* 1968;76:315.
6. NICE (National Institute for Health and Care Excellence). *Take Head Injuries Seriously.* says NICE; 2019. https://www.nice.org.uk/guidance/cg176/documents/take-head-injuries-seriously-says-nice-.
7. Paiva S, Oliveira AMP, Andrade AF, et al. Spinal cord injury and its association with blunt head trauma. *Int J Gen Med.* 2011;4:613–615.
8. NICE (National Institute for Health and Care Excellence). *Head Injury Assessment and Early Management*; 2019. Clinical guidance [CG176] https://www.nice.org.uk/guidance/cg176.
9. Steill I, Wells GA, Vandemheen K, et al. The Canadian CT head rule for patients with minor head injury. *Lancet.* 2001;357:1391–1396.
10. Mutalik S, Tadinada A. Prevalence of pineal gland calcification as an incidental finding in patients referred for implant dental therapy. *Imaging Sci Dent.* 2017;47(3):175–180.
11. Carver E, Carver B. *Medical Imaging: Techniques, Reflection, Evaluation.* 2nd ed. Edinburgh: Churchill Livingstone; 2012.
12. Denton B. Improving plain radiography of the skull: the half axial projection re-described. *Synergy.* 1998;Aug:9–11.
13. Evanson J. *Radiology of the Pituitary.* Endotext clinical endocrinology source; 2016. https://www.ncbi.nlm.nih.gov/books/NBK279161/.
14. Bell D, Gaillard F. Acute mastoiditis. Radiopaedia. https://radiopaedia.org/articles/acute-mastoiditis?lang=gb.
15. Valvassori GE, Palacios E. Magnetic resonance imaging of the internal auditory canal. *Top Reson Imaging.* 2000;11(1):52–55.
16. Kang PS, Smirniotopoulos JG, et al. Optic neuritis imaging. *Emedicine.* 2019. https://emedicine.medscape.com/article/383642-overview.
17. Zhang X, Lee Y, Olson D, et al. Evaluation of optic canal anatomy and symmetry using CT. *BMJ Open Ophthalmol.* 2018. https://bmjophth.bmj.com/content/4/1/e000302.
18. Vogl TJ, Bisdas S. Differential diagnosis of jugular foramen lesions. *Skull Base.* 2009;19(1):3–16.
19. Clark K, Swallow R, Naylor E, et al. *Clark's Positioning in Radiography.* 11th ed. Oxford: Heinemann; 1986.
20. Eisenberg R, Dennis C, May RTC. *Radiographic Positioning.* 2nd ed. Boston: Little, Brown; 1995.

13 Facial Bones and Paranasal Sinuses

ELIZABETH CARVER and LUCY BANFIELD

The most frequent reason for radiological examination of the facial bones is trauma to the region; plain radiographic imaging of the area remains a popular and appropriate method of initial assessment in the acute setting, providing information relatively quickly and with a relatively low radiation dose compared to computed tomography (CT), which is the other imaging method best suited for providing information on bony injury to the area. Low-dose CT is considered a suitable method for demonstration and assessment of orbital fractures, as plain radiographic images can sometimes be inconclusive. CT also allows for the added benefit of multiplanar reconstruction which provides greater accuracy in detection of fractures and planning for treatment of facial injury.[1] For many years it has been suggested that plain radiography may only be useful in cases showing clinical signs that clearly suggest surgical intervention,[2] but guidelines still show that plain radiography has a place in the assessment of facial and orbital injury.[3] Magnetic resonance imaging (MRI) may also be considered, but as scans are undertaken supine, the teardrop effect of the herniating orbital tissue may not be as well demonstrated as in the prone CT scan with coronal sections. CT will also provide better bony definition on the images.

CT may also be required to provide information in trauma cases when plain images in the general facial bones survey are inconclusive, or are difficult to produce at a high enough standard; this is often due to difficulties associated with patient condition in severe trauma when excessive oedema may reduce image contrast.

The facial bones can be demonstrated by a general plain radiographic survey that includes the maxilla, mandible, orbits, nasal bones and zygomae. However, provision of specific information on some of these areas requires alternative or additional projections so that a diagnosis can be made. The mandible and zygomae both require individual examination in case of injury, and plain radiography is the initial examination method of choice for these areas. In non-trauma-related indications the mandible may require CT examination to assess the progress of dental implants.

The temporomandibular joints (TMJs) can also be imaged by plain radiography, which will provide information on condylar dislocation and loss of joint space. MRI will give more useful information regarding the joint itself and, since internal disruption is the most commonly encountered problem in the joint, MRI is most suitable. Arthrography will provide dynamic information regarding the joint.

Injury to the nasal bones is not considered a reason for routine radiographic examination, but clinical specialists (e.g. for ear, nose and throat, and maxillofacial follow-up) may consider special nasal bones projections to be useful.[3] This would be the case when assessing fragment displacement and septal deviation.

Although a proportion of patients presenting with facial trauma will attend on a trolley, the majority arrive as a 'walk-in' case and can be examined erect with antiscatter device. Erect examination with a horizontal beam is essential for some projections where it is necessary to demonstrate air–fluid levels, and must be attempted whenever possible. This is particularly relevant in the case of blow-out fractures of the orbital floor, where fluid level in the maxillary sinus is used as an indicator of this type of injury.

Similarly to requirements for imaging the cranium, the severely injured patient will present on a trolley and any occipitomental (OM) projections must be modified to a mento-occipital position, with angle direction opposite to that for OM. Laterals can be undertaken with the image receptor (IR) supported vertically at the side of the face. A description of a modified projection for zygomatic arches on the trolley-bound patient is also given. In the majority of cases, however, if the patient is severely injured, then trauma CT is likely to be the examination of choice for the evaluation of any injuries. Facial examinations in the emergency situation are also covered in Chapter 17.

The choice of projections for facial bones appears to vary according to referring clinical or individual hospital protocol, but rarely includes the lateral facial bones projection. It is common to find that at least two OM projections are used, with tube angle or no angle, and there have been studies in the past to investigate whether a single projection can be used;[4,5] the most likely projection that can be suggested for this is referred to as the OM 30° in related articles, but it is necessary to ask whether this means that the orbitomeatal baseline (OMBL) lies at 30° to the IR and using a central ray perpendicular to the IR, or if a true OM with OMBL at 45° is used with a caudal tube angle of 30°? Fortunately, one article does include an image that shows the petrous ridge clearly level with the middle of the maxillary sinuses, indicating that the projection required an OMBL at 30° to the IR but with no tube angle.[4] This position is familiar as the routine OM for orbits,[6] which is collimated to include only the orbital outlines and maxillary sinuses for that area; clearly, if this projection is used for full facial bones assessment then all facial bones must be included in the primary beam. Investigation of the idea of one 'ideal' projection for facial bones assessment has involved consideration of articles and textbooks relating to radiographic positioning or recommendation of projections in facial trauma, and has yielded some additional interesting results that give rise to some very pertinent points when discussing imaging and referral.

All radiographers use eponymous terms for a few projections, for example Towne's projection of the skull, Judet's views of the acetabulum and Garth's projection of the shoulder. Unfortunately, this makes the actual technique used less memorable than the name. In the last 30 years UK textbooks have aimed to use nomenclature that indicates the actual position for the projection, rather than the name of the projection's designer, with addition of the eponymous title next to the descriptive title. Unfortunately this is not necessarily the case internationally and eponymous titles are frequently used, leading to a varying range of projection names which are then incorporated into journal articles, potentially creating confusion or even misinterpretation. A search for a list of all eponymously named projections showed that there are a large number in existence,[7] although many are supplementary specialist projections that have been largely superseded by additional imaging modalities. Many of these are not universally familiar.

An example of variation in nomenclature when discussing radiography of the facial bones can be centred around the OM projection and therefore has particular relevance to this chapter. In the UK OM tends to refer to a position with the OMBL at 45°, to ensure that the petrous ridge is just cleared from the bases of the maxillary sinuses[6,8,9]; in the United States the same projection is named PA axial, transoral, Waters' or even parietocanthal projection.[10,11] Position descriptors for this same projection also vary, with UK texts indicating an OMBL angle of 45°[6,7,9] and US texts stating 37°,[10,11] yet all who provide image evaluation criteria insist that their position will see the petrous ridge in the same place, just clear of the lower borders of the maxillary sinuses. One point to raise is that, although it is fairly easy to judge a 45° OMBL to IR angle, can anyone actually claim to accurately judge 37°? US authors do use an alternative way to ensure their positioning is accurate, by referring to alignment of the meatomental line (MML) at 90° to the IR.[10] The MML is a line joining the external auditory meatus and the chin, and it is not clear whether it can be relied on as accurate in patients with developmental deformities of the mandible, such as mandibular prognathism.

It is also noted that the way the relationship of OMBL to IR is described can also vary, with texts giving the suggested OMBL angle either related to the IR[6,8] *or* related to the perpendicular.[10] This is very confusing, even for experienced authors in radiography, but probably almost impossible for students to understand.

Even articles written in the UK cause confusion: another article exploring the concept of a single projection assessment in trauma investigated the potential of either 'the OM 15° and OM 30° projection' but did not make it clear what the actual positioning for the projections entails (again, is the OMBL at 45° for each, with caudal angle, or does the angle refer to the OMBL position?). Study of the article reveals that the OM 15° is referred to thus:

The occipitomental film with a 15° tilt (OM 15°) was considered to be the most useful view because it projects the orbital floor separate from the petrous ridge and displays the zygomatic arches.[12]

Unfortunately this means little in the search for an explanation of the actual projection details, since the tilt referred to is not explained as either tube angle or OMBL angle. Clearance of the petrous ridge to below the inferior orbital margins is seen in any OM projection with more than 20° chin lift (i.e. when the OMBL starts at 90° to the IR and the chin is raised so that the OMBL is moved through 20°), and so information on the petrous ridge in the quote above does not help clarify the situation. There is no positional information provided for the OM 30° projection in the article.

A word of warning: ensure you know the correct relationship of baselines and IR before proceeding (see Chapter 11). To conclude, much work has been written by maxillofacial surgeons on appropriate projections in facial trauma; in the absence of extensive *radiographic* experience on their part, how can we expect these articles to be consistent in their meaning for everyone?

General Survey of Facial Bones

Requests that define the desired examination as 'facial bones' require a general OM and (rarely) lateral survey of the area. OM projections are based on a position with the OMBL at 45°, using a range of caudal beam angles. More than one OM projection may be included in the survey, and two examples are shown of the 45° OM: without angulation in Fig. 13.2B and with 30° caudal angulation in Fig. 13.2C. Although discussion in the previous section shows that a 30° elevation of the OMBL from a perpendicular relationship to the IR has been suggested as a standalone projection for survey of facial bones,[4] it does not appear to be universally adopted as such.

The IR is vertical for all projections of facial bones, orbits and nose unless the patient presents supine on a trolley. An antiscatter grid is required, with the exception of lateral nasal bones.

Throughout this chapter a suggested FRD is given for each examination description; however, in practice a range of FRDs may be used (typically 100–120 cm), dependent on local protocol.

PCE COMMENTS – FACIAL BONES

There are several lines that can be followed on the OM and OM 30° projections in order to aid in interpretation of facial trauma; these are the lines of Dolan[13] (a collective name for the three lines as described by Dolan and Jacoby) and McGrigor–Campbell lines (Fig. 13.1). These lines can be used independently or as an adjunct to each other.[14]

Dolan's Lines (Fig. 13.1A)

1. Orbital line: Starting at the inner surface of the orbit above the zygomaticofrontal (ZMF) suture of one side, follow a line along the orbital surface of the zygoma, the orbital surface of the maxilla, the frontal process of the maxilla and the arch produced by the nasal bones, extending round to the ZMF on the contralateral side.
2. Zygomatic line: Beginning at the outer surface of the ZMF suture, run down along the lateral border of the zygoma and along the upper and outer process of the zygomatic arch to the TMJ on each side.
3. Maxillary line: From the midline, begin at the lateral and inferior margin of the maxilla and extend laterally to follow the lateral wall of the maxillary antrum and the inferior surface of the zygomatic arch. Repeat on the opposite side.

The zygomatic and maxillary lines together are likened to the appearance of an elephant's head and this is sometimes referred to as 'Dolan's elephant'.[14,15]

McGrigor–Campbell Lines (Fig. 13.1B)

(a) Trace from one ZMF suture to another, passing over the superior margin of the orbits.
(b) Trace the zygomatic arch, across the zygoma, the inferior orbital margins to the zygomatic arch on the opposite side.
(c) Trace a line connecting the condyle and coronoid process of the mandible, and across the maxillary antra on both sides.

It is important to scrutinise these lines in order to look for any evidence of bony injury. In addition, there are some key areas which should be considered in the interpretation process:

- Cortical disruption: pay close attention to the orbital margins, walls of the maxillary sinuses and zygomatic arches, looking for any steps or breaks in the cortex.
- Displacement of bone fragments – increased areas of density due to impacted fragments of bone.
- Opacification of sinuses, which may be due to:
  - haemorrhage
  - mucosal thickening/polyps
  - air/fluid level
  - overlying soft tissue swelling

Remember, symmetry is usual – asymmetry is not.

OCCIPITOMENTAL (OM) FACIAL BONES – BASIC PROJECTION (FIG. 13.2A–C)

Positioning

- The patient is seated, facing the IR
- The chin is placed in contact with the midline of the IR and the chin position is adjusted until the OMBL has been raised 45° from the horizontal
- The median sagittal plane (MSP) is perpendicular to the IR, which is assessed by checking that the external auditory meati (EAMs) or lateral orbital margins are equidistant from it

Beam Direction and FRD

1. Horizontal, at 90° to the IR and making an angle of 45° with the OMBL *or*
2. Initially horizontal, with caudal angulation applied according to requirements of the examination
100 cm FRD

Centring

Above the external occipital protuberance (EOP), to emerge half way between the level of the superior orbital margins and angles of the mandible

When using caudal angulation, the description for centring is unchanged, as the beam must always emerge through the middle of the area of interest; the point of entry for the central ray will become higher as angulation increases.

The centre of the IR must always be adjusted to ensure that the image is included within its boundaries.

Collimation

Orbits, zygomatic arches, mandible

Criteria for Assessing Image Quality

- Orbits, zygomatic arches and mandible are demonstrated
- Symmetry of the facial bones on each side; equal distance of the lateral orbital margins from the outer table of temporal bones
- Odontoid process is visible between the angles of the mandible

Horizontal Beam/0° Beam Angulation

- Upper border of the petrous portion of the temporal bone is level with the apices of maxillary antra
- Zygomatic arches seen as a tight 'C' and reversed tight 'C' laterally
- Sharp image demonstrating the zygomae, nasal bones, orbits and mandible in contrast to the cranial vault, and the air-filled regions of the paranasal sinuses

15–20° Caudal Angle

- Zygomatic arches are more gently curved and elongated than with the perpendicular (horizontal) central ray
- Petrous ridge falls below maxillary antra and is likely to be indistinguishable
- TMJs are clearly demonstrated either side of the coronoid processes of the mandible
- Exposure factors are assessed as for the horizontal beam projection

30° Caudal Angle

- Zygomatic arches are slightly curved and elongated, when viewed from this inferior, half-axial, perspective
- Orbits appear almost closed
- Sharp image demonstrating contrast between the inferior orbital margins, maxillary sinuses and the zygomatic arches overlying the cranial vault. The frontal bone and upper orbital area may appear over-blackened but the nasal bones are clearly seen

Common Errors: OM Facial Bones

Common Errors	Possible Reasons	Potential Effects on PCE or Report
Asymmetry of facial structures	Rotation about MSP	May be difficult to assess: zygomatic arches lateral orbital margins ZMF suture *Remember the importance of assessing symmetry (see PCE Comments) – if asymmetry is due to poor positioning, accurate assessment of traumatic asymmetry may not be possible. This is especially relevant for patients with subtle fractures*

Common Errors	Possible Reasons	Potential Effects on PCE or Report
Position of petrous ridge too high	Chin not raised enough. It has been noted that radiographers frequently ask patients to put their nose and chin onto the erect IR for this projection; this will only serve to raise the chin approximately 30°. It has also been noted that some imaging departments use this method with a 15° caudal angle, which only serves to clear the petrous ridge to the inferior margins of the antra; an almost identical image to the true OM 45° with horizontal beam will result, but there will be some distortion caused by application of the angle	Difficult to assess: maxillary antra for the presence of fluid levels fractures of the lateral wall of the maxillary antra could be obscured

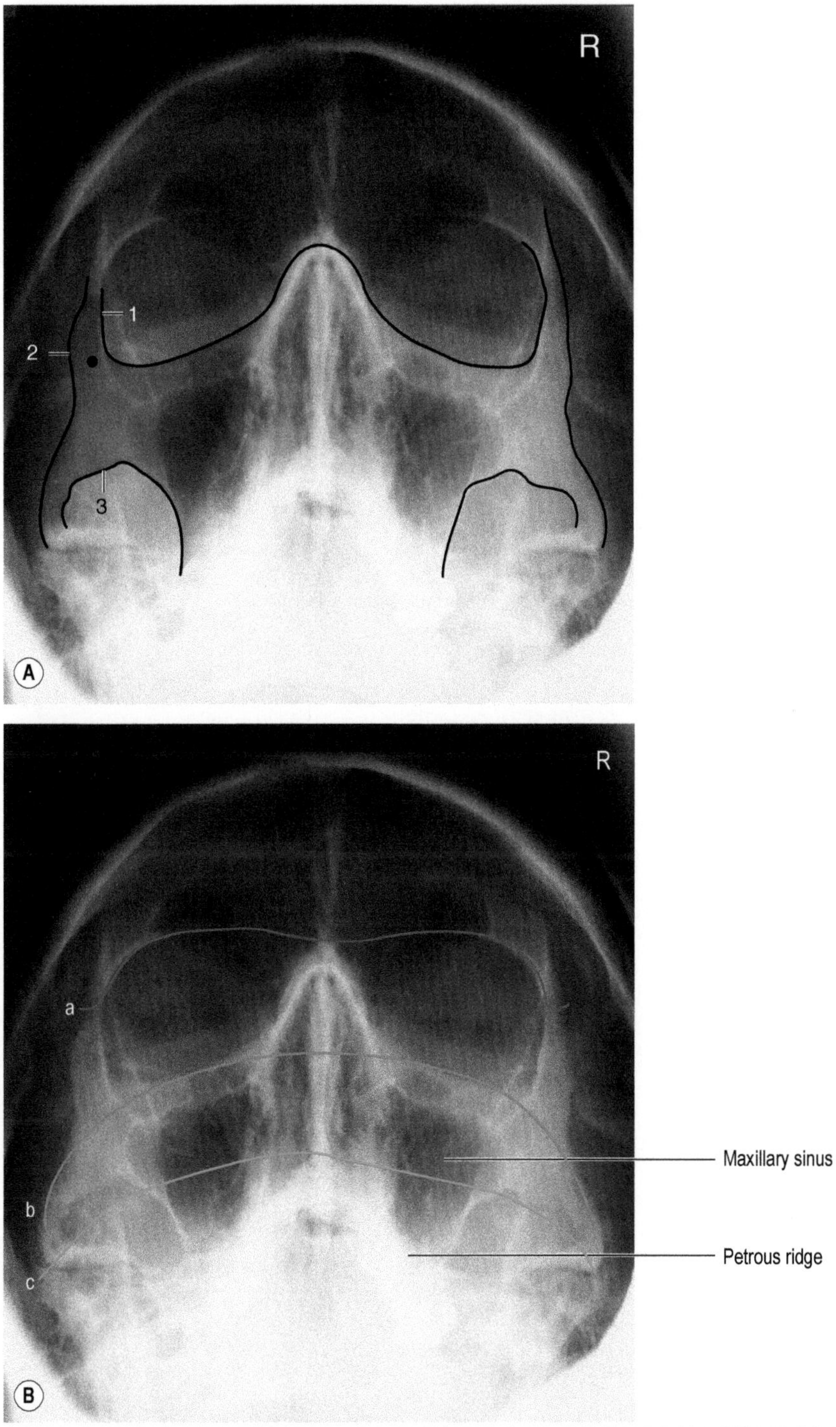

Fig. 13.1 Lines used to assess the facial bones. (A) Dolan's 'elephant' lines. 1 = orbital line; 2 = zygomatic line 3 = maxillary line. Note: patient's right side is shaded to illustrate the elephant shape. (B) McGrigor–Campbell lines: *a*, passes over the superior orbital outlines and joins ZMF sutures bilaterally; *b*, traces from the zygomatic arches, across the zygomae and inferior orbital margins; *c*, traces from each condyle through to the associated coronoid process, and across the maxillary sinuses.

LATERAL FACIAL BONES (FIG. 13.3A–C)

This projection is largely considered of little or no value[4] but may still be used in some centres.

Positioning

- The patient is initially seated, facing the IR
- The trunk is brought as close as possible to the receptor unit and the patient is asked to sit with their spine as erect as possible. This helps the patient turn their head more easily into the required lateral position
- The head is turned through 90° to bring the affected side in contact with the IR
- The MSP is parallel to the IR; there should be no tilt or rotation of the head. This can be assessed by checking the midline of the cranium over the top and symmetry of the frontal bone and orbits
- Asking the patient to gently close their eyes will assist in maintenance of the position; as the radiographer leaves the receptor unit the patient will often follow this movement with their eyes and this can result in altering the position of the head

Beam Direction and FRD

Horizontal, at 90° to the IR
100 cm FRD

Centring

To the inferior border of the zygoma

Collimation

Superior orbital margins, symphysis menti, TMJs, nasal bones

Criteria for Assessing Image Quality

- Superior orbital margins, symphysis menti, TMJs and nasal bones are demonstrated
- Superimposition of the malar processes of maxilla, orbital outlines and TMJs
- Sharp image demonstrating the malar processes of maxilla in contrast to the air-filled maxillary sinuses, and the orbits in contrast to other bones of the face. The mandible is seen in contrast to the soft tissues of the face. Nasal bones are over-penetrated

Common Errors: Lateral Facial Bones

Common Errors	Possible Reasons	Potential Effects on PCE or Report
Non-superimposition of the floor of the anterior cranial fossa; malar processes seen as one above the other; orbital outlines seen as one above the other	MSP tilted, usually with the upper part of the head tilted towards the IR. If a patient cannot comply with the required position, a compensating caudal angle can be used to reduce the effects of the tilt	More difficult to assess for posterior displacement of midface structures (although patients with significant facial trauma are likely to undergo CT examination)
Lateral orbital margins seen side by side and not superimposed; malar processes seen displaced in a horizontal direction	Head is rotated; this is often encouraged when the patient 'slumps' in their chair rather than sitting with their spine erect, as described in 'positioning' for this projection	As above

Orbits

The orbits are examined for trauma or the presence and position of intraocular foreign bodies (IOFB). IOFB assessment may be made after penetrating injury or prior to MRI scanning as a safety measure to exclude the presence of ferrous material in the eye if the patient reports a penetrating eye injury in the past.

A horizontal beam should be used wherever possible, as air–fluid levels in the maxillary sinuses can be an indicator of orbital floor fracture. Air in the top portion of the maxillary antrum will also serve to provide contrast with any soft tissue teardrop appearance of a herniating inferior rectus muscle down through the fractured orbital floor. Clearly the OM orbital projection cannot be undertaken erect with a horizontal beam on a seriously injured patient: at the very least a lateral with horizontal beam can be attempted while this type of patient is supine.

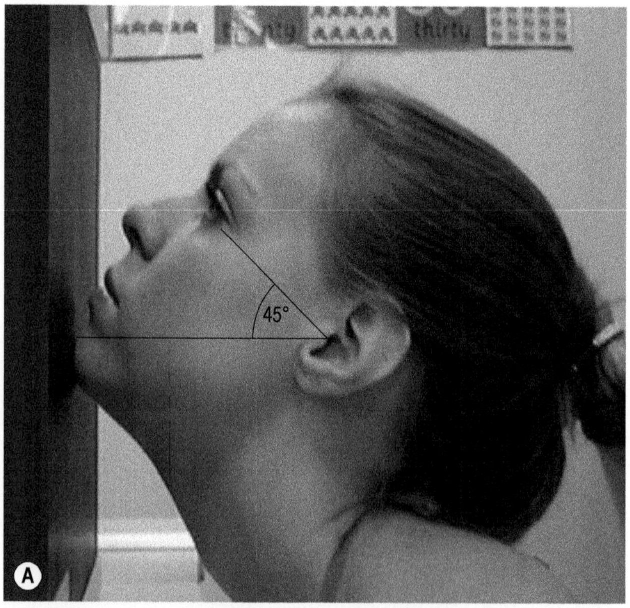

Fig. 13.2 (A) OM facial bones

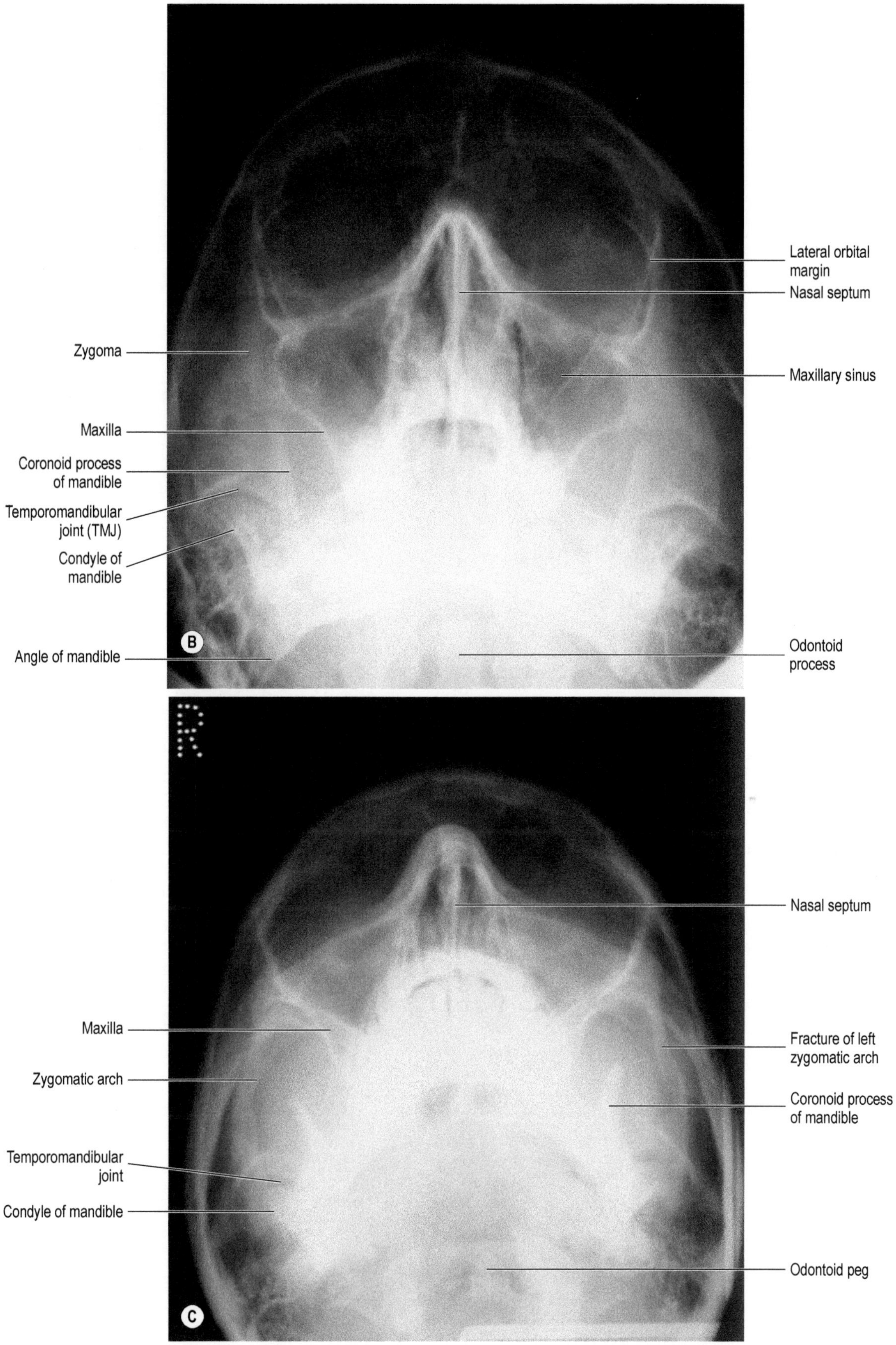

Fig. 13.2, cont'd (B) OM facial bones; (C) OM facial bones with 30° caudal angulation.

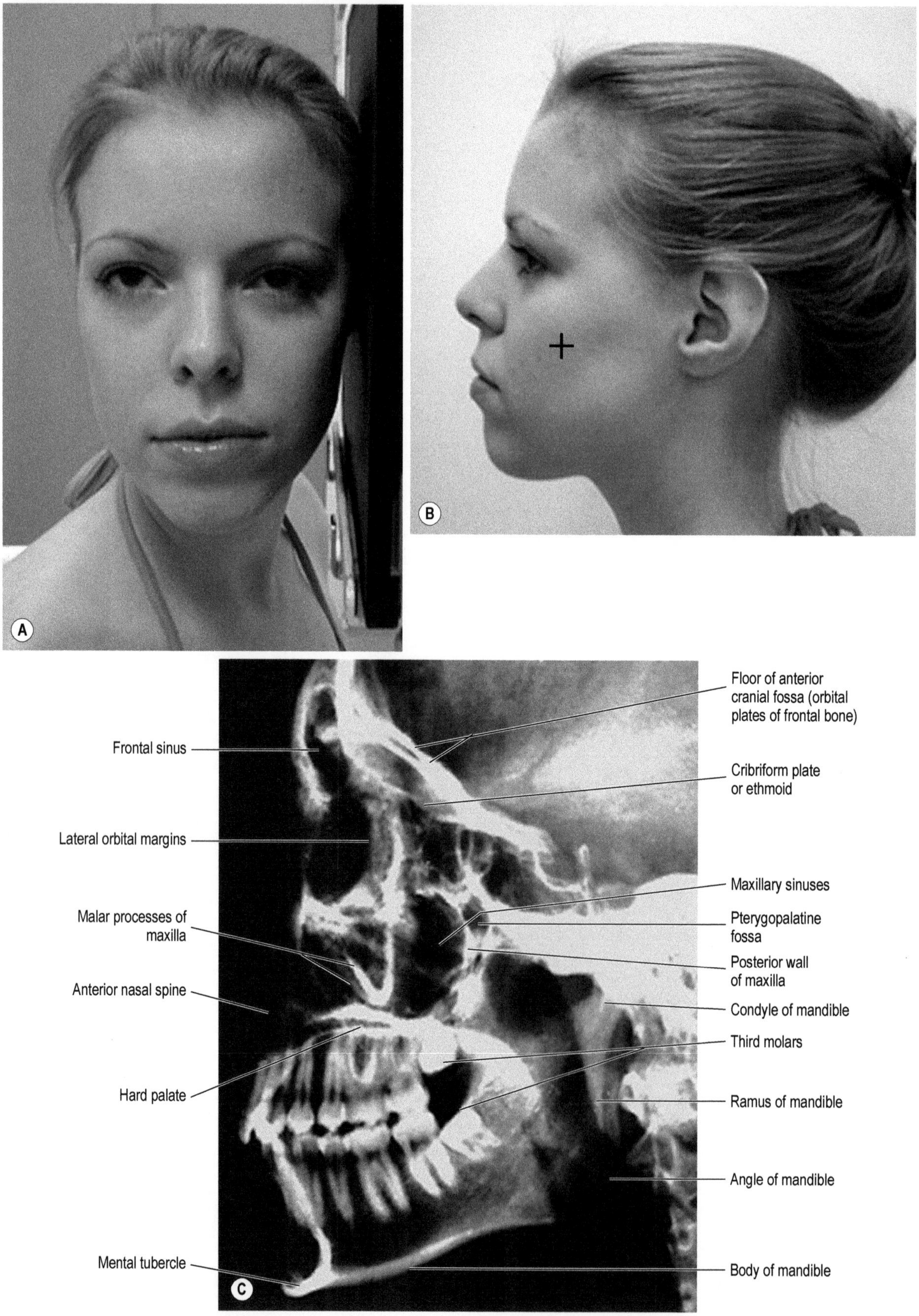

Fig. 13.3 **(A) Lateral facial bones; (B) centring for lateral facial bones; (C) lateral facial bones.** (C, Reproduced with permission from Bryan GJ. *Skeletal Anatomy*. 3rd ed. Edinburgh: Churchill Livingstone; 1996 and Gunn C. *Bones and Joints*. 4th ed. Edinburgh: Churchill Livingstone; 2002.)

PCE COMMENTS – ORBITS

Orbital emphysema (also known as the 'black eyebrow' sign) is often an indicator of a blow-out fracture of the orbital floor. Herniation of the medial orbital wall can also occur and air from the maxillary or ethmoid sinuses can escape into the orbit giving the appearance of an 'eyebrow' on the image.

'Teardrop' sign – a blow-out fracture of the orbit is more likely to be comminuted which often results in a depressed fragment that can be hinged, acting somewhat like a trapdoor. As a result, intra-orbital contents, periorbital fat and the inferior rectus muscle can herniate downwards through the orbital floor through the 'trapdoor' and become trapped, appearing as a soft tissue 'teardrop' or bulge in contrast to air in the maxillary sinus, just below the inferior orbital margin.

OM ORBITS/OM 30° ('MODIFIED OCCIPITOMENTAL'[8]) (FIG. 13.4A,B)

The orbital floor is not well demonstrated on the true 45° OM and this projection will show blow-out fractures more reliably than the true OM.

Positioning

- The patient is seated, facing the IR
- The chin is placed in contact with the midline of the IR and the chin position is adjusted until the OMBL has been raised 30° from the horizontal
- The MSP is perpendicular to the IR, which is assessed by checking that the EAMs or lateral orbital margins are equidistant from the IR

Beam Direction and FRD

Horizontal, at 90° to the IR
100 cm FRD

Centring

Above the EOP, to emerge level with the middle of the orbits

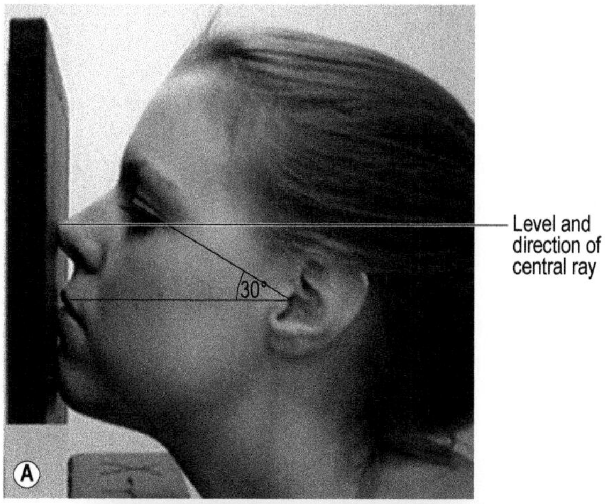

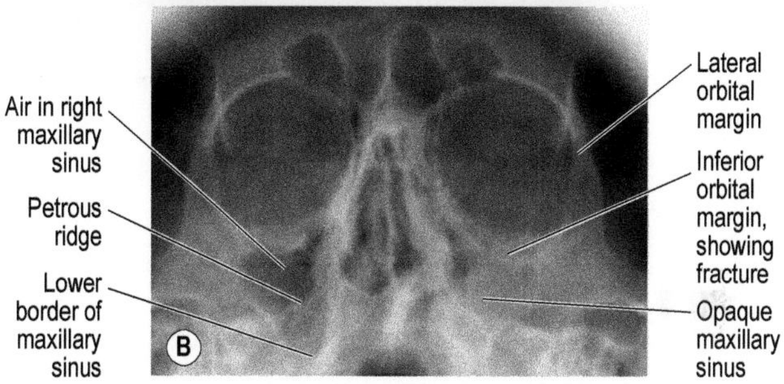

Fig. 13.4 OM orbits.

Collimation

Orbits, maxillary sinuses

Criteria for Assessing Image Quality

- Orbits and maxillary sinuses are demonstrated
- Orbital margins are equidistant from the outer table of the temporal bones
- Petrous ridge seen halfway to two-thirds down the maxillary sinuses
- Sharp image demonstrating contrast between the orbital outlines, the cranial vault, air-filled frontal and maxillary sinuses. Fine detail of the orbital floor is seen at the top of the maxillary sinuses

Common Errors: OM Orbits/OM 30°

Common Errors	Possible Reasons	Potential Effects on PCE or Report
Asymmetry of facial structures	Rotation about MSP	Difficult to assess: zygomatic arches lateral wall of orbit ZMF suture Asymmetry in facial bones radiographs is suspicious for trauma, so it is important not to erroneously introduce asymmetry
Petrous ridge level with inferior orbital margins or within orbital outline	Chin not raised enough	Difficult to assess: inferior orbital margin for fracture superior border of maxillary antrum for soft tissue 'teardrop' sign; evidence of orbital floor fracture
Petrous ridge in the lower half of the antrum, or even at its lower margin	Chin elevated too high	Difficult to assess: for orbital floor (blow-out) fractures with elevation of chin >30° maxillary antra for fluid levels

This 'modified' OM projection is suggested as ideal for a single facial bones projection[4]; to adjust this projection and utilise for positioning is the same as for full facial bones assessment. The area of interest should include mandible, TMJs and orbits. The central ray will be in the midline, to emerge level with the lower borders of the zygomae.

LATERAL ORBITS (FIG. 13.5A,B)

Positioning

- The patient is initially seated, facing the IR and positioned with their head turned as for a lateral facial bones projection

Beam Direction and FRD

Horizontal, at 90° to the IR
100 cm FRD

Centring

Over the outer canthus of the eye

Collimation

All orbital outlines, maxillary sinuses

Criteria for Assessing Image Quality

- Orbits and maxillary sinuses are demonstrated
- Orbital outlines are superimposed
- Sharp image demonstrating orbital outlines in contrast to the air-filled maxillary sinuses and ethmoid sinuses

Common Errors: Lateral Orbits

Common Errors	Possible Reasons	Potential Effects on PCE or Report
Orbital plates of frontal bone not superimposed	MSP tilted	If the lateral projection is being undertaken for FB demonstration, obliquity of the image may give a misleading impression of the position of the FB If trauma, the degree of displacement could be either under- or overestimated dependent on position
Lateral orbital margins not superimposed	Head is rotated	As above

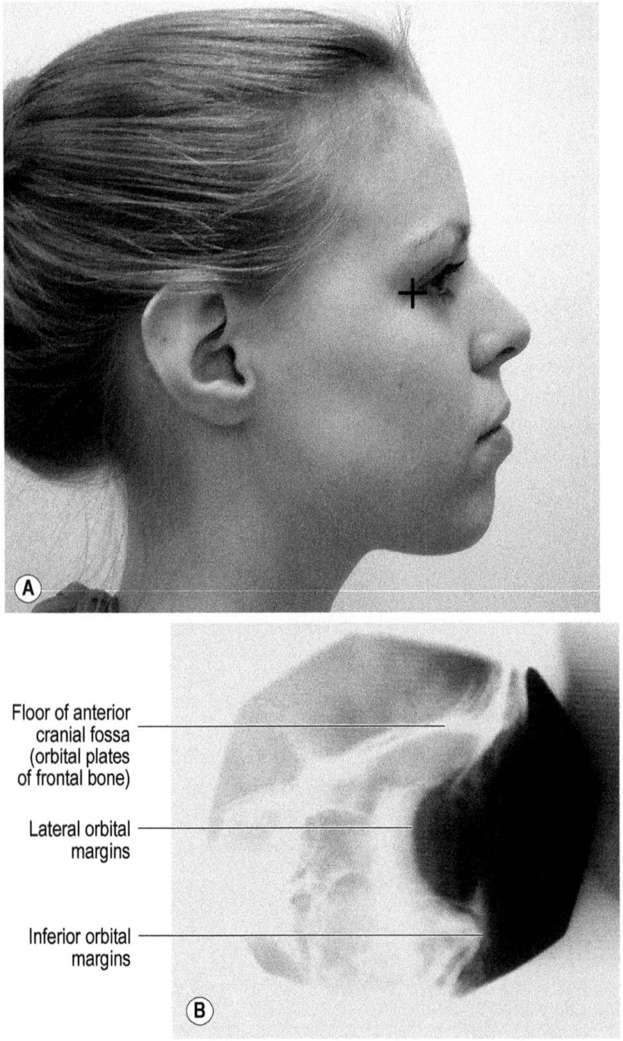

Fig. 13.5 (A) Centring for lateral orbits; (B) lateral orbits.

Nasal Bones

The IR is vertical for all projections of the nose.

OCCIPITOMENTAL (OM) NASAL BONES (FIG. 13.6A,B)

Positioning

- The patient is seated, facing the IR and positioned as for OM facial bones

Beam Direction and FRD

Horizontal, at 90° to the IR
100 cm FRD

Centring

Above the EOP, to emerge through the centre of the nasal bone

Collimation

Nasal bone, anterior nasal spine

Criteria for Assessing Image Quality

- Nasal bone and septum are demonstrated; there is evidence of frontal and maxillary sinuses superiorly and laterally
- Petrous ridge is evident as level with inferior maxillary antra
- Sharp image demonstrating the nasal septum centrally and the nasal bones laterally, in contrast with the air-filled ethmoid sinuses

LATERAL NASAL BONES (FIG. 13.7A,B)

Positioning

- The patient is initially seated, facing the IR (no anti-scatter grid), and positioned as for a lateral facial bones projection

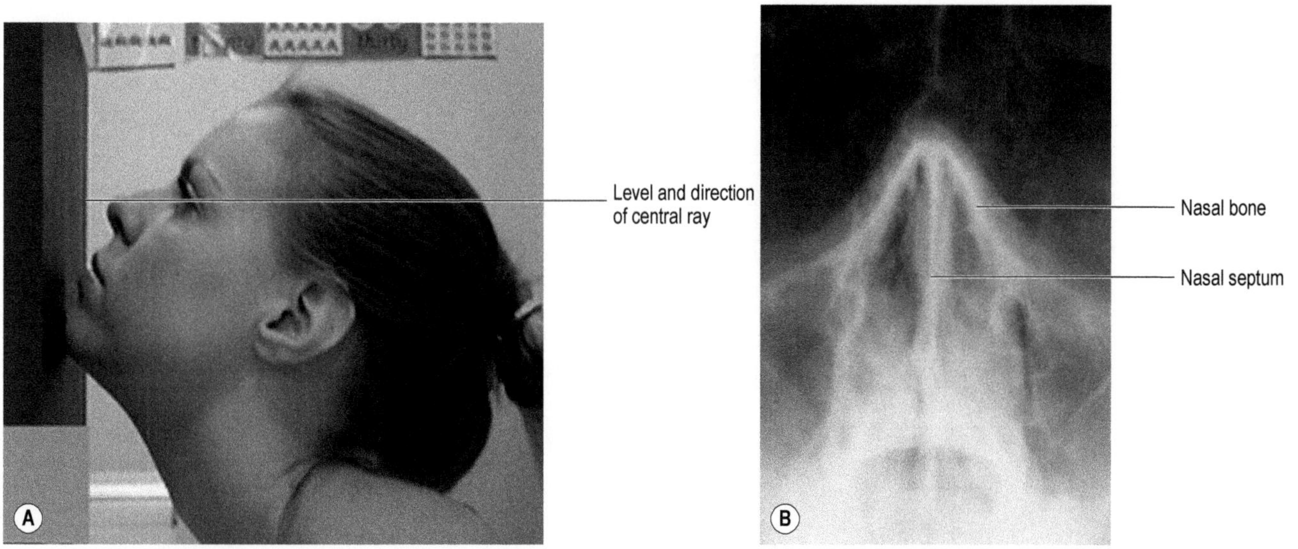

Fig. 13.6 OM nasal bones.

Beam Direction and FRD

Horizontal, at 90° to the IR
100 cm FRD

Centring

Over the nasal bone

Collimation

Nasal bone, anterior nasal spine, soft tissue of the nose

Criteria for Assessing Image Quality

- Nasal bone, anterior nasal spine and soft tissue of the nose are demonstrated
- Sharp image demonstrating bony detail of the nasal bone and anterior nasal spine, in contrast to the soft tissues of the nose and air-filled sinuses

Common Errors: Lateral Nasal Bones

Common Errors	Possible Reason	Potential Effects on PCE or Report
Omission of anterior nasal spine	Incorrect collimation and/or incorrect centring are obvious culprits	Full region cannot be assessed; the anterior nasal spine can be fractured when there is impact to the area (and often during a fight)
Poor detail over the area of interest	Most commonly this is either due to overexposure or inadequate collimation (which will mean scatter contributes to over-blackening)	Fracture may be missed

Mandible

The structure of the mandible makes it difficult to image accurately using the usual approach of obtaining two images at 90° to each other. As a result, several projections are available for demonstration of this bone, none of which individually demonstrates it adequately in its entirety:

1. The PA mandible projection, which shows the rami relatively well but causes foreshortening over the body
2. The lateral, which superimposes both sides of the mandible
3. The lateral oblique, which clears the body on the side under examination from the opposite side but foreshortens the ramus. Both lateral obliques are undertaken in any one case, as the mandible is a recognised site for contrecoup fractures

A combination of all, or any, of these projections is used to provide information on the mandible as a whole.

Alternatively, panoramic radiography can be used to demonstrate the mandible (see Chapter 14, Dental Radiography). This is a method that clearly requires specialised equipment, which is not always available. Some units are unsuitable for patients in wheelchairs and the image does have some unsharpness. The main benefit of this method is its ability to demonstrate the whole mandible and TMJs on one image, but it still may not be easy to see fractures; other projections may be required as supplements.[16]

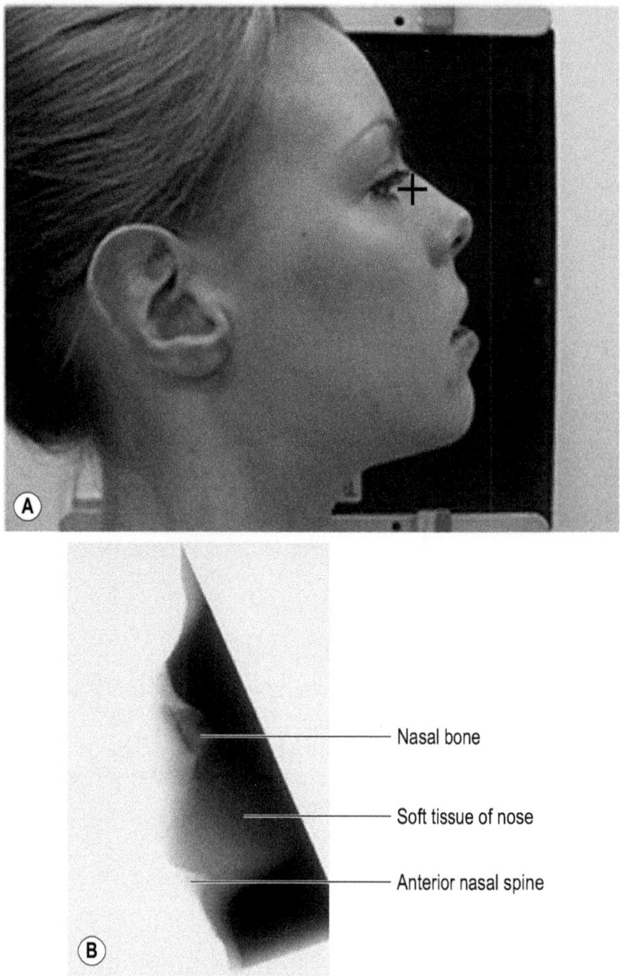

Fig. 13.7 Lateral nasal bones.

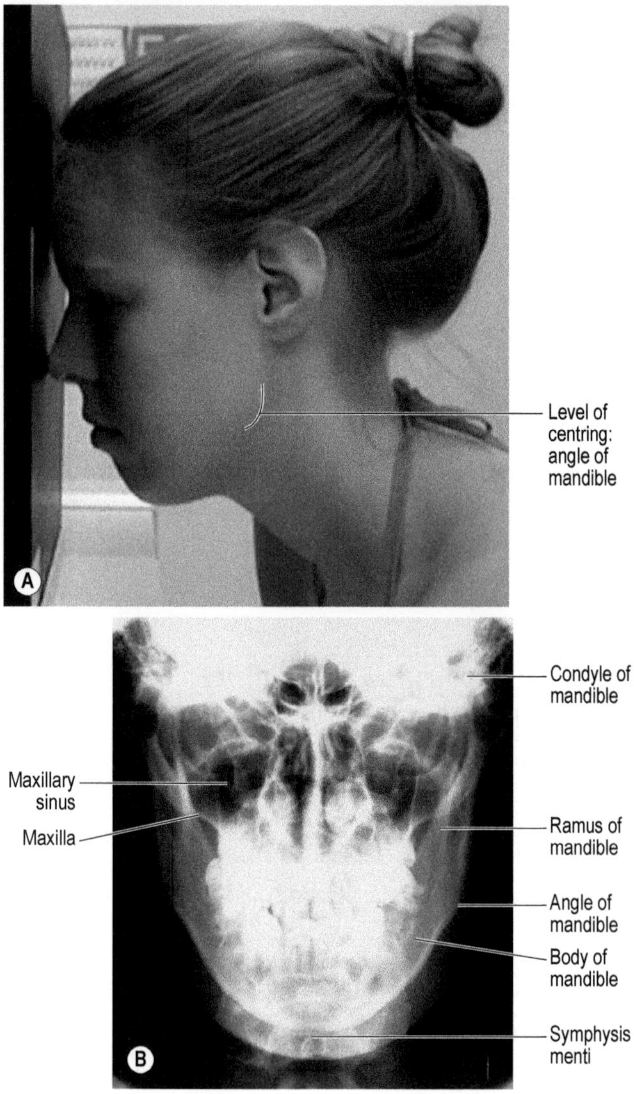

Fig. 13.8 PA mandible.

PCE COMMENTS – MANDIBLE

When reviewing the mandible for evidence of trauma, it is important to remember that it should be regarded as a 'ring bone' and therefore prone to contrecoup fractures. In other words, if you see a fracture or dislocation in one part of the mandible then you should look for a potential second, or even third fracture elsewhere in the bone. However, the mandible does have a degree of flexibility afforded by the TMJs, which means that a single fracture is possible.

The same rules apply when reviewing the PA mandible as with all radiographs of the skeleton. Assessment should be made of the adequacy of the image, then a review of the bony cortices, looking for any breaks or steps in the margins of the bone. Assess alignment of the TMJs and review for any signs of soft tissue swelling.

IR is vertical for all projections of the mandible

POSTEROANTERIOR (PA) MANDIBLE (FIG. 13.8A,B)

Positioning

Note that, although this is described as a PA projection, the patient's head is actually positioned as for an occipitofrontal (OF) projection; because the beam will not travel through the occiput or frontal bone, the projection cannot actually be named as OF.

- The patient is seated, facing the IR
- The forehead is placed in contact with the midline of the IR and the chin position is adjusted until the OMBL is perpendicular to it
- The MSP is perpendicular to the IR, which is assessed by checking that the EAMs or lateral orbital margins are equidistant from it

Beam Direction and FRD

- Horizontal, at 90° to the IR
- 100 cm FRD

Centring

In the midline of the neck, midway between the angles of the mandible

Collimation

TMJs, angles of mandible, symphysis menti

Criteria for Assessing Image Quality

- TMJs, angles of the mandible and symphysis menti are demonstrated
- Petrous ridge is level with the top of the orbits
- Condyles are superimposed over the inferior aspect of the petrous bones laterally
- Symmetry of the mandible either side of the face and neck
- Mandible is seen as a 'U' shape
- Sharp image demonstrating the entire mandible in contrast to the soft tissues of the face and neck, and the bones of the cervical vertebrae

Common Error: PA Mandible

Common Error	Possible Reason	Potential Effect on PCE or Report
Increased density where the mandible overlies cervical vertebrae, but contrast over rami may be acceptable	kVp too low to penetrate the area over the cervical vertebrae; mAs may need to be reduced if kVp increased	Difficult to assess the symphysis menti for evidence of trauma or subtle pathology

LATERAL MANDIBLE (FIG. 13.9A,B)

Positioning

- The patient is seated, facing the IR
- The head is turned through 90° to place the affected side in contact with the IR
- The chin is raised very slightly to reduce the density of the soft tissues of the throat which lie over the body of the mandible
- The MSP* is parallel to the IR, which is assessed by checking that the angles of the mandible are in alignment or superimposed

*Using the MSP of the head may not be appropriate for the lateral projection as the mandible may not lie in continuous alignment with the skull. It is suggested that, for this projection, the mandible should be considered to have an MSP that runs vertically down its midline and midway between the angles.

Beam Direction and FRD

Horizontal, at 90° to the IR
100 cm FRD

Centring

Over the angle of the mandible

Collimation

TMJs, angles of mandible, symphysis menti

Criteria for Assessing Image Quality

- TMJs, angles of mandible and symphysis menti demonstrated
- Condyles superimposed over each other; angles of mandible superimposed
- Mandible clear of the cervical vertebrae
- Sharp image demonstrating the entire mandible in contrast to the soft tissues of the neck and mouth

Common Errors: Lateral Mandible

Common Error	Possible Reason	Potential Effect on PCE or Report
Non-superimposition of required structures	a) It is tempting to use the upper facial structures to assess the lateral position of the patient; see comments at end of the Positioning section b) There may be some magnification of the side furthest from the IR on patients with wider mandibles, which will effectively take its outline outside that of the opposite side; this cannot be considered as radiographer error. Consider increasing FRD to compensate	May obscure a fracture line

LATERAL OBLIQUE MANDIBLE (FIG. 13.10A,B)

Both obliques are undertaken in order to demonstrate the whole mandible. An antiscatter grid is not used for the projection.

Positioning

- The patient is seated alongside the IR with the side under examination nearest to it
- The chin is raised very slightly, to reduce the density of the soft tissues of the throat which lie over the body of the mandible
- The MSP is initially parallel to the IR and the head then tilted towards it until the MSP is approximately 15° to it. Care must be taken not to rotate the head during the manoeuvre
- The chin is elevated as far as possible to clear the mandibular condyle from the neck

Beam Direction and FRD

Initially horizontal, then directed 10° cranially
100 cm FRD

Centring

Midway between the angles of the mandible

Collimation

TMJ and angle of mandible on the side under examination, symphysis menti

Once collimation is complete, the IR position may require adjustment until the radiation field lies within the

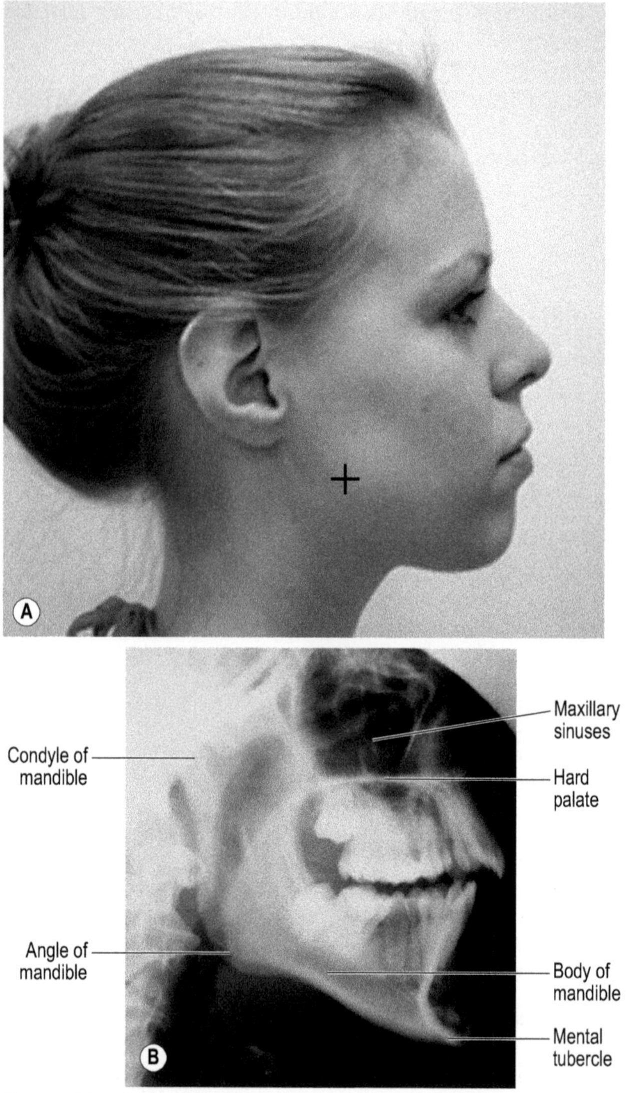

Fig. 13.9 (A) Lateral mandible – centring; (B) lateral mandible.

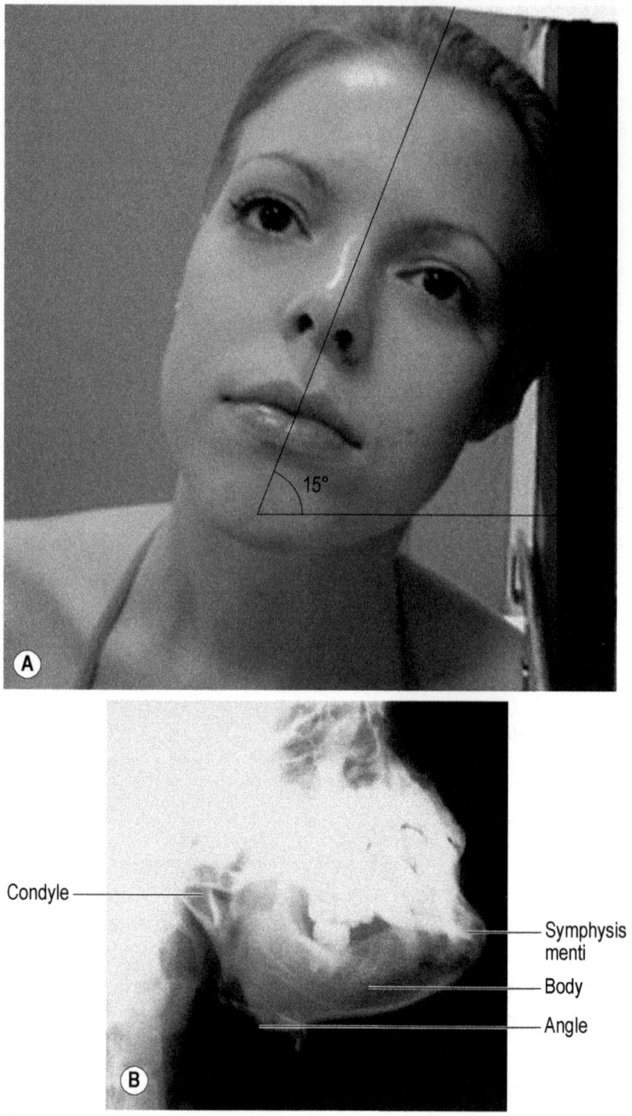

Fig. 13.10 Lateral oblique mandible.

boundaries. The outline of the soft tissues overlying the mandible should be shown as a shadow within the light beam (and within the borders of the IR).

Unfortunately the combination of angle and obliquity for this oblique method does distort and foreshorten the ramus in particular. The body of the mandible is not in contact with the IR, and this has implications for magnification and unsharpness of the body and lower portion of the ramus.

Because the lateral oblique position of the mandible itself will foreshorten the ramus of the mandible, an alternative method is to use a true lateral position of the head, with an increased cranial angle. For this the patient has been described as prone, with the head turned into the lateral position and a cranial beam angle of 25°.[17] Supine with the head turned laterally has also been described, with a 35° cranial central ray.[18] However, a prone lateral position often proves difficult for the patient, especially if injured. The supine turned lateral head position can be equally difficult but the patient's trunk can be obliqued to improve the situation; for both these supine and prone positions there is the potential for increased object receptor distance (ORD) which affects magnification of the image, although this could be improved by supporting the IR on a pad on the table-top.[17] An increase in focus receptor distance (FRD) will also reduce magnification.

Use of a 25° cranial angle in conjunction with a true lateral (seated patient position) requires the tube head to be in a relatively low position and the beam is frequently attenuated by the shoulder in larger patients; an attempt to clear the shoulder can be made by posterior rotation of the shoulder nearest the tube, but this often causes rotation of the head. The shoulder can often lie within the primary beam and be superimposed over the mandible, even with the prone lateral position.

The oblique position with cranial angulation can be deemed a general survey of the mandible and modifications have also been described which will provide more specific information on different aspects of the mandible.[10]

30° rotation towards the side under examination will demonstrate the body more adequately.

45° rotation demonstrates the symphysis menti.

It is also claimed that a rotation of 15° will give a general survey of the mandible,[10] but surely this rotation will cause the condyle to overlie the neck on the image?

Criteria for Assessing Image Quality

- TMJs, angles of the mandible and symphysis menti are demonstrated
- TMJ, condyle, ramus and body on the side under examination are cleared from the cervical vertebrae
- Sharp image demonstrating the entire mandible in contrast to the soft tissues of the neck and mouth

Common Error: Lateral Oblique Mandible

Common Error	Possible Reason	Potential Effect on PCE or Report
Condyle on the side under examination not cleared from the cervical vertebrae	Chin too low *or* forehead is rotated towards the IR	Difficult to assess affected condyle for evidence of fracture if obscured by cervical vertebrae

PANORAMIC TOMOGRAPHY FOR MANDIBLE

Please refer to Chapter 14 for this examination.

Temporomandibular Joints (TMJs)

PCE COMMENTS – TMJS

Check for the mandibular condyles and also the associated joint spaces:

Is the condyle flattened in appearance? Is there narrowing, or even fusion, of the joint space?
Is there evidence of osteophytes or erosion, or sclerosis? These are all indications of OA.
Is there evidence of joint space size on both sides?
Does the position of the condyle (lateral obliques) lie within normal range of the joint, or is there evidence of excessive anterior movement?

Don't forget to check bony integrity of the ramus just below the condyle.

LATERAL OBLIQUE TMJs (FIG. 13.11A,B)

In the lateral position the TMJs are superimposed and an oblique central ray is used to clear the image of one TMJ to reveal the other. Both sides are examined for comparison and images taken with mouth open and then closed. An erect technique is more comfortable for the patient than using a table technique.
IR is vertical. No antiscatter grid is used.

Positioning

- The patient is initially seated, facing the IR, and is then positioned as for the lateral facial bones; the TMJ under examination is in contact with the IR
- The MSP is parallel to the IR; there should be no tilt or rotation of the head. This can be assessed by checking that the interpupillary line is perpendicular to the IR
- A legend is applied to the IR to indicate whether the mouth is open or closed

Beam Direction and FRD

Initially horizontal, then angled 25° caudally
100 cm FRD

Centring

Above the TMJ remote from the IR, with the beam emerging through the TMJ under examination

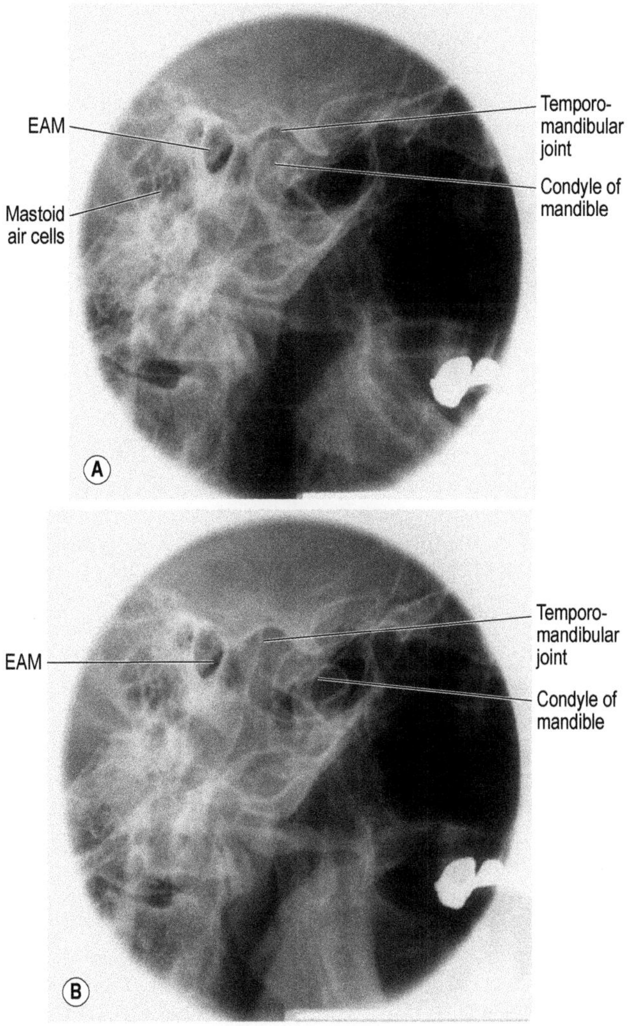

Fig. 13.11 Lateral oblique TMJs: (A) mouth closed; (B) mouth open.

The TMJ is palpable anterior to the tragus of the ear. If the patient is asked to open their mouth the radiographer's finger will feel a depression over the mandibular fossa as the mouth opens, as the mandibular condyle moves forwards from the mandibular fossa.

Collimation

TMJ, condyle of mandible

Criteria for Assessing Image Quality

- TMJ and condyle of mandible are demonstrated
- Other TMJ is clear from the area of interest
- TMJ under examination anterior to EAM
- Indication of whether the mouth is open or closed is clearly seen on the image
- Sharp image demonstrating the mandibular fossa in contrast to the temporal bone and condyle of mandible

Common Errors: Lateral Oblique TMJs

Common Errors	Possible Reasons	Potential Effects on PCE or Report
Mastoid air cells of unaffected side overlying TMJ	MSP rotated, face turning towards IR	Difficult to assess TMJ due to busy appearance of air-filled mastoids
TMJ or ramus of mandible closest to tube not cleared from TMJ under examination	1. Inadequate angle used *or* 2. Head is tilted with its vertex towards the IR, which effectively reduces the effects of angulation	Unable to adequately assess the TMJ under examination due to superimposed bony structures

OCCIPITOFRONTAL (OF) 30–35° TMJs (FIG. 13.12A,B)

IR is vertical

Positioning

- The patient is seated, facing the IR
- The forehead is placed in contact with the midline of the IR and the chin position adjusted until the OMBL is perpendicular to it, as for the basic OF position
- The IR may require displacement after accurate tube centring to ensure that the area of interest is included in its boundary
- The MSP is perpendicular to the IR, assessed by checking that the EAMs or lateral orbital margins are equidistant from it

Beam Direction and FRD

Initially horizontal, with 30–35° cranial angulation

A specific angle has not been suggested here as it does appear that there is some variation in practice.[8,9] Selection of optimum exposure factors will ensure that the joints will be well demonstrated, regardless of a 5° difference in angle.
100 cm FRD

Centring

In the midline of the neck, to travel through the TMJs

Collimation

TMJs

Exposure is made with the mouth open, and a legend should be applied to indicate this.

Most texts describe the fronto-occipital (FO) projection rather than the OF[6,7,9,10] but, as outlined in Chapter 11, the OF position is easier for the patient, especially if they can sit in an erect position. The OF position will also help reduce dose absorbed by the lenses of the eyes and the thyroid, although the close collimation required for TMJs does ensure that dose is minimised, even in the FO position. It is unlikely that the joints will lie significantly closer to the IR on either the OF or the FO projections, therefore image sharpness should be similar on both.

FRONTO-OCCIPITAL (FO) 30–35° TMJs

IR is vertical, an antiscatter grid is used. (Supine technique may be used, but the FO position is difficult to achieve with the patient supine.)

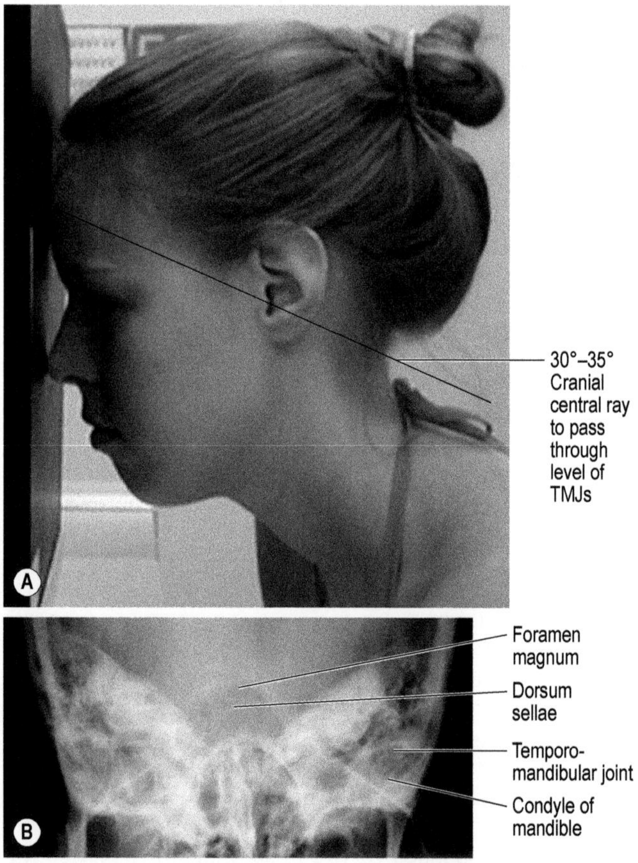

Fig. 13.12 TMJs – OF 30–35°.

This projection is essentially the same position as the 30° FO projection (Towne's) used for the cranial vault, with collimation to the area of interest and alteration of height of centring.

Positioning

- The patient is seated, with their back to the IR
- The back of the occiput is placed in contact with the midline of the IR and the chin position is adjusted until the OMBL is at 90° to it
- The MSP is perpendicular to the IR, which is assessed by checking that the EAMs or lateral orbital margins are equidistant from it
- It will be necessary to adjust the height of the IR after centring

Beam Direction and FRD

A horizontal central ray is angled 30–35° caudally
100 cm FRD

Centring

In the midline above the glabella, with the beam travelling through the TMJs and then the lower occiput

Collimation

Mastoid bones, TMJs, condyles of mandible, upper rami of mandible

Criteria for Assessing Image Quality

- Mastoid bones, TMJs, condyles of mandible and upper rami of mandible are demonstrated
- Symmetry of the petrous portion of the temporal bones on either side of the foramen magnum; the condyles of mandible are an equal distance from the lateral portions of the skull
- Dorsum sellae seen within the foramen magnum; arch of C1 may be demonstrated if a 35° angle has been used
- Sharp image demonstrating contrast between the TMJs and the denser petrous temporal and mastoids

Common Errors: OF/FO 30–35° TMJs

Common Errors	Possible Reasons	Potential Effects on PCE or Report
Asymmetry of petrous temporal bones around the foramen magnum	Rotation about MSP	Difficult to assess TMJs – distortion due to rotation and superimposition of overlying structures
Pale image over the TMJ	Inadequate penetration	Joint spaces cannot be assessed

PANORAMIC TOMOGRAPHY

As in the case of the mandible, the TMJs are seen on the panoramic examination of the mandible (see Chapter 14) but the joints are shown closed in the conventional mouth position (teeth closed over a bite guide). Open-mouth exposure should also be made in order to demonstrate the joint adequately. This is a difficult manoeuvre for patients with dislocation, and examination with the TMJ open and closed may not be possible.

Zygomatic Arches

The zygomatic arches are demonstrated reasonably well in contrast to the cranium on the OM facial bones projections, and can be shown in profile over the soft tissues of the cheeks in the FO 30° projection.

FRONTO-OCCIPITAL (FO) 30° ZYGOMATIC ARCHES (FIG. 13.13A,B)

As mentioned for the TMJ examination in this position, a technique with the patient supine may be used but is not recommended unless absolutely necessary (for example, when the patient is injured seriously enough to present supine on a trolley).

An alternative OF projection is not described, as the zygomatic arches must show some magnification in order to demonstrate them laterally at either side of the cranial vault. To undertake an OF projection would minimise magnification of the arches since they lie closer to the IR in this position; the posterior half of the vault will be magnified and potentially overlie part, or all, of the zygomatic arches.
The IR is vertical

Positioning

- The patient is seated with their back to the IR and positioned initially as for the FO 30° TMJ projection
- It will be necessary to adjust the height of the IR after centring, to ensure the area of interest lies within its borders

Beam Direction and FRD

A horizontal central ray is angled 30° caudally
100 cm FRD

Centring

In the midline above the glabella, with the beam travelling through the zygomatic arches

Collimation

Mastoid bones, zygomatic arches, zygomae, upper rami of mandible

Exposure Factors

Exposure factors must be set significantly lower than for other FO 30° projections of the cranial vault, mastoids and TMJs. This is because of the low density of the arches and the fact that no grid is necessary for the examination.

MODIFIED SUBMENTOVERTICAL (SMV) ZYGOMATIC ARCHES FOR THE INJURED PATIENT (FIG. 13.14)

This should not be attempted when there are other suspected injuries that may be exacerbated by the positioning required for the projection.

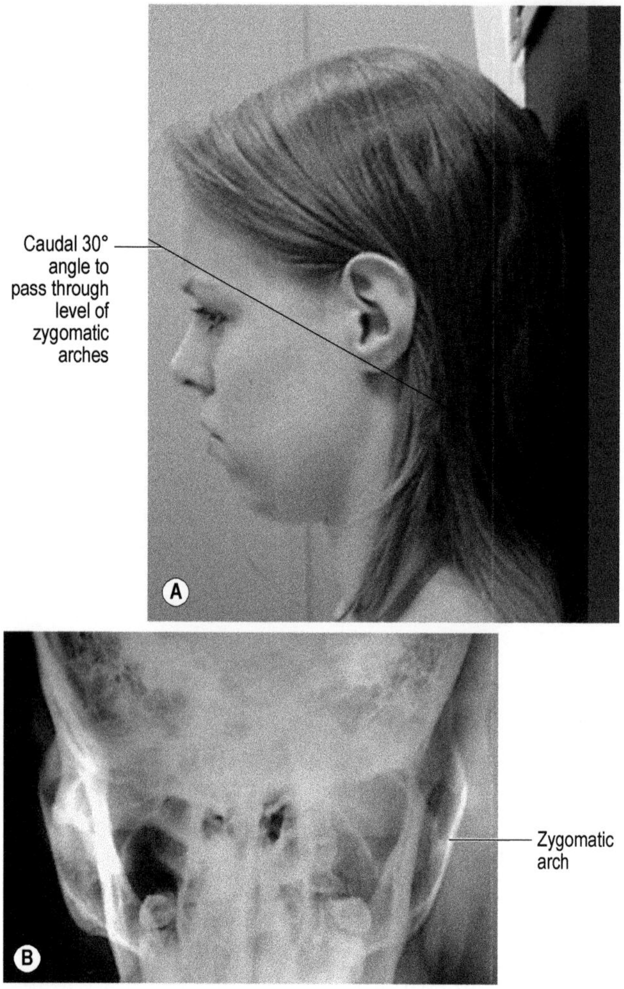

Fig. 13.13 (A) FO 30° zygomatic arches; (B) OF 30° zygomatic arches. (B, Reproduced with permission from Ballinger PW, Frank ED. *Merrill's Atlas of Radiographic Positioning and Radiologic Procedures*. 10th ed. St Louis: Mosby; 2003.)

The projection works best with a cassette type IR rather than a fixed plate detector.

Positioning

- The patient lies supine on the table or trolley; it may be necessary to place a pillow under the patient's shoulders to elevate the area of interest

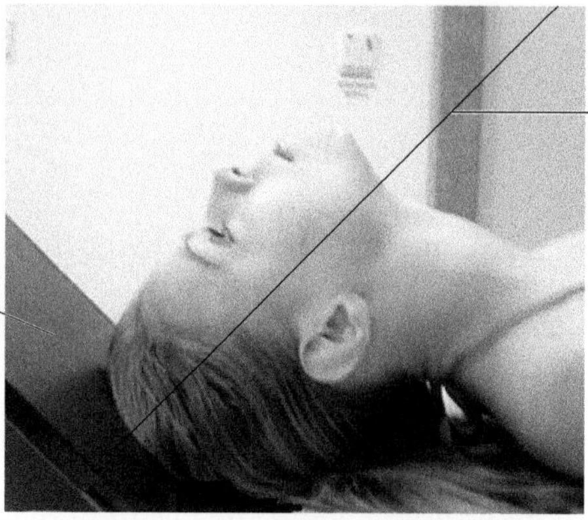

Fig. 13.14 Modified SMV zygomatic arches.

- The neck is flexed back as far as possible and the IR placed vertically in contact with the top of the head, its long axis resting on the table-top
- The IR position is adjusted (angled) until parallel to the long axes of the zygomatic arches, then supported in this position by pads and sandbags
- The MSP is perpendicular to the IR and coincident with its midline

Beam Direction and FRD

The beam should be perpendicular to the IR and zygomatic arches

FRD 120 cm, or slightly more for patients with a large abdomen, which may lie in the way of the tube head at shorter FRD

Centring

In the midline, to travel through the midpoint of the zygomatic arches

Collimation

As for the FO 30° projection

Criteria for Assessing Image Quality – FO 30°

- Mastoid bones, zygomatic arches, zygomae and upper rami of mandible are demonstrated
- Symmetry of the petrous portion of the temporal bones on either side of the foramen magnum
- Dorsum sellae seen within the foramen magnum
- Sharp image demonstrating contrast between the low density zygomatic arch and the soft tissues of the face

Common Errors: FO 30° Zygomatic Arches

Common Errors	Possible Reasons	Potential Effects on PCE of Report
Asymmetry of petrous temporal bones around the foramen magnum	Rotation about MSP	Would result in obliquity and possible foreshortening of zygomatic arch making assessment of bony anatomy difficult
Dark image with poor contrast	Quite obviously, selection of mAs and kVp is too high. Density of the arch is frequently overestimated and it should be remembered that this density is less than that of a phalanx. There is an air gap between the zygomatic arch and the IR which will need consideration when selecting exposure factors	Inadequate demonstration of bony detail due to exposure error makes assessment of subtle fractures difficult

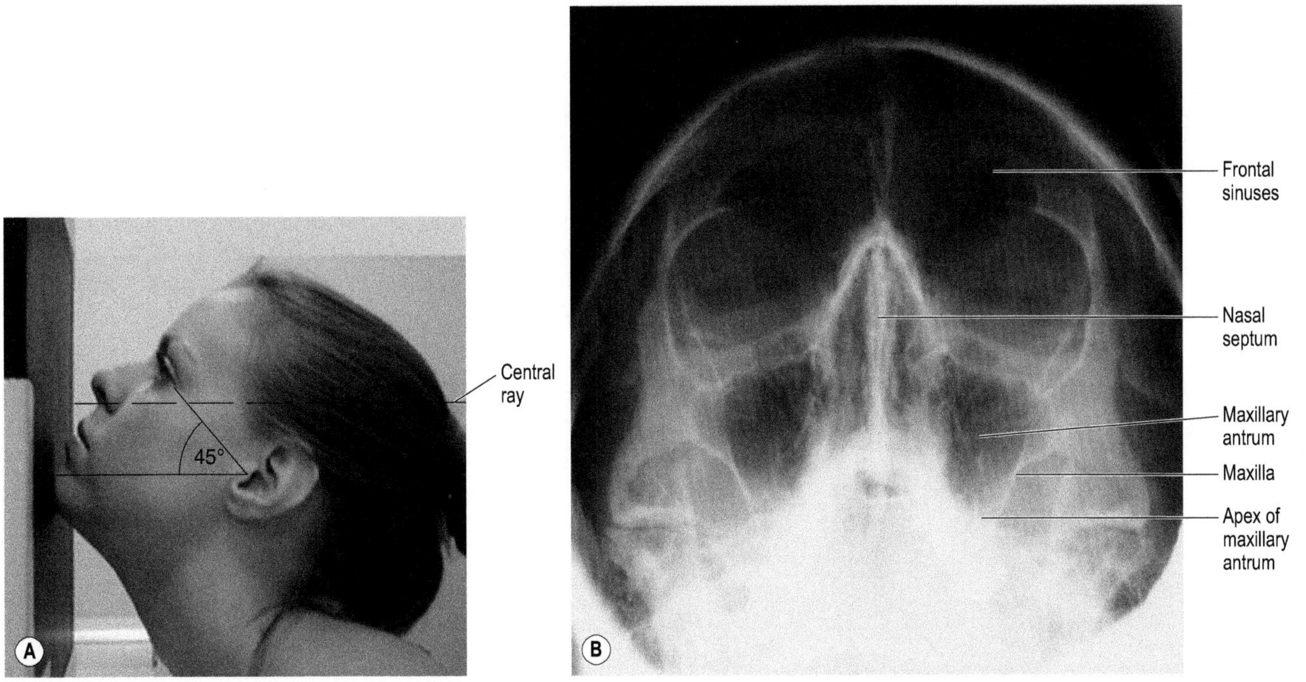

Fig. 13.15 OM sinuses.

Essentially the FO 30° zygomatic arches projection uses a tangential approach to demonstrate the area; other methods that employ the tangential approach have also been described as:

1. SMV projection with the beam centred under the chin at the level of the midpoint of the zygomatic arches. Collimation includes both sides
2. SMV with a 15° tilt of the head (the vertex turned away from the side under examination) and centring over the apex of the arch. Each side is exposed in turn[8]

Use of the SMV may prove difficult for the patient, especially those who present supine on a trolley. Maintenance of the position is also difficult for the patient. A more comfortable position is used in the modified SMV.

Criteria for Assessing Image Quality – SMV

As for the FO 30° projection.

Paranasal Sinuses

X-ray examination of the sinuses is rarely undertaken in the 21st century as acute symptoms should be diagnosed and treated clinically; CT and MRI have largely superseded plain radiography as imaging techniques, but only when treatment has proved ineffective (or if malignancy is suspected). The projections must be undertaken erect with horizontal beam, to demonstrate any fluid levels that might be present in the sinuses.

Projections are included in this text to ensure that information is made available in areas globally where CT and MRI are not readily accessible.

PCE COMMENTS – PARANASAL SINUSES

It is essential that, in OM projections, the petrous ridge does not cross the bases of the maxillary sinuses, since fluid levels in these sinuses should be visible if present, and consequently reported. Fluid levels may be noted in the frontal sinus on OF projections, and/or on the OM (in the OM fluid may appear as a vague opacity rather than a definitive fluid level).

Soft tissue bulges, apparent fluid levels and unusual densities within the antra should be commented upon, as should any loss of normal anatomical contours or apparent reduction in volume (when compared to the contralateral side). Fluid levels are most commonly noted in the maxillary antra but occasionally can be seen in the frontal sinus. Because of this it is very important to make sure that the OM position is correct, in that the petrous ridge does not cross the maxillary antra.

IR is vertical for all projections of the sinuses and post-nasal space.

OCCIPITOMENTAL (OM) SINUSES (FIG. 13.15A,B)

Positioning

- The patient is seated, facing the IR
- The chin is placed in contact with the midline of the IR and the chin position is adjusted until the orbitomeatal baseline (OMBL) has been raised 45° from the horizontal
- The median sagittal plane (MSP) is perpendicular to the IR, which is assessed by checking that the external auditory meati (EAMs) or lateral orbital margins are equidistant from it

Beam Direction and FRD

Horizontal, at 90° to the IR and making an angle of 45° with the OMBL
100 cm FRD

Centring

Above the external occipital protuberance (EOP), to emerge at the level of the inferior orbital margins

Collimation

Frontal sinuses (the upper borders of these sinuses vary with each individual and a specific border description cannot be given), maxillary sinuses

Criteria for Assessing Image Quality

- All paranasal sinuses are demonstrated
- Symmetry of facial bones on each side; equal distance of lateral orbital margins from outer table of temporal bones
- Upper border of the petrous portion of the temporal bone is level with the apex of the maxillary antra
- Images of premolars and molars are medial to, and clear of, the medial aspects of the maxillary sinuses
- Zygomatic arches are seen as tight 'handles' laterally
- Sharp image demonstrating the air-filled regions of the paranasal sinuses in contrast with the bones of the skull

Common Errors: OM Sinuses

Common Errors	Possible Reasons	Potential Effects on PCE or Report
Asymmetry of the facial structures	Rotation about MSP	Sinuses will not be adequately demonstrated, asymmetry due to positioning may falsely imply pathology
Position of the petrous ridge is too high; it is seen through the maxillary sinuses	Chin is not raised enough	Obscures maxillary antra and potential pathology, especially fluid levels or polyps
Petrous ridge is below the maxillary sinuses; image of crowns of premolars overlying the medial aspects of the maxillary sinuses	Chin is raised too high	Teeth may obscure some of the maxillary antrum and potential abnormality The frontal sinuses are foreshortened and may appear over-dark and lacking contrast, limiting diagnosis of subtle pathology
or Position appears acceptable; frontal sinuses are over-darkened and digital manipulation does not improve contrast and detail	Collimation might not be tight enough around the area of interest, thus scatter may blacken the upper anterior aspect of the frontal bone	Possible subtle bony changes or pathological processes could be masked if exposure is inappropriate

LATERAL SINUSES

It is not likely that this projection will add useful information to the OM, as the two sides of the head are superimposed.

LATERAL POSTNASAL SPACE (FIG. 13.16)

UK guidelines no longer suggest X-ray examination of this area, but some anecdotal comment suggests that this may still be used for children who snore or have difficulty breathing through their nose.

Positioning

- The patient stands or sits with the side of their head next to the IR and their MSP parallel to it
- There should be no tilt or rotation of the head. This can be assessed by checking the midline of the cranium over the top and symmetry of the frontal bone and orbits
- The chin is raised slightly, to reduce the density of the soft tissues of the throat and clear as much of the mandible as possible from the air-filled regions

Beam Direction and FRD

Horizontal, at 90° to the IR
100 cm FRD

Centring

Below the midpoint of the OMBL, half way between the level of the TMJ and angle of the mandible

Collimation

Angle of the mandible and 3–5 cm, according to size of patient, anterior to this, TMJ, pharynx and down to the level of the thyroid cartilage

Criteria for Assessing Image Quality

- Postnasal space, the posterior wall of the maxillary sinuses, the TMJ and thyroid cartilage are demonstrated
- Clear joint spaces are shown between the cervical vertebrae
- Sharp image demonstrating the darker air-filled pharynx in contrast with the soft tissues of the surrounding area and the mandible. Cervical vertebrae appear pale and low in contrast

OCCIPITOFRONTAL (OF) MAXILLARY AND ANTERIOR ETHMOID SINUSES (FIG. 13.17A,B)

Positioning

- The patient is seated, facing the IR
- The forehead is placed in contact with the IR and the chin position is adjusted until the OMBL is at 90° to it
- The MSP is perpendicular to the IR, which is assessed by checking that the EAMs or lateral orbital margins are equidistant from it

Beam Direction and FRD

Horizontal, at 90° to the IR
100 cm FRD

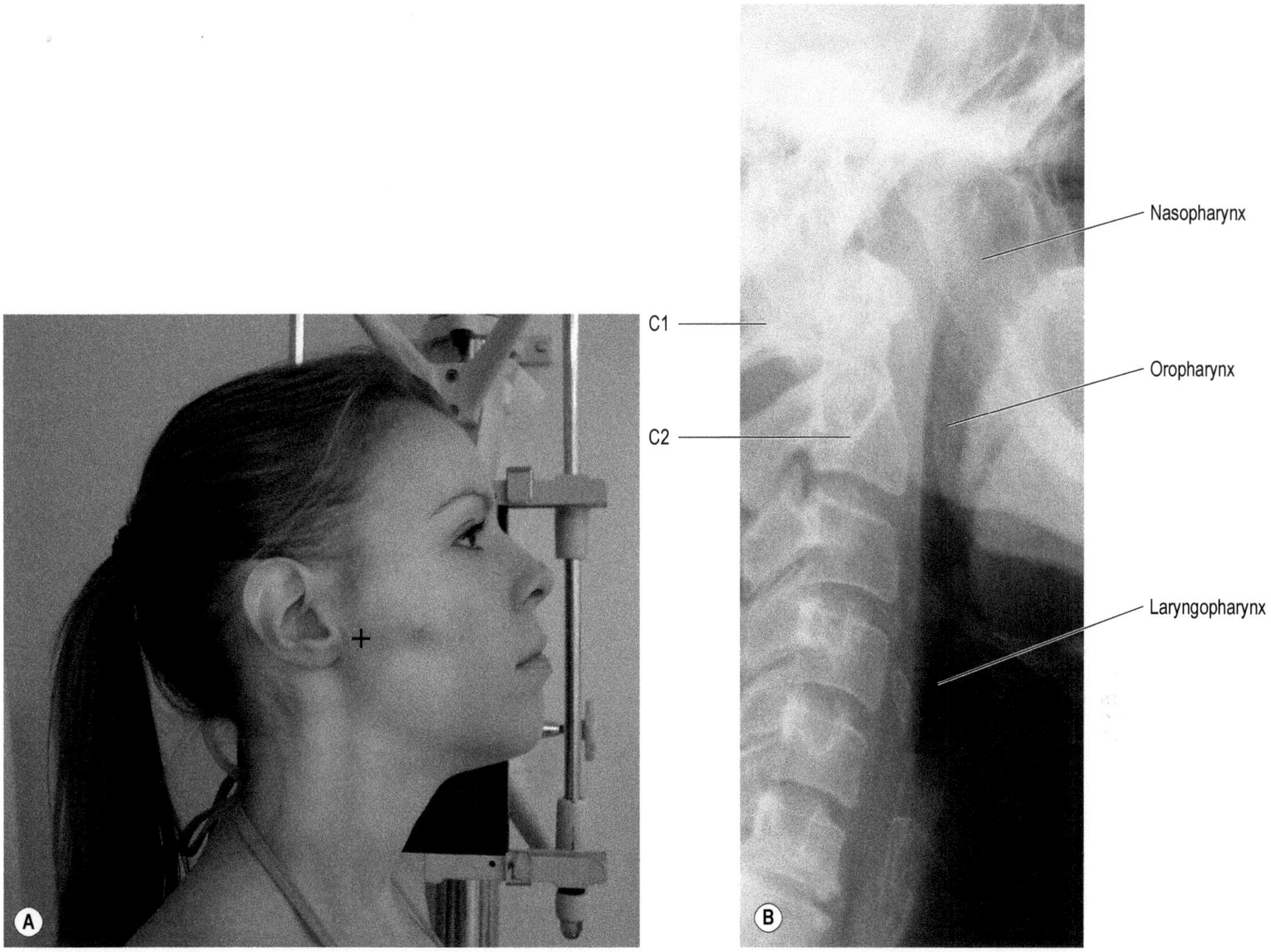

Fig. 13.16 Lateral postnasal space.

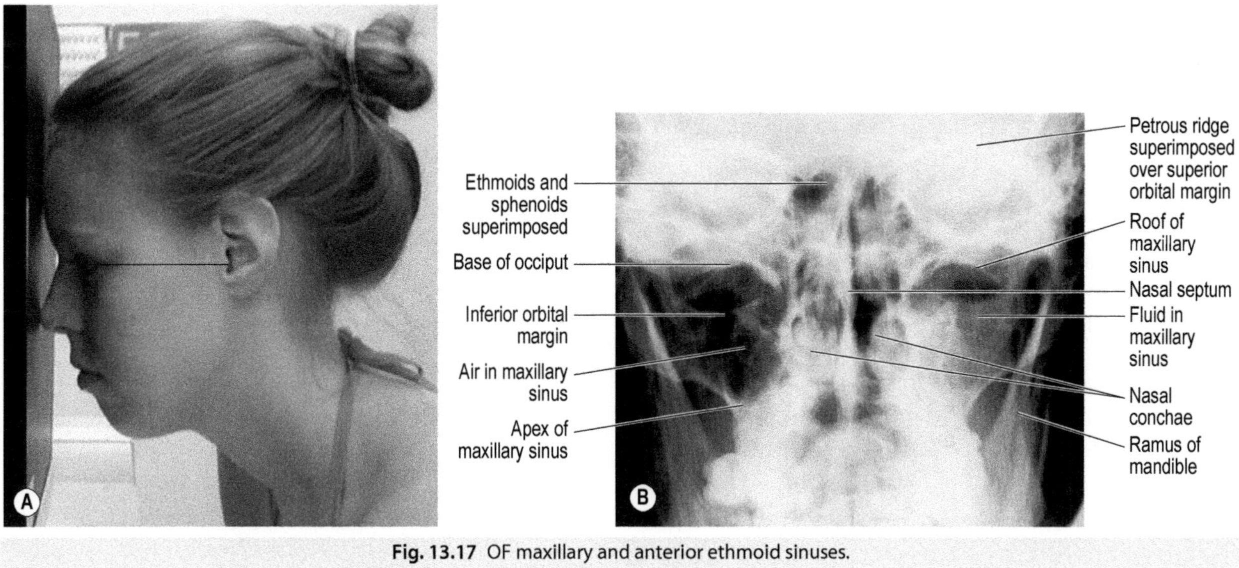

Fig. 13.17 OF maxillary and anterior ethmoid sinuses.

Centring

In the midline of the occiput, to emerge at the level of the inferior orbital margins

Collimation

Frontal sinuses (the upper border of these sinuses varies with each individual and a specific border description cannot be given), maxillary sinuses

Criteria for Assessing Image Quality

- All paranasal sinuses are demonstrated
- Equal distance of the lateral orbital margins from the outer table of the temporal bones on each side
- Upper border of the petrous portion of the temporal bone is level with the superior orbital margins
- Sharp image demonstrating the air-filled regions of the paranasal sinuses in contrast with the bones of the skull. The petrous portion of the temporal appears under-penetrated

Common Errors: OF Maxillary and Anterior Ethmoid Sinuses

Common Errors	Possible Reasons	Potential Effects on PCE or Report
Distance of the lateral orbital margins from the lateral borders of skull differs on each side	Rotation about MSP	Difficult to fully appreciate the sinuses – may falsely imply potential asymmetry of anatomy
Position of the petrous ridge is too high; it is seen above the superior orbital margins	OMBL is not perpendicular to the IR; chin is too far down	Sinuses will be inadequately demonstrated due to superimposition of bony structures. It may not be possible to identify fluid levels or polyps
Petrous ridge is too low; it is seen within the outline of the orbits	OMBL is not perpendicular to the IR; the chin is raised slightly	As above
Maxillary sinuses are over-blackened with poor contrast between the air-filled sinuses and maxilla. Petrous temporal shows good contrast and detail	Over-penetration. The maxilla itself is not a particularly dense bone and this is often overlooked	Any subtle pathology will be missed, such as small polyps

OCCIPITOFRONTAL (OF) (10°) FRONTAL SINUSES (FIG. 13.18A,B)

In the OF projection for maxillary and anterior ethmoid sinuses the frontal sinuses are foreshortened, whereas in the OM projection they are magnified and distorted. For a more accurate representation of these sinuses, the OMBL is raised to bring the vertical axis of the frontal sinus into a position where it is more parallel to the IR. 10° caudal angulation will achieve the required effect, but a horizontal beam is advised in order to demonstrate fluid levels more accurately.

Positioning

The patient is positioned initially as for the OF maxillary sinuses projection

The chin is raised 10° and a radiolucent pad placed between the forehead and IR for immobilisation

Beam Direction and FRD

Horizontal, at 90° to the IR

If the chin is to be elevated 10° then a guide must be used to assess this accurately; it is arguable whether the human eye can estimate a small angle such as 10° accurately. Use of a 10° radiolucent pad for immobilisation would be appropriate. Alternatively a large protractor, or a large piece of clear plastic marked with angles, can be placed against the OMBL.

100 cm FRD

Centring

In the midline of the occiput, to emerge through the nasion

Collimation

Frontal, ethmoid, sphenoid sinuses

Criteria for Assessing Image Quality

- Frontal, ethmoid and sphenoid sinuses are demonstrated
- Symmetry of structures around the midline
- Upper border of the petrous portion of the temporal bone half-way down the orbits
- Sharp image demonstrating the air-filled frontal and ethmoid sinuses in contrast with the frontal and ethmoid bones

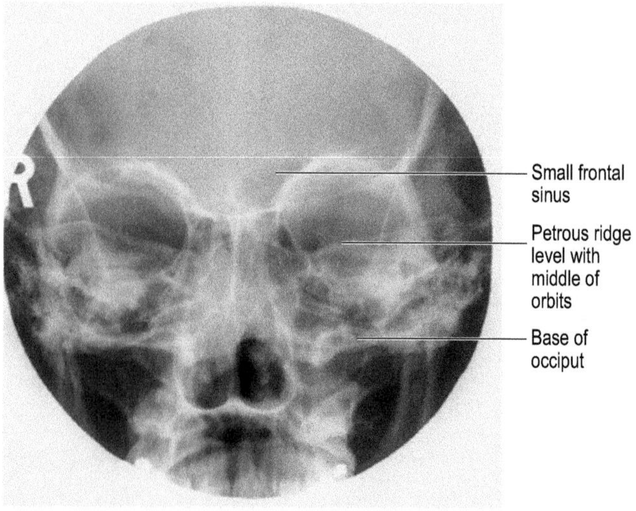

Fig. 13.18 Frontal sinuses.

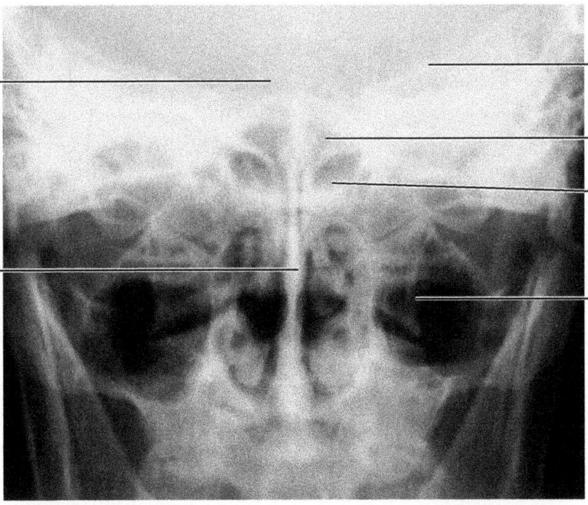

Fig. 13.19 OF sphenoid and ethmoids.

OCCIPITOFRONTAL (OF) ETHMOID AND SPHENOID SINUSES (FIG. 13.19)

Positioning

As for the frontal sinuses, these sinuses can be seen on an *OF projection*, this time with *the chin lowered* until the *OMBL moves through 10°*.

Beam Direction, Centring and Collimation

As for the OF for frontal and anterior ethmoid sinuses.

Criteria for Assessing Image Quality

- Ethmoid and sphenoid sinuses are demonstrated
- Symmetry of structures around the midline
- Upper border of the petrous portion of the temporal bone is shown above the superior orbital margins; the petrous ridges start to elevate obliquely towards the outer table of the vault, rather than appearing horizontal
- Sphenoid and ethmoid sinuses seen in the midline, slightly above the orbits and between the petrous portions of the temporal bones
- Sharp image demonstrating the air-filled ethmoid and sphenoid sinuses in contrast with the bones of the vault and petrous portions of the temporal bones

References

1. Raju NS, Ishwar P, Banerjee R. Role of multislice computed tomography and three-dimensional rendering in the evaluation of maxillofacial injuries. *J Oral Maxillofac Radiol.* 2017;5:67–73.
2. Bhattaychara J, Moseley IF, Fells P. The role of plain radiography in the management of suspected orbital blow-out fractures. *Br J Radiol.* 1997;70:29–33.
3. Royal College of Radiologists. *iRefer: Making the Best Use of Clinical Radiology.* 8th ed. London: RCR; 2017. https://www.rcr.ac.uk/clinical-radiology/being-consultant/rcr-referral-guidelines/about-irefer.
4. Pogrel M, Podlesh SW, Goldman KE. Efficacy of a single occipitomental radiograph to screen for midfacial fractures. *J Oral Maxillofac Surg.* 2000;58(1):24–26.
5. Goh S, Low B. Radiologic screening for midfacial fractures: a single 30 degree occipitomental is enough. *J Trauma.* 2002;24(4):688–692.
6. Carver E, Carver B, eds. *Medical Imaging: Techniques, Reflection and Evaluation.* 2nd ed. Edinburgh: Churchill Livingstone; 2012.
7. Sheriff I. Alphabetical list of named radiographic projections. https://www.scribd.com/document/278025168/Alphabetical-List-of-Named-Radiographic-Projections.
8. Whitley AS, Jefferson G, Holmes K, et al. *Clark's Positioning in Radiography.* 13th ed. Boca Raton, FL: CRC Press; 2015.
9. Unett E, Royle A. *Radiographic Techniques and Image Evaluation.* London: Nelson Thornes; 1997.
10. Lampignano JP, Kendrick LE. *Bontrager's Textbook of Radiographic Positioning and Related Anatomy.* 9th ed. St Louis: Elsevier Mosby; 2018.
11. McQuillen-Martenson K. *Radiographic Image Analysis.* 5th ed. St Louis: Elsevier; 2019.
12. Sidebottom AJ, Sissons G. Radiographic screening for midfacial fracture in A & E. *Br J Radiol.* 1999;72:523–524.
13. Dolan KD, Jacoby CG. Facial fractures. *Semin Roentgenol.* 1978;13(1):37–51.
14. Sciacca F et al. McGrigor–Campbell lines. Radiopaedia. https://radiopaedia.org/articles/mcgrigor-campbell-lines?lang=gb.
15. Department of Radiology, University of Washington. *Facial and Mandibular Fractures;* 2018. [online] https://rad.washington.edu/about-us/academic-sections/musculoskeletal-radiology/teaching-materials/online-musculoskeletal-radiology-book/facial-and-mandibular-fractures/.
16. Scally P. *Medical Imaging.* Oxford: Oxford University Press; 1999.
17. Frank E, Long BW, Smith BS. *Merrill's Atlas of Radiographic Positioning and Procedures.* 12th ed. St Louis: Mosby; 2011.
18. Eisenberg R, Dennis C, May RTC. *Radiographic Positioning.* 2nd ed. Boston: Little, Brown; 1995.

14 Dental Radiography

REBEKAH GOULSTON and ELIZABETH CARVER

Dental radiography is still a widespread imaging technique required by dentists and oral surgeons in dental surgeries and hospitals. Intraoral techniques in particular are low dose in relation to examinations undertaken elsewhere in the body, but this does not mean that dose should be considered irrelevant in examinations of the teeth and mouth.

Dose Reduction and Radiation Protection

Guidelines for the safe use of dental X-ray equipment[1] states that there are several things that radiographers can do to ensure that the patient receives a radiation dose that is as low as reasonably practicable when taking dental radiographs.

When taking intraoral radiographs:

- **Use paralleling technique** when taking periapicals whenever possible.
- **Use beam aiming devices** and image receptor (IR) holders whenever possible.
- Ensure that the **longest spacer cone** provided with the intraoral equipment is fitted to the machine, and that it is as close to the patient's skin as possible when the exposure is carried out. All spacer cones should be a minimum of 200 mm long. However, the longer the spacer cone, the better the resultant image quality will be. There will also be lower radiation dose as the X-ray beam will be less divergent when it comes into contact with the patient.
- **Use rectangular collimation** when taking intraoral exposures. Rectangular collimation should reduce the size of the X-ray beam to at least 40 mm by 50 mm and as such could reduce the radiation dose to the patient by as much as 50%.[2] Depending on the age and model of the equipment being used, rectangular collimation can be an integral part of the tube head or a bespoke retrofitted accessory via a universal fitting that can be positioned on the end of the spacer cone. It can also be an additional component to an IR holder.
- Use kilovoltage in the **60–70 kV** range to reduce radiation skin dose to the patient.

When taking extraoral radiographs:

- **Use AECs if fitted on the machine** but ensure that you position the patient correctly for the examination so that they work effectively. For Cone Beam Computed Tomography (CBCT) examinations, where an AEC is fitted on the unit, ensure that any thyroid collar used is put on *after* the scout projection has been taken; failure to do so may result in a higher radiation exposure than is necessary during the actual scan.
- **Use the smallest field of view/collimate as much as possible** so that only the area of clinical interest is covered on the image, for example if there was a need to image a third molar prior to extraction, a collimated dental panoramic tomography (DPT) image to show just the posterior mandibular region on the affected side could be taken (rather than DPT of the whole jaw).

Additional radiation protection points for any dental radiography examination:

- **Select the relevant technique with the lowest associated radiation dose to image the area:** for example, taking a periapical rather than DPT when there is a need to image a single tooth because the patient presents with localised odontalgia, and dental caries is suspected.
- **When manual exposures are used, select and alter exposure factors based on the size of the patient, and imaging system speed:** as with conventional X-ray machines, the use of phosphor storage devices and solid state detectors as the image receptor can usually result in a decrease of exposure factors needed to produce a quality image (when imaging-processing software algorithms are set up correctly).
- **Only use a thyroid collar for examinations in which the thyroid gland is in the line of the primary X-ray beam.** The most common of these examinations are maxillary occlusal projections and periapicals of the upper incisors (if bisecting angle technique is the only option). The thyroid collar should be positioned out of the primary X-ray beam, so as not to negatively affect image quality.

Difficulties in Providing Accuracy of Dental Assessment

The teeth themselves provide the radiographer with problems of accurate imaging, owing to the nature of their various shapes. This, added to their positions within the alveolar ridges of the maxilla and the mandible, their arched arrangement in the mouth and the varying positions of the teeth in each individual, shows that the implications for accurate representation of dentition are complex.

TABLE 14.1 Dental Terminology

Buccal/labial (Fig. 14.1)	The (outer) aspect of the teeth that lies between the teeth and the cheeks or lips
Lingual/palatal (Fig. 14.1)	The (inner) aspect of the teeth that lies between the teeth and the tongue
Distal (Fig. 14.2)	The direction of the dental arch towards the molars, posteriorly and outwards away from the MSP. Used to describe beam shift, tube shift or angulation
Mesial (Fig. 14.2)	The direction of the dental arch towards the incisors, anteriorly and inwards towards the MSP. Used to describe beam shift, tube shift or angulation and is in the opposite direction to distal movement
Alatragal line (Fig. 14.3)	An imaginary line from the tragus of the ear to the middle of the ala of the nose (the flare of soft tissue around the nostril)
Occlusal plane (upper) (Fig. 14.3)	The line joining the biting surfaces of the upper teeth. When the mouth is closed this is deemed to be the occlusal plane rather than the upper occlusal plane. The line lies parallel to the anthropological baseline and the alatragal line. It lies approximately 4 cm below the alatragal line
Occlusal plane (lower)	With the mouth open, this line lies parallel to, and approximately 2 cm below, the line which lies between the tragus of the ear and the outer canthus of the mouth. Because all radiography of the teeth should be undertaken with the mouth closed around an IR holder or occlusal film, this plane is not actually used in this text and is therefore not illustrated
Median sagittal plane (MSP) (Fig. 14.4)	Plane running vertically down the middle of the face, separating the left and right sides

Terminology Associated with Dental Radiography

Dental techniques require an understanding of some terms that are not encountered in radiography of the rest of the body; these are outlined in Table 14.1.

Techniques Used in Dental Radiography

Intraoral Techniques

Bitewings: Demonstrate the crowns and interproximal surfaces of the teeth.

Periapicals: Demonstrate the whole tooth.

Occlusals: Demonstrate a range of structures and aspects of the mouth, including the hard palate, incisors and canines, unerupted canines, premolars, mental foramen, submandibular salivary glands and ducts, and the symphysis menti.

Extraoral Techniques

Dental panoramic tomography (DPT): Demonstrates the whole mouth, including dentition, mandible, maxillary sinuses and temporomandibular (TMJ) joints.

Lateral cephalometry: Mainly used to assess the extent of malocclusions and facial deformities prior to and post surgery.

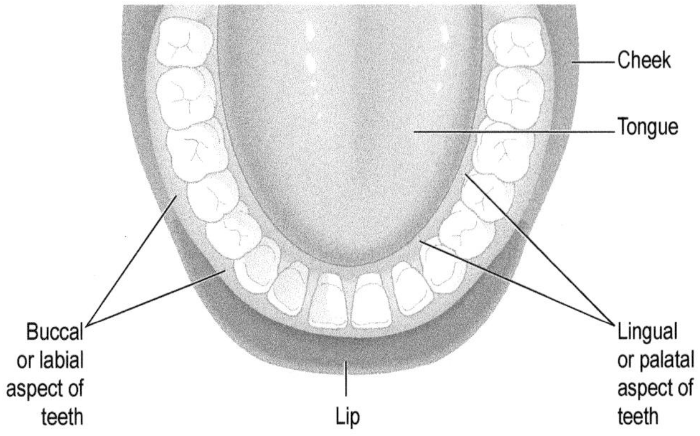

Fig. 14.1 Buccal/labial, lingual/palatal aspects of the teeth.

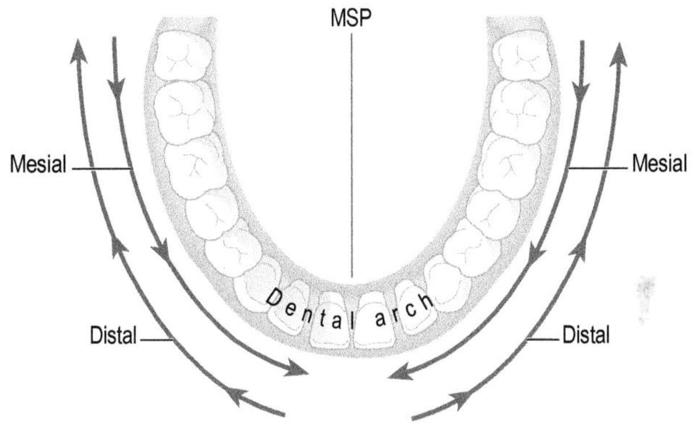

Fig. 14.2 Distal and mesial.

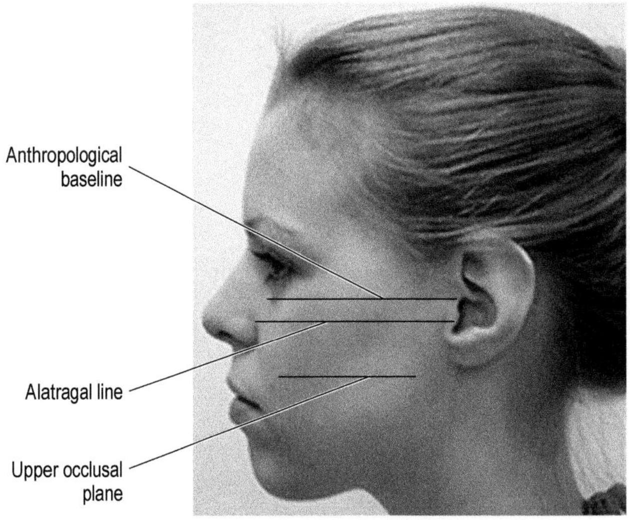

Fig. 14.3 Reference lines used in dental radiography.

Recording and Displaying the Image

Since the previous edition of this book there has been an increase in use of digital imaging for dental examinations, but there still exists a proportion of film-based radiography in dental units;[2] this is likely to continue to decrease as dental surgeries replace ageing equipment. It is therefore still necessary to give direction on the use of film and display of film images.

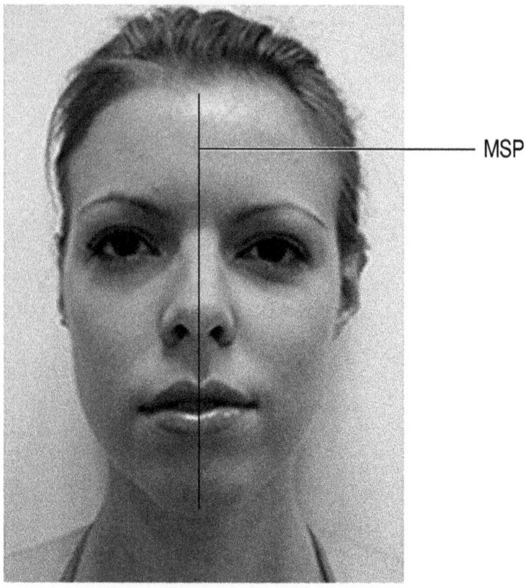

Fig. 14.4 Median sagittal plane (MSP).

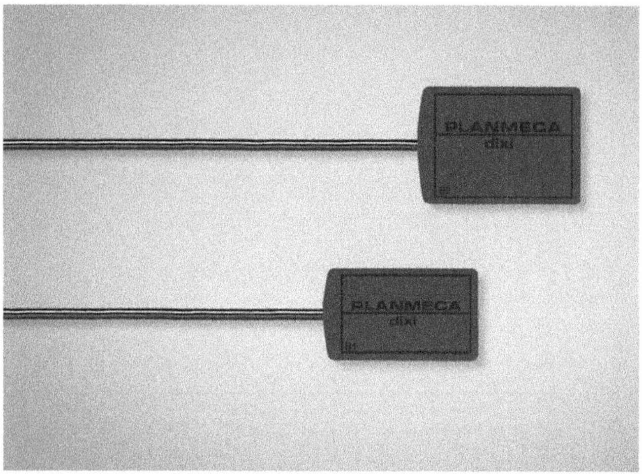

Fig. 14.5 Digital dental image receptors. (Reproduced with permission from Xograph Imaging Systems.)

As with other 2D radiography, an interim computed radiography system where a phosphor storage device is used to capture the image, and then downloaded via reader onto a computer where contrast and other qualities can be manipulated, can be used to provide 'digital' images without having to replace the existing X-ray unit. As phosphor is poisonous, and the image can be erased if it comes into contact with light, the plate should always be covered with a specially designed disposable opaque plastic bag before it is put in the patient's mouth.[3,4]

Digital dental units use solid state receptors which are connected to the digital unit (Fig. 14.5). While similar in length and height to the phosphor storage receptors and films used in dental radiography, solid state receptors can be a wider depth and/or have connecting leads attached to the back; as a result, some patients may complain that they feel very bulky in the mouth.[4]

RECEPTOR SIZES (FIG. 14.6)

A range of film/receptor sizes are available: *size 0* is the smallest and is usually used in periapical and bitewing examinations for children as well as to image the incisors and canines in adults. *Size 2* is usually used for intraoral imaging of the posterior teeth in adults. *Occlusal* receptors (size 4) are larger than size 0 and 2, as they are designed to cover a larger area of dentition. Intraoral techniques do not use a film/screen system as the area under examination is of low density and exposure factors used are relatively low, so that intensifying screens are not necessary even in the non-digitised situation.

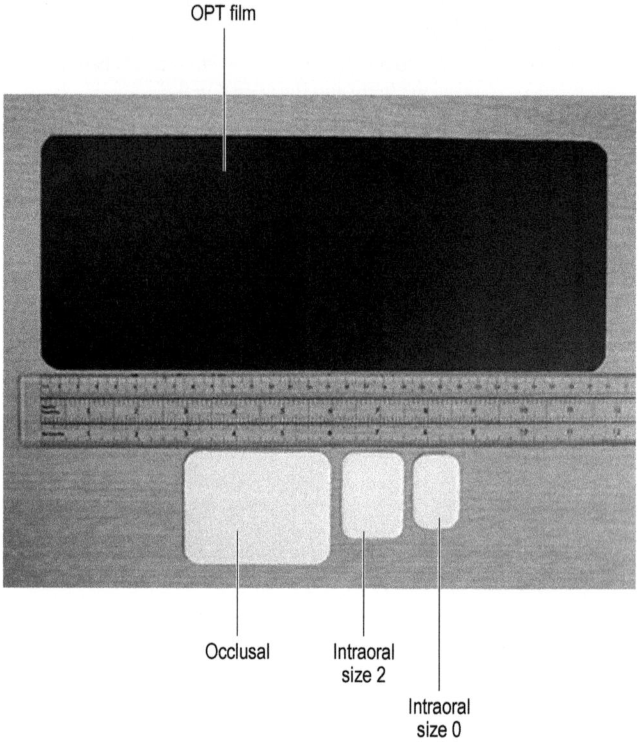

Fig. 14.6 Dental film sizes.

Cassettes and film or phosphor storage devices used in DPT are usually of a specific size designed solely for this examination, approximately 14–15×30 cm. They are used in conjunction with intensifying screens, as the area under examination is significantly denser than individual teeth. Lateral cephalometry film is 18×24 cm or similar. Digital units for both DPT and cephalometry incorporate the solid state receptor into the X-ray unit.

RECEPTOR ORIENTATION

A consistent method must be used to orientate the film in the mouth, since it is impossible to tell whether teeth are from the left or right side, from the mandible or the maxilla. The most familiar method was to use the orientation 'pimple' when using film; this is a tiny but palpable raised lump on the tube side of the film (Fig. 14.7). The 'pimple' is always positioned towards the crowns of the teeth in periapical and occlusal examinations. For bitewings the 'pimple' is usually orientated towards the roots of the upper teeth. Usually dental phosphor storage devices have a radiopaque virtual marker printed into the phosphor layer which can be used in the same way as the 'pimple' is on film to orientate the plate in relation to the tooth anatomy. Digital IRs are always used with the lead leaving the edge of the receptor, which is outside the mouth, and identification must be annotated onto the resulting image at the post processing stage.

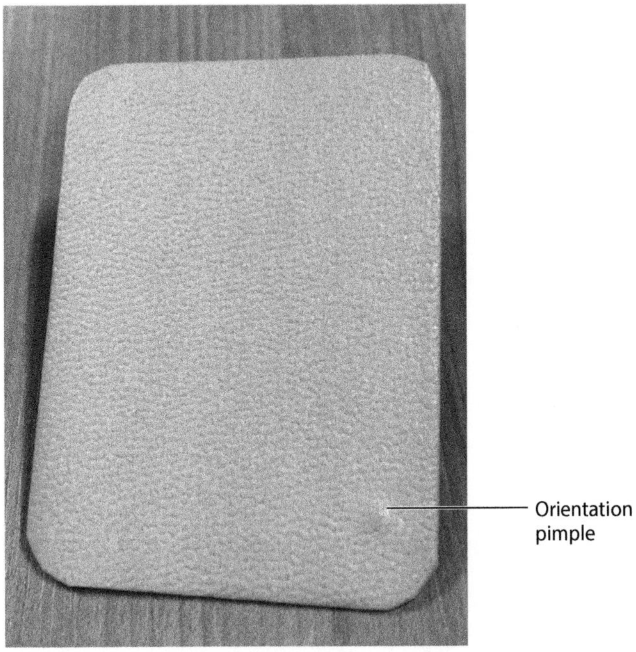

Fig. 14.7 Orientation pimple.

DISPLAYING FILM IMAGES

Films are usually mounted with patient and tooth/projection identification in clear holders or stapled to clear film or translucent mounting medium. The 'pimple' must face outwards, towards the viewing radiographer. All intraoral images are displayed following the layout of the mouth, as if looking at the patient.[3,5]

Intraoral Techniques

BITEWINGS

These demonstrate the crowns, interproximal surfaces and gingival margins of the premolars and molars. Bitewing film is available, which is a small dental film with a centralised flap of paper on the tube side of the film. The patient's teeth bite on the flap in order to immobilise and maintain position (Fig. 14.8A). Bitewing holders are used more often: these are a device into which the IR is inserted; a plastic flap/bite block at 90° to the film is placed between the patient's teeth. The standard IR size used for this examination on adults and children above the age of 6 years is equivalent to size 2 and should be used in the transverse orientation (unless clinical examination by a dental professional suggests that there is more than 6mm of bone loss around the teeth, in which case the IR should be positioned vertically in the mouth).[5,6]

Positioning

- The patient is seated with their neck leaning on a support
- A bitewing film or bitewing holder is placed with its tube side in contact with the lingual surface of the teeth under examination and the flap/bite block between the occlusal surfaces of the teeth
- The patient closes their teeth over the flap/bite block
- The median sagittal plane (MSP) is vertical and the upper occlusal plane horizontal

Beam Direction

If using dental film with a centralised flap of paper or a plastic flap holder: initially horizontal, then angled 5° caudally
If using a paralleling bitewing holder: the beam is aligned to the centre of the indicator on the paralleling holder, in the direction indicated by the holder

Centring

To the middle of the IR, over the occlusal plane

Collimation

A rectangular collimation device should always be used wherever possible, and positioned so that it is in the same orientation as the IR in the mouth

Include

The crowns of the teeth under examination and the alveolar crests, from the mesial surface of the first premolar to the distal surface of the second molar so that these are visualised on the resultant image. If the patient has an erupted third molar then an additional image will be needed, taken with the IR mesial edge in line with the distal surface of the second premolar; this shows the interproximal space and cusp contact points between the second and third molars.[6]

Criteria for Assessing Image Quality[6]

- Crowns of both maxillary and mandibular teeth and alveolar crests are demonstrated
- The occlusal plane is in the middle of the image such that equal amounts of the maxillary and mandibular anatomy can be visualised on the image
- No evidence of elongation or foreshortening of teeth
- No overlap of adjacent teeth
- Slight separation of occlusal surfaces of teeth
- Sharp image demonstrating enamel in contrast with pulp cavity and the alveolar crests

Common Errors: Bitewings

Common Errors	Possible Reasons	Potential Effect on Image Interpretation[6–8]
Overlap of the crowns at their interproximal surfaces	Beam not perpendicular to the arch of the teeth and/or the IR in the mesiodistal direction IR not parallel to the dental arch	If interproximal spaces are not visible then bone levels cannot be assessed Carious lesions may be hidden leading to a failure to treat at an early stage, thus allowing further development of the caries. Ultimately causing more pain for the patient However, it should be noted that this error may be unavoidable in some areas of the mouth if the dentition is overcrowded, causing some teeth to overlap
Foreshortening of the teeth	Beam not perpendicular to the dental arch and/or not perpendicular to IR in the vertical plane IR not parallel to the vertical axis of the teeth	Bone levels may be distorted Secondary caries (under restorations) may be missed Both of the above points may result in inappropriate treatment and carry the possibility of pain for the patient

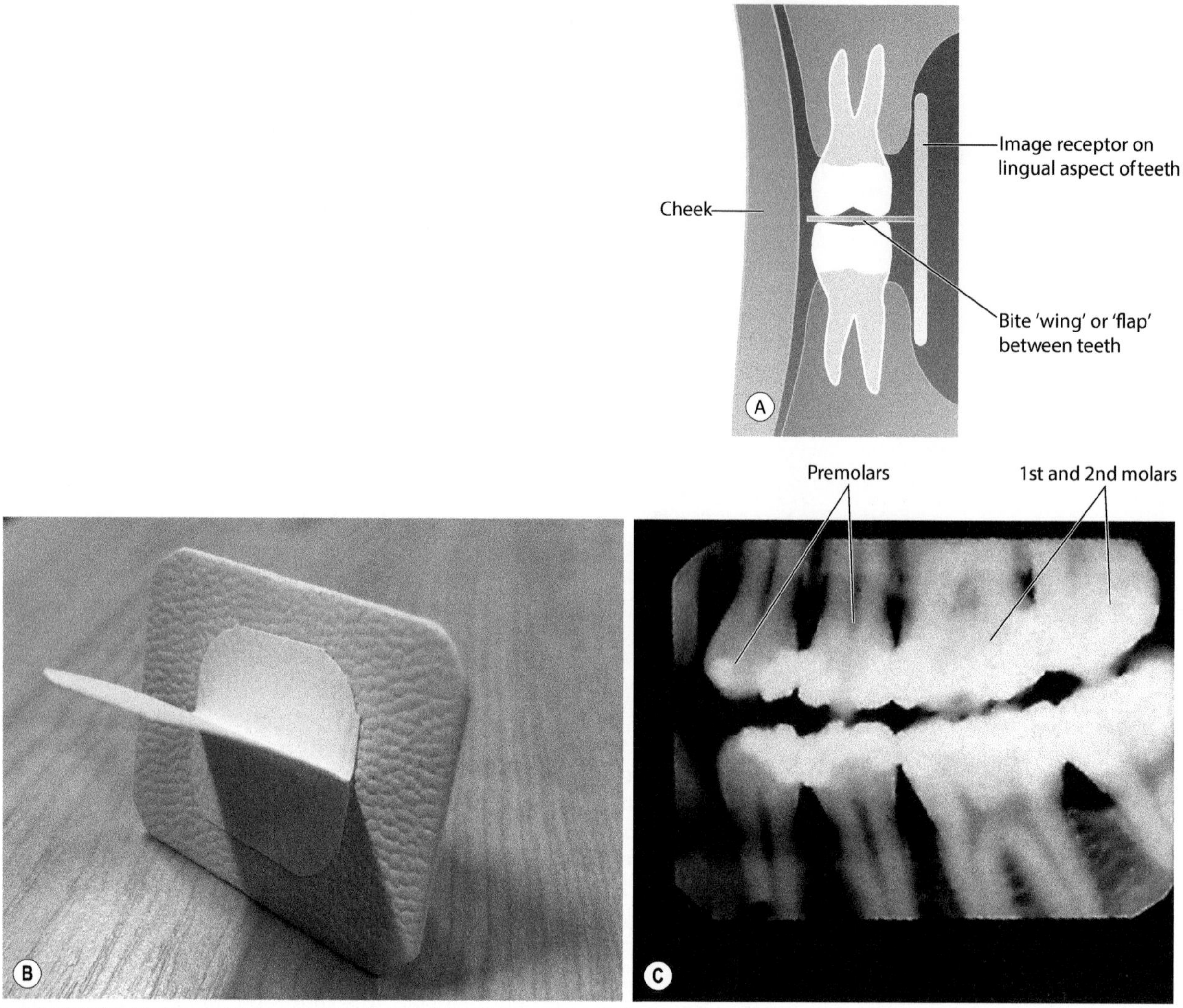

Fig. 14.8 (A) Position of IR for bitewings and relationship to teeth; (B) bitewing film; (C) Bitewing image. (C, From Whaites E. *Essentials of Dental Radiography and Radiology*. 3rd ed. Edinburgh: Churchill Livingstone; 2002.)

PERIAPICALS

Periapical examinations are generally used to demonstrate individual or small groups of teeth with images mounted following the layout of the dentition.[3]

As already mentioned in the introduction to this section, the structure and position of teeth cause problems for the radiographer when attempting to provide high-quality images of the area. Ideally, the radiographer places any body part so that its long axis is parallel to the IR and the X-ray beam is 90° to the body part and the IR.

More specifically, the most significant problems can be identified as:

1. The teeth are surrounded at their neck and root by the bones of the maxilla or mandible, which are themselves surrounded by the gum. This reduces the proportion of the tooth that can be placed in close contact with the IR. When added to the arched construction of the hard palate, positioning of the IR parallel to the tooth becomes problematic. The teeth themselves are arranged in a variation of angles in the mouth, the incisors being at a much greater angle than the molars.
2. The size of the patient's mouth will affect the possibility of positioning the IR, since a narrow dental arch may not accommodate the IR.
3. Overlapping teeth when the dentition is overcrowded will mean that it is impossible to provide images of some teeth without some superimposition.

Two techniques are available for periapicals: *paralleling* and *bisecting angle*. Each aims to reduce effects of the obliquity of the teeth and the problems outlined in the introduction to this section.

Paralleling versus Bisecting Angle Techniques

The two periapical techniques described each have advantages and disadvantages: these are briefly outlined in Table 14.2 but, as stated at the beginning of the chapter, the latest dental radiation protection guidelines specify that the best method for reduced radiation dose to the patient and

TABLE 14.2 Advantages and Disadvantages of Periapical Techniques*

Bisecting Angle	Paralleling
Object receptor distance (ORD) varies along the length of the teeth, as the IR becomes more remote from crown to root; however, at no point is it as distant from the tooth as in paralleling technique. Magnification (and therefore unsharpness) increases towards the root	Relatively long ORD along the entire length of the tooth has implications for magnification and unsharpness. Also, large teeth may not fit within the periphery of the IR
Some image distortion as beam is not perpendicular to any structure	Minimum image distortion as the receptor is always parallel to the long axis of the tooth and the beam perpendicular to the IR
Selection of angle is less likely to be as accurate as for paralleling technique, since it requires estimation of the bisecting angle. Centring may also be less accurate	Use of the alignment and centring indicator on the paralleling holder ensures accuracy of beam centring and angulation
Holders are relatively small compared to the paralleling holders	Holders are more bulky for patients; however, the rigidity and inclusion of an aiming device means that there is less chance of repeats being needed and it is easier to reproduce an image when monitoring teeth. There is therefore a lower overall radiation dose to the patient associated with this method and it is seen as the gold standard[1,6]

*Comparison of Figs 14.13 and 14.14 will help illustrate these points.

image reproducibility and quality is the paralleling technique.[1] However, the final decision may simply be based on the size of IR and holder that the patient can tolerate in the mouth and/or availability of equipment. In addition, some digital units may not provide equipment that offers a choice.

PARALLELING TECHNIQUE (FIGS 14.9–14.13)

This technique attempts to tackle the problems associated with producing accurate images of the teeth in this difficult body area. It makes use of holders that maintain the position of the IR parallel to the long axis of the tooth and enables accurate selection of the central ray at 90° to the IR.

Positioning

- The patient is seated with their neck supported
- The IR is placed in a paralleling holder – usually a size 0 longitudinally for incisors and canines, and a size 2 transversely for premolars and molars (Figs 14.9, 14.10)
- The holder is placed in the mouth with the tube side of the IR facing the lingual surface of the teeth and an IR marker near the crown surface of the teeth
- The IR is parallel to the long axes of the teeth under examination but is distant from the surface of the teeth; this may appear to be a significant distance to the radiographer, being toward the soft palate for incisors and towards the MSP for premolars and molars
- The tooth under examination is centred to the IR, or the midpoint of the range of teeth intended for inclusion is centralised
- The patient closes their mouth over the holder to immobilise the IR and maintain its position (Figs 14.11, 14.12)

Beam Direction and Centring

The beam is aligned to the centre of the indicator on the paralleling holder, in the direction indicated by the holder

Collimation

A rectangular collimation device should always be used wherever possible and positioned so that it is in the same orientation as the IR in the mouth

Include

Crowns, roots and apices of the teeth under examination, as well as 3–4 mm of bone laterally to the roots and also 3–4 mm below the lowest point of the root (known as the apex)[6]

Common errors and their impact are found after description of the bisecting angle technique.

BISECTING ANGLE TECHNIQUE

Clearly an angle is made between the long axis of the IR and the long axis of a tooth if the IR is placed on the labial aspect of any tooth and gum. Rather than directing the beam at 90° to either the tooth or the IR, in this technique the beam is aimed 90° to the *bisector* of the angle made between the tooth and IR – in other words, a compromise is reached (Fig. 14.14).

For this method, the angle of the individual patient's teeth must be estimated before commencing the examination. Although texts and dental radiography units list suggested beam angulation for this technique,[3,9] human dentition varies widely and each patient must be assessed individually. Visual examination of the dentition in a mesiodistal direction will give the radiographer an idea of beam direction in order to ensure that it will pass through the teeth at 90° and avoid overlap of the crowns at their interproximal surfaces. When assessing the angle of the long axis of the tooth in premolars, the centre of the crown must be assessed rather than the longest (labially positioned) cusp, which is usually curved and does not give an accurate indication of the tooth as a whole.

It is usual to use an IR of equivalent to a size 2 for this examination technique. When film or a phosphor storage device is used, a bisecting angle holder (Figs 14.15–14.17) should be used,[1] and using the patient's finger for support must be a last resort.

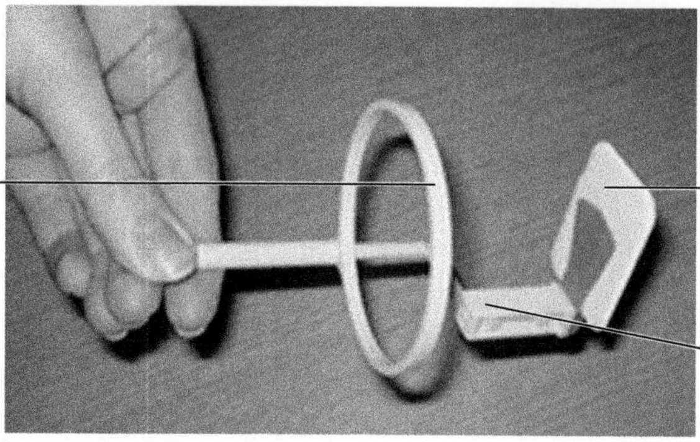

Fig. 14.9 Paralleling technique holder – film (incisors and canines).

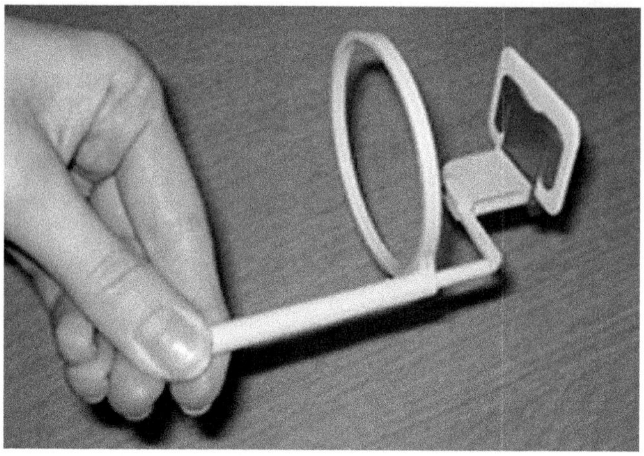

Fig. 14.10 Paralleling technique holder – film (molars and premolars).

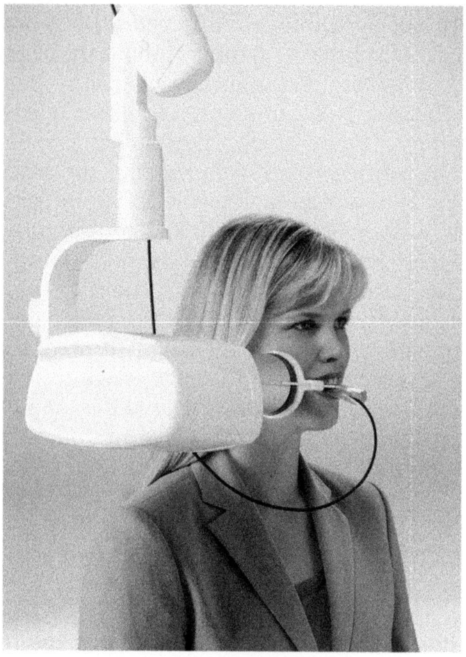

Fig. 14.11 Paralleling technique – digital receptor. (Reproduced with permission from Xograph Imaging Systems.)

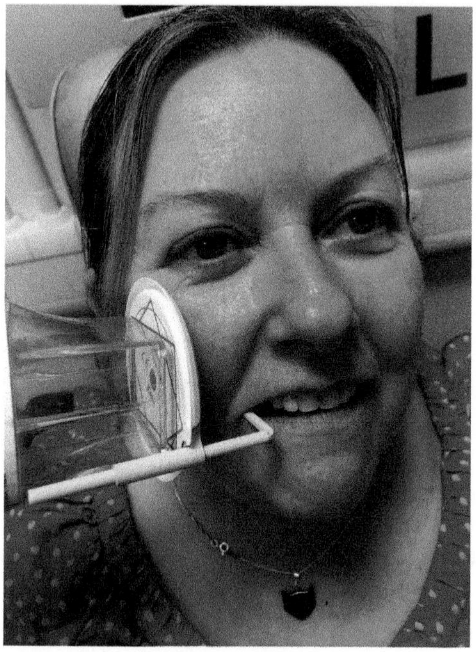

Fig. 14.12 Tube aligned with paralleling holder.

Positioning

- The patient is seated with their neck supported
- The IR has its tube side in contact with the lingual aspect of the crowns of the teeth and should always be used with the 'pimple' or other marker facing outwards towards the X-ray tube, orientated closest to the crowns of the teeth under examination. The IR is aligned longitudinally for incisors and canines and transversely for premolars and molars
- The tooth under examination is centred to the IR, or the midpoint of the range of teeth intended for inclusion is centralised
- The patient closes their teeth over the holder for incisors and canines, and closes their lips over the holder for the other teeth, to immobilise the IR and maintain its position
- The head is adjusted until the MSP is vertical and the occlusal plane is horizontal

Beam Direction

Initially horizontal, then adjusted until at 90° to the bisector of the angle formed between the long axis of the tooth and the long axis of the IR *and* 90° to the IR mesiodistally

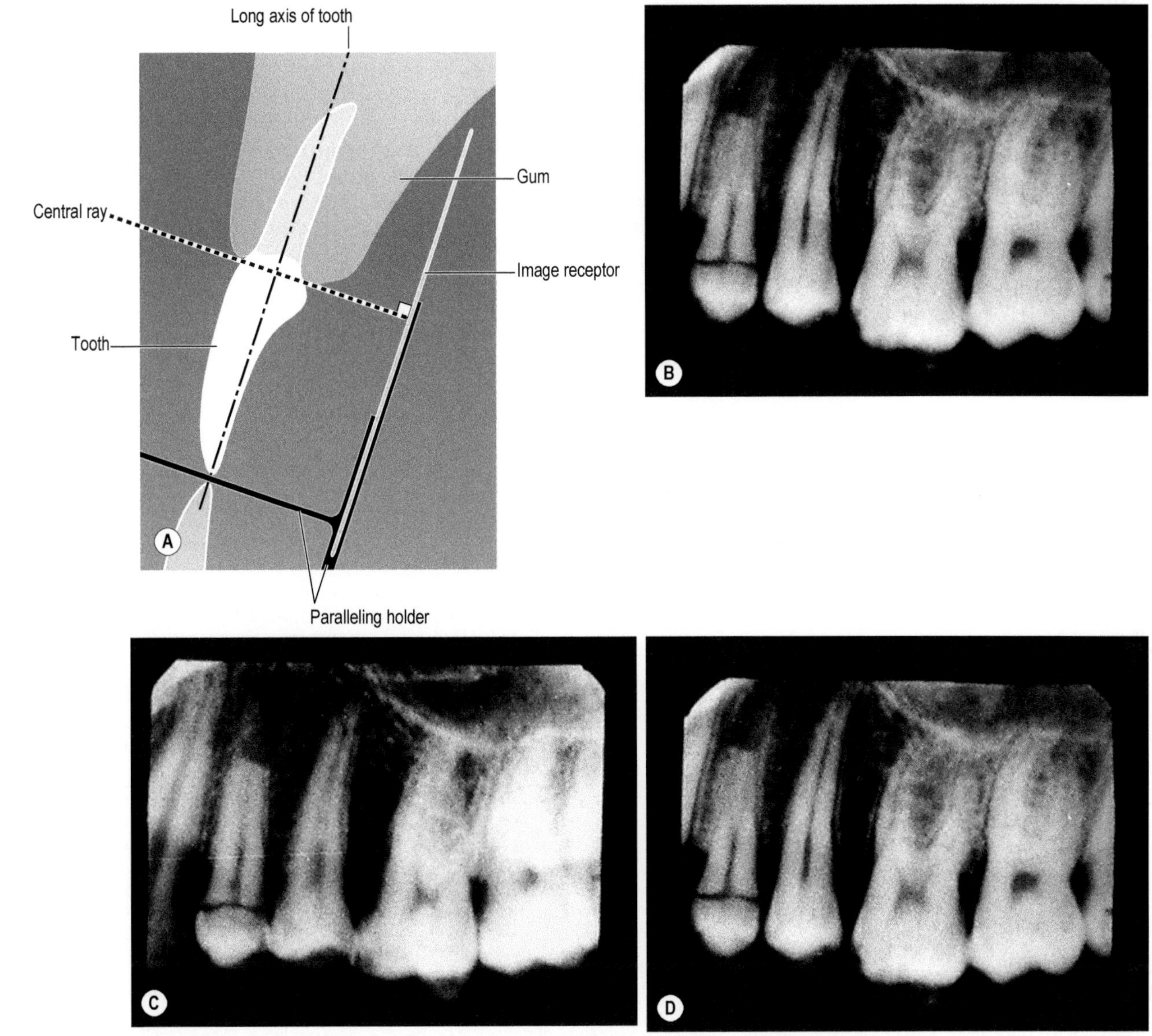

Fig. 14.13 (A) Position of IR for paralleling technique; (B) paralleling periapical. (C,D) Comparison of bisecting angle (C) and paralleling (D) technique on periapical images. (B–D, From Whaites E. *Essentials of Dental Radiography and Radiology*. 3rd ed. Edinburgh: Churchill Livingstone; 2002.)

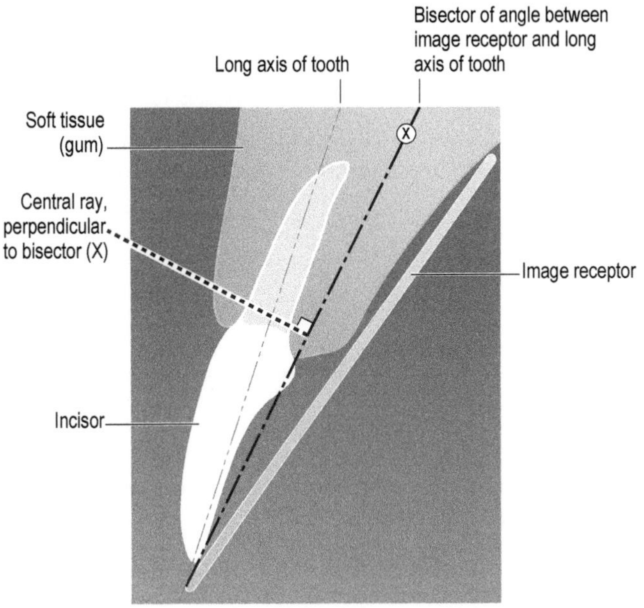

Fig. 14.14 The bisecting angle.

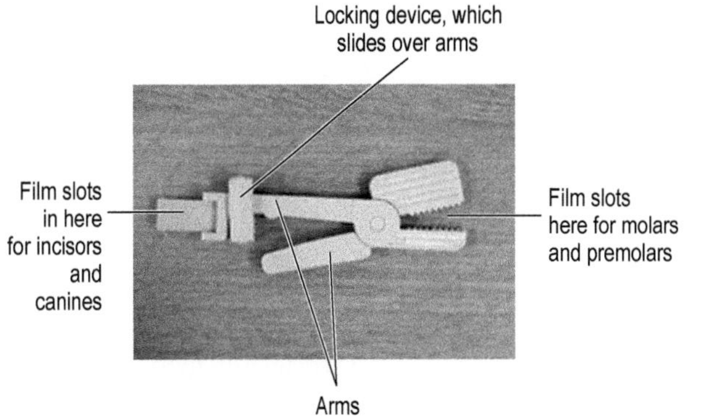

Fig. 14.15 Holder for bisecting angle technique.

Centring

Over the buccal surfaces of the teeth, to the centre of the IR

A guide for *approximate* angles for 'normally positioned' teeth is given in Table 14.3.

Collimation

A rectangular collimation device should always be used wherever possible and positioned so that it is in the same orientation as the IR in the mouth

Include

Include the crowns, roots and apices of the teeth under examination, as well as 3–4 mm of surrounding bone (and including below the apex)[6]

Criteria for Assessing Image Quality – Both Periapical Techniques[6]

- Crowns, roots of the teeth and 3–4 mm of surrounding bone (and including below the apex) are demonstrated
- Minimal evidence of elongation or foreshortening* of tooth/teeth; no overlap of adjacent teeth *if there is no overcrowding of teeth in that region*
- Sharp image showing contrast of the alveolar bone and its trabeculae, pulp cavity and enamel of the tooth/teeth

*Ideally there would be no evidence of foreshortening or elongation, but as there will always be some evidence of this owing to the arrangement of the teeth and gums, their exclusion cannot be expected.

Common Errors: Periapical Techniques

Common Errors – Both Periapical Techniques	Possible Reasons	Potential Effects on Image Interpretation[6–8]
Tooth apex and/or 3–4 mm of surrounding bone not visible on image	*Paralleling*: IR not positioned deeply enough in the patient's mouth and/or beam not perpendicular to the IR and arch of the teeth *Bisecting angle*: IR not positioned deeply enough in the patient's mouth and/or beam not perpendicular to the bisecting angle in the craniocaudal direction	Cannot differentiate health and disease in this region, in particular periapical inflammation. Other lesions may also be missed. This may result in missed or incorrect diagnosis (and possibly inappropriate treatment). These in turn carry potential for increased pain The root canal length of a tooth cannot be estimated for endodontic treatment planning if the whole tooth apex is not visible May miss root curvatures or close anatomical relationships (to neurovascular canals or the maxillary atrium, for instance) which may impact on surgical planning
Elongation of the teeth	*Paralleling*: Beam not perpendicular to the IR or arch of the teeth *Bisecting angle*: Not perpendicular to the bisecting angle in the craniocaudal direction	Periodontal bone loss can be exaggerated, potentially resulting in inappropriate treatment Signs of periapical problems can be magnified and/or appear larger than actual size, potentially resulting in inappropriate treatment It may not be possible to estimate root canal length if the whole tooth including the apex is not visible and/or it may be estimated as longer than it actually is. Either of these outcomes would impact on the effectiveness of any endodontic treatment
Foreshortening of teeth; cusps of premolars and molars seen en face and crown appears 'squat'	*Paralleling*: Beam not perpendicular to the IR or arch of the teeth *Bisecting angle*: Beam not perpendicular to the bisecting angle in the craniocaudal direction	Periodontal bone loss can be underestimated, potentially resulting in inappropriate treatment and avoidable patient pain Early signs of periapical problems can be hidden or appear smaller than actual size which may result in delayed treatment and possibly pain for the patient The root canal length of a tooth may be estimated as shorter than it actually is and therefore impact on the effectiveness of any endodontic treatment
Overlap of crowns at their interproximal surfaces	*Paralleling*: Beam not perpendicular to the IR *Bisecting angle*: Beam not perpendicular to bisecting angle in the mesiodistal direction – *unless* there is actual overlap of teeth in the mouth (both techniques)	If interproximal spaces are not visible then bone levels cannot be assessed Carious lesions may be hidden leading to a failure to treat at an early stage and further development of the caries, potentially causing pain for the patient Recurrent carious lesions may also be missed, potentially causing pain for the patient However, it should be noted that this error may be unavoidable in some areas of the mouth if the dentition is overcrowded and therefore some teeth overlap in the mouth

OCCLUSALS

As identified at the start of this chapter, occlusals have many uses, which are more specifically identified in Table 14.4.

There is one basic patient position used for most occlusals and this is described first, followed by the modification in position for true mandibular occlusals. Relevant tube displacements and angulations are listed after the description of the basic position, alongside the area demonstrated for each (Table 14.5).

IR suitable for occlusals is selected for all these examinations.

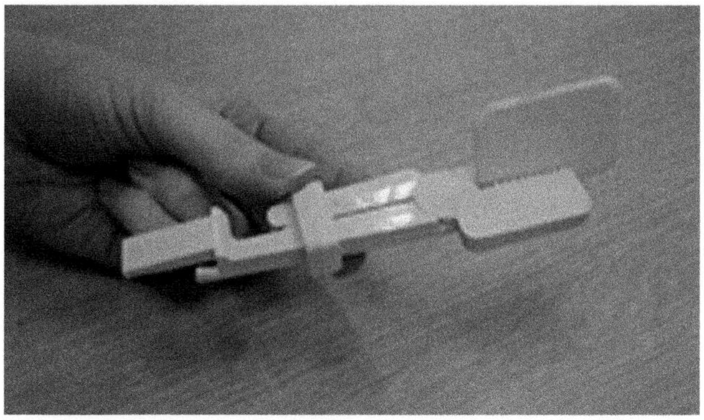

Fig. 14.16 Bisecting angle holder – film in holder for molars and premolars.

TABLE 14.3 Suggested Approximate Angulations for Bisecting Angle Periapical Technique*

Upper Teeth		Lower Teeth	
Incisors	55–60° caudal angle	Incisors	25–30° cranial angle
Canines	45–50° caudal angle	Canines	15–20° cranial angle
Premolars	35–40° caudal angle	Premolars	10° cranial angle
Molars	25–30° caudal angle	Molars	Horizontal beam

*The alatragal line must be horizontal for use with these angles.

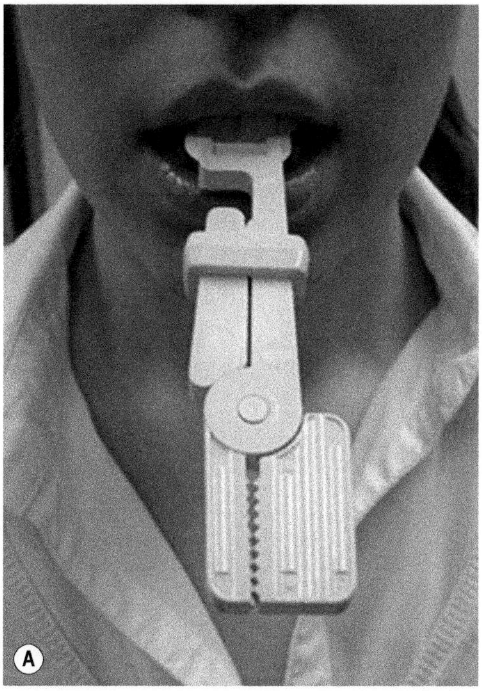

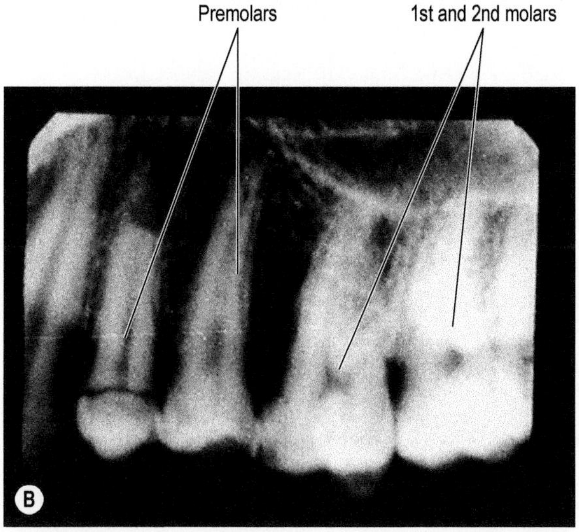

Fig. 14.17 (A) Bisecting angle holder – film in position for incisors; (B) bisecting angle periapical. (B, From Whaites E. *Essentials of Dental Radiography and Radiology*. 3rd ed. Edinburgh: Churchill Livingstone; 2002.)

TABLE 14.4 Occlusal Projections

Projection	Demonstrates
Standard maxillary occlusal (also known as upper anterior maxillary or 70° maxillary)	Upper incisors, canines, hard palate
Anterior oblique maxillary occlusal (also known as upper oblique)	Unerupted upper canines, upper premolars
Posterior oblique maxillary occlusal (also known as upper oblique or lateral maxillary)	Upper premolars and molars, floor of the maxillary antrum
Oblique mandibular occlusal (also known as lower oblique occlusal)	Unerupted lower canines, lower premolars and molars; the submandibular gland and the middle and posterior sections of the floor of mouth
45° submandibular occlusal (also known as anterior oblique mandibular)	Lower incisors, symphysis menti of mandible
Posterior true mandibular occlusal	Premolars, molars, mandible body
True submandibular occlusal (also known as anterior true mandibular or lower 90°)	Lower incisors, submandibular and sublingual ducts

Occlusal Positioning (Basic Head Positions)

- The patient is seated with their neck leaning on a support
- The IR is in the mouth, tube side upwards for maxillary teeth and down for mandibular teeth
- The IR is pushed back as far as possible, at least to the first molars and to include the incisors
- The midline of the IR is coincident with the MSP
- The teeth are closed over the IR and the MSP is vertical
- The *occlusal plane is horizontal* for most examinations
- *True mandibular occlusals* require extension of the neck as far as possible to bring the occlusal plane towards the vertical. In the case of the posterior oblique mandibular occlusal the patient's head also needs to be rotated away from the side of interest as much as possible. The head and neck are supported in this position

The basic positions are shown in Figs 14.18–14.22.

TABLE 14.5 Occlusal Projections: Beam Direction and Centring, and Criteria for Assessment of Image Quality

Area to Be Examined	Projection	Beam Direction and Centring
Upper incisors, canines, hard palate	Standard maxillary occlusal (Fig. 14.18A,B)	*Beam direction* 1. Initially vertical central ray; the tube head is in front of the patient's face, coincident with the MSP 2. The tube is then angled 20–25° towards the face, making a 20–25° angle with the IR *Centring* Over the nasal bone in the midline, to emerge over the middle of the IR
Unerupted upper canines, upper premolars	Anterior oblique maxillary occlusal (Fig. 14.19A,B)	*Beam direction* 1. Initially a horizontal central ray; the tube head is at the side of the head under examination, next to the eye and perpendicular to the MSP 2. The tube is angled 65° caudally, and then angled distally 45° until at 45° to the MSP *Centring* Over the edge of the ala of the nose on the side under examination, to emerge over the middle of the IR
Upper premolars and molars, floor of maxillary antrum	Posterior oblique maxillary occlusal	*Beam direction* 1. Initially a horizontal central ray; the tube head is at the side of the head under examination, next to the eye and perpendicular to the MSP 2. The tube is angled 65° caudally through the cheek *Centring* At the height level with the pupil, around 5 mm in front of the outer canthus of the eye[3]
Unerupted lower canines, lower premolars and molars; the submandibular gland and middle and posterior sections of floor of mouth	Oblique mandibular occlusal (Fig. 14.20A,B)	*Beam direction* 1. Initially a horizontal central ray; the tube head is at the side of the head under examination, next to the corner of the mouth and perpendicular to the MSP 2. The tube is angled 45° cranially, and then angled distally 45° until at 45° to the MSP *Centring* 2 cm below the angle of the mandible
Lower incisors, symphysis menti of mandible	45° submandibular occlusal (Fig. 14.21A,B)	*Beam direction* 1. Initially a horizontal central ray; the tube head is in front of the patient's face, coincident with the MSP 2. The tube is then angled 45° cranially *Centring* Under the symphysis menti, to emerge over the middle of the IR
Premolars, molars, mandible body	Posterior true mandibular occlusal	*Beam direction* The tube head is at the side of the head under examination; initially horizontal, the central ray is angled cranially until 90° to the occlusal plane, then displaced laterally approximately 1 cm along with the IR so that the buccal aspect of the dental arch can be demonstrated *Centring* Under the body of the mandible of the side to be imaged to emerge over the middle of the IR
Lower incisors, submandibular ducts	True submandibular occlusal (Fig. 14.22A,B)	*Beam direction* Initially horizontal, central ray is angled cranially until 90° to the occlusal plane *Centring* Under the symphysis menti to emerge over the middle of the IR

CRITERIA FOR ASSESSING IMAGE QUALITY

Standard maxillary occlusal	Anterior arch of the maxillary teeth back to the first molars are demonstrated. Incisors and canines are foreshortened; premolars and molars are demonstrated axially. Symmetry of the maxillary arch
Anterior oblique maxillary occlusal	Full length of incisors, canine and premolars including alveolar bone surrounding roots is demonstrated (on the side under examination). Incisors, canines and premolars are elongated (on the side under examination). Dental arch on the side under examination appears flattened. Superimposition of teeth on the side that is not under examination
Posterior oblique maxillary occlusal	Full length of canine, premolars and at least the first molar including alveolar bone surrounding roots is demonstrated (on the side under examination). The teeth demonstrated are elongated (on the side under examination). The anterior wall and floor of the maxillary antrum and some of the maxillary sinus space are demonstrated. Dental arch on the side under examination appears flattened. Superimposition of teeth on the side that is not under examination if demonstrated on the image
Oblique mandibular occlusal	Canines, premolars and at least the first molar of the side under examination are demonstrated. Mandibular arch on the side under examination appears flattened. Superimposition of teeth on the side that is not under examination. If the aim is to image the submandibular gland, then all molars should be visible and the lingual aspect of the floor of the mouth also. A soft-tissue exposure in such cases will improve the detection of small radio-opaque calculi in the duct and/or gland[3]
45° submandibular occlusal	Symphysis menti and mandibular arch back to first molars are demonstrated. Foreshortening of lower incisors. Superimposition of the teeth over the mandible
All projections except true mandibular occlusals	Sharp image demonstrating detail of the teeth under examination and their roots, in contrast to alveolar bone, pulp cavity and enamel

TABLE 14.5 Occlusal Projections: Beam Direction and Centring, and Criteria for Assessment of Image Quality—cont'd

Area to Be Examined	Projection	Beam Direction and Centring
Posterior true mandibular occlusal	Mandibular arch from canines to last molar on the side under examination is demonstrated. Mandibular arch is demonstrated axially (i.e. from below); all teeth included are foreshortened. Both the buccal and lingual aspect of the mandible body are demonstrated so that any expansion of the bone can be identified. Sharp image demonstrating the soft tissues of the floor of the mouth in contrast with the mandible	
True submandibular occlusal	Mandibular arch from incisors to first molars is demonstrated. Mandibular arch is demonstrated axially (i.e. from below); incisors and canines are foreshortened. Medial aspect of distal premolars overlying lingual aspect of the mandible. Sharp image demonstrating the soft tissues of the floor of the mouth in contrast with the mandible	

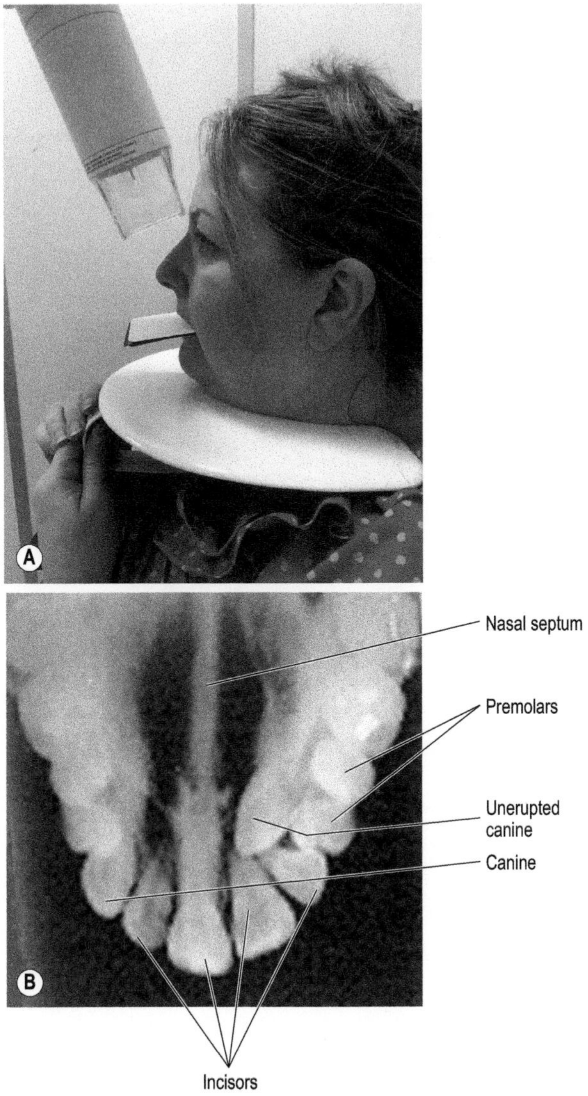

Fig. 14.18 65° standard maxillary occlusal.

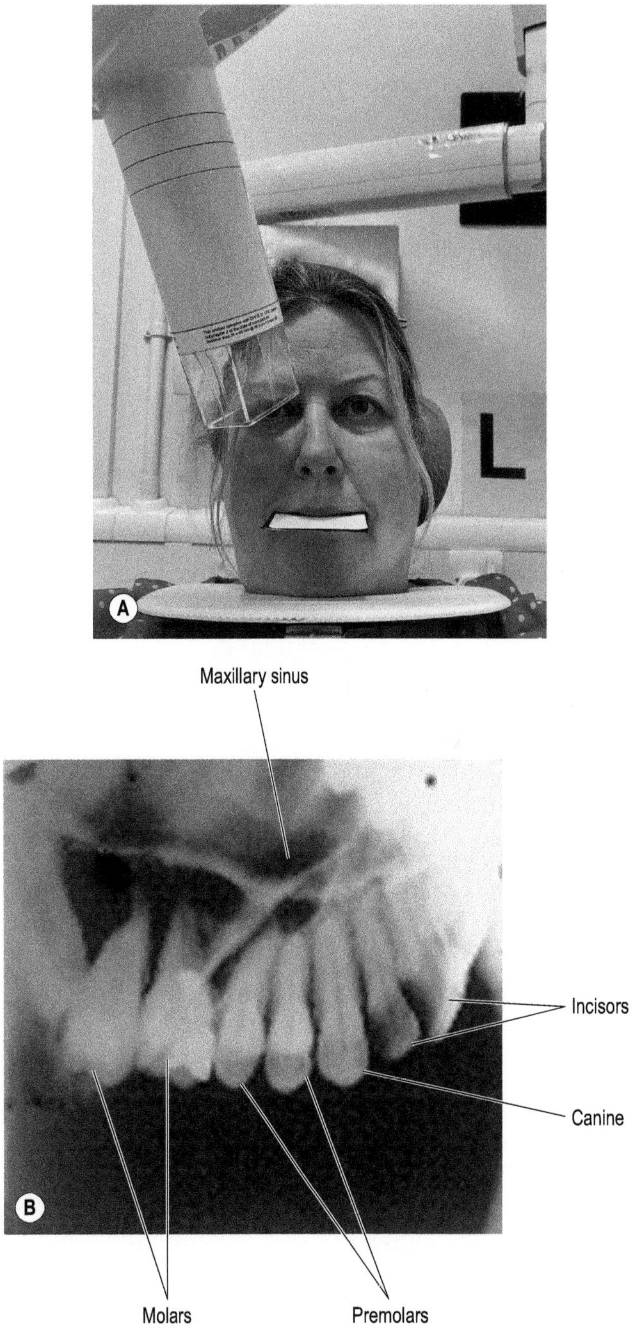

Fig. 14.19 Anterior oblique maxillary occlusal.

GENERAL COMMENT ON ERRORS– OCCLUSALS

Errors most commonly occur when the occlusal plane is not maintained in the correct relationship to the beam, or when the IR slips from the position prepared by the radiographer. For this reason it must be emphasised that initial patient preparation must include an explanation of the procedure to follow, reinforced by stressing the importance of immobilisation. The radiographer should also express understanding that the procedure may be uncomfortable for a short time.

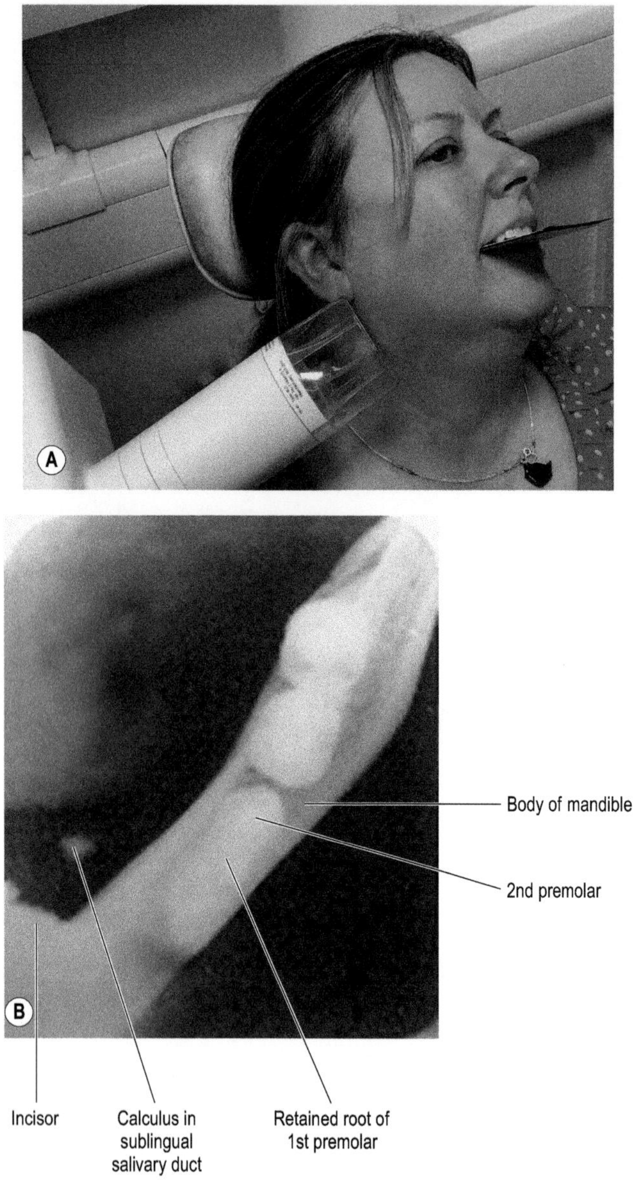

Fig. 14.20 Oblique mandibular occlusal.

PARALLAX PROJECTIONS FOR LOCALISATION

Despite the structure and position of teeth, which can cause problems for the radiographer when attempting to provide high-quality images of the dental area, the parallax principle can be applied in a number of ways to localise the position of unerupted teeth or individual roots on multi-rooted teeth in the mouth. The parallax principle states that two objects when viewed from different positions appear to alter their relative position to each other[10] and therefore, if the position of one of these objects is known, the position of the other can be identified via how it appears to move in relation to the X-ray tube head when two images of both objects are taken at different angles (Fig. 14.23).[7] Using the laws of geometry in conjunction with the rectilinear behaviour of the X ray beam, it is possible to assess direction of mislocation despite only having 2D information. In dental radiography this principle is applied using what is referred to as the *SLOB* rule in order to interpret radiographic appearances.

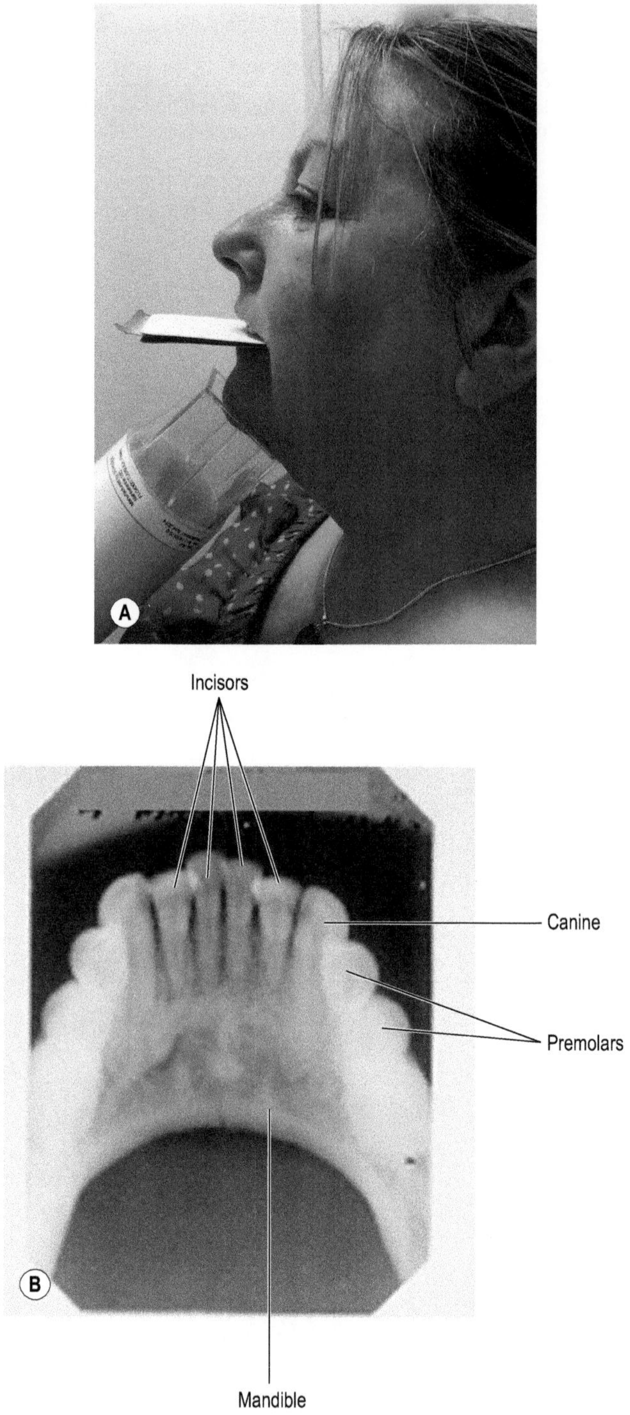

Fig. 14.21 45° submandibular occlusal.

SLOB Rule. If the object of unknown position appears to move in the same direction as the tubehead (on the image) then it is lingual/palatal to the object of known position; however, if it appears to move in the opposite direction to the tubehead then it is buccally/labially placed to the object of known position on the image.[7,8]

To summarise:

Same direction movement of object to tube head =
Lingual (palatal) tooth position
Opposite direction movement of tooth to tube head =
Buccal (labial) tooth position

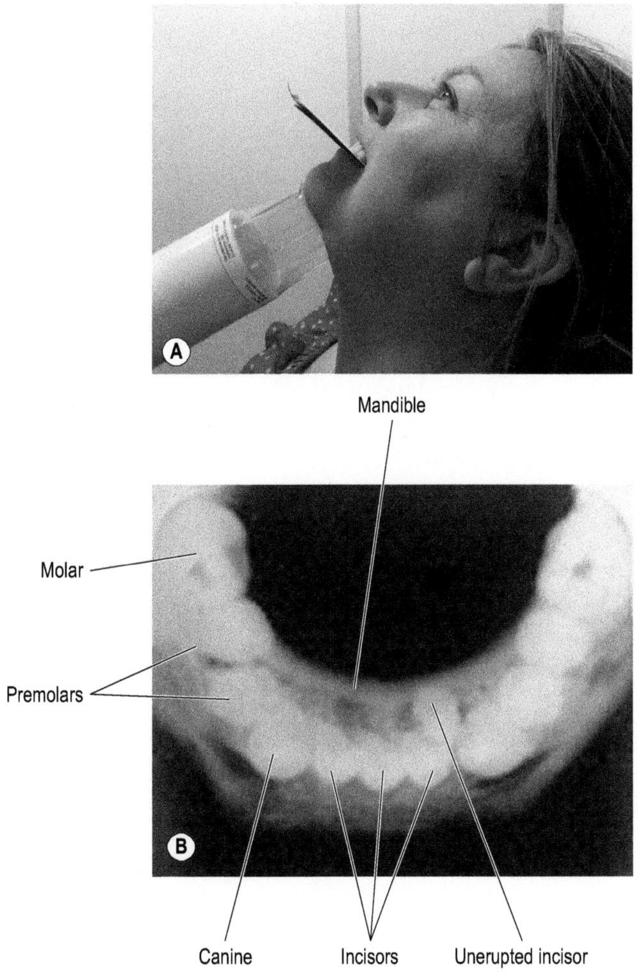
A
Mandible
Molar
Premolars
B
Canine
Incisors
Unerupted incisor

Fig. 14.22 (A) True submandibular occlusal. (B) Posterior true mandibular occlusal.

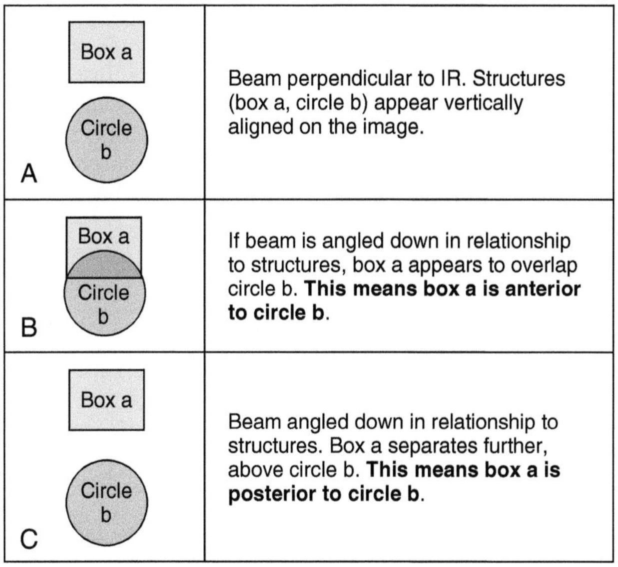
Box a
Circle b
A
Beam perpendicular to IR. Structures (box a, circle b) appear vertically aligned on the image.
Box a
Circle b
B
If beam is angled down in relationship to structures, box a appears to overlap circle b. This means box a is anterior to circle b.
Box a
Circle b
C
Beam angled down in relationship to structures. Box a separates further, above circle b. This means box a is posterior to circle b.

Fig. 14.23 Effects of beam angle change.

Identification and/or Separation of Root Canals in the Multi-rooted Tooth Using Parallax Technique

If a multi-rooted tooth (most commonly a molar) is to be endodontically (root-canal) treated, and treatment to be successful, then all roots need to be visualised and their length measured so they can be successfully filled. This may not be possible on a paralleling periapical if some roots are 'in line with each other' and perpendicular to the MSP (but buccally and lingually positioned in the tooth). In such cases parallax should be implemented using a paralleling approach wherever possible. A paralleling holder is used to position the IR; special holders are available for use during mid-endodontic procedure to ensure that the tooth surface is not used to bite on. However, it is recognised that bisecting angle may be needed, especially if the images are being taken mid-endodontic procedure when there is additional dental equipment in the mouth.[8] Two images are taken so that comparison can be made between the two beam directions used and show different positions of the tooth.

Positioning

- The patient is seated with their neck supported
- The IR is placed in a paralleling holder, the holder is placed in the mouth with the tube side of the IR facing the lingual surface of the teeth and an IR marker near the crown surface of the teeth *or*, if bisecting angle technique is being used, the IR has its tube side in contact with the lingual aspect of the crowns of the teeth. With either method, the IR is vertically aligned for incisors and canines and transversely for premolars and molars
- The tooth under examination is centred to the IR
- The patient closes their mouth over the holder to immobilise the IR and maintain its position
- The head is adjusted until the MSP is vertical and the occlusal plane is horizontal

Beam Direction

First image: Paralleling holder technique – the beam is aligned to the centre of the indicator on the paralleling holder, in the direction indicated by the holder

Bisecting angle technique – initially horizontal, which is then adjusted until at 90° to the bisector of the angle formed between the long axis of the tooth and the long axis of the IR

Second image: From the angle and direction selected for the first image, the tube is shifted 25–30° in a distal direction (to form a mesially directed angle of 25–30° to the beam used for the first image). For images taken with a paralleling holder this will result in the distal edge of the cone spacer/rectangular collimation still being in contact with the holder aiming device but the mesial edge will not be so.

Centring

Bisecting angle – over the buccal surfaces of the teeth to the centre of the receptor

When using either method – for the second image, the IR is displaced slightly in a mesial direction to ensure its centre is coincident with the central ray

Locating the Position of Unerupted Canines

Another common use of the parallax principle is to identify the position of an unerupted canine in relation to erupted anterior teeth. In these cases the principle can be applied in a number of ways depending on: the suspected position of the unerupted tooth; what previous imaging of the dental area, if any, has been carried out; and the familiarity with one technique or preference for a particular type of projection combination by the radiographer, referrer or reporter. However, given that most patients being imaged for this developmental abnormality are young, the chief intent of all involved should be to get the best quality images to identify the position of the canine, whilst exposing the patient to the lowest overall radiation dose possible.[11]

Often, DPT may have already been taken if the patient is to undergo orthodontic treatment. In such cases, a standard maxillary occlusal (if the unerupted canine appears to be nearer to the incisors on DPT), or an anterior oblique maxillary occlusal (if the unerupted canine appears to have a close relationship with the pre-molars), can be used to provide a vertical parallax.[8,11] The DPT/occlusal approach may also be advisable if the unerupted tooth is suspected to have a horizontal orientation and lies high within the maxilla in relation to the erupted teeth.[8] The use of one of the aforementioned occlusal projections in conjunction with a periapical in the canine region can also provide a vertical parallax, via which the unerupted canine can be localised if the unerupted tooth is closer to the erupted teeth.[11] Another way in which the parallax principle can be used to locate an unerupted canine is by taking two periapicals to produce a horizontal parallax: the first periapical should be centred over the central incisor region, while the second should be centred in between the lateral incisor and the first premolar, i.e. where an erupted canine would be in the mouth.[8]

Identification of Images and Location of Position of Parallax Images

Although it is essential that procedures for correct identification and image orientation are followed for all dental and other imaging procedures, parallax images need special attention to detail. It is vital that each image produced for the parallax examination is identified as to whether it is the initial image or the second image with tube shift. Only with accurate identification can the position of the tooth root or unerupted tooth be assessed. Images taken using film should be mounted or displayed side by side (for horizontal parallax) or one above the other (for vertical parallax), following the direction of the tubehead used in the examination, e.g. if the tubehead has been moved distally in the horizontal plane the second image should be mounted to the left of the first.[7] Digital images should be annotated with text indicating the direction of the tube head in relation to the tooth under examination and/or the X-ray beam. In order to assess the relative positions of the teeth both/all images taken during a parallax examination should be viewed thus: side by side for horizontal parallax, one above the other for vertical parallax.[7]

Dental Panoramic Tomography (DPT)

This technique requires the use of a specialised DPT unit (Fig. 14.24A,B), the tomographic principle being that which is used to produce the image of the full mouth and its dentition. The moving tube effectively blurs out the shadow of overlying structures by placing the dental arch in the axis of the tomographic movement. Structures not lying within this axis are effectively blurred, and so their detail does not overlie the image of the teeth and mandible. However, the area of interest does show some element of unsharpness compared to radiographic images of other body parts when a non-moving tube is used.

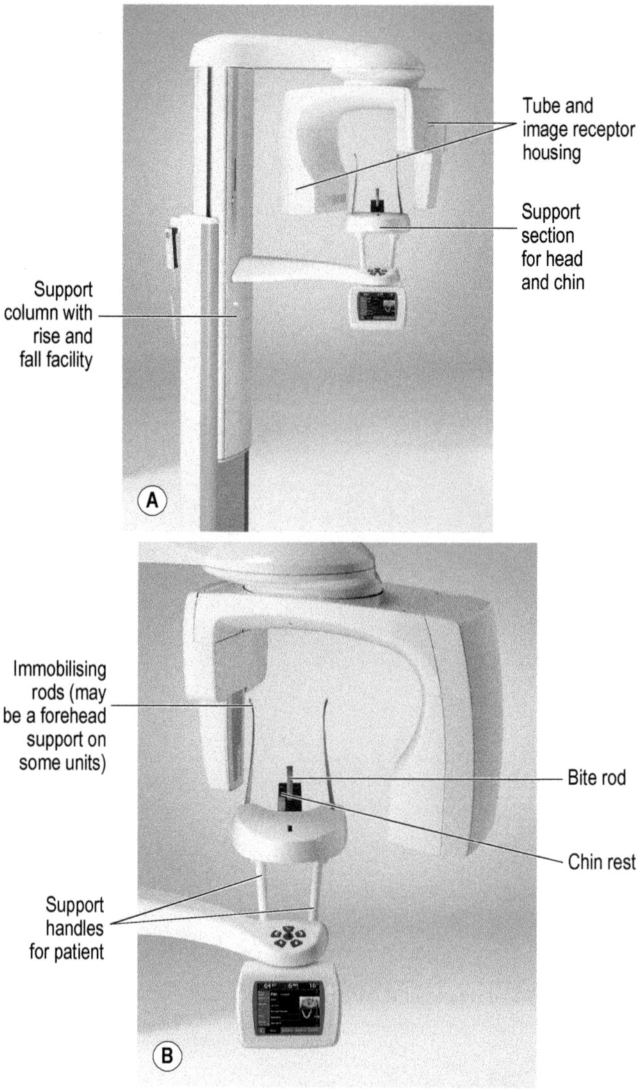

Fig. 14.24 DPT unit. (Reproduced with permission from Xograph Imaging Systems.)

The technique opens out the image of the dental arch to appear in a linear arrangement on the final image. In the dental setting DPT is most commonly taken prior to orthodontic treatment or oral surgery to remove wisdom teeth or multiple grossly carious teeth.[5] As mentioned in Chapter 13, the DPT examination can be used to demonstrate the temporomandibular joints and mandible.

The tomographic movement of the unit attempts to follow the dental arch, which it keeps within the tomographic axis of the beam as it travels around the patient's face – this is generally referred to as the focal trough. Accurate positioning is needed to place the dental arch in the focal trough and keep unwanted structures such as the cervical vertebrae clear of it.

Due to the range of DPT machine manufacturers and options available on purchase, the exact operator instructions will differ for each machine. However, to ensure good image quality a DPT machine usually includes:

- A chin rest
- A bite rod

- Head supports
- Positioning lights

The X-ray beam leaves the tube housing via a slit collimator and the thin beam moves around the dental arch and across the IR; this arrangement reduces the inevitable penumbra that would be caused by a wider beam. However, some penumbral effect is unavoidable.

The tomographic movement travels around the head with a horizontal beam, in opposition to traditional tomographic units that move over the supine patient and use a beam which is initially vertical and moves longitudinally or in a circular, elliptical or helical course.

Owing to the nature of this horizontal movement the use of the DPT unit may be distracting for the patient and so they should always be warned of it in advance of the exposure. Patient preparation, especially important for children and those with additional needs, may also include a demonstration of tube movement, using the 'test' setting if available. The unit is then returned to the start position.

If used, a DPT cassette is inserted into the erect cassette holder on the unit. Digital equipment incorporates the IR into the unit and DPT is selected on the unit.

Most DPT equipment now has the ability to collimate the images so that if the image is being used prior to dental surgery only one side, or even one quadrant/area of the mouth need be exposed to radiation, reducing overall radiation dose to the patient. Positioning for such examinations is identical to positioning for a full DPT and usually the machine will still make a full rotation of the patient although the exposure time is shorter, it is therefore crucial that the patient is prepared for this prior to exposure.

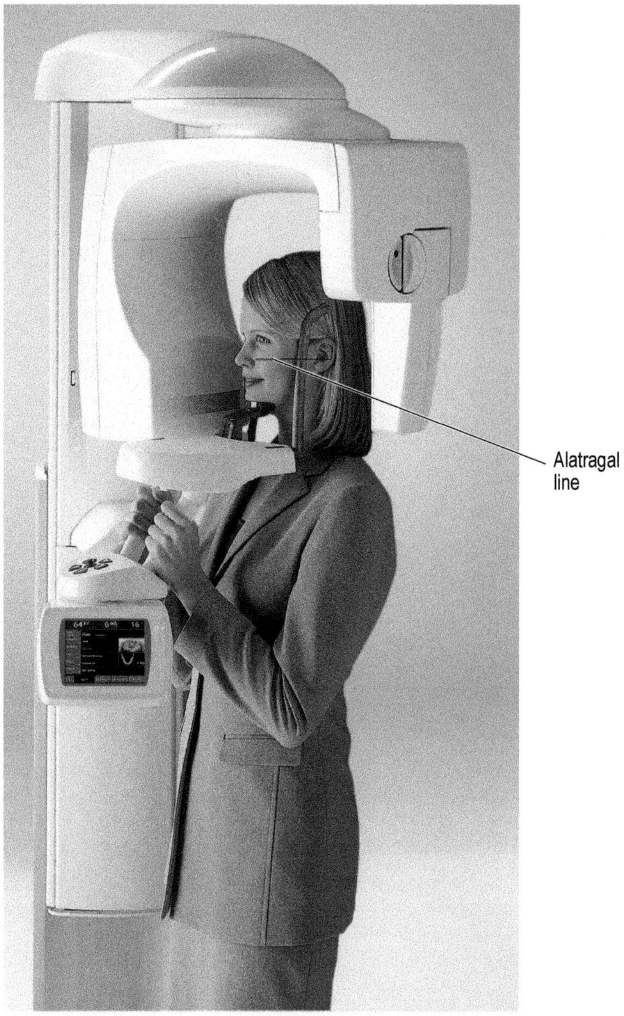

Fig. 14.25 Patient positioned in DPT unit. The patient's MSP is vertical and there must be no rotation. The alatragal line is horizontal, as indicated by the black line on the model. Note how the patient has stepped forward to bring the cervical vertebrae into the correct position. (Reproduced with permission from Xograph Imaging Systems.)

Positioning (Fig. 14.25)

- The patient is asked to remove all artefacts from the head and neck area – jewellery, dentures, removable orthodontic appliances, etc.
- A clean bite rod is inserted into the chin rest, or a disposable plastic cover is applied to the permanent bite rod
- The patient is seated or standing with their chin resting on the chin support
- The patient bites with their central incisors in the groove on the bite rod, to effect separation of teeth on the image
- The patient holds onto the support handles and is asked to step forward slightly to bring the cervical spine vertical. If seated, their chair is pulled forward by the radiographer
- The radiographer then uses the positioning lights to ensure that:
  - The MSP is vertical and perpendicular to the bite rod
  - The height of the unit is adjusted until the anthropological baseline is parallel to the floor
  - The final third light is positioned over the interproximal space between the upper lateral incisor and the canine teeth – to do this the radiographer needs to ask the patient to open their lips so the teeth can be seen, if the patient is edentulous this light should be lined up with the corner of the mouth
- Throughout this manoeuvre the head must not tilt or rotate and the chin must not lift or drop
- The head clamp is applied for immobilisation
- The patient is then asked to close their lips and press their tongue forwards against the teeth and the roof of the mouth for the duration of the exposure
- Exposure is made after a reminder to the patient to keep still during tube movement

Criteria for Assessing Image Quality (Fig. 14.26)[6]

For a full DPT:

- All of the mandible, including symphysis menti inferiorly and condyles superiorly, is demonstrated. The hard palate and lower part of the maxillary sinuses are demonstrated
- Dentition is demonstrated in a horizontal line
- Bite rod is shown between upper and lower central incisors with separation of occlusal surfaces of all teeth
- All teeth are seen relatively sharply
- Slightly blurred shadow of the anterior aspect of the neck structures is superimposed over images of the incisors; sharper image of bodies of the cervical vertebrae seen at both lateral edges of the image, cleared from the area of interest
- Mandible outline is continuous and not 'stepped'

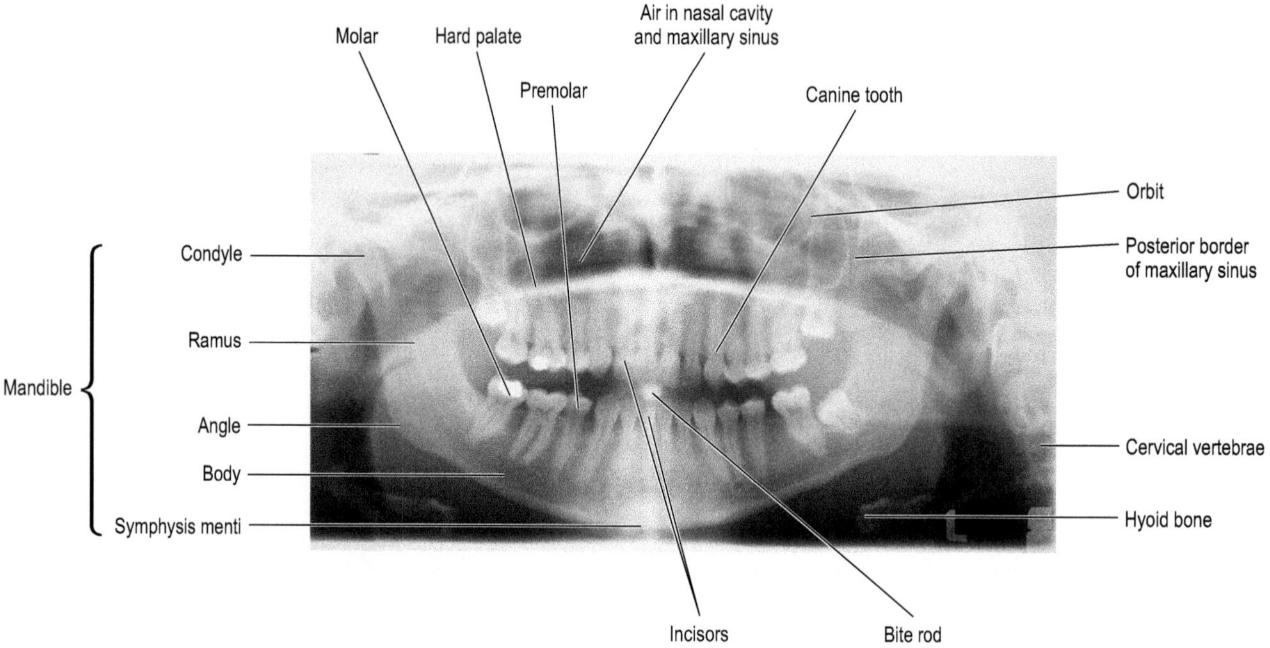

Fig. 14.26 DPT image.

Common Errors: Dental Panoramic Tomography

Common Errors	Possible Reasons	Potential Effects on Image Interpretation[8,12]
Dark band seen across the roots and upper aspect of crowns of upper teeth	Tongue not depressed against roof of mouth during exposure; lips may not be closed	Hard tissue structures may not be visible as the air shadow is overlying them Periapical inflammation on maxillary teeth can be masked or mimicked An extensive air image may also conceal or mimic caries
Step appears in the image, particularly noticeable over the mandibular outline	Patient may have moved their mandible during exposure	Not possible to rule out fracture of the mandible or anomalous morphology Cannot differentiate health and disease in affected area
Part of the image is blurred whereas the rest appears sharp	Patient movement at some point during exposure, but not throughout exposure	Cannot differentiate health and disease in blurred area
Dentition layout not seen as horizontal, occlusal plane appears to 'smile'; mandibular incisors may be blurred and slightly magnified; complete TMJ region may not be shown if full DPT image is required	Occlusal plane not horizontal; chin is lowered slightly	Cannot differentiate all health and disease in mandibular anterior area If the complete TMJ region is not visible then it is not possible to assess and report on the health of this area
Dentition layout not seen as horizontal, mouth appears upturned (sulking); maxillary incisors may be slightly blurred and magnified	Occlusal plane not horizontal; chin is raised slightly	Cannot differentiate health and disease in maxillary anterior area
Dentition layout not seen as horizontal, appears tilted. Unsharp posterior teeth	MSP not vertical	Cannot differentiate all health and disease in unsharp area
Middle section of the mandible not seen sharply Unequal magnification of the teeth, one side of the jaw appears much larger or smaller than the other; mandibular condyles are at different levels relative to the edge of the image if full DPT image taken	MSP rotated; some or all of the patient's teeth and alveolar bone do not lie within the focal trough, being asymmetrically related to it	It may appear that the patient has facial asymmetry when they do not Cannot differentiate health and disease in the condylar or anterior regions of the jaw
Very narrow incisors; cervical vertebrae may be seen centrally	Patient's chin too far forward into the unit so the teeth and alveolar bone do not lie within the focal trough, but are anterior to it	Cannot differentiate health and disease in anterior region
Broad, unsharp incisors; these are sometimes likened to 'piano keys'; large white ghost shadows of the opposite mandible visible over posterior teeth	Patient's chin not far enough into the unit so the teeth and alveolar bone do not lie within the focal trough, but are posterior to it	Difficult to differentiate health and disease in any area as central area blurred and ghost shadows can overlie structures and pathology in the focal trough more posteriorly
Prominent image of cervical vertebrae superimposed over the incisors	Patient is not standing erect in the machine. Instead the patient is leaning forwards and the upper part of the cervical spine lies more anteriorly than the lower part	Cannot differentiate health and disease in anterior region

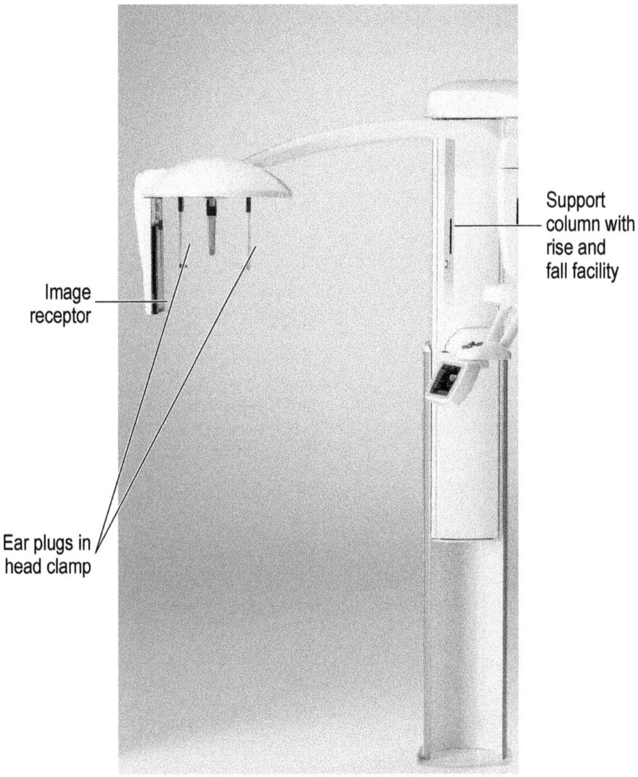

Fig. 14.27 Cephalometry unit. (Reproduced with permission from Xograph Imaging Systems.)

Cephalometry

Prior to maxillofacial surgery and orthodontic treatment it is usually necessary to examine the relationship of the soft tissues of the face to facial bones and teeth. This is most commonly done using a lateral cephalograph projection. After treatment, further assessment is made and it is therefore essential that all images in the series are comparable. To ensure that this is the case, specialised equipment is used to produce consistent images.

The unit can be independent or form part of a unit that has dual function for DPT and lateral cephalometric applications. An example of a cephalometry unit is shown in Fig. 14.27. Whether the cephalometry unit is combined, or not, its structure usually includes:

1. Fixed focus receptor distance (FRD): this is most often 180 cm but in any case a minimum 150 cm should be used to minimise magnification and geometric unsharpness. If the object receptor distance (ORD) can be altered in a unit, the distance of the MSP from the IR must be registered to allow accurate assessment; a measurement facility may be found on the nasion support (see point 3, below).
2. Head clamps with ear plugs. These are inserted into the external auditory meati (EAMs) to ensure accurate and consistent positioning.
3. Nasion support, which slides in an anteroposterior direction in relation to the patient. This ensures that different-sized heads can be immobilised in the unit. The nasion support also usually contains a radiopaque ruler which can be used by the orthodontic/surgical team to measure the magnification in the image and therefore take account of this when using the image to take measurements for surgical planning. If a ruler is not built into the machine then a radiopaque object or distance of known size needs to be on the images so magnification can be calculated.
4. A filter that is used to compensate for the range in density from facial soft tissue to facial bones. If a digital IR system is being used the soft tissue filter will probably be added as part of the image post processing after exposure. For film or CR systems the filter can be permanently situated in the tube head (both free-standing and DPT units) or, in older equipment, an aluminium wedge is attached to the light beam diaphragm.
5. If used, a 24×30 cm cassette is placed longitudinally in the erect cassette holder on the unit. For digital units, the cephalometry option is selected on the unit.

In newer cephalometry units it is possible to change the size of the field of view and exposure factors depending on the size of the patient; this should be used whenever possible to reduce radiation dose. Additionally, many digital cephalometry units use a scanning method, in which a narrow X-ray slit beam slowly moves past the patient to build up an image. While it is recognised that this method can reduce the patient radiation dose considerably,[2] it should also be noted that movement artefact is more likely because the overall exposure time will be longer than a static method. Movement of the machine past the patient can be unnerving, so they need to be warned of this in advance of exposure.

LATERAL CEPHALOMETRY (FIGS 14.28, 14.29)

Positioning

- The patient is erect with their MSP parallel to the IR
- The height of the unit is adjusted until the earplugs can be placed in the EAMs to immobilise the head
- The occlusal plane is horizontal
- The nasion support is positioned in contact with the nasion
- If not applied at the post processing stage or permanently situated within the tube housing, a wedge filter is inserted over the light beam diaphragm with its thicker end aligned over the soft tissues of the face
- The patient is asked to close their back teeth and relax the lips; this is maintained during exposure

Beam Direction

Horizontal, at 90° to the IR; this is fixed for most units

Centring

Over the earplugs and the middle of the IR; this is fixed for most units

Collimation

Smallest field of view possible should be selected but resultant images should show ear plugs and all facial features including soft tissue outlines of the forehead, face/nose and mandible

Criteria for Assessing Image Quality[6]

- Soft tissue outline of face including forehead, nose, lips and chin are demonstrated
- Whole of mandible and ear plugs are demonstrated
- Superimposition of both the ear plugs and of the right and left facial structures
- Anthropological baseline is horizontal
- Sharp image demonstrating detail of the facial bones *and* soft tissues of the face

Common Errors: Lateral Cephalometry

Common Errors	Possible Reasons	Potential Effects on image interpretation[3,8]
Patient not biting together in centric occlusion and/or lips are not relaxed	Patient was not instructed to do so or has released their bite. However, it should be noted that if cephalometry is being carried out mid-treatment, some patients, typically those using functional appliances, may be unable to achieve a centric occlusion[8]	As measurements for treatment planning are taken from all cephalograph images, any error may have an impact on the effectiveness of resultant patient treatments
Radiopaque markers in the ear plugs appear separated and/or lack of superimposition of craniofacial bones that is not consistent with patient's appearance and clinical information	Patient is rotated/MSP is not parallel to the IR; if the ear plugs are not inserted fully this is also likely to impinge upon positioning of the MSP	
Nasion ruler or object of known size not visible	Nasion support not touching the nasion; field of view not big enough	
Nose and/or chin missing off image	Field of view not big enough; ear plugs are not inserted fully and/or nasion support not in position and patient has moved forward	
Soft tissues of the face too dark	Filter not applied, or not selected on the unit	
Chin too high	Anthropological baseline not horizontal	
Denser soft tissues below the chin in comparison with the other soft tissues of the face	Anthropological baseline not horizontal; the chin is down and increases the density of the soft tissues under the mandible	

Cone Beam Computed Tomography

Cone beam computed tomography (CBCT) has been developing for dental and maxillofacial applications since the end of the 20th century. It is also sometimes referred to as digital volume tomography, cone beam volumetric tomography or cone beam imaging. CBCT provides a high-resolution 3D dataset of the region of interest. This is achieved via an imaging technique in which the patient is positioned in the centre of an imaging gantry. It uses an X-ray source that generates a cone-shaped beam on one side and an IR, usually a silicon flat panel detector, on the other (Fig. 14.30). The patient is immobilised using head supports and, if standing or sitting erect, a chin rest. Most commonly, two initial scout views are then taken (lateral and PA) so that the exact size and position of the field of view (FoV) to be included can be set. The gantry then moves around the patient, 180° or 360°, to collect hundreds of 2D images, which in turn are then reformatted via computer software algorithms to create 3D images. The resultant image display usually shows series images in axial, coronal and sagittal planes as well as a 3D 'volume-rendered' image. Secondary multiplanar reconstruction can then be used to produce cross-sectional images in other planes, such as following the dental arch, to provide further diagnostic information.

While the radiation dose to the patient of CBCT is significantly lower than conventional CT it is still higher than standard dental imaging techniques, it should therefore not be used routinely as a dental imaging technique.[1,3,5,8,11] Most CBCT machines have the ability to limit the size of the FoV covered by the circular beam, sometimes to as small as 40×40 mm. Small FoV can cover single teeth and/or small regions of the jaws; medium FoV are designed to cover most of the dental region, while large FoV usually include the whole craniofacial region, including cranial base and skull vault.[3,8] As previously stated at the beginning of the chapter, the smallest FoV possible should be used that will still provide all the clinical information needed, whilst keeping the radiation dose to the patient to a minimum.[1,5,11,13] European guidelines[13] do, however, acknowledge that CBCT may provide additional clinical information at a lower dose than other conventional methods for planning orthognathic surgery and dental implant placement. Several guideline documents[5,11,13] also state that small field CBCT may also help plan treatment in the following situations when standard dental imaging projections have proved inconclusive:

- Following dental trauma
- Assessment of the position of unerupted teeth
- Localisation of multiple roots prior to endodontic procedures

Advantages and disadvantages of CBCT imaging can be seen in Table 14.6.

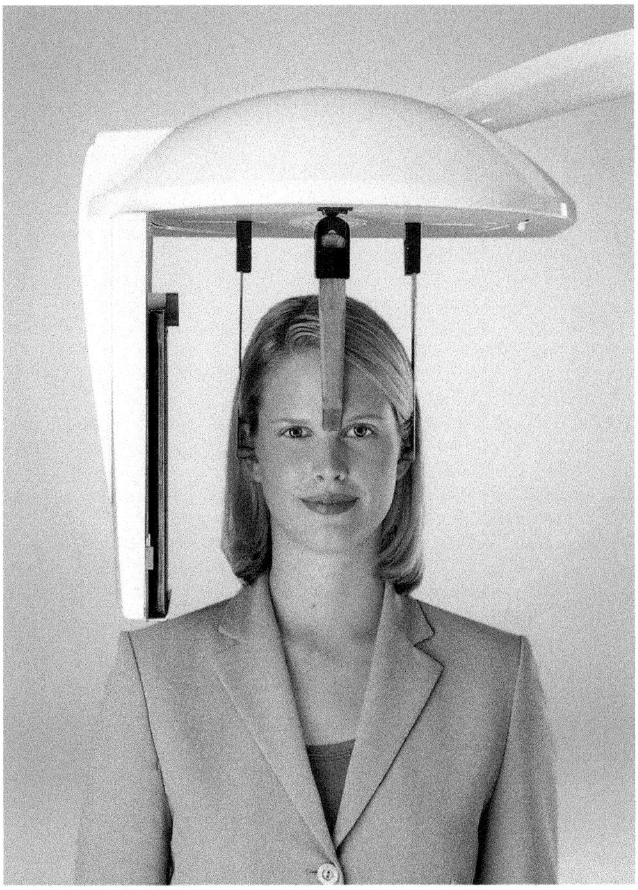

Fig. 14.28 Positioning the patient for lateral cephalometry.

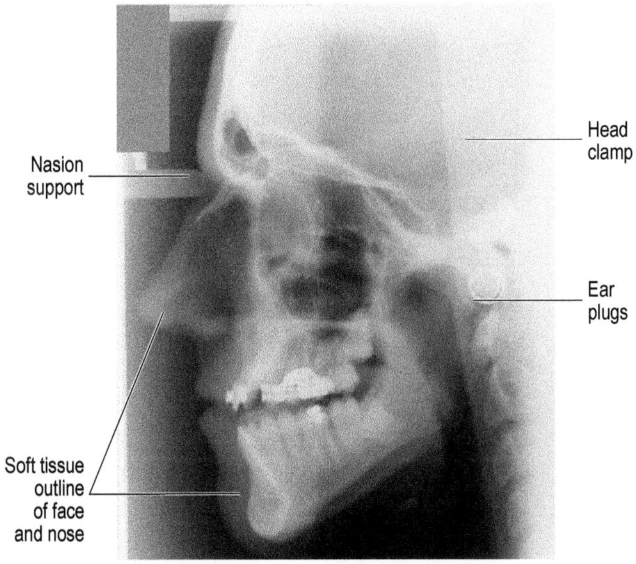

Fig. 14.29 Lateral cephalometry image.

Patient Positioning

Like DPT and cephalometry equipment, there is a large range of CBCT machines available and so operator instructions and patient positions will differ. Supine systems are available but most systems require the patient to sit or stand in the gantry. Positioning is similar to that of a conventional DPT examination. Thyroid collar use is considered good practice[8,11] (except for scout projections if the unit is fitted with AEC,[1] as previously stated). If the CBCT machine has a chair attached as part of the imaging system this will have a weight limit which should be taken into consideration. Some manufacturers now provide so called 'hybrid' units that can perform CBCT as well as conventional 2D DPT and cephalometry examinations.

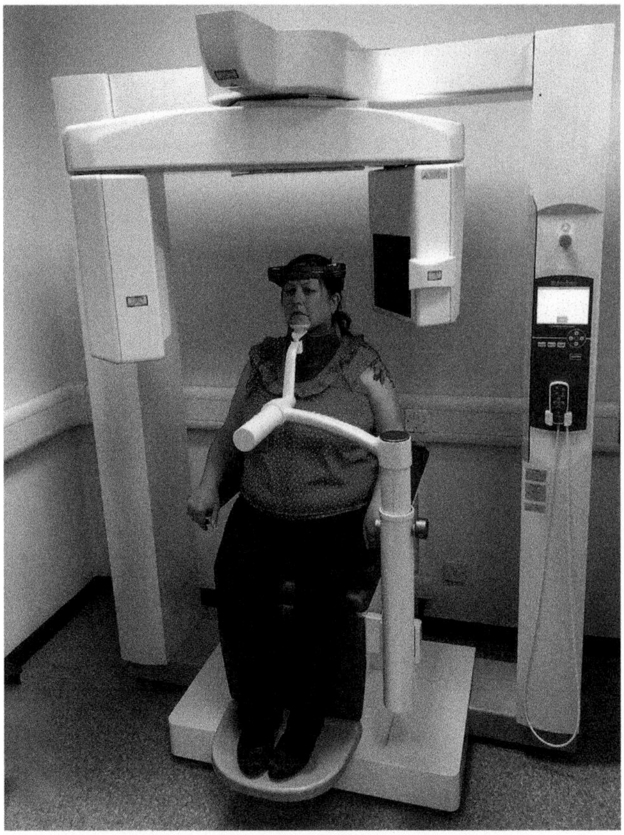

Fig. 14.30 Patient positioned in cone beam CT unit.

TABLE 14.6 Advantages and Disadvantages of Cone Beam Computed Tomography of the Dental and Maxillofacial Region

Advantages	Disadvantages
3D dental-specific imaging provided	Units are expensive when compared with conventional DPT units
High contrast resolution allowing excellent depiction of bony detail	Soft-tissue contrast is limited
Short exposure time	Even slight patient movement can result in blurred images
Multiplanar reconstruction possible	Few or no FoV options on some systems
Resultant images are highly accurate so bone and tooth related measurements can be easily made	Metal-related streak and beam hardening artefacts from dental restorations may result in clinical information being hidden
Lower radiation dose than conventional CT in most cases	Limited availability compared with conventional CT

Criteria for Assessing Image Quality[13]

- All of the area of interest included in the scan volume
- Minimal streak artefacts over the area of interest
- No blurring on the resultant images
- Adequate contrast and brightness

In Europe all CBCT examinations should be carried out under the supervision of a dentist, dental specialist or dental and maxillofacial radiologist who has 'adequate theoretical and practical training' in CBCT, it is also the responsibility of this person to ensure that the resultant CBCT images are adequately reported.[13] Therefore, if the radiographer is in any doubt about CBCT image quality they should always seek the advice of the supervising clinician.

References

1. Public Health England (PHE) and Faculty of General Dental Practice (UK) (FGDP[UK]). *Guidance Notes for Dental Practitioners on the Safe Use of X-ray Equipment.* 2nd ed. London, UK: PHE and FGDP(UK); 2020.
2. Holroyd JR, Smith JRH, Edyvean S. *PHE-CRCE-51: Dose to Patients from Dental Radiographic X-ray Imaging Procedures in the UK – 2017 Review.* London: Public Health England (PHE); 2019.
3. Whitley AS, Jefferson G, Holmes K, et al. *Clark's Positioning in Radiography.* 13th ed. Boca Raton, FL: CRC Press; 2015.
4. Horner K, Drage N, Brettle D. *21st Century Dental Imaging.* London: Quintessence Publishing; 2008.
5. Horner K, Eaton KA, eds. *Selection Criteria for Dental Radiography.* 3rd ed. London: Faculty of General Dental Practice (UK); 2018.
6. European Commission Directorate-General for the Environment. *Radiation Protection No. 136: European Guidelines on Radiation Protection in Dental Radiology: The Safe Use of Radiographs in Dental Practice.* Luxembourg: Office for Official Publications of the European Communities; 2004.
7. Horner K, Rout J, Rushton VE. *Interpreting Dental Radiographs.* London: Quintessence Publishing; 2002.
8. Whaites E, Drage N. *Essentials of Dental Radiography and Radiology.* 5th ed. London: Churchill Livingstone Elsevier; 2013.
9. Unett EM, Royle AJ. *Radiographic Techniques and Image Evaluation.* London: Chapman and Hall; 1997.
10. Harty FJ. *Concise Illustrated Dental Dictionary.* 2nd ed. Oxford: Butterworth Heinemann; 1994 (reprint 2001).
11. Isaacson KG, Thorn AR, Atack NE, et al. *Guidelines for the Use of Radiographs in Clinical Orthodontics.* 4th ed. London: British Orthodontic Society; 2015.
12. Rushton VE, Rout J. *Panoramic Radiography.* London: Quintessence Publishing; 2006.
13. European Commission Directorate-General for Energy. *Radiation Protection No. 172: Cone Beam CT for Dental and Maxillofacial Radiology. Evidence-Based Guidelines.* Luxembourg: Office for Official Publications of the European Communities; 2012.

15 Chest and Thoracic Skeleton

ELIZABETH CARVER and PETER SUTTON

Plain radiographic examination of the chest, in particular the posteroanterior (PA) projection, is considered to be the most commonly performed examination in the imaging department and is still used every day. Current guidelines suggest chest X-ray is useful in the following cases:

- Acute chest pain
- Suspected aortic dissection
- Suspected pulmonary embolism
- Suspected pericarditis/pericardial effusion, myocarditis, heart failure
- Chronic angina (stable)
- Suspected heart valve disease
- Congenital heart disease
- Pneumonia
- Pleural effusion
- Haemoptysis
- Insertion or removal of devices in the very sick[1]

Since the late 20th century there has been a reduction in referrals for X-ray imaging due to evolving referral guidelines but there still exists a wide range of referral reasons that are still considered valid. Plain radiography of the chest was used more extensively in the 20th century than today and is no longer justified in the following cases:

- Non-cardiac-related chest pain
- Screening medicals (with exception of high-risk immigrants and those who need employment-specific imaging; for example, 'deep sea divers')
- Upper respiratory tract infection[2,3]
- 'Routine' preoperative chest[4]

Common Findings on the Chest Image

Common findings on the chest image include abscess; atelectasis; bullae; calcifications; cardiomegaly; consolidation; emphysema; empyema; fibrosis; haemothorax; hiatus hernia; hilar enlargement or displacement; mastectomy; mediastinal enlargement (including lymph node enlargement); metastasis; neoplasm; pleural effusion; pleural plaques; pneumonectomy; pneumonia; pneumoperitoneum; pneumothorax; pulmonary oedema; raised diaphragm/s; rib fractures; thyroid goitre; tracheal shift; vertebral collapse.

Note that this is not a fully comprehensive list of all indications for referral for chest radiography; it is a resumé of commonly encountered appearances.

The Chest X-ray and Infectious Patients

The chest X-ray is commonly undertaken on patients who carry serious infection risk for hospital staff and other patients. If the infection risk relates to disease that can seriously affect morbidity and mortality, then special measures must be followed in order to avoid cross-infection.

Radiographers should be familiar with, and closely follow, the cross-infection policy that is provided by their hospital infection prevention and control team.

Examples of diseases that will require special measures:

- Pulmonary tuberculosis (TB)
- SARS-CoV-2 (COVID-19)
- Extended spectrum beta lactamase (ESBL)-producing coliforms
- Methicillin-resistant *Staphylococcus aureus* (MRSA)
- Viral diarrhoea and vomiting
- Other multi-resistant organisms
- H1N1 influenza
- Chicken pox
- *Clostridium difficile*
- Meningitis
- *Escherichia coli*

On infectious patients the majority of chest radiography is undertaken using a mobile X-ray unit, most often on the ward; to bring the patient to the imaging department would extend the risk to patients and staff in that department. In situations where there is an epidemic, dedicated rooms may be made available just for X-ray examination of infection risk patients; these may be either a dedicated permanent X-ray room that has temporarily been commissioned for the duration of the epidemic, or a dedicated room that houses a mobile X-ray unit (consideration for the latter must be made with regard to radiation protection, in that there should be no direct risk to personnel immediately outside that room). A DR mobile unit is most suitable for the second option, rather than CR, to ensure that there are as low a number of stages possible that could potentially transfer infection.

Regarding undertaking the examination safely, specific hospital protocols will vary, but advice will reflect the following principles:

Personal protective equipment (PPE) must be worn by the health professional during the examination, and removal/disposal of that equipment will in itself carry guidance. The infection type will dictate the level of required PPE but the most serious infections will require medical mask, gown, gloves and eye protection to be worn. For some infections N95 or FFP3 masks are likely to be mandatory and staff must undergo a mask fitting procedure prior to use of these. Donning and doffing of PPE must be done in accordance with standard operating procedures and staff must be familiar with these to ensure safe use of PPE.

Imaging examinations require the presence of two radiographers: one to position the IR (and therefore handle the patient) and one who handles equipment that is not in contact with the patient. All equipment should be cleaned after use. The IR should be in a cover that can be disposed of in an appropriate clinical waste bag after the examination.

PPE must be removed in a designated room/area outside the examination room, and disposed of in the appropriate clinical waste bags as designated by the cross-infection policy. Guidance on the order in which to remove PPE is also given in any policy, but usually all items are removed before gloves are removed. Hands are then washed thoroughly with soap and water.

The Erect PA Chest Projection and Comments on Its Implementation

The erect posteroanterior (PA) chest projection is the primary method for demonstration of the thoracic contents and it is universally acknowledged that this is the gold standard for demonstrating the chest. Reasons for this are straightforward and logical.

Erect

1. Undertaking the projection in the erect position allows for demonstration of unnaturally located fluid, which finds its natural level within the thoracic cavity and is well demonstrated as more dense in appearance than the air-filled lung tissue. In the supine position this pleural fluid will lie posteriorly in a layer that will show as an increased density over the hemithorax in which it lies; this density may overlie other pathology.[5] Wherever possible, radiographers should undertake chest radiography erect; in the case of the infirm patient an erect sitting projection is a suitable alternative and this can be achieved using a stool or, preferably, a commercially built chair designed for stability and versatility. These chairs have wheels for manoeuvrability, wheel locks for stability, and removable back and arms for versatility. A PA erect chest can therefore be undertaken with the chair back removed but chair arms in place (Fig. 15.1A–D). For patients who must remain in a wheelchair, on a trolley or bed, an erect anteroposterior (AP) projection can be undertaken.
2. Inspiratory effort is more effective when the thorax is in the erect position.

Posteroanterior (PA)

1. The PA projection allows forward tilt of the thorax to elevate the lung apices above the clavicles. TB frequently manifests itself in the lung apex, thereby indicating the importance of clearing this area from the image of the clavicles (although a lordotic projection will clear the clavicles entirely above the apices, allowing visualisation of the lung apex without superimposition of the clavicles over the lower apical portion). Numbers of reported cases of TB in the 21st century are relatively insignificant in the UK compared to incidence historically (up until the first half of the 20th century), but it is by no means non-existent and World Health Organization (WHO) reports show that TB is still very much considered to be a challenge globally.[6] In addition to revealing the lung apices, forward tilt also avoids a lordotic appearance of the image; lordosis affects the accuracy of cardiothoracic ratio (CT ratio) assessment for cardiomegaly and reduces the apparent position of the diaphragm.
2. The chin can easily be supported clear of the apices by resting it upon the upper border of the IR.
3. As the heart lies anteriorly within the thorax (Fig. 15.2) the degree of magnification of this organ is minimised in the PA position; again, in assessment of the CT ratio, minimal magnification is preferred.
4. In an adult woman, compression of breast tissue against the IR will reduce body thickness and ensure the lowest exposure factor settings can be used.
5. It is acknowledged that the use of PA projections reduces the radiation dose to anteriorly positioned radiosensitive organs, owing to the higher average beam energy after travelling through the posterior portions of the chest (thereby producing less absorption in these anterior organs). The sternum and female breasts lie within the field of primary radiation and will also benefit from reduction of dose in the PA position.
6. Obliquity of the X-ray beam at the periphery of the thorax will assist projection of the scapulae away from the area of the lung fields. The angle of this obliquity is likely to vary, as the distance of the scapulae from the central ray will differ according to the width of the chest, but it is likely that this angle will be quite small, even in the patient who has a wide chest. Examples of such angles of obliquity of the beam at 2 m focus receptor distance (FRD), at different points around the beam centre (when using a central ray at 90° to the IR) and using geometric calculations, are given below as approximate figures (figures are given to the nearest decimal point).

Distance from Centring Point (cm)	Angle of Oblique Rays at This Point (2 m FRD)
12	3.4°
17	4.8°
21.5	6.2°

Comments on Exposure Technique Selection

In order to image the lung tissue adequately in contrast to air within the thorax, for the most part of the 20th

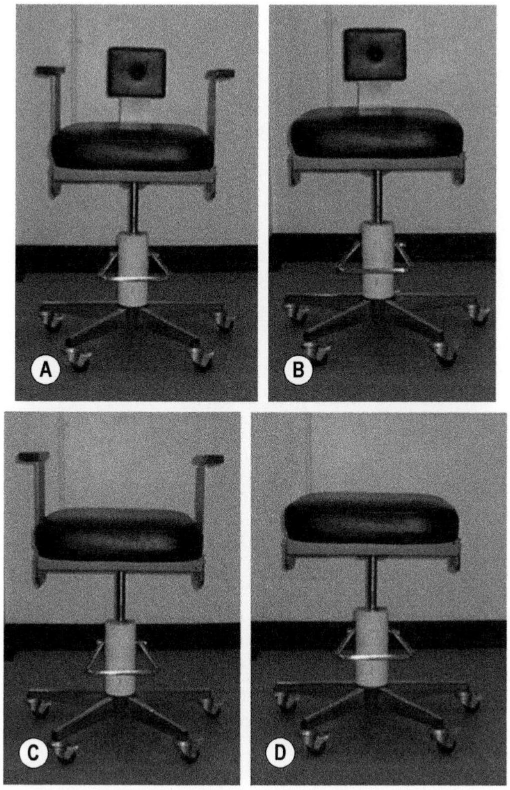

Fig. 15.1 Versatile chair with removable back and arms.

century exposure factors with a fairly low kVp were traditionally selected for chest radiography. These were usually in the range of 60–75 kVp and accompanied by values of 6–12 mAs. However, structures overlying dense areas such as the heart failed to be demonstrated owing to the low penetration of the beam. As long ago as 1996, European guidelines not only stressed the importance of using a high-energy beam in order to penetrate such areas, but also emphasised the reduction of absorbed dose by using high kVp techniques, namely 125 kVp.[7] These high kVp techniques may well require the use of an antiscatter grid or bucky, and use of automatic exposure devices (AEDs) is recommended in the 1996 EC guidelines, as is selection of the right AED chamber.

Positioning Choices for the PA Projection

There have been relatively few published comments in the past regarding actual positioning techniques (although there has been reasonably frequent comment on exposure factor techniques, radiation protection and dedicated chest radiology systems).

Historically, and internationally, descriptions for PA chest techniques included a confusing range of centring points (T4–T7), suggestions for caudal angulation or use of the horizontal beam. This range of techniques should be questioned, especially as consistency of approach is desirable when aiming to provide a quality-led service.

Direction of Central Ray

It appears that, internationally, beam angulation has never been in widespread use and the UK appeared to be

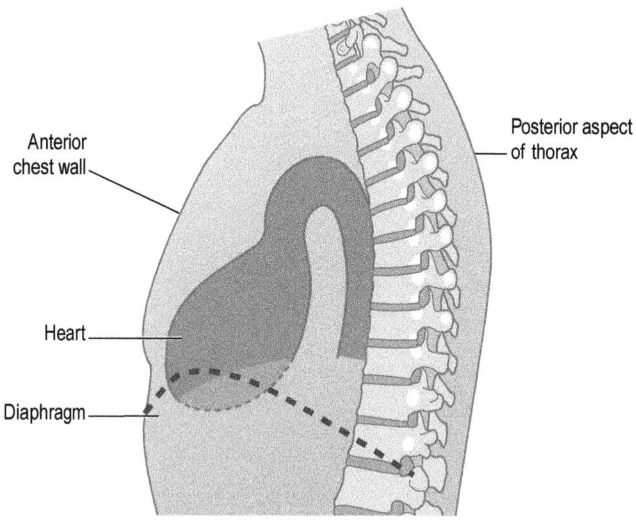

Fig. 15.2 Heart in relationship to anterior chest wall.

the area most likely to have used it.[8] Anecdotally it does seem that use of caudal angulation in the UK is less than at the end of the 20th century, but there seems to be no empirical research to support this. Caudal angulation has been suggested as inappropriate as the (minimal) obliquity of the beam used is actually likely to reduce the amount of posterior inferior lung tissue demonstrated above the diaphragm on the image (this is despite the common belief that its use 'opens out the lung fields' or maximises the amount of lung tissue seen above the diaphragm).[9] The effectiveness of small angles has also been challenged.[10] In addition, caudal angulation takes the beam direction towards the abdomen, thereby potentially increasing radiation dose to this region. To summarise, the use of caudal angulation does not offer improvements in image quality, may reduce the amount of lung tissue seen above the diaphragm, and potentially adds to the radiation burden for abdomen and gonads; it is can therefore be considered pointless.

Centring Point

In the last few decades suggestions for centring varied from T4 to T7,[11–14] with the middle of the IR, chest or thorax also mentioned in some texts.[13–15] In some cases more than one suggestion is given. So which is most appropriate? An additional question is: do texts specifying a vertebral level mean the body *or* the spinous process of that which is indicated? This is an important point when it is remembered that the body of a thoracic vertebra lies level with the spinous process of the one above it. It is also important that a suggested centring point be located as a palpable surface marking, so in this chapter the relevant spinous process will be referred to.

One suggestion for accurate assessment of the centring point involves using a ruler to measure the radiographer's hand span in order to help locate a centring point (given in centimetres and inches from T1) for use on the 'average' male and 'average' female,[16] but how can this be standardised or accurate when the assessment (and opinion) of 'average' is likely to vary from radiographer to radiographer,

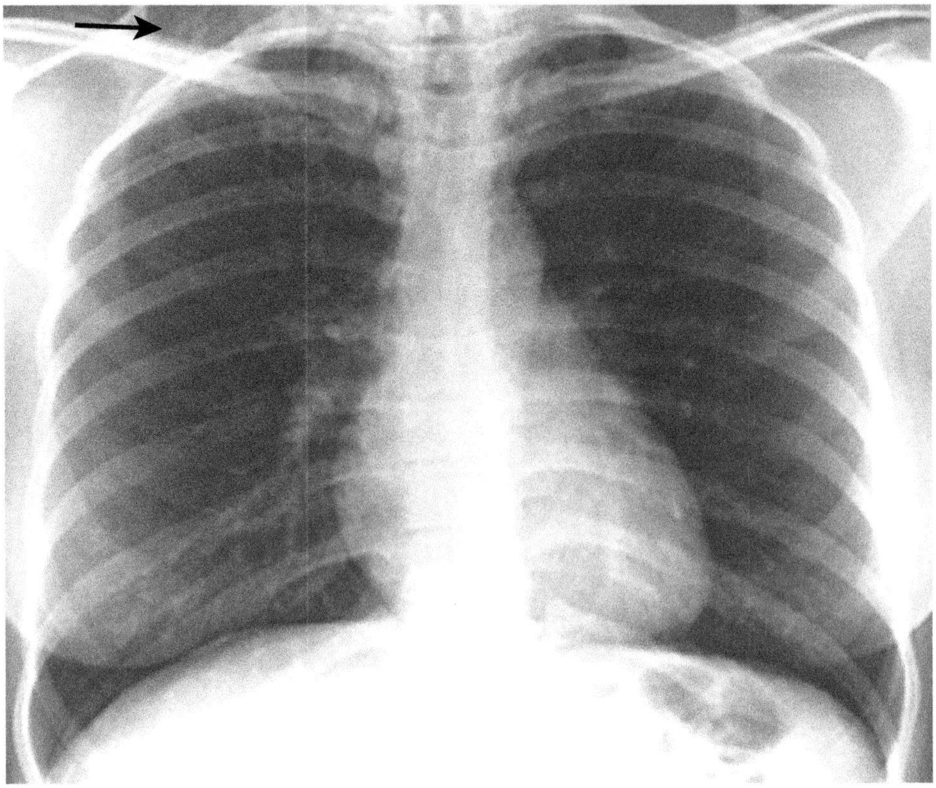

Fig 15.3 Subtle lucencies seen over the right neck and upper shoulder region are hair.

and any set measurement in centimetres or inches varies in its distance down each individual spine from a given point?

Centring points are most effective when simply in the centre of the area of interest, whether or not tube angle is used, and this should similarly apply to the chest region. Considering the issue of using a sensible centring point for the chest, previous editions of this book suggested a move from traditional centring points as high as T6 (which lies only one-third of the distance from apices to costophrenic angles) after research showed that this point almost never lies in the middle of the area of interest: indeed, study of PA chest images has shown that the vertebral body that most frequently lies level with the midpoint of the lungs is the body of T8 (spinous process of T7).[17]

Yet the reality of actually visualising this centring level accurately at a distance of 2 m (when centring the beam) can also be questioned, despite accurate palpation at the skin surface before walking the 2 m to the X-ray tube. Of course, a mark can be made at the appropriate level on the patient's gown after palpation, but realistically, only female patients undergo chest radiography in an examination gown. Would marking of the skin on a male patient be ethical? Probably not. Alternatively, a removable sticker could be applied to the back of male patients, but this may also not be acceptable to every individual.

In support of the question regarding the ability to accurately select a centring point from 2 m, it was found that radiographers frequently believed that they used a specific centring point for PA projection of the chest but in reality they ensured that the area of interest lay centrally over the IR. They then centred to the middle of the IR and the area of interest.[18] This provides a well-centred image and suggests that radiographers are accurate at centring appropriately at 2 m, but *not* at selecting the point they believe they use. For this reason the description of technique and centring point in this book reflects a combination of this second method and selection of a specific centring point.

Potential Impact of Artefacts

Removal of artefacts such as bras, jewellery and body piercings is vital, as for all other examinations in medical imaging, but there are additional risks of non-metallic artefacts that may mimic pathology; buttons, clips and even motifs on shirts can all be mistaken for abnormality, and lead the patient to have unnecessary further medical tests. Digital viewing stations are highly sensitive and are potentially capable of showing absolutely every aspect of clothing, or other artefacts, however low in density they may seem. Loose hair draped over a patient's back can produce streaking over the image, as seen in Fig. 15.3 (mimicking tracking at the base of the neck that can be associated with pneumomediastinum).[19] Pigtails and plaits are dense and can mimic cavitary lesions typically seen in tuberculosis and some tumours. The dark arrows on Fig. 15.4 illustrate a hair plait. This could easily be mistaken for a cavitary mass and lead to unnecessary high radiation dose examinations such as computed tomography (CT).

Impact of Errors Related to the Examination

As in any imaging procedure the quality of the chest X-ray examination directly affects the ability of a reporter to interpret the resultant image and produce an accurate report,

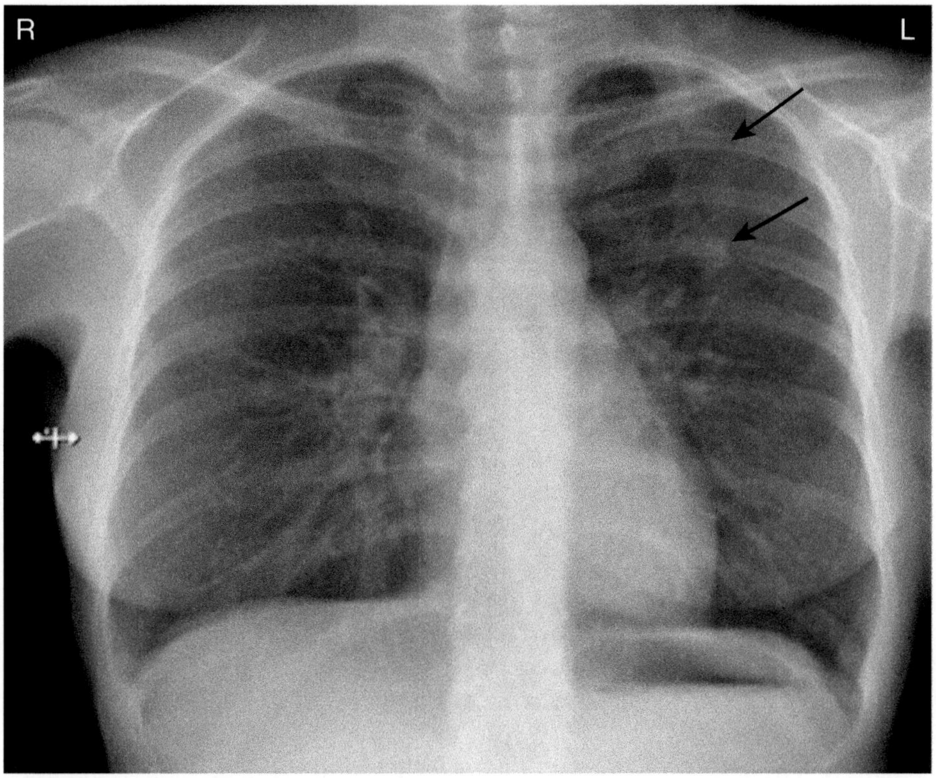

Fig. 15.4 Hair plait showing on area of interest (see arrows for outline).

but the complexity of interpreting chest images means that errors also have a complicated impact on many different aspects of interpretation. All radiographers must aim for an image that is of optimal quality but is it possible to accept a suboptimal image for reporting or preliminary clinical examination (PCE)? The answer is simple: if an image is not of optimum quality but does answer the clinical question then it should not be repeated. The way to understand how to decide if a suboptimal image still answers the clinical question is by understanding how errors impact upon the radiographer's ability to provide PCE or full report. Remember, the radiographer examining the patient will provide PCE but the image will still be forwarded for full report by a reporting radiographer or radiologist. It is the examining radiographer who must bear the responsibility of ensuring that adequate information is provided in order that the clinical question is indeed answered. More detail on impact of specific errors is included in common errors tables in this chapter.

PCE COMMENTS

The plain (non-contrast) chest X-ray has long been considered by radiologists, clinicians and reporting radiographers to be the most difficult examination to interpret.

'Image analysis and interpretation is a complex multi-step process with anatomical, physiological, neuropsychological and psycho-emotional components. Errors are therefore common and interpretation of chest X-rays is notoriously difficult, with false negative rates of 20–30% and false positive rates of 2–5%.'[20] As with all general radiographic projections, there are limitations to commenting on what is essentially a 3D structure with only 2D information. To compare, a simple area of the body such as a wrist or a finger often has two or three radiographic views yet a chest with its multiple internal structures often has only one, the PA.

Using a systematic approach to assess images, a level can be reached where it is possible to provide PCE. Clearly, the start point for understanding how to approach PCE is a sound knowledge of the thorax and its contents, including radiographic appearances of the anatomy of the area.

Many different pathologies share the same features on a chest X-ray, providing challenges for both reporting radiographers and those providing initial PCE for referrers. An accurate clinical history and sound knowledge of pathology is paramount to obtaining an accurate diagnosis. An example of situations where similar features are shared are given in Fig. 15.5 – one of the most commonly asked clinical questions is: Does the patient have an infection or does he/she have pulmonary oedema? Note that similar appearances are identified on Fig. 15.5A and 15.5B, yet the patient in pulmonary oedema presented with shortness of breath and pedal oedema and the second patient with widespread pneumonic infection exhibited a fever with a productive cough and green sputum. Things *look* the same. Very often clinical history will dictate diagnosis, supporting the need for referrers to provide adequate medical history on requests for imaging. This is absolutely key and this will be the factor in determining diagnosis as chest appearances manifest themselves in the same way for many different pathologies.

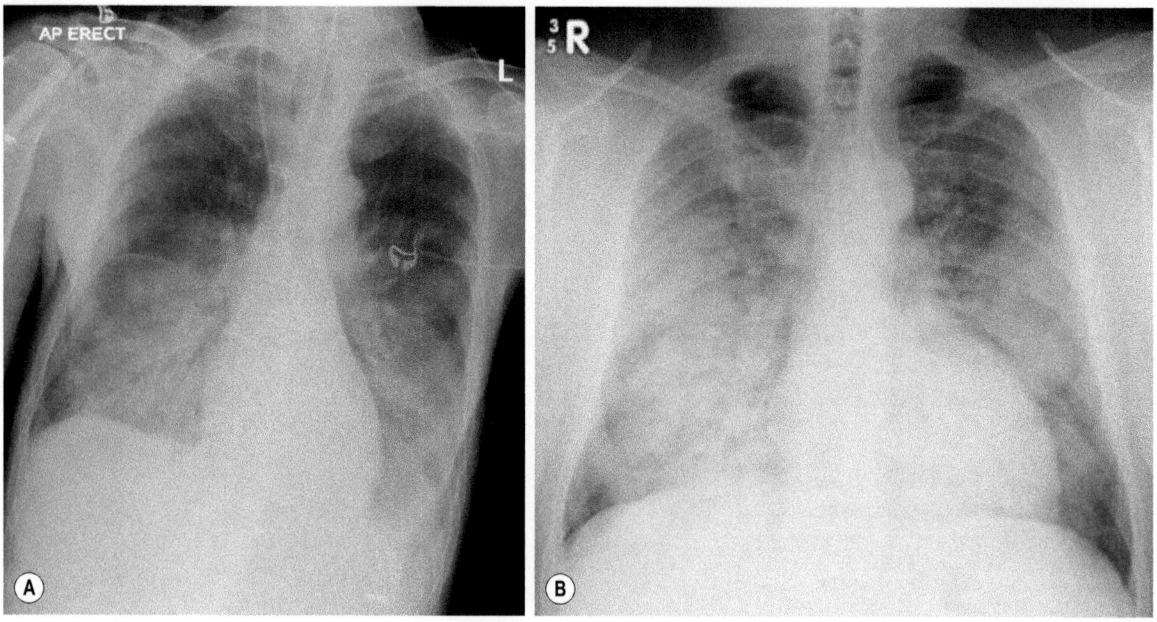

Fig. 15.5 Similar appearances may be shared by different pathologies, highlighting the importance of providing adequate clinical history for the radiographer. (A) Pulmonary oedema; (B) widespread pneumonic infection.

Assessing and Describing Abnormalities

Appearances on a chest radiograph can be described without actually providing a *diagnosis*. On initial viewing do not try to reach a diagnosis but do use easy descriptive terms that describe appearances. This, accompanied by sound knowledge of pathology, will provide the foundation for useful PCE. Even the most experienced radiologists don't always know what radiographic appearances represent.

It is absolutely imperative to have a systematic approach to viewing chest radiographs as in every other part of the body. Find a system and stick to it, since failure to do this will likely result in missed abnormalities/pathologies. The aim of this section in this chapter is to provide a sound foundation for approaching PCE for chest radiography, and the following information offers an example of how to approach image viewing in a suitably systematic way.

Interpretation

Before viewing the chest image:

- Always address the clinical question
- Adopt an inquisitive approach
- Be aware of areas where mistakes are often made
- Adopt a systematic approach and feel comfortable with it[21]

Viewing the Image

1. Check patient details, markers and legends.
2. Check image quality. Image quality will have a direct effect on your ability to interpret the resultant image, so make sure that you have checked out the impact of errors in the 'common errors' section relating to the PA chest image. Don't forget your systematic approach so that nothing is omitted.
3. Assess the anatomy: is everything in its normal anatomical position? Has anything been pushed or pulled out of position?
4. Borders and outlines: are they crisp and sharp? Are any missing?
5. Are there any unusual radiolucent or radiodense areas, or hidden abnormalities?
6. Record PCE for submission to referrer. If no abnormality is detected, this should be recorded.

Example of a standard PCE process used to comment on a chest image:

> 'The cardiomediastinal contours are unremarkable.
> Normal hilar appearances.
> The lungs are well expanded and clear.
> No collapse, consolidation or effusion.
> The visualised bony thorax is intact and unremarkable.'

This provides an in-depth example of how the findings on a chest X-ray examination should be reported clearly. It shows the referrer a systematic approach to both viewing and producing a chest X-ray evaluation. Of course, in terms of abnormality a more targeted approach may be desirable: e.g. 'There is a large right pleural effusion.'

Anatomical Assessment of Key Areas

Heart

- The heart should not take up more than half the width of the cardiothoracic diameter to be considered within normal range (Fig. 15.6). Modern viewing equipment has measuring tools and the heart should be measured at its widest point, and the thoracic measurement is taken from measuring chest wall to chest wall. There should be adequate penetration through the heart

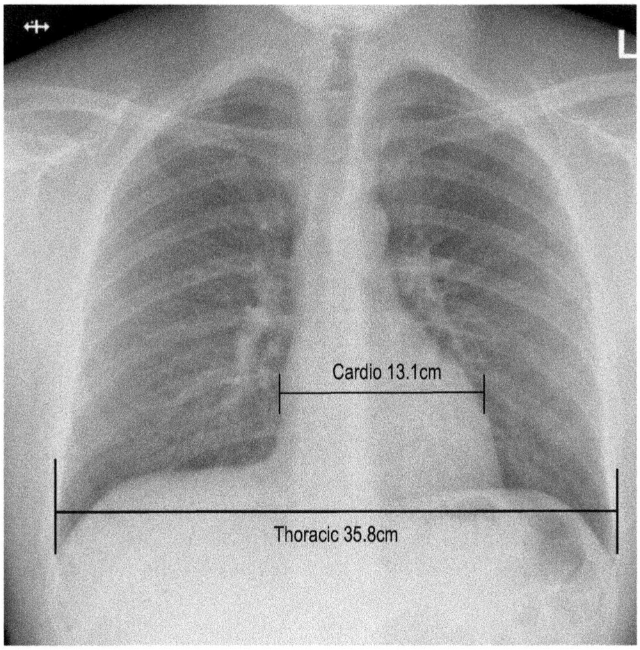

Fig. 15.6 Measuring the cardiothoracic (CT) ratio.

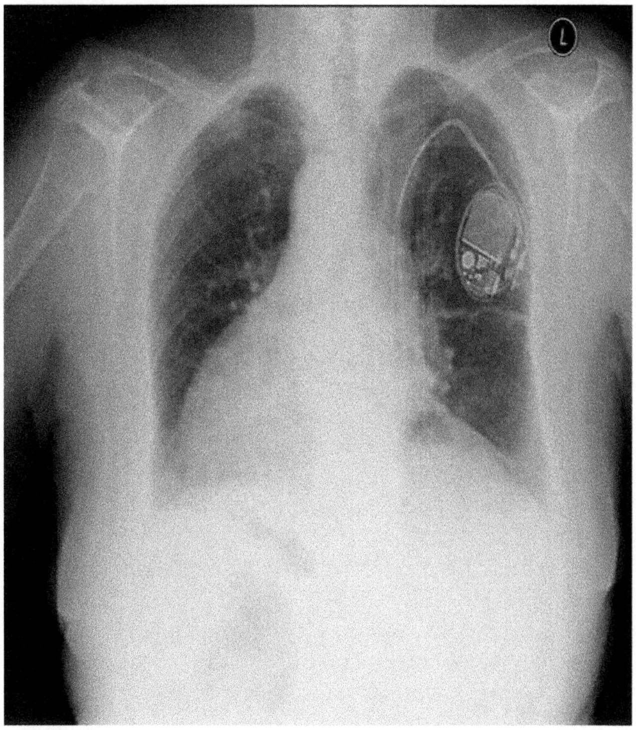

Fig. 15.7 Situs inversus.

border. Any retrocardiac opacity/opacification may be indicative of underlying pathology.

- Heart borders should be sharp. Hazy opacity at the apex or right cardiophrenic angle is usually a prominent fat pad.
- Check the heart is on the correct side. If it appears with the ventricular apex pointing to the right rather than to the left this indicates dextrocardia, which occurs in approximately 1 in 10,000 cases. Accompanying features are: superior vena cava seen on the left rather than the right, and the horizontal fissure seen on the left rather than the right. It is also important to note if this normal variant also shows transposition of other organs such as the liver and stomach; this is known as situs inversus (Fig. 15.7) and for this variant there is an incidence of 1 in 12,000 cases. Check for air in the stomach fundus on erect or semi-erect images; if it appears below the right diaphragm this supports a diagnosis of situs inversus rather than just dextrocardia. The left diaphragm will, in most cases, appear slightly higher than the right since the liver will sit on the left rather than the right. It is vital that a correct anatomical marker is used so that dextrocardia and situs inversus are not incorrectly diagnosed, or even missed simply because it is assumed that an image has not been flipped horizontally during post processing procedures.

Aortic and Mediastinal Contours

- Be familiar with the normal appearances of the cardiomediastinal contours. Check for lumps, bumps and changes in size and position. Mediastinal shift can indicate underlying pathology.
- Be familiar with normal age-related differences or changes.

Hila

Each hilar shadow is composed mainly of vessels, mainly the pulmonary system. There are wide variations in appearances for each individual.

- Hilar contours should be smooth and well defined. Check for any lumps or bumps as these may indicate underlying pathology.
- Position. The left hilum should never be lower than the right. If it is lower than the right something has pulled it down or, conversely, something may have pulled the right hilum up.
- Penetration should show information through the hila. Any increased radiopacity can indicate underlying pathology.

Note: Hila are a very difficult structure to interpret and even the most experienced examiners often ask for a second opinion on this area.

Lung Fields

- Check from apices down to the hemidiaphragms.
- Inflation: Check for depth of inspiration. An adequately inspired chest X-ray should show nine posterior and six anterior ribs above the level of the hemidiaphragms; although lower than this does not necessarily indicate hyperexpansion. If the hemidiaphragms are depressed more than this *and* they are flattened, then conditions such as COPD can be considered.
- Symmetry: Lungs should be approximately the same size.
- Density: Are the lungs or areas of lungs hyperdense or over-blackened (hypodense/hyperlucent)?

Abnormal hyperdense appearances in the lungs:

Alveolar: Is there air space opacity? Words that can be used to describe this are 'fluffy' or patchy. This appearance may represent infection or pulmonary oedema. Complete 'white out' may reflect a huge collapse, effusion or pneumonectomy

Nodular: tumours, infection or inflammatory changes
Reticular: 'mesh- like'. These are interstitial changes found in interstitial lung disease or interstitial oedema
Abnormal *hypodense* appearances in lungs can be due to hyperexpansion or true hyperlucency. Common causes can be COPD, emphysema, air trapping, bullae, cysts or pneumothorax

Diaphragm

- Hemidiaphragms should be smooth.
- Are diaphragms elevated?
- Are there any lumps or bumps?
- Are there any signs that indicate free air below them which may indicate a perforation?

Pleura

The pleura should not be visible unless there is an abnormality/underlying disease process. The most common abnormality of the pleura is pneumothorax, which can be caused by a number of things:

- Chest trauma. Any blunt or penetrating injury to the chest can cause lung collapse.
- Lung disease. Examples are COPD or pulmonary fibrosis. Any process that damages the lung parenchyma makes the patient more susceptible to a pneumothorax.
- Small air blisters (pleural blebs) can develop on the top of the lung. These can burst, causing a pneumothorax.
- Mechanical ventilation due to increased positive pressure. Common in pneumonia and acute respiratory distress syndrome.
- It is important to be able to spot the difference between a simple pneumothorax and a tension pneumothorax, which is a life-hreatening condition. In a tension pneumothorax the pressure of the air is so great it causes mediastinal shift, effacement of the heart border and depression of the hemidiaphragm. This can block venous return and put the patient at risk.
- The pressure of the air should be relieved by a drain/venflon as soon as possible; this highlights the importance of accurate and speedy PCE.

Bones of the Thorax

All bones of the thorax should be checked:

- Is anything missing?
- Check size, shape and position. Remember that some abnormalities may be congenital.
- Check for fractures. Minor rib fractures are easily missed. It is important to adopt a systematic approach to viewing the bony thorax. This reduces the incidence of missing small fractures. It is often useful to flip the image through 90° and change the windowing to obtain better visualisation of the bones, thus nulling the soft tissues.
- Are there any artefacts that may indicate previous surgery?
- Check bone density. Are the bones hyperdense or hyperlucent? Are there localised hyperdense or hyperlucent areas within individual bones? These appearances may indicate metastatic or metabolic bone disease.

Soft Tissues

- Should have a normal configuration.
- Check for lumps, bumps or masses.
- Is there anything missing? For example, mastectomy patients will have absence of breast shadow, most often unilaterally.
- Is there air in the soft tissues, such as in surgical emphysema?

Leads, Lines and Devices

A common reason for undertaking chest X-ray examinations is post insertion of leads, lines and devices. It is extremely important that the clinician or healthcare professional knows that the inserted artefact has gone into the intended location, and if there are any associated complications present.

Create a small log book or portfolio of any leads, lines or devices that are encountered. Research their correct position and associated complications. Find out what happens if they are positioned in the wrong place. This is where radiographers can play a vital role in the patient's management. A simple comment will help inexperienced clinicians immensely and improve the confidence and effectiveness of the radiographer as an independent practitioner.

Suggested Structure for PCE in Event of Suspected Abnormality

1. Are unusual appearances bilateral or unilateral? If unilateral identify the side.
2. Any displacement of anatomy: structures should be named.
3. Unusual radiolucent or radiodense appearances – identify anatomical areas affected. Include comment if sharpness or absence of anatomical outlines are affected.
4. Identify relative size of the abnormality, e.g. small, medium or large. If possible, provide measurement in centimetres.
5. Shape of the abnormality, e.g., 'round', 'crescent like', 'stellate' are good words to use. Are the borders crisp/well defined/ill defined?
6. If there are multiple appearances of the same type, state number. Are the abnormalities widespread or contained in one area?
7. How dense is the abnormality? Does it have a calcified or cavitary area?

Commonly Encountered Situations where PCE Plays an Important Part in Effective Diagnosis and Patient Management

Tension Pneumothorax (Fig. 15.8A,B)

The image in Fig. 15.8A shows a large left-sided tension pneumothorax, depressed left hemidiaphragm, mediastinal shift to the right and the left heart border is pushed away. After drain insertion the mediastinal shift, diaphragm position and heart border have returned to normal (Fig. 15.8B).

Pleural Effusion

A pleural effusion is fluid in the pleural space and therefore shown in contrast with the rest of the lung tissue as dense white areas on the radiograph – these appearances can vary from minor blunting of the costophrenic angles to complete

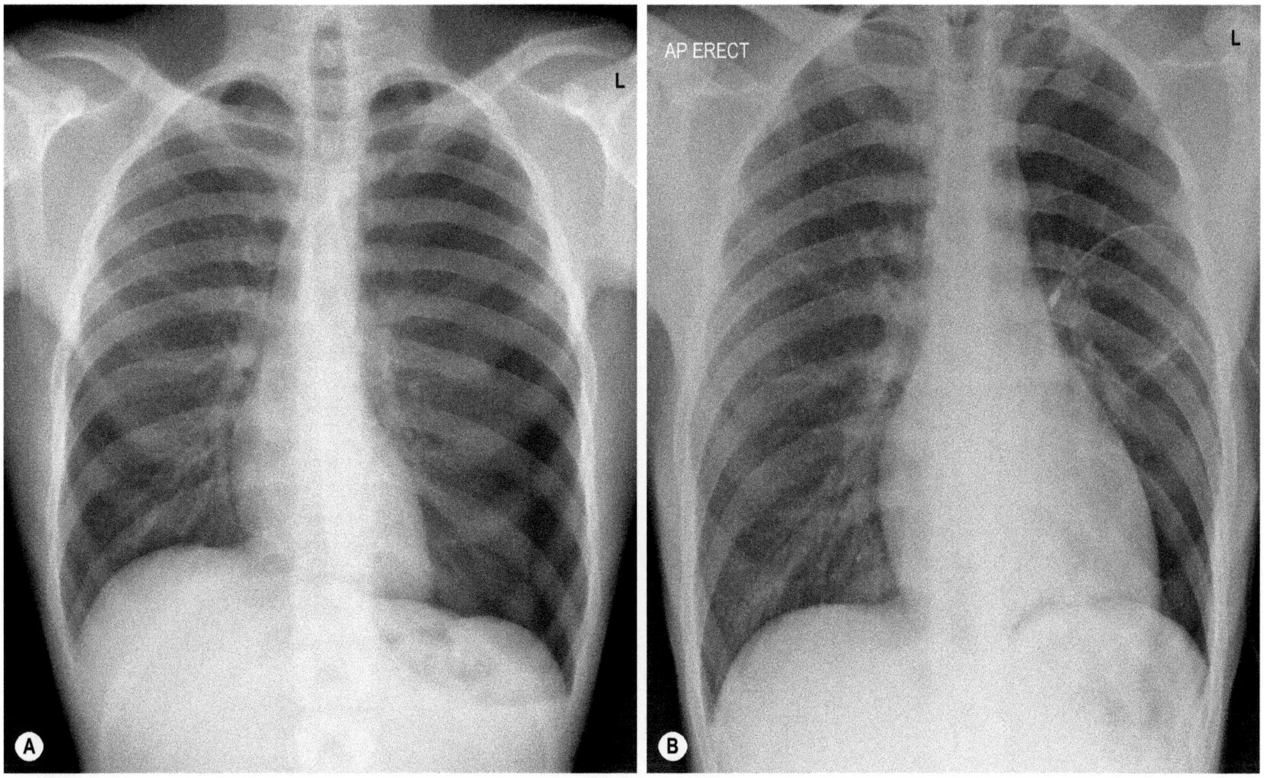

Fig. 15.8 (A) Large left-sided pneumothorax; (B) image taken after drain insertion.

'white out' of the lung fields. A large effusion can result in up to 3 litres of fluid collection in the patient's chest, often resulting in mediastinal shift.

- Small pleural effusion (Fig. 15.9)
  - Note minor blunting of the left costophrenic angle
  - Volume of the pleural effusion will be approximately 250 mL. (The lungs extend down posteriorly to the hemidiaphragms, therefore minor changes on the examination equals a significant amount of pleural fluid)
- Moderate pleural effusion (Fig. 15.10)
  - There is a moderate left-sided pleural effusion
  - There is complete effacement of the left hemidiaphragm
  - Volume of pleural fluid is approximately 400 mL
- Large pleural effusion (Fig. 15.11)
  - Large left-sided pleural effusion
  - Notice the midline shift of the trachea to the right due to volume of fluid
  - There is approximately 1 litre of pleural fluid
  - It is not known what is causing such a large amount of pleural fluid, or if the fluid is masking any underlying pathology.
  - CT or ultrasound may be appropriate

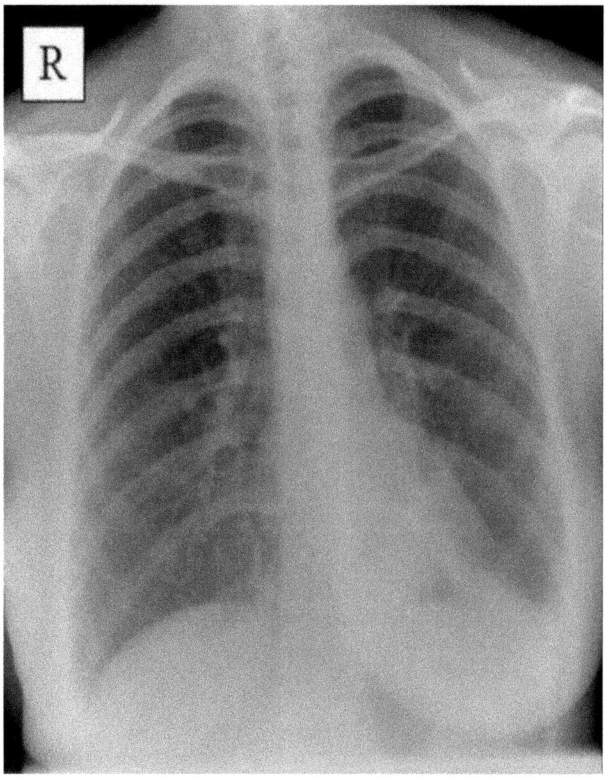

Fig. 15.9 Small left-sided pleural effusion.

Abnormal Appearances of the Ribs

Check ribs for sclerotic or lytic lesions, and any apparent fractures.

- In Fig. 15.12 most of the bones of the thorax cage are affected by sclerotic lesions; the ribs have a hyperdense, cotton-wool-like appearance, described as sclerotic

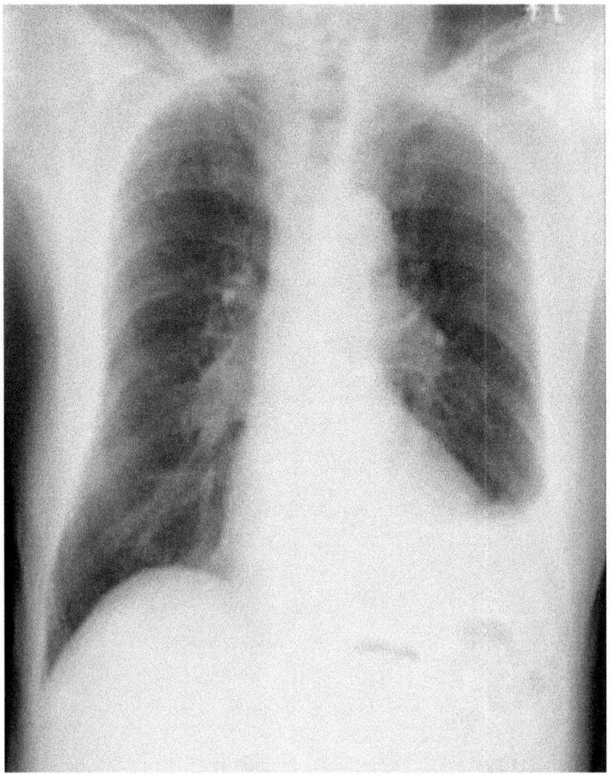

Fig. 15.10 Moderate pleural effusion.

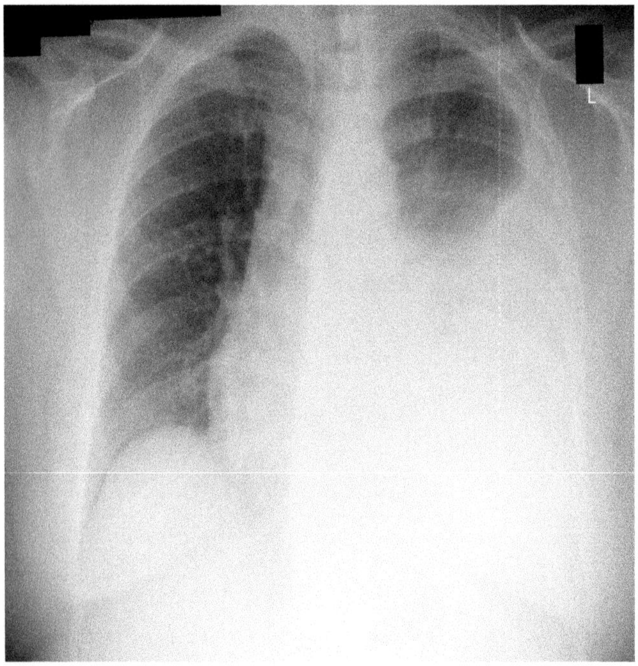

Fig. 15.11 Large pleural effusion.

as the bone constantly tries to heal itself. These are sclerotic bony metastases from prostate cancer.

- A lytic appearance would show lucent areas, giving a hole-like appearance in the bones.
- Fractures may be subtle or clearly displaced.

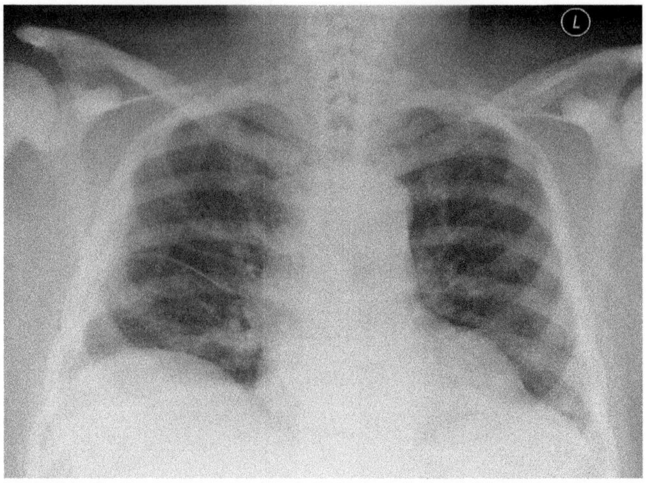

Fig. 15.12 Dense sclerotic lesions in the ribs are so extensive that they cause total loss of normal bone appearances (see ribs on Fig.15.13 for comparison of rib density).

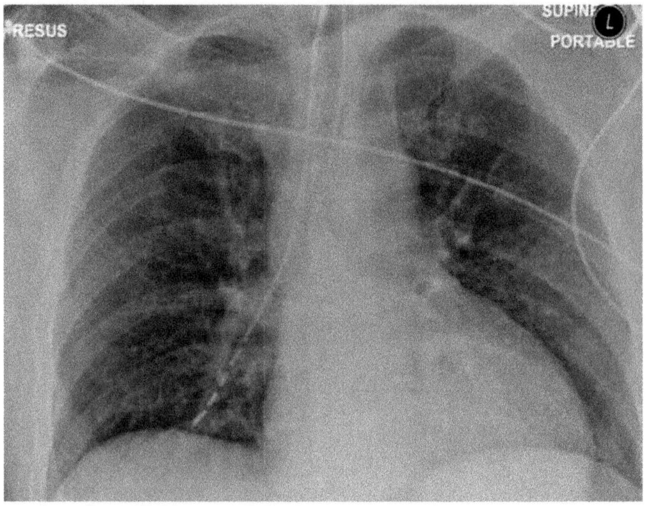

Fig. 15.13 Malpositioned NG tube. The same image also shows an endotracheal tube down the right main bronchus. Both tubes should be repositioned immediately.

Position of Leads, Lines and Devices

Referrals are most likely for assessment of position of devices that are intended to assist patient treatment. The most common examples are: positions of drains for pneumothoraces (Fig. 15.8B), nasogastric tubes (Fig. 15.13), central venous catheters (CVC) (Fig. 15.14) and central venous pressure (CVP) lines (Fig. 15.14). In these post procedure examinations referrers are looking for accuracy of position of the devices, and also to exclude pneumothorax, a recognised complication of CVP line insertion in particular.

Fig. 15.13 shows a nasogastric tube in the right main bronchus; this needs to be removed immediately, as feeding the patient can cause aspiration pneumonia. In addition, an endotracheal tube is seen in the right main bronchus. This will lead to aeration of the right lung only and eventually the left lung will collapse. A simple call to the clinician from the radiographer carrying out the examination could avoid serious risks associated with these issues.

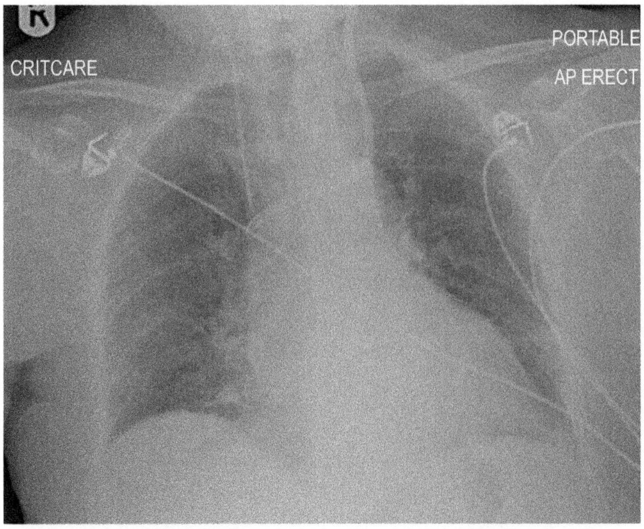

Fig. 15.14 Right and left venous catheters with both tubes correctly positioned with the tips in the region of the superior vena cava.

Note on image quality: In Fig. 15.13 the ECG leads are lying across the lung fields, rather than cleared from them and the lower left lung and ribs are not included in the image.

Examples of central venous pressure (CVP) line, central venous catheter (CVC) on one image are shown in Fig. 15.14:

- A right-sided CVP line is positioned with the tip in the superior vena cava.
- A left-sided venous catheter crosses the midline and the tip is also positioned in the superior vena cava.
- ECG leads have not been adequately cleared from the area.

POSTEROANTERIOR (PA) ERECT CHEST (FIG. 15.15A–C)

IR is vertical

Positioning

- The patient stands erect, with the anterior aspect of their chest placed in contact with the IR
- The height of the IR is adjusted until the whole of the thorax is included in its perimeter. The beam is collimated to the patient's thorax
- The patient's feet are separated slightly, for stability
- The patient leans forward and the chin is raised slightly and rests against the IR, or upon its upper border if a cassette-type IR is used
- The median sagittal plane (MSP) is perpendicular to the IR; this is checked by ensuring the sternoclavicular (SC) joints are equidistant from the IR. The MSP is coincident with the long axis of the IR
- The elbows are flexed and the backs of the hands are placed on the sides of the waist, resting on the lateral aspects of the iliac crests. The elbows are then gently pressed forward towards the IR, to clear the scapulae from the lung fields on the image. Ensure that the hands are actually on the *lateral* aspect of the waist, as this maximises forward movement of the shoulders; positioning of the hands on the posterior aspect significantly reduces the range of forward movement
- This projection can be undertaken with the patient seated if the patient has difficulty standing
- A PA marker is most frequently used, on the relevant upper corner of the radiation field

Beam Direction and FRD

Horizontal
2 m FRD

Centring

Positioning as described should ensure that centring is over the middle of the thorax, coincident with the spinous process of T7 (body of T8)

Collimation

First thoracic vertebra, first rib, lateral margins of ribs 2–10, costophrenic angles

Expose on arrested inspiration; maximum effort required

Before exposure the radiographer should check that the shoulders are not raised during the inspiratory effort, or that the arms and shoulders have not relaxed backwards. The time lapse between initially pressing the arms forward during positioning and exposure may seem relatively short, yet patients frequently, and usually imperceptibly, relax their arms enough to superimpose at least some scapular outline over the upper lung fields during this short time.

Criteria for Assessing Image Quality

- First thoracic vertebra and first rib, lateral rib margins and costophrenic angles are demonstrated. The costophrenic angles must be demonstrated above the collimated field
- 3–5 cm of apical tissue is projected above the clavicles
- Posterior aspects of the ribs are slightly inclined from the thoracic spine down towards their lateral borders
- Anterior aspects of the ribs are inclined more steeply than the posterior aspects, from their lateral borders down towards the midline
- Medial ends of the clavicles are equidistant from the midline of the thoracic vertebrae
- Scapulae are cleared from the lung fields
- Six anterior or nine posterior ribs are demonstrated above the diaphragms
- Sharp image demonstrating the vascular pattern of the lungs to the periphery in contrast with the air-filled lung tissue and dense structures of the hila and mediastinum (heart, aorta). Trachea and proximal bronchi should be visible, as should the retrocardiac lung and mediastinum. The thoracic vertebrae (intervertebral disc spaces) should be evident through the cardiac image. Diaphragms and costophrenic angles should be clearly seen. These exposure factor criteria relate to high kVp technique.[3] For images produced with kVp lower than 85–90, penetration is assessed by checking that the spinous process of T4 is adequately seen in the midline, as in Fig. 15.15C. (Note that the patient positioning in Fig. 15.15C is superior to that in Fig. 15.15B.)

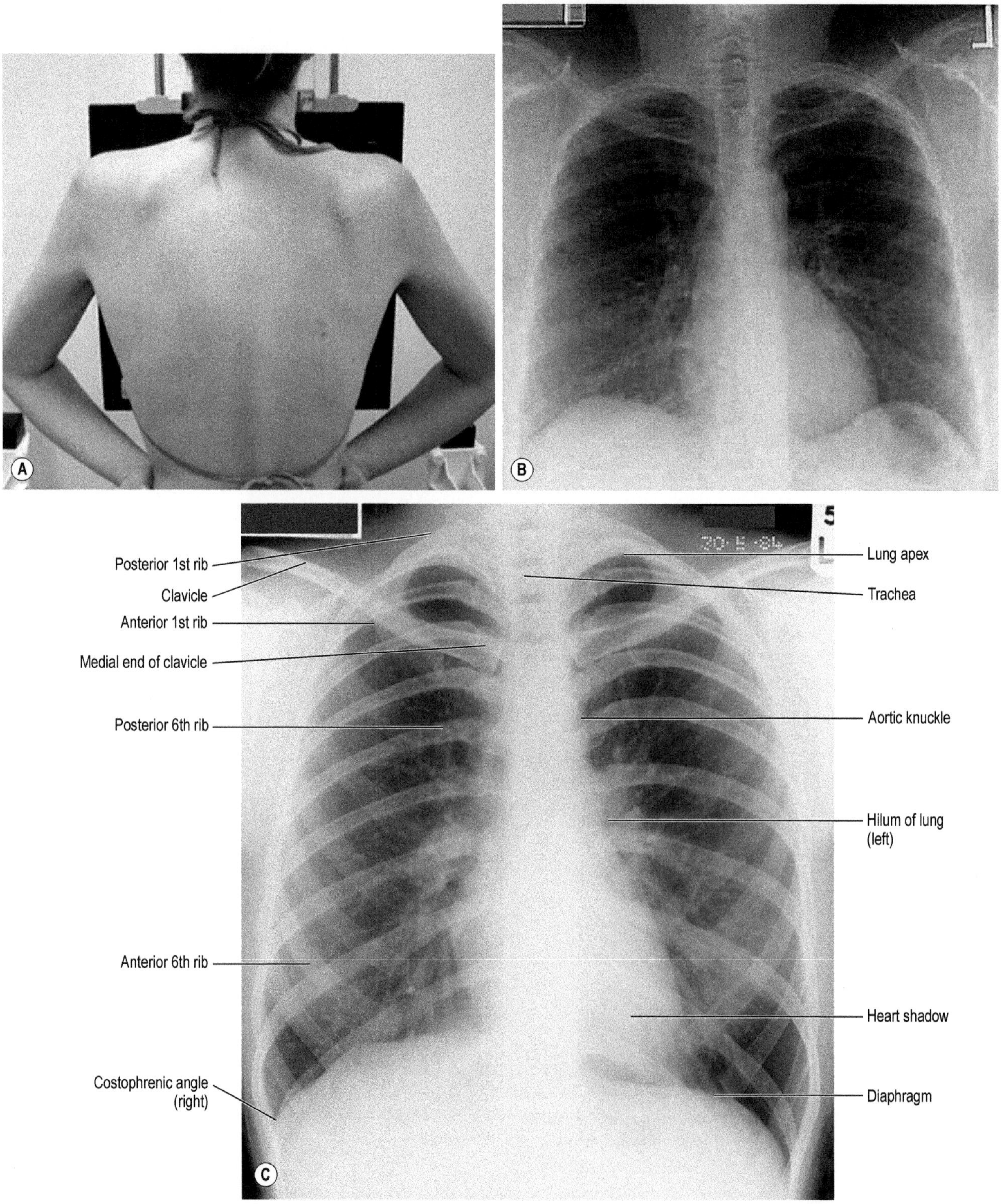

Fig. 15.15 (A) PA chest; (B) PA chest using high kVp; (C) PA chest (labelled to show anatomical structures) using lower kVp.

Common Errors: PA Erect Chest

Common Errors	Possible Reasons	Potential Effects on PCE or Report
Area of interest not included adequately	Poor centring, excessive collimation, digital cropping during post processing, patient size may exceed boundaries of IR, IR may be in inappropriate orientation	All lateral rib outlines above the costophrenic angles *must* be shown on the final image. Not including the lateral chest wall means that soft tissue masses and bony pathology/trauma can be missed. When 'post processing' images *do not* digitally crop them so closely that bones and soft tissue information is lost to make the examination look more 'presentable', or to disguise the fact that collimation was inadequate during the examination. Digital cropping may crop off a rib fracture, or tumour in a rib or peripheral lung tissue Although the lateral radiograph is more sensitive than the PA when demonstrating pleural effusions, most often a good-quality PA is the first indication that the lateral will be necessary.[22] **All of each sharp point of both costophrenic angles *must* be clearly visible.** Indeed, up to 250 mL[23] of fluid may be present before blunting on the costophrenic angles is noted
Medially positioned soft tissue shadow, between and/or overlying the apices	Chin not raised adequately	Soft tissue may obscure medial aspects or all of the lung apices, a common area where pathology is found. Most commonly these include Pancoast tumours, small apical pneumothoraces and TB, which can be missed if apices are not clearly shown
Scapulae overlying upper, lateral aspects of lung fields	Elbows and shoulders not pushed forward adequately, or patient has relaxed their arm position Patients with limited shoulder movement may not find it possible to fully comply with the required action; try extending the patient's arms in forward abduction, with internal rotation at the shoulder	In an image that shows adequate lung detail, this may not be an issue but the scapulae potentially can mask subtle pathology, the most common being pneumothorax
Apices inadequately cleared above the clavicles; posterior and anterior aspects of the ribs flattened	Patient is lordotic, i.e. not leaning forward towards the IR	Failure to clear the apices will have the same effects as under 'chin not raised adequately' Accurate assessment of CT ratio not possible. Although the clavicles are projected above the lung apices and will produce excellent visualisation of the lung apices, there will be poor characterisation of other structures The heart and mediastinal contours are elongated, affecting apparent cardiothoracic ratio Vascular structures are enhanced and their contours appear as changed from normal anatomy The hemidiaphragms are projected up, mimicking lower zone consolidation
Medial ends of the clavicles not seen at an equal distance from the thoracic vertebrae	Patient is rotated. The medial end of the clavicle furthest from the vertebrae corresponds to the side rotated away from the IR. Any evidence of scoliosis? If the patient has scoliosis, it may not be possible to ensure the clavicles lie equidistant from the midline[24]	Accurate assessment of CT ratio not possible Hilar markings will appear more prominent on one side of the thorax and potentially mimic the suggestion of pathology Mediastinum will appear widened and the trachea will appear shifted laterally[5,22] Rotation may cause lung asymmetry or a difference in lung densities when compared to each other. Apparent reduced size or volume loss on one side can suggest pathology such as fibrosis or scarring; a largely increased apparent size on one side may suggest asthma or COPD. Differing lung densities may lead to false-positive for infection or pulmonary congestion One hilum will appear more prominent than the other on the image – it will not be possible to decide if the prominence is due to pathology or is just 'projectional' Medially positioned lesions in lungs may be obscured by mediastinal structures Difficult to assess mediastinal abnormalities or reasons for tracheal shift Soft tissue outlines may be changed or enhanced

Common Errors: PA Erect Chest—cont'd

Common Errors	Possible Reasons	Potential Effects on PCE or Report
Fewer than six anterior ribs or nine posterior ribs are demonstrated above the diaphragms	Poor inspiratory effort. Bariatric patients or patients with dyspnoea may find improvement difficult Miscounted ribs. Check again. The first and second ribs cross over superiorly on the image and can sometimes be erroneously counted as one, rather than two. A tip when checking rib numbers is to assume that the posterior aspects of the first and second ribs appear to cross over, like a kiss on a birthday card – so always 'count the kiss' first and remember that the kiss = ribs one and two. Counting the thoracic vertebrae is another method that can be used to identify posterior ribs and confirm rib number Any evidence or history suggestive of infective or cardiac disease, lobar collapse, lobectomy, subphrenic abscess, phrenic nerve paralysis or upper abdominal mass? These are likely to affect diaphragm height and improvement may not be possible	Suboptimal inspiratory effort can cause the hila to appear pathologically enlarged, when in reality it is due to overcrowding of the vasculature. This can lead to false-positive decisions such as pulmonary hypertension or lymphadenopathy Lung bases are less aerated and produce increased density, and it is not possible to ascertain if infection is present as a result Accurate assessment of CT ratio not possible. Poor inspiratory effort gives the impression of cardiomegaly. This is because the fibrous sac of the pericardium is connected to the diaphragm by a central tendon; during inspiration the diaphragm is pushed down and the central tendon pulls the heart down too, almost stretching it. This leads to a reduced cardiac diameter when compared to the expiratory phase in which the diaphragm moves up, causing the central tendon to relax and leading to a greater cardiac diameter. This therefore affects the apparent CT ratio. However, a simple chest image is not necessarily an accurate indicator of heart size, which can vary by approximately 2 cm, depending on whether the image is taken in systole or diastole Hilar enlargement. A suboptimal inspiratory effort can cause the hila to appear pathologically enlarged when in reality it is due to crowding of the vasculature. This can lead to inaccurate diagnosis of conditions such as pulmonary hypertension or even lymphadenopathy
High contrast image with failure to show spinous processes through the mediastinum, unable to manipulate image to show required detail	kVp too low	May cause retrocardiac opacity to be suspected, suggesting an abnormality that is not present With digital equipment it is often possible to manipulate the image in order to assess retrocardiac appearances. However, should the exposure index show readings in the unacceptable range, it is not likely that digital manipulation will clarify the situation adequately (see Chapter 3, Table 3.1)

Other Chest Projections

ANTEROPOSTERIOR (AP) ERECT CHEST (FIGS 15.16, 15.17)

The AP erect chest is undertaken when a patient is too ill or frail to stand or sit PA erect.

IR is vertical

Positioning

- A patient who can sit on a chair sits with their back to the IR (Fig. 15.16)
- For a patient who presents on a trolley or bed the IR is (a) brought to the back of the patient (digital plate technique), or (b) placed in the erect holder or (c) supported by a large 45° pad which rests on the raised back of a trolley or bed (Fig. 15.17)
- The posterior aspect of the chest is placed in contact with the IR
- The height of the IR is adjusted until the whole of the thorax is included in its perimeter. Ensuring that the first thoracic vertebra is below the upper border of the receptor will ensure that the lung apices are included at the top of the image
- The patient sits, supported with their back against the IR
- The beam is collimated to the patient's thorax and its upper border positioned level with the upper border of T1
- A small radiolucent pad is placed behind the shoulders to reproduce the slight elevation of the lung apices above the clavicles achieved in the PA position. The chin is raised slightly and the MSP is coincident with the long axis of the IR

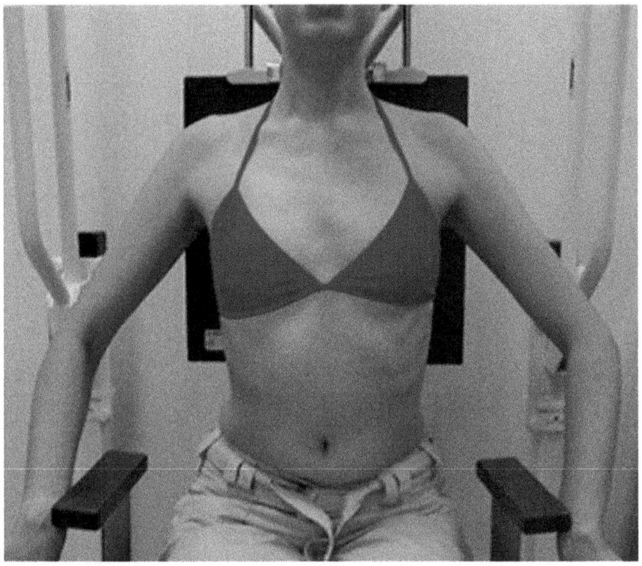

Fig. 15.16 AP chest for patient in chair.

- The MSP is perpendicular to the IR; this is checked by ensuring the SC joints are equidistant from the receptor
- For the patient who is sitting on a chair, the elbows are flexed and the backs of the hands are placed on the sides of the waist, resting on the lateral aspects of the iliac crests. The elbows are then gently pressed forward

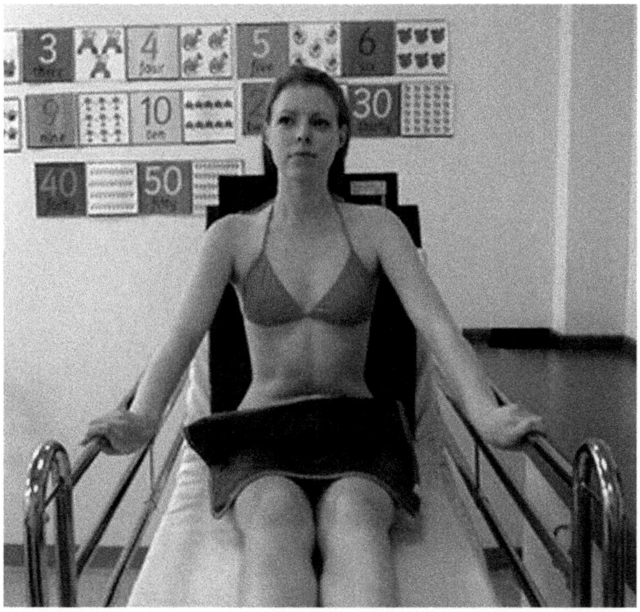

Fig. 15.17 AP chest for patient on trolley.

towards the IR, to clear the scapulae from the lung fields on the image. This is exactly the same action as that required for the PA projection. Some patients in bed or on a trolley may also be able to achieve this position

- For patients unable to clear the scapulae by the above method, the arms are abducted and, if possible, rotated internally at the shoulders until the thumbs are directed to the floor. Resting the forearms on the trolley or bed sides, while maintaining some internal rotation, is an effective method of achieving and maintaining this position (Fig. 15.17)
- An AP marker is used, within the relevant upper corner of the radiation field
- If the patient has electrocardiogram (ECG) leads attached to their chest, or is using an oxygen mask, care must be taken to clear these artefacts from the field. ECG leads should leave the chest area by the 'shortest route' if they cannot be temporarily detached (Fig. 15.18)
- An 'erect AP' legend is applied next to the anatomical marker

Beam Direction and FRD

Horizontal
2 m FRD

A caudal angle may be used to reduce the effect of lordosis if the patient (unavoidably) is leaning back. The angle should be selected by assessing the degree of recumbence, although approximately 5° has been suggested.[18] Use of such an angle should be carefully considered, as significant deviation from the use of a horizontal beam may affect demonstration of fluid in the chest cavity.

Centring

To the middle of the thorax (approximately midway between the sternal angle and xiphisternum)

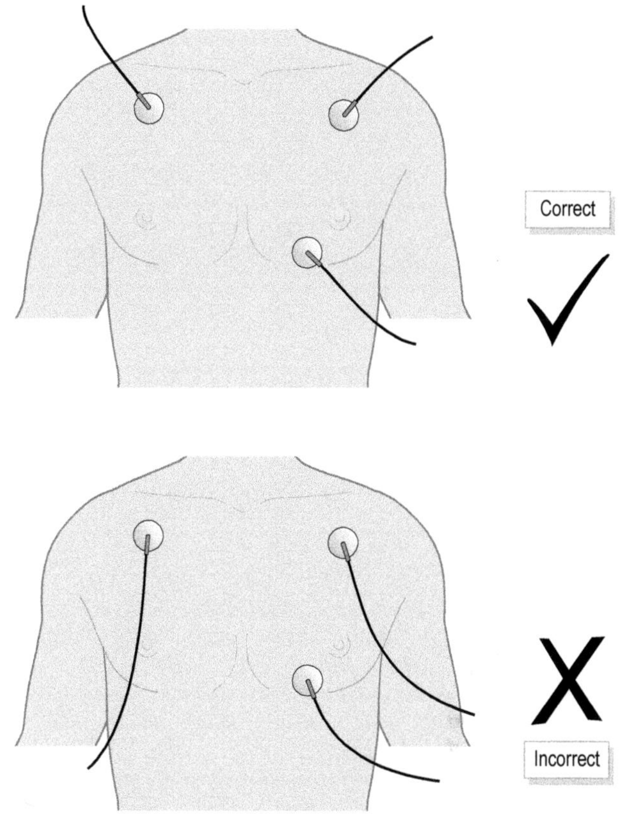

Fig. 15.18 Position of ECG leads for chest radiography.

Collimation

First thoracic vertebra, first rib, lateral margins of ribs, costophrenic angles

Expose on arrested inspiration; maximum effort required

Criteria for Assessing Image Quality

Criteria are identical to those for the PA projection, but it should be remembered that elevation of the apices above the clavicles may be less successful than on a PA image, despite use of the radiolucent pad suggested in the positioning description. It is likely that there will still be some lordosis, as it is tempting for the infirm patient to lean back, using the IR for support. This is potentially made worse when the patient attempts good inspiratory effort. Elevation of the chin is often difficult for the infirm patient and is made more difficult if the thorax is tilted slightly forward by the radiolucent pad. Forward tilt will also cause some magnification of the upper thorax.

Lordosis is more likely to occur in bed or trolley-bound patients, where the IR is supported by a sponge and the patient's legs extend forward, increasing the tendency of the thorax to lean back. The possibility of lordosis increases further when pillows are substituted for the pad. The potential risk of lordosis in the AP position does not validate approval of its presence on the image, and maximum effort should be made to avoid its incidence.

Common Errors: AP Erect Chest

Common Errors*	Possible Reasons	Potential Effects on PCE or Report
Lordosis	Patient using IR as support for their back. If lordosis cannot be improved, a compensating caudal angle may be effective in reducing the effect	As for effects of lordosis in PA projection
Soft tissue shadow over lower lung fields	Abdominal tissue may be superimposed; usually seen in lordotic patients on a trolley or bed. It is especially prevalent in patients who have a large abdomen	Impacts upon key information required to assess lung bases and CT ratio assessment (see Potential Effects for PA projection)

*See also errors outlined for PA projection.

SUPINE ANTEROPOSTERIOR (AP) CHEST

This is undertaken on the very sick patient, most often in the mobile situation. Two people are required to facilitate safe manual handling while positioning the patient on the IR.

Positioning

- The patient's trunk is elevated from the bed or trolley and the IR is placed underneath the chest, to include the whole of the thorax within its boundaries
- MSP is perpendicular to the IR and coincident with its long axis
- The chin is raised slightly
- The arms are abducted and, if possible, rotated internally at the shoulders
- An AP marker is used, on the relevant upper corner of the radiation field
- A 'supine AP' legend is applied next to the anatomical marker
- Artefacts should be moved as described for the AP erect projection

Beam Direction and FRD

Vertical; however, a caudal angle of 5° will reduce the appearance of lordosis on the image

FRD as high as possible – up to a maximum of 2 m; FRD can be maximised by lowering the bed

Centring

To the middle of the thorax, as for erect AP chest

Collimation

First thoracic vertebra, first rib, lateral margins of ribs 2–10, costophrenic angles

> Expose on arrested inspiration; maximum effort required
>
> For patients on a ventilator it may be necessary to ask for suitably designated staff to facilitate suspension of respiration by controlling the ventilator.

Consideration for Radiation Protection – Mobile Radiography

Although some patients will be examined in the supine position on a trolley in the imaging department, the majority of supine chest examinations are undertaken as mobile examinations on the ward or Emergency Department recovery, i.e. in a radiation supervised area rather than a controlled area. Therefore, the radiographer's responsibility regarding radiation exposure is of paramount importance, particularly regarding protection of personnel and other patients in the vicinity.

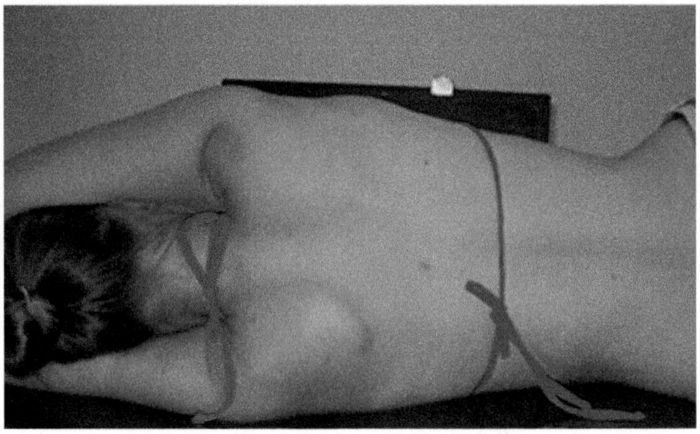

Fig. 15.19 Lateral decubitus PA chest.

Criteria for Assessing Image Quality

Criteria are identical to those for the PA and AP projections, with the risk of lordosis similar to that for the AP projection. Suspension of adequate inspiration is likely to be more difficult in the case of the unconscious patient who is breathing independently, therefore a maximum attempt to achieve an adequately inspired, sharp image must be made.

Unfortunately, it is often not possible to achieve the optimum FRD of 2 m for the supine projection, owing to equipment or environment restrictions. This will cause magnification that is greater than for examinations undertaken at 2 m FRD. With the additional consideration of the fact that the heart is already magnified in the AP position, assessment of CT ratio is further compromised. The mediastinum will also appear enlarged.

LATERAL DECUBITUS POSTEROANTERIOR (PA) CHEST (FIG. 15.19)

This projection should be employed when it is vital that a horizontal beam is used to demonstrate pleural effusions but the patient cannot sit or stand; ultrasound can also be used to confirm or exclude this condition.[5] Occasionally, small pneumothoraces require demonstration using this method.[16]

IR is vertical

Positioning

- The patient lies on a radiolucent pad: (a) *on their affected side*, to allow for the settlement of pleural fluid in the lateral portion of the lung or (b) *on their unaffected side* to allow the demonstration of air in the pleural cavity. The knees are flexed for comfort and stability and the arms raised to clear them from the area of interest and primary beam
- The IR is placed vertically, its long axis parallel to the long axis of the table-top, trolley or bed
- The anterior aspect of the chest is placed in contact with the IR and the position is adjusted until the whole of the thorax is included in its perimeter, with the first thoracic vertebra included. The MSP is coincident with the longitudinal axis of the receptor
- The chin is raised slightly to clear it from the lung apices. The MSP is perpendicular to the IR; this is checked by ensuring the SC joints are equidistant from the IR
- A PA marker is applied

Beam Direction and FRD

Horizontal
2 m FRD

Centring

To the middle of the thorax, over the spinous process of T7 (body of T8)

Collimation

First thoracic vertebra, first rib, lateral margins of ribs 2–10, costophrenic angles

Criteria for Assessing Image Quality

Criteria follow those for the PA erect chest. However, if the suspected pathologies outlined as reasons for use of this projection are found, it may not be necessary to repeat the examination in the case of rotation, poor inspiration, poor scapular clearance or lordosis. The most important criterion for this projection is the inclusion of the whole area of interest, especially the lateral border of the hemithorax related to the pathology in question.

LATERAL CHEST (FIG. 15.20A,B)

Unless there is known pathology related to a particular side of the chest, the PA projection should be examined to determine the pathology site before taking the decision to use this projection. Decision on the appropriate lateral is made on the basis that the side with the most significant pathological feature is selected for positioning closest to the IR. Use of the lateral projection has declined since the late 1980s with the increased use of computed tomography.

Under no circumstances should a lateral projection be undertaken as 'routine' or without relevant clinical reason. An acceptable exception for use of the lateral chest projection, even when the PA shows no abnormality, is to undertake the projection after pacemaker insertion in order to show anterior configuration of the pacemaker leads. Although this may on the surface appear to be a routine request, there is still a clinical reason for performing the examination.

As for the PA chest, EC guidelines also recommend use of an antiscatter grid in conjunction with 125 kVp exposure technique and use of an AED,[7] although this is not currently widespread in practice. Commonly, a grid is used only for larger patients and kVp is often lower than 125.

IR is vertical

Positioning

- The arms are raised and the lateral aspect of the chest is placed in contact with the IR
- The height of the IR is adjusted so the thorax lies within its perimeter and the beam is collimated to include the whole of the thorax
- The feet are slightly separated for stability
- The elbows are flexed and the hands clasped at the back of the head; the humeri are adducted medially until parallel. Upper arm tissue and humeri must be cleared from as much of the apices and upper lungs as possible

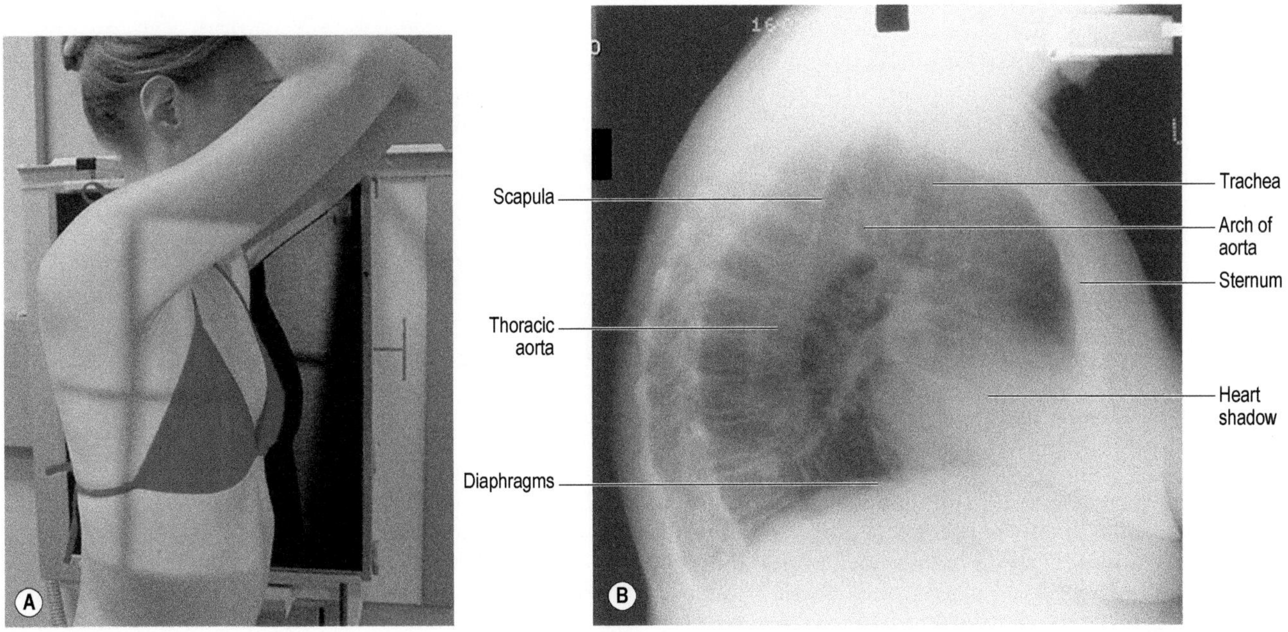

Fig. 15.20 Lateral chest.

- A slight forwards tilt of the trunk will bring the thorax into a vertical position
- The MSP is parallel to the IR

Patients who cannot comply with the positioning described above can be examined with the modifications listed below.

Difficulty	Modification or Adaptation
Patient cannot maintain position of raised arms, cannot raise arms or cannot flex elbows comfortably	Patient holds vertical structure with raised hands. Commonly a drip stand is used for this
Patient cannot stand	Projection can be undertaken using a stool or chair (Fig. 15.21)
Patient needs support at their back (if sitting)	A radiolucent pad can be placed behind the patient's back, as in Fig. 15.22

Beam Direction and FRD

Horizontal
2 m FRD

Centring

Midway between the sternum and posterior ribs antero-posteriorly, level with a point midway between the sternal angle and the xiphisternum

Collimation

Shoulder, sternum, spinous processes of thoracic vertebrae, posterior and anterior costophrenic angles

Criteria for Assessing Image Quality

- Shoulder, sternum, spinous processes of thoracic vertebrae, posterior and anterior costophrenic angles are demonstrated
- Shoulder and soft tissue of upper arms overlying lung apices only
- Condyles on posterior aspect of thoracic vertebrae are superimposed; posterior aspects of ribs are superimposed
- Intervertebral joint spaces are clear
- Image of left diaphragm seen slightly above right
- T11 is demonstrated above the posterior diaphragm
- Sharp image demonstrating lung markings in contrast with the heart, aorta, air-filled trachea and ribs. The sternum, posterior heart border, diaphragms, anterior and posterior costophrenic angles and thoracic vertebrae should also be demonstrated

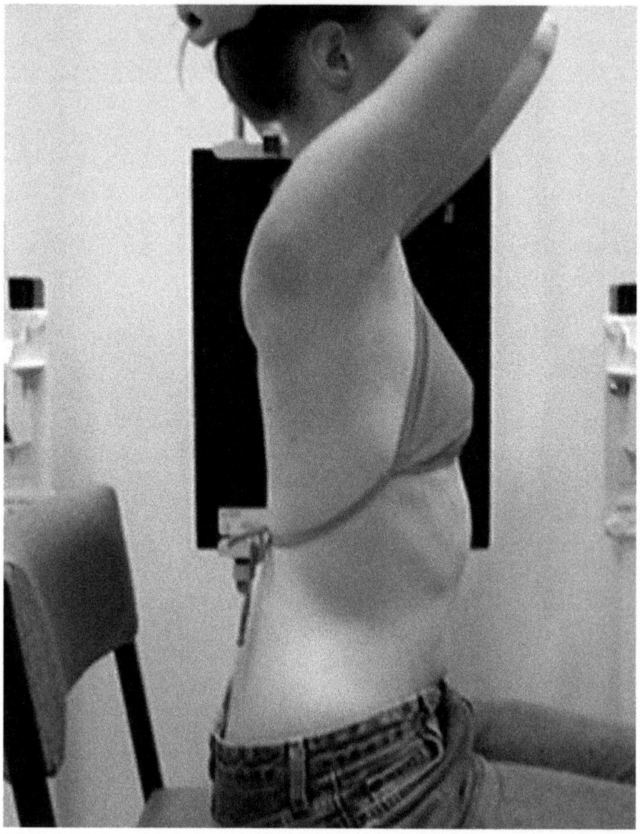

Fig. 15.21 Lateral chest in chair.

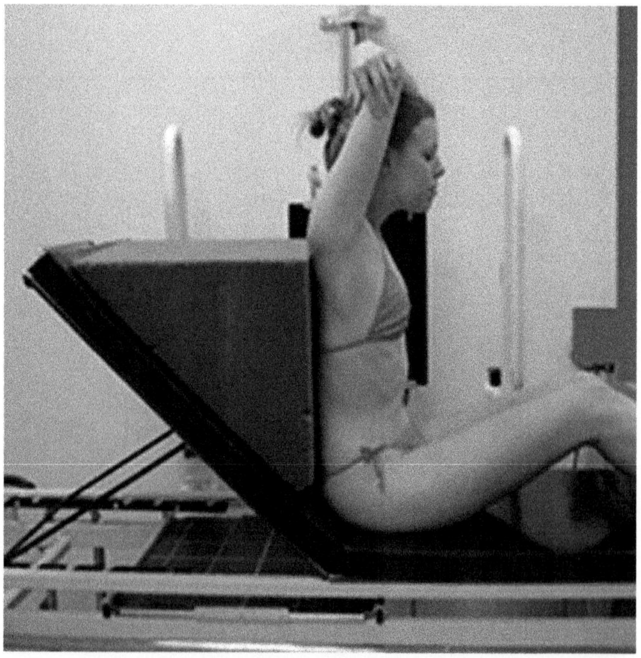

Fig. 15.22 Lateral chest on trolley.

PCE COMMENTS – LATERAL CHEST

Using a preferred systematic review is mandatory; check key areas before offering comment and ensure quality criteria are met.

Follow the airway from the neck to the hilum. The trachea, of course, is the upper portion of the airway and is generally tilted posteriorly as it descends into the thorax. Check for impingement or a position that may suggest something is pushing, pulling or overlying the trachea.

Lungs: The lateral projection provides a better assessment of the lungs/lung volumes than the PA as the costophrenic gutters are hidden behind the diaphragm on a PA projection. Check for any opacifications or abnormalities that differ from the normal appearance.

Fissures: Oblique fissures in the normal patient are seen from T4/5 posteriorly, travelling through each hilum; the left should finish around 5 cm behind the costophrenic angle (anteriorly) and the right immediately behind the costophrenic angle (anteriorly). They are often superimposed for most of their length, as seen on the image.

The horizontal fissure separates the right upper and right middle lobe, travelling anteriorly from the hilum.

Fissures that appear displaced or accompanied by increased density over adjacent lung tissue (and contained within the margin of the fissure) should be commented upon.

Hemidiaphragms: The lateral provides a good opportunity to assess the shape of the hemidiaphragm. Indeed, loss of diaphragmatic doming in conditions such as COPD is very easy to spot in the lateral. Are there signs of elevation, irregular outlines, unusual densities or fluid levels (which may suggest pleural effusion)?

The *costophrenic angles* should be sharp but blunting is not always an indicator of pleural effusion; it can be attributed to other lung or pleural pathology, or even hyperinflation. However, comment should be made if blunting is seen.

Cardiac shadow: Check size, position and if the outlines are crisp.

Hilum: As previously described, the hilum consists mainly of vascular structures. Check for position, distortion, increased opacity or lobulation.

Dark areas: There are areas on the lateral chest radiograph where there is not significant overlying soft tissue from organs or musculature. These areas show areas of normal lung and lie posterior to the sternum, superior to the aortic arch and in the inferior/posterior part of the chest. As you travel inferiorly over the thoracic spine, appearances should become darker as we lose the overlying soft tissues. Any increase in opacification in these areas must be considered pathological for pathologies such as infection or malignancy.

Bones: Sternum, thoracic spine and ribs. Compression fractures in the thoracic spine are very obvious on a lateral projection. Any change in density, or position should be noted. The lateral provides visualisation of the sternum impossible in a PA projection. Check for sternal fractures or changes in density which may suggest malignancy. Check for position; depression of the sternum is illustrated in trauma and also pectus excavatum.

Check soft tissues for any 'lumps or bumps' that should not be present.

Familiarity with normal radiographic anatomy will help with the decision as to whether unusual densities are normal or abnormal. Often a lateral is only performed if abnormality is suspected on the PA projection, giving clues as to where abnormalities may be seen.

Devices: One of the most common requests from referrers for lateral examinations is to identify position of devices or leads, e.g. post pacemaker insertion. This will identify an anterior configuration of the pacemaker leads impossible in a PA projection. The lateral projection in this instance also provides a view posterior to the inserted pacemaker/defibrillator which may mask pathologies such as a tumour on the PA projection.

The following is a systematic synopsis of common pathologies and where they may manifest on a lateral projection:[25]

1. Retrosternal space/anterior clear space – mediastinal tumours, lymphoma, retrosternal goitre, thymoma, teratoma
2. Upper middle mediastinum: trachea and retrotracheal space (Raider triangle). Endothoracic goitre, enlarged paratracheal lymph nodes, oesophageal tumours, vascular abnormalities
3. Central middle mediastinum – hilar area: lymphadenopathy, pulmonary arterial hypertension, bronchogenic cyst, pulmonary lesions that mimic hilar pathology
4. Lower area – retrocardiac space: hiatus hernia, pulmonary consolidation, lung carcinoma
5. Posterior costodiaphragmatic angles – posterior clear space: pleural effusion, Bochdalek hernia
6. Interlobar fissures: lobar collapse with displacement of the fissures, fluid in the fissures
7. Thoracic spine and posterior mediastinum: vertebral body metastases, pathological vertebral fractures, neurogenic tumours
8. Sternum: metastatic lesions, trauma
9. Cardiac shadow: cardiac calcifications, pericardial calcifications, pericardial effusion.

Common Errors: Lateral Chest

Common Errors	Possible Reasons	Potential Effects on PCE or Report
Non-superimposition of condyles of vertebral bodies; non-superimposition of posterior aspects of ribs	Rotation; MSP not parallel to IR	For both rotation and tilt (below) it becomes more difficult to assess fissures accurately, or the exact location of any lesions spotted on the PA projection
Intervertebral joint spaces not cleared	Patient tilt; MSP not parallel to IR *or* patient has scoliosis. The PA chest image will confirm this	
Pale shadow over upper lungs	Unavoidable at extreme upper lung area (apices); soft tissue shadow lower than this is almost certainly due to the upper arms dropping from their required position. Take care not to confuse the appearance with pathology	Upper lung fields cannot be assessed

Lung Apices

As with the lateral projection, modern imaging methods have largely superseded the use of apical projections, but it may be a low radiation dose approach to use apical projections to clarify whether a suspicious appearance needs further investigation. Indeed, use of the lordotic projection to characterise apical or upper zone opacities may negate the need to use computed tomography with its higher radiation dose.

Suspected lesions in the lung apex may well be seen above the clavicle on a PA chest image, but there is some risk that the clavicle itself will overlie some appearances. The lung apex can be cleared from the clavicle in one of the following ways:

1. With the patient initially AP or PA, the thorax is tilted in extreme lordosis to elevate the clavicles above the lung apices. A horizontal beam is used (see Figs 15.23A,B, 15.24).
2. With the patient initially PA, a horizontal beam is angled 30° caudally to project the lung apices below the clavicles (see Fig. 15.25).
3. With the patient initially AP, a horizontal beam is angled 30° cranially to project the clavicles above the lung apices. An appropriate method to clear the clavicles from the apices should be chosen after consideration of imaging principles and dose implications

When undertaking apical projections it is important to consider image quality, radiation dose and patient tolerance.

Method 1 (Lordotic AP or PA with Horizontal Beam)

The horizontal beam image has less distortion than methods using angulation, but the AP position has implications for increased dose to the thyroid, eye lens, breast and sternum compared to the PA position. In the AP position the patient can lean back onto the IR for support, but unless there are suitable structures for the patient to hold on to, the PA method can be unstable. In the AP position the apical region is closer to the IR, whereas there is increased lung-apex-to-film distance in the PA position, which has implications for magnification unsharpness of the area. An air gap will also exist, requiring some increase in exposure. However, the air gap will have the effect of some reduction in scatter and hence improved image quality.

Method 2 (PA Position with 30° Caudal Angulation)

The benefits of the PA position are as those for method 1 but the 30° angulation will cause some image distortion.

Method 3 (AP Position with 30° Cranial Angulation)

Disadvantages of using the AP position are as those outlined in method 1, but in addition to this the angulation will cause some image distortion, as in method 2. Because the angle is directed cranially, the dose to the lenses of the eyes and thyroid will be greater than with AP method 1.

This method will be more acceptable to patients who cannot comply with requirements for sitting or standing in a PA position, as for the routine chest PA projection. It can be used in the supine position, with a vertical central ray directed 30° cranially.

A lordotic projection can also be used to demonstrate right middle lobe collapse, using the PA position described in method 1, and inclusion of all thoracic anatomy as for the routine PA chest projection, centring at the level of T8.

Apparent lesions adequately seen above the clavicle on the PA projection can be demonstrated in a different plane by using a lordotic apical projection, since information on lung apices cannot be gleaned from a lateral chest image. Beam angulation will provide a more distorted image and is therefore of limited value. The current recommendation for investigation of suspicious lesions in this region is to use CT, whenever readily available.

Exposure Factors

As the apices are not overshadowed by dense structures such as the mediastinum, in apical projections it is not necessary to use a high kVp technique or antiscatter grid. A lower kVp will help reduce scatter and increase contrast quality. The projections should be well collimated, which will reduce dose and therefore also ensure optimum contrast by assisting with scatter reduction.

LUNG APICES: ANTEROPOSTERIOR (AP) LORDOTIC (FIG. 15.23A,B)

IR is erect

Positioning

- The patient initially sits erect in the AP position, with their seat approximately 25–35 cm from the IR. Distance varies according to patient height: taller patients will need to sit further away than shorter patients
- The patient leans back to rest the backs of their shoulders upon the IR; the clavicle should lie horizontally level with the C7/T1 region
- The IR is adjusted until the area of interest lies within its boundaries
- The MSP is perpendicular to the IR
- The SC joints are equidistant from the IR
- Scapular clearance is required as for the PA chest projection
- An AP marker is used

Beam Direction and FRD

Horizontal
2 m FRD

Note that magnification reduction is not as great an issue as in the full PA chest projection, since the CT ratio is not relevant to the projection. Therefore it is not inappropriate to use a shorter FRD.

Centring

Over the sternal angle

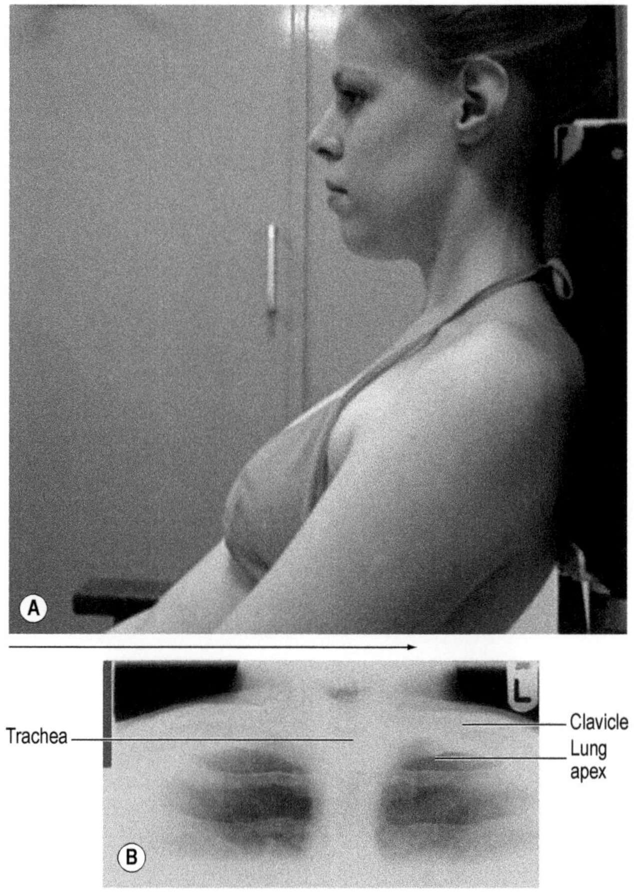

Fig. 15.23 AP lung apices with lordosis.

A visual check that the shadow of the upper border of the soft tissue above the shoulder and clavicle lies within the light beam field and within IR boundaries will ensure that the tops of the lung apices are included.

Collimation

Upper border of T1, clavicles, lung apices, lateral borders of ribs 1–5, fifth thoracic vertebra

LUNG APICES: POSTEROANTERIOR (PA) LORDOTIC (FIG. 15.24)

IR vertical

Positioning

- The patient initially sits erect in the PA position, with their seat directly in front of the IR
- The patient leans back, away from the IR, until their clavicles lie horizontally level with the C7/T1 region
- The patient holds onto the unit, bucky housing or handles for stability
- The SC joints are equidistant from the IR
- Scapular clearance is required
- A PA marker is used

Beam Direction and FRD

Horizontal
2 m FRD

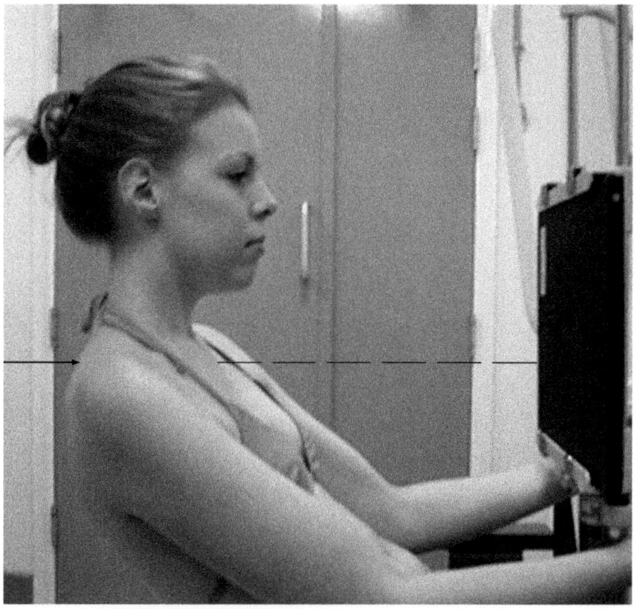

Fig. 15.24 PA lung apices with lordosis.

In contrast to the AP method, this distance is essential in order to reduce magnification and unsharpness.

Centring

Over the midline of the patient, to emerge through the sternal angle

Collimation

Upper border of T1, clavicles, lung apices, lateral borders of ribs 1–5, fifth thoracic vertebra

For both the PA and AP lordotic projections of the apices, a visual check that the shadow of the upper border of the soft tissue above the shoulder and clavicle lies within the light beam field will ensure that the tops of the lung apices are included.

LUNG APICES: PA WITH 30° CAUDAL ANGULATION (FIG. 15.25)

Most dedicated digital chest units have a fixed central ray which is perpendicular to the IR; this method, and the AP with cranial angulation, is therefore unsuitable for use with this type of unit.

IR is erect

Positioning

- The patient sits erect in the PA position
- The SC joints are equidistant from the IR
- Scapular clearance is required
- A PA marker is used

Beam Direction and FRD

Initially horizontal, which is then directed 30° caudally
2 m FRD

Centring

Over the vertebral column, to emerge at the sternal notch

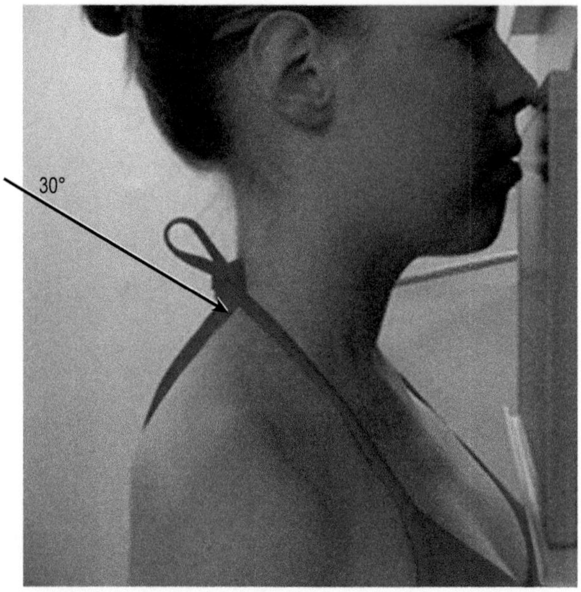

Fig. 15.25 PA lung apices with 30° caudal angulation.

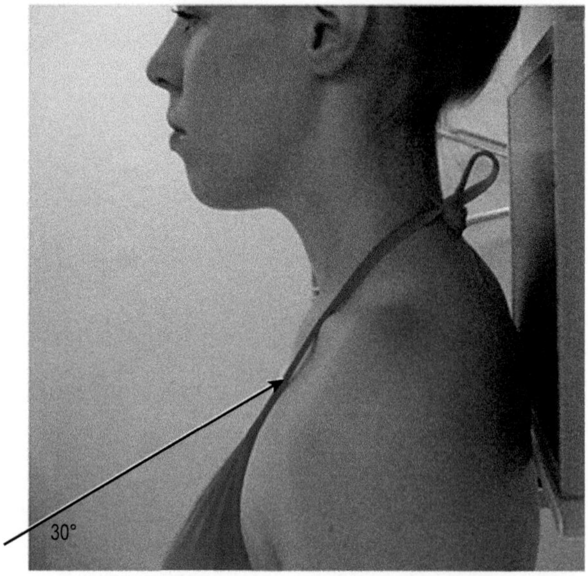

Fig. 15.26 AP lung apices with 30° cranial angulation.

Collimation

Upper border of T1, clavicles, lung apices, lateral borders of ribs 1–5, fifth thoracic vertebra

A visual check that the shadow of the upper border of the soft tissue above the shoulder and the clavicle lies within the light beam field will ensure that the tops of the lung apices are included.

LUNG APICES: AP WITH 30° CRANIAL ANGULATION (FIG. 15.26)

IR is vertical

Positioning

- The patient sits erect in the AP position
- The SC joints are equidistant from the IR
- Scapular clearance is required
- An AP marker is used

Beam Direction and FRD

Initially horizontal, which is then directed 30° cranially
1 m FRD

Centring

To the sternal angle

Collimation

Upper border of T1, clavicles, lung apices, lateral borders of ribs 1–5, fifth thoracic vertebra

A visual check that the shadow of the upper border of the soft tissue above the shoulder and clavicle lies within the light beam field will ensure that the tops of the lung apices are included.

All methods: Expose on arrested inspiration

Criteria for Assessing Image Quality

- Upper border of T1, clavicles, lung apices, lateral borders of ribs 1–5 and fifth thoracic vertebra are demonstrated on the image
- Clavicles cleared above the tops of the lung apices
- Flattened appearance of the ribs
- Medial ends of clavicles equidistant from the midline of the thoracic vertebrae
- Scapulae cleared from the lung fields

Common Errors: Lung Apices with 30° Angulation

Common Errors	Possible Reasons
Overall image density low, unable to compensate during post processing	Insufficient exposure given; the projection requires an increase from that used for the PA projection as the beam travels through an increased thickness due to lordosis or beam angulation. If PA lordotic method used, has the increased air gap been considered?
One lung apex more dense than the other	Rotation
Clavicles overlying lung apices	Lordosis or beam angle is insufficient

Potential Effects on PCE or Report

The most important aspect of this image is its ability to show lung apices clear of the clavicles, in order to assess subtle lesions that may lie behind the clavicles. Sub-standard images related to exposure factors or clearance of clavicles from lung tissue will clearly impact on accurate assessment of this area

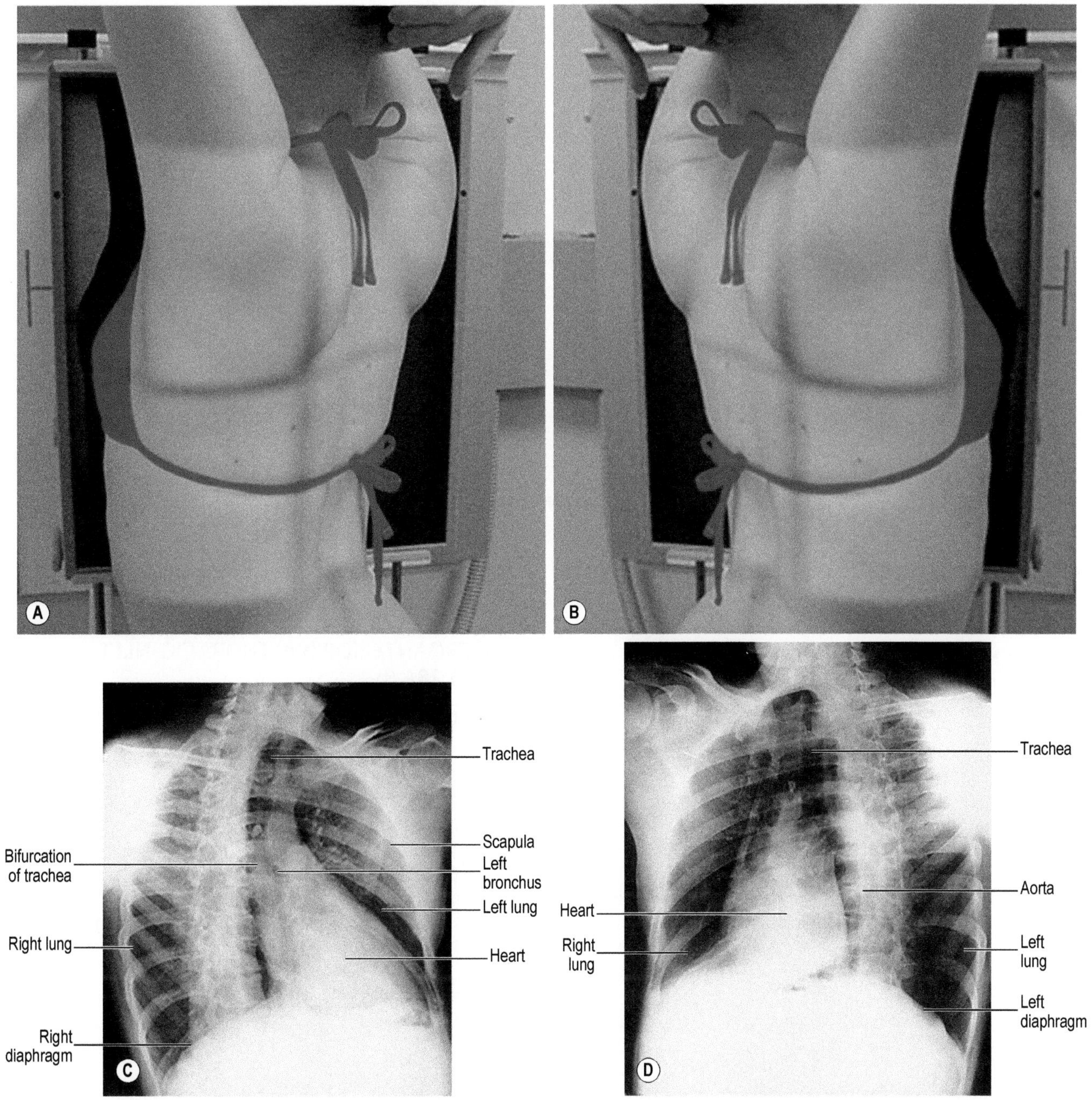

Fig. 15.27 (A) RAO chest; (B) LAO chest; (C) RAO chest; (D) LAO chest. (C and D, Reproduced with permission from Ballinger PW, Frank ED. *Merrill's Atlas of Radiographic Positioning and Radiologic Procedures.* 10th ed. St Louis: Mosby; 2003.)

Oblique Projections of the Chest

Prior to the widespread use of CT, oblique projections of the chest were valuable for demonstrating the estimated 40% of lung tissue obscured by dense structures in the chest.[26] In addition, oblique projections can be used to demonstrate the mediastinum, heart and great vessels, trachea, hila and pleural plaques evident in cases of mesothelioma.

45° ANTERIOR OBLIQUE CHEST (RAO, LAO) (FIG. 15.27A–D)

IR is vertical for all oblique projections of the chest

Positioning

- A horizontal beam is collimated to the size of the patient's thorax, with the patient standing with the front of their chest in contact with the receptor
- The IR height is adjusted until the area of interest lies within its boundaries
- From a PA position, the patient rotates 45° to the left for the RAO or 45° to the right for the LAO projection
- The feet are slightly separated for stability
- The arms are raised at the sides of the head and then flexed at the elbows; the forearms are then rested across the top of the head. This clears the arms from the field

- Without leaning forward, the patient is immobilised by resting the shoulder nearest the IR against the IR
- A PA marker is most frequently used on the upper aspect of the IR. The RAO should bear a right marker and the LAO a left marker, which should always lie above the side nearest the IR

Beam Direction and FRD

Horizontal
2 m FRD

Centring

To the middle of the IR, at the level of the spinous process of T7 (body of T8), midway between the vertebral column and the lateral borders of ribs on the side furthest from the IR

Collimation

First thoracic vertebra, first rib, lateral margins of ribs 2–10, costophrenic angles

Criteria for Assessing Image Quality

- First thoracic vertebra and first rib, all rib outlines and diaphragms are demonstrated
- Arms are cleared from the lung fields
- Vertebral column shown closer to the lateral border of the thorax on the side positioned nearest the IR
- Heart shown in its entirety over the vertebral column and side positioned furthest from the IR
- Seven anterior ribs are demonstrated above the diaphragms. These should be counted on the side positioned nearest to the IR
- Sharp image demonstrating the dense mediastinal structures in contrast with air-filled lungs

Common Errors: 45° AO Chest

Common Errors	Possible Reasons	Potential Effects on PCE or Report
Heart shadow slightly overlapping onto side nearest IR	Less than 45° rotation on the thorax	Retrocardiac space cannot be assessed
Appearance of space between heart shadow and vertebral column on side furthest from IR	More than 45° rotation on the thorax	As above

OTHER ANTERIOR OBLIQUE CHEST POSITIONS

The 45° obliques described are probably the most useful obliques today, as they are most appropriate for a general oblique survey of the chest and adequate for demonstrating pleural plaques when ongoing assessment may not require CT at every stage. Other obliques are suggested for demonstration of more specific structures:

1. Trachea, great vessels and cardiac outline will best be seen with a greater angle of rotation (60°) on the RAO projection.[13,16] The structures are seen well clear of the vertebral column, as is the descending aorta.
2. Bifurcation of the trachea and arch of aorta can be demonstrated by using a 70° rotation on the LAO projection.[13] Structures are seen cleared from the vertebral column but the descending aorta is seen to overlie it.

Thoracic Inlet

The trachea can appear deviated or compressed on plain radiographic images, owing to tumour or thyroid goitre, goitre being the most common finding. Goitre can also cause medicinal widening. It can also deviate from the midline towards the side of lobar collapse on AP or PA projections. Rotation when positioning the patient will cause apparent deviation of the trachea from the midline. In the 21st century, the area covered by the thoracic inlet is largely examined by MRI, CT or radionuclide imaging (RNI) studies.

IR is erect for all projections of the thoracic inlet

POSTEROANTERIOR (PA) THORACIC INLET (FIG. 15.28A,B)

Positioning

- The patient faces the IR; the feet are slightly separated for stability
- The MSP is coincident with, and perpendicular to, the long axis of the IR
- The chin is raised until the occiput and mandible are superimposed, to maximise the amount of upper trachea demonstrated on the image
- A PA marker is most frequently used, on the upper aspect of the IR

Beam Direction and FRD

Horizontal
100 cm FRD

Centring

Through T2 to emerge through the sternal notch

Expose on arrested inspiration

Collimation

C4–T6 longitudinally, lateral soft tissue outlines of the neck

Criteria for Assessing Image Quality

- Trachea down to its bifurcation and lateral soft tissue outlines of the neck are demonstrated
- Spinous processes of vertebrae and the trachea are demonstrated down the centre of the vertebral bodies and medial ends of clavicles equidistant from the spinous process
- Mandible and occiput are superimposed
- Sharp image demonstrating air-filled trachea in contrast to the soft tissue of neck and vertebral column

Common Errors: PA Thoracic Inlet

Common Errors	Possible Reasons
Symmetrical dense white shadow of occiput obscuring upper trachea	Chin raised too high
Symmetrical shadow of mandible obscuring upper trachea	Chin not raised enough
Asymmetrical shadow of occiput and/or mandible superimposed over upper neck	Head is rotated. If appearances are accompanied by rotation of the trunk (see next comments below) the whole of the MSP is incorrectly positioned
Trachea not centralised over vertebral column	MSP not perpendicular to IR *or* some deviation may be due to external common compression (for example in cases of thyroid enlargement). This, of course, is not due to radiographer error

Potential Effects on PCE or Report

The most important aspect of this image is its ability to show the air-filled thoracic inlet in contrast with the soft tissues of the neck. Sub-standard images related to exposure factors or clearance of other body tissues from the trachea will clearly impact on accurate assessment of this area

LATERAL UPPER RESPIRATORY TRACT AND THORACIC INLET (FIG. 15.29A,B)

Positioning

- The patient stands erect with their MSP parallel to the IR; the feet are slightly separated for stability. This projection may be undertaken with the patient sitting
- The chin is raised until the mandible is cleared as far as possible from the upper trachea
- The shoulders are relaxed downwards to clear them from the inlet into the thorax

Beam Direction and FRD

Horizontal
200 cm FRD

This is an increase from the 100 cm used for the PA projection. It aims to reduce magnification of the trachea, which lies further from the IR owing to the shoulder's position against the IR

Centring

To the middle of the neck, at the level of the thyroid eminence

Collimation

Nasopharynx and down to include medial end of clavicle, anterior soft tissue outline, vertebral bodies of cervical vertebrae, T1

Good collimation, avoiding irradiation of the orbits, can be improved by slightly rotating the light beam diaphragm so that its long axis follows the angle of the neck.

Expose on arrested inspiration

Criteria for Assessing Image Quality

- Nasopharynx, oropharynx, upper trachea, medial end of clavicle and anterior aspect of soft tissues of neck are demonstrated
- Mandible is elevated to clear it from as much of the trachea as possible (but there will still be some superimposition)
- Sharp image demonstrating air-filled trachea in contrast to the soft tissue of the neck. The vertebral column will be under-penetrated

Common Error: Lateral Upper Respiratory Tract and Thoracic Inlet

Common Error	Possible Reason	Potential Effect on PCE or Report
Soft tissue shadow obscuring clavicle and trachea	Poor patient posture during exposure (shoulders not relaxed). This may be a problem with kyphosed patients	The most important aspect of this image is its ability to show the air-filled trachea inlet in contrast with the soft tissues of the neck. Sub-standard images related to exposure factors or clearance of other body tissues from the trachea will clearly impact on accurate assessment of this area

LATERAL LOWER TRACHEA AND THORACIC INLET (FIG. 15.30A–C)

A grid may be used for this technique

Positioning

- The patient stands erect with their MSP parallel to the IR; the feet are slightly separated for stability. This projection may be undertaken with the patient sitting
- The arms are extended and raised either side of the head, until vertical. The chin is raised to further effect this manoeuvre, which aims to clear the humeral heads from the retrosternal area of the trachea

The method described for clearance of humeral heads from the area of interest is contrary to those previously described,[15] where the hands are clasped behind the back and the shoulders pulled back (Fig. 15.30B). This method is difficult for many patients, particularly those with degenerative disease of the joints and some who are overweight. The method using raised arms has previously been suggested as an alternative for patients with stiff shoulders[17]

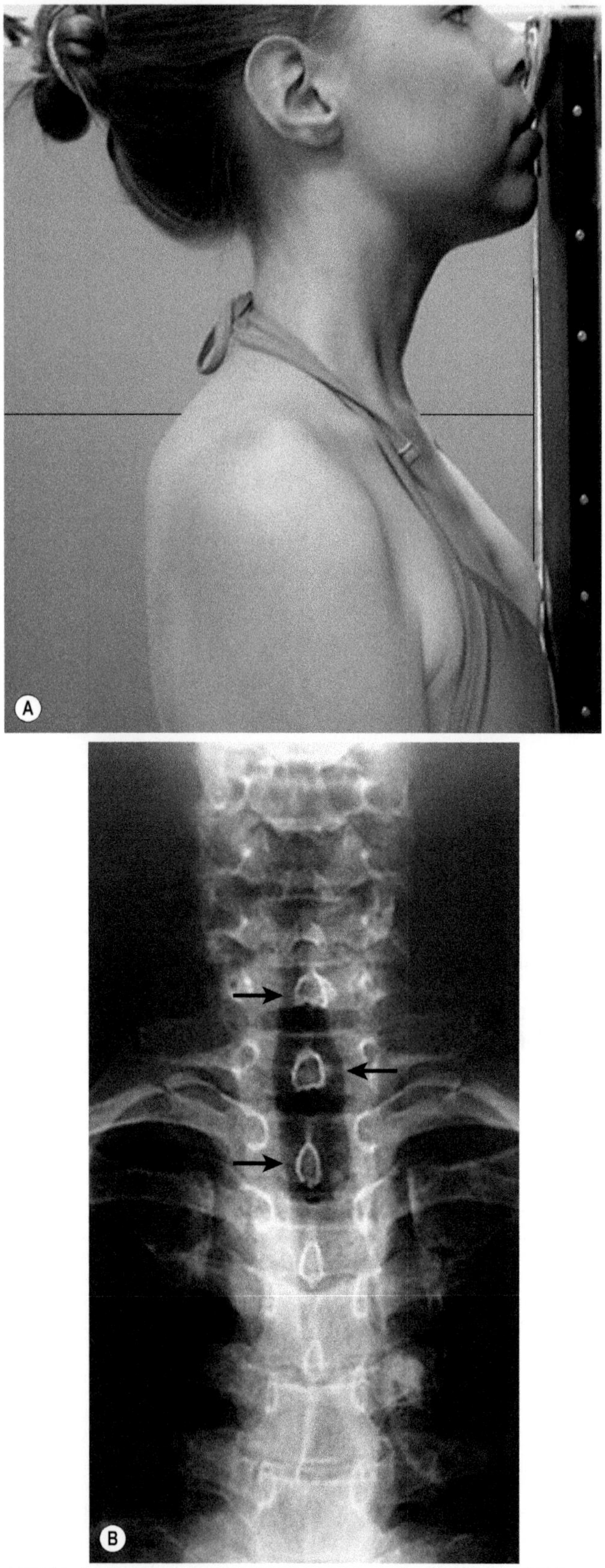

Fig. 15.28 PA thoracic inlet. (B) The arrows outline the lateral margins of the air-filled trachea. (B, Reproduced with permission from Ballinger PW, Frank ED. *Merrill's Atlas of Radiographic Positioning and Radiologic Procedures*. 10th ed. St Louis: Mosby; 2003.)

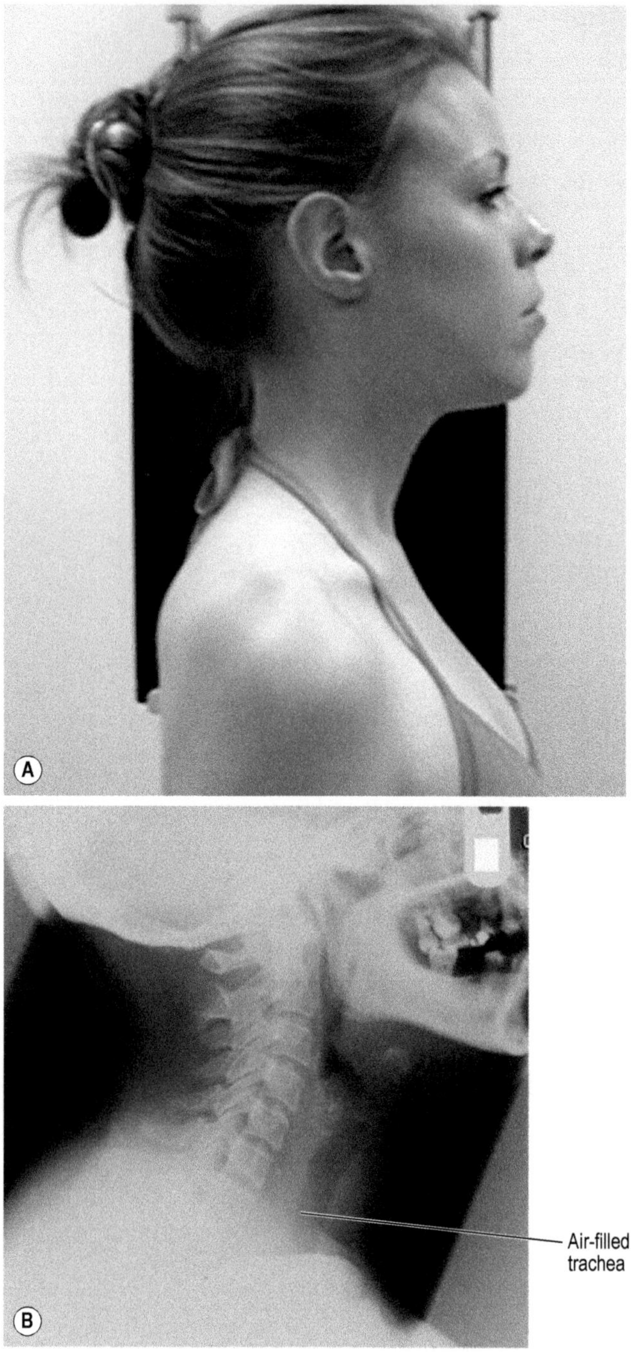

Fig. 15.29 Lateral upper respiratory tract.

and is a viable first choice owing to its easy implementation. It must be remembered, however, that failure to raise the chin adequately and bring the arms vertical will limit the effectiveness of the manoeuvre.

Beam Direction and FRD

Horizontal
200 cm FRD

As for the lateral of the upper region, this FRD is selected to counteract magnification caused by increased object receptor distance (ORD).

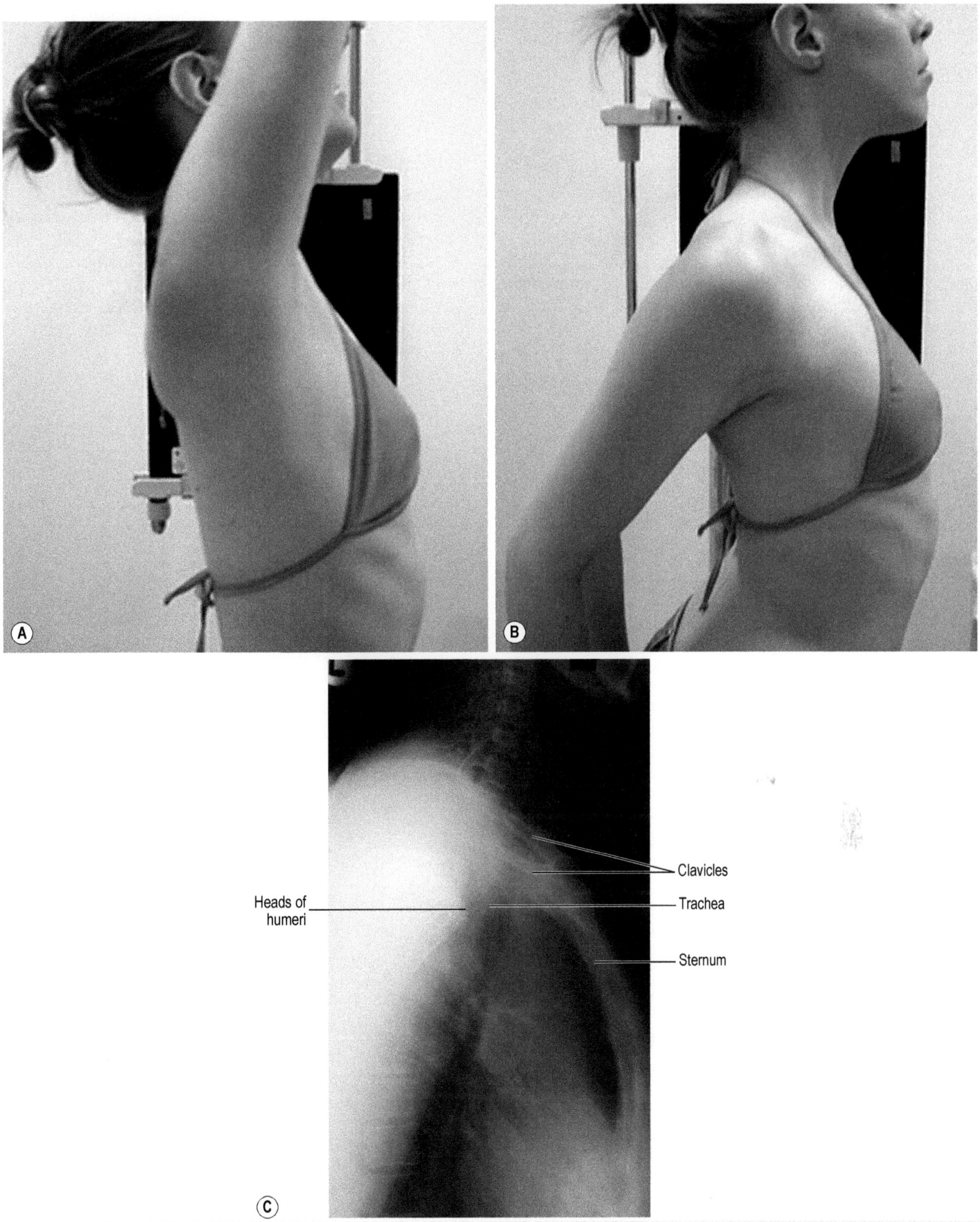

Fig. 15.30 Lateral lower trachea and thoracic inlet with (A) arms raised and (B) arms pulled back. (C) Lateral lower trachea and thoracic inlet.

Centring

Below the sternal notch, at the level of the sternal angle

Collimation

Thyroid eminence and carina of trachea, soft tissue anterior to trachea in neck and thorax, bodies of cervical vertebrae, lung tissue posteriorly

It is important that the whole of the trachea is demonstrated by the combination of the two lateral projections described for the trachea and thoracic inlet. As a result, the crossover area, which is that of the inlet of the trachea into the thorax level with the sternal notch, must be seen adequately on both images. Because two exposures are made this has implications for dose to the patient; it is possible to undertake one projection of the whole area, using a high kVp technique and centring at the level of C6–C7 while collimating to include the whole of the trachea.[16]

Expose on arrested inspiration

Criteria for Assessing Image Quality

- Trachea from above the sternal notch down to its bifurcation, manubrium sterni, lung tissue anterior and posterior to the trachea are demonstrated
- Soft tissue of shoulders and heads of humeri are cleared from the trachea
- Sharp image demonstrating air-filled trachea in contrast to the lung tissue, clavicle and manubrium

Common Error: Lateral Lower Trachea and Thoracic Inlet

Common Error	Possible Reason	Potential Effect on PCE or Report
Density overlying trachea on image	Arms and shoulders inadequately raised or not pulled back	The most important aspect of this image is its ability to show the air-filled thoracic inlet in contrast with the soft tissues of the lungs and ribs. Sub-standard images related to exposure factors or clearance of other body tissues from the trachea will clearly impact on accurate assessment of this area

Thoracic Skeleton

The rib series has long been considered a non-justified projection by many experts in the field.[1,27] Although painful, rib fractures are treated conservatively unless displacement causes fracture fragments to penetrate the soft issue of the thorax and induce pneumothorax or haemothorax. Evidence of these conditions is definitely required via radiographic examination, and the PA chest projection is considered to be the most appropriate means for demonstration of these appearances.[28]

The bones of the thorax consist of the ribs and sternum, but radiographic examination of the area also involves demonstration of the sternoclavicular joints, as the most important aspect of diagnosis is that of assessing the effect injury may have had on thoracic contents. The PA chest image is also very likely to demonstrate the fractured rib and fragments causing a pneumothorax, haemothorax or evidence of visceral damage.[1,29] Ribs positioned below the diaphragm on the PA image are those that are less likely to penetrate the pleura, thus reducing or eradicating the need for separate X-ray examination of these. The PA chest image also shows ribs 1–6 reasonably well in their entirety, but not ribs 7–12.

Metastatic deposits may be demonstrated by X-ray but are better located via scintigraphy; however, as metastases in the rib may lead to pathological fracture it may be necessary to undertake plain radiography. In addition to fractures and metastasis, other rib lesions seen on plain radiography include fibrous dysplasia, aneurysmal bone cysts, myeloma and granuloma,[30] but it is questionable whether X-ray would be the method of choice to demonstrate them.

OBLIQUE RIBS

The oblique projection is designed to turn the lateral portions of the ribs away from their profiled position as seen on the PA chest radiograph. Of course, this means that other aspects of the ribs will not be well demonstrated on the oblique projection. For this reason, oblique ribs projections must always be accompanied by a PA chest radiograph.

It is more than obvious that exposures should be made on arrested respiration, but the phase varies according to the ribs under examination owing to the position of the diaphragm in relation to individual rib height. Because the diaphragm effectively splits the area covered by ribs into two different densities, this has implications for adequate demonstration of ribs on the radiograph. As a result, exposure for oblique projections of the upper ribs (1–6) is made on arrested inspiration to facilitate their demonstration over the air-filled lung tissue, and ribs 7–12 on expiration to demonstrate them over abdominal tissue below the diaphragm.

In addition to the phase of respiration, angulation can be used to maximise the number of ribs shown above or below the diaphragm. Caudal angulation will project the image of the diaphragm lower in the case of the upper ribs, as can cranial angulation to project it higher and maximise the number of lower ribs shown below the diaphragm.

PCE COMMENTS – RIBS (ALL PROJECTIONS)

Unless shown already via chest X-ray, assess lung markings to exclude pneumothorax.

Check bone density. Are the bones hyperdense or hyperlucent? Are there localised hyperdense or hyperlucent areas within individual bones? These appearances may indicate metastatic or metabolic bone disease.

Is there evidence of expansion of the localised area when a lesion is suspected within the rib?

Where cortical outlines can be clearly assessed (more usually clearer on upper ribs), check these for continuity. If a suspicion of fracture, assess if subtle or clearly displaced.

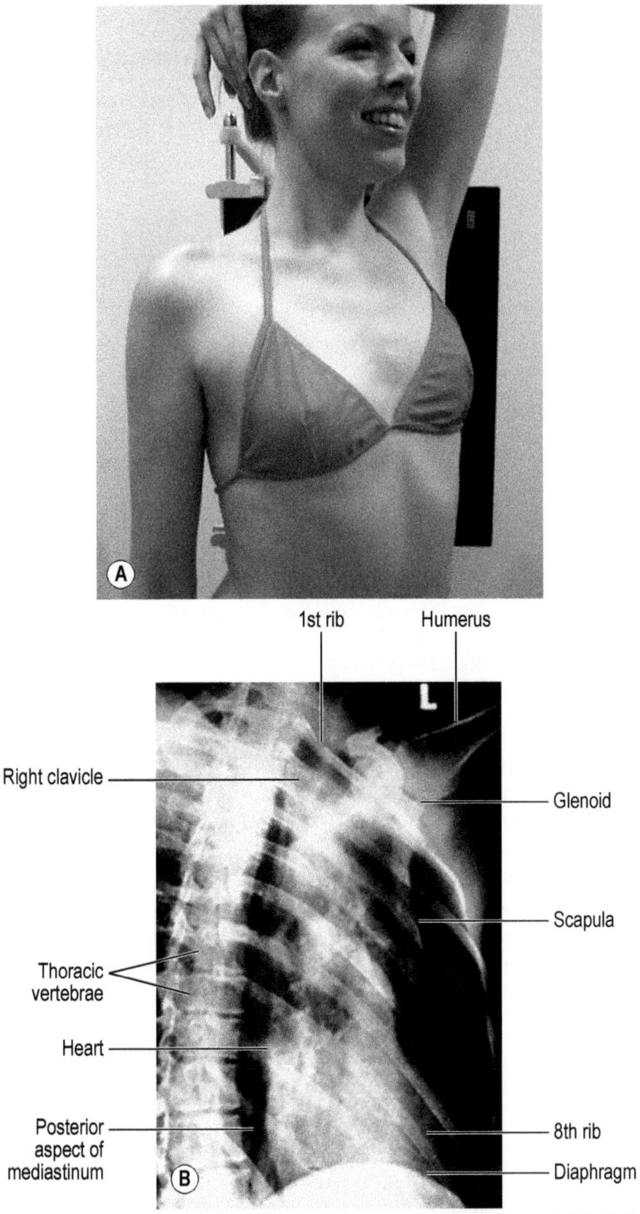

Fig. 15.31 Posterior oblique – upper ribs. (B, Reproduced with permission from Bryan GJ. *Skeletal Anatomy*. 3rd ed. Edinburgh: Churchill Livingstone; 1996 and Gunn C. *Bones and Joints*. 4th ed. Edinburgh: Churchill Livingstone; 2002.)

POSTERIOR OBLIQUE FOR UPPER RIBS (FIG. 15.31A,B)

IR is vertical for projections of the ribs unless otherwise stated, an antiscatter grid is often required for lower ribs

Positioning

- The patient stands with their back to the IR and faces the X-ray tube; the side under examination is positioned with the lateral borders of ribs 1–6 well within the IR border
- The arm on the side under investigation is raised and the forearm rested on the head; this will clear the arm from the area of interest
- The patient is rotated 30–45° towards the side under examination; the thorax on the side of interest rests against the IR

Beam Direction and FRD

Beam is initially horizontal, with 12° caudal angulation
100 cm FRD

Centring

Two-thirds of the way down the line adjoining sternal notch and xiphisternum

IR displacement may be required to ensure that the area of interest lies within its boundaries

Collimation

C7 to T12, lateral margins of ribs on affected side, midclavicular line on the opposite side

It is not necessary for this projection to be undertaken erect, but it is described thus as it is more comfortable for the patient who has painful ribs, as their weight does not lie on their injured thoracic ribcage. Supine oblique positioning can still be adopted for patients who cannot sit or stand erect.

Upper rib oblique projection were often described using an antiscatter grid and in some cases still are,[16] but as ribs 1–6 lie superior to the diaphragm in a low-density area, direct exposure is possible without an antiscatter device. This allows reduction in exposure factors and therefore affords less radiation dose to the patient.[28] In the case of larger patients it is possible that provision of adequate contrast may be compromised by an increase in tissue density. This, coupled with the higher density over the mediastinum, may require the use of a grid.

Expose on arrested inspiration

Criteria for Assessing Image Quality

- The entire length of ribs 1–6 are demonstrated above diaphragm
- Arm is cleared from thorax
- Heart shadow may overlie medial aspect of sixth rib in the case of right-sided ribs, or most of the sixth rib in the case of left-sided ribs
- Oblique appearance of thoracic vertebrae
- Image of anterior ribs moved laterally in comparison to their position as seen on the PA chest image
- Sharp image demonstrating ribs in contrast to air-filled lung tissue and viscera of the mediastinum and heart

Common Errors: Posterior Oblique for Upper Ribs

Common Errors	Possible Reasons	Potential Effects on PCE or Report
Contrast or detail of image is poor	AEC and central ray may be lying over the mediastinum, due to positioning error Since there is a wide range of tissue densities in the area of interest, this will have a potential impact on selection of exposure factors. This is especially difficult in patients who have dense body tissue or excess adipose tissue Exposure factors selected are inappropriate. Useful guidance on this is given in Chapter 3, Table 3.1	It may not be possible (and indeed this is most likely) to assess the cortical detail needed to spot subtle fractures or lytic lesions

Common Errors: Posterior Oblique for Upper Ribs–cont'd

Common Errors	Possible Reasons	Potential Effects on PCE or Report
Pale shadow overlying lateral ribs	Arm not cleared from area	This will render the image unsuitable for assessment of fractures and lesions
Lower ribs (4–6) pale and shown below diaphragm	Exposed on expiration	This will render the image unsuitable for assessment of fractures and lesions

POSTERIOR OBLIQUE FOR LOWER RIBS (FIG. 15.32A,B)

Positioning

- The patient stands with their back to the IR and faces the X-ray tube; the side under examination is positioned with the lateral borders of ribs 7–12 well within the IR boundaries
- The arm on the side under investigation is raised and the forearm rested on the head; this will clear the arm from the area of interest
- The patient is rotated 30–45° towards the side under examination; the thorax on the side of interest rests against the IR

Beam Direction and FRD

Central ray is initially horizontal, with 12° cranial angulation
100 cm FRD

Centring

Midway between the lower costal margin and xiphisternum

IR displacement may be required to ensure that the area of interest lies within its boundaries.

Collimation

2.5 cm below lower costal margin to midway between the sternal notch and xiphisternum, lateral margins of ribs on the affected side, midclavicular line on the opposite side

Expose on arrested expiration

Note that the oblique for lower ribs is described as for the upper ribs, with the patient erect. This is in contrast to older methods,[31] which suggest this projection be undertaken with the patient in a supine oblique position. The erect position has been used here simply for reasons of patient comfort.

Criteria for Assessing Image Quality

- The entire length of ribs 7–12 demonstrated below the diaphragm; ribs 7 and 8 are frequently shown above the diaphragm but, since the heart shadow tends to overlie these ribs in the oblique position, contrast over these ribs is usually similar to those seen below the diaphragm
- Arm cleared from thorax
- Oblique appearance of thoracic vertebrae
- Ribs appear less curved than in a PA or AP image
- Sharp image demonstrating ribs in contrast to abdominal and heart tissue

Common Errors: Posterior Oblique for Lower Ribs

Common Errors	Possible Reasons	Potential Effects on PCE or Report
Pale shadow overlying lateral ribs	Arm not cleared from area	This will render the image unsuitable for assessment of fractures and lesions
Ribs 7–8 dark and shown above diaphragm	Exposed on inspiration; more likely to affect the right side than the left due to there being less heart tissue superimposed over the ribs on this side	As above

Sternum

The mechanism for injury to the sternum is most likely to be that of a significant crush injury, as in a road traffic accident when the steering wheel impacts upon the driver's chest and can be undertaken with the patient seated or supine on a trolley.

LATERAL STERNUM (FIG. 15.33A,B)

IR is vertical, an antiscatter grid may be required for larger patients

Positioning

- The patient stands or sits erect with the lateral aspect of their chest placed in contact with the IR. If standing, their feet are separated for stability
- The height of the IR is adjusted to coincide with the sternum
- The MSP is parallel to the IR
- The arms are raised above the head to clear from the area of interest as for the chest lateral; the chin is raised *or*
- The shoulders are pulled back (this may be difficult for some patients)

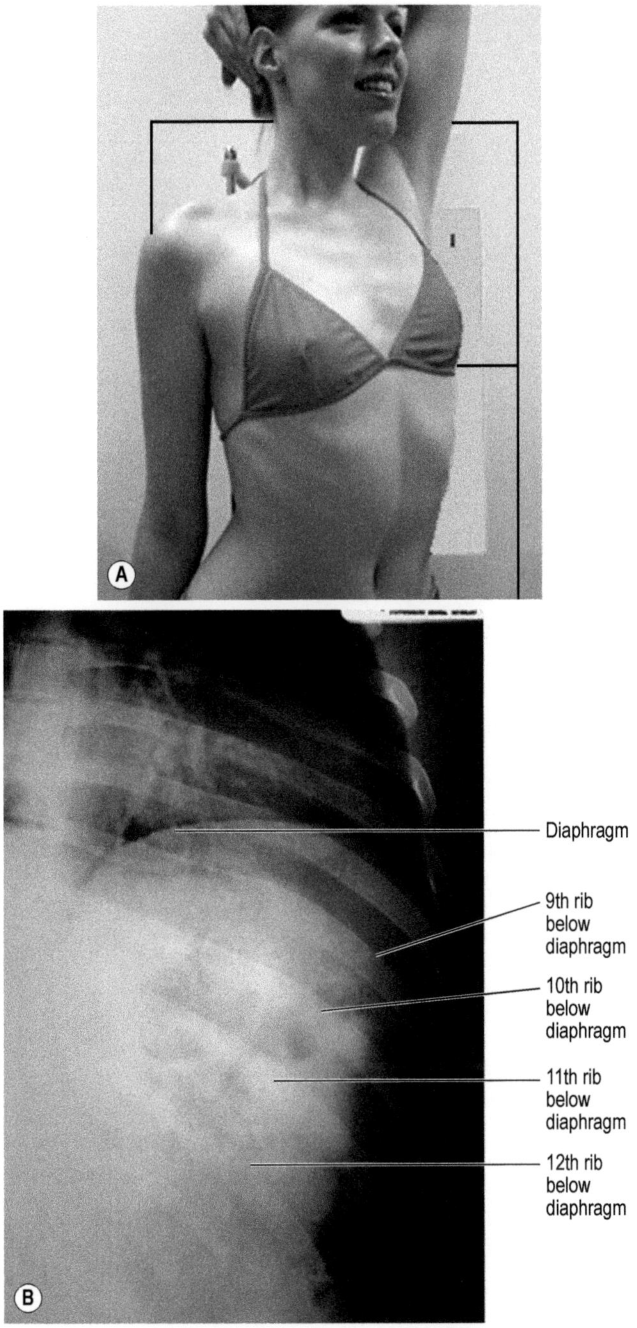

Fig. 15.32 Posterior oblique – lower ribs.

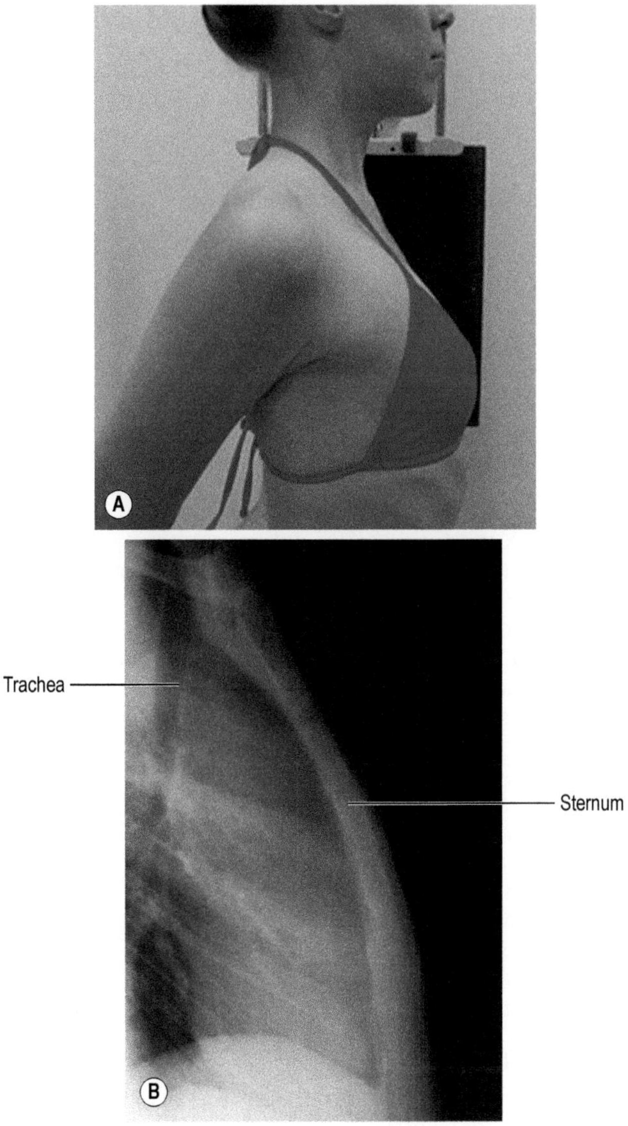

Fig. 15.33 Lateral sternum.

Expose on arrested respiration

Arrested respiration avoids movement unsharpness on the image, which is the primary function of the manoeuvre. However, arrested inspiration will serve to press the sternum further forward, which is especially beneficial when the arms are pulled backwards rather than raised.

Beam Direction and FRD – lateral sternum

Horizontal, at 90° to the IR
100 cm FRD

Centring

Midway between the sternal notch and xiphisternum

Collimation

SC joints, manubrium, sternal body and xiphisternum, soft tissues of anterior sternal area, retrosternal lung tissue

Rotation of the light beam diaphragm housing to coincide with the long axis of the sternum will maximise efficiency of collimation to the field.

Criteria for Assessing Image Quality

- SC joints, manubrium, sternal body and xiphisternum, soft tissues of anterior sternal area, retrosternal lung tissue are demonstrated
- Arms are cleared from the area of interest
- SC joints are superimposed
- Sharp image demonstrating bony trabeculae in contrast with anterior soft tissues and retrosternal lung tissue

Common Errors: Lateral Sternum

Common Errors	Possible Reasons	Potential Effects on PCE or Report
Pale density over upper sternum and SC joints	Arms not cleared from field	Loss of contrast and density will render information inadequate for assessment
White sternum with no bony detail evident	kVp too low. Also see Chapter 3, Table 3.1	Superimposition of body tissue and loss of contrast and density will render information inadequate for assessment
Lower aspect of sternum not included on image	During inspiration the patient may lean back or elevate the lower chest during the manoeuvre, moving the lower sternum outside the field of collimation or off the receptor completely. Care should be taken to observe the patient during the manoeuvre	Comment cannot be made on all of the sternum; therefore PCE or report is incomplete

ANTERIOR OBLIQUE STERNUM (FIG. 15.34A,B)

This projection is not recommended for trauma cases as it involves a prone position if the patient cannot stand, and in any case it provides no valuable additional information to the lateral. However, it has been recommended for demonstration of inflammatory conditions.[30]

The oblique position clears the sternum from the vertebral column; some texts describe a right anterior oblique,[18,31] but consideration must be given to the fact that the majority of the heart shadow lies over to the left. For this reason, the left anterior oblique is described here, where the right side is moved away from the IR to position the sternum over the right lung. The right atrium of the heart will also move to the right, but this forms a significantly lower proportion of heart tissue than that which would be projected if a right anterior oblique were performed.

The projection can be undertaken erect or prone and therefore IR orientation will depend on which is selected. An antiscatter grid is often required.

Positioning

- The patient lies prone *or* stands facing the IR
- The IR position should be checked to ensure the sternum lies within its boundary
- The patient is rotated 45° towards the right, into the LAO position; the right arm is raised onto the pillow if semi-prone, or on the top of the IR if erect. A 45° radiolucent pad will assist in accurate positioning for both methods, with the added advantage of immobilisation for the semi-prone position. For the semi-prone patient the knee on the raised side is flexed and used as additional immobilisation
- The sternum should lie coincident with the long axis of the IR
- A PA anatomical marker is usually used for this projection

Expose on gentle respiration, using low mA and long time selection

This will blur the rib shadows on the image.

Beam Direction and FRD

Perpendicular to the IR
100 cm FRD

Centring

To the centre of the IR, over the raised side of the thorax

Collimation

The sternum, SC joints

Criteria for Assessing Image Quality

- Sternum and SC joints are demonstrated
- Sternum and SC joints are clear of the vertebral column, and superimposed over the right lung
- Sharp image of the sternum in contrast with the soft tissues of the lung. Blurred rib shadows

Common Error: Anterior Oblique Sternum

Common Error	Possible Reason	Potential Effects on PCE or Report
Sternum partially overlying vertebral column and mediastinum	Inadequate obliquity. This most frequently occurs in the semi-prone position, when the 45° pads used to assess rotation (and aid immobilisation) are not pushed far enough under the thorax. Use of these pads to achieve a 45° rotation can be more effective if the patient lies in a lateral position initially, with the thin edge of the sponge wedge placed closely against the lowered side. The patient then lowers their right side down onto the pad, rather than raising this side from the prone position The weight of the patient can also compress the pad sufficiently to affect angle of obliquity. Use of two pads or one long pad placed under the thorax may prove more effective	Overlying structures will obscure required information related to the sternum

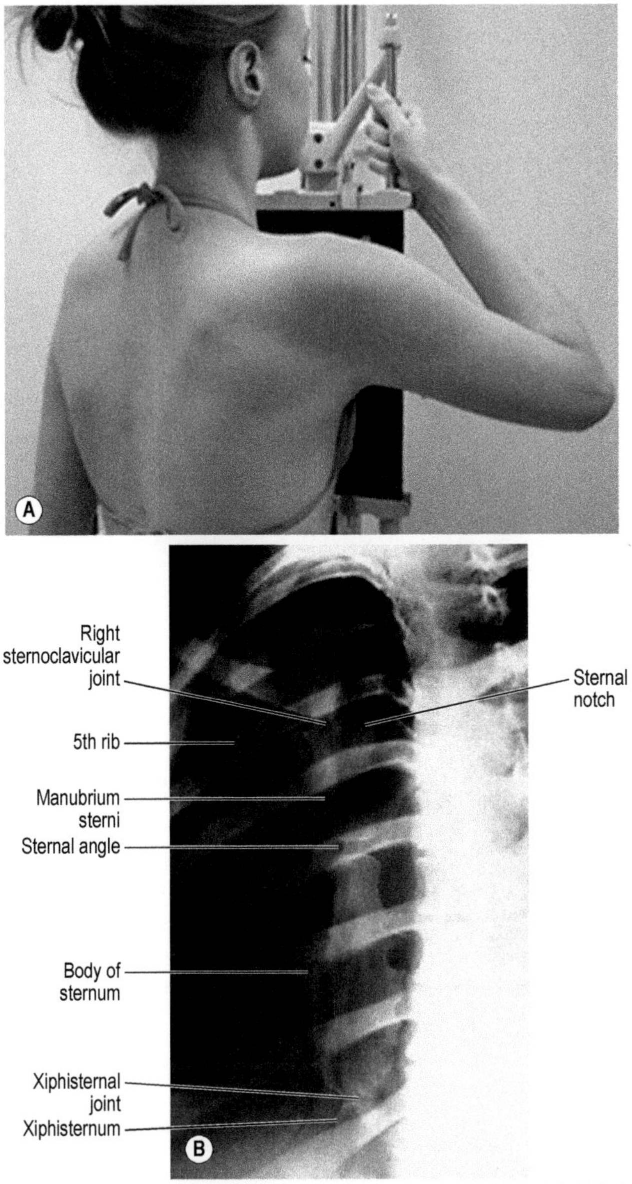

Fig. 15.34 (A) Anterior oblique sternum; (B) oblique sternum. (B, Reproduced with permission from Bryan GJ. *Skeletal Anatomy*. 3rd ed. Edinburgh: Churchill Livingstone; 1996 and Gunn C. 4th ed. *Bones and Joints*. Edinburgh: Churchill Livingstone; 2002.)

Sternoclavicular (SC) Joints

The SC joints are examined for evidence of subluxation of the joints.[16]

POSTEROANTERIOR (PA) STERNOCLAVICULAR JOINTS (FIG. 15.35A,B)

IR is vertical, an antiscatter grid is not required

Positioning

- The patient stands facing the IR
- The feet are separated for stability

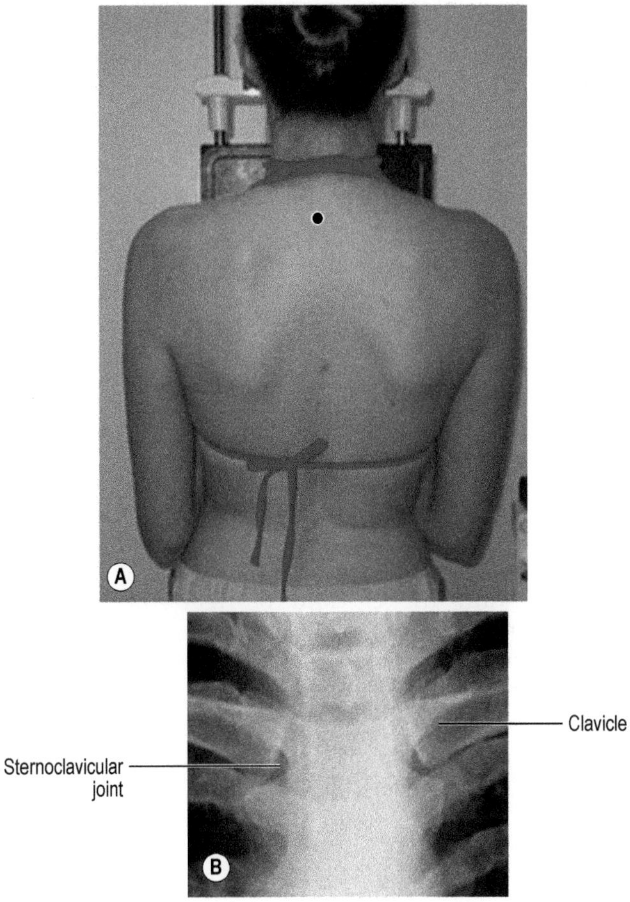

Fig. 15.35 PA sternoclavicular joints.

- The MSP is perpendicular to the IR, assessed by ensuring that the medial ends of the clavicles are equidistant from the IR
- A PA anatomical marker is usually used for this projection

Expose on arrested respiration

Beam Direction and FRD

Horizontal, 90° to the IR
100 cm FRD

Centring

Over the middle of the body of T2 and to emerge through the sternal notch

Collimation

Both SC joints

Criteria for Assessing Image Quality

- Both SC joints are demonstrated
- Medial ends of the clavicle are equidistant from the spinous processes of the thoracic vertebrae
- Sharp image demonstrating joints either side of the vertebral column in contrast to the vertebrae, medial ends of the posterior ribs, soft tissue of the lungs and sternum

Common Error: PA Sternoclavicular Joints

Common Error	Possible Reason	Potential Effect on PCE or Report
Medial ends of clavicle not equidistant about the vertebral column; one joint only demonstrated	MSP not perpendicular to IR; the medial end of clavicle furthest from the vertebrae corresponds to the side rotated away from the IR	Information on both joints will not be available

OBLIQUE STERNOCLAVICULAR JOINTS (FIG. 15.36A,B)

Both joints are examined for comparison.
IR is vertical

Positioning

- The patient stands facing the IR
- *To demonstrate the left SC joint* the patient is rotated 45° towards the right, into the left anterior oblique position
- *To demonstrate the right SC joint* the patient is rotated 45° towards the left, into the right anterior oblique position
- The feet are separated for stability
- A PA anatomical marker is usually used for this projection. To avoid confusion, the PA anatomical marker should indicate the side of the joint under examination *and* be placed over to the relevant side on the IR

Expose on arrested respiration

Beam Direction and FRD

Vertical, 90° to the IR
100 cm FRD

Centring

Level with T2, over the side of the thorax furthest from the IR, to emerge through the sternal notch

Collimation

Both SC joints

Criteria for Assessing Image Quality

- Both SC joints are demonstrated
- Sharp image demonstrating joint under examination contrast with clavicle and sternum

For the left SC joint

- Both joints are cleared from the vertebral column and shown overlying the lung apex on the right
- The right joint is shown with the medial end of the clavicle overlying the joint
- The left joint space is demonstrated as open

For the right SC joint

- Both joints are cleared from the vertebral column and shown overlying the lung apex on the left
- The left joint is shown with the medial end of the clavicle overlying the joint
- The right joint space is demonstrated as open

Common Error: Oblique Sternoclavicular Joints

Common Error	Possible Reason	Potential Effect on PCE or Report
One or both joints are not seen clear of the vertebral column	Inadequate obliquity. A 45° pad assists in assessing angle of rotation more accurately	Joint space assessment will not be possible

Anterior obliques have also been described with significantly less rotation – as little as 10° – the reason for this being that there will be clearance of the spine with minimum distortion of the joint.[32] However, it is noted from resulting images that this obliquity does not adequately clear the joint from the relatively high density of the upper mediastinum.

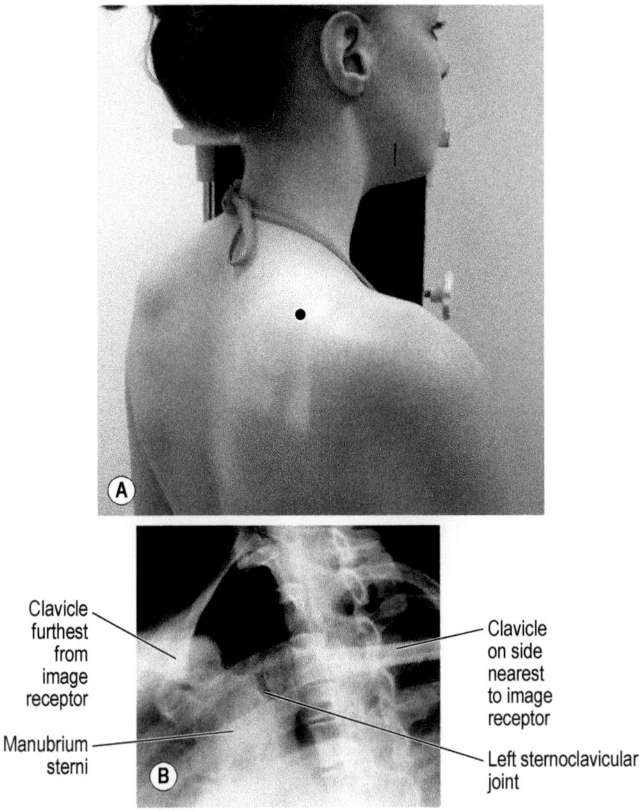

Fig. 15.36 (A) Anterior oblique sternoclavicular joints; (B) oblique sternoclavicular joints.

References

1. Royal College of Radiologists. *iRefer: Making the Best Use of Clinical Radiology*. 8th ed. London: RCR; 2017. https://www.rcr.ac.uk/clinical-radiology/being-consultant/rcr-referral-guidelines/about-irefer.
2. *The Ionising Radiation (Medical Exposure) Regulations*. UK Statutory Instrument 2017 No. 1322; 2017. [IR(ME)R]. https://www.legislation.gov.uk/uksi/2017/1322/contents/made.
3. European Commission Directorate-General for the Environment. *Radiation Protection 118: Referral Guidelines for Imaging*. Luxembourg: Office for Official Publications of the European Communities; 2000.
4. NICE (National Institute for Health and Care Excellence). *Routine Preoperative Tests for Elective Surgery*; 2016. [NG45] https://www.nice.org.uk/donotdo/do-not-routinely-offer-chest-x-rays-before-surgery.
5. Scally P. *Medical Imaging*. Oxford: Oxford University Press; 1999.
6. Global WHO. *Tuberculosis Report*. Geneva: World Health Organization; 2019. https://www.who.int/tb/publications/global_report/en/.
7. European Commission Directorate-General for Research and Innovation. *European guidelines on quality criteria for Diagnostic radiographic images. EUR 16260 Luxembourg*. Office for Official Publications of the European Communities; 1996.
8. Sjovall A. (Correspondence) PA chest films. *Br J Radiol*. 1982;55:168.
9. Smith RF. (Correspondence). *Radiography*. 1982. April:80.
10. Dimmick R. (Correspondence). *Radiography*. 1981. March:79.
11. Clark KC. *Positioning in Radiography*. 4th to 10th ed. London: Heinemann; 1945–1979.
12. Unett EM, Royle AJ. *Radiographic Techniques and Image Evaluation*. London: Chapman and Hall; 1997. 1997.
13. Swallow RA, Naylor E, Roebuck E, et al. *Clark's Positioning in Radiography*. 11th ed. London: Heinemann; 1986.
14. Ballinger PW, Frank ED. *Merrill's Atlas of Radiographic Positioning and Radiologic Procedures*. 10th ed. St Louis: Mosby; 2003.
15. Watkins P. *A Practical Guide to Chest Imaging*. Edinburgh: Churchill Livingstone; 1984.
16. Lampignano JP, Kendrick LE. *Bontrager's Textbook of Radiographic Positioning and Related Anatomy*. 9th ed. St Louis: Mosby; 2018.
17. Unett E, Carver B. The chest X-ray: centring points and central rays – can we stop confusing our students and ourselves? *Synergy*. 2001:14–17.
18. Unett E, Carver B. The chest X-ray: centring points and central rays – can we stop confusing our students and ourselves? *Synergy*. 2001:8–9.
19. Gaillard F. Pneumomediastinum. [online] Radiopaedia. https://radiopaedia.org/cases/pneumomediastinum-14 (accessed 2020).
20. Darby M, et al. *Pocket Tutor: Chest X-ray Interpretation*. London: JP Medical Publishers; 2012.
21. DeLacey G, et al. *The Chest X-Ray: A Survival Guide*. Philadelphia: Saunders; 2008.
22. Meholic A, Ketai L, Lofgren R, et al. *Fundamentals of Chest Radiology*. Philadelphia: Saunders; 1996.
23. Burgener FA, Kormano M, Pudas T, et al. *Differential Diagnosis in Conventional Radiology*. 3rd ed. New York: Thieme; 2007.
24. McQuillen-Martensen K. *Radiographic Image Analysis*. 4th ed. Philadelphia: Saunders; 2015.
25. Jovanovic P. The importance of the lateral chest radiograph – a systematic approach. *ESR. European Congress of Radiology*. 2018. https://tinyurl.com/yxjg9gz2.
26. Chotas H, Ravin C. Chest radiography: estimated lung volume and projected area obscured by the heart, mediastinum and diaphragm. *Radiology*. 1994;193:403–404.
27. Hoffstetter P, Dornier C, Schäffer S, et al. Diagnostic significance of rib series in minor thorax trauma compared to plain chest film and computed tomography. *J Trauma Manag Outcomes*. 2014;5(8):10 (eCollection).
28. Carver E, Carver B, eds. *Medical Imaging: Techniques, Reflection and Evaluation*. 2nd ed. Edinburgh: Churchill Livingstone; 2006.
29. Chan O. *ABC of Emergency Radiology*. Oxford: BMJ Books; 2013.
30. Helms CA. *Fundamentals of Skeletal Radiology*. 3rd ed. Philadelphia: Saunders; 2005.
31. Sutherland R. *Pocketbook of Radiographic Positioning*. 2nd ed. Edinburgh: Churchill Livingstone; 2003.
32. Long BW, Rafaert JA. *Orthopedic Radiography*. Philadelphia: Saunders; 1995.

16 Abdomen

SAEED ALQAHTANI, CHRISTINE EADE and ELIZABETH CARVER

Projection radiography of the abdomen is often used for assessment of gross anatomical deviation, such as displacement of organs in the case of abdominal tumours or obstruction of the alimentary tract. Information on the urinary system can be provided by the projection abdominal image, preceding other imaging procedures, also providing information on gross anatomical deviation within the urinary system. The appearance of radio-opaque calculi will be demonstrated on the image but urography, ultrasound, radionuclide imaging (RNI) or computed tomography (CT) will be required to provide information on renal function, site of urinary obstruction or extent of obstruction. The role of these imaging methods in genitourinary investigations is considered in Chapter 22. Hints and tips on preliminary clinical evaluation are contained at the end of this chapter.

Throughout this chapter a suggested FRD is given for each examination description; however in practice a range of FRDs (typically from 100 cm to 120 cm) may be used, dependent on local protocol.

SUPINE ABDOMEN (FIG. 16.1)

IR is horizontal, an antiscatter or virtual grid is employed

Positioning

- The patient is supine with the arms slightly abducted from the trunk
- The median sagittal plane (MSP) is coincident with the long axis of the table and the centre of the bucky
- Anterior superior iliac spines (ASISs) are equidistant from the table-top
  a) The iliac crests are level with the middle of the IR, *or*
  b) Using the calibrated markings on the light beam diaphragm, collimate to the IR boundary; ensure that the lower edge of collimation lies below the lower border of the symphysis pubis
- Because of magnification, owing to the significant distance from the symphysis pubis to the IR, the symphysis pubis should lie well above the lower boundary of the IR
- Central ray and the middle of IR should be accurately aligned

Beam Direction and FRD

Vertical, at 90° to the IR
100–120 cm FRD, selected to ensure magnification is at its minimum and include the maximum amount of abdominal tissue on the image

Centring

Positioning for (a) is over a point in the midline of the abdomen, level with the iliac crests

Note that this point refers to the actual *highest point of the crests at the back*, rather than the lower level palpated on the lateral aspect of the abdomen.

Positioning for (b) is to the centre of the IR

The midline of the abdomen, or MSP, can be identified by palpating the middle of the upper border of the symphysis pubis and the xiphisternum. The line joining these surface markings will represent the position of the MSP.

Collimation

Symphysis pubis, as much upper abdomen as possible, lateral soft tissue outlines

Comments on Centring, Collimation and Area of Interest

It has been stated that the 11th thoracic vertebra should be included in the collimated field as it lies above the renal outlines and at the tip of the right lower lobe of liver and spleen.[1] It is noted that in most adults this would not usually allow for the inclusion of all the upper abdominal contents; however, with the exception of examination of the upper gastrointestinal tract, ultrasound is the most appropriate imaging modality for the upper abdomen. This would negate the necessity for the inclusion of abdominal tissue immediately below the diaphragm. When the supine abdomen position is used to demonstrate the kidneys, ureter and bladder, and additional abdominal information is not required, lateral collimation can be made to the ASIS on each side to more effectively reduce radiation dose.

Traditionally, a specific centring point has been given when describing the anteroposterior (AP) supine abdomen. This has usually been stated as level with the iliac crests in the midline, as in centring (a), above.[2] Unfortunately, the continuing trend for an increase in average height, noted especially in Europe and the Western world and estimated to be increasing by between 10 and 30 mm per decade,[3] affects the amount of body tissue that can now realistically be included on the image. Although the iliac crests do appear midway between the diaphragm and symphysis pubis on the image, centring point (a) will only be useful in smaller patients, i.e. those whose abdominal tissue will actually 'fit' within the maximum receptor length. Selection of the centring point/positioning method will therefore depend upon the radiographer's assessment of the patient's size.

An additional complication occurs with larger patients, whose adipose tissue will cause further elevation of the symphysis pubis above the table-top; this increases the effect of magnification, potentially adding to the risk of the image of the symphysis being projected below the lower border of the IR. Using the suggested method (b) of centring will reduce the risk of projecting the symphysis pubis off the lower end of the image in these cases.

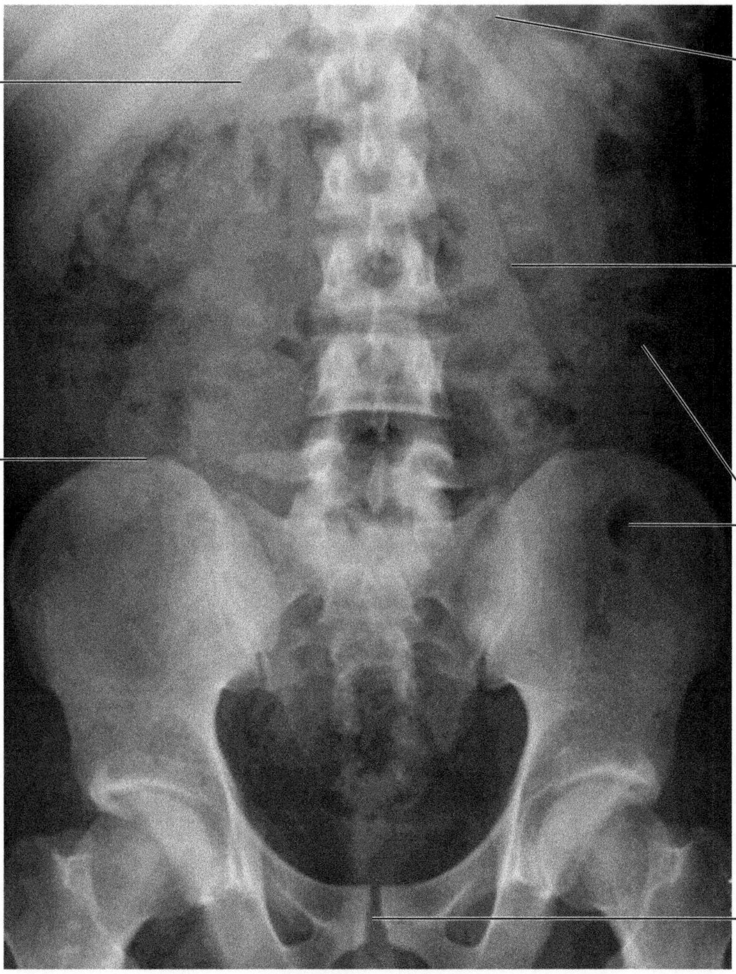

Fig. 16.1 Supine abdomen.

Compensation for magnification may be made by increasing the focus receptor distance (FRD),[4] but this may still not be effective enough for very tall patients. Unfortunately, in these cases it may be necessary to undertake an additional projection of the upper abdomen if it is essential to include this area in the examination. Indeed, it has been suggested that the hypersthenic patient requires two, separately centred, abdomen images.[5] This would result in a higher radiation dose to the patient than undertaking an additional, well-collimated, upper abdomen projection.

With regard to the increase in average height of a population, it is a positive step that larger image receptors are becoming increasingly available. Unfortunately, not all manufacturers currently offer the 35×47 cm IR as an option; hopefully this will change in the future.

Expose on arrested respiration during exposure

Exposure must be made on arrested respiration to reduce the risk of movement unsharpness on the image, caused by the shift of abdominal organs during diaphragmatic movement. There is a range of recommendations regarding the phase of respiration to suspend,[1,6] and questions regarding the most appropriate choice arise from this. Suspension of respiration after exhalation cannot be excluded as it facilitates lower density of abdominal tissue, necessitating the selection of lower exposure factors and hence reducing dose compared to exposure in the opposite phase of respiration. Unfortunately, when this issue is considered alongside that of the tall patient, as discussed above, it can be argued that exhalation will exacerbate the problems of including all the required area on the image.

Therefore, the concept of exposure on arrested inspiration to compress abdominal contents into an apparently shorter area may become more acceptable, as it reduces the area covered by the abdominal contents (i.e. the area from the diaphragm to the symphysis pubis), increasing the chance of a single exposure examination. This is clearly an opportunity for the reflective practitioner to base their decision on practice using a benefit-versus-risk approach.

Criteria for Assessing Image Quality

- Symphysis pubis, as much of the upper abdomen as possible, and lateral soft tissue outlines of the abdomen are included on the image
- Spinous processes of vertebrae seen coincident with the midline of the image and centralised and aligned down the middle of the vertebral bodies
- Symmetry of the iliac crests
- Sharp image demonstrating soft tissue in contrast with bowel gas and bony structures

Note that scoliosis will affect the symmetry of the vertebral column and position of the vertebrae coincident with the long axis of the film. It is distinguishable from rotation due to position error by the distinct lateral curve of the column and potential variation of rotation down its length.[1] If inclusion of the relevant body area on the image is acceptable, a repeat should not be considered. In the case of positional rotation it must be remembered that correction will be possible and will improve accuracy in the appearance of organ position within the abdominal cavity.

Common Errors: Supine Abdomen

Common Errors	Possible Reasons	Potential Impact on Interpretation
Symphysis pubis is not included on the image	Inaccurate centring/positioning *or* tall patient? Centring point at the level of the iliac crests may have been used. Try centring method (b)	Pelvic area will not be sufficiently visualised and pathology may be missed, for example bladder calculi
Upper abdomen is not included; symphysis pubis is well above the lower edge of the film	May have been centred using the lateral borders of iliac crest rather than the highest point at the back	Upper abdomen will not be sufficiently visualised and pathology may be missed, for example calcified gall stones, pancreatic calcifications
Vertebral column is not coincident with the midline of the film	Xiphisternum to symphysis line is inaccurately positioned *or* scoliotic patient	Lateral aspects of the abdomen may be missed, impacting on diagnosis
Spinous processes are not demonstrated in the midline of the vertebral bodies	MSP is not perpendicular to the table-top; palpate ASIS to ensure it is equidistant from the table *or* the patient is scoliosed	The image will appear rotated and make comparisons of renal size more difficult

ERECT ABDOMEN

Validity of Use of This Projection

The erect abdomen has traditionally been requested to diagnose/exclude obstruction of the bowel, alimentary perforation or the effects of stab injury. The erect position allows air to rise above fluid levels in the obstructed bowel where the inferior level of the air shadow appears flat, or under the right diaphragm in cases of perforation. Towards the close of the 20th century the validity of requests for the erect abdomen examination began to be questioned, as it was recognised that other projections demonstrate appearances suggestive of obstruction or perforation. More specifically, in the case of the supine acute abdomen, these appearances are:[7]

- *Sentinel loop sign*: an isolated loop of distended bowel indicates the effects of inflammatory processes such as appendicitis or pancreatitis, causing ileus.
- *Dilated small bowel loops*: indicate small bowel obstruction. Loops are centrally sited and there is absence of faecal matter; eventually the distal bowel becomes airless as it collapses, but the stomach may still contain air. Air in the distended small bowel may appear as a ladder or stack of coins.
- *Dilated colon*: points to obstruction. Dilation of the colon with air is noted, up to the site of obstruction. The bowel is much distended, with distended haustra, and the appearances are notable around the edges of the abdomen, rather than the more centralised loops as in the case of obstructed small bowel.
- *Volvulus*: obstruction appears as a distended portion of looped bowel. The obstruction is caused by the closed ends of the loop, which may have a 'coffee bean' appearance.

As the right hemi-diaphragm lies at a higher level than the left, in cases of perforation gas or air in the peritoneal cavity will rise to lie under the right hemi-diaphragm. The appearance is that of a dark line under the diaphragm, often following its curve, created by the contrast of the gas itself against the dense abdominal tissue. In addition, it should be remembered that heart and chest disease – myocardial infarction, dissecting aortic aneurysm, pneumonia and pulmonary embolism in particular – may give rise to symptoms that mimic an 'acute abdomen'.[7] Is there a need to irradiate the whole abdomen simply to demonstrate the subdiaphragmatic area? Probably not. This is largely supported by guidelines from the Royal College of Radiologists in their referral guidelines for imaging, where a supine abdomen accompanied by an erect chest examination is recommended for patients with symptoms suggestive of the acute abdomen; however, these guidelines do suggest that an erect abdomen examination may be considered if strongly suspected obstruction is not confirmed on a supine abdomen image. A lateral decubitus projection of the abdomen *is* suggested if the patient cannot be examined erect for the chest film in cases of suspected perforation;[8] this projection is described in Chapter 15. The erect chest radiograph itself should not be forgotten as a useful projection for this region: apparent upper abdominal pain can be due to lower lobe pneumonia and an erect chest radiograph will provide evidence of either, on one image and with one exposure, which uses lower exposure factors than those for an abdomen radiograph. Prior to positioning and exposure, the patient must always have been in an erect position for at least 5 minutes to allow air to rise to the highest point in the abdominal cavity.

For infirm patients, an erect projection of the chest can be attempted in the AP position with the patient sitting supported, in bed or on a trolley (Chapter 15). For some patients even this will prove difficult; in these cases a left lateral decubitus (right-side raised) projection of the upper abdomen can be undertaken; this is a PA projection with the IR supported vertically against the anterior aspect of the upper abdomen. Centre to the middle of the IR.

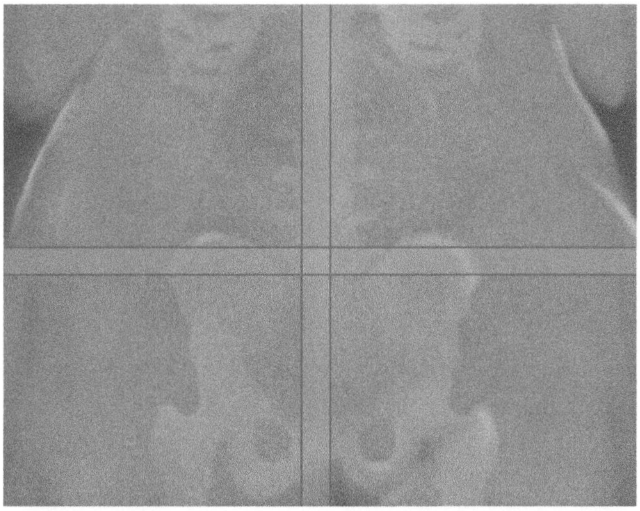

Fig. 16.2 Imaging the abdomen in obese patients – four-receptor method.

Positioning

IR is vertical, an antiscatter grid is employed

- The patient is sitting, or standing erect with legs separated for stability
- MSP is perpendicular to the IR and coincident with its long axis
- The middle of the IR is level with the iliac crests *or* its upper border should include the upper abdomen if this area is required

Beam Direction and FRD

Horizontal, at 90° to the IR
100–120 cm, FRD is selected to ensure magnification is at its minimum and include the maximum amount of abdominal tissue on the image

Centring

To the centre of the IR

Collimation

As much upper abdomen as possible, lateral soft tissue outlines

The symphysis pubis need not be included as it should be included on the supine abdomen projection.

Exposure Factors

Exposure factors will require an increase from the supine AP projection, to allow for increased density due to sagging of the abdominal tissue in this position.

Image Quality

Image quality is assessed as for the supine abdomen, but there may be a reduction in contrast compared to the AP projection, due to increased exposure factors and abdomen sag. The symphysis pubis need not be included.

Bariatric Patients

In this group of patients due consideration should be given in order to gain a diagnostic image while keeping the patient dose at a tolerable level.

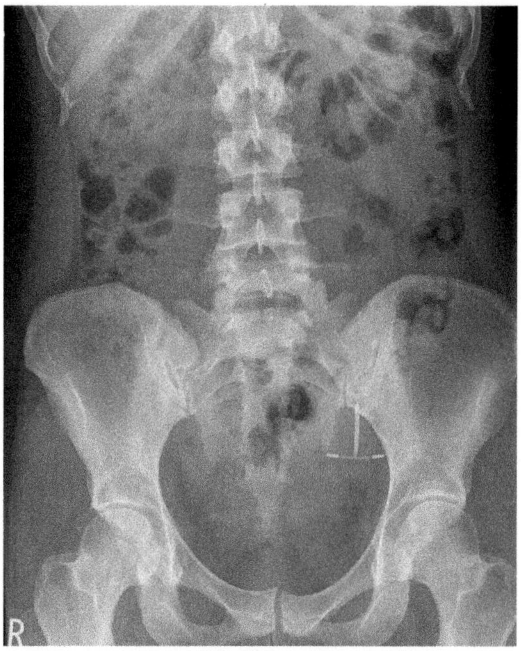

Fig. 16.3 A female with IUCD not detected on ultrasound, shown on the abdomen radiograph projected within the pelvis adjacent to the left sacroiliac joint, the important point here being that if it is not in the uterine cavity it is not doing its job as contraception.

Centring

The centring point applied in bariatric patients is exactly the same as the one applied in normal patients – midline of the abdomen and level with the iliac crest. However, identifying the iliac crest can be challenging in bariatric patients due to excessive fat. Accurate centring is crucial to avoid misalignment of the examined part and of high importance when automatic exposure control (AEC) is used; this is to eliminate image distortion. It is suggested that the patient's arms should be positioned parallel to the abdomen and the elbow level can be used as a centring marker instead of the iliac crest.[9] However, this technique of centring is a suggestive solution lacking any evidence-based research.

Collimation

As stated above, due to the excessive amount of fat in the case of bariatric patients, multiple images might be used in order to cover the abdominal region. This is been reported to be already applied in some bariatric centres where the influx of patients with obesity is high.[10] However, there is no guideline on how much overlapping should be used when multiple images are employed. This should be kept to a minimum in order to reduce absorbed dose to the internal organs where overlapping is applied. Two images to cover the upper and lower abdomen with the long axis of the receptor positioned transversely across the image may be used. However, in some cases four images will be required to cover the abdomen in a minority of very obese patients. In both cases overlap should be minimised (Fig. 16.2).

Exposure Factors

Due to the excessive fat in bariatric patients, exposure factors have to be changed compared to normal weight patients in order to gain a diagnostic image. However, there are no guidelines on exposure factors selection based on patients' size in digital radiography.[11] A few studies have investigated dose optimisation in bariatric patients in order to produce exposure factors prediction models,[12,13] However, image quality could not be assessed due to the homogeneity of phantoms used in these studies.

A preliminary study suggested the use of 75 kVp while using 130 cm FRD and 0.3 mm of copper filtration.[14,15]

PCE COMMENTS – ABDOMEN

Preliminary clinical evaluation for abdomen projection radiographs is not commonly used by radiographers in the same way as it is for musculoskeletal imaging. The non-specific findings often seen in the acute abdomen makes diagnosis difficult even for the trained eye of radiologists and reporting radiographers. Other imaging modalities, in particular CT (see Chapter 26), are far more accurate at assessing for pathologies that were traditionally imaged using abdomen radiographs, such as bowel obstruction or renal tract calcification, as the underlying cause can also be identified.

However PCE assessment by the radiographers at the time of imaging is helpful in specific circumstances where the radiographer is far more confident with a straightforward diagnosis.

Examples include query retained foreign body, misplaced intrauterine contraceptive device (IUCD) (Fig. 16.3), or musculoskeletal findings such as an unexpected hip fracture on the edge of the abdomen X-ray. Some basic guidance for PCE of the abdomen is outlined below.

Use a systematic approach to check the entire image, including:

- Bowel and other organs
  - Review the bowel gas pattern and check for free gas
  - The normal diameter of the intestines does not usually exceed:
    - 3 cm for the small bowel
    - 6 cm for the colon
    - 9 cm for the caecum[16]
  - Faeces are visualised most commonly in the colon and have a mottled appearance due to trapped gas within them
  - Bowel gas has a wide variation of distribution
- Review each of the intra-abdominal organs looking for enlargement, abnormal outlines, calcifications or intraparenchymal air:
  - The liver
  - The gallbladder for calcified gallstones and cholecystectomy clips
  - Stomach – which will contain variable amounts of air
  - Kidneys
  - Spleen
  - Bladder (will vary depending on fullness)
- Calcification and artefact
  - Confirm the origin of any calcifications
- Skeleton
  - Explore for any fractures and other pathologies

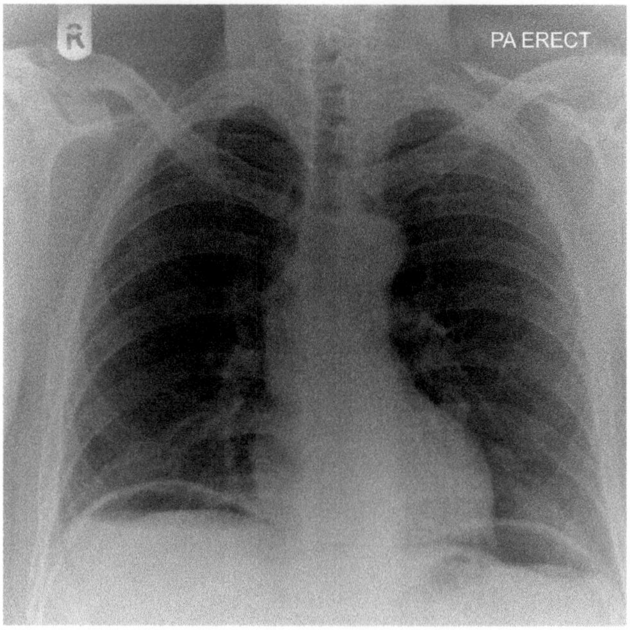

Fig. 16.4 A 57-year-old male presenting with epigastric pain who had an erect chest X-ray showing free sub-diaphragmatic air under both hemi- diaphragms, indicating bowel perforation.

- Check the lung bases if visible (see Chapter 15)
- The psoas muscle should also be visible
- A suspected perforation is better visualised on an erect chest radiograph. In these cases, the patient needs to be in the erect position for at least 10 minutes prior to the exposure (Fig. 16.4; also see Chapter 15).[16,17]

References

1. McQuillen-Martensen K. *Radiographic Image Analysis*. 3rd ed. Philadelphia: Saunders; 2010.
2. Eisenberg R, Dennis C, May RTC. *Radiographic Positioning*. 2nd ed. Boston: Little Brown; 1995.
3. Cole TJ. Secular trends in growth. *Proc Nutr Soc*. 2000;59(2):317–324.
4. Gunn C. *Radiographic Imaging: A Practical Approach*. 3rd ed. Edinburgh: Churchill Livingstone; 2002.
5. Bontrager K, Lampignano JP. *Textbook of Radiographic Positioning and Related Anatomy*. 7th ed. St Louis: Mosby; 2010.
6. Swallow RA, Naylor E, Roebuck E, et al. *Clark's Positioning in Radiography*. 11th ed. London: Heinemann; 1986.
7. Nicholson DA, Driscoll PA. *ABC of Emergency Radiology*. London: BMJ Books; 1995.
8. RCR Working Party. *Making the Best Use of a Clinical Radiology Services: Guidelines for Referrers*. 6th ed. London: Royal College of Radiologists; 2007.
9. Carucci LR. Imaging obese patients: problems and solutions. *Abdom Imaging*. 2013;38:630–646.
10. Alqahtani SJ, Welbourn R, Meakin JR, et al. Increased radiation dose and projected radiation-related lifetime cancer risk in patients with obesity due to projection radiography. *J Radiol Protect*. 2018;39(1):38.
11. Ching W, Robinson J, McEntee M. Patient–based radiographic exposure factor selection: a systematic review. *J Med Radiat Sci*. 2014;61(3):176–190.
12. Zheng X. Patient size based guiding equations for automatic mAs and kVp selections in general medical X-ray projection radiography. *Radiat Prot Dosimetry*. 2017;174:545–550.

13. Zheng X. Body size and tube voltage-dependent guiding equations for optimal selection of image acquisition parameters in clinical X-ray imaging. *Radiol Phys Technol.* 2018;11:212–218.
14. Alqahtani SJM, Meakin JR, Palfrey JM, et al. *The Impact of Different Exposure Factors on Image Quality of Lumbar Spine in Five Different Sizes Phantoms: A Factorial Design Study*. Vienna, Austria: European Congress of Radiology; 2018. 27 February – 3 March.
15. Alqahtani SJM, Meakin JR, Palfrey JM, et al. *The Impact of Different Exposure Factors on Radiation Dose of Lumbar Spine in Five Different Sizes Phantoms: A Factorial Design Study*. Vienna, Austria: European Congress of Radiology; 2018. 27 February – 3 March.
16. https://geekymedics.com/abdominal-x-ray-interpretation/.
17. James B, Kelly B. The abdominal radiograph. *Ulster Med J*. 2013;82(3):179–187.

17 Emergency Department Radiography

CHRISTINE EADE, ELIZABETH CARVER and DARREN WOOD†

This chapter will evaluate the position of the imaging professional within the multidisciplinary team, consider the advancing role of the radiographer, and review how an understanding of injury mechanisms and pattern recognition informs the choice of projection and technique adaptation in the traumatised patient. Special considerations for techniques, in addition to choice of radiographic equipment, will also be considered for this wide field of service provision.

The Role of the Radiographer in the Multidisciplinary Team

The progression of highlighting abnormalities through the use of a 'red dot' system[1] has been well documented, and by 2004 a national survey showed that 81% of hospital trusts/boards were using this aspect of role development.[2] The red dot was then replaced in 2013 with a more robust scheme – preliminary clinical evaluation (PCE).[3] This practice is used by radiographers; they assess the image and make an informed judgement on the clinical appearances that are then communicated to the referrer in an unambiguous written form.

Alongside this, the development of the Advanced Trauma Life Support (ATLS)[4] approach to dealing with the patient with multiple injuries and the inception of the four-tier system[5] of working in the UK have advanced the position of the radiographer within the Emergency Department (ED) multidisciplinary team. Gradual development of service provision through advanced training, to create the reporting radiographer, has further ensured the value of this team member in the ED.

The role of the reporting radiographer has ensured that an invaluable service can now be provided instantly in the ED. Acting as report writer, advanced ED imaging practitioner, advisor to junior radiographic staff or students and other professionals in the multidisciplinary team, the reporting radiographer keys in neatly with the advanced practitioner or consultant practitioner level of the 'four-tier' system of work that has evolved during the first part of the 21st century.

Current guidance on immediate reporting (also known as 'hot reporting') also advocates that the final written report of ED radiographs of suspected fractures is available before the patient is discharged from the ED, further strengthening the role of the reporting radiographer.[6]

Although the advanced practitioner may be seen as a key representative for imaging within the multidisciplinary team, it should be remembered that the radiographer has a responsibility to ensure they contribute fully to the trauma service. As a member of the ATLS team, the imaging practitioner must take command of their aspect of the service provided for the patient. In a stressful situation, the radiographer must control their contribution through being competent in their skills and the needs of the patient and providing leadership to the team for the imaging aspects of the care; this ensures that a good outcome is achieved while maintaining safety for patients and the wider ATLS team. The radiographer working in the resuscitation room is not only responsible for the patient, but also for the staff within the area. In this way the radiographer becomes an advocate for all those who come into contact with ionising radiation in the resuscitation room.

It is not only in the ATLS situation that the radiographer will display the versatility to cope with the demands of the varied ED patient presentations, across widely ranging age groups and varying requirements for adaptation of techniques. The radiographer also displays their value to the multidisciplinary team for all ED cases in which they are involved. However, admitting a lack of knowledge or ability should not be seen as a suggestion of general inability; examples of this are most likely to lie in unusual circumstances, for example in difficult patient presentations or difficulty with highlighting perceived abnormalities. Admission of lack of knowledge or ability, and acceptance that another more experienced or skilled member of the team may provide a better service, is the most responsible and appropriate action for this situation. This may be reflected in discussing ED images, or requests for imaging, with the referrer or radiologist so that the best patient outcome may be achieved. Human factors in healthcare are used with a primary purpose of enhancing clinical practice through the overarching understanding of the effects of teamwork, equipment and culture on human behaviour, and application of professional knowledge in the clinical setting. The principles of human factors can be applied in the identification and assessment of patient safety risks and in the analysis of incidents to identify learning and points of change.[7]

Knowledge and its application in the form of advising alternative imaging, perhaps with a protocol-driven application of the Ionising Radiation (Medical Exposure) Regulations 2017 (IR(ME)R),[8] is further evidence of the extended service provision of the radiographer within the multidisciplinary team. Indeed, acting as a gatekeeper of ionising radiation exposure to the general public is one of the more demanding roles, expected even of the newly qualified radiographer. The safety role of the radiographer also includes providing guidance on the exposure of 'carers and comforters'.[6]

Radiographers must explain the benefits and detriments to exposure and the likely direct health benefits to the patient. This process should, in compliance with the IR(ME)R, be part of the justification procedure prior to exposure.

Justification also incorporates communication of risks and benefits to patients. Radiographers must provide, wherever practicable, and prior to an exposure taking place, adequate information to the patient or their representative as to the benefits and risks associated with the radiation dose from the exposure to gain consent. Finally the radiographer should adopt the 'pause and check' approach as advised by their representative professional body to ensure all IR(ME)R requirements are met before the exposure is given.[8]

It is necessary that the radiography professional understands the following:

- Trauma mechanisms
- Most common injury presentations associated with trauma mechanisms
- How trauma mechanism and presentation may influence projection or technique selection
- How trauma mechanism and presentation may influence technique adaptation, in varied situations

Being able to draw on a wide experience base that has been developed through reflection upon practice (be this formalised or in an intuitive way) is another expectation of the ED radiographer. With this in mind, it is the professional and medico-legal responsibility of radiographers to ensure that they maintain and continually develop their skills. Ensuring participation in continuing professional development (CPD) is paramount for even the most experienced; this is reinforced by the Health and Care Professions Council (HCPC) requirements that radiographers must show evidence of ongoing CPD, in order to maintain registration with the HCPC in the UK.

The Team Role of the Radiographer: Image Interpretation

The PCE system has become an accepted norm for the practising radiographer and is a fundamental feature of undergraduate pre-registration diagnostic radiography programmes in the UK.

The radiographer's expertise in image appreciation begins with their ability to evaluate images for quality purposes, and one of the main purposes of this text is to promote a logical and systematic approach to this. During quality evaluation the radiographer will recognise pathologies or abnormalities, and so they are already effectively commenting to themselves or colleagues prior to the application of a PCE. The application of a number of basic pointers makes image review possible:

- Correct patient identifier
- Correct anatomical marker
- Correct area included (on all projections)
- Correct radiographic position
- Adequate exposure factors used (for contrast, appropriate exposure index (EI) or deviation index (DI) and sharpness)[9]

These pointers apply to all radiographic images and relate to the structures used in this text, which are projection-specific rather than broad in their application. As the image produced should be of a diagnostic standard, implementation of these checks is vital before the radiographer can clinically evaluate appearances adequately and with confidence. As for image quality assessment, there are some basic pointers to enable accurate assessment of the image for identification of any pathologies/abnormalities:

- Assess the whole area, avoiding the urge to focus on the 'obvious'
- Examine the cortical outline and trabecular pattern (follow the outline of the bone, assess for disruption)
- Look at the soft tissue (any change may indicate a subtle fracture)
- Check radiographic lines, zones and arcs (for this the radiographer needs to be aware of the basics and how to use them)
- Research any previous/recent imaging.[10–12]

Using these basic pointers will enable radiographers to expertly analyse images so as to be able to clinically evaluate them and provide the initial PCE.

The PCE must be logically presented to all involved, from referral to image retrieval, so that practitioner and referrer are aware that this is not a *final report* but rather the opinion of a professional within their own field; it should be used as an aid by the referrer in deciding on a final diagnosis. A system where all radiographers are expected to participate will give the referrers more confidence in the system when compared to the historical 'red dot' scheme where radiographers had the option to 'opt out' of making a decision, putting the onus on to the clinician/referrer. To ensure effective PCE provision will require continued review and audit.

It may be difficult to ascertain the medicolegal position of a PCE unless a test case was to be presented. Even if a radiographer is not held responsible in civil proceedings, there is no reason why disciplinary or professional conduct hearings would not find the radiographer guilty of negligent conduct in situations relating to a PCE on anatomical appearances, if the employer has implemented a suitable framework for such a scheme. Vicarious liability by the employing hospital trust expects reasonable standards of care to have been exercised when supporting its employees in the execution of their duties. This includes operating within recognised protocols, working to professional standards, and also, on the part of the employer, the provision of appropriate educational support and safe working practices agreed by all participants.[13]

Similarly, radiographers who provide a reporting service, and have necessarily undergone significant postgraduate education, should offer the same standard of report as a radiologist; it is not acceptable to provide a lower standard of report simply because they are not radiologists.[14]

If a radiographer is unsure about a case and the wider clinical picture, it is important for them to discuss the images and clinical indications with a radiologist or more experienced reporting radiographer.

The Team Role of the Radiographer: Suitable Equipment Choice

Experience also plays a significant role in the activities of service provision, especially on the ancillary equipment selection front. Frequently, this type of equipment for support to the ED imaging department is often selected without including the radiographer in the purchasing exercise. As an example, the choice of patient trolleys that are widely used across disciplines often results in difficulties not only for radiology staff but also for the patient and the wider team in the ED. In the end, a poor-quality service is often delivered because of a lack of foresight in operating as a cohesive team. Holistic care demands cooperation across boundaries seen as traditional divides; however, borders are created where they are inappropriate.[5] This is a particular problem where professions that form the minority in an area of operation are perceived as lacking in appreciation for what is best for that department area or the patient. Advocacy for the patient and service can take many different forms that are frequently not recognised. The awareness of human factors and their influence on team working and patient outcome is vitally important for the radiographer.

Mechanisms of Injury

A range of reasons exist as to why patients present in ED. Certain patterns of trauma present themselves time and again, i.e. the 'common occurrences', although some injuries present after apparently minor trauma or as a result of seemingly ridiculous circumstances. Probably the most famous of all causes of injury is the 'fall onto outstretched hand' or FOOSH. Another commonly encountered trauma involves twisting of the ankle, which generates injury patterns that are linked, as force is transmitted along the whole of the leg. Certain age groups, because of their involvement in specific activities, or alternatively as a result of pathological processes influencing bone integrity, display unexpectedly severe presentations of injury following apparently innocuous trauma forces. Table 17.1 attempts to draw together injuries linked to the mechanism so that potential skeletal imaging projections can be determined and expected injury patterns anticipated.

An awareness of the developmental anatomy of the skeleton is important, as injury patterns change with age. Young children may not yet possess the skeletal components that generate adult injury characteristics, and indeed the maturity of bone may be responsible for causing variations in presentation. With their understanding of this, the radiographer can act as a resource of information for the referrer, so that an appropriate examination is embarked upon with least detriment to the child radiologically.

Silver Trauma Pathways have been introduced into some hospitals in the UK, which recognises the potential of severe fracture from low-level trauma.[15] For example, Fuller et al reported 61% of over-50s with a cervical spine fracture has sustained their fracture from a ground-level fall and those with upper cervical spine fractures were significantly older (mean age 80.1 yr ± 11.9) than those with lower cervical spine fractures (mean age 70.7 yr ± 12.6).[16] The Silver Trauma Pathway also prompts assessment of factors important in elderly care, such as assessment of cognition and frailty.

It is with all the above in mind, and the need to deal with the psychological aspects of the traumatised patient and accompanying relatives or friends, that the role of the radiographer is a wide-ranging one, acting as the advocate for holistic imaging management. Following recognition of the above it is appropriate to consider the more esoteric projections or adaptations to projection radiography that may be considered useful adjuncts to the trauma radiographer's range of skills.

Further Projections and Adapted Techniques

Working around the patient in non-standard and trauma situations is one of the greater skills of the experienced ED radiographer, and an understanding of how radiographic equipment or body parts may safely be moved to achieve the required positions is of major importance. As well as appreciating these subtleties, the radiographer has a further responsibility for ensuring that appropriate radiation protection methods can be achieved for the patient, staff or relatives who may have to be present in these situations. Good collimation, selection of appropriate imaging equipment and radiation protection techniques – all considered 'run of the mill' aspects of good practice – will require adaptation to ensure successful application. Clean technique approaches will also be required where open wounds are present, with appropriate protection for the radiographer and supplementary considerations for equipment and the cleaning of this thereafter. Cling film is sometimes used in the ED to wrap equipment, as protection against contamination from blood and other body fluids. Alternatively, plastic sheaths may be made for foam immobilisation pads or cassettes; care must be taken to ensure that these covers are kept clean and do not cause problems through artefact generation on images.

THE UPPER LIMB

Common mistakes made in obtaining projections of the hand and fingers frequently occur as a result of the mistaken belief that the radiographer is being kinder to the patient by not causing excessive pain. Another example is when the radiographer attempts to obtain several finger projections in a single exposure. In both these instances it becomes immediately apparent that a less than acceptable image might be obtained, resulting in an increased risk of inaccurate diagnosis from the projection provided for radiological opinion. This lack of foresight and poor practice serves no purpose except to place the patient at risk and to lay the practitioner open to claims of negligent practice. Although hand injuries may not appear severe, the actual effects of the injury may be quite significant. By understanding this, the radiographer should realise that the highest standard of imaging possible must be achieved. This requires assertiveness (with respect to encouragement of achieving an ideal position when the patient may resist) in order to gain the best result, or adaptation of a technique to allow an image to be obtained in less than ideal circumstances. Further up the upper limb, towards the elbow and shoulder, similar demands surface to ensure that unambiguous radiographic representation of the traumatised limb or joint is achieved. Of particular concern are the supracondylar and radial head regions of the elbow, and adequate evidence of the relatively rare, but easily missed, posteriorly dislocated shoulder is vital.

TABLE 17.1 Mechanism of Injury Related to Examination Requirements

Mechanism	Part Injured	Projections	Additional or Alternative Projections	Alternative Imaging
FOOSH	Carpometacarpal joint	DP, DPO, lateral hand	Ball catcher's projection to show discreet fractures of the base of the fifth metacarpal	RNI or MRI for occult scaphoid fracture MRI or ultrasound (US) for suspected ligament damage
	Scaphoid Distal radius (Colles' fracture)	PA wrist/scaphoid with ulnar deviation PA oblique scaphoid Lateral wrist/scaphoid PA with forearm raised 30° (see Fig. 4.24A) PA and lateral wrist	If scapholunate dissociation stress projections similar to standard scaphoid images may be needed later, as treatment effectiveness is assessed PA oblique wrist	
	Radial head	AP and lateral elbow	Specific radial head projections (see Chapter 5)	
	Glenohumeral joint	AP shoulder Axial or Y view of scapula	Modified axials as described and discussed in Chapter 5	CT, MRI or US to evaluate for Bankart lesion of glenoid labrum or rotator cuff damage
	Acromioclavicular joint	AP A/C joint		US or MRI for long-standing injury – used also to evaluate rotator cuff
	Coracoid process	AP of shoulder region	Inferosuperior coracoid (AP with 20–30° cranial angle)	
Inversion at ankle	Ankle	AP and lateral ankle	30° internal oblique ankle (mortice) or external oblique ankle Stress projections for ligament integrity evaluation	US to examine ligament integrity
	Base of fifth metatarsal	DP and DPO foot		US may be used to evaluate peroneus brevis or related ligaments
	Neck of fibula	AP and lateral tibia and fibula		
Falls from a height	Calcaneum	Axial and lateral calcaneum	Standing axial (if possible) Subtalar oblique projections	CT to evaluate fracture fragments
	Ankle	AP and lateral ankle		CT to evaluate fracture fragments
	Pelvis	AP pelvis Lateral hip (if indicated – see related discussion, Chapter 8)	Judet's view of acetabulum Sacrum/sacroiliac joint	CT to evaluate fracture component relationship/3D reconstruction
	All spinal regions	AP and lateral of spinal region (see Chapter 9 for discussion on C-spine)	Obliques	CT to evaluate fracture component relationship/3D reconstruction
Flexion/ extension or compression of spine	Cervical spine	Odontoid process (open mouth) AP and lateral (see Chapter 9 for discussion on C-spine)	Obliques Flexion and extension laterals if neck is stable Lateral skull for ?C1 crush injury	CT and MRI to evaluate bone fracture relations and soft tissue damage respectively (see Chapter 9 for discussion on C-spine)
Flexion/ extension or compression of spine	Thoracic spine	AP and lateral		CT and MRI to evaluate bone fracture relations and soft tissue damage respectively
	Lumbar spine	AP and lateral		CT and MRI to evaluate bone fracture relations and soft tissue damage respectively
Rotation forces	Knee	AP and lateral	Intercondylar notch Internal/external obliques of knee	
	Elbow	AP and lateral	Modified AP, for the elbow in flexion as described and discussed later in this chapter	CT to evaluate fracture component relationships; US to evaluate ligament damage; MRI for longer-term soft tissue damage evaluation
	All spinal regions	AP and lateral	Oblique projections of area as required to evaluate intervertebral articulations and vertebral foramina	CT to evaluate bone relations and soft tissue damage; MRI for soft tissue damage

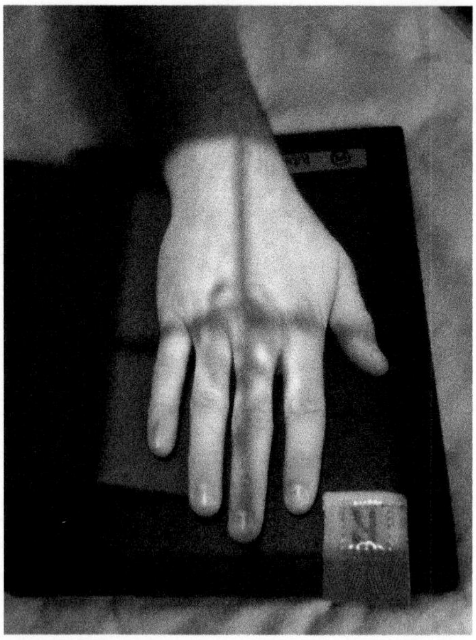

Fig. 17.1 Clear joint presentation in the injured hand. Placing a 15° pad under the fifth metacarpal enhances the joint visualisation of the injured hand.

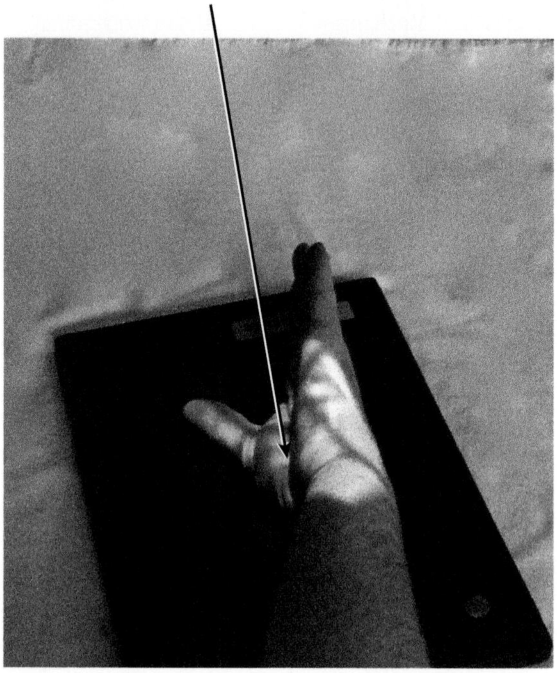

Fig. 17.2 Angulation to clear the thenar eminences of the thumb. Angulation 10° cranially along the long axis of the first metacarpal ensures the thenar eminences do not superimpose and a good projection of the articular surface of the metacarpal base is achieved.

Adapted Projections of the Hand

Frequently the patient requiring hand radiography will present to the Clinical Imaging department on a trolley, as a result of shock after experiencing trauma and being able to see the effects of the damage inflicted upon the limb. It is possible that routine projections of the hand may be undertaken with the arm extended across onto a table or platform, but adaptation may be necessary if other injuries prevent this. At this point the radiographer must consider adapting technique to ensure a diagnostic image is produced, without the serious compromise of increased radiation dose to radiosensitive tissues. However, there are other methods of providing images of the hand, and this section identifies a range of these.

Lewis[17] identified a way to address the perceived problems of the inadequacy of hand projections by suggesting that the dorsipalmar (DP) projection is obtained with the forearm medially rotated at the elbow so that the ulnar border of the hand is lifted from the cassette surface. A 15° radiolucent foam pad is placed under this aspect of the hand to immobilise the limb and raise the medial portion of the hand (Fig. 17.1), with the remainder of the technique used following that of the DP hand described in Chapter 4.

As patients are often reluctant to flatten their hand and extend their fingers following trauma, or soft tissue swelling prevents this from happening, this small change to technique allows the interphalangeal, metacarpophalangeal and carpal joints to be displayed squarely so that a true representation of the bony relationships can be gathered. The elevation of the medial aspect of the hand also places the little finger and 5th metacarpal into a DP position, rather than the oblique position in which they lie in the routine DP hand position.

Lewis continues to make further suggestions about hand radiography that would improve visualisation of certain digits.[18] Of the thumb he makes the point that, in the normal anteroposterior (AP) and lateral projections, the thenar eminence and other structures medial to the thumb are frequently superimposed over the first metacarpophalangeal joint, preventing clear visualisation owing to imperfect achievement of radiographic density. He suggests, for the AP projection, that the radiographer simply angles the central X-ray beam 10–15° along the long axis of the thumb, towards the wrist, so that the soft tissue structures are projected away from the area of interest. Using this technique helps reveal the proximal joint region without juggling with exposure factors that may overexpose the distal part of the thumb while attempting to reveal the proximal aspect (Fig. 17.2). The supine AP thumb technique described in Chapter 4 is probably most suitable, especially for the patient who presents on a trolley.

In a third suggestion about hand technique modifications Lewis describes another projection of the fifth metacarpal, a bone that is difficult to demonstrate owing to the anatomical relationship of the bones or soft tissues of the hand in the dorsipalmar oblique (DPO) or lateral projections.[19] He recommends further external rotation of the hand from the lateral position by an extra 5–10° so that the overlying second to fourth metacarpals no longer superimpose. The central ray is directed towards the middle of the fifth metacarpal and angled so that the ray is parallel with the thumb, which has been extended and abducted such that it does not overlie the fifth metacarpal (Fig. 17.3). Although an elongated projection is generated, almost the whole of the fifth metacarpal becomes visible.

Normally used for visualising the small joints of the fingers in the arthritic patient, the ball catcher's[20] projection may be used to show the extent of damage in the 'fight bite' situation (Fig. 17.4). Puncture of the assailant's skin by the victim's tooth may lead to the development of osteomyelitis.

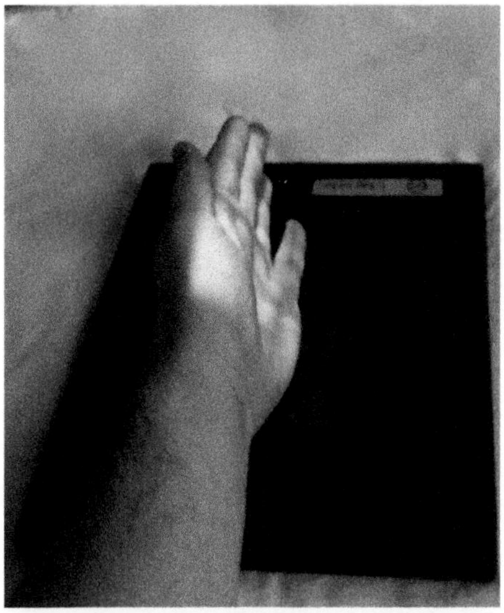

Fig. 17.3 Fifth metacarpal neck projection. Slight over-rotation of the lateral hand allows visualisation of the neck of the fifth metacarpal. The thumb is further abducted before exposure.

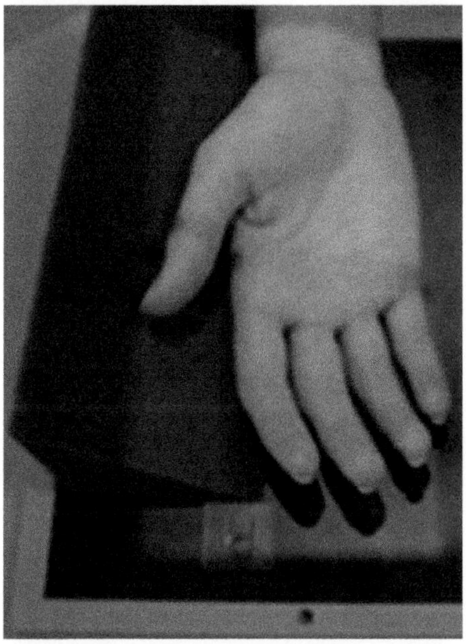

Fig. 17.4 Ball catcher's projection to show metacarpal heads tangentially.

Other than the clinical signs of the puncture wound or soft tissue swelling, little evidence of such an injury may be noted. However, the tangential representation of the metacarpal heads generated by this projection allows the viewer to see the indentation caused when the tooth has impacted with the metacarpal during a punching injury. The technique is described in Chapter 4, but it is not necessary to expose both hands and centring must be altered to coincide with the head of the third metacarpal, collimating to the single hand.

Adapted Projections of the Thumb

Injuries to the thumb are highly debilitating, as the ability to grip is compromised. Assessment of the integrity of the ulnar and radial collateral ligament at the metacarpophalangeal joint is achievable through the use of self-applied stressing forces in the posteroanterior (PA) thumb projection. This is achieved by using the index finger of the affected hand to generate adduction and abduction forces. The patient is asked to adduct the thumb by placing their index finger over the distal surface of the tip of the thumb and pulling it medially towards the finger; abduction is achieved by placing the tip of the index finger against the medial aspect of the tip of the thumb before pushing the tip of the thumb laterally, away from the index finger (Fig. 17.5A,B). Through stressing in a horizontal direction, the ulnar and radial collateral ligaments are strained to reveal their integrity. Rupture is revealed by widening of the respective side of the metacarpophalangeal joint that is associated with the damaged ligament.

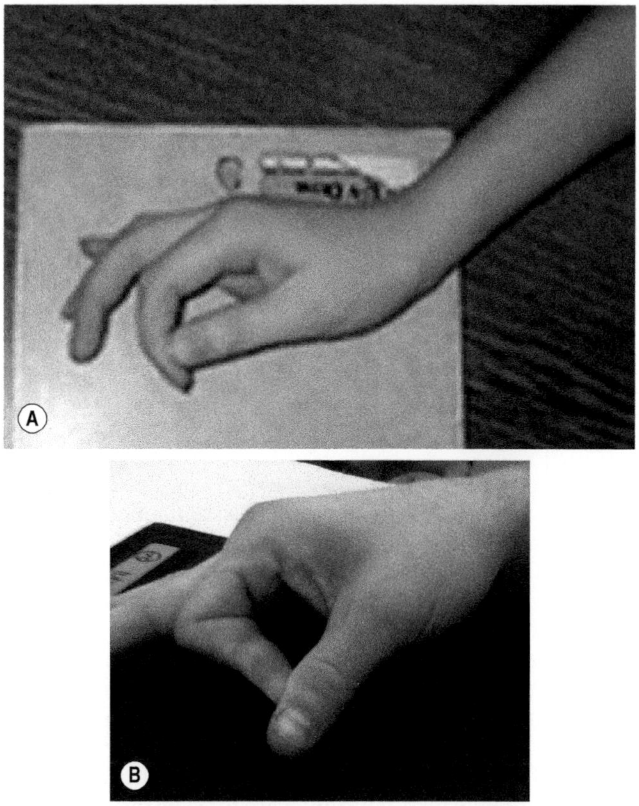

Fig. 17.5 Stress projections of the thumb. (A) The stressed thumb is being pulled towards the hand by the index finger while (B) shows the opposite stressing force. These projections are used to show radial and ulnar collateral damage, respectively, around the first metacarpophalangeal joint.

Should a true lateral projection of the base of the first metacarpal be required to reveal subtle fractures, the Gedda–Billings projection can be used.[21] Position as for the lateral thumb projection and angle the central ray 10° along the axis of the metacarpal, towards the forearm. This will free the articular surface from any superimposition over the trapezium (Fig. 17.6).

Adapted Projections of the Wrist and Forearm

As noted with the hand, occasionally it is necessary to adapt the positioning of the patient to achieve the correct projection. One of the neatest tricks that may be used to obtain

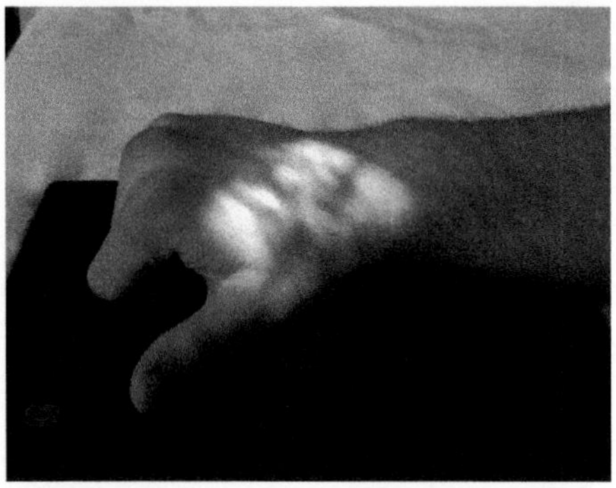

Fig. 17.6 The Gedda–Billings lateral projection of the thumb. This projection gives an uninterrupted lateral perspective of the base of the first metacarpal.

PA and lateral projections of the wrist is to encourage the patient to extend their arm and abduct it; this makes external rotation for the lateral projection easier. If the patient cannot externally rotate to a lateral position, the pronated hand and wrist can be raised onto a radiolucent pad, with the image receptor (IR) supported vertically against the medial aspect of the wrist; a horizontal beam is used lateromedially. Appropriate upper arm support may also be required with this technique. A mediolateral approach may be used if the arm cannot be abducted sufficiently to achieve the lateromedial technique, but care must be taken to avoid irradiating the trunk unnecessarily. If it is not possible to move the forearm into a pronated position for the PA wrist projection, place the wrist in the lateral position and raise it onto a radiolucent pad with an IR supported vertically against the anterior aspect of the wrist, using a horizontal beam technique for the central ray. Where independent cassette-type IRs are not available and direct digital units are used, the arm and pad can be supported on a small table placed next to the vertical detector; if the patient is on a trolley then the trolley must be at 90° to the digital unit and the patient's arm fully abducted, to ensure that the trunk is not near the primary beam. An AP approach will be necessitated in this instance.

With an injury to the forearm it can be extremely difficult for the patient to assume the standard (anatomical position) attitude required for radiography. If this is the case the forearm is best treated as two separate objects for imaging, although the individual joint aspects will manifest themselves as correct radiographic presentations on the resultant images. Handling of the limb is recommended as follows (this requires shoulder movement, and the radiographer should ascertain that this is safely possible):

- At the commencement of positioning ensure the table is level with the shoulder
- Abduct the limb from the trunk at the shoulder, while encouraging the patient to extend their elbow so that the whole arm may be rested on the table-top
- Externally rotate the shoulder to bring the elbow joint into a true AP position as the arm is supinated
- Often when in this position the patient will naturally want to rest the arm, with the wrist very close to the lateral position; this will allow an AP elbow and lateral wrist projection to be obtained on one image. Clearly there will be crossover of the shaft of radius over the ulna
- After obtaining the previous image, the arm is internally rotated at the shoulder and the elbow flexed. The medial aspects of the upper arm and elbow are placed in contact with the table-top. The positions of radius and ulna in relation to the humerus do not alter. The forearm thus assumes a position that now generates lateral elbow and, through natural pronation of the hand, PA wrist projections. Again, there will be crossover over the radial and ulnar shafts
- For both positions described, centre to the mid forearm and collimate to include the whole of the lower forearm

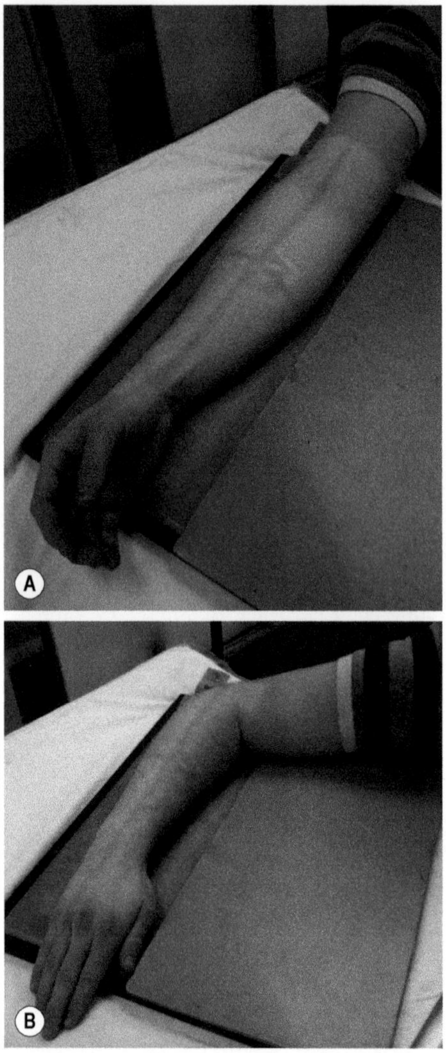

Fig. 17.7 Trauma projections of the forearm. Non-standard positions of the forearm to aid the patient who is injured by obtaining projections that are (A) lateral wrist with AP elbow and (B) vice versa.

Although this is not an anatomically correct approach, at least two projections of the injured forearm at 90° to each other are obtained so that some approximation of the anatomical relationship can be gleaned (Fig. 17.7A,B).

Shoulder injury is likely to affect the ability to achieve some of the positions described above, and a horizontal beam technique (as those described for the wrist) may be required. This technique is highly valued in such limiting situations but is very dependent upon the position in which the patient's forearm and the IR can be supported. The approach must be taken from the perspective that minimal patient movement is required, and similar results can be obtained as indicated above with the least pain to the patient. However, care must be exercised with respect to achieving these projections without unnecessary exposure to primary radiation from the horizontal beam technique, as there are implications for its direction towards the trunk. Careful use of an appropriate thickness of lead rubber over the trunk, collimation and turning the patient's head away from the X-ray tube are all essential measures that must not be ignored.

Adapted Projections of the Elbow and Humerus

The elbow is one of the most difficult areas to examine adequately following trauma, owing to concerns about exacerbating possible neurovascular damage. Frequently the patient will present with the elbow partially flexed and will resist attempts to extend it for an AP projection because of pain. To negotiate this problem individual images of each half of the elbow joint, i.e. proximal radius and ulna or distal humerus, should be obtained. In this way a relationship between major elbow components is noted and the articular surfaces are shown to advantage.[21] For AP images the posterior aspects of forearm and humeral portions of the elbow should be placed in contact with the IR in turn, thus allowing the radial and ulnar joint surfaces to be seen tangentially, or the trochlear/capitellar surfaces of the humerus to be displayed clearly, for each projection (Fig. 17.8A,B). A vertical central ray, or beam perpendicular to the joint portion of interest if a horizontal beam technique has to be used, is centred in turn at a point in the middle of the two articulation areas, i.e. over the proximal radioulnar joint for the proximal forearm and through the coronoid/olecranon fossa region for the distal humerus.

Patients with significant elbow injury may also present with the elbow held in full flexion as this guards against excessive pain. There is an association between this position and the likelihood of there being a fracture to the supracondylar region of the humerus, particularly in the younger patient. In these instances any attempt to extend the arm would be inappropriate, as it could cause further damage to the soft tissue structures in the area. The worst case scenario would be permanent disability, as in Volkmann's ischaemic contracture. Instead of extending the elbow for the AP projection, take an image of the elbow with the arm still flexed but held in an AP distal humerus position, resting the posterior aspect of the upper arm on the cassette, which has been placed on the examination table. The upper arm should be positioned with the elbow level with the shoulder (Fig. 17.9A) and the vertical beam is centred midway between the humeral epicondyles. Collimate to the area of interest, but use exposure factors modified (increased) to allow for the greater thickness of the tissue overlying the elbow; higher kVp should be used to even out the range of densities that are required for demonstration. The distal radius and ulna can be similarly demonstrated in the flexed elbow by positioning the posterior aspect of the forearm in contact with the IR. This time the elbow and wrist lie in the same plane (Fig. 17.9B). Centring remains as for the projection for distal humerus, as do considerations

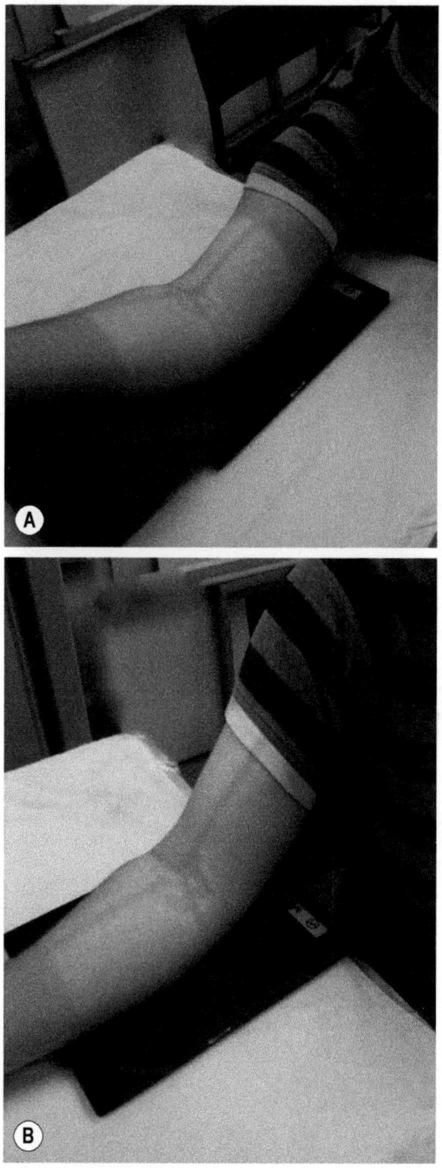

Fig. 17.8 The semi-flexed projections of the elbow. Obtaining the semi-flexed elbow image from the frontal aspect as two separate projections allows the tangential viewing of the articular surfaces to be achieved thus providing a detailed examination of the injured joint.

for exposure factor selection (see Chapter 5).[22] Use of both projections may be necessary to demonstrate the elbow adequately (Figs 17.9C,D), but justification for this must be ascertained, as there are implications for radiation dose owing to the use of two exposures. It must be noted that the image of the elbow joint will not be as accurate as in the routine AP projection. However, elbow flexion *is* required for the lateral projection of the joint, and this projection is less likely to be compromised by the flexed elbow position. Positioning the arm into the correct position for the lateral is also relatively easy, thereby lessening the risk of further injury to the joint, but it must be remembered that the optimum flexion in this projection is 90° and incorrect flexion will affect fat pad appearance. Using an adapted technique to demonstrate the radial head, as described later in this chapter and in Chapter 5, is also possible with the elbow retained in a flexed position.

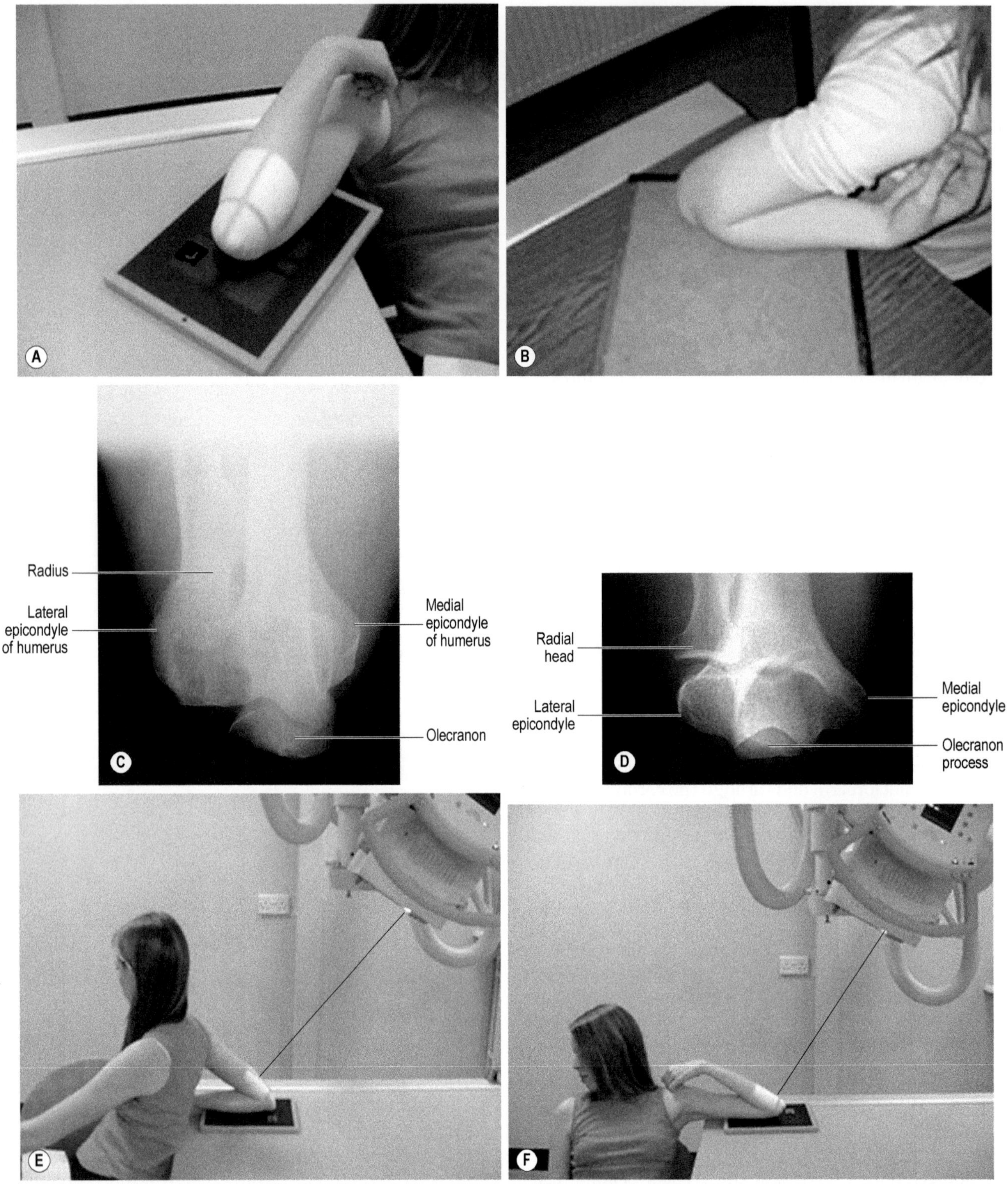

Fig. 17.9 (A,B) Fully flexed projections of the traumatised elbow show (A) the position to demonstrate the distal humerus and (B) the proximal radius and ulna; (C) X-ray image of flexed elbow projection to demonstrate humerus; (D) X-ray image of flexed elbow projection to demonstrate radius and ulna; (E) elbow in flexion – upper arm in contact with receptor, with beam angulation – this projection will show proximal radius and ulna; (F) elbow in flexion – forearm in contact with IR, with beam angulation – this projection will show distal humerus.

Still considering examination of the elbow in flexion, if the patient is unable to place the appropriate aspect of the arm in contact with the cassette (e.g. if information on radius and ulna is required, the patient is supine and cannot sit to put their forearm in contact with the IR, or if information on distal humerus is required and the posterior aspect of the upper arm carries significant abrasion), then the flexed elbow position can be modified. For proximal radius and ulna, when the posterior aspect of the forearm cannot be placed in contact with the IR, place the posterior aspect of the humerus in contact with the IR and use a beam angle perpendicular to the long axis of radius and ulna (Fig. 17.9E). For distal humerus, when it is not possible to place the posterior aspect of the upper arm in contact with the IR, place the posterior aspect of the forearm in contact with the IR and angle the central ray until it is perpendicular to the humerus (Fig. 17.9F). The centring point for each is midway between the humeral epicondyles. Note that the angle for either will vary greatly with each patient, due to variations in upper arm build, the degree of elbow flexion the patient holds the injured arm in, and the amount of abduction achievable at the shoulder.

Clearly the patient who presents on a trolley is unlikely to be able to sit next to a table for flexed elbow projections, but it is possible to reproduce them with the patient supine and the flexed joint positioned on the trolley, the arm abducted from the supine trunk (if cassette type IRs are used). In order to achieve projections, fixed horizontal direct digital receptors should be used alongside the trolley and the arm abducted over the receptor. A horizontal beam technique may be necessary if the shoulder rotation needed to bring the elbow into the correct position is not possible; this would be appropriate for both AP and lateral projections. The elbow is supported on a radiolucent pad and the IR vertically positioned against the posterior aspect of the humerus, as described for the modified projections of the wrist and forearm.

With more specific reference to the lateral projection for the injured elbow, obtaining a satisfactory lateral image frequently demands ingenuity in adaptation if the patient is unable to sit at the end of the table. The general rule, however, is to ensure that the elbow is supported on the IR so that the shoulder and elbow are at the same level, as in the routine lateral elbow position. This may be quite easy in a supine patient if the shoulder is mobile. However, it may not be possible to achieve this, even in a patient who is able to sit at the table, and often it is the extent of required external rotation at the shoulder that limits positioning; often the patient is limited to a position where their wrist and elbow joints lie lower than their shoulder. To reduce the effects of this, the lateral elbow projection can be modified by supporting the IR and arm with wedge-shaped pads and using a beam angle that will strike the IR at 90° (Fig. 17.10). Erect digital plate detector units are often versatile in that they can be angled to accommodate such modification. Similarly, the AP projection can be adapted so that it does not require the extent of external rotation at the shoulder. This is a horizontal beam approach where the elbow lies in a lateral position in relation to the table-top, but has the IR vertically behind its posterior aspect (Fig. 17.11). Again this may require the support of several foam immobilisation pads, and care should be taken to ensure that the arm lies parallel to the table-top.

When the patient cannot move their upper arm, but can stand or sit, a useful alternative technique for the lateral elbow projection is to position them erect PA and facing a vertical IR as if for a full lateral humerus projection. The flexed elbow, supported at the forearm by the hand of the uninjured side, should be abducted away from the body so that, viewed from the posterior aspect of the patient, the medial aspect of the elbow is visible (Fig. 17.12). This approach may also be adopted for the patient who might present on a trolley but is able to sit with their legs over the side. With the trolley placed close to the erect IR a similar result to that described may be obtained.

Elbow injury that also involves the bones of the forearm is relatively common and frequently creates damage

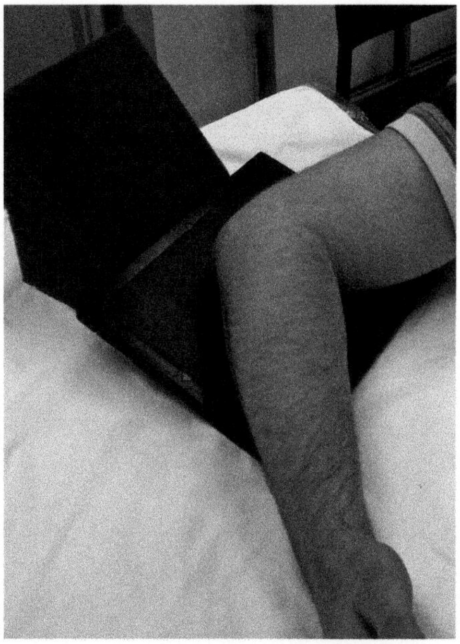

Fig. 17.10 Reduced movement lateral projection of the elbow. Note the IR is supported obliquely to ensure a comfortable but accurately positioned limb. The hand and shoulder are in the same plane and the hand supported to maintain this. In this case a slight mediolateral angle will ensure that the beam is perpendicular to the IR. This projection can be used for trolley-bound patients.

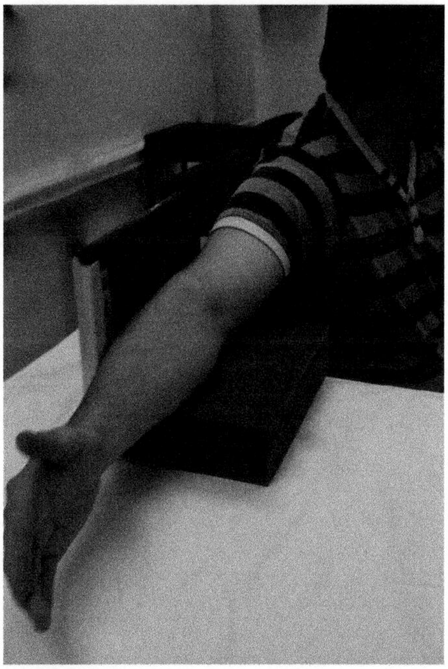

Fig. 17.11 Horizontal beam AP projection of the elbow. This is used when the patient cannot externally rotate the shoulder for a routine AP, in conjunction with horizontal beam. This figure shows how the projection can be used for partially flexed elbows as well as extended elbows. The projection can be achieved for trolley-bound patients.

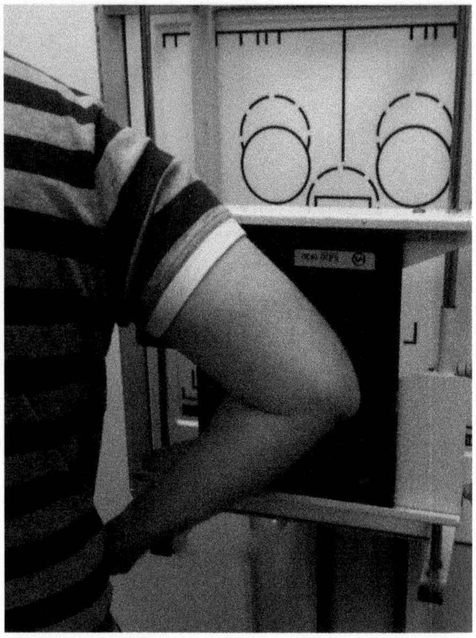

Fig. 17.12 The PA erect lateral elbow projection, performed in much the same way as the lateral full-length humerus.

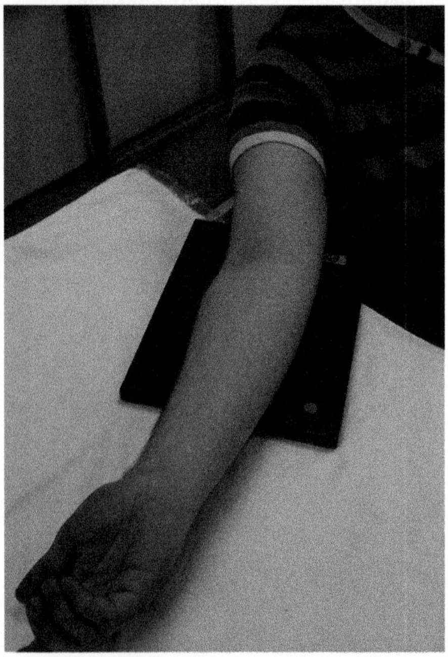

Fig. 17.13 External rotation to reveal proximal forearm details. Further external rotation from the AP elbow position will allow visualisation of the radial head, neck and tuberosity.

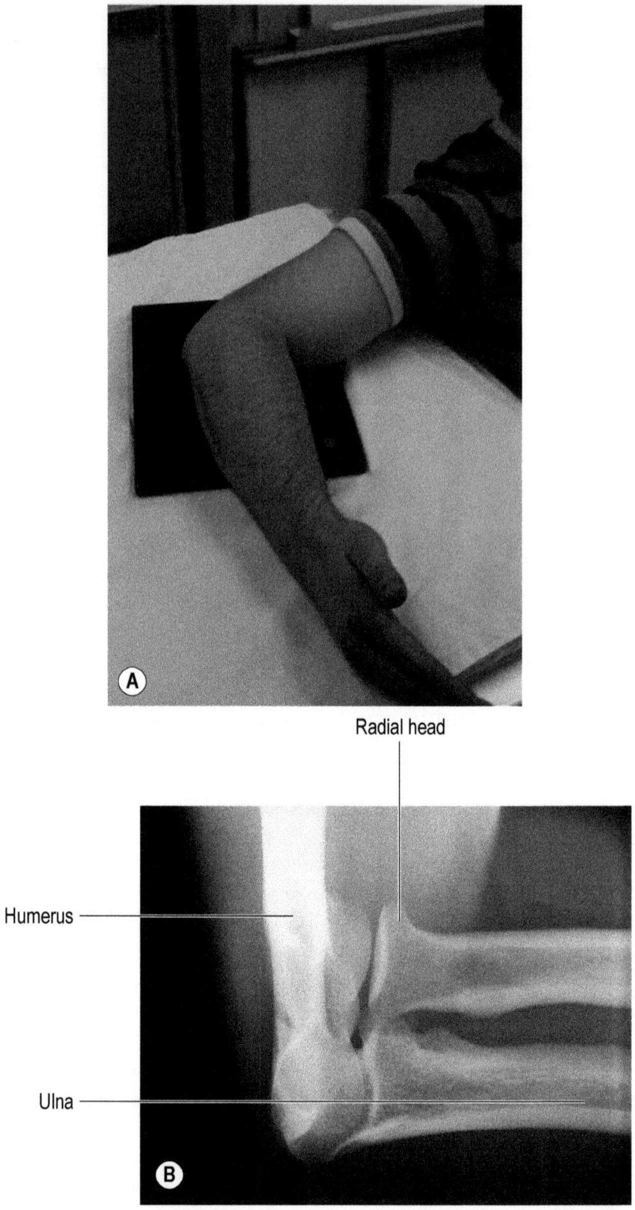

Fig. 17.14 (A) Coyle radial head projection; by angling 40–45° lateromedially, this projection separates the radial head from the superimposing ulna for suspected radial head/neck fractures; (B) Coyle radial head X-ray; by angling 40–45° lateromedially, this projection separates the radial head from the superimposing ulna for suspected radial head/neck fractures.

that may not be identified. Rotating the elbow externally from the true AP position so the humeral epicondyles lie at 45° relative to the IR cassette allows visualisation of the *radial head, neck and tuberosity* without superimposition of other bones (Fig. 17.13). An image of this is shown in Chapter 5 (Fig. 5.5B). The humeral capitellum will also be clearly displayed with this projection. Internal rotation of the elbow from the AP position will advantageously display the coronoid of the ulna, the trochlea and an elongated medial epicondyle of the humerus (see Fig. 5.8A,B).

The radial head can also be further visualised in the lateral position by rotating from the lateral elbow position start point. Four exposures can be made with the forearm in this lateral position: displaying maximum supination; lateral with the ulnar border of the forearm in a comfortable position; pronation of the hand and hyperpronation of the hand with the hand positioned as if attempting an AP projection of the thumb. This gradually rotates the radial head so that aspects of the proximal radial profile are displayed (see Figs 5.6A,B and 5.7A,B). Finally, the Coyle projection[23] of the radial head employs lateromedial angulation of 45° across the forearm, which is in a lateral position (Fig. 17.14A,B). This projection separates the radial head and capitellum from superimposing structures to reveal indistinct injuries that may be too subtle to detect on the normal lateral image.

Fractures of the *humerus* often appear dramatic owing to deformation of the limb, and these demand the utmost care from the imaging practitioner. In cases like this the patient is best examined erect so that the most information can be obtained using a single projection, in the same way as follow-up images would be achieved. However, if the patient presents on a trolley or has to be examined on the X-ray table, an immobilisation pad support will be necessary to obtain a true projection of the limb. Although images reveal their best information by being taken with the IR in close proximity to the limb, using an IR tray or under-trolley tray may be a desirable option to minimise movement of the arm and reduce patient discomfort. The associated projection at 90° to the first can be obtained using a combination of overlapping horizontal beam projections from the shoulder down and elbow up. Moving the arm away from the body and elevating it on supporting pads to allow clear visualisation of the limb may be necessary for these projections. The required arm positions can be achieved with (non-cassette type) fixed digital receptors in the same way as described for the forearm and elbow above. Good communication techniques and appropriate analgesia are the most helpful additions that can be offered in this setting – as in most trauma imaging approaches (Fig. 17.15A–C).

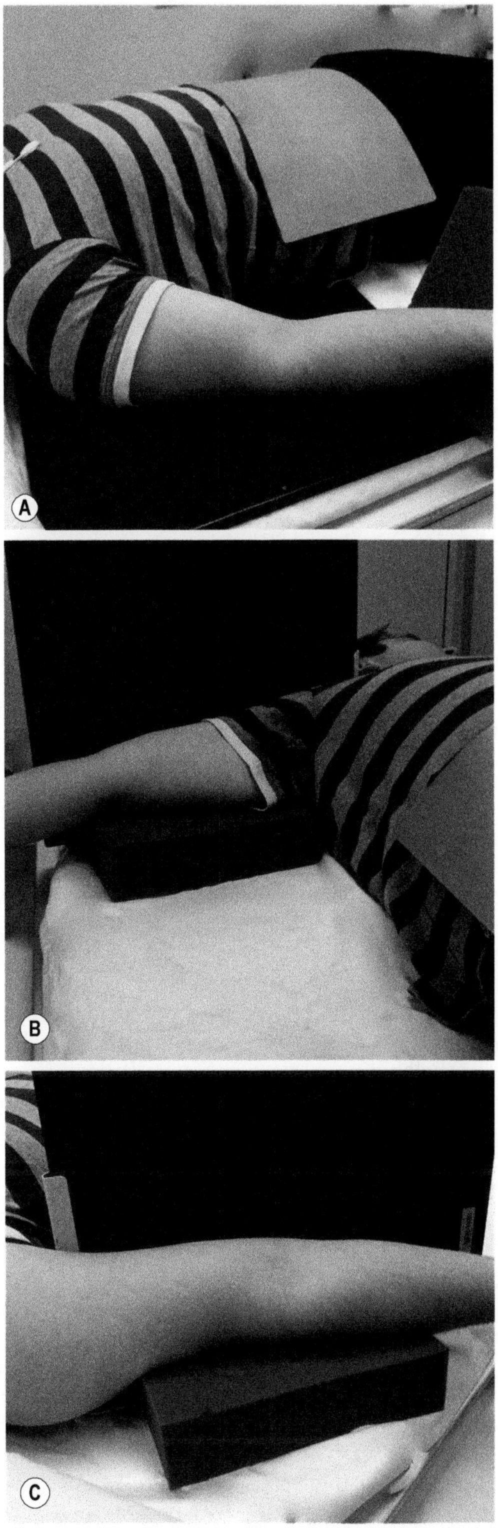

Fig. 17.15 Supine projections of the injured humerus. Several options are available for obtaining images of the injured humerus with differing impacts on the patient from a movement (A,B) and potential radiation dose (C) perspective.

Adapted Projections of the Shoulder Joint

The shoulder joint (specifically the glenohumeral joint) has been the source of the generation of many tailored projections to prove various injury and degenerative processes. This section will consider the supplementary projections of value following trauma.

Confusion is occasionally apparent regarding the degree of external rotation required for the AP projection of the shoulder. Ideally, appropriate clinical evaluation will result in the indication by the referrer; for example, if the *clavicle* is the injured component for which a radiological opinion is sought, this would necessitate a clavicular projection. Where this is not the case, and foreshortening of the clavicle is not a consideration, appropriate external rotation of the trunk to the affected side should be attempted so that the glenoid edge will be projected in profile. This will allow the viewer to scrutinise the *glenohumeral joint* effectively so that the image can be correctly evaluated for the presence of subtle dislocation or fracture characteristics. This rule also applies for patients who present in a supine position, depending of course on the potential for causing further injury by rotating the patient. The suitability of different alternatives to the axial shoulder projection must be considered before a technique is selected; discussion on this is given in Chapter 5.

The modified axial projection is one that can be used in any situation. Essentially, the projection is obtained by positioning the patient as for an AP shoulder, as seen in Chapter 5, with 30–45° caudal angulation from the original perpendicular beam direction (Fig. 5.19); it is easily undertaken on the supine patient (Fig. 17.16). This can also be undertaken with 45° rotation on the trunk; this is sometimes known as the Garth projection or Garth apical oblique,[24] and is used to assess dislocation by examining the position of the humeral head relative to the glenoid of the scapula. The projection can also be undertaken erect or supine. On the resulting images for either of these angled AP projections, if the humeral head lies inferiorly to the glenoid then the dislocation is anterior, with the positions of the anatomical structures reversed for posterior dislocations, i.e. the glenoid edge

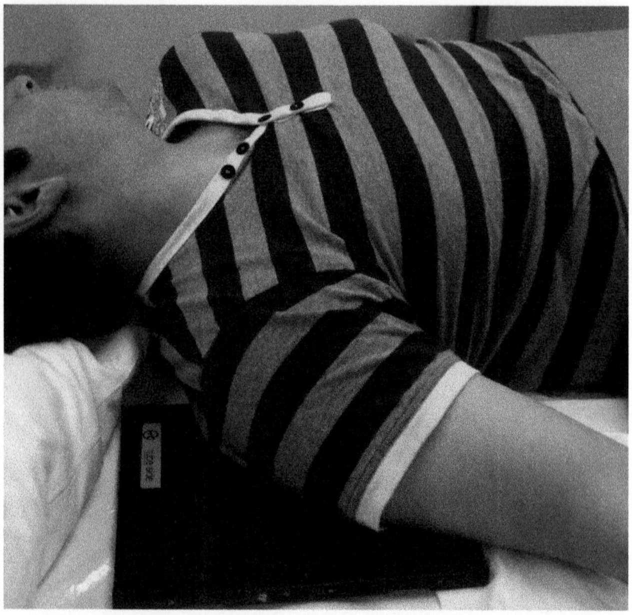

Fig. 17.16 The Garth projection. The Garth projection to reveal dislocation of the glenohumeral joint. This projection produces a half axial projection of the shoulder and is one option to consider where a true axial image might not be possible. It can also be undertaken sitting or standing.

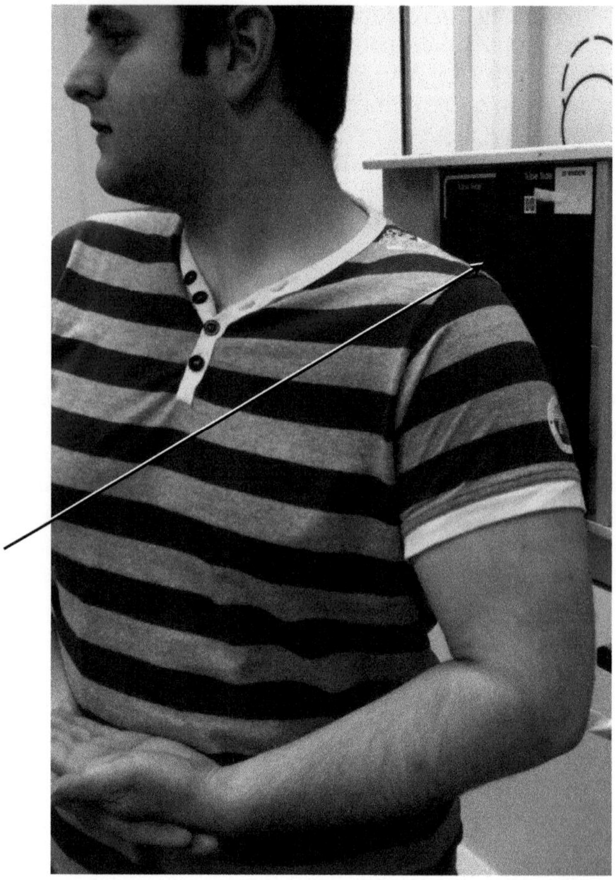

Fig. 17.17 Inferosuperior projection to show the coracoid of the scapula. The coracoid projection also allows good visualisation of the acromioclavicular joint, projected clear of other shoulder structures.

is lower in relation to the humeral head. Where the patient is unable to be seated and presents on a trolley, true inferosuperior or superoinferior projections may be achieved by gently encouraging the patient to abduct the arm so that an IR can be placed in the axillary space. Alternatively, the IR is placed above the shoulder and the central ray directed from below the joint. This may be feasible, while minimising pain, as relatively small amounts of movement are required following the performance of the AP projection that complements the above.

Further discussion on the options for shoulder projections, including considerations for implementation in trauma situations, can be found in Chapter 5.

Owing to the structure of the shoulder, the *coracoid process* has other structures superimposed over it on the image. This may be a particular problem in younger patients, where secondary ossification of the coracoid tip could mimic a fracture; this necessitates clear visualisation of this aspect of the shoulder.

If any kyphosis of the thoracic region is present, simply angle 20–30° cranially with the patient in the normal AP shoulder position (Fig. 17.17). Greater kyphosis will require greater angulation. This image can also be helpful in the evaluation of the *acromioclavicular joint.*

THE LOWER LIMB

Adapted Projections of the Foot, Ankle and Leg

Where injuries of the *foot* are concerned, radiographers frequently have to work around the patient, depending heavily at times on the versatility of the radiographic equipment. This means that, although projections are standardised or similar, the equipment must be manoeuvred into various positions, rather than moving the patient's limb. Horizontal ray techniques are often used to create a projection that is at least similar to the standard projection in the less injured patient.

When the patient presents in a *wheelchair* for foot examinations, consider placing the IR on the floor or on a small step for the patient to place the injured foot upon. In this way the frail patient does not have to be moved and a standard projection is possible. Slight extension of the ankle, required to clear the tibia and fibula from the majority of the tarsus, is also easier in this position. The *trolley-bound patient* can be examined with the leg fully extended or with the hip and knee slightly flexed. The cassette-type IR can be supported on a pad under the plantar aspect of the foot, or the fixed digital plate angled and brought into contact with the plantar aspect of the foot; it does not matter at what angle the IR and foot lie, as long as the central ray is correctly angled until it is perpendicular to the IR. In some cases it may be necessary to elevate the foot slightly by resting the back of the heel on a radiolucent pad, so that the knee and lower leg are not projected over the image. This would be most likely in the patient whose leg is fully extended. The practitioner's skills are of paramount importance here, with respect to angling the beam and accurately positioning the IR.

Working in this way indicates that the patient probably requires no more than the equivalent of the basic 'two projections at right-angles' series. That said, orthopaedic colleagues may request further projections, such as those of the *subtalar joints*. The best projections to reveal the most information on the whole region are the medial and lateral

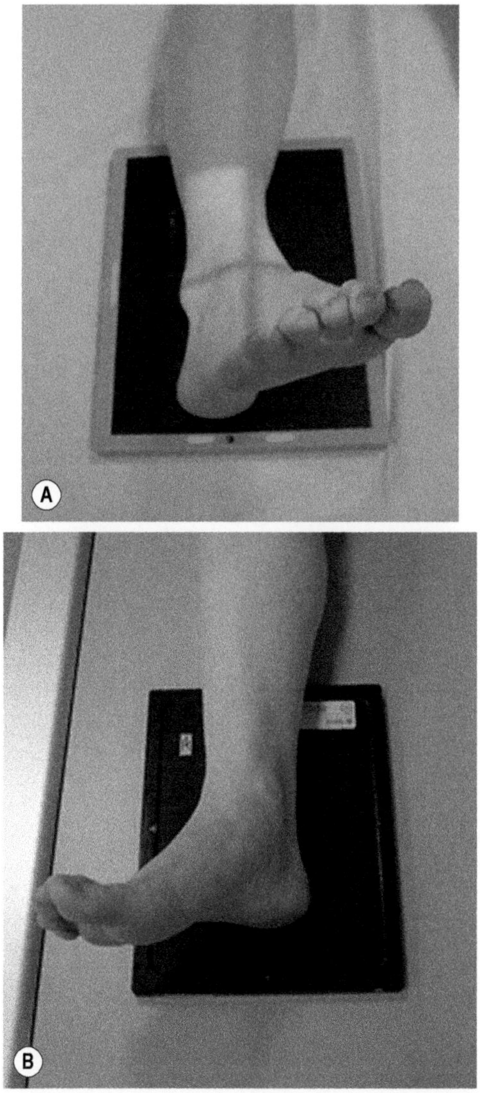

Fig. 17.18 (A) The 'common' subtalar projection – the 'common' subtalar view, whereby a midpoint angle of 45° internal and external rotation of the ankle is accompanied by 20° cranial angulation of the central ray to reveal the majority of the subtalar articulation in a pair of images; (B) 45° external oblique ankle.

ankle obliques, where the foot is rotated respectively internally and externally from the AP ankle position to form an angle of 45° to the IR (Fig. 17.18A,B). The central ray is angled 20° cranially and directed towards the talus. Collimate to include the ankle joint, talus calcaneum and both malleoli.

Examinations for injury related to areas proximal to the ankle can usually be obtained by using a combination of routine and horizontal ray techniques. Splinting devices may be present and, where possible, these should be removed to avoid artefact generation. Should the leg be so badly injured that gross rotation of one part relative to another is displayed (e.g. shaft of tibia and fibula rotated in relation to the ankle joint), then obtain projections that ensure that at least one part of the limb is projected with its joint in the correct orientation, so that the associated portion of the injured part can be assessed relative to the part that is correctly projected. Using the lower leg as an example, this would mean AP knee and lateral ankle obtained by vertical X-ray beam; lateral knee and AP ankle obtained by horizontal ray technique.

Not all leg injuries will be as remarkable as the example above. When the patient is able to climb onto the examination table, further simple projections may be helpful in elucidating subtle injuries. Internal and external oblique projections of the ankle can be performed with the foot rotated through the axis of the ankle to form the required angle of 45° to the table-top for the respective projections. The vertical central ray is centred on the ankle joint and collimated as described for the AP ankle in Chapter 6. The internal oblique will show the *distal tibiofibular joint* and *lateral malleolus* clearly, with the external oblique displaying the *medial malleolus* and *talus* to advantage. Under- and over-rotation of the ankle joint in the lateral position are also useful images to obtain from the perspective of displaying (a) the posterior tibial lip in the under-rotated lateral and (b) the posterior margin of the fibula in the over-rotated lateral.

Stress projections to reveal ligament integrity in the ankle may also be required. The inversion stress projection shows the integrity of the *lateral collateral complex*, whereas the eversion stress projection is helpful for showing the integrity of the *medial collateral complex*. As the referring clinician is normally responsible for the action of stressing the joint in each direction, the radiographer must control the situation by taking care to ensure any lead rubber protective devices used do not impinge on the region being imaged. One such example would be to ensure that the clinician's hands and the lead rubber gloves, worn while applying stress to the joint, do not overlie the area of interest. It is also relatively easy for the clinician to inadvertently move the ankle from the AP position, which is adopted as a baseline, so that the area under examination is projected incorrectly; this would make detection of subtle injury difficult. Alternatively, some radiology departments have developed stressing devices as a variation on the Thomas wrench, which the patient may control manually, though usually this device is operated by the medical practitioner.[25] This may produce the desired result, but care is required so that the patient does not overstress the joint and cause more injury. More likely, however, is the chance that the patient will not exert enough force on the joint to achieve a diagnostic result.

To assess the *tibiotalar* and *talofibular ligaments* of the ankle using the lateral projection, the anterior draw stress projection can be attempted without the presence of the clinician; this is a variation on that described by Horsfield and Murphy.[25] The back of the heel of the patient's affected limb is rested on a wooden block that has been placed on the table or trolley-top; the ankle joint is therefore raised above the table or trolley (Fig. 17.19). An IR is positioned on the medial aspect of the ankle and a horizontal X-ray beam is centred over the lateral malleolus. A medium-sized sandbag should be placed on the mid-shaft of the tibia so that the ankle joint is gently stressed for approximately 1 minute before exposure. Collimation must include the whole of the ankle joint as well as at least 5 cm of the distal tibia. Be sure the malleoli are equidistant from the *block*, as for the AP position (malleoli are positioned relative to the *block* rather than to the IR). A positive response to stressing the joint shows the talus to have subluxed anteriorly, indicating damage to the ligaments indicated. Remember to remove

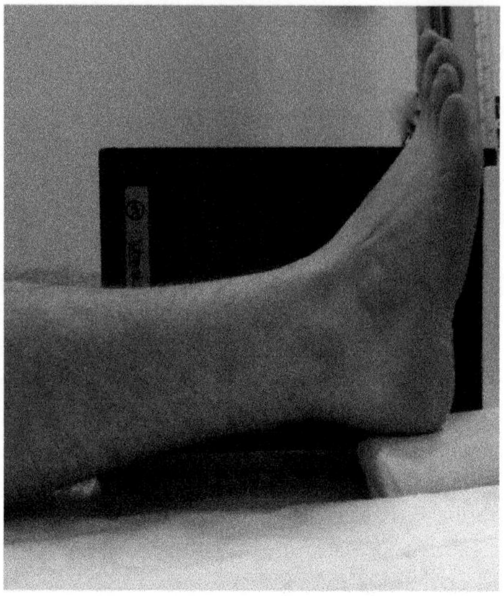

Fig. 17.19 The anterior draw stress projection.

the weight as soon as possible after exposure as this examination is often uncomfortable for the patient.

Adapted Projections of the Knee, Thigh and Hip

Knee injuries are usually best evaluated via the routine AP and horizontal ray lateral so that subtle soft tissue signs such as lipohaemarthrosis may be detected. This has added advantages in that (a) the patient need not be moved in more serious trauma situations, and (b) any radiographic evidence that may indicate an effusive collection in the suprapatellar region will not be disturbed. That said, the presence of an effusion should merely prompt the search for an underlying, more serious, bony cause.

Fractures of the *patella* are most commonly in a transverse direction, which should not be disturbed by bending the knee to achieve a lateral projection. However, the vertical fracture pattern that may not be obvious on the AP projection may require a tangential/inferosuperior skyline projection to reveal its nature. In these situations a projection with a small (around 30°) angle of flexion at the knee, the degree of flexion probably being governed by the extent of compliance attainable by the patient in conjunction with clinical history, should be attempted. Unfortunately this minimal flexion will require the central ray to be directed quite closely towards the body and head of the patient; however, this problem may be navigable by asking the patient to lie on the affected side with the slightly flexed knee resting in a lateral position close to the edge of the examination table (see patellar projections in Chapter 7). The head should be tilted back to clear the eyes as far as possible from the primary beam. In this way a grazing angle tangential to the patella is achieved which allows the patient to lean back from the track of the central ray, thereby reducing the likelihood of exposing the torso and head. Flexion must not be considered if derangement of the knee complex is suspected, or in the case of suspected tibial plateau fracture.

Femoral fractures are normally the result of significant force and are often accompanied by other injuries, so that adapted techniques are frequently required to obtain the images necessary for patient management. As with earlier examples, the use of horizontal beam techniques is vital in these situations, as is negotiating around splinting devices. The lateral is best undertaken with a horizontal beam and IR supported vertically at the side of the thigh. Lateromedial projections are favoured when it is difficult or inadvisable to raise the other leg to clear it from the femur under examination, although the lateromedial approach will involve the primary beam being directed towards the leg not under examination. AP projections can be obtained with the IR in a trolley tray, so that the limb is not moved unnecessarily. Image magnification is likely to be a problem if the IR is placed in a tray for this projection, and an increase in focus receptor distance (FRD) will be required to help compensate for this. The approach to the lateral projection will mean that the IR may not extend sufficiently far along the thigh to include the injury site for evaluation in a single projection. The long femur may also not actually fit within the boundary of the IRs available (see Chapter 7 where the issue of patient length is discussed), and the only option in this instance is to obtain overlap images so that minimal movement of the patient is maintained. Also note that the femur is an area with a range of densities along its length, necessitating the use of a higher kVp non-gridded technique. To summarise these suggestions, an acceptable compromise must be reached that may result in some loss of the contrast and detail in the image but allow a single projection to be obtained, with concomitant reduction in radiation dose to the patient.

Adapted Projections of the Pelvis and Hips

Most hip fractures are found in the elderly, but some younger patients may present with conditions such as slipped upper femoral epiphysis (SUFE), or after involvement in high-energy accidents that may have caused dislocation at the hip. Patients who have undergone total hip replacement may present with dislocation of the femoral portion owing to such simple manoeuvres as standing from a seated position in a low chair. Occasionally, young athletes may present with stress injury to the neck of femur or, more rarely, a true fracture of the same region.

When the neck of femur has been fractured, two projections at right-angles are often required: a full AP pelvis, to allow full evaluation of the pelvic girdle for other injuries, and a horizontal beam lateral (HBL) of the hip (although some centres accept that if an obvious fracture is seen on the AP then a further projection is unnecessary; Chapter 8 provides further comment on the need for a lateral hip projection). A common error with the horizontal ray lateral projection is to allow the thigh of the unaffected side to obstruct the X-ray beam, thereby creating a soft tissue artefact. Proprietary devices are available to help the patient keep the uninjured limb suitably raised; the hip and knee are flexed until the thigh is as near vertical as possible, so that the thigh is cleared from the beam path. See Chapter 8 and Figs 8.7 and 8.8A for description of this technique, using a proprietary device to keep the thigh raised. A less expensive alternative is to use a large radiolucent foam pad, which can be positioned appropriately under the leg; this does not allow for visualisation of the centring point and must be positioned after centring and collimation have taken place.

These methods of producing a HBL are possible only when the patient is able to elevate the unaffected limb. An example of such a situation is when the patient has had a

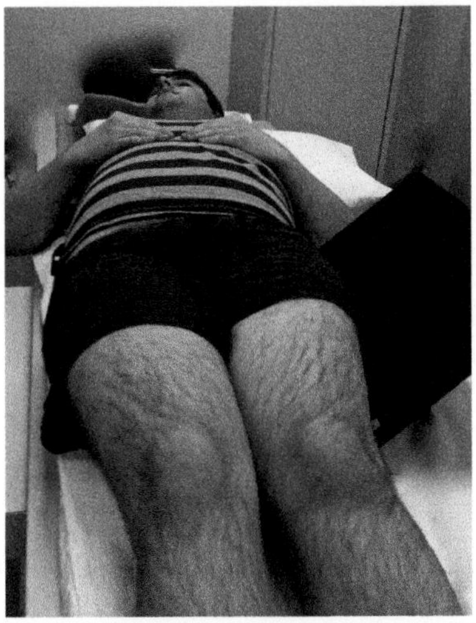

Fig. 17.20 The half-axial hip projection. The half lateral/semi-axial hip projection for patients unable to elevate the opposite side to produce a horizontal ray lateral. Use of a larger IR will facilitate inclusion of the upper third of femur to provide a lateral projection of the shaft.

recent hip replacement in the uninjured hip, and there is a risk that the movements described above might cause dislocation of the unaffected side, which would be a disastrous result. When this is the case an axial oblique that will give lateral orientation information can be attempted. For this the patient remains supine with the IR initially positioned as for the HBL. From this position the cassette is tilted backwards 25° and supported with sandbags and foam pads. The horizontal central ray is angled 25° caudally and then rotated on the ceiling mount until the central ray is perpendicular to the IR. This tip beam is centred over the medial aspect of the upper thigh at the level of the greater trochanter, to pass through the hip level with the femoral pulse (Fig. 17.20). Collimate the beam appropriately and select exposure factors slightly lower than those indicated for the HBL.

Regarding major trauma, an AP examination of the pelvis is standard in the major trauma series associated with the ATLS protocols. However, in a trauma situation there are likely to be inherent problems that will require additional care in undertaking the examination. The fractured pelvis carries serious risks associated with unstable bony components and vascular damage, requiring movement of the patient to be minimised, especially until haemodynamic stability is achieved. As a result the patient must be examined on the trauma trolley, using an IR with grid in the tray beneath the trolley. Often, accurate centring of the IR to coincide with the median sagittal plane (MSP), area of interest and central ray is difficult, as the IR is positioned under the patient by 'guess' or estimation. Patients rarely present perfectly centralised on a trolley and often lie obliquely across its central long axis. Some practitioners peer down the gap between the trolley-top and the cassette tray to assess the alignment of the IR and MSP; unfortunately this is not the most accurate way of assessing the situation, as the narrowness of the gap means that the IR and the patient cannot be seen at the same time. Where space permits, the following are useful in ensuring accurate alignment:

- Ensure the trolley is parallel to the wall of the X-ray room and the tube ceiling track
- At the head end of the trolley, find the midpoint of the trolley-top or central handle (not the mattress, which is often not centralised on the trolley) and position the vertical central ray over this point
- Move the tube down the trolley towards the patient's pelvis, without any crosswise shift of the tube
- When the tube is level with the pelvis, assess the distance between the patient's MSP and the central ray; this will give a good indication of how far to displace the IR laterally if the MSP is displaced from the midline of the trolley; it may be necessary to turn the IR slightly if the patient's pelvis is lying diagonally
- Reposition the tube to lie over the midline of the pelvis and the correct centring point
- Collimate as for routine pelvis or hips AP

This tip can prove useful for any supine AP projection of the spine, abdomen or pelvis.

Less severely traumatised trolley-bound patients may also be examined on the trolley; attention to detail will ensure the correct projection is obtained and that the body part is centralised to the IR. Some imaging departments prefer to move the patient on the trolley mattress across to the examination table to ensure that a degree of imaging standardisation is achieved. However, this does expose practitioners and patients to risk of injury through manual handling.

When the resuscitation room is not being used as the examination area, other projections beyond the AP pelvis may be requested if the patient has been stabilised haemodynamically. These include:

- Judet's iliac oblique acetabulum (may be performed as a whole pelvis examination)
- Judet's obturator oblique acetabulum (may be performed as a whole pelvis examination)
- Posterior oblique of ilium
- AP pubis
- Inlet projection of pelvis
- Outlet projection of pelvis

Judet's projections involve 45° rotation of the patient, (a) towards the affected side to reveal the *iliac* portion of the hemipelvis and (b) away from the affected side to show the *obturator* aspects. Respectively, the projections show (a) the posterior or ilioischial column and anterior acetabular rim (when the affected side is lowered) and (b) the anterior or iliopubic column and posterior acetabular rim. When undertaken in order to show each half of the pelvis the whole hemipelvis should be included and the central ray directed to the acetabulum in both projections.[26] See Chapter 8 and Figures 8.9 and 8.10 for a full description of the obliques.

Good visualisation of the anterior portion of the iliac bone and the crest is achieved by positioning as for the iliac oblique (Chapter 8), but centring the vertical central ray over the iliac wing and remembering to collimate and adjust exposure as appropriate. A supplementary projection of the *pubis* may be helpful, especially where the syndesmosis is 'bobbly' or it is unclear as to whether or not a fracture is present. Position the patient as for the AP projection of both hips. Apply 20° cranial beam angulation for males and 30° cranial angulation for females (to allow for the differences in pelvic shape). Centre to the lower border of the symphysis pubis and collimate to include the pubic and ischial rami, ensuring that the image lies within the boundaries of the IR. The projection gives an apparently elongated (although in fact more accurate) projection of the pubic and ischial rami compared to the AP pelvis, as the effects of the natural tilt of the pelvis are countered by the cranial angle, thereby preventing foreshortening.

The pelvic inlet and outlet projections provide added information for the evaluation of the degree of pelvic component movement after a fracture to the area.[27] For the *inlet* projection, position the patient as for the AP pelvis. Use a central ray angled 40° caudally, centred to the level of the ASIS, along the midline. Collimate the beam to include the whole of the pelvis and ensure that the image lies within the boundaries of the IR. This projection is used to assess the degree of posterior displacement of the hemipelvis or inward/outward rotation of the anterior pelvis following trauma. The pelvic ring should be clearly demonstrated when exposure factors are selected to demonstrate the anterior and posterior structures; if this is the case, then the iliac wings are usually overexposed. For the *outlet* projection, position as above but angle the central X-ray beam 40° cranially, centring the central ray to a point at the inferior border of the symphysis pubis. As with the pubic bone AP projection, the effect of pelvic tilt is countered, so the projection shows these unforeshortened bones clearly. Visualisation of the iliac wings is poor because of superimposition of the acetabula.[28]

Finally, SUFE presentation requires the use of the trauma frog lateral in conjunction with the AP pelvis projection. Starting in the position for AP pelvis, flex the knees and externally rotate the hips through approximately 40–60° and bring the soles of the feet into contact with each other. Support the legs at the knees with foam immobilising pads and sandbags. Using a vertical X-ray beam, centre at a point 1–2.5 cm proximal to the symphysis pubis (according to the size of the child) in the midline, and collimate the beam to include both hips/femoral necks. In this projection the pelvis is shown as an AP projection. The proximal femora are projected laterally as for the 'turned' lateral projection; however, when visualised together this projection may be called the modified Cleaves projection.[29]

THE SPINE

Although this section will consider the adapted projections of the spine, it should be apparent that the majority of regions of the spine require just AP and lateral projections to be obtained following trauma. In practice, computed tomography (CT) is used in most departments as the frontline investigation where the index of suspicion is high,[30] as clinical answers can be readily achieved and its sensitivity is far greater than that of projection radiography.[31] Although CT is used more frequently today, the following techniques are still an important adjunct and still as a frontline investigation in many circumstances.

Adapted Projections of the Cervical Spine

Standard AP and lateral projections are often requested following whiplash-type injuries; the patient is frequently able to sit or stand for the lateral projection as they often present 24–48 hours after the accident. A supine lateral is required for the patient who is at risk from movement, and the lateral image must always be examined before a decision on further patient management is made. The common belief is that the lateral cervical projection must take preference as the first projection undertaken in the cervical spine; this is appropriate if there is serious concern that significant neck trauma has occurred. Current National Institute for Health and Care Excellence (NICE) guidelines advocates that those over the age of 65 with a history of trauma to suspect fracture, should be transferred to CT for cervical spine imaging, negating the need for projection radiography that has a low sensitivity for fracture detection in the degenerate spine.[30] A cervical spine fracture will always need CT, so if a lateral radiograph shows a fracture, there is limited benefit doing any additional projections and the patient should be referred directly to CT by the referring clinician or the radiographer depending on local protocols.

The problems of shoulder shadow obscuring the cervicothoracic region are typically similar to those encountered in the patient attending for examination of the cervical spine to evaluate degenerative changes and, as such, may be treated with similar techniques. Where more severe injuries necessitate patient presentation on a trolley, either in the imaging department or in the resuscitation room, then adaptation will be necessary to negotiate the shoulder superimposition problem. Frequently, where the patient is conscious, explaining what the radiographer is attempting to achieve enables the patient to reach down towards their feet with their arms and clear the soft tissue of the shoulders from the lower cervical vertebrae. This is especially effective if coupled with an expiration breathing technique prior to exposure.

The supine patient may be advised to use an arm folding technique, if this is considered safe; for this the arms are extended and crossed at the wrists, with the medially rotated hands clasped together (Fig. 17.21A,B). Many departments will immediately adopt the swimmer's position, which can be undertaken supine as well as erect, as described in Chapter 9 (Fig. 9.4A–C),[32] but the validity of its use can be questioned as it necessitates significant movement of the shoulders for the neck-injured and multiply-injured patient, carries somewhat confusing information due to overlying structures, and is often low in quality due to scatter produced by area density and increased exposure factors. All these factors make interpretation more difficult; unsurprising, then, that it has been found that almost half of the swimmer's projections studied in one piece of research were inadequate for use as a diagnostic tool.[33] There is additional discussion on the validity of the swimmer's projection in Chapter 9.

A dichotomy exists in more difficult cases with respect to how some kind of adequate projection might be obtained to reveal possible injuries to the cervical spine. Suggestions have been made regarding the performance of trauma obliques,[34,35] but unfortunately this is often met with resistance from some, usually inexperienced, personnel, who imply that reading the images is 'difficult'.[36] To produce images for the oblique cervical projection, the patient is supine on the examination table (but usually on a trolley). An IR is placed in the trolley tray or directly on the tabletop next to the patient's neck. When the trolley-top method is used this may mean the IR is pushed partially under the

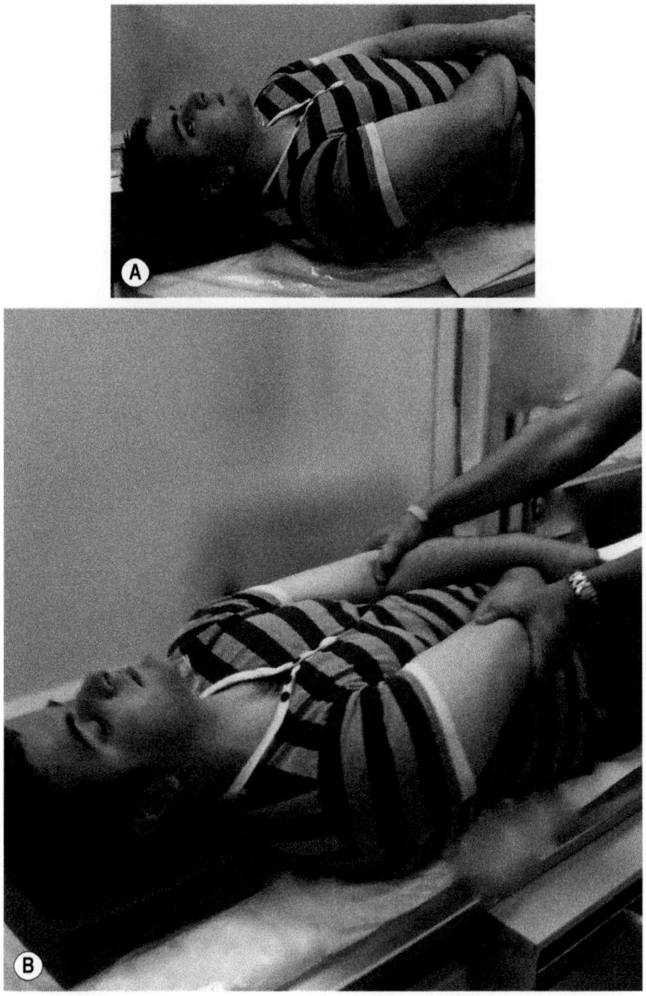

Fig. 17.21 Arm folding may help reveal the cervicothoracic junction.

head. This should be done only under supervision, but will not be a problem with the tray method. Angle the X-ray tube 45° in a lateromedial direction, the central ray entering the side of the neck furthest from the IR at the level of C4 (Fig. 17.22A–C). Both obliques are undertaken. No grid is necessary, but if one is required for a large patient ensure that the grid lines are running parallel to the direction of the central ray. This avoids grid 'cut-off'. To produce a more elongated image of the posterior spinal elements and the vertebral bodies, perform the same projection as above but with the lateromedial angulation at 60°. Although the bodies will not be projected in good relief, the posterior elements will be shown to advantage, so that injury to these regions will be revealed. In both techniques, images should be obtained from each side of the neck.

See Chapter 9 for useful additional discussion on the cervical spine and the spine in trauma.

Adapted Projections of the Thoracolumbar Spine

Generally speaking, most images of these regions can be obtained by appropriate use of AP vertical ray techniques with the patient on the trolley or examination table. Horizontal ray techniques allow the lateral projections to be obtained without the need to move the patient. Care is required, however, to ensure the IR is in the appropriate position without risk of injury to the patient and the projection of table- or trolley-top artefacts onto the image. The latter is most problematic as objects built into the trolley or table impinge upon the posterior spinal elements.

THE CRANIOFACIAL SKELETON

Chapters 12 and 13 indicate techniques that were once the mainstay of craniofacial imaging in the radiology department. The trolley-top skull technique is mentioned in this chapter as it shows necessary adaptation of technique; the reality is that the likelihood of its use for the cranial vault is very low, as CT is now the imaging modality of choice.[37]

All skull and facial examinations can be achieved using the trolley-top method when embarked upon with a logical approach that uses the vital skills of understanding patient anatomy and the principles of angulation and geometry. Whereas many projections are described in this book (see Chapters 12 and 13) as being obtained from a PA direction to enhance radiation protection considerations, simply reversing angles through 180° allows images to be obtained from the AP perspective. Obviously, magnification will cause differences in the appearances of some projections: for example, the orbits are particularly affected by magnification. Care must also be taken where the IR has to be placed directly under the head, which is usually impossible for patients with neck injury; in these cases the IR can be placed in the IR tray under the trolley, if suitable for the technique required.

Adapted Projections of the Cranial Vault

As with the descriptions in earlier chapters, the ability to achieve skull projections hangs on the fact that the orbitomeatal baseline (OMBL) is perpendicular to the IR. If this is not possible, and when the patient can be safely moved, a large radiolucent support under the neck or spine can be an advantage. This is particularly useful for kyphotic individuals. Placing this wedge beneath the shoulders will aid patient comfort and encourage the head to fall naturally into a position that will place the OMBL perpendicular to the IR, which is placed directly under the skull (Fig. 17.23). The radiographer should avoid placing the IR under any support as this increases the object receptor distance (ORD). The central ray must be angled to ensure that it forms the required angle to the OMBL. If it is still not possible to position the OMBL at 90° to the IR, compensation can be made by initially aligning the central ray with the OMBL and then adding the appropriate angle for the relevant projection before centring the beam. As a more specific example, consider a patient whose chin is raised so that the OMBL is raised 10° from the perpendicular: for a projection that requires a 20° cranial angle the central ray will initially be selected as 10° caudally to coincide with the OMBL and then angled 20° cranially from this point to achieve the correct 20° to the OMBL. On examination the beam will be 10° cranially. An alternative is to position the external auditory meatus level with the lower border of the orbit and use a vertical central ray; the petrous ridges will lie at the bottom of the orbits on the resulting image, as if a 20° cranial angle had been used in conjunction with an OMBL relationship of 90° to the IR.

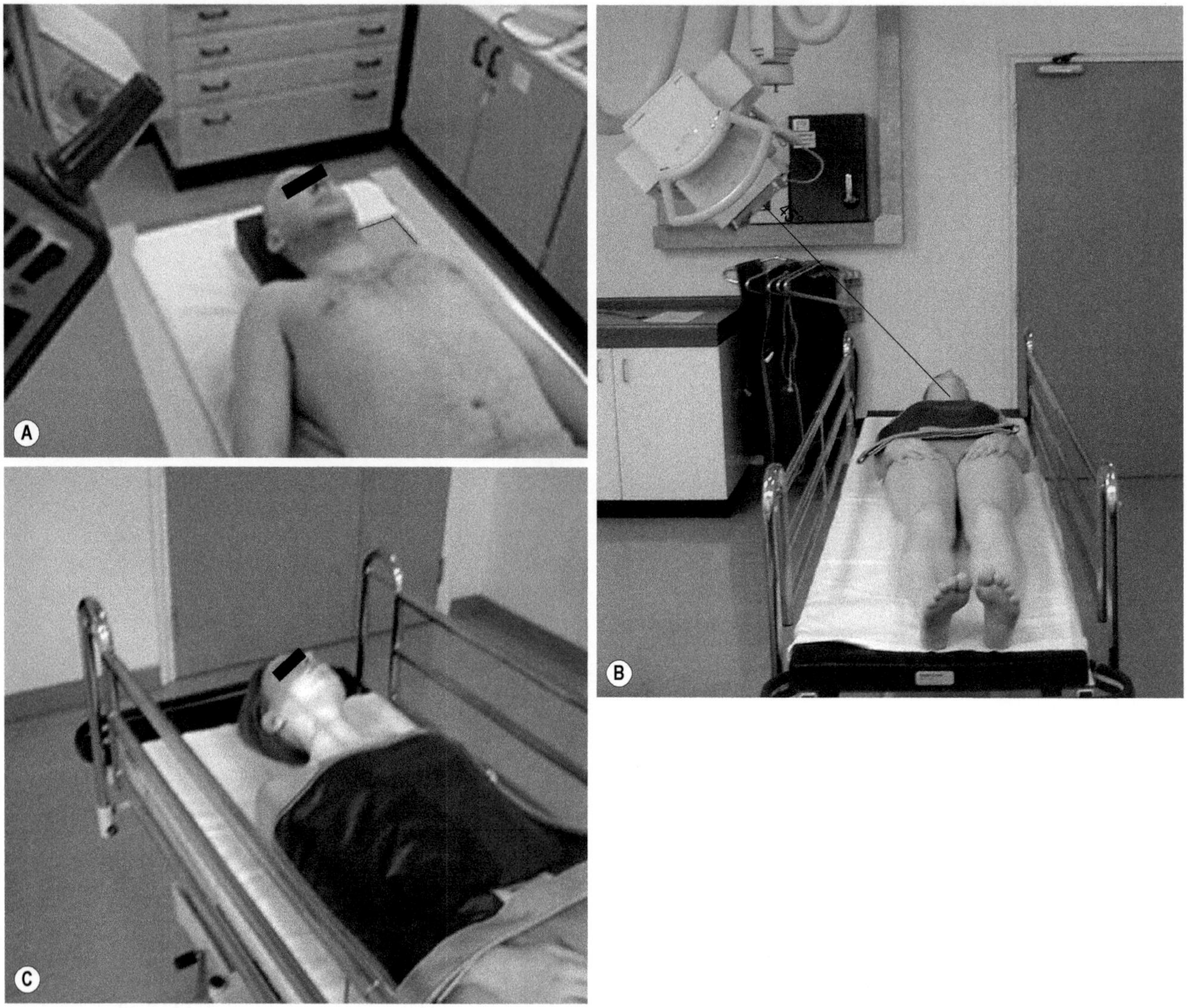

Fig. 17.22 The trauma oblique cervical spine projection.

The fronto-occipital (FO) 30° (Towne's) projection of the occipital region is essentially an AP projection anyway, and the OMBL is positioned by the use of pads as for other FO projections. As mentioned, pads must never be placed under the head and must be placed under the IR.

Lateral projections are fairly straightforward, with the IR supported vertically at the side of the head, which is supported on a radiolucent pad (Fig. 17.24). If a neck-injured patient cannot be moved to raise the head on a pad, the IR must be positioned alongside the trolley with its lower edge well below the occiput; this will create an increased ORD and the FRD should be increased to compensate for magnification and unsharpness.

Adapted Projections of the Facial Bones

Facial projections can almost always be obtained when the patient is compliant and can be examined in an erect sitting position; for those who are severely injured the likelihood is that CT will be the frontline investigation, although plain radiography does yield useful information in this area.

For the supine patient the occipitomental (OM) projections are replaced by AP mento-occipital positions, with the chin raised to place the OMBL either 45° or 30° from the vertical, depending on the required projection. If it is too difficult for the patient to lift the chin adequately, one solution, where presentation permits, is to place supports under the shoulders so room is made for the head to be tilted backwards to allow the OMBL to form an appropriate angle relative to the IR (see Fig. 17.25A,B). The centring point is in the midline, level with the midpoint of the facial structures required for inclusion on the image. When this modification is not possible, an alternative has been described[38] where the head is supported on a radiolucent rectangular pad and the IR is supported vertically at the vertex of the skull. The OMBL is parallel to the IR. The X-ray tube is initially horizontal and the caudal angle is then applied according to the requirements of the projection. For this the tube has to be positioned close to the chest of the supine patient for some angulations, and this may be difficult with units having bulky tube housings. Increasing FRD with the adjustment of exposure factors will act to overcome this. Another alternative involves slight tilting of the IR in conjunction with chin adjustment (if possible) to ensure the OMBL lies parallel to the IR. This allows the tube to be used in a higher

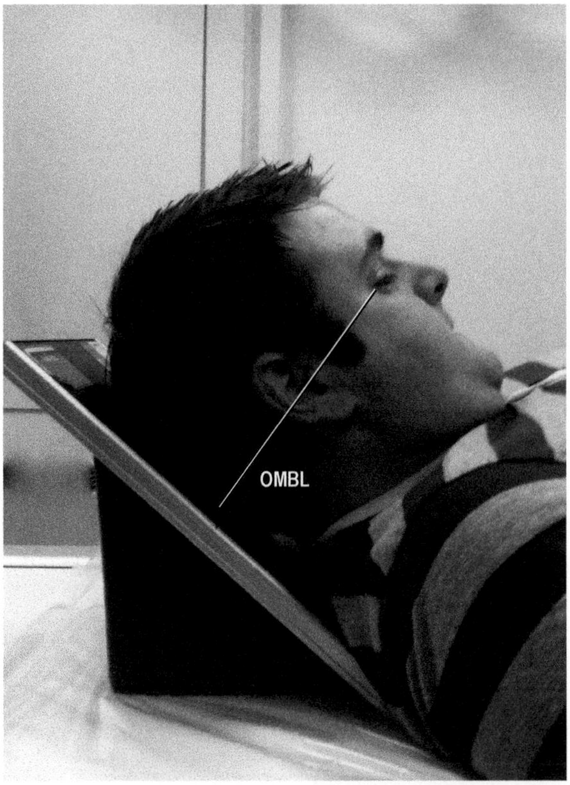

Fig. 17.23 An adaptation for the FO skull. The AP table-top projection of the skull, where the patient is unable to lie flat. Note the pad lies under the IR and patient, rather than under the head and on top of the IR.

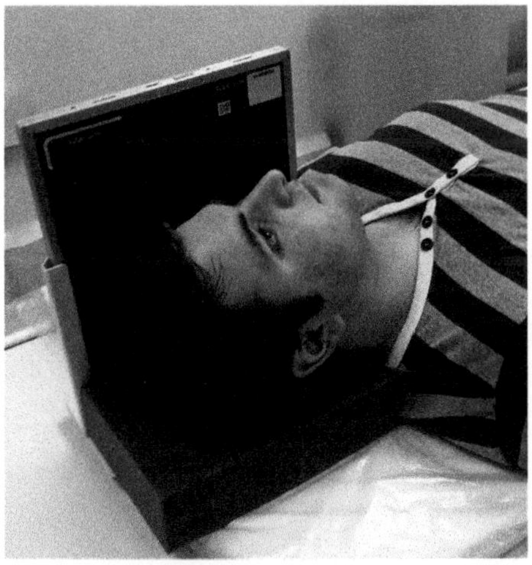

Fig. 17.24 Continuing to work around the patient to generate a table-top lateral skull. The horizontal beam lateral (HBL) projection of the skull with the head elevated on a radiolucent pad.

position; the initial tube position will of course change from horizontal to 90° to the IR.

Selection of Trauma Imaging Equipment

ED and its associated imaging department should ideally be sited as close neighbours, if not in the same departmental

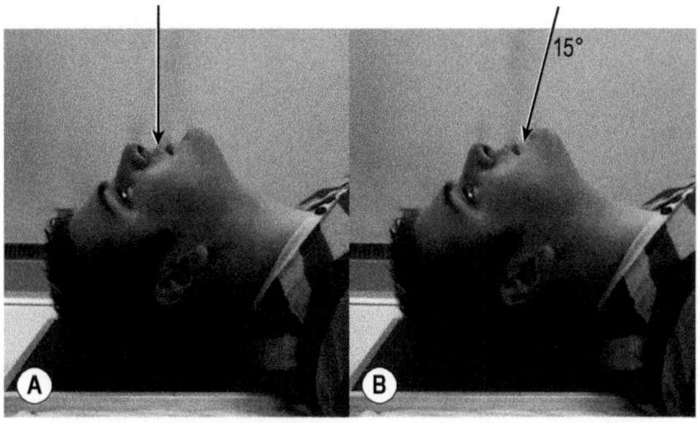

Fig. 17.25 Adapted facial techniques where patient can extend the neck. Tilted head projections to show the facial bone structures as equivalent (A) OM and (B) OM 15° projections.

area. The rooms themselves should display features that will enable them to handle the wide variation in patient presentation that spans ages from cradle to grave. X-ray rooms should be spacious, with a large 'footprint', so that enough room is available for practitioners to work around the patient in relative ease, while using X-ray equipment capable of performing the maximum range of movement possible. This is often in the face of fairly tight budgetary constraints. However, despite likely restrictions on cost, the use of a rise and fall table is a must for the range of patients who may be examined in ED (many of the projections identified in the earlier sections necessitate this versatility), and who must be worked around to obtain the required images.

As stated earlier, ancillary equipment should be chosen to meet the demands of adaptability and ease of use,[38] and support equipment must also be robust and available either as static units in the examination room, or reliably mobile if the decision is made to share facilities. Piped gases and suction should be provided in any newly built department, and all staff should be trained in the use of this and other general equipment. Short-handedness through lack of education in a moment of demand will not carry any weight in a court of law, should litigation be instigated as a result of neglect.

Some ED imaging departments will show signs of age owing to the degree of obsolescence of X-ray equipment in use. Initiatives such as the guidelines generated by NICE[37] for evaluation and treatment of head and some neck injuries have contributed to the death of projection radiography assessment in these situations.

If equipment breaks down the versatility of the experienced practitioner comes to the fore, with their ability to instantly translate static techniques to mobile equipment. Therefore, patients can still expect to receive a service that, although adapted, will provide the answers needed in a traumatic situation. Advances in mobile X-ray unit technology have enabled the mobile ward service, breakdown situations in ED or in some departments the imaging service in the resuscitation room, to move from good to excellent. Indeed, the use of mobile equipment support in the resuscitation room is seen by many to be an advantage over static units. By offering versatility and manoeuvrability, with an X-ray tube and generator that can provide almost identical qualities to those offered by static equipment, the mobile unit can be perceived as superior. Another bonus for mobile radiography is the availability of digital mobile units, with versatile IR sizes and wireless digital IRs. Although state of the art equipment may be built into a new establishment, the anecdotal experience of the authors and others has shown that implementation of this does not always meet the demands of the service or its users. Much depends upon the activity of the hospital and how assertive staff may be in the resuscitation area. Resuscitation is for just that – for very ill patients; radiation protection issues and the impact of image quality on performing radiographic examinations in an area not fully designed for X-ray imaging makes us ask why radiography is performed in an area out of context. Even so, many radiographers appreciate the fact that their needs are being recognised by commissioning of such equipment; however, they are able to perform perfectly well when a breakdown occurs and mobile machinery has to be employed.

References

1. Snaith B, Hardy M. Radiographer abnormality detection schemes in the trauma environment. An assessment of current practice. *Radiography*. 2008;14(4):277–281.
2. Price RC, Le Masurier SB. Longitudinal changes in extended roles in radiography: a new perspective. *Radiography*. 2007;13(1):18–29.
3. Lockwood P, Pittock L. Multi-professional image interpretation: performance in preliminary clinical evaluation of appendicular radiographs. *Radiography*. 2019;25(4):e95–e107.
4. American College of Surgeons. *Advanced Trauma Life Support Student Manual*. 10th ed. Chicago: American College of Surgeons; 2018.
5. Hargadon J, Staniforth M. *A Health Service of All the Talents: Developing the NHS Workforce*. London: Department of Health; 2000.
6. NICE (National Institute for Health and Care Excellence). Fractures (non-complex): assessment and management. NICE guideline [NG38] https://www.nice.org.uk/guidance/ng38; 2016.
7. Karsh B, Holden R, Alper S, et al. A human factors engineering paradigm for patient safety: designing to support the performance of the healthcare professional. *BMJ Qual Safety*. 2006;15(suppl 1):i59–i65.
8. The Ionising Radiation (Medical Exposure) Regulations 2017 [IR(ME) R]. UK Statutory Instrument 2017 No. 1322. https://www.legislation.gov.uk/uksi/2017/1322/contents/made.
9. Seibert JA, Morin RL. The standardized exposure index for digital radiography: an opportunity for optimization of radiation dose to the pediatric population. *Pediatr Radiol*. 2011;41(5):573–581.
10. Chan O. *ABC of Emergency Radiology*. 3rd ed. Oxford: BMJ Books; 2013.
11. Hardy M, Snaith B, eds. *Musculoskeletal Trauma: A Guide to Assessment and Diagnosis*. Edinburgh: Churchill Livingstone; 2011.
12. Raby N, Berman L, Morley S, et al. *Accident and Emergency Radiology: A Survival Guide E-Book*. Elsevier Health Sciences; 2014.
13. Dimond B. *Legal Aspects of Radiography and Radiology*. Oxford: Blackwell Science; 2002.
14. Dimond B. Red dots and radiographers' liability. *Health Care Risk Rep*. 2000;6:10–12.
15. Murali M, Bolton L, Bhaktal S. Silver Trauma Pathway: a new gold standard in elderly trauma care. *BMJ Leader*. 2018;2(suppl 1):A32. https://bmjleader.bmj.com/content/2/Suppl_1/A32.1.
16. Fuller N, Knapp K, Stokes O, et al. Cervical spine fractures in the elderly: are there missed opportunities for prevention? *Osteoporosis Int*. 2018;29:638.
17. Lewis S. New angles on the radiographic examination of the hand – I. *Radiogr Today*. 1988;54(617):44–45.
18. Lewis S. New angles on the radiographic examination of the hand – II. *Radiogr Today*. 1988;54(618):29.
19. Lewis S. New angles on the radiographic examination of the hand – III. *Radiogr Today*. 1988;54(619):47–48.
20. Eyres K, Allen T. Skyline view of the metacarpal head in the assessment of human fight-bite injuries. *J Hand Surg*. 1993;18(1):43–44.
21. Long BW, Rafert JA. *Orthopaedic Radiography*. Philadelphia: Saunders; 1995.
22. Swallow RA, Naylor E, Roebuck E, et al. *Clark's Positioning in Radiography*. 11th ed. London: Heinemann; 1986.
23. Coyle G. *Radiographing Immobile Trauma Patients – Unit 7*. Denver: MultiMedia Publishing, Inc; 1980.
24. Garth Jr WP, Slappey C, Ochs C. Roentgenographic demonstration of instability of the shoulder: the apical oblique projection. A technical note. *J Bone Joint Surg Am*. 1984;66(9):1450–1453.
25. Horsfield D, Murphy G. Stress views of the ankle joint in lateral ligament injury. *Radiography*. 1985;51(595):7–11.
26. Monks J, Yeoman L. Judet's views of the acetabulum: a demonstration of their importance. *Radiogr Today*. 1989;55(628):18.
27. Foster LM, Barton ED. Managing pelvic fractures, Part 2: physical and radiologic assessment. *J Crit Illness*. 2001;16(5):255.
28. Hunter JC, Brandser EA, Tran KA. Pelvic and acetabular trauma. *Radiol Clin North Am*. 1997;35(3):559–590.
29. Hardy M, Boynes S. *Paediatric Radiography*. Chichester: John Wiley & Sons; 2008.
30. NICE (National Institute for Health and Care Excellence). Spinal injury: assessment and initial management. NICE guideline [NG 41] https://www.nice.org.uk/guidance/ng41; 2016.
31. Bailitz J, Starr F, Beecroft M, et al. CT should replace three-view radiographs as the initial screening test in patients at high, moderate, and low risk for blunt cervical spine injury: a prospective comparison. *J Trauma Acute Care Surg*. 2009;66(6):1605–1609.
32. Carver B. Cervical spine. In: Carver E, Carver B, eds. *Medical Imaging: Techniques, Reflection and Evaluation*. 2nd ed. Edinburgh: Churchill Livingstone; 2012:121–135.
33. Rethnam U, Yesupalan RS, Bastawrous SS. The swimmer's view: does it really show what it is supposed to show? A retrospective study. *BMC Med Imaging*. 2008;8(1):2.
34. Ireland AJ, Britton I, Forrester AW. Do supine oblique views provide better imaging of the cervicothoracic junction than swimmer's views? *Emerg Med J*. 1998;15(3):151–154.
35. Fell M. Cervical spine trauma radiographs: swimmers and supine obliques; an exploration of current practice. *Radiography*. 2011;17(1):33–38.
36. Daffner RH. Radiographic interpretation of cervical vertebral injuries. *Adv Emerg Nurs J*. 1997;19(3):11–25.
37. NICE (National Institute for Health and Care Excellence). Head injury: assessment and early management. Clinical guideline [CG 176] https://www.nice.org.uk/guidance/cg176; 2019.
38. Ponsford A, Clements R. A modified view of the facial bones in the seriously injured. *Radiogr Today*. 1991;57(646):10–12.

18 Principles of Theatre and Mobile Radiography

JAMES HUGHES

Radiographic examinations performed outside the imaging department can be challenging for radiographers, as normal techniques and methods may not be practicable in the ward, theatre, or Emergency Department. Mobile imaging equipment may lack features or options that are used on static units found within the department, and radiation protection becomes a more complex issue when working in an area not set up exclusively for radiographic examinations. There may be other staff and patients present, as well as medical equipment that it is necessary to work around; therefore a calm considered and professional attitude is required in order to safely produce high-quality images in what may be a stressful and complex multidisciplinary environment.

Theatre Radiography

A working operating theatre can be an intimidating place; there are local rules and guidelines for working in theatres that the radiographer must be familiar with, including both safety of the patient, (for avoiding injury and infection/contamination), and staff (from bodily fluids and sharps). Local infection control rules apply, and include wearing scrubs and theatre shoes rather than uniform or personal clothes, and containing hair in hairnets and beard snoods before entering the theatre area. It is important to be aware of any sterile surfaces and fields throughout the procedure. If in doubt, the radiographer should ask members of the surgical team if any equipment is sterile or if there are any potential hazards nearby before moving equipment. It is also a good idea to become familiar with the theatre department's sharps/splash injury procedures in case of such an occurrence.

Positioning

Theatre radiography requires production of the highest-quality diagnostic images possible with minimum radiation dose and within the restrictions required by the surgical procedure under way. Imaging in theatre requires compromises for the sake of practicality, however with good technique and experience it is almost always possible to produce good-quality images. Patient positioning is normally optimised for the surgical procedure rather than imaging, and the sterile field means that it is not possible to get close to or palpate the region of interest, nor adjust the patient's position mid-procedure. As such, it is necessary to move the imaging equipment around the patient rather than position the patient on the receptor, whilst avoiding the sterile fields and other equipment. However, as imaging is a key part of the procedure, positioning can often be adjusted for ease of access with the C-arm. It should be remembered that a multidisciplinary team approach is vital in this environment, and a spirit of collaboration and mutual assistance should be encouraged.[1]

For upper limb procedures the limb may be abducted from the torso, while for lower limb procedures the contralateral limb may be repositioned to allow C-arm access. For abdominal procedures the patient can be moved on the table-top away from the centre column of the table. The radiographer should be aware of any anatomy that may be overlying or will prevent moving the C-arm to acquire images. For example, if working on the right knee, the left knee would overlie it on the lateral projection unless either: (a) the left leg is lowered so that it is below the right, or (b) the right leg is raised. Surgical tables give a wide range of options for adjusting the position of the patient, and it is best to discuss these at the start of the case with the surgical team to evaluate how imaging will be performed before the patient is draped and the case commences.

The C-arm should preferentially be used in an 'under-couch' orientation, with the receptor head above and the X-ray tube below. As shown in Fig. 18.1, in this position scattered radiation isodose curves show exposure is greatest below the table.[2] This configuration causes backscattered radiation to be reflected downwards to the floor rather than into the surgeon's face or torso. It also allows the receptor to be brought close to the patient without striking the table

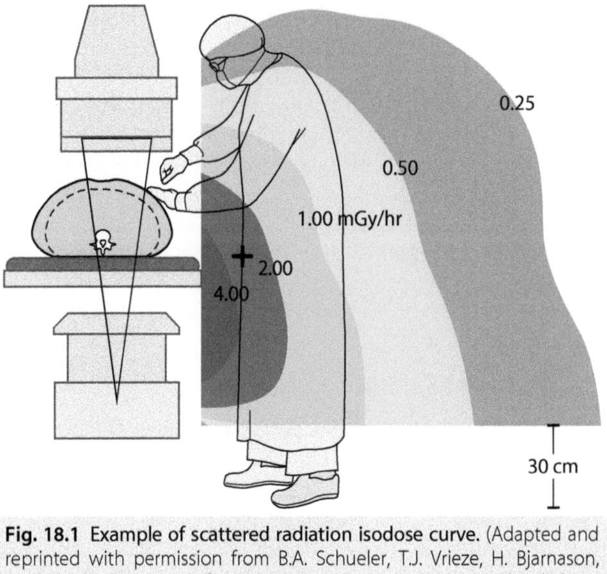

Fig. 18.1 Example of scattered radiation isodose curve. (Adapted and reprinted with permission from B.A. Schueler, T.J. Vrieze, H. Bjarnason, et al. An investigation of operator exposure in interventional radiology. RadioGraphics, 26 (2006), pp. 1533–1541.)

or supports. Most C-arms are set up to be used in this configuration and will produce a reversed image if changed into the 'over-couch' configuration. However, they can be used 'over-couch' for procedures where magnification needs to be avoided and dose minimised to the patient (e.g. manipulation of paediatric limb fractures).[3]

It should be kept in mind that the receptor head is not designed to be a weight-bearing structure, and so can be damaged if used as an operating surface (e.g. during a closed manipulation of a wrist fracture). The receptor head should never be allowed to be used as an operating surface if any drilling or insertion of hardware is to take place, as the receptor can be damaged and the drill de-sterilised.[4]

It is good practice to bring the C-arm in from the opposite side to where the surgeons will be working. For example, if working on the right knee it is standard practice to bring in the C-arm from the left. Lateral projections are typically required and are obtained by rotating the C-arm so that the beam is horizontal. Other procedures may also require the C-arm to be repositioned in order to demonstrate surgical hardware or joints. For example, the insertion of an intramedullary nail will require the whole length of the bone to be demonstrated in two projections as the case progresses, and as such the C-arm will be moved along the shaft. Check at the start of the case that there will not be any potential collisions between the C-arm and supports when moving, as it is preferable to make any adjustments to positioning before the sterile drapes are applied.[5]

Supports used around the region should be made of radiolucent material. The radiographer should be aware of sandbags or other supports placed under regions, which may not be radiolucent, and negotiate removal or replacement where these might impede imaging the required areas. Similarly, many sections of operating tables (such as hinges) are beam-occluding. If these are used, the patient should be positioned so that the relevant anatomical areas are not overlying them. Beam blocking artefacts that do not cover relevant anatomy but are within the image field may affect the exposures given by the C-arm system and cause overexposure/increased dose. Careful positioning and collimation can avoid the major effects of these.

Correctly centring the C-arm over the desired region without exposing can be difficult as the area will typically be in the sterile field. By looking across the receptor head at the widest point from two or more directions, it is often possible to get a good idea of where the receptor is centred. Remember that due to the gap between the receptor and the patient, the image (and any movements made to the C-arm or patient) will be magnified. As such, small adjustments of positioning are preferable to large ones. This is especially true if electronic magnification is used. Once an image is taken, it can be used as a guide to adjust the C-arm position to improve the centring.

Imaging and Radiation Protection

Radiographers are responsible for radiation protection for both the patient and the staff present in theatre when equipment is live. Radiation protection for the patient is similar to that used in department, requiring correct identification and pregnancy status and minimising exposure. Good collimation and accurate centring will lessen the dose to the patient and improve the quality of images. As discussed in Chapter 3, lead equivalent shielding for the patient is no longer recommended; if deemed necessary, it should not be used around the area of interest, as poorly placed shielding can increase the dose to the patient and/or obscure relevant anatomy.[6] As such, careful collimation is recommended to avoid irradiating radiosensitive anatomy.

The team should be protected by lead equivalent shielding in the form of aprons or barriers. Avoid exposing when the surgeon's hand is in the beam path. Announcing exposures before taking them keeps everyone informed that X-rays are in use. If anyone is not shielded or there are any other issues, the radiographer must not expose until they are corrected. Staff who routinely work in the vicinity of the C-arm (such as surgeons) should also have their own dosimeter or dose monitoring system.[7]

Modern C-arms use an automatic exposure system with a pre-set range of exposures to regulate the intensity of the X-ray beam. This allows for continuous exposure compensation throughout the procedure. However, the system can get confused by large areas that are more or less dense than the region under interest. Collimation should be used to shape the beam around the relevant anatomy and cone off areas of higher or lower density. These actions also have the advantage of reducing the dose to the patient and scattered radiation to the surgical team. However, it is very easy to clip off relevant anatomy, especially if the body part or C-arm is moved.[8]

It may be possible to pre-set the exposure system to the type of procedure: newer C-arm systems have settings for orthopaedic, paediatric, abdominal and other procedures, and will calibrate exposure from both the examination setting and the signal returned from the receptor. Most systems will also have options for pulsed fluoroscopy that can reduce the frame-rate of image acquisition. As each image in a fluoroscopy examination requires a radiation exposure to produce it, reducing the frame rate can significantly reduce radiation dose by lowering the number of exposures performed (e.g. from 24 frames/exposures per second to 12); however there is a greater risk of producing blurred images if there is any movement.[9] Consequently this should not be used when live fluoroscopic imaging runs are required.

Electronic magnification modes are present on C-arms; these will increase the spatial resolution of the image, allowing smaller detail to be visualised more clearly across a smaller area. Image intensifier (II) systems amplify images by receiving a large incident image signal at the input phosphor and condensing it onto a small detector. In these systems electronic magnification will reduce the size of the incident image signal, so they require greater radiation exposure to generate a good image to compensate for the loss of amplification within the II. As such, electronic magnification will increase the radiation dose to the patient. Flat panel receptors increase the exposure significantly less than II systems when using magnification modes since they do not amplify the image signal in the same manner.[10]

At the end of the procedure the cumulative dose and screening time should be recorded along with saved images in order to allow dose audit and identify any issues with the C-arm system,[11] as well as ensuring compliance with the Ionising Radiation (Medical Exposure) Regulations.[12]

When to Image

Typically, the surgeon will state when imaging is needed, although it is good practice to be able to anticipate this as the surgeon will also be busy with the procedure. The radiographer should be aware that the surgeon may not state when to stop screening during live fluoroscopy. This can result in unjustified exposure to the patient and team. A good technique is for the radiographer to watch the surgeon's eyeline during live screening and to stop the exposure when their attention is away from the C-arm monitors.

In orthopaedics or spinal surgery imaging is typically needed when:

- Achieving reduction of a fracture
- A fixator is being implanted
- The stability of a reduction or fixation is being checked.

The path of any implant or device being inserted into bone will need to be checked to ensure that it is following the desired path and not penetrating structures that are not required for the fixation. The integrity of joints around the fracture/fixation sites will also often be checked, sometimes under dynamic imaging to check the functioning and range of movement of the joint. Often imaging is needed at the end of a case (especially post plaster) to ensure that the reduction has not been compromised.

For abdominal procedures imaging may be needed when:

- Catheters or guidewires are being advanced or positioned
- Contrast agent is injected to highlight structures.

These may require live screening and movement of the C-arm (e.g. to follow a catheter from the bladder to the kidney). When an injection of contrast is made, e.g. to demonstrate blockages etc., it can be important to save a non-contrast image beforehand. Many modern C-arms feature digital subtraction angiography (DSA) settings; these can significantly increase the radiation dose compared to standard fluoroscopy modes and so should be used only where necessary, e.g. for vascular procedures.

Modern systems have a large capacity for storing images, allowing the radiographer to regularly save images during a case for later reference or to avoid re-exposing. It is good technique to save key images throughout a procedure, especially when switching between projections or regions (going from an anteroposterior to a lateral projection, for example). Images that do not need archiving can be discarded at the end of the procedure, while key images should be annotated if required and archived.

Mobile Radiography

Mobile examinations are typically performed when the patient is not stable or well enough to be transferred to the radiology department for imaging. Mobile X-ray equipment is produced with additional functions to ensure mobility and ease of adjustment; they have typically been designed to be used at shorter focus receptor distances (FRD) than fixed location departmental equipment (especially for chest X-rays where it may not be possible to achieve the recommended distance). A shorter FRD causes magnification of structures not in contact with the image receptor (IR), which if care is not taken could cause a failure to include all the required anatomy on the resulting image. Increasing the FRD to reduce magnification is desirable but, due to restrictions of layout of the room in which the examination is being performed, may not be feasible (particularly for projections performed with the patient supine). Note also that the light beam used to check collimation will become less visible on the patient at greater FRD, and/or if there is greater than desirable ambient light at the location.

Chest X-ray

The most commonly performed mobile examination is the chest X-ray (CXR) which, due to patient condition, may need to be performed anteroposterior (AP) instead of the standard posteroanterior (PA) projection. If practicable, an erect PA projection will produce an image with more diagnostic information; however, if the patient is not well enough to attend the radiology department, it is often the case that they are unable to achieve and maintain the positioning needed for a PA CXR. An erect AP CXR can demonstrate air and fluid levels within the chest as well as aiding detection of free air within the abdomen, a sign of hollow organ perforation. The supine CXR will not allow visualisation of small amounts of free air or fluid, and offers less diagnostic information than an erect CXR; however, it may be the only feasible examination in the unstable or intubated patient. Further detail and explanation of these projections, and circumstances in which they may be performed, can be found in Chapter 15.

Other Examinations

Other examinations, such as abdominal and pelvis images, can also be produced with mobile equipment. However, they will typically require a greater mAs than the CXR, and with a mobile unit may require greater exposure times due to the limited mA output of the units compared to departmental equipment. As such, respiratory artefact can become an issue. The best approach to reduce respiratory artefact is for the radiographer to ask the patient to hold respiration (either in or out, depending on the examination performed), then to let them breathe normally once the exposure has taken place. In the unstable or non-communicative patient however this will not be feasible and so the next best approach is to observe their breathing with the equipment prepared for exposure and expose once they are in full inspiration/expiration. For the ventilated patient, it may be possible to ask one of the team to hold the patient's respiration while the exposure takes place.

Examinations requiring greater exposure may also necessitate the use of a grid to cut down on scattered radiation on the image. These may cause issues with grid cut-off if not correctly positioned and used (for example, the use of a focused grid at an incorrect FRD, or a parallel grid that is angled). They will also produce grid-lines on the resulting image as generally only static grids are available for mobile examinations. Finally, higher exposures may also cause backscatter into the IR, which can cause loss of detail or artefacts on the image from metallic items such as the bed frame or even the detector circuitry.[13]

Entering the Ward/Department

When arriving in the ward/department with a mobile machine, the radiographer should let the ward/department team know that they are there, and confirm which patient and which examination is to be performed with them. The radiographer must be respectful and bear in mind that they are in another department, where there may be methods of working that they are unfamiliar with. It is possible that the patient may not be able to identify themselves, and so the department team may have to confirm the patient's identity. Equipment may be present that cannot be moved, either around the patient or attached to them. If possible, all artefact-producing material (such as necklaces) should be removed from the patient at the start of the examination, however it is best to check with the team what equipment they are willing/able to remove (e.g. ECG leads may be able to be removed if measurements are not currently taking place).

Additional requirements are detailed in Chapter 15 in the section 'The Chest X-ray and Infectious Patients'.

Positioning the Equipment

The radiographer should ensure that the mobile machine is positioned such that the tube can be correctly positioned and the beam centered, and that it is not blocking any important access points (such as a doorway). It is important to consider not just the immediate area around the patient, but also the surrounding areas where other patients and staff may be present. For example, if the team are performing a care procedure on a patient in an adjacent bay, it may be best to wait until they are finished before setting up for the exposure. Similarly, other patients may have visitors with them who are unaware of the requirements of radiation protection, and will need to be advised to leave the area during the performance of the examination. The radiographer should take particular care to check for any staff or members of the public who may be behind curtains or other non-protective barriers.

Consider also the beam direction. The IR is not a radiation barrier, and will allow some beam through. For an erect AP CXR on a patient with their back towards a solid wall, the transmitted beam will most likely be absorbed by or scattered from the wall. However, for a horizontal-beam lateral hip, the beam can continue on through the receptor, possibly towards a patient/staff in an adjacent bay. In such cases, consider using additional lead equivalent shielding behind the receptor, or use lead equivalent screens if available. With higher exposures, the amount of scattered radiation also increases. Distance from the tube, primary beam and patient is the most common form of radiation protection in mobile examinations. Protection in the form of lead rubber aprons can be used for those staff that cannot leave the patient during the exposure. This normally will include the radiographer, and may include any other staff who need to remain present. All other staff should withdraw away from the area by at least 2 m during the exposure.[14]

The exposure on the X-ray unit should be set to the correct examination setting; these settings are often preprogrammed into the machine, or there should be an exposure chart available with exposure ranges categorised by anatomy and projection. The exposure must of course in all cases be adjusted, e.g. to adapt for the patient's body habitus, or variations in FRD.

Positioning the Patient

If possible the patient should be positioned erect for a CXR. Most beds and trolleys have controls that can raise the patient into an upright sitting position, or to tilt the whole bed so the patient is more upright, but care must be taken that they do not slide down the mattress. This is a good time for the radiographer to check for and remove any artefact-causing items from around the area under examination. The radiographer should then position the X-ray tube so that it is pointing at the correct area of interest with the correct angulation of the central ray. See chapters relevant to each area of anatomy for further information on positioning requirements.

Positioning the Receptor

For erect chest AP images the receptor can be placed directly behind the patient. This can be aided with the use of slide-sheets or a radiolucent cushion to aid positioning and make the examination more comfortable for the patient. For supine examinations the receptor can be placed under the mattress if using an X-ray trolley with a radiolucent mattress, but the effect of increasing the distance between patient and receptor needs to be considered. Alternatively (if the patient is on a non X-ray compatible bed for example) the receptor may be positioned directly under the patient. This will require several staff to assist with turning/lifting the patient and placement of the receptor, where moving the patient in this way is appropriate.

For other projections the receptor may be placed into a separate holder or supported in position with radiolucent supports such as foam pads. The receptor should be positioned central to the relevant anatomy and covering the entire area that will need to be demonstrated. It should also be positioned so that it is parallel to the area under examination in order to prevent distortions on the image. This is especially important if an antiscatter grid is being used.

However the receptor is placed, the radiographer should never attempt to move a patient on their own, especially if the patient has any attachments or monitoring in place. Bear in mind that a receptor (especially one with a grid attached) can be extremely uncomfortable to lie on, and patients may struggle to maintain the correct position. Do not attempt to move the receptor if it is in contact with the patient's skin, as this may cause abrasions and injury to the patient. It may also cause folds in the skin that can mimic pathology on the resulting image.[15]

Collimating

The radiographer should then re-check the centring and collimate to the region of interest, making sure that the beam will not be projected beyond the region of the receptor as this will give extra radiation dose without contributing to the image. If it is hard to see the light-beam, the radiographer can ask if it is possible to lower the lighting in the bay or area. If the receptor is placed in a tray underneath the patient on an X-ray compatible trolley, the radiographer should ensure that it is appropriately aligned to the central ray. Once the collimation and centring is satisfactory, the radiographer should announce to the ward/department that they are ready to expose.

Expose

The radiographer should make a final check that the exposure settings and positioning are correct, and that all required preparations have been made. The exposure should be announced at the last moment before making the exposure (typically by calling out 'X-rays'), and one last check should be taken that all other staff have either moved away from the area or are wearing suitable protection. The radiographer should then prep the X-ray machine, and expose once the patient is on full inspiration (for chest) or expiration (for abdomen), by either prompting the patient or by watching their respiration. When the exposure is complete the radiographer should announce that X-ray exposure is ended and that the team may return to the patient.

If using a digital radiography (DR) system where the images are immediately visible, the radiographer should review the image on the monitor before removing the receptor; otherwise, the receptor should be removed for digital processing, ensuring that it is kept separate from any unexposed receptors. If multiple examinations are being performed and a DR system is not being used, it is a good idea to mark each receptor with the patient and examination details for ease of processing.

The radiographer should make a note of the exposure factors and radiation dose, and remove the X-ray machine. Both the machine and receptor should be cleaned before performing any further imaging with them. Finally, the radiographer should ensure the image or images have been sent and archived, and record the exposure factors and dose with the exam information on the local Radiology Information System.

References

1. Hughes J. *Introduction to Intra-operative and Surgical Radiography*. Ch 7: p. 47. Oxford: Oxford University Press; 2018.
2. Schueler BA. Operator shielding: how and why. *Techn Vasc Intervent Radiol*. 2010;13(3):167–171.
3. Tremains M, Georgiadis G, Dennis M. Radiation exposure with use of the inverted-C-arm technique in upper-extremity surgery. *J Bone Joint Surg Am*. 2001;83:674–678.
4. Waseem M, Kenny NW. The image intensifier as an operating table – a dangerous practice. *J Bone Joint Surg Br*. 2000;82-B:95–96.
5. Hughes J. *Introduction to Intra-operative and Surgical Radiography*. Ch 13: pp. 100–107. Oxford: Oxford University Press; 2018.
6. Marsh RM. Hallway Conversations in Physics: what considerations should be made when performing fluoroscopy guided examinations on pregnant patients? *AJR Am J Roentgenol*. 2017;209:195–196.
7. Rehani MM, Ciraj-Bjelac O, Vañó E, et al. Radiological protection in fluoroscopically guided procedures performed outside the imaging department. *Ann ICRP*. 2010;40:1–102.
8. Hughes J. *Introduction to Intra-operative and Surgical Radiography*. Ch 4: pp. 18–29. Oxford: Oxford University Press; 2018.
9. Newman B, John S, Goske M, et al. Pause and pulse: radiation dose in pediatric fluoroscopy. *Pediatric Rev*. 2011;32:83–90.
10. Nickoloff EL. AAPM/RSNA Physics Tutorial for Residents: Physics of flat-panel fluoroscopy systems. *Radiographics*. 2011;31:591–602.
11. Wang J, Blackburn T. AAPM/RSNA Physics Tutorial for Residents – X-ray image intensifiers for fluoroscopy. *Radiographics*. 2000;20(5):1471–1477.
12. *The Ionising Radiation (Medical Exposure) Regulations 2017 [IR(ME) R]*. UK Statutory Instrument; 2017. No. 1322. https://www.legislation.gov.uk/uksi/2017/1322/contents/made.
13. Walz-Flannigan AI, Brossoit KJ, Magnuson DJ, Schueler BA. Pictorial review of digital radiography artifacts. *Radiographics*. 2018;38:833–846.
14. Abrantes A, Rebelo C, Sousa P, et al. Scatter radiation exposure during mobile X-ray examinations. *Health Manag*. 2017;17(1):68–72.
15. Dixon A. Skin fold mimicking pneumothorax. [online] Radiopaedia.org. https://radiopaedia.org/cases/skin-fold-mimicking-pneumothorax?lang=us.

19 Paediatric Imaging in General Radiography

DONNA JANE DIMOND and TIM PALARM

Introduction

Paediatric patients presenting for radiographic imaging range from the very small, such as neonates and premature babies, to adolescents. Regardless of age, each group has unique differences and presents separate challenges for the examining radiographer. Despite the presence of numerous specialist paediatric units throughout the country, most children will first encounter imaging examinations through an attendance at the Emergency Department (ED) of a local general hospital. Therefore, children are quite likely to meet radiographers who are more at home examining adults and with equipment and surroundings designed for that purpose.

In this chapter, key examinations have been chosen that are likely to be encountered in independent practice in addition to those regularly carried out in dedicated paediatric imaging departments. Some of the radiographic techniques explored will need to be cross-referenced with the relevant chapter elsewhere within this textbook. Details of invasive procedures and specialised examinations are therefore not included, and readers are encouraged to refer to paediatric texts, peer-reviewed articles and guidance from professional bodies for in-depth information. There are also numerous specialist interest groups, such as the Association of Paediatric Radiographers[1] and the Children's Imaging Taskforce,[1] affiliations of the Society and College of Radiographers (SCoR) that can be accessed via their dedicated social media group or websites. This chapter is not designed to be definitive or exhaustive but to provide a general overview of techniques, which from both professional experience and published literature have been shown to work well. It is recognised that alternative methods may be used which can also achieve the required level of diagnostic quality. Radiographers are encouraged to formulate collaborative approaches through interprofessional working with other healthcare professionals and contact with colleagues at dedicated paediatric units throughout the country. Not only will this be of direct benefit to patients, but it will also contribute to the radiographer's continuing professional development. The niche specialty of paediatric imaging provides potential scope for the introduction of advanced and consultant radiographer practitioner roles for those aspiring to a career in this area within hospitals supportive of such development.

Throughout this chapter a suggested FRD is given for each examination description; however in practice a range of FRDs (typically from 100 cm to 120 cm) may be used, dependent on local protocol.

Special Considerations When Imaging Children

A key factor in gaining high-quality diagnostic images is undoubtedly the gaining of the child's trust,[2,3] and to a lesser extent that of the parent/carer, prior to the commencement of the examination. With such trust follows the development of the patient–radiographer relationship that should result in compliance by the child and upbeat thoughts about the imaging experience. Positive feelings are invaluable in the paediatric age group as a large proportion of children are likely to return for X-rays in their formative years (Fig. 19.1), particularly those with conditions that require ongoing monitoring. An unpleasant experience involving an unfriendly member of staff may jeopardise not only the current examination but may also cause bad memories to resurface during future visits.

The National Imaging Board, within the report 'Delivering Quality Imaging Services for Children',[4] advises that all children should be treated in a paediatric environment by paediatric specialists and healthcare professionals. Clearly this is unachievable in many general hospitals. Therefore, it is recommended that imaging departments should have at the very least a named lead radiographer and a core team of staff that are specially trained, competent and enthusiastic about undertaking paediatric examinations.[3] It is the lead author's opinion that all undergraduate diagnostic radiography students should be provided with learning opportunities in a dedicated paediatric imaging department in keeping with advice offered by the Society of Radiographers.[3] Most radiographers will examine children as early as their first clinical position upon graduation and evidence suggests that 1:5 of their patients will fall under 16 years of age. Therefore, a sound knowledge and understanding of the specialty and relative issues, such as parent/carer management, immobilisation, radiation protection, safeguarding and legal considerations, gained during undergraduate training both practically and academically, will be of great benefit to all radiographers commencing their careers.

Anxiety is a common emotion in patients of any age, but one that is often heightened in children due to unfamiliar surroundings, unknown adults and sometimes the reactions of their parents/carers.[5] Such feelings are often heightened by accompanying pain from an injury or illness. The radiographer needs to appear friendly, positive and self-assured and able to instil a sense of confidence in both the child and the parent/carer whilst deftly managing the examination.

Ensuring that the physical environment is favourable to imaging children is an important factor,[6] although this is often dependent upon additional funds and the backing of management. Child-friendly décor, furnishings with toys and books and suitable entertainment ideally away from the adult waiting area helps to achieve a welcoming, relaxed and warm atmosphere (Fig. 19.2).

Understanding the different stages of child development,[7] physical, social, emotional and cognitive, is vital in order to tailor the examination for the patient. In short, the examination should fit the child rather than vice versa. Some helpful tips are as follows:

- Having realistic expectations is essential. A 3-year-old child cannot be expected to perform/maintain the same positioning/actions as a 13-year-old.
- Enabling the child to make choices, such as which parent/carer they prefer to accompany them or the selection of a lead rubber gown for their parent/carer, will give them a degree of feeling in control over their surroundings.
- Allowing the child to bring a favourite toy or comforter into the examination room helps dispel fears. On occasions, taking an X-ray of the toy can prove a worthwhile venture to help the child understand what the examination involves.

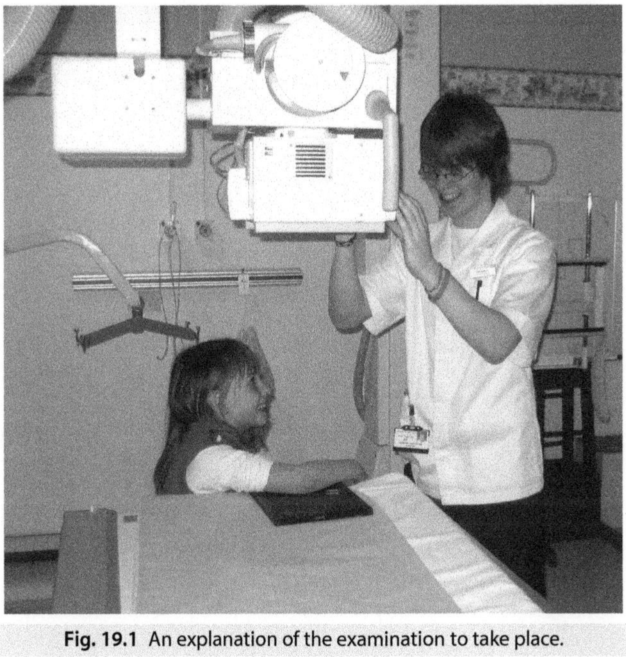

Fig. 19.1 An explanation of the examination to take place.

- Likening the patient's position for the examination to a normal everyday occurrence can be extremely advantageous. For example, asking a child to breathe in as they would do to blow up a balloon or swim under water is likely to result in a better effort than the sole instruction to breathe in.
- Rewards, be it stickers or certificates, have proven to be excellent incentives, particularly for children likely to return for regular imaging. Children who regularly attend the Imaging Department look forward to receiving another sticker for their collection.
- Consideration should always be given to each child's privacy and dignity during the examination. This needs to be balanced alongside the requirement to obtain images of maximum diagnostic quality with no artefact and at the lowest dose as reasonably practicable. This includes removal of nappies for abdominal and pelvic imaging and any clothing, particularly that which incorporates diamante and/or sequin embellishment or transfers, likely to overly the area of interest.
- An uncooperative child may be so as a result of being in pain. This possibility should always be considered, and an examination halted should the radiographer feel additional relief is needed.

Parents/carers play a pivotal role in the imaging of the young child, particularly the pre-school age group. Babies and toddlers have very strong attachments to family members and resent any form of separation.[8] When examining older children, the radiographer may need to make a decision regarding the degree of involvement of the parent/carer and their location within the X-ray room. In addition to any anxieties, the older child is likely to be more aware of him/herself and understand how refusal to cooperate can control a situation according to their liking. In the authors' experience there is a risk that some parents will assert themselves and attempt to orchestrate the proceedings. It is important that the radiographer carefully manages the imaging environment and examination, making the role of the accompanying parent/carer clear to them at the outset.

Radiation Protection and Dose Limitation

In keeping with the Ionising Radiation (Medical Exposure) Regulations 2017 (IR(ME)R),[9] all doses to patients should

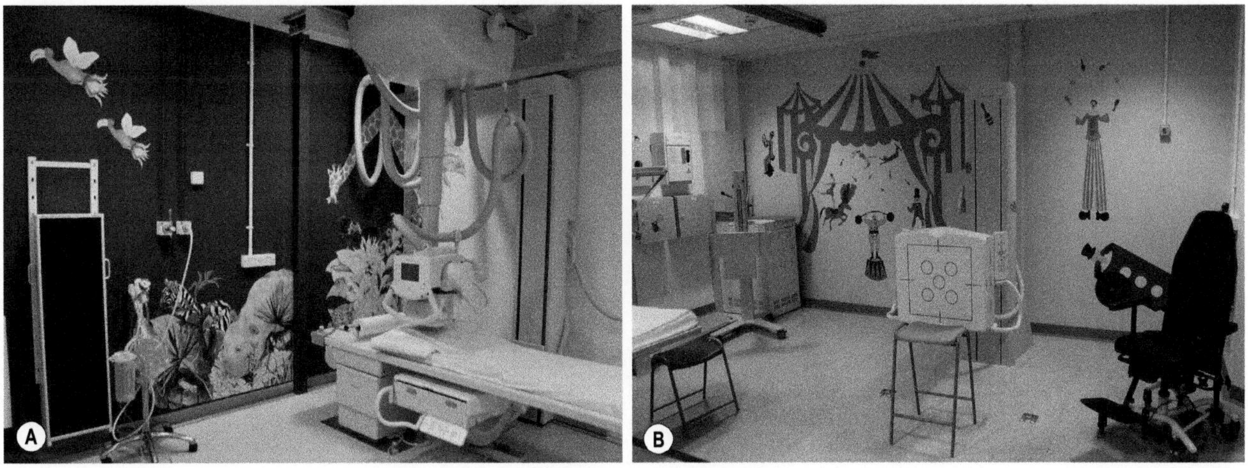

Fig. 19.2 (A,B) Examples of a child-friendly X-ray room.

be kept as low as reasonably practicable (ALARP concept). For paediatric patients, it is vital that departments use examination-specific protocols that consider the patient's size, weight and age, the clinical indication(s) and region of imaging.[10] Over the years numerous directives, such as Image Gently, have sought to improve awareness regarding the radiation protection of children.[11]

Children have a marked higher radiation sensitivity than adults and as such there is a greater opportunity for potential harmful effects to manifest themselves. As future parents, they also are at risk for passing on radiation-induced genetic defects to their offspring. It should be remembered that many children will have conditions that require monitoring throughout their tender years, hence the cumulative effect of X-rays should also be considered. Neonates and infants have significant levels of haematopoietic bone marrow throughout the body and owing to the child's body proportions differing from those of an adult, there is the potential for larger areas of the body to be included within the primary beam or be affected by scattered radiation. Therefore, effective collimation of the beam is essential.

The author's rationale is to offer suggestions for radiation dose reductions; however, optimisation of exposure factors may be more realistic.

For examinations conducted on larger children using the X-ray table and bucky, automatic exposure devices may be used. The radiographer needs to carefully consider the size of the selected chamber in comparison with the child's anatomical size. In these instances, it is important that the correct ionisation chamber and X-ray tube potentials are selected. Information on exposure factors should be readily available throughout the department, including mobile apparatus. It is essential that there is close working alongside clinical scientists and radiologists to ensure that the appropriate balance between dose and image quality are maintained.

In keeping with IR(ME)R,[9] prior to carrying out a diagnostic radiographic examination, all requests must be clinically justified. It is not uncommon for junior clinicians and triage staff more familiar with adult patients to over-request X-rays on children through inexperience of image interpretation or difficulties encountered during the initial assessment. IR(ME)R 2017 indicates that a discussion should take place regarding the risks and benefits from imaging directly with the patient involved and/or the parent/carer depending upon the age of the child. Ideally this should be undertaken by the referrer, but radiographers should ensure that they fulfil this requirement should it be apparent that no conversation has taken place regarding the potential hazards and gains of the examination.

Checking previous images is an essential part of any radiographer's role regardless of the discipline. In paediatrics, such an assessment can provide useful information regarding the technique employed, in addition to the exposure used and the exact image series obtained. The author recommends the use of facilities on the Radiology Information System (or similar) to record any specific approaches that worked well or issues that staff should be aware of when undertaking an examination in the future.

Radiographers will need to confirm the pregnancy status of any patient of child-bearing age before undertaking a radiographic examination.[9] The lower age limit for pregnancy status is currently 12 years; however, some patients commence menstruation as young as 10, prompting some departments to extend the lower end of the age range. The issue of ascertaining the pregnancy status is a complex and delicate issue. A simple and uncomplicated approach is recommended by the author to achieve an honest answer. Firstly, the radiographer should question whether the patient has started their monthly periods. If the answer is confirmatory, the radiographer needs to ask whether there is any possibility that the patient could be pregnant. Ideally this conversation should take place away from the parent/carer and made clear to the patient that it is an important part of the radiographer's responsibility to ask such questions. Proof of pregnancy status/their response to the question should be retained and permanently documented by electronic or paper means.

A common error by radiographers who do not X-ray children regularly is the failure to sufficiently collimate the primary beam. This may be through fear of missing the area of interest off the image. The use of effective clinical holding (immobilisation), be it with devices or a parent/carer/member of staff, coupled with ongoing learning and skill development, should enable the radiographer to feel confident to collimate appropriately and therefore limit radiation. A holder can be defined as anyone who supports and immobilises a patient during a radiographic exposure. Different centres may employ varying approaches in their recommended choice or preference of holder – be it the child's parent/carer or healthcare worker. The author encourages both debate and appropriate recommendations/guidance from the professional body on this subject.

Care should be taken to ensure that any parent/carer remaining within the X-ray room and/or providing clinical holding, is consented for the role (documented) and is adequately protected (lead or equivalent apron). There must also be clear instruction by the radiographer how to put the apron on properly and the importance of good posture and use of an appropriate X-ray table height to avoid injury. Prior to enlisting the assistance of any parent/carer or healthcare professional of childbearing capacity, the radiographer should consider the possibility of pregnancy and should provide the holder with clear instructions to avoid the need for repeat exposures.

The holder's fingers should always be excluded from the primary beam. Should the fingers be close to the primary beam, lead rubber gloves/mittens should always be worn though these will not provide complete protection at higher beam energies (Fig. 19.3). It is recommended that records are kept of any radiographers or healthcare personnel who hold children for X-ray examinations to avoid the same individual regularly undertaking this role.

Radiographic Examinations

This chapter will examine standard imaging requested on paediatric patients. It will provide the undergraduate and less experienced radiographer with a fundamental understanding using a common-sense approach. Depending upon the area examined, it will be necessary to offer specific descriptions of techniques that differ in the approach for adult examinations of the same area. Other examinations may require only an observation on possible differences that may be relevant to immobilisation strategies and positioning that requires a supine approach for babies and very young children.

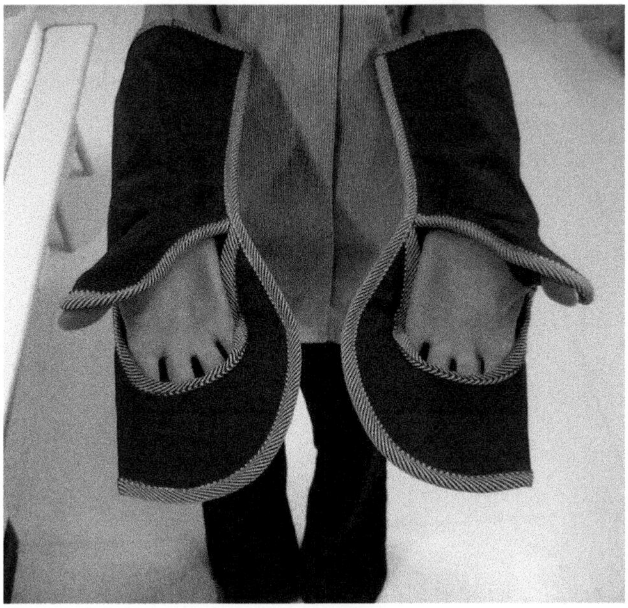

Fig. 19.3 Lead rubber mittens.

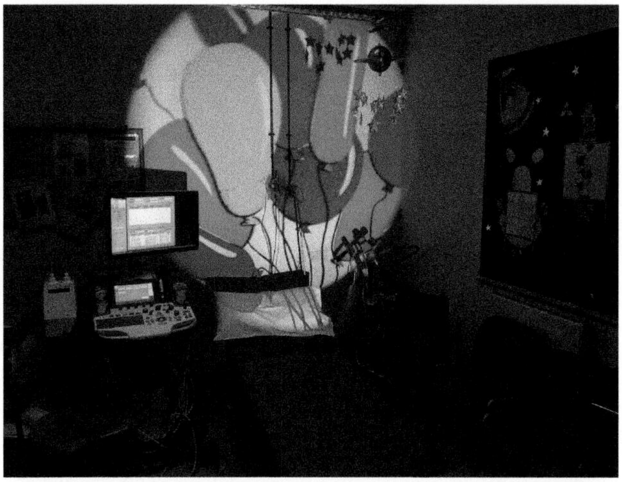

Fig. 19.4 Image projector to distract patients from the examination.

Body regions included in this chapter are as follows:

- Chest (including ingested/inhaled foreign bodies)
- Abdomen
- Appendicular skeleton
  - Upper limb
  - Lower limb
- Axial skeleton
- Skeletal survey

Facilitating the Radiographic Examination

Prior to commencing any imaging examination, the radiographer must undertake a holistic assessment, considering the child's physical state, their emotional, cognitive and educational needs. Often talking to the child is enough in itself as a distraction technique. A positive identification of the patient should have been obtained in keeping with the employer's documented procedure specifically relating to children.[12] It is also essential the radiographer establishes who is accompanying the child as part of a safeguarding approach.[13]

As previously mentioned, immobilisation or clinical holding is sometimes unavoidable to obtain diagnostic images in a safe and controlled manner. Most hospitals will have a patient immobilisation policy document and it is important that a copy is kept in the imaging department. It is essential that all radiographers likely to be involved in the clinical holding of children are adequately trained and aware of the occasions that merit they themselves immobilising the child (e.g. skeletal survey for non-accidental injury/suspected physical abuse).

An awareness of different approaches to gaining a child's cooperation (Fig. 19.4) is vital. This may include distraction techniques, play therapy, improved explanation, or simple persuasion. Non-cooperation may be due to the child simply having a bad day or sensing their parent/carer's anxieties. On occasions having a break or 'time out' can work wonders. Children who have undergone a seemingly endless series of examinations may benefit from returning on another day providing this does not jeopardise their clinical management.

Samples of tried and tested techniques are as follows:

- Prepare the examination room with several sizes of image receptor (if using CR), immobilisation pads and sandbags, protective lead aprons.
- Employ appropriate methods to reduce the potential for cross-infection.
- Select a preliminary imaging exposure prior to inviting the child into the room.
- Introduce yourself to the child and their family using your first name and role. Make eye contact and smile. Asking who the child has brought with them will make them feel important and act as a means of establishing the identity of the adult without mistake or embarrassment while considering safeguarding guidance.
- Upon entering the examination room, ask them how they are today, whether they have had an X-ray before. Encourage them to talk about it if they are happy to do so.
- Look for conversation topics such as birthdays, holidays, festive seasons, school, sports (particularly if a sports shirt is being worn), or favourite television programmes (characters are often featured on clothing).
- Demonstrating the position required is often more effective than a description. Enlisting the help of the parent/carer can be particularly beneficial.
- Consider a practice run to limit the need for a repeat examination, for example, for chest X-rays to avoid overinflation of the lungs.
- The child watching the light beam diaphragm and announcing when the light has gone out has proved to be a useful game. The child feels important in being given a job and is likely to be more compliant.
- Encourage the child to count whilst the X-ray is being taken. This may assist in maintaining the correct position.
- Children requiring comfort and reassurance from their parent/carer are best examined close to these adults. Clinicians carrying out patient assessment and examinations on children undertake as many required tests as possible while the child is seated upon the lap of their

parent/carer.[14] This approach works equally well with children in the X-ray room.
- If two projections are required and one is likely to be easier or less distressing than the other, it often pays to perform this projection first utilising the position that the child finds more comfortable.

Common Mistakes and Errors

General errors that can occur in paediatrics and the reasons for them are detailed below.

Common Errors: Paediatric Imaging

Common Errors	Possible Reasons	Potential Effects on PCE or Report
Too large an X-ray field size	Overestimation of a child's anatomical proportions/area of interest. Concern that the child may move out of the usual collimated area	Increased scatter and noise on the image: may make interpretation of subtle changes more difficult
Insufficient demonstration of anatomical area	Incorrect centring points – appropriate for adults, but not for children	Omission of part/all of area of interest can result in abnormalities being overlooked
Images of the parent's/holder's hands, or other parts in the region of interest	Presence of the parent/holder within the primary beam Insufficient communication from the radiographer and/or the parent/holder not understanding their role.	Obscuring of anatomical detail that can result in abnormalities being overlooked or misinterpreted
Blurring of anatomical structures (movement unsharpness)	Patient movement, crying, respiration, inadequate immobilisation technique employed, too long an exposure time Increased cardiac motion in babies for chest imaging Inappropriate choice of generator unable to support short exposure times. This may be more evident where mobile equipment is used	Loss of sharpness will obscure anatomical detail, increasing the possibility of abnormal appearances being overlooked
Under- or overexposure of the resultant image through employing the use of an automatic exposure device (upright bucky and/or table)	Similar to adults, incorrect selection of the ionisation chamber Movement of the child outside of the ionisation chamber	Limited demonstration of subtle changes that can indicate injury or disease
Additional radiographic artefacts	Clothing image artefact Jewellery (inc. body piercing items) in situ Foam support pads/sandbags not radiolucent	Obscuring of anatomical detail increasing the possibility of abnormal appearances being overlooked

Chest

The chest X-ray is one of the most commonly requested radiographic images in children but is often difficult to obtain and of poor quality, particularly in the younger age group.[15]

It is imperative that any clothing is removed to avoid the presence of artefact (embroidery, gemstone decoration, transfers on garments) on the resulting image. Long hair should be moved away from the area of interest as should any monitor wires or leads, providing it is not detrimental to the patient to do so.

The posteroanterior (PA) erect projection is preferred by radiologists, although in practice the anteroposterior (AP) is more readily performed in infants and young children as they are more likely to cooperate with this style of examination. This patient preference can be attributed to the need to visualise their surroundings and their parent/carer. The choice of technique relies heavily upon the confidence of the radiographer; the less capable individual may elect to use the AP projection when careful assessment and communication will have established that a PA projection may have been achievable. It may be more convenient for the radiographer to undertake a supine AP projection in preference to an erect AP. It should be remembered that the majority of children reach their sitting milestone at approximately 6 months of age.[7] The inference here is that at the very least erect projections should be performed from this age, or even before.

METHOD 1 – POSTEROANTERIOR (PA) ERECT CHEST

Please refer to the appropriate chapter on adult chest radiography (Chapter 15), as this technique is used for older children.

METHOD 2 – ANTEROPOSTERIOR (AP) ERECT CHEST (FIG. 19.5)

- An appropriately sized IR should be selected and placed into the chest stand.
- A stool is placed in front of the chest stand. A rubberoid material, e.g. Dycem®, can be placed on the seat to prevent the child slipping.
- The child is encouraged to sit on the stool with their back against the IR (in the chest stand). The upper border of the receptor should be visible above the shoulders.
- A 15° radiolucent pad (if using digital radiography check the pad does not cause an artefact) may be placed behind the child's shoulders and head, in front of the receptor, to limit the degree of lordosis and to act as a soft cushion to protect the back of the head.

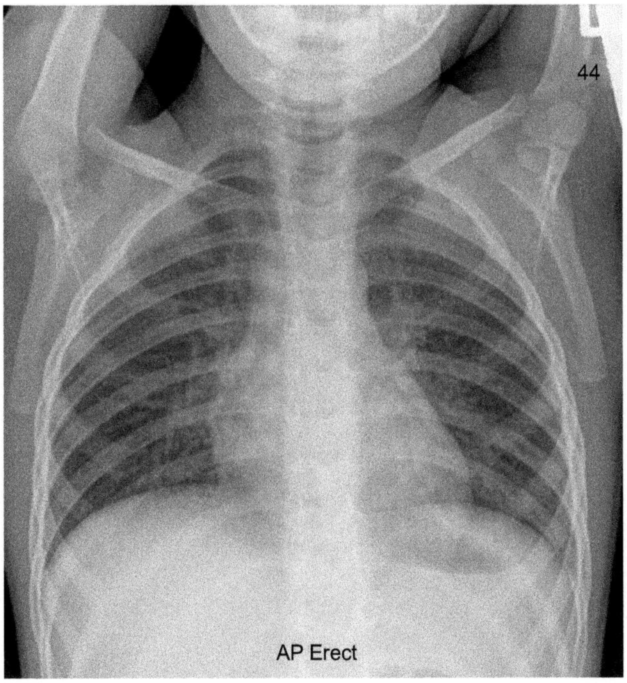

Fig. 19.5 AP chest X-ray.

- A Velcro® band may be useful to assist in maintaining the optimum position – this can be likened to a seat-belt.
- Both arms should be flexed at the elbow and raised to the side of the head where they may be supported by the child's parent/carer or holder.

Beam Direction and FRD

A caudal angle of 5–10° at a distance of 180 cm is universally used

Centring Point

In the midline between the sternal angle and the xiphisternum

Collimation

Apices, lateral margins of both lungs as well as the cardiophrenic sulci and costophrenic sulci

Respiration

If the child is able to cooperate, encourage them to take a big breath in and to hold it

Observe the child's breathing and make the exposure on inspiration if they are unable to comply with instructions

METHOD 3 – SUPINE CHEST

This may be performed in the imaging department or other setting. Requests for a portable chest and abdomen should be performed separately. Tempting though it may be to take one projection to include both chest and abdomen, this must be avoided as this method produces an image of poor quality with a lordotic chest and utilises an exposure suitable only for one area. The only exception is in the case of a 'central line' placement assessment, and for this purpose collimation should be refined to a rectangular area that demonstrates the line only.

- An appropriately sized receptor is placed on the examination table, or in the cot/bed/incubator. Incubator sides should be opened for the absolute minimum of time to avoid temperature changes that adversely affect the patient. Neonates are also susceptible to noise and vibration, which should be kept to a minimum. Please be aware that incubators need to be separated by a distance of at least 2 feet or 0.6 metres in order to reduce the cumulative scatter dose to neighbouring patients.[16]
- The child is placed upon the IR with the shoulders and head resting upon a 15° pad, for identical reasons to those stated in Method 1.
- If not detrimental to the child's well-being, the arms should be extended, abducted anteriorly, raised and immobilised by the side of the head. Most efficient immobilisation is achieved by the arms held against the head by the elbows.
- Some assistance/additional immobilisation may also be required to avoid rotation of the child's lower body.
- When examining a child in an incubator, strips of lead rubber can be arranged to form a 'window' over the top of the incubator providing radiation protection to the child and holder whilst improving image quality.

Beam Direction and FRD

A caudal angle of 5–10° at a distance of 100 cm. Larger FRDs should be utilised but this is usually unachievable owing to available tube height and incubator limitations

Centring Point

For babies, in the midline at the level of the sternal angle or nipples

For older children, consider the same centring point as for adults

Collimation

Apices and lateral margins of both lungs, to include the cardiophrenic sulci and costophrenic sulci

A baby's diaphragm is anatomically higher than that of older children and adults. The bifurcation of the trachea occurs at the level of T3/4 as opposed to T5/6.

Respiration

Observe the child's breathing and make the exposure on inspiration if they are unable to comply with instructions. Care should be taken to avoid obtaining a hyperinflated image.

Criteria for Assessing Image Quality (Methods 1 and 2)

The criteria for assessing a paediatric chest image are the same as for that of an adult, with additional considerations. It is essential, particularly in the neonatal group, that reproducible exposure factors are consistently used.

- Image is as free as possible from artefact
- Sharp visualisation of the heart and lungs
- Mandible and chin must not obscure the lung apices
- Adequate penetration (appropriate kVp) to demonstrate the retro-cardiac area
- No evidence of rotation – scrutiny of rib symmetry
- The chest does not appear lordotic

For general errors, please refer to the 'Common Mistakes and Errors' section of this chapter above.

Common Errors: Paediatric PA/AP Chest

Common Errors	Possible Reasons	Potential Effects on PCE or Report
Lordotic image – anterior ribs appear horizontal or lie above the posterior ribs	Hyperextension of the child's arms Child has arched their back during exposure	Obscuring of the lung bases and diaphragm along with widening of the superior mediastinum increasing the possibility of abnormalities being overlooked or appearances being misinterpreted
Left to right asymmetry of the anterior and posterior ribs	Child is rotated – small children are far more 'cylindrical' in shape	Heart size may appear enlarged or diminished depending on direction of rotation, increasing the possibility of abnormalities being overlooked or misinterpreted
Soft tissue opacification over one or both apices	Neck is insufficiently extended; the soft tissues of the chin or mandible are overlying the area of interest	Obscuring of anatomical detail Changes in the apices may be overlooked (e.g. pneumothorax)
Hyperinflated chest	Exposure has been made during a large intake of breath by the child during crying or overenthusiasm	Misinterpretation of appearances as an indication of reactive airways disease (e.g. asthma)
Excessive amount of abdomen included on the chest image	Incorrect centring as performed for adults	Subtle changes may be overlooked owing to the nature of the diverging beam (e.g. rib fractures)
Spine appears curved/scoliotic	Poor positioning of patient (slouching to one side)	Misinterpretation of the existence of a scoliosis in a normal spine
Vertical streaking artefact	Hair artefact	Obscuring of anatomical detail increasing the possibility of abnormalities being overlooked or misinterpretation of 'lines' as pathology (e.g. pneumothorax)

LATERAL CHEST

Please refer to the appropriate chapter on adult chest radiography (Chapter 15) as this technique is used for older children.

Positioning

- Children where possible should be imaged erect, either standing or sitting, as for adults
- Very young children should be examined lying on their left side upon the IR with their head supported on a foam pad
- Infants being nursed in incubators may require a horizontal beam lateral whilst the receptor is safely supported vertically at one side
- Arms should be raised to either side of the head away from the area of interest
- The neck needs to be adequately extended as to prevent superimposition of the soft tissues of the chin or mandible upon the resultant image

Beam Direction and FRD

Horizontal or vertical at 90° to the image receptor

FRD issues are as for the AP chest but it is likely that a 180 cm FRD will be achievable for an older child examined erect

Centring Point

Young children – midway between the anterior and posterior margins of the thorax at the level of the sternal angle

Older children – as for adults

Collimation

As for adults

Criteria for Assessing Image Quality

As for adults

INGESTED OR INHALED FOREIGN BODIES

Young children and sometimes those with special educational needs and disabilities may attend Emergency Departments following the swallowing or inhalation of small objects. Usually clinicians will have taken a detailed history and excluded the presence of the item within clothing or other body cavities prior to referral for imaging. Ideally a duplicate of the item believed to have been inhaled/ingested will have been brought by the parent/carer to hospital but unfortunately this does not always occur. Items commonly ingested or inhaled include coins, batteries and Lego bricks.

A common sense approach to the radiographic management of such patients is recommended. The ED staff will have already made a clinical decision regarding patient management and some units employ the use of a metal detector to localise objects if they are ferrous in nature. This assists in prioritising the order and number of images required. Images need to be obtained and re-projectioned prior to carrying out the next, if required.

For suspected inhaled foreign bodies, a chest X-ray is required. Even if the item is not purported to be radiopaque, the chest X-ray is still of value in identifying any possible associated collapse or air-trapping and/or consolidation of the lung.[17]

For ingested foreign bodies a chest and upper abdominal X-ray should be performed only if there is the suspicion of a swallowed foreign body that is sizeable, sharp, toxic, or where leakage is a possibility. It must be ensured that there is an area of anatomical overlap.

On the chest image it is useful to include the neck (patient's head turned to one side) to ensure the foreign body is not located in the nasopharynx or oropharynx.

Abdomen

The abdominal X-ray is routinely requested either alone or in conjunction with imaging modalities such as ultrasound and magnetic resonance imaging. Although undertaken frequently on neonatal units, this practice is not recommended on the ward for older children due to image quality and reasons pertaining to radiation protection. Owing to the marked radiation dose imparted to the patient, all requests for abdominal imaging must be clinically justified and consideration given to the other imaging investigations that may be more appropriate as the primary examination. The lateral decubitus (right side uppermost) technique are sometimes undertaken in specific cases, such as a suspected perforation, when an erect chest is not feasible. Occasionally imaging of both the chest and abdomen are requested simultaneously. This can be justified due to the reasons outlined in the chest section in this chapter, although the effective dose has been reported to be 5% greater.[15]

Prior to carrying out abdominal radiography, the child must always be undressed, including the nappy and any potential artefacts removed from the area. Particular care should be taken with baby vests that have poppers, both the front and the back need to be removed from the area of interest.

ANTEROPOSTERIOR (AP) ABDOMEN

An appropriately sized IR is positioned with the long axis in line with the child's MSP. For smaller children it is not necessary to utilise a scatter reduction device or grid.

Positioning

- The child is positioned supine on the examination table as for the equivalent adult examination
- For babies who do not require a secondary radiation reduction device (grid), the child is placed in direct contact with the IR
- For children unable to remain still, the femora and upper torso are supported (holding arms and legs) by an assistant to prevent rotation and lateral flexion of the trunk
- The arms are raised onto the pillow to enable the humeri to be shielded from the primary beam
- For portable examinations on the neonatal unit, the incubator lid can be used as placement for lead rubber strips (see procedure for paediatric chest examination)

The exposure should be made on arrested respiration

Radiation Protection

Do not use secondary radiation grids for small children

Employ X-ray tube potentials between 60 and 65 kVp with short exposure times

Beam direction and FRD

Perpendicular central ray at 100 cm FRD

Centring Point

In the midline at the level of the iliac crests

The umbilicus is at the same level and is a reliable centring point for babies

Collimation

Employ shadow shielding wherever possible

The beam should be collimated to include the entire diaphragm and upper border of the symphysis pubis. The lateral walls of the abdomen must also be included

Criteria for Assessing Image Quality

- The diaphragm, upper border of the pubic rami and lateral abdominal walls should be included
- There should be symmetry of the pelvic structures and the spinous processes should be demonstrated down the centre of the vertebral bodies
- There should be clear contrast between the skeleton and soft tissues, enabling clear demonstration of bowel gas

Common Error: Paediatric AP Abdomen

Common Error	Possible Reason	Potential Effects on PCE or Report
Hemidiaphragms and/or superior borders of the pubic rami absent	Radiographer underestimation of size in assessment of child's anatomical proportions	Omission of required anatomical area Abnormal appearances may be overlooked, e.g.: hemidiaphragms – hiatus hernia, pneumothorax pubic rami – foreign body, fracture

Please also refer to the 'Common Mistakes and Errors' section of this chapter.

Appendicular Skeleton: Upper Limb

HAND AND FINGERS

The same principles are applied here as for adult radiography. The only differences relate to the variations in technique due to the child's age and level of cooperation. Hand and finger imaging are regularly undertaken to rule out a bony injury or the presence of a foreign body in the soft tissues.

As previously mentioned, small children are more likely to be content sat upon their parent/carer's lap, where they can feel secure as well as be able to see around them. However, some circumstances may dictate that the child is happier being examined in a supine position.

The greatest challenge of examining this area is ensuring that the fingers remain fully extended and the correct position is maintained. Various methods have been described to gain an optimum dorsipalmar (DP) image. The author recommends a small radiolucent ruler to immobilise the fingers (Fig. 19.6) but equally having the parent/carer hold the child's hand in the desired position and remove the restraint at the moment of exposure can be successful and less traumatic for the child.

A lateral projection can prove equally as challenging. The use of a foam pad to gently separate the affected finger from its fellows can be utilised to maintain the position for the image to be obtained.

Suggested Projections for Conditions Affecting the Hands in Children

Polydactyly. (Presence of additional digit(s), usually arising from the first or fifth metacarpal)

- DP to assess the number of metacarpals present

Bone Age

- DP to include the wrist to assess the stage of epiphyseal development in order to establish an 'age' to compare to the child's chronological age

DP, Obliques and Lateral Projections of the Finger(s)/Hand

- Positioning should be as for adults whenever possible
- Beam direction, FRD, centring point, collimation and criteria for assessing image quality are as for adult radiography (see Chapter 4)

Common Errors: Paediatric Fingers/Hands

Common Errors	Possible Reason	Potential Effects on PCE or Report
Difficult to tell the fingers apart on the lateral projection	Insufficient detraction of unaffected fingers from the area of interest	Obscuring of area of interest Abnormal appearances may be overlooked (e.g. fracture)
Metacarpals superimposed on oblique projection	Over-rotation from the DP position	Abnormal appearances may be overlooked, e.g. fractures involving the base of the proximal phalanx or metacarpal-phalangeal joint
Fingers overexposed and metacarpals/carpals underexposed	Differential thickness between the anatomical areas Inaccurate selection of image parameters	Abnormal appearances may be overlooked through loss of anatomical detail. Consider retaining two copies with appropriate window settings for both areas separately

Please also refer to the 'Common Mistakes and Errors' section of this chapter.

FOREARM AND WRIST

Alongside falls onto outstretched hands (FOOSH), a significant number of upper limb injuries in all ages are associated with recreational activities. Such is the case with the inappropriate use of trampolines[18] and falls from monkey bars.[19]

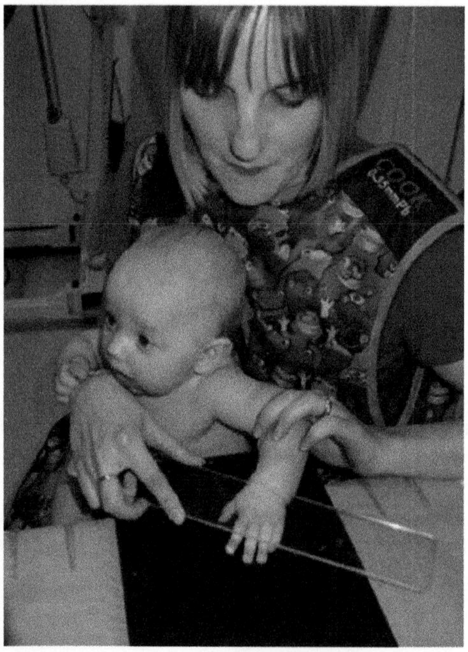

Fig. 19.6 Positioning for a hand X-ray utilising plastic ruler for immobilisation.

It is regarded as poor practice to obtain one image of the entire upper limb, even in cases where clinical examination has been difficult.[20] The only exception to this rule is for surveys undertaken to assess and characterise skeletal dysplasias. Should any abnormalities be present they will be neither visualised easily nor accurately owing to compromises in positioning and centring of the beam. The author recommends that such entire limb requests should come from senior clinicians only.

For forearm requests, both wrist and elbow joints should be visualised on one image. This is particularly relevant in cases where there is a seemingly isolated fracture of either the radius or ulna. Scrutiny of the wrist and elbow is essential to rule out a Monteggia or Galeazzi injury. Overlooking such injuries can have considerable impact on the child's prognosis and result in a negligence claim against the hospital.

Suggested Projections for Conditions Affecting the Wrist in Children

Scaphoid

- DP and lateral projections of the wrist should be obtained prior to additional scaphoid projections

Scaphoid injuries are relatively rare in children compared to wrist injuries and the radiation burden can be significantly reduced by taking this approach.

Rickets. DP wrist to demonstrate the metaphysis, which in positive cases will appear frayed and 'cupped' in positive cases (Fig. 19.7)

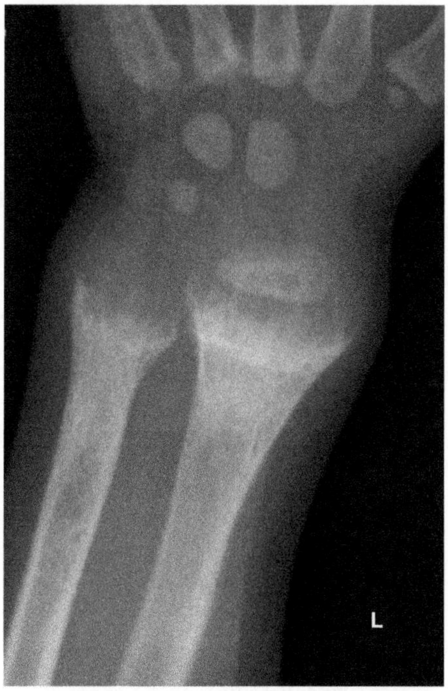

Fig. 19.7 DP wrist projection of a patient with rickets.

AP and Lateral Projections of the Forearm

- Positioning should be as for adults whenever possible
- Beam direction, FRD, centring point, collimation and criteria for assessing image quality are as for adult radiography (see Chapter 5)

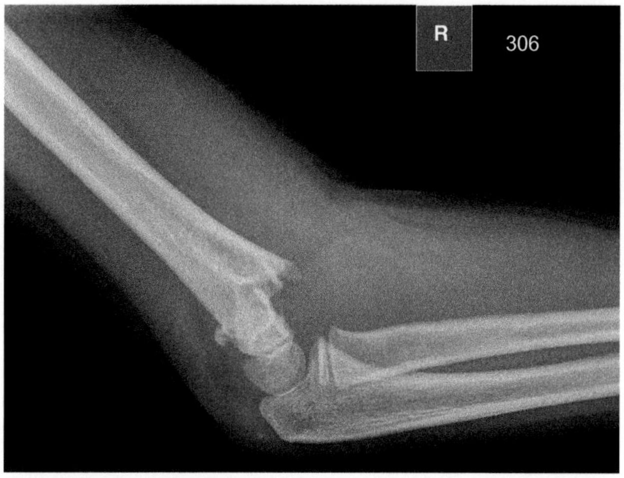

Fig. 19.8 Lateral elbow demonstrating an incomplete supracondylar fracture with accompanying soft tissue effusion.

DP and Lateral Projections of the Wrist

- Positioning should be as for adults whenever possible
- Beam direction, FRD, centring point, collimation and criteria for assessing image quality are as for adult radiography (see Chapter 4)

Common Error: Paediatric Wrist

Common Error	Possible Reason	Potential Effect on PCE or Report
Radius and ulna not superimposed on the lateral projection	Incorrect positioning for the lateral projection due to under- or over-rotation from the DP The result of the X-ray table height being inappropriate to facilitate patient positioning	Abnormal appearances may be overlooked, e.g. subtle torus (buckle) fracture

Please also refer to the 'Common Mistakes and Errors' section of this chapter.

ELBOW

The elbow remains one of the most complex areas injured in the paediatric age group, a source of great concern to radiographers and clinicians alike. Complications from injuries can range from brachial artery damage manifesting as a compartment syndrome and Volkmann's ischaemic contracture to median nerve damage, malunion and myositis ossificans.

The technique employed will depend upon the age of the child and the nature of the injury if trauma is involved. Most elbow injuries occur in the 3–10 year age group[21] (Fig. 19.8) and involve the supracondylar area of the distal humerus proximal to the trochlea and capitellum. Fractures may be complete or incomplete but involve a break in the anterior cortex with posterior displacement of the distal fragment. Other elbow injuries involve avulsion of the epicondyles and dislocations. In dislocations, the distal humerus slides over the coronoid process, often with associated fractures.

The paediatric elbow is notoriously difficult to interpret due to the six centres of secondary ossification. The order and timing of the appearance of the ossification centres is listed in Table 19.1. Careful assessment of the image and identification of the ossification centres present should identify most fractures, but the expert opinion of a consultant orthopaedic surgeon or consultant radiologist is often required. Requests for comparison projections of the unaffected elbow should never be accepted unless cleared by a consultant radiologist.

In cases where the child is in severe pain it is advisable to proceed only if they have had sufficient pain relief. The child may prefer to sit alone, on the lap of their parent/carer, or to lie down. It is good practice to obtain the lateral of the elbow before attempting the AP projection. The reason for this is to enable the radiographer to be aware of the extent and severity of the injury prior to positioning for the often difficult and painful AP projection. The positioning of the lateral projection needs to be accurate to enable evaluation of the soft tissue anterior and posterior fat pads of the distal humerus that will indicate the presence of a fracture

TABLE 19.1 Centres of Ossification in the Paediatric Elbow

	Approximate Age in Years	Ossification Centre
C	1	Capitellum
R	3	Radial head
I	5	Internal (medial) epicondyle
T	7	Trochlea
O	9	Olecranon
L	11	Lateral external epicondyle

Data from Children's Orthopaedics and Fractures.[22]

in the absence of bony signs. An AP projection may be achieved by externally rotating the arm from the shoulder joint which will move the elbow into the desired position. An axial projection of the joint if held in a flexed position may be used as an alternative to the AP projection, as is described in Chapter 5.

A common misconception is that injuries to the proximal radius will involve the head of the bone. Although common in adults, paediatric injuries in this region are more likely to affect the radial neck owing to the presence of the epiphysis and are reported to account for 10–15% of all presenting elbow injuries.[23]

AP and Lateral Projections of the Elbow

- Positioning: If feasible the child should be positioned similarly to adults, utilising supine and erect (sitting or standing) positioning and a horizontal beam direction when deemed to be appropriate
- Assistance may be required to support the limb should foam pads and sandbags be insufficient
- Beam direction, FRD, centring point, collimation and criteria for assessing image quality are as for adult radiography (see Chapter 5)

Common Errors: Paediatric Elbow

Common Errors	Possible Reasons	Potential Effects on PCE or Report
True lateral projection not obtained	Incorrect positioning involving the level of the forearm being at a different height to the humerus	Abnormal appearances may be overlooked (e.g. presence of a dislocated proximal radius forming part of a Monteggia injury)
Poor visualisation of one or both fat pads	Inappropriate exposure utilised Poor positioning for lateral projection	Abnormal appearances may be overlooked (e.g. presence of raised fat pad indicating an occult fracture)

Please also refer to the 'Common Mistakes and Errors' section of this chapter.

SHOULDER, CLAVICLE AND PROXIMAL HUMERUS

Injuries of the shoulder and humerus are common in the older child, particularly those engaged in sporting activities. In the first instance, trauma cases should be examined in an AP and lateral position. As with adults, axial projections of the shoulder are only of benefit to the child if he or she is able to cooperate and may be better suited to non-trauma situations when the patient is sufficiently comfortable and is able to abduct the shoulder joint.

The clavicle remains one of the most frequently injured areas in children, accounting for 7–15% of all paediatric fractures.[24] It is often diagnosed clinically owing to the superficial position of the clavicle and the degree of local swelling that occurs immediately post injury. The majority of injuries are midshaft, either complete (overlapping of the two fragments) or incomplete (superior apical angulation). They are commonly caused by a direct fall onto the front of the shoulder. An audit of clavicle injuries at the author's previous workplace demonstrated that a single 20° degree cranially angled projection of the clavicle will demonstrate most injuries. APs of the shoulder are only undertaken should this initial projection show no abnormality. The justification for this protocol is that more clavicle injuries are easily identified than on the conventional AP projection, though further research needs to be undertaken with respect to the efficacy of this protocol. Requests for specialised projections of the acromio-clavicular and sterno-clavicular joints should be discussed with a consultant radiologist as they seldom yield additional diagnostic information.

AP Projection of the Shoulder and Humerus

Positioning

- Wherever possible, position in a similar technique to adults (see Chapter 5)
- Patient can be seated on a stool or stand depending upon their level of cooperation
- The amount of shoulder or proximal humerus to be included depends on nature of injury and clinical examination
- The arm of the injured side can be supported by the patient's other arm or held by the parent/carer
- A small radiolucent pad may be placed between the trunk and the arm of the affected side to abduct it sufficiently and avoid superimposition of adjacent structures
- Ideally, the exposure is made on arrested respiration

Beam Direction, FRD and Centring Point. As for adults, but these may be modified to accommodate the clinical information

Collimation

For the humerus – as for adults

For the shoulder – include the entire shoulder girdle and proximal third of the humerus. On some occasions the entire length of the humerus will need to be visualized, including the gleno-humeral and elbow joints (for injuries that extend to include the midshaft, e.g. spiral fractures)

Common Errors: Paediatric Shoulder and Humerus

Common Errors	Possible Reasons	Potential Effects on PCR or Report
The shaft of the humerus cannot be fully visualised	The arm has not been sufficiently abducted, if the patient's collar and cuff support is in situ. Appropriate advice should be sought from medical personnel	Abnormal appearances may be overlooked
The clavicle is overlapped by the lung apices and 1st ribs	Requires cranial angulation of the beam	Abnormal appearances may be overlooked as the clavicle is obscured (e.g. subtle fractures)
The clavicle appears foreshortened	Patient is over-rotated towards the affected side.	Abnormal appearances may be overlooked

Please also refer to the 'Common Mistakes and Errors' section of this chapter.

Appendicular Skeleton: Lower Limb

FEET AND TOES

Dorsiplantar and dorsiplantar oblique projections are routinely undertaken for trauma and orthopaedic referrals. Young children are examined either seated upon the examination table or supine with a parent/carer supporting the child to remain correctly positioned for the examination.

The toes need to remain fully extended and the correct position maintained. The author suggests the use of a small radiolucent ruler to immobilise the toes but equally having the parent/carer hold the child's foot in the desired position and remove the restraint at the moment of exposure can be successful and less traumatic for the child.

The lateral projection may be required for the assessment of the foot for specific conditions or a suspected foreign body. On occasions, standing projections will be requested to demonstrate the foot when weight bearing.

Axial projections of the calcaneum may be indicated following trauma when the patient lands on their feet from a significant height. These are performed in the same way as for adults.

Suggested Projections for Conditions Affecting Feet in Children

Congenital Talipes Equino Varus (Club Foot)

- DP with the patient standing or simulated standing if non-ambulant. It is essential that the talus remains vertical for accurate assessment
- Two lateral projections, one taken in maximum dorsiflexion, one in extension to assess the mobility of the mid and hind foot. These can be achieved with the use of a ruler

Polydactyly. (Presence of additional digit(s), usually arising from the 1st or 5th metatarsal.)

- DP to assess the number of metatarsals present

Hallux Valgus (Bunion)

- DP with the patient standing to enable accurate evaluation of the deformity when weight bearing

Pes Planus (Flat Foot)

- DP projection and a standing lateral to assess loss of the medial longitudinal arch and degree of rigidity

Tarsal Coalition

- DP, DP oblique and lateral projections, sometimes with modified axial calcaneum projection (Harris Beath), with the patient in an erect axial calcaneum position, with the sole of the foot flat on the IR and the central ray in angles between 35° and 55° (see Fig. 6.17A)[25] to demonstrate any abnormal join(s) between the tarsal bones

DP, Oblique and Lateral Projections of the Foot and Toes

- Position is as for adults (see Chapter 6). The parent/carer will need to support or immobilise younger children and babies
- Beam direction, FRD, centring point, collimation and criteria for assessing image quality are as for adult radiography (see Chapter 6)

Common Errors: Paediatric Foot and Toes

Common Errors	Possible Reasons	Potential Effects on PCE or Report
Difficult to tell toes apart on the lateral projection	Insufficient detraction of unaffected toes from the area of interest	Abnormal appearances may be overlooked, e.g. fracture
Toes and metatarsals too superimposed in the oblique projection	Over-inversion of the foot	Abnormal appearances may be overlooked, e.g. fractures involving the base of the proximal phalanx or metatarsal-phalangeal joint
Phalanges overexposed out and tarsal bones underexposed	Due to differential thickness between the anatomical areas Inaccurate selection of image parameters	Mitigate by retaining two copies with appropriate window settings for both areas separately

Please also refer to the 'Common Mistakes and Errors' section of this chapter.

KNEE

Unlike adults, there is little to be gained by performing radiographic examinations of the child's knee in a standing position, unless directed by an orthopaedic specialist. Standing projections are appropriate for demonstrating the extent of degenerative changes, of which there is a low incidence in paediatrics.

The patella does not commence ossification until the age of 3 years and specific projections such as the axial or skyline are of limited value unless in cases of skeletal dysplasia that directly affect the development of the knee joint, such as nail–patella syndrome (Fong's disease).

A bipartite patella can sometimes mimic a fracture and may be discovered coincidentally. They occur in the upper outer quadrant of the patella, are smooth-edged and will not be accompanied by the soft tissue signs of swelling, an effusion or lipohaemarthrosis (fat–blood interface) which would be seen alongside the majority of fractured patellae. Occasionally, tripartite patellae are found.

Should images for knee pain prove normal, consideration should be given as to whether the origin of the pain is within the hip, as in cases of Legg–Calve–Perthes disease and slipped upper femoral epiphysis.[26]

AP and Lateral Projections of the Knee

- Positioning is as for adults (see Chapter 7). The parent/carer will need to support or immobilise younger children and babies
- Always use a horizontal beam to obtain the lateral projection to demonstrate a potential lipohaemoarthrosis in any history of trauma
- Beam direction, FRD, centring point, collimation and criteria for assessing image quality are as for adult radiography (see Chapter 7)

Additional Projections

Additional projections are sometimes required, usually requested by orthopaedic specialists needing to visualise specific aspects of the knee and patello-femoral joint.

Osteochondritis of the Tibial Tuberosity (Osgood–Schlatter's Disease)

- A traction apophysitis involving the tibial tuberosity and in essence should be a clinical diagnosis.
- A lateral projection only should be undertaken.

Osteochondral Defect or Osteochondritis Dissecans

- The formation of a loose body within the joint space which initially appears as a flattened area of the distal femur, usually the lateral aspect of the medial condyle. Occasionally, this may also result from trauma to the area.
- The intercondylar notch (tunnel) projection (see Chapter 7) is effective at demonstrating the stage of abnormality and amount of bone involved as well as confirming the donor site.

Common Errors: Paediatric Knee

Common Errors	Possible Reasons	Potential Effects on PCE or Report
On the AP projection the patella does not lie in the midline	Over- or under-rotation of the lower limb	Misinterpretation of the existence of a subluxed or dislocated patella in a normal knee
On the AP projection a lucent line is present traversing the proximal tibia	This is the tibial tuberosity projected as such due to over- or under-rotation of the lower limb	Misinterpretation of the existence of a fracture in a normal knee
On the lateral projection the femoral condyles are not superimposed	Over- or under-rotation of the lower limb into the lateral position	Anatomical detail obscured increasing the possibility of overlooking an abnormality, e.g. fracture, loose body
The intercondylar notch is not adequately demonstrated	Over-flexion or under-flexion of the knee joint	Obscured area of interest increasing the possibility of overlooking an abnormality, e.g. fracture or loose body presence

Please also refer to the 'Common Mistakes and Errors' section of this chapter.

TIBIA, FIBULA AND ANKLE

It should be remembered that it is regarded as poor practice to obtain one image of the entire lower limb. Should abnormalities be present they will be neither visualised easily nor accurately, owing to compromises in positioning and centring of the beam. As with the upper limb, the author recommends that such entire limb requests should come from senior clinicians only.

Toddler's Fracture

- A minimally displaced fracture of the midshaft of the tibia seen in young children that occurs after low-energy trauma, such as jumping off a sofa.[27]

AP and Lateral Projection of the Tibia/Fibula

- Positioning is as for adults. The parent/carer will need to support or immobilise younger children and babies
- Consider using a horizontal beam to obtain a lateral projection in cases of obvious deformity through trauma
- Include both joints on the initial visit or in cases of trauma. This may be reduced to the joint nearest the site of injury on subsequent visits, provided the referrer is in agreement

- Beam direction, FRD, centring point, collimation and criteria for assessing image quality are as for adult radiography (see Chapter 6)

AP and Lateral Projection of the Ankle
- Positioning is as for adults. The parent/carer will need to support or immobilise younger children and babies
- Consider using a horizontal beam to obtain a lateral projection in cases of obvious deformity through trauma
- Beam direction, FRD, centring point, collimation and criteria for assessing image quality are as for adult radiography (see Chapter 6)

Common Errors: Paediatric Tibia, Fibula and Ankle

Common Errors	Possible Reasons	Potential Effects on PCE or Report
AP projection of a young child's lower limb appears oblique	Inadequate rotation of the child's trunk	Obscured area of interest increasing the possibility of overlooking an abnormality, e.g. fracture
Lateral projection of young child's lower limb is either over- or under-rotated	Inadequate rotation of the child's trunk	Obscured area of interest increasing the possibility of overlooking an abnormality, e.g. fracture

Please also refer to the 'Common Mistakes and Errors' section of this chapter.

Axial Skeleton: Vertebral Column

The newborn spine is relatively straight, developing its curvatures as the child reaches the relevant milestones of holding up his/her head and beginning to weight bear.[7]

The vertebral column may require imaging following significant trauma or in the event of the development of deformity, known complications or pain of a chronic nature. Chronic pain is managed conservatively in adults, but in children any spinal tenderness or discomfort is treated as a genuine and serious ailment until proven otherwise.[28] Imaging is undertaken to rule out causes such as leukaemia, osteomyelitis, discitis or spondylolysis.

Most trauma cases are now routinely examined by CT scanning. However, on the occasions that plain film X-ray is required radiographers must ensure that precautionary measures, cervical collar (if used), sandbags and tape, are undertaken to the same extent as with adults until possible fractures have been excluded. Paediatric injuries are more likely to involve C3 and above.[29]

CERVICAL SPINE

AP and Lateral Projections of the Cervical Spine

- Positioning should be as for adults, whenever possible
- For younger children and babies, secondary radiation grids are not required
- It is advisable to sit the ambulant child on a stool as opposed to undertaking the lateral projection in a standing position
- In small children a supine position (horizontal beam) is recommended as a means of obtaining a lateral projection
- An AP (C1–C2) open mouth projection should always be obtained in cases where acute injury is suspected
- Beam direction, FRD, centring, collimation and criteria for assessing image quality are as for adult radiography (see Chapter 9)
- To ensure the rami of the mandible do not overlie the anterior vertebral bodies, the chin should be gently lifted and supported in that position with the assistance of a parent/carer if necessary

Torticollis (Wry-neck)
- AP (C3–C7/T1) and lateral projections (C1–C7/T1)

Atlanto-occipital Instability. Seen in some patients with trisomy 21 (Down syndrome) and mucopolysaccharidosis (Morquio syndrome).

- Lateral projections should be obtained, in both flexion and extension
- Care should be taken to ensure that neither position is forced

Fixed Rotary Subluxation
- Three AP projections of C1 and C2, one taken with the neck in a neutral position and the remaining two with the head turned 15° in both directions

THORACIC SPINE

AP and Lateral Projections of the Thoracic Spine

- Positioning should be as for adults whenever possible
- For younger children and babies, secondary radiation grids are not necessary
- Beam direction, FRD, centring, collimation and criteria for assessing image quality are as for adult radiography (see Chapter 9)

LUMBAR SPINE

AP and Lateral Projections of the Lumbar Spine

- Positioning should be as for adults whenever possible
- For younger children and babies, secondary radiation grids are not necessary
- A lumbo-sacral junction (L5/S1) is not routinely undertaken unless specifically requested as the area is adequately demonstrated on the lateral projection
- Beam direction, FRD, centring, collimation and criteria for assessing image quality are as for adult radiography (see Chapter 10)

Spondylolisthesis/Spondylosis.
Anterior displacement of one vertebral body upon another.

- A tightly collimated projection of the lumbosacral junction (L5/S1) will demonstrate any abnormalities specific to this area

Common Errors: Paediatric Vertebral Column

Common Errors	Possible Reasons	Potential Effects on PCE or Report
AP/lateral projection demonstrates oblique vertebra	Over- or under-rotation of the child's trunk	Subtle abnormal appearances may be overlooked, e.g. spondylolisthesis
Bony anatomy on AP projection not sufficiently demonstrated	Overlying bowel gas present, particularly in babies	Obscuring of anatomical detail may increase the possibility of abnormal appearances being overlooked
Metallic artefact demonstrated over lumbar spine in teenagers	Navel piercing ring/bar in situ	Obscuring of anatomical detail may increase the possibility of abnormal appearances being overlooked, e.g. vertebral fractures
Longitudinal artefact demonstrated over spine on neonates	Umbilical clip in situ	Obscuring of anatomical detail may increase the possibility of abnormal appearances being overlooked e.g. developmental anomalies such as hemi vertebra
Lower region of cervical spine not visualised on lateral projection	Shoulders obscuring vertebra	Obscuring of anatomical detail may increase the possibility of abnormal appearances being overlooked, e.g. vertebral fractures
Odontoid peg/process not visualised on C1/C2 projection	Insufficient opening of the patient's mouth Artefact caused by orthodontic braces	Obscuring of anatomical detail may increase the possibility of abnormal appearances being overlooked, e.g. vertebral fractures Seek advice from a radiologist regarding alternative imaging

Please also refer to the 'Common Mistakes and Errors' section of this chapter.

WHOLE SPINE FOR SCOLIOSIS

Scoliosis is a lateral curvature and rotation of the spinal column, often alongside a thoracic hypokyphosis. Non-structural curves can be postural or caused through habit, others as a complication of a leg length discrepancy or pelvic obliquity.

The presence of a vertebral malformation, such as a hemi- or butterfly vertebra, will produce a sharp scoliosis at the site of the deformity. A structural scoliosis can be metabolic, neuropathic, myopathic and idiopathic in origin. Most scoliosis cases are believed to be idiopathic with an incidence of 85%[30] primarily affecting adolescent girls.

Scoliosis imaging must demonstrate the spine in its functional state and include C3 to the sacroiliac joints. Visualisation of the iliac apophyses or Risser's sign[31] is essential to demonstrate the amount of growth remaining for the patient. Although increasing numbers of departments are utilising the EOS X-ray System to gain 3D images of the spine, conventional radiography is still very much in use, particularly when imaging children who are unable to support themselves and require holding by a parent/carer.

Patients able to stand should be positioned for a PA projection in order to limit radiation exposure to the developing breast tissue, thyroid gland and gonads. For those unable to stand, every attempt must be made to obtain the image in an AP sitting position with the legs apart to avoid artefact from the knees. Specialist spinal chairs are rapidly becoming an essential tool for imaging scoliosis and kyphosis in the more significantly affected patients. Depending upon the degree of kyphosis and lordosis connected with the scoliosis, a lateral projection may also be required. By definition a scoliosis exists wherever the coronal curve has a measurement of greater than 10.[32,33] It is essential that the images are reliable and reproducible. Treatment is driven by the curve magnitude and currently includes bracing to arrest the progression of developing curves and surgical rodding or fixation for curves of >40°.[33]

Axial Skeleton: Pelvis and Hips

X-ray examinations of the pelvis and hips are a frequent investigation in children. Although the amount of radiation absorbed by the body for a single X-ray is relatively small, paediatric patients with hip problems are likely to be monitored for a considerable period into adulthood, thereby becoming more susceptible through the cumulative effect of regular X-rays.

Advances in technology and current evidence of radiation exposure risks has prompted a review of the use of patient gonad shielding with key groups, such as the American Association of Physicists in Medicine and the Institute of Physics and Engineering in Medicine[34] supporting the discontinuation of such practice. However, UK guidance suggests that gonad shielding may be appropriate in males in certain examinations, but departmental protocols must be followed.[35] Radiographers should be prepared for questioning regarding this change in practice from patients and parents/carers who may express anxiety about radiation exposure to the gonad area. The use of shielding may allay the fears of some patients and parents/carers and this should be considered when developing revised shielding policies.

Should shielding be deemed as necessary, the author recommends shields made of solid lead encapsulated within plastic that it is both resilient and easily cleaned. Initial AP projections of the pelvis and hips in emergency scenarios and orthopaedic referrals should always be imaged without shielding to ensure that no bony or soft tissue injury or pathology is overlooked.

Fractures of the hip account for less than 1% of all paediatric fractures and are usually only caused by significant trauma.[36] Traumatic dislocations are also unusual and only occur when a considerable amount of force is involved, such as that encountered in some road traffic incidents. Depending upon the history given it may be pertinent to perform a lateral projection, which may take the form of a horizontal beam approach as opposed to a turned lateral.

X-rays of the hips to assess development in neonates are of limited value owing to the ossification of the femoral capital epiphysis not commencing until the age of 4–6 months. Ultrasound is the preferred means of assessing the hip in this age group. Radiography should only take place should there be a suspicion of osteomyelitis or septic arthritis and under the direction of a consultant orthopaedic surgeon.

Developmental Dysplasia of the Hip (DDH)

Developmental dysplasia of the hip covers a spectrum of hip problems ranging from the frankly dislocated hip at birth to a dislocatable hip, general hip laxity or abnormalities of the acetabulum that render it insufficient to contain the femoral head in a correct position. Risk factors documented include a positive family history, female gender, breech presentation, first pregnancy (to term) and the presence of other skeletal abnormalities such as neck torticollis and congenital talus equines varus (club foot).[37] Usually a single AP projection is sufficient for monitoring purposes.

Irritable Hip

This is an acute onset of hip pain and stiffness in the 3–9 years age group. Hip X-rays are often unremarkable, and the visualisation of effusions is best demonstrated by ultrasound. X-rays should only be performed should an ultrasound be normal and to exclude other causes of hip pain, such as Perthes' disease.

Legg–Calve–Perthes Disease (LCP) or Perthes' Disease

Normally referred to in its shortened form, Perthes' disease is an idiopathic hip disorder involving ischaemia and necrosis of the femoral epiphysis with eventual remodelling, though joint congruency is often compromised. It is usually seen in the 4–8-year age group but can occur as early as the age of 2 or as late as 10. Bilateral Perthes' occurs in 10–12% of cases, though such patients demonstrate different stages of the disease on each side.[38] Boys are affected more than girls and often show signs of a delayed bone age. AP and frog lateral projections should always be obtained.

Slipped Upper Femoral Epiphysis (SUFE)

A slipped upper femoral epiphysis is the movement in which the proximal femoral metaphysis moves anteriorly and externally rotates, giving the illusion that the epiphysis has 'fallen off' the proximal femur. A SUFE can be either acute or chronic in nature and is seen predominantly in boys in the 9–15-year age group. Twenty-five per cent of cases will have a slippage of the other side within 6 months,[37] therefore it is essential that all examinations include an AP pelvis and frog lateral of both hips, including follow-up examination.

ANTEROPOSTERIOR (AP) PELVIS AND HIPS

Positioning

- The child is positioned in a similar fashion to adults with the legs extended
- The knees should be placed to together with the patella anterior
- To aid immobilisation the parent/carer should be instructed to place a hand over the knees to prevent the child from bending their knees and twisting of the trunk
- For younger children and babies, secondary radiation grids are seldom necessary

Beam Direction and FRD

Perpendicular central ray
110 cm FRD

Centring Point

In the midline, at the level of the femoral heads. Accurate location is described in the technique for the AP projection of the adult hip. Sensible modification will be necessary for small children

Collimation

Ensure the entire pelvis is demonstrated, to avoid missing avulsion fractures of the anterior superior iliac spine

Criteria for Assessing Image Quality

- No rotation of pelvis
- Optimum demonstration of the soft tissues and bony anatomy
- Periarticular soft tissue planes should be demonstrated
- Obturator foraminae should be symmetrical
- Greater trochanters should be symmetrical and not foreshortened

FROG LATERAL FOR HIPS

Positioning

- The child is positioned in a supine position with the legs straight
- The knees are flexed to draw the feet towards the trunk
- Keeping the feet in position the hips are then abducted to open the knees until the lateral aspects of the femora are in contact with the table-top
- After such external rotation the plantar aspects of both feet should be in contact
- Should the child experience discomfort and be unable to abduct the affected hip to the same extent as the unaffected hip, care must be taken to avoid compensatory pelvic tilt. In severe cases separate laterals of each hip are preferable
- For younger children and babies, secondary radiation grids are not necessary

Beam Direction and FRD

Perpendicular central ray
100 cm FRD

Centring Point

As for the AP projection detailed above

Collimation

The hip joints and proximal femora

Criteria for Assessing Image Quality

- No rotation of the pelvis (if unachievable, single lateral projections should be performed)
- Optimum demonstration of the soft tissues and bony anatomy
- Periarticular soft tissue planes should be demonstrated
- Obturator foraminae should be symmetrical

Common Errors: Paediatric Pelvis and Hips

Common Error	Possible Reasons	Potential Effects on PCE or Report
Asymmetry of iliae and obturator foraminae of the pelvis	Rotation of patient to one side – pelvic tilt introduced	Abnormal appearances may be overlooked, e.g. limited femoral head coverage by the acetabulum
Asymmetry of obturator foraminae, greater trochanters and femoral necks on frog lateral projections	Overabduction of one of the limbs, usually the non-affected side, resulting in the patient being lopsided	Obscuring of anatomical detail may increase the possibility of abnormal appearances being overlooked, e.g. fractures, lesions
The femoral neck appears foreshortened	This may be due to the patient flexing their knee and lifting the leg	Obscuring of anatomical detail, in particular, poor demonstration of the femoral neck

Please also refer to the 'Common Mistakes and Errors' section of this chapter.

Axial Skeleton: Skull and Facial Projections

The incidence of skull imaging in paediatrics has largely diminished since the advent of the NICE guidelines[39] and acknowledgement that the absence of a skull fracture does not rule out an intracranial injury.

Although CT has largely taken the place of traditional X-rays, skull radiography is still requested as part of a skeletal survey for non-accidental injury/suspected physical abuse, skeletal dysplasia and oncology referrals. It may also be requested for the assessment of ventriculo-peritoneal shunts (lateral projection only) for the portion present in the skull and soft tissues of the cervical spine.

Despite the increased radiation dose to the lens of the eyes, for younger children it is normal practice to produce a fronto-occipital (FO) projection as opposed to the reverse projection. Children are less anxious and disorientated by not having the image receptor close to their face. The positioning described below is aimed at smaller children and may involve the use of two holders.

Craniosynostosis

The premature closing of skull sutures may lead to the development of an unusual-shaped head. Generally, an FO with a cranial angle of 20° and lateral projections are required, though occasionally a FO 30° (Towne's) is added depending upon the sutures being scrutinised.

Cochlear Implant(s)

Patients with newly fitted cochlear implants will require imaging to demonstrate the petrous portion of the temporal bone to ensure the structure, particularly the electrode placement, is correctly positioned. An oblique projection (modified Stenvers) can be taken as follows to demonstrate the bony anatomy and position of the implant electrodes whilst minimising radiation to the orbits.

With the patient being seated laterally with their affected side closest to the IR with the OMBL perpendicular to the IR, the patient's head is rotated 45° to bring the cheek of the affected side in contact with the image receptor. The beam should be centred with 12° cranial angulation midway between the external occipital protuberance and EAM of the unaffected side.[40] For older children the positioning is in keeping with that employed for adults and Chapter 12 should be consulted.

FRONTO-OCCIPITAL (FO) SKULL

Positioning

- The child is placed supine. For babies and to prevent movement of the arms, legs and trunk, the child can be swaddled in a blanket and supported. The OMBL should be perpendicular to the IR
- A secondary radiation grid is not required for small children
- Care should be taken to ensure that the head does not tip forward placing the jaw in contact with the chest. This will produce a 30° FO (Towne's) view as opposed to a FO
- To assist and maintain the position a holder wearing protective mittens/gloves may use two 45° pads placed on either side of the head

Beam Direction and FRD

Perpendicular central ray
100 cm FRD

Centring Point

In the midline of the glabella so the emergent beam passes through the occiput

Collimation

Effective collimation acknowledging the need to protect the holder's hands

Criteria for Assessing Image Quality

- The fontanelles should be adequately demonstrated in babies
- Optimum demonstration of the bony anatomy and soft tissues
- No rotation should be evident as demonstrated by the distance between the lateral borders of the orbits and lateral margin of the skull being equidistant
- The petrous ridges should be horizontal and visible through the lower third of the orbit

LATERAL SKULL

Positioning

- From the supine positioning the child's head should be gently turned to the affected side (if an injury is involved). Limited rotation of the trunk will assist in positioning of the head
- To assist and maintain the position a holder wearing protective mittens/gloves may use a 45° pad to support the back of the head and apply gentle pressure to the child's jaw using their thumb

- Ensure that the median sagittal plane is parallel to the image receptor

Beam Direction and FRD

Perpendicular central ray
100 cm FRD

Centring Point

Midway between the glabella and the occiput

Collimation

Effective collimation to include the whole cranial vault acknowledging the need to protect the holder's hands

Criteria for Assessing Image Quality

- The fontanelles should be adequately demonstrated in babies
- Optimum demonstration of the bony anatomy and soft tissues
- Rotation should not be evident as demonstrated by the superimposition of cranial floor and both aspects of the occiput

Common Errors: Paediatric Skull

Common Errors	Possible Reasons	Potential Effects on PCE or Report
FO angle needed here unless there isn't one projection resembles a Towne's projection demonstrating foramen magnum as opposed to frontal bone	The chin has been allowed to drop onto the chest Child's cranial vault is misshapen due to delivery (e.g. Ventouse method)	Overlapping of structures increase the possibility of overlooking abnormalities, particularly fractures involving the frontal area
Lateral projection demonstrates an oblique sella turcica of the sphenoid bone. The cranial floor is not superimposed with both aspects of the occiput	Insufficient or excessive rotation of the head and neck from the AP position	Obscuring of anatomical detail may increase the possibility of abnormalities being overlooked, e.g. subtle fracture lines may be confused with sutures

Please also refer to the 'Common Mistakes and Errors' section of this chapter.

PARANASAL SINUS AND POSTNASAL SPACE PROJECTIONS

Sinus projections may be occasionally requested for children with a history of acute infection not suitable for CT or MRI assessment.

Formation and pneumatisation of the sinuses occurs gradually during early childhood and are not complete until puberty. Therefore, particular care must be taken to ensure that any requests for sinus projections are clinically justified.

A single occipitomental (OM) projection with 15° caudal angulation taken with the mouth open provides the best overall assessment of the four groups of sinuses.

The lateral postnasal space (see Chapter 13) is very occasionally examined by conventional X-ray for children with histories of snoring, adenoidal speech and/or difficult nasal breathing. The mouth should remain closed at the time of exposure. The soft tissues of the adenoidal pad should be clearly demonstrated to enable assessment of their size.

Skeletal Surveys

NON-ACCIDENTAL INJURY/SUSPECTED PHYSICAL ABUSE

The term non-accidental injury (NAI) of children has recently been retitled suspected physical abuse (SPA), though many departments have continued to use the original term. The skeletal survey undertaken as part of the workup remains a topic at the forefront of paediatric radiography. The continued impact of national reports of several high profile cases[41,42] and speculation that the incidence of child abuse is on the rise, have led to an increased awareness amongst clinical professionals, culminating in the publication of a revised guidance document from the RCR and SCoR.[43]

Although skeletal fractures seldom pose an immediate threat to an ill-treated child, they remain the most robust radiological indicator of abuse in babies and toddlers.

The aims of carrying out such a skeletal survey are threefold: the diagnosis of known or suspected injuries, the demonstration of any damage to the child as yet undetected by the health professionals in charge of the child's care, and the justification of moves (if necessary) to stop a child being returned to a dangerous environment. In addition to providing the imaging of such patients, radiographers are required to call upon interpersonal skills to manage angry and/or distressed parents/carers whilst maintaining a child-friendly environment in a potentially volatile atmosphere.

It is recommended that departments undertaking such examinations should have a written protocol outlining the entire procedure from the clinical referral to the radiological report.[43] The current process at the author's previous workplace is outlined below.

Referral. Requests for skeletal surveys may only be accepted by consultant radiologists. The parents/carers should have had an explanation of the skeletal survey and the reasons for it explained to them by the clinical team prior to the examination.

Prioritisation. Although NAI/SPA cases are not clinical emergencies, it is recommended that the skeletal survey should only be performed during the normal working day and within 24 hours of the time of the request, and no later than 72 hours.[43]

Medico-legal Issues. It should be remembered that all skeletal surveys in cases of suspected abuse could be presented as evidence in a court of law. It is essential that all images are of optimal diagnostic standard with correct centring, exposure, appropriate collimation and accurately marked

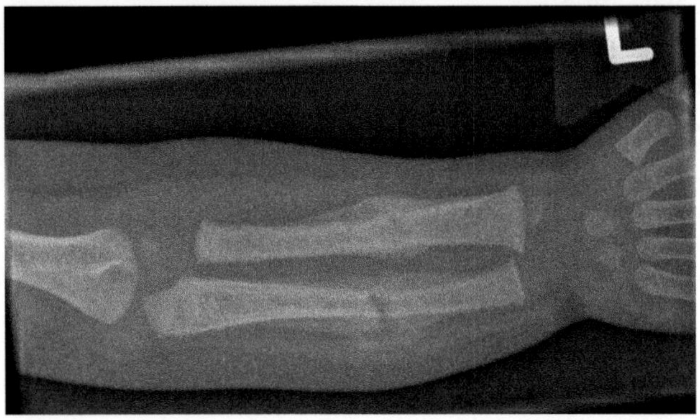

Fig. 19.9 AP forearm demonstrating healing fractures of the radius and ulna in a patient with suspected physical abuse / non-accidental injury.

with the patient's demographic details and date with correct side markers[44] placed within the primary beam at the time of the examination (Fig. 19.9). Ideally, two radiographers with training in paediatric techniques will undertake the survey. Additionally, a health professional (usually a qualified nurse) should be present to act as a witness to the proceedings and assist with any immobilisation when required.

Image Quality. Babygrams or whole body images are not acceptable under any circumstances. The imaging of the right and left lower limbs together in one exposure should also be avoided. It is vital that image quality is at the highest possible level to enable the easy detection of subtle injuries, particularly metaphyseal fractures and rib injuries.

Projections. Recommended included projections for a skeletal survey of NAI/SPA differ slightly on the age of the child (Table 19.2).[43]

Upon completion of the examination, the projections should be checked by a consultant radiologist prior to the child leaving the department. Any suspicious appearances, such as a periosteal reaction, will require additional projections. All children are required to return for follow-up surveys to enable a review of key areas within 11–14 days and no later than 28 days after their initial survey.[43] This examination should take place regardless of the initial survey findings. All skeletal surveys undertaken for suspected abuse are required to be reported by two radiologists with at least 6 months' specialist paediatric radiology training.

The use of a checklist/record is recommended, with specimen located within the RCR and SCoR guidance document.[43] It should be completed by the examining radiographer(s) to ensure that all the appropriate image checks are carried out. It may also act as a record of who was present, the types of immobilisation used (consent for this given and by whom), exposures, dose, examination room, final number of images and the radiologist reporting the skeletal survey images.

TABLE 19.2 Projections for Skeletal Survey of NAI/SPA

Area	Projection (Baby)	Projection (Older Child)
Chest	PA/AP, left and right posterior obliques (include all ribs 1–12 both sides)	
Abdomen	AP to include the entire pelvis and hips	
Hands	DP of left and right	
Forearm	AP of left and right whole arm centred on the elbow	AP of left and right
Humeri		AP of left and right
Wrist	Coned lateral of left and right	
Elbow	Coned lateral of left and right	
Whole spine	Lateral	Lateral (separate projections depending on size of child)
Skull	OF/FO and lateral projections	
Feet	DP of left and right	
Tibiae/fibulae	AP of left and right whole arm centred on the knee	AP of left and right
Femora		AP of left and right
Ankle	Coned lateral left and right	
Knee	Coned lateral left and right	

TABLE 19.3 Projections for Skeletal Survey of Skeletal Dysplasia

Area	Projection
Chest	PA/AP
Pelvis	AP
Hand	DP to include wrist for bone age assessment
Upper limb	AP of humerus and forearm
Whole spine (cervical, thoracic and lumbar regions)	AP and lateral
Skull	Lateral
Lower limb	AP of femur and tibia/fibula
Foot	DP

DYSPLASIA

Skeletal dysplasias are a heterogeneous group of over 200 disorders characterised by abnormal cartilage and bone growth. Many forms are detectable antenatally during routine ultrasound screening or at clinical examination at birth. A significant number will not become apparent until the child is older. Patients will have an abnormally structured skeleton, sometimes in conjunction with disorders of other systems, such as the VACTERL group of defects (vertebral defects, anal atresia, cardiac defects, tracheo-esophageal fistula, renal anomalies and limb abnormalities). Cases vary from the minimally affected, such as the epiphyseal dysplasias, to those with high mortality and morbidity such as osteogenesis imperfecta. Radiology plays an important role in the diagnosis and classification of skeletal dysplasias by scrutinising the child's bone density and growth plates.

Suggested projections for survey of skeletal dysplasias are demonstrated in Table 19.3.

For any projections of the long bones, both associated joints must be demonstrated to enable thorough scrutiny.

Occasionally a skeletal survey may be carried out for oncology (e.g. Langerhans cell histiocytosis) and rheumatology referrals. Image series will be as listed as in Table 19.3 with the addition of an AP of the skull.

Acknowledgement

The invaluable contribution to this chapter of Mr Jonathan Green, Superintendent Radiographer (CT), Bristol Royal Hospital for Children, University Hospitals Bristol, is gratefully acknowledged.

This chapter is dedicated with love and affection to my father, Stanley Peerless (1928–2019), a source of unwavering strength and inspiration (DJD).

References

1. Society and College of Radiographers. [homepage online] 2019. https://www.sor.org/practice/paediatrics.
2. Thukral B. Problems and preferences in pediatric imaging. *Ind J Radiol Imaging*. 2015;25(4):359–364.
3. Society and College of Radiographers. *Practice Standards for the Imaging of Children and Young People*. London: SCoR; 2009.
4. National Imaging Board. Delivering Quality Imaging Services for Children. 2009. Gateway reference 13732. [online] 2019. http://www.sor.org/sites/default/files/images/Delivering%20Quality%20Imaging%20Services%20for%20Children.pdf.
5. Harding J, Davis M. An observational study based on the interaction between the paediatric patient and the radiographer. *Radiography*. 2015;21:258–263.
6. Mathers S, Anderson H, Macdonald S. A survey of imaging services in England, Wales and Scotland. *Radiography*. 2011;17:20–27.
7. Meggitt C. *Child Development, an Lllustrated Guide: Birth to 19 Years*. 3rd ed. Harlow: Pearson Educational; 2012.
8. Bretherton I. The origins of attachment theory: John Bowlby and mary Ainsworth. *Develop Psychol*. 1992;28(5):759–775.
9. The Ionising Radiation (Medical Exposure) Regulations 2017 [IR(ME)R]. UK Statutory Instrument 2017 No. 1322. https://www.legislation.gov.uk/uksi/2017/1322/contents/made.
10. International Atomic Energy Agency. Radiation protection of children in radiology. [online] 2019. https://www.iaea.org/resources/rpop/health-professionals/radiology/children.
11. Boylan J. Image Gently® at 10 years. *J Am Coll Radiol*. 2018;15(8):1193–1195.
12. Society and College of Radiographers. Patient identification: guidance and advice. [online] 2019. https://www.sor.org/sites/default/files/document-versions/patient_identification_guidance_and_advice_1.pdf.
13. Royal College of Paediatrics and Child Health. Safeguarding children and young People: roles and competencies for healthcare staff. [online] 2011. https://www.rcpch.ac.uk/resources/safeguarding-children-young-people-roles-competencies-healthcare-staff.
14. Barrett T, Booth I. Sartorial eloquence: does it exist in the paediatrician–patient relationship? *Br Med J*. 1994;309:1710–1712.
15. Tschauner S, Marterer R, Gubitz M, et al. European Guidelines for AP/PA chest X-rays: routinely satisfiable in a paediatric radiology division? *Eur Radiol*. 2016;26(2):495–505.
16. Jones N, Palarm T, Negus I. Neonatal chest and abdominal radiation dosimetry: a comparison of two radiographic techniques. *Br J Radiol*. 2001;74(886):920–925.
17. Elloy M, Worley G, Bailey C. Foreign body inhalation: a case of mistaken identity? *J Emerg Med*. 2010;38(4):499–501.
18. Klimek P, Stranzinger E, Wolf R, et al. Trampoline related injuries in children: risk factors and radiographic findings. *World J Paediatr*. 2013;9(2):169–174.
19. Migneault D, Chang A, Choi E. Pediatric falls: are monkey bars bad news? *Cureus*. 2018;10(11):e3548.
20. Gyll C, Hardwick J. *Radiography of Children: A Guide to Good Practice*. Edinburgh: Churchill Livingstone; 2005.
21. Greenspan A. *Orthopaedic Imaging: A Practical Approach*. 5th ed. Philadelphia: Lippincott Williams & Wilkins; 2010.
22. Benson M, Fixsen J, Macnicol M, et al. *Children's Orthopaedics and Fractures*. Berlin: Springer-Verlag; 2010.
23. Eberl R, Singer G, Schalamon J, et al. Galeazzi lesions in children and adolescents: treatment and outcome. *Clin Orthop*. 2008;466(7):1705–1709.
24. Rennie L, Court-Brown CM, Mok JYQ, et al. The epidemiology of fractures in children. *Injury*. 2007;38:913–922.
25. Wheeless' Textbook of Orthopaedics Online. Radiographic evaluation: calcaneal fractures. https://www.wheelessonline.com/orthopaedics/radiographic-evaluation-calcaneal-fractures/; 2018.
26. Staheli L. *Fundamentals of Pediatric Orthopaedics*. 5th ed. Philadelphia: Lippincott Williams & Wilkins; 2015.
27. Schuh A, Whitlock K, Klein E. Management of toddler's fractures in the pediatric emergency department. *Pediatr Emerg Care*. 2016;32(7):452–454.
28. Brooks T, Friedman L, Silvis R, et al. Back pain in a pediatric emergency department: etiology and evaluation. *Pediatr Emerg Care*. 2018;34(1):e1–e6.
29. Wheeless' Textbook of Orthopaedics Online. Radiology of the pediatric cervical spine. http://www.wheelessonline.com/ortho/pediatric_c_spine; 2018.
30. Manaster B. *Diagnostic Imaging: Musculoskeletal Non-traumatic Disease*. 2nd ed. Elsevier; 2016.
31. Risser J. The iliac apophysis: an invaluable sign in the management of scoliosis. Clin Orthop. 11:111–119.
32. Cobb JR. Scoliosis– quo vadis? *J Bone Joint Surg Am*. 1958;40:507–510.
33. Mo F, Cunningham M. Pediatric scoliosis. *Curr Rev Musculoskelet Med*. 2011;4:175.
34. Institute of Physics and Engineering in Medicine. Radiation protection specialist interest group Updates. [online]. 2019. ipem.ac.uk/Members/CommitteesGroups/Science,ResearchInnovationCouncilandSIGs/RPSIGUpdates.aspx.
35. The British Institute of Radiology. Guidance on using shielding on patients for diagnostic radiology applications. [online]. 2020. https://www.bir.org.uk/media/414334/final_patient_shielding_guidance.pdf.
36. Papalia R, Torre G, Maffulli N, et al. Hip fractures in children and adolescents. *Br Med Bull*. 2019;129(1):117–128.
37. Pollet V, Percy V, Prior H. Relative risk and incidence for developmental dysplasia of the hip. *J Pediatr*. 2017;181:202–207.
38. Kannu P, Howard A. Perthes' disease. *Br Med J*. 2014;349:g5584.
39. NICE (National Institute of Health and Care Excellence). Head injury – triage, assessment, investigation and early management of head injury in infants, children and adults. Clinical guideline [CG56] 2007. https://www.nice.org.uk/guidance/CG56.
40. Murphy A, Hacking C. Modified Stenvers view. [online]. Radiopaedia.org. https://radiopaedia.org/articles/modified-stenvers-view-1?lang=us.
41. Department of Health. The Victoria Climbié Inquiry. Report of an inquiry by Lord Laming. [online] January 2003. https://www.gov.uk/government/publications/the-victoria-climbie-inquiry-report-of-an-inquiry-by-lord-laming.
42. Care Quality Commission. Care quality Commission publishes report on the NHS care of baby peter. [online] May 2009. https://www.cqc.org.uk/news/releases/care-quality-commission-publishes-report-nhs-care-baby-peter.
43. Royal College of Radiologists and Society and College of Radiographers. The radiological investigation of suspected physical abuse in children. *Ref BFCR*. 2017;17:4. https://www.rcr.ac.uk/publication/radiological-investigation-suspected-physical-abuse-children.
44. Royal College of Radiologists and Society and College of Radiographers. Imaging for non-accidental injury: use of anatomical markers. *Ref BFCR*. 2011;11:5. https://www.rcr.ac.uk/publication/imaging-non-accidental-injury-nai-use-anatomical-markers.

20 Contrast Media

SUSAN CUTLER and FIONA MACGREGOR

Contrast media are substances used to highlight areas of the body in radiographic contrast to their surrounding tissues. Contrast media enhance the optical density of the area under investigation so that the tissue/structure absorption differentials are sufficient to produce adequate contrast with adjacent structures, enabling imaging to take place. There are numerous types of radiographic contrast media used in medical imaging, each of which have different applications depending on their chemical and physical properties. When used for imaging purposes, contrast media can be administered by injection, insertion, or ingestion.

History of Radiographic Contrast Media

Radiographic contrast has been used for over a century to enhance the contrast of radiographic images. In 1896, in the year after X-rays were discovered, inspired air became the first recognised contrast agent in radiographic examinations of the chest. In 1898, the first contrast studies were carried out on the upper gastrointestinal tract of a cat using bismuth salts. These salts were very toxic and safer agents were required; by 1910 barium sulphate and bismuth solutions were being used in conjunction with the fluoroscope, barium sulphate having been used with differing additives ever since for imaging of the gastrointestinal tract.

Images of the urinary system were achieved in the early 1920s. At this time syphilis was treated with high doses of sodium iodide; during treatment the urine in the bladder was observed to be radio-opaque due to its iodine content. In 1923 the first *angiogram* and opacification of the urinary tract was performed using sodium iodide. Sodium iodide was too toxic for satisfactory intravenous use, again necessitating the need to find a less toxic iodinated compound.

The first iodine-based contrast used was a derivative of the chemical ring pyridine, to which a single iodine atom could be bound in order to render it radio-opaque. Iodine-based contrast media have been used ever since. These media, however, produced varying adverse reactions, and it was realised that a contrast agent was needed that was both safe to administer and which enhanced the contrast of the radiographic image. Modern ionic contrast agents were introduced in 1950 and were derivatives of triiodobenzoic acid; this structure enabled three atoms of iodine to be carried, rendering it more radio-opaque. However, the agents still caused adverse effects, as they were still of high osmolarity; which is explained below.

Ionic media dissociate in water; their injection into the blood plasma results in a great increase in the number of particles present in the plasma; this has the effect of displacing water. Water moves from an area of greater concentration to an area of lesser concentration by the process of osmosis, the physical process that occurs whenever there is a concentration difference across a membrane and that membrane is permeable to the diffusing substance. Osmolality (which is generally considered interchangeable with the term 'osmolarity') is defined as the number of solute particles, i.e. the contrast medium molecules, dissolved in 1 litre of water. These media exert tremendous osmotic activity on the body. The osmolality of normal human blood is around 290–300 mOsm/kg (milliosmoles per kilogram), the osmolality of ionic contrast is 5× this figure, as detailed later in this chapter.

There remained a need to find a water-soluble, iodine-based, contrast agent with reduced toxicity but which still produced satisfactory radio-opacity on images. In the 1970s and 1980s non-ionic low-osmolality contrast media (osmolality approximately 2× that of blood), became widely available; the first non-ionic contrast medium being introduced in 1974, representing a major advancement in diagnostic imaging. Most recently the non-ionic dimers have emerged, these media are highly hydrophilic, resulting in lower chemotoxicity, and they are iso-osmolar with the respective body fluids, meaning they can be used for examinations such as angiography and computed tomography (CT) arteriography, which require high doses of contrast media to be administered and where low toxicity is essential.

Requirements of the 'Ideal' Contrast Medium and Types of Contrast Agent

There is currently no contrast medium on the market that is considered to be ideal, but the ideal contrast medium should fulfil certain requirements for safe and effective application. It should be:

- Easy to administer
- Non-toxic
- A stable compound
- Concentrated in the required area when injected
- Rapidly eliminated when necessary
- Non-carcinogenic
- Of appropriate viscosity for administration
- Tolerated by the patient
- Cost-effective

Contrast media are divided into two main categories. The first is *negative* contrast media, which are radiolucent and of low atomic number, causing the part in which they are placed to be more readily penetrated by X-rays than the surrounding tissue; as they attenuate the X-ray beam less effectively than body tissue, they appear darker on the X-ray image. Gases are commonly used to produce negative contrast on radiographic images. The second type is *positive* contrast media; these are radiopaque and of a high atomic number, causing the part in which they are placed to be less readily penetrated by X-rays than the surrounding tissue. Consequently, this contrast agent-filled area appears denser than body tissue. Barium sulphate- and iodine-based solutions are used in medical imaging to produce positive contrast.

NEGATIVE CONTRAST MEDIA

The following gases create negative contrast on radiographic images:

- *Air*: Introduced by the patient during a radiographic examination, e.g. inspiration during chest radiography, *or* can be introduced by the radiographer as part of the examination in a double-contrast barium enema
- *Oxygen*: Introduced into cavities of the body, for example in the knee during arthrography to demonstrate the knee joint
- *Carbon dioxide*: Although not routinely used, carbon dioxide can be introduced into the gastrointestinal tract in conjunction with a barium sulphate solution to demonstrate the mucosal pattern. Carbon dioxide can also be introduced into the colon when performing a double-contrast barium enema. It has been recommended that carbon dioxide be used as the negative contrast agent in a double-contrast barium enema, rather than air, as it causes less immediate abdominal pain[1] as well as less post procedural pain and discomfort.[2] However, some studies have shown that carbon dioxide produces inferior distension and additional insufflations are required to maintain adequate quality distension.[3]

POSITIVE CONTRAST MEDIA

Barium and iodine solutions are used to create positive contrast on radiographic images.

Barium Sulphate Solutions ($BaSO_4$) Used in Gastrointestinal Imaging

Barium solutions were the universal contrast media used for radiographic examinations of the gastrointestinal (GI) tract for decades. Barium examinations of the GI tract have been in the main superseded by CT colonography and endoscopy.[4] The cross-sectional images generated by CT can be reformatted in multiple planes to generate detailed 3D images. The procedure is quick to perform and is generally well tolerated by patients.

On occasion barium examinations of the GI tract are still undertaken and the following characteristics make barium solutions suitable for imaging of the GI tract:

- High atomic number (56) producing good radiographic contrast
- Insoluble
- Stable
- Relatively inexpensive
- Excellent coating properties of the gastrointestinal mucosa.

Barium suspensions are composed of barium sulphate mixed with additives and dispersing agents, held in suspension in water. Compounds to stabilise the suspension are added; these act on the surface tension and increase the viscosity of the solution. A dispersing agent is added to prevent sedimentation, ensuring an even distribution of particles within the suspension. Also added to the suspension is a defoaming agent, used to prevent bubbles that may mimic pathology in the GI tract. Flavourings are usually added to oral solutions, making them more palatable for patients. There are many varieties of barium suspension available and the type used depends on the area of the GI tract being imaged. It also depends greatly upon the individual preferences of the practitioner.

Patients rarely have allergic reactions to barium sulphate but may react to the preservatives or additives in the solutions. Barium sulphate preparations are usually safe as long as the GI tract is patent and intact. A severe inflammatory reaction may develop if it is extravasated outside the GI tract; this is most likely to occur when there is perforation of the tract. If barium sulphate escapes into the peritoneal cavity, inflammation and peritonitis may occur. Escaped barium in the peritoneum causes pain and hypovolaemic shock and, despite treatment that includes fluid replacement therapy, steroids and antibiotics, there is still a 50% mortality rate; of those who survive, 30% will develop peritoneal adhesions and granulomas.[5] Aspiration of barium solutions during upper GI tract imaging is considered to be relatively harmless, most frequently affecting the elderly patient. Physiotherapy is usually required to drain the aspirated barium and should be performed before the patient leaves the department. Sedated patients should not undergo radiological examinations of the upper GI tract as their swallowing reflex may be diminished, increasing the risk of aspiration. Oral barium sulphate should not be administered in cases of obstruction as it may inspissate (congeal) behind an obstruction, compounding the patient's condition.

When preparing barium solutions for administration it is important to check expiry dates and ensure the packaging is intact. Solutions administered rectally should be administered at body temperature to improve patient tolerability and also reduce spasm of the colon. It is important that the administrator knows the patient's full medical history and checks for any contraindications prior to administration. Barium sulphate solutions are contraindicated for the following pathologies:

- Suspected perforation
- Suspected fistula
- Suspected partial or complete stenosis
- Paralytic ileus
- Haemorrhage in the gastrointestinal tract
- Toxic megacolon
- Prior to surgery or endoscopy
- If the patient has had a recent gastrointestinal wide bore biopsy (usually within 3–5 days) or recent anastomosis

When barium sulphate solutions are contraindicated for gastrointestinal imaging, a water-soluble iodine-based contrast medium (e.g. Gastrografin or Gastromiro) should be used. These can be administered orally, rectally or mechanically, e.g. via a stoma. The iodine concentration of Gastrografin is 370 mg/mL and of Gastromiro 300 mg/mL. When used for imaging the GI tract, water-soluble contrast produces a lower contrast image than barium owing to its lower atomic number.

The patient's consent must be given prior to the administration of barium contrast solutions.

The patient should be given a full explanation, be reassured about the examination and given the opportunity to ask questions. It is important when using barium sulphate solutions that associated pharmacological agents such as buscopan and glucagon, used in conjunction with barium solutions, are fully understood and the indications and contraindications ensuring their safe application adhered to.

Iodine-Based Contrast Media Used in Medical Imaging and Their Development

The largest group of contrast media used in imaging departments are the water-soluble organic preparations in which molecules of iodine are the opaque agent. These compounds contain iodine atoms (atomic number 53) bound to a carrier molecule. This holds the iodine in a stable compound and carries it to the organ under examination. The carrier molecules are organic, containing carbon, and are of low toxicity and high stability. Iodine is used as it is relatively safe and the K edge = 32 keV (binding edge of iodine K-shell electron), is close to the mean energy of diagnostic X-rays. Selection of kVp for imaging examinations using iodine-based contrast plays a part in providing optimal attenuation. The absorption edge of iodine (35 keV) predicts that 63–77 kVp is the optimal range.

Iodine-based compounds are divided into four groups (Fig. 20.1) depending on their molecular structure, as follows:

1. Ionic monomers
2. Ionic dimers
3. Non-ionic monomers
4. Non-ionic dimers

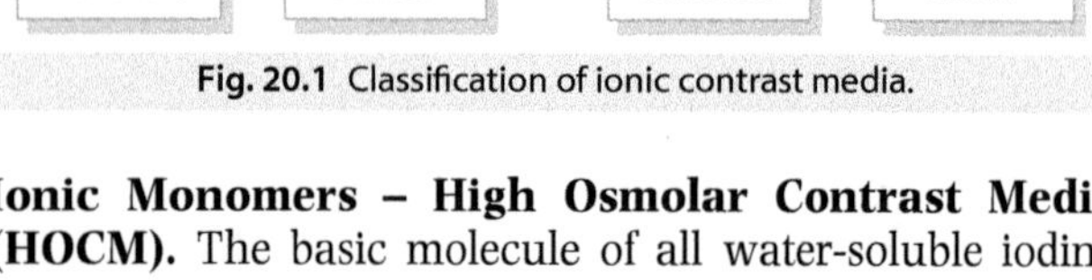

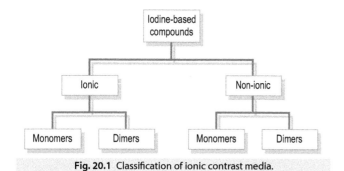

Fig. 20.1 Classification of ionic contrast media.

Ionic Monomers – High Osmolar Contrast Media (HOCM). The basic molecule of all water-soluble iodine containing contrast media is the benzene ring. Benzene itself is not water-soluble; to make it soluble, carboxyl acid (COOH) is added. Three of the hydrogens in this molecule are replaced by iodine, rendering it radioopaque, but it still remains quite toxic. The remaining two hydrogens (R_1 and R_2 in Fig. 20.2) are replaced by a short chain of hydrocarbons, making the compound less toxic and more acceptable to the body. The exact nature of these compounds differs between different contrast media, but they are usually prepared as sodium or meglumine salts as these help to provide solubility.

Ionic compounds dissociate (dissolve) into charged particles when entering a solution. They dissociate into positively charged cations and negatively charged anions. For every three iodine molecules present in ionic media, one cation and one anion are produced when it enters a solution. Their 'effect' ratio is therefore 3 : 2. These solutions are highly hypertonic, with an osmolality approximately five times higher than human plasma (1500–2000 mOsm/kg H_2O compared with 300 mOsm/kg H_2O for plasma).

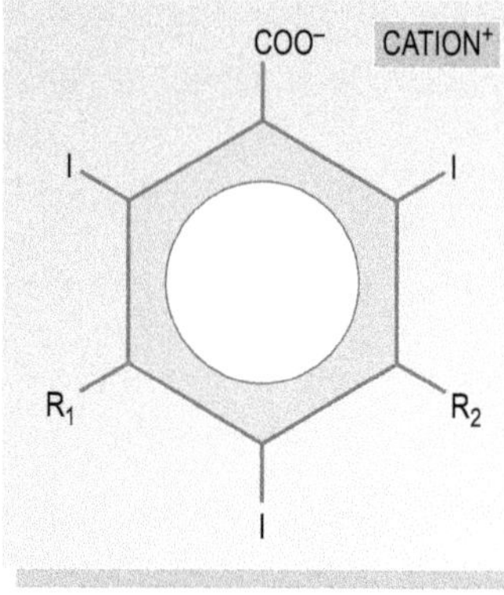

Fig. 20.2 Molecular structure of an ionic monomer (HOCM).

Ionic Dimers – Low Osmolar Contrast Media (LOCM). As contrast agents developed in the 20th century, it was acknowledged that a contrast medium with reduced osmotic effects was needed. As previously stated, the higher the 'effect' ratio the lower the osmolarity of the contrast media. An attempt was made to increase the 'effect' ratio and produce a contrast medium with lower osmolarity. This was achieved by linking together two conventional ionic contrast media molecules. The resulting dimeric ionic contrast medium was an improvement on the HOCM. Reduced osmolality (600 mOsm/kg H_2O) made the contrast more tolerable for patients. The ionic molecule still dissociates into two particles, a positive cation and a negative anion. However, there are now twice as many particles in solution with twice the osmolarity. Each molecule carried six iodines (as opposed to three in the HOCM), hence there is an iodine atom-to-particle ratio of 6 : 2; so only half the number of molecules are needed to achieve the same iodine concentration. This means a lower volume of contrast medium is therefore required for an examination. (See Fig. 20.3 for molecular structure.)

Non-ionic Monomers (LOCM). These are low osmolar agents and do not dissociate into two particles in a solution, making them more tolerable and safer to use than ionic contrast. For every three iodine molecules in a non-ionic solution, one neutral molecule is produced. Non-ionic contrast media are therefore referred to as 3 : 1 compounds. They substitute the sodium and meglumine side chains with non-ionising radicals $(OH)_n$. Two major advantages arise through the change in chemical structure: the first is that

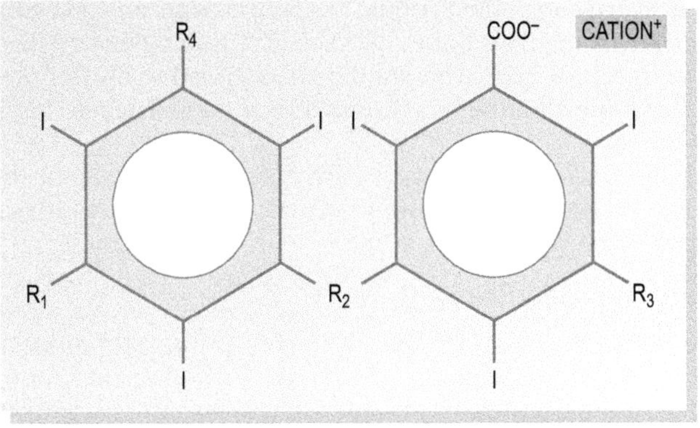

Fig. 20.3 Molecular structure of an ionic dimer (LOCM).

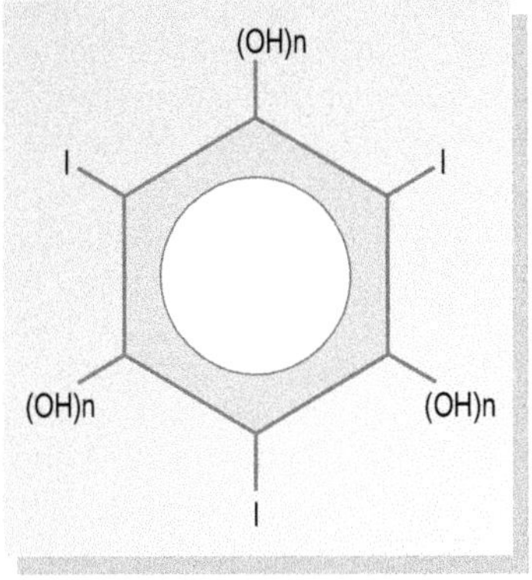

Fig. 20.4 Molecular structure of a non-ionic monomer.

the negative carboxyl group is eliminated, thereby reducing the neurotoxicity; and the second is that the elimination of the positive ion reduces osmolality to 600–700 mOsm/kg H_2O. Non-ionic LOCM is recommended for intrathecal and vascular radiological procedures. (See Fig. 20.4 for molecular structure.)

Non-ionic Dimers (Isotonic) – the Gold Standard. Clearly, a contrast agent in solution with similar osmolality to blood plasma (approximately 300 mOsm/kg H_2O) is the ideal option. Non-ionic dimers are dimeric non-dissociating molecules; for every one molecule there are six iodine atoms. The ratio is therefore 6 : 1, double that of the non-ionic monomers. An important feature of these is that they are *isotonic*. Their iso-osmolality, combined with a slower diffusion of the larger molecules across vessel walls from the vascular space, plays a significant role in imaging venous phase images following arterial injections (and arterial phase images following venous injections). These compounds represent a gold standard water-soluble iodine contrast medium. (See Fig. 20.5 for molecular structure.)

The Percentage Solution

The percentage solution indicates the amount of solute in the solvent. The percentage solution does not indicate the percentage iodine content, as demonstrated in Table 20.1.

The solvent affects the viscosity of the contrast agent. Viscosity is the resistance to flow of a contrast medium and relates to the concentration, molecular size and temperature of the contrast. The volume and density of contrast used is dependent upon the examination being undertaken, the pathology being investigated, the age of the patient and the patient's medical status.

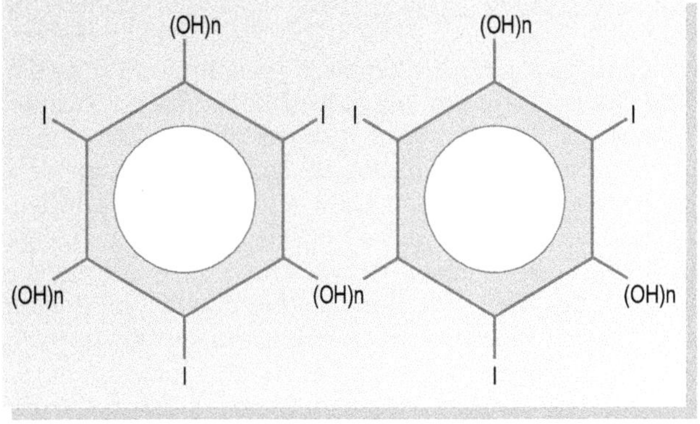

Fig. 20.5 Molecular structure of a non-ionic dimer.

TABLE 20.1 Percentage Iodine Content in Contrast Media

Contrast Media	Percentage Solution	Iodine Concentration of Solution
Urografin 370	76	370 mg/mL
Gastrografin	76	370 mg/mL
Niopam 370	75.5	370 mg/mL

Essential Criteria for the 'Ideal' Intravenous Contrast Agent

- Water-soluble
- Heat/chemical/storage stability
- Non-antigenic
- Available at the right viscosity and density
- Low viscosity, making them easy to administer
- Persistent enough in the area of interest to allow its visualisation
- Selective excretion by the patient when the examination is complete
- Same osmolarity as plasma or lower
- Non-toxic, both locally and systemically
- Low cost

Possible Side-Effects of Ionic-Based Contrast Media

Any water-soluble ionic contrast introduced into the vascular system can potentially cause physiological adverse effects. These effects are caused by the high osmolarity and chemotoxic effects of the medium. Although both ionic and non-ionic iodine media have physiological effects on the body, ionic media are of higher osmolarity and potentially cause more side-effects in the patient. Ionic contrast media have approximately five times the osmolarity of human plasma. Water-soluble organic iodine contrast media have two effects: the desirable primary effect of attenuating X-rays and providing the radiographic image with adequate contrast, and the unwanted secondary effect of inducing potential side effects in patients.

PRIMARY EFFECT – IMAGE CONTRAST

Optimum attenuation is achieved by selecting the appropriate concentration of iodine in solution for the planned examination. Two solutions with the same iodine content should provide the same iodine concentration in blood after intravenous injection. This is not the case, however, and the concentration may be affected by small molecules diffusing out of the blood vessel lumen, or by solutions of high concentration within the blood vessel drawing water out of adjacent cells by osmosis (therefore diluting the solution), as mentioned in the introduction to this chapter. To illustrate this, remembering that osmolality is defined as the number of solute particles (e.g. the contrast media molecules) dissolved in 1 litre of water, a comparison between normal blood plasma osmolality and different contrast agents is shown below:

- Normal blood plasma ~300 mOsm/kg water
- Ionic monomer ~1200–2400 mOsm/kg water, making it very hypertonic
- Ionic dimers, and non-ionic monomers and dimers (LOCM), are still hypertonic but to a much lesser degree, reducing the osmotic activity. They are, however, more expensive. Isotonic iodixanol (Visipaque) has approximately a third the osmolality of the non-ionic media and a sixth of that of the monomeric ionic media.

When comparing two contrast media with the same iodine concentration, a higher venous concentration of iodine is obtained when diffusion of contrast medium is slowed down by using large molecules (dimers) and osmotic effects are reduced by reducing the number of molecules/ions in solution (monomers).

SECONDARY EFFECT – ADVERSE EVENTS

Contrast media are specifically designed to minimise secondary effects or adverse reactions. The 'perfect' contrast agent would cause no adverse effects at all. Although reactions to contrast media are rare, it is essential that every effort is made to minimise the risk. Acute adverse reactions do occur and are defined as reactions that occur within 1 hour after administration of contrast medium. Adverse reactions to contrast media or drugs are generally classified into two categories:

- Idiosyncratic reactions are dose-dependent and usually anaphylactoid in nature. These are unpredictable, having a prevalence of 1–2% (0.04–0.22% severe), and are fatal in 1 in 170 000.[6]
- Non-idiosyncratic reactions are divided into chemotoxic and osmotoxic. Chemotoxic effects can be minimised through the use of LOCM. As LOCM are available at a reasonable cost the use of higher-toxicity substances could be challenged ethically, and medicolegally.[7] These reactions are predictable and more likely to occur in debilitated patients or those in poor medical health. They are dose-dependent and are caused primarily by osmotic effects causing shifts in fluids from the intracellular to extracellular structures, leading to cell dehydration and dysfunction.

The onset of these reactions is variable, but 70% of reactions occur within 5 minutes of injection; latest guidance states that the patient should not be left alone for the first 5 minutes and should not leave the department/observation within 15 minutes, this should be extended to 30 minutes if the patient has been assessed as being at a higher risk of reaction.[8]

Contrast media affect specific organs or systems of the body; the following is a summary of some of the major systemic effects of contrast media.

Cardiovascular Toxicity

Pain can occur at the injection site during intravascular contrast administration. Thrombus formation and endothelial damage may occur, and contrast may impair platelet aggregation and blood clotting, possibly provoking a painful sickle cell crisis. Osmotic effects of the contrast media can also cause vasodilatation with associated hot flushing. Fluid shifts, as already discussed, can produce an intravascular hypervolaemic state, systemic hypertension and pulmonary oedema. Contrast media can lower the ventricular arrhythmia threshold and precipitate cardiac arrhythmias or cause an angina attack. In rare cases this may lead to cardiac arrest, necessitating urgent medical intervention.

Nephrological Toxicity

Ionic contrast may affect renal output, causing renal impairment; this is usually temporary. Contrast-induced acute kidney injury (CI-AKI), previously known as contrast-induced nephropathy (CIN) and contrast nephrotoxicity, is defined as an impairment in renal function, resulting in an increase in serum creatinine by more than 25% from the baseline or 44 μmol/L increase in absolute value following the intravascular administration (within 48–72 hours) of contrast medium in the absence of an alternative aetiology. Although the risk factors for CI-AKI are not yet fully understood, the following conditions may increase the incidence of nephrotoxicity in patients who receive an intravascular contrast medium:

- Pre-existing kidney disease
- Diabetes mellitus
- Multiple myeloma
- Hypertension
- Dehydration
- Large volume of contrast injected
- Age of patient
- Anaemia
- Renal transplant

The risk factors associated with the procedure to be undertaken must also be considered:

- Intra-arterial administration of contrast media
- Multiple administrations of contrast media within a few days
- Large doses of contrast media administered

Nephrotoxic effects can be minimised by ensuring that the patient is hydrated and by using low or iso-osmolar contrast media. In patients with known renal impairment alternative imaging strategies need to be considered that do not require the administration of iodinated contrast media.

Special consideration must be given to diabetic patients on oral metformin (Glucophage). These patients may have associated renal impairment resulting in being more prone to developing lactic acidosis if iodine-based contrast media are administered. Advice has suggested that metformin is not recommended in diabetic patients with renal impairment.[9] Continued intake of metformin after the onset of renal failure results in a toxic accumulation and subsequent lactic acidosis. However, if serum creatinine levels are within the normal range a low volume of contrast medium (up to 100 mL) can be administered intravenously. The recommendations use eGFR as a measure, this is 'estimated glomerular filtration rate' which is mathematically derived from serum creatinine measurement. There is no need to stop metformin after contrast administration in patients with eGFR >30 (>45 for intra-arterial injection), but if eGFR is unknown or below these levels, then metformin must be withheld 48 hours before and 48 hours after the administration of the iodinated contrast media.[8] Renal function should then be assessed after contrast administration, and if it is within normal limits after 48 hours, metformin intake can be resumed. Anecdotal evidence shows that in many imaging departments *all* patients taking metformin are advised to withhold this medication for 48 hours prior to and after administration of contrast agents, it is suggested that this protocol be revisited in light of later advice.[10] It is important to be aware of Trust and hospital policies when administering contrast media as the literature regarding both iodinated and gadolinium-based contrast agents is ever-changing.

Neurotoxicity

The incidence of serious neurotoxic effects is low following the administration of intravascular contrast media; neurotoxicity of contrast media is related to the osmolality of the solution. Entry of contrast media into the central nervous system is normally limited, but may be increased by the osmotic opening of the blood–brain barrier. The blood–brain barrier provides protection for the brain by acting as a selective barrier; it regulates the amount and composition of the brain's cerebrospinal fluid, in order that exchanges across the barrier between the blood and cerebrospinal fluid, which would harm the brain, are reduced, whereas exchanges of essential substances are facilitated. Ionic media are hyperosmolar with respect to human plasma and may dehydrate the cerebral endothelial cells, causing them to dysfunction and breach the barrier, resulting in depolarisation of cerebral neurons and leading to possible seizures. Seizures are more likely to occur in patients with brain tumours, abscesses and other processes that disrupt the blood–brain barrier. Convulsions may also occur as secondary to cerebral hypoxia (caused by hypotension), cardiac arrest or anaphylaxis, which may be induced after administration of a contrast medium. Neurotoxicity can be reduced by using a low osmolar contrast medium as these are less likely to breach the blood–brain barrier.

What Happens During a Reaction and How Reactions May Be Prevented

Improvements in the chemical structure of modern contrast medium molecules have resulted in a significant reduction in the number of acute reactions. Severe reactions are a rare occurrence and previous allergic reactions to contrast material, asthma and known allergies are factors associated with an increased risk of developing a reaction. An injection of contrast medium causes the release of histamine from the basophils and mast cells in the blood. Some patients release more histamine than others, and the reason for this is still not fully understood. Another possible mechanism for reactions to contrast media is thought to be the inhibition of enzymes, e.g. cholinesterase, which deactivates and hydrolyses acetylcholine, causing symptoms of vagal overstimulation resulting in bronchospasm and cardiovascular collapse.

Patients must be assessed and past medical history ascertained before any contrast medium is administered. Any patient with a medical history that raises concern can be given prophylactic treatment to prevent potential reactions. Intravenous administration of a hydrocortisone may be given before the contrast agent to suppress inflammatory and allergic responses. This reduces the chance of allergic reactions, including anaphylaxis, renal failure or a possible life-threatening emergency. Prophylactic drugs should be administered in a separate syringe as they may cause crystallisation when they come into contact with contrast media. Serious reactions still occur, and awareness of, and treatment for, the different types of reaction is paramount for any staff member involved in intravenous administration of contrast media. Owing to the unpredictable nature of contrast reactions it is essential that appropriate resuscitation drugs are available in the examination room. In addition, professional guidelines and departmental protocols also recommend a clinician be available to deal with any potential severe reaction that may occur, if the contrast medium is being administered by a radiographer.

Non-ionic versus Ionic Contrast Media

As already discussed, ionic media dissociate in solution, altering the sodium balance in the body, whereas non-ionic media, which are made of compounds, do not dissociate in solution. Non-ionic contrast agents do not give the extra ion load that ionic contrast media do and are therefore more 'in tune' with body homeostasis and physiology. Non-ionic contrast media are usually safer to administer and better tolerated by patients. Ionic contrast is less expensive and is usually used for examinations such as cystograms, when contrast is introduced into a body cavity and not directly into the circulatory system. Non-ionic contrast is used primarily in examinations where the contrast is administered directly into the circulatory system. Advantages of non-ionic contrast media include:

- Reduction in the number of side-effects; reactions prove to be 3–10 times lower with non-ionic contrast, owing to the fact that it stimulates less histamine release
- Decreased vasodilatation, producing less alteration in the body haemodynamics and causing less damage to the vessel endothelium
- Reduced effect on the blood–brain barrier
- Improved tolerability for the patient

Administration of Intravenous Contrast Media

All personnel involved in the administration of contrast media as part of a radiological examination must be aware of the relevant legal and professional regulations; they should have the required training/qualifications, and hospital Trusts and departments should have appropriate protocols and procedures in place to ensure the safe and effective examination of all patients.

LOCM should be the medium of choice for intravenous administration, but *especially* to:

- Infants
- The elderly
- Those with cardiac or renal impairment
- Diabetics
- Patients with a history of asthma or severe allergy
- Patients with a history of a previous reaction to contrast media

If a patient presents with a history of a previous reaction to a contrast agent, there is a serious danger of producing a severe and possibly fatal reaction if the examination is undertaken. Patients with an allergy, who have previously tolerated an injection of contrast media, may have become sensitised, and great care must be taken on any subsequent examination. The referrer should evaluate the risk involved against information to be gained from the examination being undertaken, and alternative imaging modalities used if deemed more appropriate.

Use of Intravenous Contrast Media during Pregnancy and Breast Feeding

During pregnancy, iodinated or gadolinium-based agents may be used where the radiographic examination with use of intravenous contrast media is deemed absolutely essential. In the case of iodinated agents, during the first week post delivery the child will require thyroid function tests; no such tests are required after administration of gadolinium-based agents. Post administration of intravenous iodinated contrast media to a lactating mother, she may continue to breast feed normally; with gadolinium-based contrast agents as high-risk agents are generally not used in clinical practice, there is no requirement to stop but it is recommended that breast feeding cessation/continuation be at the discretion of the mother in consultation with the clinician.[11]

PRECAUTIONS TAKEN IN THE ADMINISTRATION OF CONTRAST MEDIA

Reactions to the administration of contrast medium are not predictable and all patients should be monitored closely during the procedure. The importance of assessing the patient before the procedure cannot be over emphasised. This will give the radiographer a baseline value from which to measure the patient's condition throughout the procedure. The radiographer should be familiar with the symptoms of the various adverse events that may occur. The following is a summary of general advice and precautions to be taken before, during and after the administration of an intravenous contrast medium.

Before Injection

- Know the patient and their medical history
- Reassure the patient and obtain their consent
- If the patient is a high-risk patient administer a LOCM
- Consider the following high-risk factors which are associated with the administration of intravenous contrast medium:
  - A previous severe adverse reaction to contrast medium
  - Asthma or a significant allergic history
  - Proven or suspected hypersensitivity to iodine
  - Severe renal or hepatic impairment
  - Severe cardiovascular disease
  - Epilepsy
  - Hyperthyroidism
  - Multiple myeloma
  - Pre-existing thyrotoxic symptoms
  - Severe respiratory disease
  - Diabetes
  - Sickle cell anaemia
- Check the batch number and expiry date of the contrast medium
- Ensure the contrast medium is administered at body temperature
- Check the correct contrast volume, dose and strength for the procedure being undertaken
- Check the sterility of the packaging and that the contrast agent does not contain crystals or is cloudy
- Know the procedure and be aware of the possible adverse effects that might occur
- Check emergency equipment and be familiar with its application
- Obtain a positive identification check on the patient

During the Injection

- Know where the radiologist/administering doctor may be reached
- Evaluate the patient's vital signs and observe respiration, pulse, patient colour and level of consciousness, being aware of any changes

After the Injection

- A suitably qualified person should remain with the patient for at least 15 minutes
- All relevant documentation regarding the contrast agent used should be correctly completed upon completion of any contrast administration. All relevant information regarding the contrast agent and its administration must be included in the patient's permanent medical record:
  - Contrast medium used
  - Volume administered
  - Density
  - Batch number
  - Who performed the injection
  - Any adverse effects and any treatment or drug therapy given
- In the event of any serious adverse reactions this should be reported to the manufacturing company to coordinate worldwide data collection on similar recent reactions. This ensures a global perspective
- On completion of the examination check that the patient is fit to travel home and do not allow them to leave if there is any doubt. If any concerns are identified the patient should be checked by a doctor before leaving the department

RADIOGRAPHERS PERFORMING INTRAVENOUS ADMINISTRATION OF CONTRAST MEDIA

It is well documented that the clinical role of the radiographer has been evolving rapidly in recent years. Given the drive for role expansion in radiography, it is now common practice for radiographers to administer intravenous contrast media in their clinical roles. Although these extended roles bring increased job satisfaction and responsibility for radiographers, they equally bring associated legal and professional accountability. It is paramount that radiographers undertaking this role be adequately trained and aware of the professional issues. They must operate under an agreed protocol and a written scheme of work. The employing authority should be informed in writing and be assured of the competency of any radiographer undertaking this role; it is recommended that intravenous training should lead to a nationally recognised qualification that allows transferability between employers.

Before performing any intravenous administration it is important that the radiographer is aware of the:

- Related anatomy, physiology and pathology
- Correct choice and disposal of any equipment used
- Criteria for choosing the vein, aseptic techniques
- Indications and contraindications for any contrast media used
- Potential problems that may arise, including management of adverse reactions
- Health and safety issues relating to intravenous administration

Aseptic technique must be maintained throughout the procedure. The circulation is a closed sterile system and venepuncture can provide a method of entry for pathogens into the system. Intravenous-related infection is a major cause of mortality and morbidity in hospitalised patients. A reduction in hospital-acquired infections is at the forefront of government policy, as the majority of these infections are preventable and expensive. Patients with cannulae in situ are prone to developing nosocomial infections, and as the majority of acute patients in hospital are cannulated,[12] the potential to develop an infection is high if careful technique and protocols are not observed. Any intravenous cannulation can potentially cause infection to the patient; pathogens can be transmitted from contaminated equipment such as the distal tip of the needle or cannula, hubs or connectors or from the healthcare worker's hands. All departments have a hand-washing policy that must be adhered to in order to minimise risks, as bacteria can invade the site where the needle is inserted and local infection may develop in the skin around the needle. Bacteria can also enter the blood through the vein and cause a generalised systemic infection. These potential harmful infections can be reduced by:

- Being aware of touch contamination of equipment
- Ensuring all packaging is intact before opening
- Checking expiry dates
- Choosing insertion sites carefully
- Minimal manipulation of connections
- Following handwashing procedures
- Investigating mild pyrexias that may develop and treating them immediately
- Observing and recording intravenous sites regularly

HEALTH AND SAFETY

Owing to the prevalence of blood-borne viruses it is necessary for the professional administering the contrast medium to protect themselves from any potential blood spills. Good-quality gloves should be worn when performing venepuncture; these will protect from blood spillage but will not prevent a needlestick injury. Needlestick injuries account for a high number of accidents to staff in hospitals; hepatitis B is more easily transmitted than human immunodeficiency virus (HIV), so any healthcare professional working with body fluids and performing intravenous injections should be vaccinated for hepatitis B and have their antibody levels checked as recommended. The impact for a staff member who suffers a needlestick injury can be devastating in terms of health effects, and the waiting period for results of blood tests following such injury can be psychologically traumatic.

Needlestick injuries most often occur when:

- The needle misses the cap (sheath) and accidentally enters the hand holding it
- The needle pierces the cap and enters the hand holding it
- The poorly fitting cap slips off of a recapped needle and the needle stabs the hand

As recapping can account for 25–30% of all needlestick injuries there is no substitute for careful technique when performing any venepuncture procedure. Used needles should be discarded directly into a sharps container without being re-sheathed.

Treatment of Needlestick Injuries

Campaigns targeting improved infection control, better management and staff training to reduce exposure to blood-borne pathogens can remove human error, but they cannot remove the primary risk – the needle or sharp itself.

If a needlestick injury occurs, departmental safety policy should be followed, and in any case the following steps should be followed immediately:

- Bleed the puncture site immediately
- Wash the needlestick injury site under running hot water
- Report the incident to your supervisor and occupational health department
- Seek medical treatment if necessary

INTRAVENOUS CONTRAST INJECTION

Vein Choice

The choice of vein is vital when performing an intravenous contrast injection. Painful, sore or bruised sites should be avoided as these may be irritated as a result of previous use, or they may be sclerosed. Always use veins with the largest diameter possible: these are easily palpable and have good capillary refill. If at all possible, use veins on the non-dominant side; veins that cross joints or bony prominences or have little skin cover (e.g. the wrist) should be avoided if at all possible. The area selected should have no broken skin, infection, lymphoedema, arteriovenous shunts or fistulae.

There are also some practical considerations to consider: for example, the purpose of the cannulation and the length of time the needle is to remain in situ. Always choose the injection device after assessing the condition and accessibility of the individual patient's veins. The sites of choice on the upper limb are branches of the basilic, cephalic or median cubital vein. Preference should be given to veins that are patent and healthy and are easily detectable, visually or by palpation, as already discussed.

Preparation of Injection Site

Care should be taken in preparing the site for injection. Asepsis is vital, as the skin is being broken and a foreign device introduced into the sterile circulatory system. The two major sources of microbial contamination are:

- Cross-infection from the practitioner to the patient
- Skin flora of the patient

Good hand-washing and drying techniques are essential and gloves must be worn for each patient. The skin around the injection site should be cleansed with a preparation such as isopropyl alcohol or 1% iodine. In practice, alcohol swabs are usually used, and several types are available. To reduce the risk from the patient's own flora, the area should be cleansed for at least 30 seconds and it is important that swabbing is in one direction only. Once the site is swabbed it should not be touched again and should be allowed to dry for approximately 30 seconds before insertion of the needle to facilitate coagulation of organisms ensuring disinfection. Allowing the area to dry also prevents stinging. The injection site should not be touched after disinfection.

Cannulation Insertion Technique

- Ensure all the equipment required is available prior to commencement of the procedure.
- Approach the patient in a confident manner and explain the procedure; ensure that the patient is comfortable and is aware of the procedure – this reduces anxiety
- Allow the patient to ask questions
- Obtain consent
- Ascertain medical history and check allergies
- Support the chosen limb on a pad
- Apply a tourniquet to the upper arm on the chosen side to assess the injection site (tourniquets and pads are potentially a mechanism for cross-infection that staff need to be aware of). The patient may assist by clenching and unclenching their fist
- Select a vein using the criteria already discussed
- Wash and dry hands
- Put on gloves
- Clean the skin carefully for at least 30 seconds using the appropriate preparation. Do not palpate the vein or touch the skin after cleansing
- Anchor the vein by applying manual traction to the skin a few centimetres below the chosen injection site
- Insert the cannula ('Venflon') smoothly at a 20–30° angle; look out for blood flashback into the chamber of the cannula and then advance the cannula 2–3 mm slowly. Next withdraw the needle 5–10 mm so that it does not go through the wall of the vein, and then advance the plastic cannula along the vein
- Remove the needle and dispose of it correctly
- Do not attempt repeated insertions with the same cannula. If the first insertion is not successful the procedure should be repeated with a new cannula
- Release the tourniquet
- A saline 0.9% flush is then undertaken through the cannula. Fluid from a saline bottle is drawn into the syringe and air bubbles within the syringe removed
- Inject the contrast medium. The cannula should stay in situ until completion of the examination
- Place a sterile cotton wool ball over the site to remove the needle
- Apply pressure to the site after the cannula has been removed and continue to apply pressure for approximately 1 minute until bleeding has stopped
- Ensure the patient has no allergy to plasters; inspect the injection site before firmly applying a dressing
- Discard waste in the correct manner
- Remove gloves and wash hands

TREATMENT OF ADVERSE REACTIONS TO INTRAVENOUS CONTRAST MEDIA

It has already been stated that all patients must be kept under constant observation during and after contrast medium administration and emergency drugs and oxygen should be available. Staff working in the area should be trained in cardiopulmonary resuscitation and know how to initiate an emergency call. Before initiating any treatment, the severity of the event should be carefully evaluated; this ensures the appropriate treatment can be given. Reactions to intravenous administration of contrast media can be classified into three categories – mild, moderate and severe.

Mild Reaction

Mild reactions simply require careful observation of the patient. Most of the symptoms will pass within a few minutes. It has been suggested that a great many mild adverse effects are the result of the patient's fear and apprehension.[13] Mild adverse reactions are encountered in as many as 15% of patients after administration of intravenous ionic HOCM and up to 3% of patients after non-ionic LOCM.

Signs and symptoms of a mild reaction include:

- Nausea
- A warm feeling that may be associated with hot flushing
- Sneezing
- Rhinorrhoea
- A metallic taste in the mouth
- Headache
- Pallor
- Pruritus (itching)
- Diaphoresis (sweating)

Treatment of mild reactions usually only involves observation of the patient and reassurance. Usually no medical treatment is required and the reaction does not interfere significantly with the examination procedure being undertaken.

Moderate Reaction

This is a more severe reaction in which medical treatment is necessary and/or where the examination procedure is delayed or otherwise affected. Signs and symptoms of a moderate reaction include:

- Erythema
- Urticaria
- Pruritus
- Chest pain
- Abdominal pain
- Vasovagal syncope
- Facial swelling due to oedema

Treatment of a moderate reaction may vary. Compression and tight clothing should be released and the patient reassured. The patient will need to be seen by a clinician, and the adverse reaction should be documented in the patient's permanent medical record. All documentation should be completed according to department protocols. Drug therapy may be required, such as antihistamine (e.g. Piriton 10 mg) intravenously, or adrenaline (epinephrine) 0.5 mL 1:1000 solution subcutaneously, to reduce the symptoms.

Severe Reaction

Seek medical advice immediately; medical treatment with hospitalisation is necessary. The examination is terminated. The management of severe adverse reactions, including drug treatments, should be handled by the resuscitation team.[14] Signs, symptoms and effects of a severe reaction may include:

- Paralysis
- Seizures
- Pulmonary oedema
- Bronchospasm
- Laryngeal oedema
- Anaphylactic shock
- Respiratory arrest
- Cardiac arrest

It is important that the radiographer recognises the significance of certain signs:

- *Pulmonary oedema*: dyspnoea and cyanosis; the patient develops a cough with white frothy sputum, accompanied by dyspnoea
- *Anaphylactic shock*: dramatic onset; pallor, sweating, nausea, syncope. A weak pulse due to hypotension, bradycardia or tachycardia may be observed. In severe cases cardiac arrest may occur[15]
- *Cardiac arrest*: dramatic onset; absence of palpable pulse, dilated pupils, pallor, cyanosis
- *Respiratory arrest*: abrupt onset of cyanosis with cessation of breathing
- *Cerebral oedema*: the accumulation of excessive fluid in the substance of the brain leading to convulsions and possible coma

Administration of oxygen by mask (6–10 L/min) is vital and should be performed as soon as possible when a severe reaction occurs, as hypoxia may develop. Severe reactions require immediate recognition and evaluation of the patient's cardiopulmonary status. Cardiopulmonary resuscitation (CPR) equipment should be readily available in any area where contrast media are used. The radiographer should be trained in the techniques of CPR. Treatment of a severe reaction should follow the 'ABCD system':

Airway open
Breathing restored
Circulation maintained
Drug and definitive therapy

Contrast media should never be injected by anyone unfamiliar with resuscitation procedures. Radiology staff and management should continually review departmental protocols to ensure all staff are aware and are able to carry out their roles should an event occur.

Other Potential Complications

Any patient who undergoes intravenous cannulation has the potential to develop any of the following complications. Some are preventable, others are not:

- Infection
- Phlebitis and thrombophlebitis
- Emboli
- Vasovagal response
- Pain
- Haematoma/haemorrhage
- Extravasation
- Unintended arterial cannulation
- Allergy

Tissue damage from extravasation of contrast material is caused by the direct toxic effect of the agent. The contrast is usually absorbed fairly quickly; cream such as Lasonil, which is anti-inflammatory, can be applied to the injection site to aid the process. Compartment syndrome may occur if enough contrast material leaks into surrounding tissue. Compartment syndrome occurs when swelling takes place within a compartment of a limb and increases pressure on arteries, veins and nerves. In addition to causing extreme pain, this may lead to impaired blood flow and muscle and nerve damage. Compartment syndrome is a medical emergency requiring immediate treatment to prevent tissue death and/or permanent dysfunction.

Arterial Administration of Contrast Media

In arteriography, a contrast medium is introduced via a catheter into an artery, rendering the lumen of the vessel opaque to X-rays. As the contrast is delivered as a bolus under high pressure, a pressure injector is usually used for administration. In angiography the femoral artery is the most frequent approach to the arterial system, using the Seldinger technique. Low osmolar contrast media should be used for all angiographic studies and isotonic contrast is recommended as it has improved tolerability for patients when high doses are administered. The quantity and strength of the contrast used is dependent upon the area of the vascular system being investigated.

Magnetic resonance angiography (MRA) is an emerging modality that examines blood vessels, using magnetic resonance imaging (MRI) technology to detect, diagnose and aid the treatment of heart disorders, stroke and vascular disease. MRA can provide detailed images of blood vessels without using any contrast medium, although contrast may be administered if necessary to enhance image quality, as discussed later in the chapter.

Use of Contrast Media in Other Examinations

Contrast Media in Biliary and Hepatic Imaging

Contrast examinations of the biliary system are very rarely undertaken, having been superseded by cross-sectional imaging techniques such as CT, MRI and ultrasound.

Endoscopic Retrograde Cholangiopancreatography (ERCP)

This examination is a collaborative technique undertaken by an endoscopist but requires radiological screening and imaging. After the endoscope has been introduced, the ampulla of Vater is located and the contrast introduced. Low-density water-soluble contrast is used to prevent any calculi that may be present in the biliary system being obscured. Strictures can be accurately identified and, if required, interventional procedures such as stenting or stone removal can be performed. Other biliary examinations requiring contrast media are listed in Table 20.2.

Magnetic resonance cholangiopancreatography (MRCP) has superseded ERCP as it is not invasive and does not require the use of a contrast agent.

IODISED OILS AS A CONTRAST MEDIUM

These are used very infrequently in the imaging department today. The examinations that use these contrast media have in the main been superseded by cross-sectional imaging modalities. They are used in examinations where water-soluble agents are contraindicated or where a viscous compound is required:

- Sialography 0.5–2 mL of Lipiodol per side
- Dacrocystography 0.5–2 mL of Lipiodol per side

These contrast agents are not easily absorbed and in some cases may carry a risk of oil embolus.

Table 10.3 gives details of other radiographic examinations that make use of contrast media.

CONTRAST MEDIA USED IN ULTRASOUND

Contrast agents can improve the image quality of sonography, either by reducing the reflectivity of undesired interfaces or by increasing the back scattered echoes from the desired regions. Use of contrast media in ultrasound has been well established for cardiac imaging since the 1980s, for example, air being used to demonstrate atrial septal defects. Blood was taken from the patient, shaken to introduce air bubbles and then reinjected and imaged. The problem with this technique was the reproducibility and homogeneity of the contrast effect owing to variations in bubble size. This led to the development and manufacture of specialised products, e.g. Echovist; an echo-rich

TABLE 20.2 Contrast Media Used in the Biliary System

Examination	Contrast Media	Rationale for Use
Preoperative cholangiography	HOCM or LOCM 150 5 mL and then 20 mL usually used	Low iodine content to avoid obscuring any stones
Postoperative cholangiography (T-tube)	HOCM or LOCM 150 approx. 20–30 mL	Low iodine content to avoid obscuring any stones
Percutaneous transhepatic cholangiography	LOCM 150 20–60 mL	Low iodine content to avoid obscuring any stones
Biliary drainage	LOCM 200 20–60 mL	Low iodine content to avoid obscuring any stones

TABLE 20.3 Contrast Media Used in Other Examinations

Examination	Contrast Media, Dose, Strength and Volume	Comments
Hysterosalpingography	HOCM or LOCM 10–20 mL	LOCM has no advantage. Using non-ionic dimers is associated with decreased procedural and delayed pain[8]
Contrast venography	Approx. 30 mL LOCM	Use to image possible deep vein thromboses. It is invasive and is dependent upon cannulation of a vein often in a swollen foot
Arthrography	4–10 mL HOCM or LOCM. Air or oxygen can also be used to create a double contrast image	Volume of contrast used dependent upon joint under investigation
Cystography and micturating cystourethrography	HOCM or LOCM can be used	Volume used dependent upon the size of the structure and also patient tolerance
Renal imaging including retrogrades, nephrostomy, percutaneous nephrolithotomy	LOCM is frequently used	IVU: 50 mL 370 mg/mL standard for adult.[4] Other areas: volume dependent upon anatomical area. HOCM can be used dependent upon radiologist

microbubble, microparticle suspension. The gas microbubbles reflect ultrasound almost totally, resulting in a strong echo enhancement.[16] The use of contrast media in abdominal ultrasound is still in its infancy; it is particularly useful in demonstrating portal vein thrombosis, alleviating the need for conventional, more invasive angiographic examinations. Also, intravenous vascular contrast agents can aid the imaging of malignant tumours in the liver, kidney, ovary, pancreas, prostate and breast. Tumour angiogenesis and Doppler signals from small tumour vessels may be detectable after an injection of contrast medium. As already discussed, however, these contrast media can cause adverse reactions.

CONTRAST MEDIA USED IN MRI

MRI generates high natural contrast in images but contrast media may still be used to improve tissue characterisation, image quality as well as the sensitivity and specificity of abnormalities and pathologies identified. In some brain pathologies little difference exists in signal intensity between healthy and diseased tissue, hence the need for a contrast medium to enhance image quality. The most common agent used is gadolinium, a rare earth metal and a paramagnetic agent, enabling it to provide contrast between the lesion or pathology and the surrounding tissue by shortening the T1 relaxation time. Clinical indications for MRI contrast are discussed in Chapter 27.

Gadolinium has to be chelated with diethylenetriamine penta-acetic acid, as free gadolinium ions are highly toxic. It is hydrophilic, having very low lipid solubility, and so does not cross the blood–brain barrier, however recent evidence has shown that small quantities of gadolinium can be deposited in the brain, no ill effects have been seen but this has led to recommendations by the European Medicines Agency (EMA), suspending the use of some formulations of gadolinium contrast agent, and restricting the use of others.[17]

Nephrogenic Systemic Fibrosis

Gadolinium has had a relatively favourable safety profile, but research has identified that, rarely, patients can develop nephrogenic systemic fibrosis (NSF) with clinical symptoms developing anywhere from day of administration to several years post exposure to gadolinium. NSF is a rare multisystemic fibrosing disorder that mainly affects the skin, but may affect other organs in patients with renal insufficiency. Links have been made in the literature between the administration of gadolinium and NSF.[18] Together with the concerns mentioned above changes in both the agents used and screening of patients prior to contrast administration have been introduced,[11] including the use of eGFR checks prior to administration of gadolinium agents in a similar fashion to those previously discussed for iodinated media earlier in this chapter. Details of both withdrawal of marketing authorisation, and recommended use of the remaining gadolinium-based agents can be found via both EMA and RCR guidance publications.[11]

CONTRAST MEDIA USED IN CT

Contrast media are used to enhance the quality of images produced during CT examinations. The contraindications, which have already been discussed, apply to the use of contrast in these examinations. Contrast media for CT examinations are administered in four different ways:

- Intravenous injection
- Oral administration
- Rectal administration
- Inhalation: This is a relatively uncommon procedure in which xenon gas is inhaled for a highly specialised form of lung or brain imaging. The technique, xenon CT, is only available at a small number of locations worldwide and is used only for rare cases.

Almost all CT examinations of the abdomen and pelvis require the administration of oral contrast agents to opacify the gastrointestinal tract. Good bowel opacification helps differentiate between the lymph nodes, tumour masses and unopacified loops of bowel. Contrast enhancement in CT scanning of the abdomen and pelvis requires the patient to ingest oral contrast medium; either a dilute barium sulphate solution or alternatively an oral water soluble iodine-based contrast medium, e.g. Gastrografin. Patients usually need to drink at least 1000–1500 mL to fill the stomach and intestines sufficiently. Scanning is usually performed 1 hour after drinking the contrast to allow time for it to pass into the intestine. Although this may seem inconvenient, the oral contrast makes an essential improvement in the quality of the CT study and results in a more accurate diagnosis by providing delineation of low contrast structures. Contrast can be administered rectally to help distinguish anatomical areas in the lower abdomen.

Water can be used as a negative agent, which is useful for assessment of carcinoma of the stomach. Another approach to negative contrast is, when scanning a female pelvis, to place a tampon in the vagina, which allows radiolucent air to distend the vagina, creating additional contrast between the reproductive organs. Air is used in CT colonoscopy for contrast purposes and to distend the bowel to unfold the mucosa; this procedure produces 3D images of the entire colonic mucosa similar to those obtained during colonoscopy. Additional information on CT colonoscopy is found Chapter 21.

Non-ionic water-soluble isotonic contrast agents are used in CT to highlight blood vessels and to enhance the tissue structure of various organs such as the brain, spine, liver and kidneys. CT angiography has developed rapidly and increased greatly since the early to mid-1990s, and most UK imaging departments undertake CT angiography as an adjunct to axial scanning. With CT contrast examinations the ability to time image acquisition to coincide with peak contrast enhancement was in the past a challenge for practitioners working in this imaging modality. The use of a pressure injector, coupled with current CT software, addresses this issue while ensuring that the radiographer is distanced from the CT scanner during exposure. As previously discussed the requirements for eGFR apply for the administration of iodinated contrast in CT as elsewhere in imaging, however the potential for costly cancellations of appointments and delays to patient treatment has been identified as a particular potential problem for outpatient CT appointments in particular. This has led to investigation of point of care creatinine testing being carried out by the National Institute for Health and Care Excellence (NICE).[19,20]

References

1. Farrow R, Stevenson GW. In: Armstrong P, Waistie ML, eds. *A Concise Textbook of Radiology*. London: Arnold; 2001.
2. Farrow R, Jones AM, Wallace DA, et al. Air versus carbon dioxide insufflation in double contrast barium enemas: the role of active gaseous drainage. *Br J Radiol*. 1995;68:838–840.
3. Holemans JA. A comparison of air, carbon dioxide and air/carbon dioxide mixture as insufflations agents for double contrast barium enemas. *Eur Radiol*. 1998;8:274–276.
4. Pickhardt PJ, Kim DH. CT colonography: pitfalls in interpretation. *Radiol Clin North Am*. 2013;51(1):69–88.
5. Chapman S, Nakielny R. *A Guide to Radiological Procedures*. 5th ed. London: Saunders; 2009.
6. Lalli AF. Urographic contrast media reactions and anxiety. *Radiology*. 1974;112:267–271.
7. Bush WH, Albright DE, Sather JS. Malpractice issues and contrast use. *J Am Coll Radiol*. 2005;2005(4):344–347.
8. Royal Australian and New Zealand College of Radiologists. *Iodinated Contrast media Guideline*. Sydney: the Royal Australian and New Zealand College of Radiologists; 2018.
9. Royal College of Radiologists. *Standards for Intravascular Contrast Agent Administration to Adult Patients*. 2nd ed. London: RCR; 2011.
10. Royal College of Radiologists. *Standards for Intravascular Contrast Agent Administration to Adult Patients*. 3rd ed. London: RCR; 2015.
11. Royal College of Radiologists. *Guidance on Gadolinium-Based Contrast Agent Administration to Adult Patients*. London: RCR; 2019.
12. Stuart RL, Cameron D, Scott C, et al. Peripheral intravenous catheter-associated *Staphylococcus aureus* bacteraemia: more than 5 years of prospective data from two tertiary health services. *Med J Aust*. 2013;198(10):551–553.
13. Lalli AF. Urographic contrast media reactions and anxiety. *Radiology*. 1974;112:267–271.
14. Thomsen HS, Morcos SK. Management of adverse reactions to contrast media. *Eur Radiol*. 2004;14(3):476–481.
15. O'Neil JM, Bride KDM. Cardiopulmonary resuscitation and contrast media reactions in a radiology department. *Clin Radiol*. 2001;56(4):321–325.
16. Harvey CJ, Blomley M, Eckersley R, et al. Developments in ultrasound contrast media. *Eur Radiol*. 2001;11(4):675–689.
17. European Medicines Agency. *EMA's Final Opinion Confirms Restrictions on Use of Linear Gadolinium Agents in Body Scans*. European Medicines Agency; 2017. EMA/635217/2017.
18. Markmann P, Skov L, Rossen K, et al. Nephrogenic systemic fibrosis: suspected causative role of gadodiamide used for contrast-enhanced magnetic resonance imaging. *J Am Soc Nephrol*. 2006;17(9):2359–2362.
19. Nixon F, Albrow R. *Point-of-care Creatinine Tests to Assess Kidney Function before Administering Intravenous Contrast for Computed Tomography (CT) Imaging*. London: National Institute for Health and Care Excellence; 2018.
20. NICE (National Institute for Health and Care Excellence). *Point-of-care Creatinine Devices to Assess Kidney Function before CT Imaging with Intravenous Contrast*. Diagnostics guidance [DG37]; 2019. https://www.nice.org.uk/guidance/dg37.

21 Gastrointestinal Imaging

MICHAEL SMITH, SUE RIMES, KELLEY OCHILTREE, LISA BROWN, GEORGIA WILLMOTT and DARREN WOOD†

Radiological examination of the gastrointestinal (GI) tract was originally undertaken using fluoroscopy, with barium sulphate suspension and gas as contrast agents to provide a double-contrast study. Accessory organs of the tract have traditionally been examined using iodine-based contrast agents. However, in the rapidly changing field of medical imaging, the development of faster image acquisition, higher resolution, better computing power and improvements in post processing software, we now see the tract examined by a variety of methods, some of which supersede conventional contrast radiography.[1,2] Advances in the technology of multidetector computed tomography (CT) systems have increased the use of CT for diagnosis in the small bowel.[3] CT enterography and magnetic resonance (MR) enterography are now considered to be more accurate in defining the extent and severity of small bowel inflammation, identifying neoplasms and detecting extraluminal pathology. Capsule endoscopy is another imaging modality used to examine the GI tract. It is highly sensitive but has a lower specificity, and there is also the risk of capsule retention.[4–6] Computed tomography colonography (CTC) is now the radiological imaging of choice when looking at the large bowel.[7] In addition, endoscopic ultrasound is used by some centres to examine the lining of the upper GI tract and adjacent organs such as the biliary system, lymph nodes and pancreas. It is also possible to carry out interventions such as biopsy, stent insertion and drug therapies at the same time.[8,9] Positron emission tomography (PET) or combined PET/CT scanning is also used to diagnose and monitor GI tract malignancy.[9,10] Often these newer imaging techniques are undertaken in addition to barium studies. The demand for videofluoroscopy or the 'modified barium swallow' is increasing, due in part to NICE guidance on the management of dysphagia as part of the rehabilitation of stroke patients.[11] Another growth area in GI imaging is in the management of bariatric patients who have surgery or gastric band placement for weight loss management. As a result of this growth, imaging for these examinations is included in this text for the first time.

Besides examination of the tract itself, other contrast-enhanced X-ray imaging procedures provide studies of the abdominal region, namely angiography and arteriography. Angiography is an injectable contrast agent-based technique used to provide a 'road map' that shows the arterial or venous supply to the entire abdominal cavity. Arteriography is mainly used to assess tumour resectability or demonstrate suspected GI haemorrhage. The superior mesenteric artery, inferior mesenteric artery and coeliac axis are filled with a contrast agent in order to show the entire region. Venography can be used in assessment of the portal venous system and is generally used for preoperative demonstration of varices. The use of CT and MR angiography and Doppler ultrasound has negated the need for these procedures in most circumstances.

Notes on Position Terminology for Fluoroscopic Examination

In the UK, positioning terminology has tended to describe positions in relation to the image receptor (IR). This concept is generally easily understood when the traditional position of the IR is described (e.g. under the examination table) but can become confusing when over-couch IRs are used; fluoroscopic units often fall into this category. Further confusion occurs when it is realised that fluoroscopy units may have over- or under-couch IRs; this then makes it even more difficult for an author to ensure that their readers fully understand position descriptions.

For example, if a patient is initially supine on a *conventional radiography examination table* (*over-couch tube, under-couch IR*) and their right side is then raised, the position is described as a left posterior oblique (LPO), as the patient is oblique with the posterior aspect of their trunk still in contact with the table-top (Fig. 21.1); on a *fluoroscopy table* with *under-couch tube* and *over-couch IR*, this same body position is usually described as a right anterior oblique (RAO) as the right anterior aspect of the body is nearest the IR. Simpler projections such as anteroposterior (AP) change to postero-anterior (PA) with over-couch receptor and under-couch tube. Students in particular become very confused by this, and many radiographers resort to describing the positions as 'right side raised' or 'left side raised' to avoid confusion.

For the purpose of this chapter and to avoid this confusion, the authors have decided to use the *traditional under-couch IR and over-couch tube descriptor*, identical to that used for general under-couch IR, over-couch tube radiography. Figure 21.1 identifies the positions in full. We hope that this proves less confusing than using the traditional fluoroscopy description technique.

Upper GI Tract

The upper GI tract consists of the oropharynx, hypopharynx, oesophagus, stomach and first part of the duodenum (for a general appraisal of the layout of this part of the GI tract see Fig. 21.2). The aim of a contrast examination is to outline these structures in single and/or double contrast to obtain optimum visualisation. The most common contrast

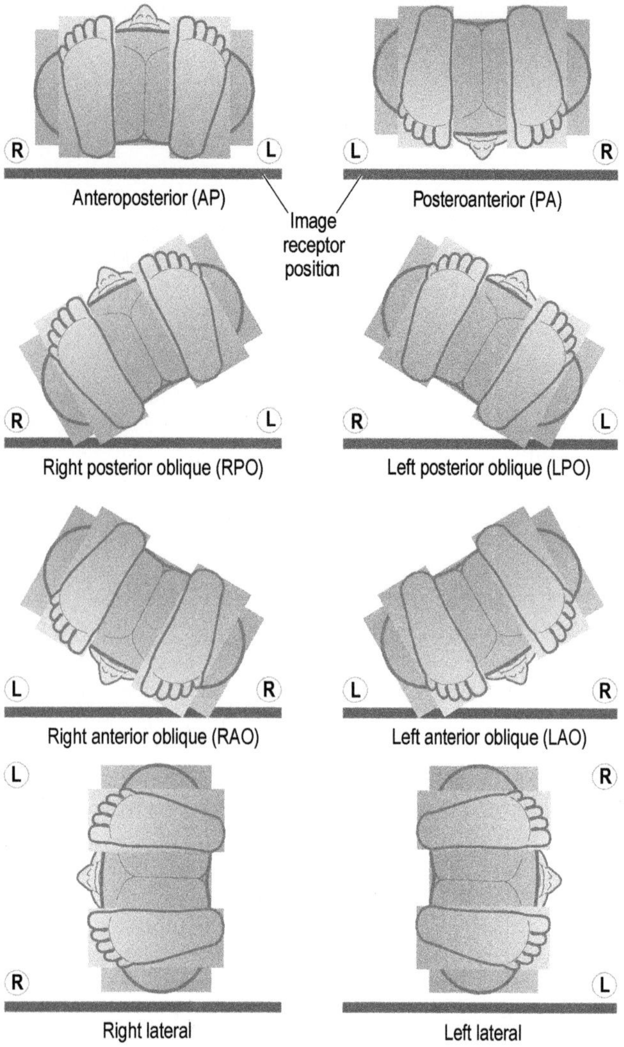

Fig. 21.1 Positioning descriptions for use in this chapter.

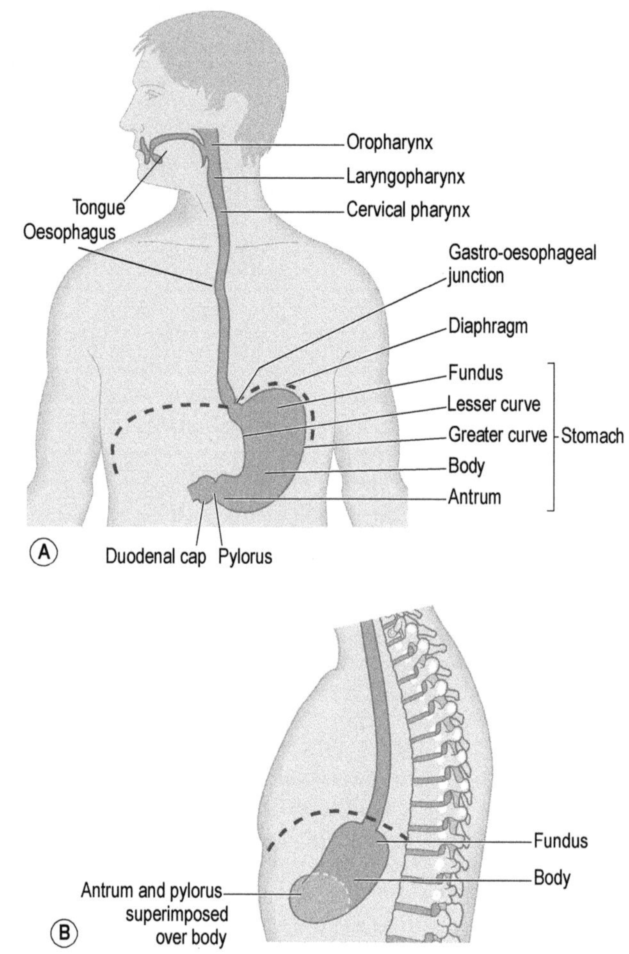

Fig. 21.2 (A) Upper GI tract – diagrammatic representation from AP view; (B) position of stomach – lateral view from left.

agent used is a barium sulphate suspension, although ionic and non-ionic contrast agents can be used.

Most patients who have upper GI symptoms are referred primarily for oesophago-gastro-duodenoscopy (OGD), but this may be used in conjunction with other tests so that a 'gold standard' approach is applied.[12] For some symptoms there is, as yet, no acknowledged standalone gold standard.[13] There are, however, sometimes reasons why contrast-enhanced X-ray studies are required: for example, when patients cannot tolerate an OGD due to medical constraints; when patients simply refuse an OGD procedure; or when their symptoms persist after OGD results are found to be negative. Contrast examinations are the examination of choice in suspected cases of high dysphagia (above the sternal notch) and when motility issues such as achalasia are suspected.[14]

REFERRAL CRITERIA FOR EXAMINATION OF THE UPPER GI TRACT

Barium Swallow

- Sensation of 'lump in throat' (globus)
- Regurgitation of unaltered food
- Dysphagia
- Gastro-oesophageal reflux (GOR)
- Assessment of oesophageal perforation (water-soluble contrast must be used)
- Known hiatus hernia – anatomical roadmap required prior to surgery
- Assessment of anatomy prior to stent placement
- Patient refuses OGD

Barium Meal

- Anaemia
- Suspected carcinoma
- Upper abdominal mass
- Normal OGD but persistent symptoms of dyspepsia, weight loss, recurrent vomiting or epigastric pain
- Patient refuses OGD
- Assess transit to small bowel postoperatively
- Anastomosis check postoperatively

PATIENT PREPARATION – ALL EXAMINATIONS OF THE UPPER GI TRACT

The patient should be starved for at least 6 hours before the examination,[15] but 5 hours has been considered adequate.[16] It is suggested that this should be the case even if only a barium swallow is indicated, in case views of the stomach are found to be required; this avoids the patient having to return for a second examination. However, medications must be taken as normal. This is because some diseases affect the swallowing process and effective medication often improves the mechanism of swallowing. One example of this is in the case of Parkinson's disease. If drug therapy is suspended, swallowing may be compromised, resulting in inadequate imaging of the swallowing process.

- The patient should cease smoking for 6 hours. Smoking can increase the amount of stomach secretions, which can prevent the barium sulphate from coating the stomach mucosa adequately
- All jewellery or artefacts (e.g. hearing aids) should be removed
- Patient clothing should be removed and a radiolucent gown should be worn
- The patient should then be informed of the procedure (they should have received information with their appointment prior to attending) so they can give their consent
- Compliance with preparation instructions should be checked

BARIUM SWALLOW AND MEAL

Historically, this examination has been carried out on patients as a complete examination. With the development of radiographer-led procedures there is a move towards giving a direct answer to a set of clinical indications and questions and so tailoring the examination to fit this need. The barium swallow and meal can therefore reasonably be split into two discrete procedures when the clinical picture has a definite direction.

BARIUM SWALLOW

This examination is used for patients who have high dysphagia or definite oesophageal symptoms, or quite often have had a normal OGD but are still symptomatic; often a motility disorder may be the cause.

A barium swallow examination will include images of the oropharynx, pharynx, oesophagus and stomach and will assess for structural and motility abnormalities.

Contraindications

- Known aspiration during ingestion (although this can be overcome by using non-ionic water-soluble contrast)
- Gastrografin should be avoided due to risk of chemical pneumonia; its use should also be avoided in cases of bronco-oesophageal fistula
- Suspected perforation

Contrast Agent

- Barium sulphate suspension 250% w/v[15,16] or water-soluble contrast medium

Additional Equipment

- Disposable cup
- Straw for prone swallow reflux assessment
- Tissues

Technique

The initial imaging should always be a lateral view of the pharynx. The technique described assumes the patient is mobile and able to follow instructions. If not, the technique should be modified and fortunately most fluoroscopy equipment can be positioned to compensate for a patient who struggles to comply.

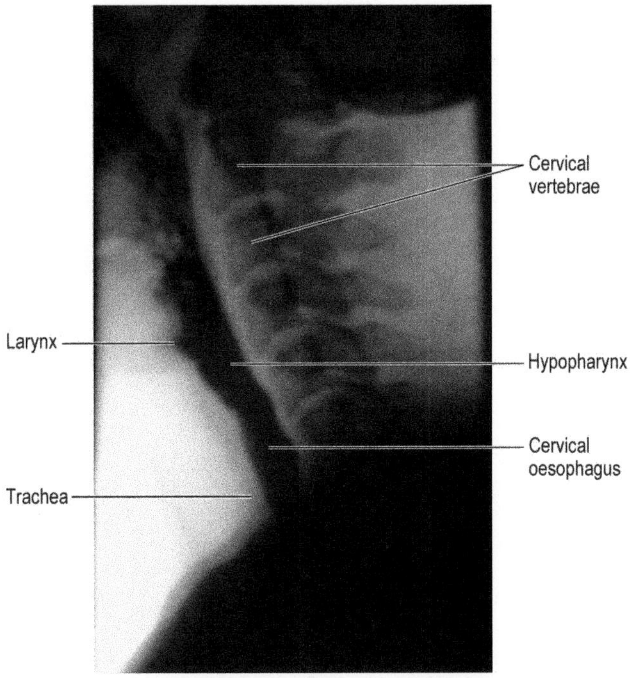

Fig. 21.3 Lateral view of hypopharynx and cervical oesophagus.

If there is any query that the patient may aspirate the contrast agent, the initial swallow is best carried out using a water-soluble contrast, although aspiration of barium sulphate has been considered by some to be relatively harmless.[16] Aspiration may not be suspected but unsuspected 'silent aspiration' may be found. Otherwise use the following technique (ensure that you have understood the notes on fluoroscopic examination positioning descriptors earlier in this chapter before considering technique descriptors):

- The patient is initially asked to stand erect in the AP position on the fluoroscopic table and hold the cup of barium sulphate in their hand, usually the left, as further turning of the patient is usually to the left. The arm will then lie clear of the trunk, without the patient having to negotiate its movement around the intensifying screen carriage.
- The patient is turned into the left lateral position in order to commence with routine assessment of possible aspiration. They are asked to take a 'normal' (for them) mouthful of the liquid and hold it in their mouth until asked to swallow. This is to give the practitioner a chance to centre on the area of interest, the pharynx, and optimise the collimation. This view allows the posterior wall of the hypopharynx to be optimally viewed (Fig. 21.3). It also clearly shows the larynx and trachea, thereby allowing demonstration of laryngeal penetration and/or aspiration should it occur
- If the radiographic equipment allows, a fluoroscopy pulse rate or digital spot image frame rate (DSI) of 3 per second is suggested as an initial choice. The pulse rate is the number of pulses per second selected for fluoroscopy.

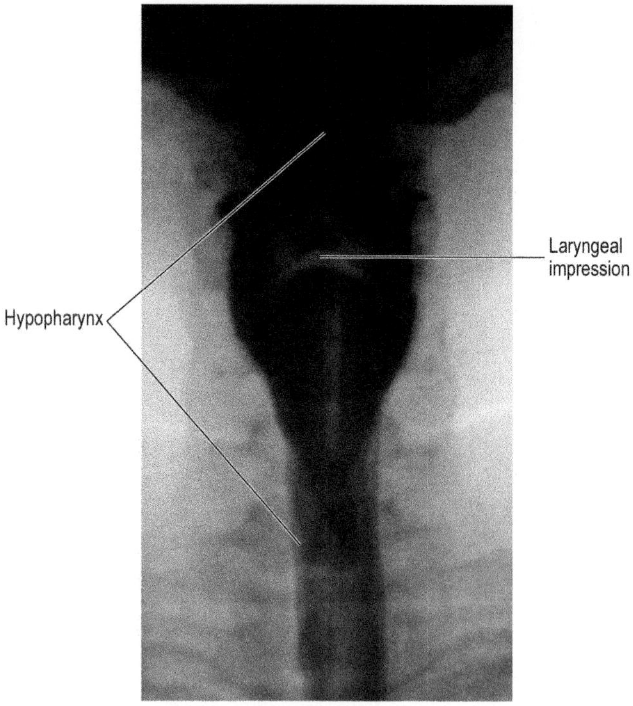

Fig. 21.4 AP barium swallow showing normal hypopharyngeal anatomy.

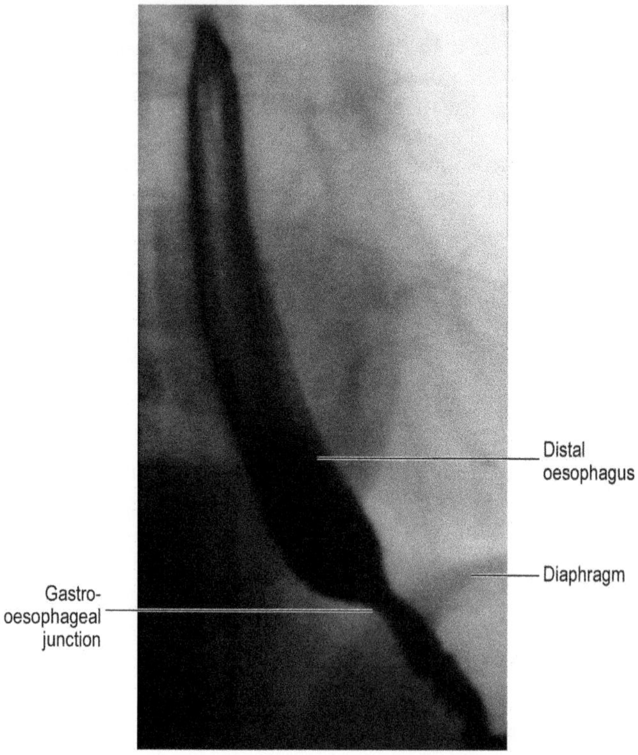

Fig. 21.5 Distal oesophagus and gastro-oesophageal junction (GOJ) (LPO).

The frame rate refers to the number of frames per second selected for taking an imaging run. Modern digital equipment can allow recording of a single fluoroscopy image or a run of images at a chosen pulse rate. This offers a reduction in radiation dose by allowing retrospective and repeated study of the patient's swallowing action without returning to rescreen missed actions, and also allows a more real-time assessment to take place. Where investigation of motility is the only indication these captured fluoroscopy images will be adequate for the study. Where pathology is suspected a series of digital spot images (DSI) should be taken at up to 3 frames per second in order to produce images of higher quality

- The patient is then asked to swallow and exposure is initiated. The exposure is terminated when the barium bolus passes beyond the screened image or point of interest. This lateral pharynx view may be repeated, as some pathologies such as cricopharyngeal spasm may be transient and thus not occur on every swallow
- The patient is then turned back to AP, ideally standing with their chin raised so that their symphysis menti is superimposed over the occiput. The AP view is the optimum for hypopharyngeal anatomy;[17] it will be seen in both single- and double-contrast images (Fig. 21.4). A series of images are captured, as described above, and again this view may be repeated at least once more to ensure there is consistency in the images, making it easier to definitively identify pathology
- A view of the mid and distal thirds of the oesophagus is taken in the erect LPO position, taken after the patient is asked to swallow. In this position the oesophagus does not lie over the thoracic spine and the gastro-oesophageal junction (GOJ) is opened out, thereby ensuring clearer visualisation. The barium bolus is imaged as a column and a series of images are taken to show the distal third of the oesophagus. The frame rate may be reduced to 2f/sec for this series as the bolus progresses more slowly. This allows mucosal rings and peptic strictures to be shown well.[18] As the column passes and the mucosa relaxes, spot films can be taken; this may show oesophagitis (Fig. 21.5)

Barium Swallow including Reflux Assessment

Patients for this study often present with clinical symptoms of GOR. They often have a feeling of retrosternal discomfort and no other symptoms. The National Institute for Health and Care Excellence (NICE) offers guidance on the management of gastro-oesophageal reflux and gives recommendations on the use of endoscopy, Helicobacter testing, the role of radiological imaging and when to consider surgery.[12] The barium study can still be useful as an adjunct to other tests, as some GOR patients may have small hiatus hernias that are not seen on endoscopy. These patients may have mucosal changes in the distal third of the oesophagus, such as oesophagitis or Barrett's oesophagus, a premalignant condition known to be caused by GOR.[19] The barium swallow is used to view the region closely and observe the fundus to check for herniation.

- To detect signs of a hiatus hernia, GOR or dysmotility, the fluoroscopic couch is placed horizontally and the patient turned to their right to assess reflux. Spot images of the area are taken
- A prone swallow is then undertaken. The patient lies either completely prone with their head turned to one side or in the RAO position, which throws their oesophagus away from their spine. The patient then drinks some barium through a straw and the barium bolus is screened

as it travels along the oesophagus. Spot films are taken or fluoroscopy images are captured (to reduce radiation dose). This view maximises oesophageal distension and can also produce well-coated views of the oesophagus and gastro-oesophageal junction. It is a particularly good view to demonstrate oesophageal varices. As this series of images primarily assesses motility it is appropriate to capture a run of fluoroscopy rather than initiate a DSI run. A prone swallow must *never* be attempted if aspiration or laryngeal penetration is evident when erect
- The patient is then asked to rotate through 360° at their own pace; this will ensure that all aspects of the gastric mucosa are coated ready for assessment of the stomach
- A supine AP view and an erect AP view of the stomach is taken
- To complete the examination an image is taken to demonstrate gastric emptying and to show the first and second part of the duodenum. If gastric pathology is suspected a full barium meal or OGD should be considered

Common abnormalities in the pharynx include persistent cricopharyngeal impressions or diverticula, the most common diverticulum type being Zenker's; this occurs in the mid-hypopharynx and is more common in the older population. They are quite often termed hypopharyngeal pouches.[18] The pouches can become quite large, often causing patients to be referred because of regurgitation of undigested food. They are also often difficult to endoscope, as the scope enters the pouch and cannot be passed further; the barium swallow can often be the most appropriate test for confirming the presence and extent of this pathology.

Oesophageal webs are also best seen on the lateral projection, shown on the anterior wall, although they are best viewed with rapid imaging sequences; they have been noted in 1–5% of asymptomatic patients and 12–15% of dysphagia patients.[18]

Common findings in the oesophagus include carcinoma, dysmotilty, reflux, hiatus hernia and achalasia.

BARIUM MEAL

This examination is performed to show the stomach and duodenum. It is rarely requested due to the increased use of endoscopy as the front-line examination, and is recommended for use in a very limited number of circumstances. These include: if endoscopy proves negative and symptoms persist; after (healed) surgery to assess afferent loop, narrowed anastomoses and closed loops or internal hernias,[20] or to assess complications after bariatric surgery.[20] It can also still be useful for those patients who are not considered fit for, or refuse, OGD.[21]

Patient Preparation

Patient preparation is as for all upper tract examinations

Contraindications

- Complete large bowel obstruction[16]

Contrast Agents and Pharmaceutical Aids for the Examination

- Barium sulphate suspension 250% w/v
- Effervescent granules and citric acid, or other gas-producing agent
- An antispasmodic agent such as hyoscine-*N*-butyl bromide (Buscopan) may be used intravenously. This helps to reduce peristalsis in the stomach and prevent rapid progress of the barium into the small bowel[16]

Additional Equipment

- Disposable cup
- Small cup for effervescent agent
- Tissues
- A straw may be required for ingestion of barium sulphate when the table is horizontal (if needed)

Technique

(Ensure that you have understood the notes on fluoroscopic examination positioning descriptors earlier in this chapter before considering technique descriptors.)

If required, the patient may be given the antispasmodic agent immediately prior to commencing the examination, although some practitioners prefer to give the antispasmodic during the examination when the barium is just beginning to leave the pylorus. Administration of an antispasmodic should not give false results during the reflux check.

- The patient is asked to stand on the step of the fluoroscopic couch and then the procedure for ingesting the gas-producing agent is explained. The importance of keeping the gas in the stomach is emphasised, and an explanation of a strategy to prevent belching (dry swallowing) is given
- The patient is given the effervescent agent (dry, or mixed with a small amount of water if this is more tolerable for the patient); they are then asked to drink the citric acid, to produce carbon dioxide and distend the stomach
- The patient is turned slightly to their left and asked to swallow a mouthful of the barium; the barium column is screened and spot images are taken of the distal oesophagus with single and double contrast
- After three or four reasonable mouthfuls of barium have been ingested, the table is tilted horizontally and the patient asked to rotate (at least once) through 360° to enable the barium to coat the stomach mucosa. A prone swallow may also be undertaken at this point. Periodic screening during this movement allows for images to be taken if the radiographer feels it is necessary, especially if a small hiatus hernia or GOR are noted. This also enables the operator to note which positions show the anatomy most effectively, in preparation for other spot images. Quite often the most difficult region to image well can be the duodenal cap, owing to the peristaltic action of the small bowel (which can occur even after administration of intravenous muscle relaxant); therefore, if the duodenal cap is well visualised during the patient's initial movements, there may be an opportunity to obtain the spot images required
- Once the patient has completed their rotation and good mucosal coating and distension of the stomach have been noted, it is possible to obtain the spot images. If coating is poor, give the patient more barium or ask them to perform another 360° rotation; if distension is inadequate

then repeat the dose of effervescent agent. Because this is a dynamic investigation it is best to take the spot images as quickly as possible, and if the chance arises and an area is well shown while moving the patient, take the opportunity

The following positions are a general guideline to how best to show the anatomy of the stomach and duodenum in double contrast:

1. The patient with their right side raised (LPO) demonstrates the antrum and the greater curve (Fig. 21.6)
2. If the patient is supine this demonstrates the antrum and the body of the stomach and also the lesser curve (Fig. 21.7A,B)
3. Turning the patient into the RPO position demonstrates the lesser curve en face (Fig. 21.8)
4. Moving the patient into the right lateral position with head tilted up shows the fundus (Fig. 21.9A,B)

A combination of the following positions will help to best demonstrate the duodenal loop and duodenal cap. It may be necessary to use magnification at this point to optimise the view:

1. LPO (Fig. 21.10)
2. Supine
3. RPO, centred on and collimated to the duodenal loop
4. Prone

The patient can then be tilted erect and turned slightly to the left to show the fundus (Fig. 21.11). If visualisation of the duodenal cap has been poor during the earlier (table horizontal) stages of the examination, turning the patient in both directions (while they are standing) may provide better views of the duodenal cap.

Patient Aftercare

- A damp tissue should be provided for the patient to clean their mouth
- The patient should be informed that their stools will be paler or white for a few days, and to keep their fluid intake

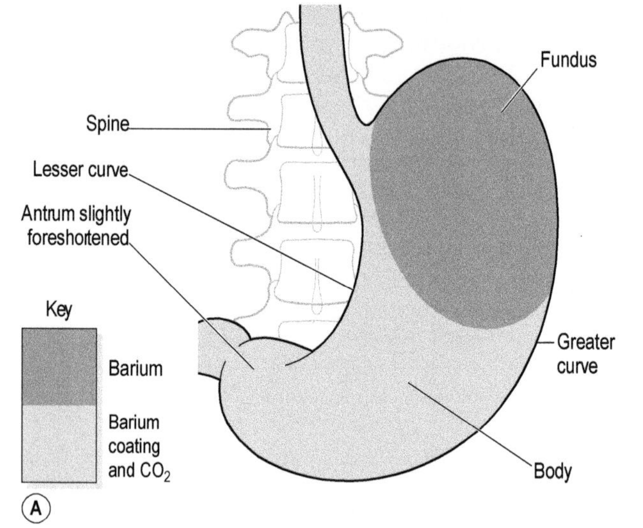

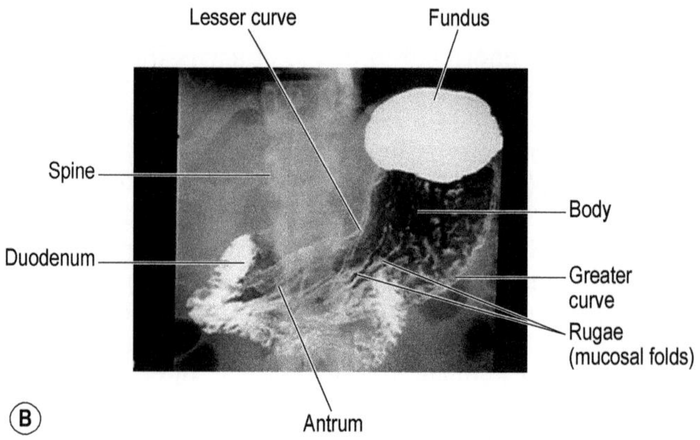

Fig. 21.7 (A) Supine position for antrum, body and lesser curve – barium pools in the lowest point, which in the supine position is the fundus, allowing CO_2 to rise into the body and antrum which are coated with barium; (B) supine stomach.

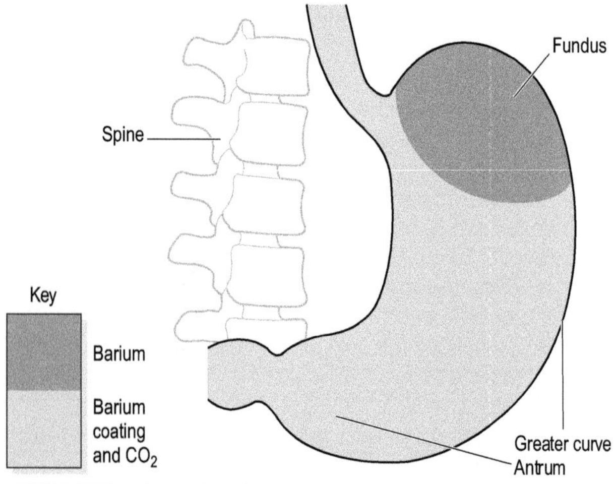

Fig. 21.6 LPO position for antrum and greater curve. The stomach is turned to the left: the barium drops into the fundus and obscures it; CO_2 rises into the body and antrum to act as double contrast for good visualisation of these areas. The greater curve is also visualised.

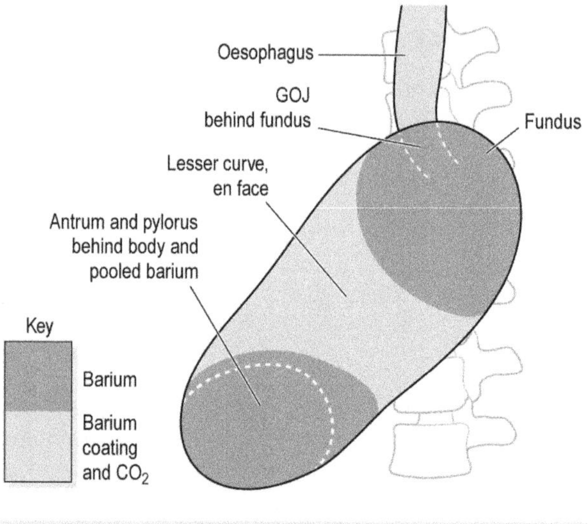

Fig. 21.8 RPO position to show lesser curve en face. Obliquity moves the lesser curve to turn it from profile to an en face position; it is seen through the CO_2-filled body. Barium will pool in the fundus and antrum as these are the lowest points of the stomach in this position.

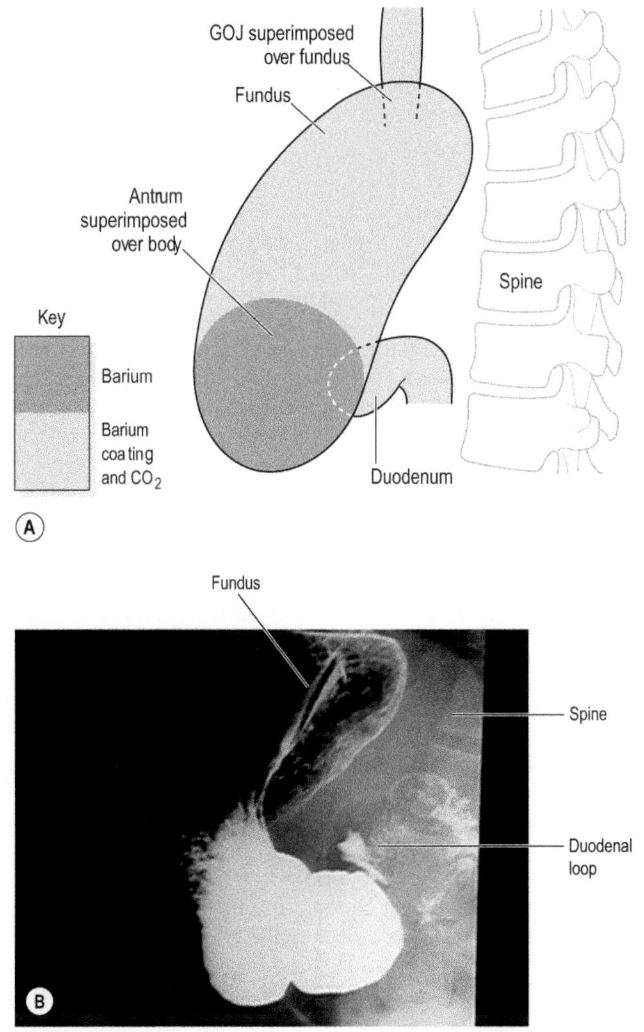

Fig. 21.9 (A) Right lateral position, head tilted up, to show fundus – barium pools in the antrum as it is now the lowest positioned part of the stomach and CO_2 rises to the fundus; (B) right lateral, head tilted up.

up to reduce any chance of constipation. Encourage a high-fibre diet for several days

- Ensure that the patient knows how to obtain their results
- If a muscle relaxant is used, the patient must be informed of the possibility of experiencing blurred vision and should be advised not to drive should this occur

Potential Complications

- Leakage of barium from an unsuspected perforation
- Constipation
- Partial bowel obstruction becoming complete obstruction due to barium impaction[16]
- Aspiration of barium: as previously mentioned, each patient must be carefully questioned before the procedure to ensure the examination is tailored for that individual. If a patient coughs during or shortly after meals, or has a recent history of chest infections, then aspiration must be considered a risk. Some patients are at a higher risk of aspiration than others. These include patients who have had a previous cerebral vascular accident, Parkinson's disease, multiple sclerosis, motor neurone disease, dementia, Huntington's chorea, previous head injury, other progressive or acquired neurological disorders, acute exacerbation of chronic obstructive pulmonary disease (COPD), history of recurrent chest infections, history of head or neck carcinoma with associated surgery or radiotherapy, or recently extubated patients. If mild aspiration occurs during an examination, encourage the patient to cough and expectorate the barium. No more barium should be given, but the examination may be continued if appropriate and safe to do so. If severe aspiration occurs then the examination must be terminated and the patient referred for physiotherapy. The patient should not leave the radiology department until a physiotherapist has assessed their condition. A referral to the speech and language therapy department for a future appointment may also be appropriate

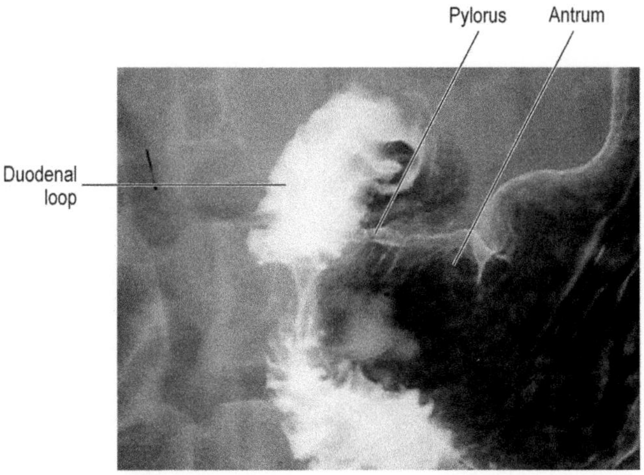

Fig. 21.10 LPO – antrum and duodenal loop.

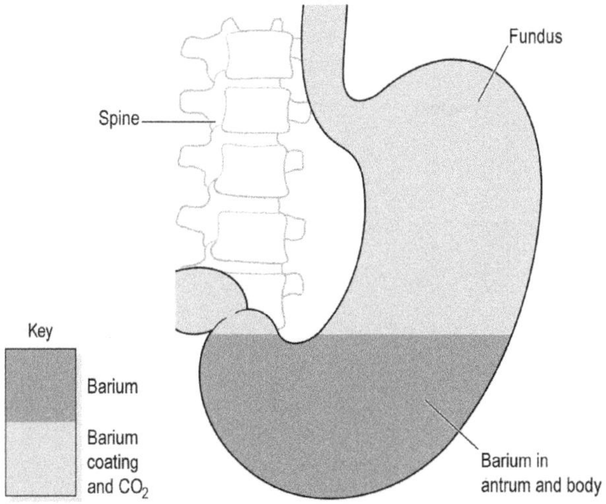

Fig. 21.11 Erect (slight LPO) position to show fundus. Barium sits in the antrum and body; CO_2 rises into the fundus.

Supplementary Techniques

For patients with dysphagia it may be necessary to undertake the swallowing section of the examination using an imitation 'food bolus', as liquid may show no abnormality. Common examples of imitation food bolus are marshmallow coated in barium or pieces of fresh bread coated in barium. If a patient is unable to ingest the barium rapidly the relaxing effect of adding ice to the barium could be used.[18]

BARIATRIC IMAGING

Increasing levels of people living with obesity in developed countries and escalating numbers of people with type 2 diabetes has resulted in guidance recommending bariatric surgery as the most effective long-term obesity management strategy.[22] Patients with a Body Mass Index (BMI) of 35 kg/m^2 or more with complications or 40 kg/m^2 without may be offered gastric bypass surgery or gastric band placement to assist them with a weight loss programme.[23]

Roux-en-Y bypass is one of the most common procedures offered and involves a surgical procedure to create a small stomach pouch and to by-pass the stomach and first part of the duodenum (Fig. 21.12). The original stomach remains in place and remains connected to the small bowel to allow gastric secretions to pass through the gut. This surgery limits both the amount of food that can be eaten and the degree of absorption of nutrients from food. This is a non-reversible procedure and should be very carefully considered. Fluoroscopic imaging of patients following gastric bypass surgery normally comprises a contrast study of the oesophagus, stomach remnant and proximal small bowel.

Common indications for referral are:

- Investigate for strictures or adhesions
- Reflux
- Possible obstruction
- Possible leak following breakdown of sutures/staples
- Possible retrograde filling of the main body of the stomach via the efferent bowel loop

More routinely offered to people living with obesity is a gastric band (Fig. 21.13). This is an inflatable cuff which is laparoscopically positioned around the fundus of the stomach to create a small stomach pouch, grossly restricting the passage of food through the gastro-oesophageal junction and through to the body of the stomach. Correct pressure on the vagus nerve promotes early and prolonged satiety with small portions of food, thus supporting weight loss and ongoing weight management. A port, attached to the abdominal wall and linked to the band via silicone tubing, allows the clinician access to inflate and deflate the band as required.

A gastric band is more flexible as it can be adjusted as required and deflated in certain situations such as before surgery or during pregnancy. However, it is not an easy solution; it demands lifelong adjustments to eating habits and reflux and obstruction can result from overeating, not chewing properly or trying to eat too fast. It is also possible to maintain and even increase weight if the patient does not engage with changing eating and lifestyle habits. Patients with gastric bands require regular review and make up a large portion of the bariatric work for fluoroscopy teams.

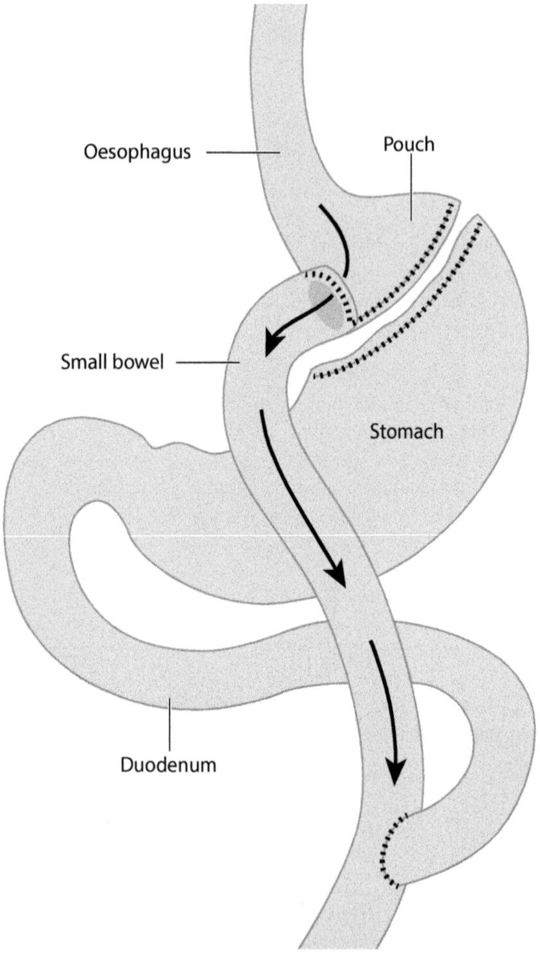

Fig. 21.12 Roux-en-Y gastric bypass and associated anatomy.

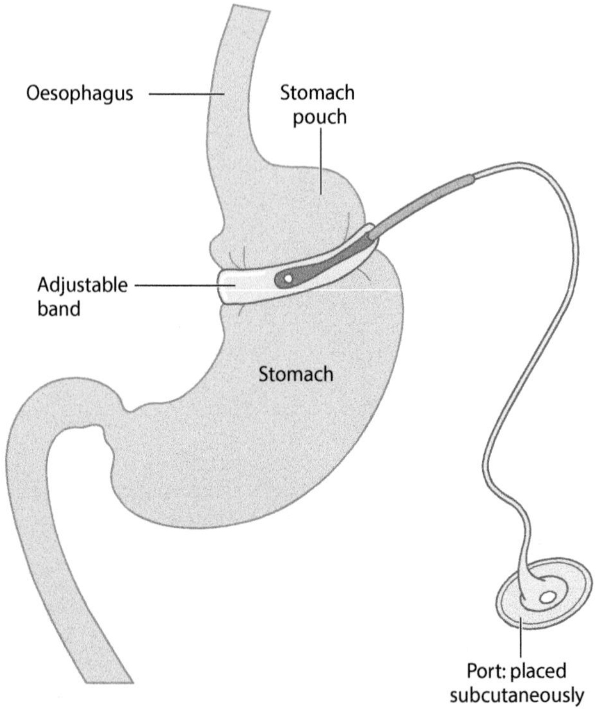

Fig. 21.13 Position of a gastric band.

Gastric band imaging comprises two patient groups: those requiring a contrast swallow and those requiring assessment of their band and port.

Contrast swallows are undertaken for the following indications:

- Assess the degree of band restriction
- Determine band position
- Check for herniation of the stomach above the band
- Check for erosion of the band into the stomach wall

Referrals taken to check the patency of the band and tubing and the position of the port will cover the following indications:

- Problems with maintaining adequate restriction and appropriate satiety
- Investigating for leaks in the band or tubing
- Checking poorly positioned ports which cannot be accessed in clinic by feeling for the port position
- Filling and de-filling gastric bands under fluoroscopic guidance. This may be required if the port is poorly positioned and difficult to access or if achieving appropriate fill has been unsuccessful.

Imaging for band systems will involve injecting a non-ionic, low osmolar iodinated contrast agent into the port, positioned just below the skin. Fluoroscopic guidance is used to access the port and images are taken to look for kinks in the tubing or leaks in the system; most common sites are at the points of attachment between the port, tubing and band, or within the cuff. An accurate assessment can also be made on the amount of fluid that is contained within the band and the band can be adjusted as part of the procedure. Oral contrast agent is then given to the patient under fluoroscopic control, to check the degree of restriction is appropriate (Fig. 21.14).

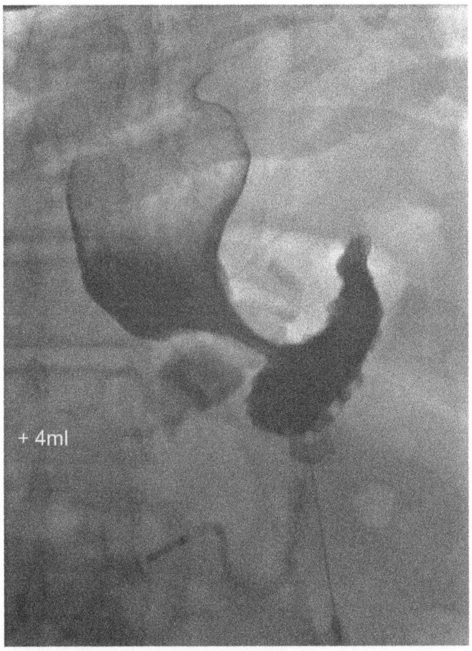

Fig. 21.14 Fluoroscopic image showing a correctly positioned gastric band with an adequate degree of restriction.

VIDEOFLUOROSCOPY

This is usually undertaken in conjunction with speech therapists. Its aim is to assess patients who have swallowing dysfunction due to mechanical or neuromuscular problems, with the result that they are at increased risk of aspiration and associated chest problems. The aim of the procedure is to decide on the best strategy, compatible with nutrition, that will help the patient cope with the swallowing disorder.

Images may be recorded on video, but most equipment now has the ability to record a fluoroscopy run at a high pulse rate (up to 10 frames per second). This is preferable as it allows images to be transferred to PACS (picture archiving and communication system) whilst minimising patient dose and allowing for relatively long screening runs. DSI runs are not advocated for videofluoroscopy as the relatively high radiation dose cannot be justified for a study looking at function rather than pathology. A single DSI image may be taken as a reference image at the start of the procedure. Fluoroscopic recording of the swallow at up to 30 frames per second can be valuable, but this often produces more images per run than can be stored within each patient study file on the room workstation. It also significantly increases patient dose and contradicts guidance to speech and language therapists to minimise dose to the eyes and thyroid.[24] This therefore may not be a workable option.[25]

Criteria for referral for videofluoroscopy include:

- When silent aspiration is suspected but not clearly confirmed on bedside assessment
- When the degree of aspiration as a result of ingestion of different food consistencies needs clarification
- When the degree of dysphagia appears mild but the patient suffers from recurrent chest infections
- When long-term non-oral feeding, e.g. percutaneous endoscopic gastrostomy, is being considered
- When postural or procedural swallowing techniques will benefit the patient

Most referrals are for patients who have suffered:

- Cerebrovascular accident
- Motor neurone disease
- Multiple sclerosis
- Parkinson's disease
- Previous head or neck surgery, e.g. partial laryngectomy

The technique requires the patient to swallow small amounts of liquid, semi-solids and solids in order to ascertain their safety in eating and drinking. The patient is screened in the lateral pharynx position while they swallow the various consistencies, and the process is recorded for later review.[25] Occasionally an AP pharynx view is taken, for example, to define asymmetries of pharyngeal residue and which side is affected.[26] As well as demonstrating aspiration at different consistencies, videofluoroscopy also allows coping strategies to be tried; for example, using a chin tuck on swallowing, or turning the head to one side, may prevent aspiration.

If the patient is able to comply, fluoroscopy is used to follow a single bolus through the pharynx and oesophagus into the stomach to exclude any obvious pathology, or hold up of passage of food into the stomach.[27]

The aim of the process is to decide on the best strategy compatible with nutrition, to help the patient cope with their problem.

Small Bowel

The small bowel (from the duodenojejunal flexure to the ileocaecal valve) can be examined by one of two methods: the barium follow-through (BaFT) or the small bowel enema. The aim is to produce a continuous column of barium suspension outlining the small bowel.[3]

In most circumstances these procedures have been replaced by MRI of the small bowel[21] as the examination is more sensitive. Barium studies may be offered to patients who cannot tolerate MRI or where MRI is contraindicated (for MRI contraindications, see Chapter 27).

REFERRAL CRITERIA FOR SMALL BOWEL IMAGING

- Anaemia
- Diarrhoea
- Persistent pain
- Crohn's disease
- Meckel's diverticulum

BARIUM FOLLOW-THROUGH (BaFT)

During this examination the patient has to drink a volume of barium sulphate suspension, and images (fluoroscopy and/or permanent image recording) are taken as the small bowel fills. The examination frequently takes 2 hours, and in some instances can take most of the day.[28]

Contraindications

- Suspected perforation
- Complete obstruction

Patient Preparation

Patient preparation is usually the same for both follow-through and small bowel enema, but local imaging department protocols may vary. Generally the patient is not allowed to eat or drink for 5–6 hours prior to the examination. Some centres may give the patient a mild laxative and/or a clear fluid diet the day before the examination.

Contrast Agent

- At least 300 mL 100% w/v barium sulphate suspension is required for an adult BaFT.[16] The constituents of the drink are:
  Barium sulphate suspension
  Effervescent agent (may be carbonated barium sulphate suspension)
  Water
  Accelerator, e.g. Gastrografin or metoclopramide hydrochloride (Maxalon®)

Additional Equipment

- Disposable cup
- Small cup for effervescent agent
- Tissues

Technique

- The patient is asked to drink the barium sulphate suspension steadily. Drinking too quickly can cause nausea; drinking too slowly causes the barium sulphate suspension to flocculate and the small bowel does not distend adequately to obtain diagnostic images
- The imaging technique used depends on the equipment available, the preference of the practitioner or local imaging department protocol. The actual timing of imaging depends on each individual patient and the motility speed of the bowel. Transit of barium through the proximal bowel (jejunum) is usually rapid, whereas transit through the distal bowel (ileum) is often less rapid[16]
- A series of prone over-couch abdominal radiographs (Fig. 21.15 – see Chapter 22 for prone positioning) may be taken at predetermined time intervals, e.g. every 30 minutes, or alternatively each image is individually assessed in order to determine the timing of the subsequent image. The radiographs are usually taken prone because the pressure on the abdomen helps to separate the bowel loops.[16] The first image is usually taken 15–20 minutes after drinking commenced. When the barium has been seen to reach the terminal ileum, fluoroscopy is used to image the ileocaecal area, although over-couch images can be taken if necessary

The terminal ileum will be shown on a prone image of the abdomen. The patient lies prone and a radiolucent pad is placed in their right iliac fossa; for the pad to be inserted correctly the patient must lie on their left side and the pad placed and held firmly in the right iliac fossa. The patient then rolls prone to prevent small bowel falling back against the caecum and obscuring the terminal ileum. Prone positioning then follows as for the prone abdomen/KUB (kidneys, ureters, bladder) as described in Chapter 22, with collimation to include the whole of the small bowel.

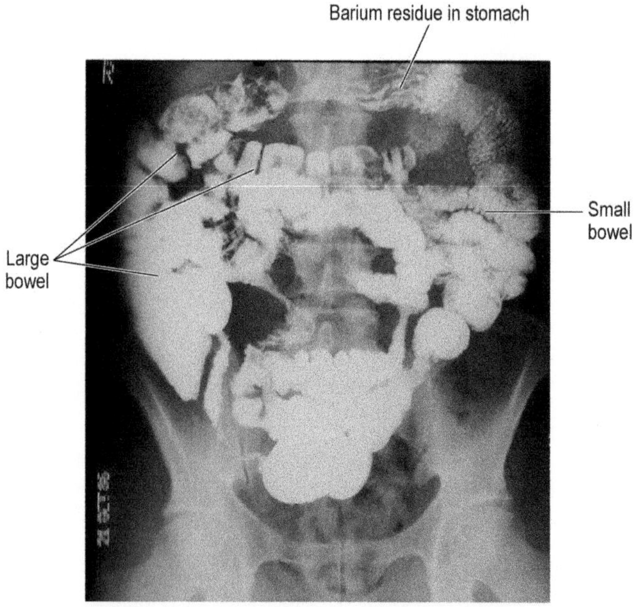

Fig. 21.15 Prone abdomen.

Alternatively, fluoroscopy may be used to image the small bowel at the necessary intervals. With fluoroscopy, the proximal jejunum is often imaged supine or in the RPO position. All the other loops are usually imaged supine until the terminal ileum is reached.

- Regardless of imaging modality, all bowel loops should be palpated (using lead rubber gloves with hands outside the primary beam) or the abdominal wall compressed with a radiolucent pad during imaging. Barium does not move into areas of adhesions, which are difficult to spot anyway, as they are often subtle and can be obscured by overlapped loops of barium-filled bowel
- Fluoroscopy of the terminal ileum frequently requires an LPO position, but sometimes RPO or prone positions are more satisfactory
- An erect abdominal view may be required to show fluid levels, usually required when jejunal diverticulosis is present.[3] This is usually imaged with fluoroscopy, but an over-couch image may be taken

Potential Complications

- Constipation
- Abdominal pain
- Transient diarrhoea (due to a large volume of fluid)

Patient Aftercare

- Ask the patient to increase their fluid intake over the next 48 hours to prevent constipation
- Warn the patient about white stools

There are certain criteria and common errors that relate to all small bowel barium studies – see below.

Criteria for Assessing Image Quality

- All barium-filled loops of bowel (area of interest) are included on the film
- Sharp image clearly demonstrating valvulae conniventes
- Adequate penetration to demonstrate detail in the contrast-filled bowel

Common Errors: Barium Follow-through

Common Errors	Possible Reasons and Strategies to Overcome These
Image is pale and valvulae conniventes are not demonstrated	Image is underexposed. Increase the kVp. A high kVp technique reduces subject contrast through increased penetration of the X-ray beam but also reduces the exposure time and radiation dose.[29] As a contrast agent is given the low inherent contrast within the abdomen is raised so a high Kv technique is appropriate
Slow barium transit of the proximal bowel	Ask the patient to lie in the right lateral decubitus position to promote gastric emptying[28]
Slow barium transit of the distal bowel	Give the patient a hot drink. If the patient has been in the department for a long time, a small snack can be given to try to encourage small bowel movement[16]
Overlying loops of bowel	If the overlying loops of bowel are deep within the pelvis ask the patient to avoid micturition, as a full bladder may push up and separate the loops of bowel. If the bladder is already full and the bowel loops are overlapping, ask the patient to empty their bladder. Alternatively, the patient can lie prone over a radiolucent pad to displace the loops[16]

SMALL BOWEL ENEMA (FIG. 21.16A,B)

During a small bowel enema the duodenum is intubated and a contrast agent introduced. This is arguably the ideal method for imaging the small bowel as it results in improved visualisation of the bowel loops.[16,17] This is because the infusion of contrast agent avoids segmentation of the barium column and the small bowel is unobstructed by the overlying barium-filled stomach and duodenum. This method also avoids pyloric control over the rate of transit.[28] However, it is invasive for the patient and time-consuming, and can be technically difficult for the operator.

The small bowel enema may also be used after a BaFT to localise a lesion or examine a particular section of small bowel.[16]

Contraindications

- Facial surgery or trauma
- The patient is prone to nose bleeds
- Active Crohn's disease (especially of the duodenum)
- Severe gastro-oesophageal reflux/hiatus hernia
- Suspected perforation
- Complete obstruction

Patient Preparation

- As for BaFT
- The procedure must be carefully explained, as it is often difficult for the patient to tolerate[16]

Contrast Agent

For single contrast, typically 1000 mL of fluid is used.[17] The mixture comprises barium sulphate suspension and water; the ratio of barium sulphate to water tends to vary according to the preferences of the examining radiographer or radiologist. For double-contrast examination 150–200 mL barium sulphate suspension is followed by up to 2 L methylcellulose 0.5%.[17]

Additional Equipment

- Nasogastric or duodenal catheter
- Lubricating jelly for the tube
- Anaesthetic spray
- Tissues
- Sterile gloves
- Swabs to wipe the tube after removal

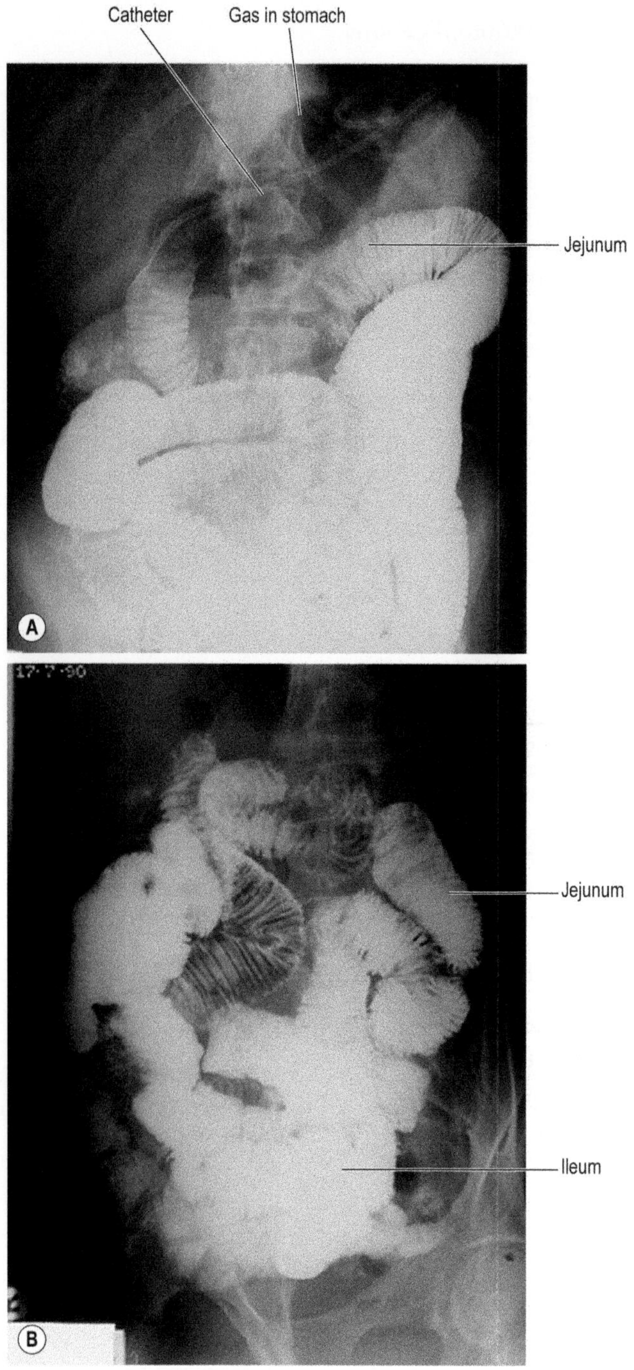

Fig. 21.16 Small bowel enema.

Technique

- The patient lies supine and, under fluoroscopic control, the duodenal or nasogastric catheter is inserted until the tip of the catheter is shown in the duodenojejunal flexure. The anaesthetic spray may be used to numb the throat, but this prevents the examination continuing by follow-through if the intubation is unsuccessful.
- The guidewire within the catheter acts as a stiffener to prevent coiling and enables manipulation into the correct position.
- The barium solution is infused by gravity or by an enteroclysis pump.
- Imaging is usually by fluoroscopy, but spot films can be taken as well. The terminal ileum may need prone imaging as for BaFT.
- For a double-contrast study methylcellulose solution is infused after the barium sulphate suspension until the terminal ileum is demonstrated in double contrast.
- During a single-contrast examination air may be introduced at the end of the examination to demonstrate the terminal ileum in double contrast. Air may be introduced via the duodenal catheter or by a rectal catheter.
- All the loops of bowel are usually imaged supine until the terminal ileum is reached and oblique views may be needed.

Potential Complications and Patient Aftercare

As for BaFT examination.

Lower GI Tract: Large Bowel

The large bowel comprises the colon, rectum and caecum and should wherever possible be imaged using computed tomography. The Special Interest Group in Gastrointestinal and Abdominal Radiology (SIGGAR) undertook a multicentre randomised trial which compared barium enema (BaE) with computed tomography colonography (CTC). The findings, first published in 2013, concluded that CTC was a more sensitive test and should be the preferred radiological test for patients with symptoms suggestive of colorectal cancer.[30,31]

REFERRAL CRITERIA FOR LARGE BOWEL IMAGING (CTC OR BaE)

- Change in bowel habit
- Iron deficiency anaemia
- Rectal bleeding
- Tenesmus
- Left iliac fossa pain
- Palpable mass
- Documented cancer on endoscopy: to exclude synchronous lesions

CONTRAINDICATIONS FOR LARGE BOWEL IMAGING (CTC OR BAE)

- Acute inflammatory bowel disease
- Colonic perforation
- Toxic megacolon
- Recent endoscopic biopsy or polypectomy (studies may be performed more than 2 days after routine biopsy and 2 weeks after full-thickness biopsy)

BARIUM ENEMA

Whilst the barium enema is no longer accepted as first-choice procedure for investigating the large bowel, an overview of the examination is provided for reference.

Prior to the procedure, patients are instructed to follow a low residue diet and take a laxative in order to cleanse the bowel.

As with other GI procedures described, barium sulphate and gas (air or CO_2) are used for this double-contrast procedure.

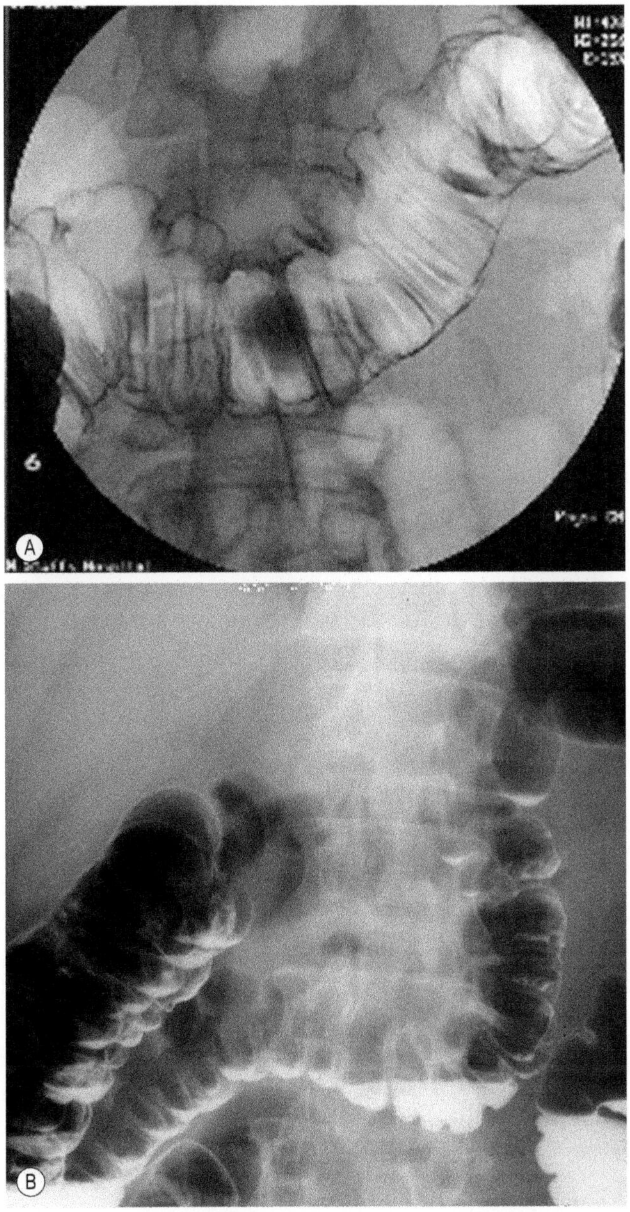

Fig. 21.17 (A) Supine transverse colon; (B) erect transverse colon.

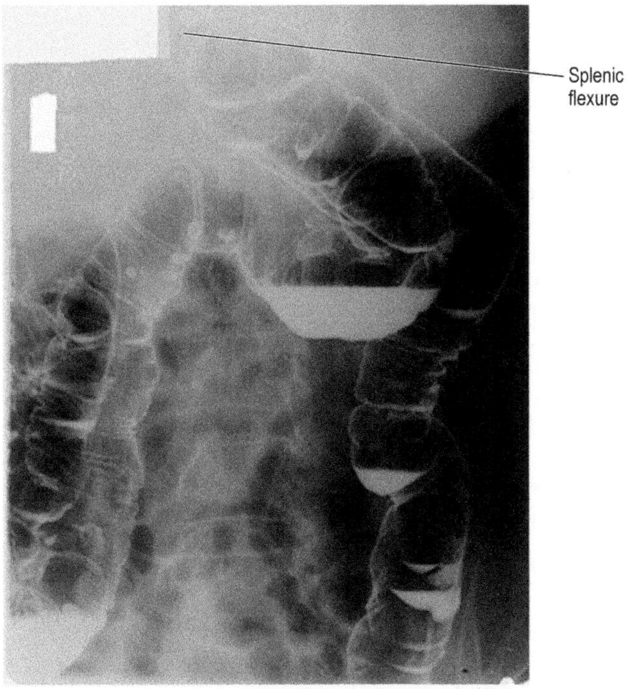

Fig. 21.18 Erect RPO splenic flexure.

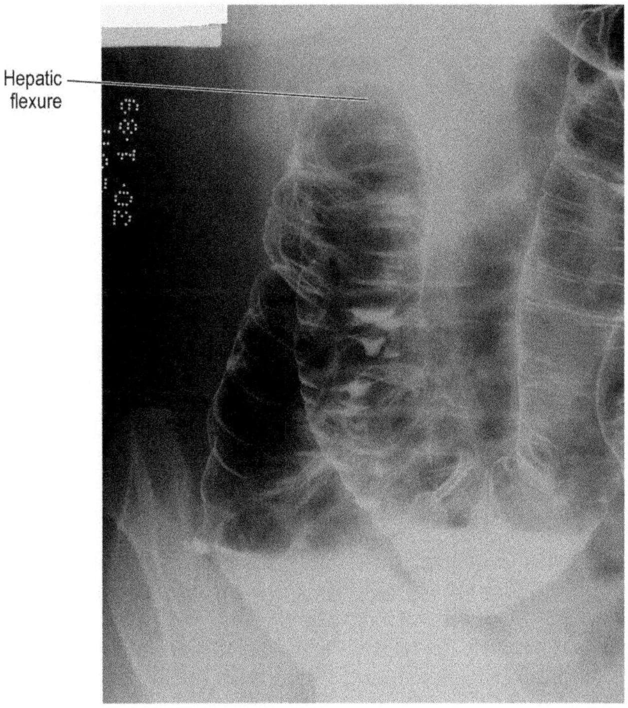

Fig. 21.19 Erect LPO hepatic flexure.

The barium is administered as an enema with the patient lying on their left side, head slightly lower than the feet. The barium is run around the bowel as far as the mid transverse colon by turning the patient from lateral to prone and then drained back out by reversing the positioning and bringing the patient back to lateral with head elevated. This action provides the barium coating which will act as the double contrast with the air/CO_2.

A hypotonic agent (a smooth muscle relaxant), e.g. Buscopan® or glucagon is frequently given during the procedure to reduce bowel spasm. Contraindications for Buscopan include cardiovascular disease and glaucoma, so glucagon may be given in these instances.[32]

Air or CO_2 is then administered via the rectal tube to fully distend the bowel before imaging.

Spot images are taken of all bowel segments to demonstrate the entire lumen in double contrast at least once (Figs 21.17–21.19). The patient is positioned supine, prone, lateral and erect in order to achieve this, thus moving the barium liquid into the different parts of the bowel; the region shown will be the gas-filled sections contrasting with the fine barium coating of the bowel. For example, if the patient is supine the transverse colon will be demonstrated in double contrast as it lies anterior in the abdomen and the ascending and descending colon will contain the barium liquid. When the patient turns prone the liquid will pool in the transverse colon allowing the ascending and descending colon to be demonstrated in double contrast. Oblique projections will be needed to show the sigmoid colon and specific spot images will be used to demonstrate the caecum and terminal ileum; erect and decubitus positions are also used to complete the examination.

Once the procedure is completed the patient is invited to use the toilet to remove any excess barium liquid, allowed to recover in a quiet area and encouraged to have something to eat and drink.

A barium enema is an invasive test requiring good patient compliance and patients need to be fit and mobile enough to move on the table. Many elderly patients find the procedure difficult to tolerate and need a high level of care both during and following the procedure. Patients should also be advised to ensure they drink plenty of fluids for the rest of the day of examination. If Buscopan is used patients should be advised to seek medical attention if they develop painful blurred vision after leaving the imaging department.

Modifications to the Barium Enema

- A water-soluble contrast agent may be used to demonstrate a recent bowel anastomosis or in cases of suspected bowel perforation. This procedure is most commonly undertaken to check the integrity of an anastomosis following bowel resection and prior to reconstruction of the large bowel and removal of a covering ileostomy.
- With the patient laying in a lateral position, a Foley catheter is placed in the rectum. Before contrast is introduced, control images to demonstrate the surgical sutures or staples are taken in AP, lateral and oblique projections. An iodine-based contrast agent is then run into the rectum using the catheter and a giving set, and a series of images are taken, focusing on the area of the anastomosis. Alternatively, contrast may be introduced manually using a bladder syringe.
- Patients with an ileostomy or colostomy may require a barium examination to examine their proximal bowel. A soft Foley catheter is gently inserted into the stoma and the barium sulphate solution is slowly infused into the colon. This procedure has, wherever possible, been replaced by CTC with the rectal insufflation catheter placed in the stoma.

CT COLONOGRAPHY (CTC)

The double-contrast barium enema (DCBE) was a long-standing first-choice radiographic investigation of the large bowel, but, as previously stated (see barium enema section above), it has largely been superseded by CTC, which is minimally invasive and better tolerated by the majority of patients.[33] Evidence has also established that CTC sensitivity to polyps >10 mm is between 91% and 100%[34] compared to DCBE, which has a variable detection rate of between 48%[35] and 81%.[36] It also has the advantage of being able to detect extracolonic lesions, particularly beneficial when the patient presents with vague symptoms relating to the large bowel.

Colorectal cancer is the third most common cancer in the UK, with 100 new cases being reported as diagnosed daily.[37] Early detection is essential to survival. The 5-year relative survival rate his risen from 50% to 59% since the first edition of this textbook and the 10-year relative survival rate is 54%.[38] This may be in part due to the improvements in the UK National Bowel Cancer Screening Programme (NBCSP). However, survival rate is still dependent on the stage of disease. CTC is widely available within the UK following improvements in both training and technology and is much better tolerated than DCBE; it can therefore be used for elderly and reduced mobility patients, from both the symptomatic and asymptomatic population. Radiation dose for CTC is comparable to that for DCBE,[39,40] and if sinister colonic pathology is detected the patient does not need to undergo dual examination (DCBE and staging CT scan), thus a radiation dose reduction is offered in such cases. It is also advantageous because patients with positive findings will not have to wait for a CT staging scan, thereby accelerating diagnosis to treatment times.

Indications

CTC is indicated for the same reasons as DCBE and, in addition:

- Incomplete optical colonoscopy[24]
- To evaluate the colon proximal to an obstruction
- If optical colonoscopy is contraindicated

Contraindications

- Immediately following colonic biopsy
- Acute inflammatory bowel disease
- Colonic perforation
- Toxic megacolon
- Recent endoscopic biopsy or polypectomy (studies may be performed more than 2 days after routine biopsy and 2 weeks after full-thickness biopsy)

Note that contraindication to contrast media is *not* a contraindication to CTC, as CTC may be performed without contrast. If findings prove positive for the colon, ultrasound may be used to exclude liver metastases. Some centres perform non-contrast CTC and only administer contrast if CTC indicates sinister colonic pathology.

Patient Preparation

Laxative use for bowel preparation prior to CTC has mostly been replaced by faecal tagging. This requires the patient to follow a low-residue diet 2 days prior to the examination and ingest oral contrast the day before (100 mL of Gastrografin in two separate doses of 50 mL, at 0800 and 1600 hours).

The faeces and contrast agent combine and help differentiate faeces from lesions in the colon when imaging takes place. The technique is also useful if the patient has had an incomplete colonoscopy, particularly due to suboptimal bowel preparation, as the patient can return for CTC the following day without having to undergo rigorous bowel preparation again. It has become more widely used in any case, particularly as both radiologists and radiographers gained more experience in assessing the scan. Because the instruction to 'follow a low-residue diet' may not be meaningful to those without a good understanding of foodstuffs and fibre, it is sensible to offer patients examples of foods they may eat, and those to be avoided (Table 21.1).

It is important to emphasise that drinking plenty of fluids is advisable, as with any bowel preparation method. Alternatively, a combination of laxative and

TABLE 21.1 Example of a Patient Dietary Information Sheet

Food Type	Foods Allowed	Foods to Avoid
Drinks	Water, coffee, tea, milk in very small amounts in hot drinks, herbal tea, cordial	Excess milk, juice with pulp, smoothies
Bread	White bread, white baps, white pitta, plain naan, plain chapati (not made with brown flour)	Wholemeal and granary bread, caraway, poppy or sesame seeds, pizza
Cereals	Rice Krispies, cornflakes, frosted flakes	Whole grain cereals, muesli, bran, Weetabix, porridge, shredded wheat
Dairy and spreads	Butter, margarine, cheese, paneer, eggs, plain salad dressing, mayonnaise, smooth yogurts (no fruit), crème fraiche, fromage frais	Yogurt or cheese containing fruit or nuts
Meat	Lean beef, chicken, white fish (no batter)	Oily fish, sausage, processed meats, fatty meat, chicken skin
Carbohydrates	White potatoes, white rice, white pasta, plain noodles	Wild grain rice, brown rice, couscous, polenta, jacket potato skin, pearl barley, wholemeal pasta, potato salad, pasta salad, quinoa, processed foods
Soup	Broth, cream soup	Vegetable soups, soup with solids
Vegetables (limit to 1–2 portions per day)	Shredded lettuce, tinned vegetables, mushrooms, tomato purée, passata	Raw vegetables, stalks, skins, seeds, peel, broccoli, Brussels sprouts, cabbage, cucumber, onion, turnip, beans, tomatoes, peppers, radish, sweetcorn, celery
Fruit (limit to 1–2 portions per day)	Avocado, ripe banana, tinned peaches, pears or apples, stewed fruit	Raw fruit with skin, berries, melon, dates, figs, pineapple, prunes, raisins, sultanas, currants, underripe bananas
Desserts	Plain jelly, low fat custard, bread pudding without nuts or fruit, rice pudding, honey, golden syrup, plain biscuits or crackers	Pastries, rich desserts, digestive biscuits, flapjacks, Hobnobs
Sweets	Boiled sweets, marshmallows, plain, milk or white chocolate in moderation	Nuts, fruits, jams, marmalade
Miscellaneous	Gravy, herbs (except garlic), spices in moderation, salt, vinegar, white sauce	Pickles, popcorn, crisps, relish, pepper, coconut, olives, ready meals (processed meals)

non-ionic oral contrast or dilute barium may be offered the day prior to the examination. Commonly used laxatives include pico-sulphate magnesium citrate (Picolax, Ferring Pharmaceuticals Ltd, UK) or magnesium citrate (Citramag, Sanochemia UK Ltd) with iohexol 350 mg/1 mL (Omnipaque, GE Healthcare) or barium sulphate 177 g 100% w/v (E-Z-Paque, Bracco UK) faecal tagging.

Contrast Agents

- Gastrografin (see section on patient preparation above)
- Non-ionic water-soluble contrast agent, e.g. Niopam 300 (iopamidol 61.2% w/v), Omnipaque 350 (iohexol 350 mg/1 mL)

Some centres do not use intravenous contrast agent unless sinister pathology is detected during CTC.

Additional Equipment

- Automatic CO_2 insufflator (Fig. 21.20) is preferable *or* air or CO_2 hand insufflation device
- Rectal catheter to attach to CO_2 insufflator
- Lubricating jelly
- Gauze swabs for application of lubricant to tip of catheter
- Vinyl or nitrile gloves
- Antispasmodic agent – hyoscine butylbromide 20 mg/mL IV, e.g. Buscopan. 2 mL syringe and filter needle

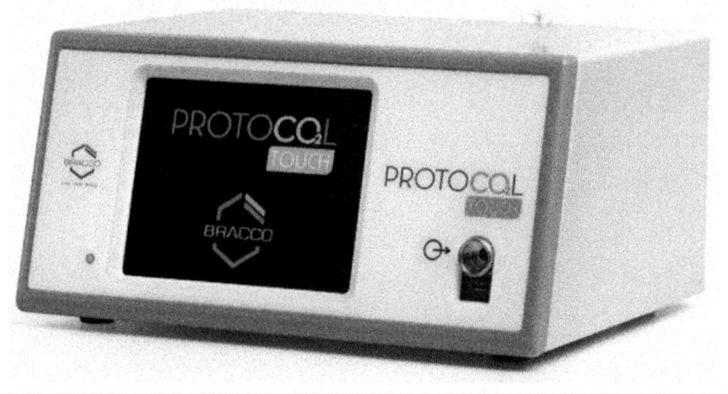

Fig. 21.20 Electronic CO_2 insufflator. (Image courtesy of Bracco UK Ltd.)

- Intravenous cannula (or 'Venflon') for administration of contrast medium and antispasmodic agent
- 10 mL saline and 10 mL syringe (optional)

Preparation Immediately Prior to the Examination

- All radio-opaque objects should be removed from the patient's chest, abdominal and pelvic region
- Check all equipment is readily available. Plug in the CO_2 insufflator and switch on. Open the valve to the insufflator using the spanner provided, ensuring that there is sufficient CO_2 in the cylinder (gauge on the insufflator) to commence the examination

- The rectal catheter is attached to the CO_2 insufflator in accordance with the manufacturer's instructions
- Informed consent should be obtained from the patient prior to the examination, therefore it is necessary to give a full and detailed account of the procedure so that the patient can make an informed decision to proceed. Their agreement to proceed should be documented. Checks should be made regarding allergies, particularly to iodine, and contraindications to Buscopan®

Technique

- The patient lies in the supine position on the CT scanner table
- An intravenous cannula ('Venflon') is inserted into a suitable vein; its position and stability can be checked using normal saline flush. An antispasmodic agent can then be administered if not contraindicated (see barium enema technique above for contraindications to Buscopan), but glucagon is not recommended as an alternative[41]
- The patient then lies on their left side with their knees and hips flexed, and the lubricated catheter is introduced and retention balloon inflated (it is important to ensure that the patient has had a per rectal examination to exclude low rectal pathology before proceeding with this). CO_2 is then insufflated automatically at a pressure of 20 mmHg until approximately 1.2 L have been administered or the pressure has reached the required setting and is maintained. Fluctuations in pressure may be indicative of spasm, however, colonic pathology such as stricture due to carcinoma or diverticular disease may be responsible, therefore care must be taken
- With the patient on their left side, CO_2 is allowed to rise into the right colon. The patient is then turned into the supine position with their arms raised above their head (to reduce the possibility of artefact)
- The scanner table is then moved into position, ensuring that the start position is above the level of the patient's diaphragm. At this point it should be ensured that the height of the scanner table has been adjusted so that the longitudinal positioning beam is level with the midpoint of the abdominal tissue
- If contrast is being administered, the tube from the contrast injector is now connected to the cannula and secured. The injector syringe is positioned to allow for maximum movement of the scanner table. A 'scout' view (terminology will vary according to the scanner manufacturer) is then performed with the patient supine, from a level just above the patient's diaphragm to a level just below the symphysis pubis. The scout view should also be assessed at this point to assess adequate colonic distension (see Fig. 21.21). This is extremely important, as distension is essential to ensure adequate visualisation on the scan (for additional information see below under 'Problem-Solving – inadequate distension'); but how is adequate distension defined? One piece of published research suggests that it should be assessed for all bowel segments, using a scale of 'no distension' (therefore totally inadequate) to the 'optimum' of 2 cm distension or more[42]
- Using the scout view as a baseline, the scan is then planned from above the diaphragm to just below the symphysis pubis and the patient scanned craniocaudally, still lying supine. A scan start delay of 50 seconds is required from initiation of the contrast injection to ensure that the liver is imaged in the portovenous phase. This is necessary, particularly if sinister colonic pathology is encountered, for the exclusion of liver metastases and to exclude extracolonic pathology[43]
- Once the supine scan has been completed, the contrast injector can be disconnected and the patient turned into the prone position. The cannula can be left in situ, but care must be taken that it is not compromised during repositioning. Patients can experience delayed reaction to contrast injections and antispasmodics therefore it is

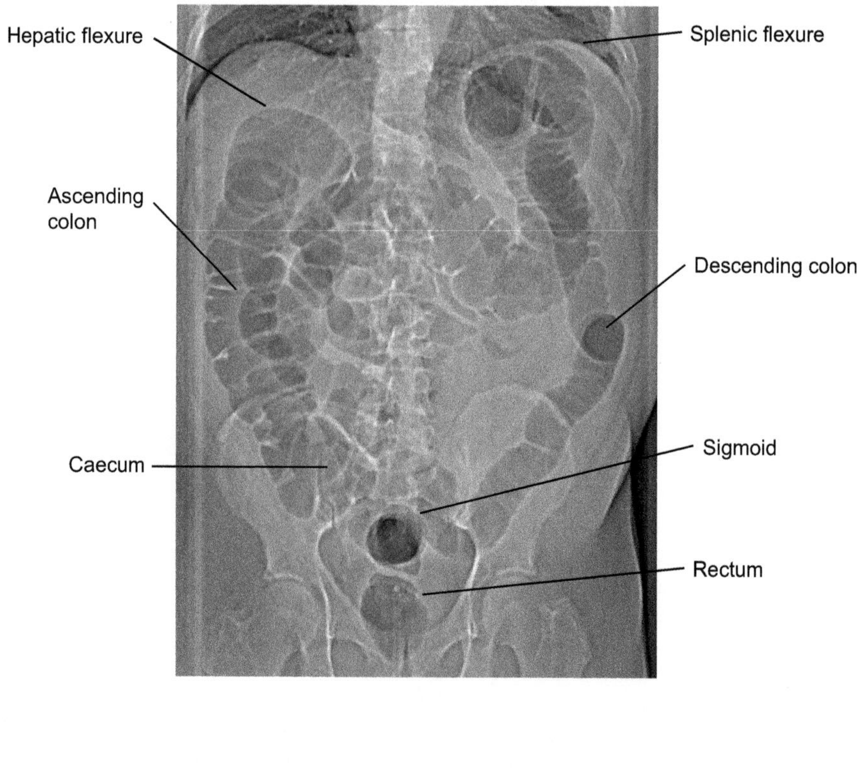

Fig. 21.21 Scout view.

important to maintain venous access for this reason, so that emergency or counteractive drugs can be administered without delay

- The patient is aligned again with a start position just above the level of the diaphragm, and terminating at a level just below the symphysis pubis. The scout view is performed and colonic distension assessed again. If the CO_2 insufflator should terminate (usually at 4.0L CO_2) this should be restarted in order to maintain colonic distension throughout the procedure. A prone scan is then planned from above the diaphragm to just below the symphysis pubis and the patient is again scanned craniocaudally. The scan parameters should be adjusted to a lower dose (e.g. effective mAs of 50). Although this results in a slight reduction in image quality it is sufficient to confirm or exclude any pathology that may have been observed on the supine component of the examination
- The total dose length product for the examination should then be recorded
- Contrast agents and antispasmodic drugs should also be recorded including batch numbers and expiry dates
- Once both scans have been completed the CO_2 insufflation should be terminated immediately and the rectal catheter removed

Acquisition Parameters

Supine: 120kV
160mAs (effective)
16 collimation × 0.7mm
Prone: 120kV
50mAs (effective)
16 collimation × 0.75mm

Image Assessment: Area of Interest

Both supine and prone scans are checked to ensure the whole of the colon, rectum and beyond the anal verge have been imaged, and that the whole of the liver is included. It is particularly important to include all solid abdominal organs so that other abdominal pathology, including metastases, can be excluded.

Problem-Solving

- *Inadequate distension.* This must be assessed on the scout view, and if the colon and rectum are not adequately distended further insufflation must take place. The initiation of the scan should be delayed until distension is sufficient. If necessary, repeat the scout view. Although this involves a small radiation dose it is extremely important that the bowel is distended fully before starting the scan. Inadequate distension will affect the ability of the observer to detect colonic lesions, particularly small polyps, and will be insufficient if a 3D 'fly-through' is required. Lateral decubitus views are also helpful, particularly if there is insufficient distension of either side of the colon (Fig. 21.22 – note the bilateral hip replacements, which can cause streak artefact – see 'Other artefacts' below). Raising one side allows CO_2 or air to rise and enhances distension.
- *Patient movement artefact.* Motion artefact is generally encountered during the examination if the patient is unable to hold their breath for the duration of the scan (although patient movement may be encountered, especially if the patient is agitated or restless). Scan times vary, but can be between 10 and 30 seconds depending on the technology of the scanner in question, which can be a particular problem for the elderly and those with existing chest conditions, e.g. COPD, asthma or pneumoconiosis. Ideally, if the patient can hold their breath for the first 15 seconds of the scan time this will enable the majority of the solid abdominal organs to be adequately visualised. It is preferable to scan the patient craniocaudally so that the abdominal section is scanned first; it is this region that is most affected by motion artefact due to respiration, and therefore it is important that it is captured sooner rather than later. In the pelvis, motion artefact due to inadequate arrested respiration is less of an issue as pelvic organs are less likely to move during respiration. It is therefore important to stress the need for the patient to remain relatively still and to hold their breath when instructed to do so, for the duration of the scan if possible.
- *Other artefacts.* Metal objects can cause streaking artefact and this can result in degradation of the resulting images.[44] It is important to ensure that patients are prepared for the examination by removing any metal objects from the area to be scanned. If the patient is unable to raise their arms above their head (see section on positioning) then all metal objects should be removed from this region. It may be that some metal objects cannot be removed, e.g. hip replacements. Streak artefact from this source is difficult to avoid, and although techniques such as gantry angulation and thinner acquisition sections can be used in some types of CT examination, this is not a recommendation for CTC.

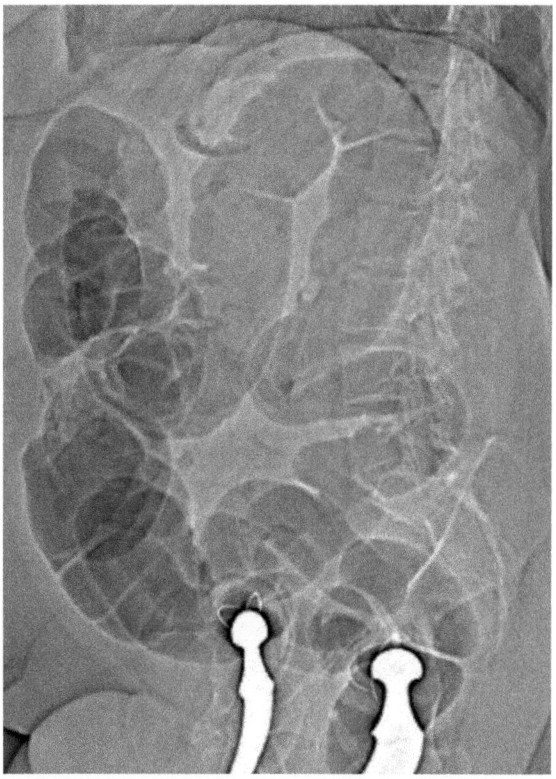

Fig. 21.22 Lateral decubitus.

Patient Aftercare

The patient should remain in the department for at least 15 minutes after contrast agent injection to ensure that no delayed adverse events occur, and during this time the cannula should be left in situ. The images should be reviewed by a suitably qualified radiographer or a radiologist prior to the patient leaving the department.

Potential Complications

With CTC there is a small risk of colonic perforation, and this should be excluded before the patient leaves the department: the CT scan is reviewed to ensure that there is no free air in the abdomen and, as the patient should remain in the department for 15–20 minutes after a contrast agent injection, they can be assessed periodically for signs and symptoms of perforation; these signs and symptoms include severe abdominal pain, nausea and, in extreme cases, fever and vomiting.

The patient may also experience mild symptoms of abdominal cramping after colonic insufflation; if this occurs they should remain in the X-ray department until the symptoms subside. Wherever possible CO_2 should have been used in the examination, as opposed to room air, to reduce or even eliminate these symptoms. CO_2 is readily absorbed, and therefore the colon is distended for a shorter period.

If Buscopan® is used, patients **must** seek medical attention if they develop painful blurred vision after leaving the imaging department, as this may be an indication of undiagnosed glaucoma.

Additional Information

It is essential that a multidetector CT scanner is used so that detailed image reconstruction can take place. Ideally there should be access to 3D software to allow the images to be reviewed and to assist with problem-solving. This technology has advanced considerably and some centres employ a 3D fly-through as a first read. Polyps can sometimes be easier to identify at this stage (Fig. 21.23).

It is also essential that dual-position scanning is used. This is vital to help distinguish between actual pathology and faecal residue. If the patient is unable to lie in the prone position, lateral decubitus imaging should be used. CTC is limited in its detection of colitis, and optical colonoscopy remains the 'gold standard' for diagnosis of ulcerative colitis.

Defaecating Proctography

The proctogram was first developed during World War Two and was used to examine soldiers infested with the whipworm parasite which was known to cause rectal prolapses. Whipworm is now commonly diagnosed via colonoscopy or lab smear tests.[45] The proctogram has evolved to include both X-ray and MRI techniques and can now diagnose many different pelvic floor conditions. Most patients referred for proctograms are women and for this reason there is reference to use of contact agent in the vagina in technique descriptions in this chapter.

When the pelvic floor is working normally, the puborectalis muscle contracts and maintains a bend in the rectum, helping with stool continence.[46] During the act of 'bearing down' the puborectalis relaxes and allows the rectum to straighten so that the stool can be passed. The urethra passes through the front section of the pelvic floor, as does the vagina in females. Bearing down is similar to a Valsalva manoeuvre.

The aim of proctography is to visualise the functioning dynamic of the pelvic floor and to show any pathologies/abnormalities that may explain the patient's symptoms. In fluoroscopic proctography a contrast agent is required in order to visualise this dynamic on the images and is usually a barium sulphate solution, which may be mixed with another form of media such as porridge or mashed potato (for coeliac patients, potato is a preferred agent, to avoid any intolerance). Patients also have to attend earlier than their actual procedure in order to drink barium. In MR proctography, ultrasound gel is used as a contrast agent to visualise the rectum.[47]

The full names for the types of defaecating proctography in use today are fluorographic defaecating proctography (FDP) and magnetic resonance defaecating proctography (MRDP). Variation in practice exists at the present time, some centres advocating MRDP whilst others use either or both FDP and MRDP. Both have advantages

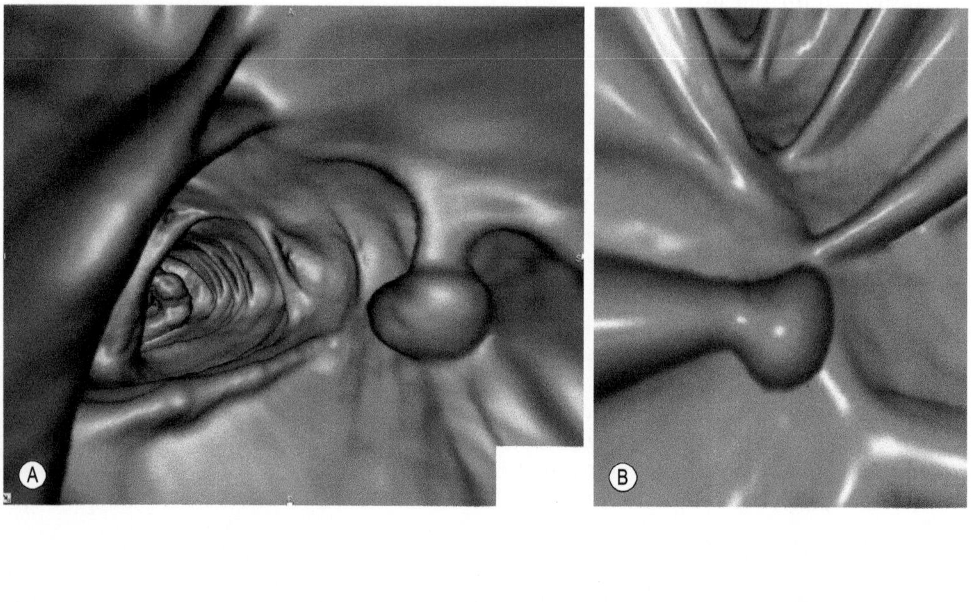

Fig. 21.23 (A,B) Polyps. (Images courtesy of Bracco UK Ltd.)

and disadvantages. For example, MRDP allows all three pelvic compartments to be evaluated in one examination with superior soft tissue assessment; it is less invasive and does not involve radiation. However, it is more expensive and MRI contraindications will exclude its use for some patients (see Chapter 27) and at least one study has found that MRDP underestimated grades of intussusception in 60% of examinations and failed to identify them in 40%. This study suggested that some patients would benefit from examination via FDP *and* MRDP.[48] Another suggestion is that there is a perceived weakness of MRDP linked with the supine positioning of the patient, resulting in underestimation of dysfunction.[49]

This examination is undertaken to demonstrate the anatomy and physiology of the rectum, anal canal and pelvic floor dynamically, during defaecation, using videofluorography or MRI dynamic scan. It is an examination performed mainly, but not exclusively, on female patients.

REFERRAL CRITERIA

- Difficult or suspected obstructed defaecation (obstructed defaecation syndrome, or ODS), incomplete rectal emptying
- Urgency
- Defect in levator ani
- Perineal swellings
- Evaluation of rectocoele, enterocoele, rectal mucosal prolapse and intussusception
- Faecal incontinence
- Post defaecation incontinence
- Pouchitis
- Pre- and postoperative evaluation for LVR (laparoscopic ventral rectopexy) surgery
- Preoperative evaluation for consideration of stapled transanal resection of the rectum (STARR) for obstructed defaecation syndrome

COMMON ABNORMALITIES SEEN WITH PROCTOGRAPHY

- *Obstructed defaecation*: a term used to describe one component of constipation, in that patients may be unable to evacuate their bowels properly. This can be identified by excess straining, incomplete emptying, multiple unsuccessful bowel movements and the feeling of a 'blockage'. It can be caused by structural abnormalities such as rectocoeles or rectal prolapses. It can also be caused by the inability to coordinate the pelvic floor muscles properly in order to produce a bowel movement.[50]
- *Rectocoele*: the anterior wall of the rectum pushes into the posterior wall of the vagina, creating a bulge. These are usually caused by a thinning of the tissue of the recto-vaginal septum between the rectum and the vagina, and weakness in the pelvic floor muscles. It can be caused by a number of factors, including trauma arising from vaginal deliveries (Ventouse delivery, forceps delivery), constipation, chronic straining or gynaecological/rectal surgeries (e.g hysterectomy). Rectocoeles can result in a number of symptoms such as difficulty in having a complete bowel movement, excess straining, multiple straining attempts, rectal pain, constipation, faeces getting stuck in the rectocoele and having to press on the rectocoele in order to empty.[51]
- *Incomplete rectal emptying*: the rectum cannot empty completely or the patient feels as if their bowels do not empty completely.
- *Intussusception:* this is where a section of intestine moves into another part of the intestine, such as in the parts of a telescope. This then creates a block for faeces, often causing obstruction. In serious cases it can also lead to a cut off of the blood supply to the intestine which can lead to bowel perforation, infection and necrosis of bowel tissue.[52]
- *Enterocoele*: the small bowel pushes onto the back wall of the vagina by dropping down within the abdominal cavity. This then forms a large bulge between the bowel and the vagina on the proctogram. It can cause obstruction and a 'dragging' sensation for patients.[53]

CONTRAINDICATIONS TO PROCTOGRAPHY

- *Allergies*: although rare, some patients may be allergic to lubricating jelly or contrast agents used during a proctogram. This will then mean the patient's referral should be reconsidered between referrer and consultant radiologist, when alternative examinations will be discussed.
- *Pregnancy*: 10 day rule/pregnancy status ascertained prior to FDP examination, MRDP should be avoided during pregnancy since the pelvic floor will be affected by the gravid uterus.
- *Postoperative rectum* (e.g. coloanal anastomosis): proceed with caution.
- *Limited mobility*: due to the limitations of manual handling aids within MRI environments, patients with poor mobility are not suitable for this type of scan. In these cases, FDP may be more tolerable for the patient.
- *Reduced compliance*: this examination requires compos mentis patients to comply with instructions. Some patients can find compliance difficult due to anxiety and/or psychological distress. This can give false-negative/positive results from the examination.[54]
- *MRI contraindications*: for example, MRI unsafe pacemaker or aneurysm clip. Since MRI proctograms carry stricter contraindicatory criteria, fluoroscopic proctograms may be the only option available to some patients.[55] For a full list of MRI contraindications see Chapter 27.

PATIENT PREPARATION FOR PROCTOGRAPHY

Proctography is a very intimate and potentially embarrassing examination for many patients, therefore it is essential that during the examination the patient's privacy and dignity are uppermost in the mind of staff at all times. It is important that the radiographer keeps the environment secure by limiting the members of staff within the area, locking doors to prevent staff members walking in and using no entry/do not disturb signs on doors.

The radiographer should try to cover the patient as much as possible when performing intimate sections of the examination, for example placing a sheet over the patient when administering contrast agent or putting a sheet over the lower half of the patient during the examination.

FDP

No bowel or dietary preparation is required before attending hospital,[56] although some centres may advocate a laxative suppository immediately prior to the examination. Medication can be taken as usual.

MRDP

Patient preparation prior to the MRI scan can vary; some centres will not have any nil by mouth instructions. Others will ask the patient to starve for 4 hours prior to the examination; this usually makes the examination more pleasant for the patient, as there is less possibility of faecal matter being present during the dynamic section of the scan. A phosphate-based enema is given 10 minutes before the examination; alternatively, glycerin suppositories can be administered 30 minutes before the examination.

Both Techniques

Patients should receive an information letter/leaflet prior to their attendance so that they can give their consent.[57] On arrival, the patient is asked to change into a radiolucent hospital gown; this will give the patient some comfort that none of their clothes will become soiled during the procedure. They should be given a summary of what to expect from the examination and what is expected of them during the procedure; it is useful to explain the stages of the examination, including the actions they will be asked to take. Patients should also be told that they have the option to stop the examination and withdraw their consent to continue at any point. A conversation should then occur between the radiographer and the patient to ascertain their symptoms, which will aid with reporting of images.

This is an intimate, invasive and sensitive examination and careful explanation of what the patient is required to do is important. Patient privacy and dignity must be a major consideration at all times. A chaperone is essential during these procedures to reassure the patient, particularly if a member of the opposite sex is performing the intimate parts of the examination.[57]

FLUOROGRAPHIC DEFAECATING PROCTOGRAPHY

Contrast Agents

1. Barium sulphate suspension, e.g. E-Z-Paque 96% w/w powder, 177 g mixed with water to 60% w/v. The patient drinks this to opacify the small bowel and to help visualise enterocoeles, 45–60 minutes prior to the examination; 10 mL of this suspension is retained for vaginal opacification
2. Barium sulphate suspension, E-Z-HD 98% w/w powder, 340 g mixed with 40 mL warm water to toothpaste-like consistency for opacifaction of the rectum. Some imaging departments mix porridge or instant mashed potato to a ratio of: 2 cups mash/porridge to 1 cup of hot water with ½ cup of barium, mixed to a smooth and fairly thick consistency

Contrast Administration Equipment

- Plastic disposable apron and vinyl gloves
- Enema air tip catheter
- 3 ×50 mL syringes with a catheter tip
- Lubricating gel with gauze swab for application of lubricant to catheter
- Filling cannula to draw up barium for vaginal opacification
- 10 mL syringe
- Incontinence pads, whole and cut into strips

Examination Area Preparation (Fig. 21.24)

- It is essential to have toilet facilities adjacent to the examination room so patient privacy and dignity is maintained
- A commode is placed in the examination area, with bed pan and disposable inserts
- Lead equivalent protective glass should be covered to give patients maximum privacy, with the radiographer monitoring their patient via the screen

Note: Essential staff only should be present in the examination room.

Admission Process

- The patient's last menstrual cycle is documented, if applicable
- Oral barium is given to the patient 45 minutes to 1 hour prior to the examination
- Full explanation of the examination procedure is given
- The patient is asked to change into a gown with the opening at the back (they may leave their clothes on from the waist up but should be asked to remove clothing from the waist down)
- The patient's identity is checked as per hospital protocol and examination history for recent studies and duplication

Procedure

- Informed verbal consent is gained by the person performing the procedure
- The practitioner will also provide information on the risk and benefit of having X-rays to the patient (or their representative or carer)
- 45–60 minutes before proctography, the oral contrast agent is given to the patient
- 45–60 minutes after the oral contrast is ingested, the radiographer revisits explanation of the examination manoeuvres with the patient and ensures that they understand the instructions fully

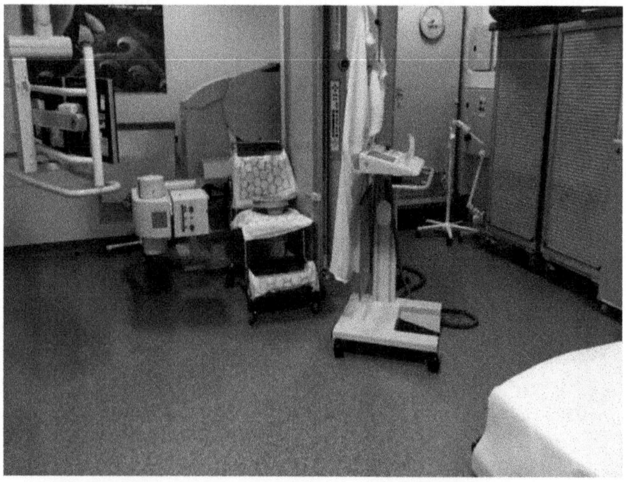

Fig. 21.24 Preparing the imaging suite for fluoroproctography.

- The patient is asked to lie in the left lateral decubitus position on a trolley in the fluoroscopy suite. For all female patients 5–10 mL of liquid barium sulphate is injected into the vagina (if consent is granted) to demonstrate the presence of an enterocoele and its effects on the vaginal wall
- A well-lubricated enema air contrast tip catheter is gently inserted until the tip is just inside the patient's anus. Approximately 150 mL of barium sulphate paste (E-Z-HD 98% w/w powder, toothpaste-like consistency) is injected slowly into the rectum via a catheter tip syringe
- The catheter is removed and the patient asked to try to retain the paste whilst moving from the trolley to the commode, then screened fluoroscopically to ensure they are in a lateral position. The collimators are manipulated so that the sacrum is seen posteriorly and at least 5 cm of the skin edge inferiorly
- A series of videofluorographic images are taken whilst the patient follows instruction on various pelvic manoeuvres. These vary slightly in selection and include a variation of actions from the following list, in order to assess the dynamic of the area before, during and after defaecation:
  a. At rest to visualise the pelvic floor in its usual position (Fig. 21.25)
  b. Squeezing their pelvic floor muscles as if trying not to defaecate (also known as a Kegel manoeuvre). This demonstrates contraction of the pelvic floor (Fig. 21.26)
  c. 'Push' or Valsalva manoeuvre, without allowing defaecation. It is explained to the patient as 'bearing down' until they feel the pressure 'down below'. This helps to visualise the pelvic floor under pressure
  d. defaecation (Fig. 21.27). The patient is encouraged to empty as much of their rectum as possible and to pass as much of the rectally inserted contrast as possible. This is to visualise the pelvic floor in its most extreme dynamic. It is very important that the patient passes as much of the contrast agent as possible before the examination is finished; not only to demonstrate incomplete evacuation but also for their own comfort. If the patient is unable to empty the paste on the commode they may retire to the privacy of the toilet and, upon emptying the rectum as much as possible, they return to have the final image taken[58]
  e. 'At rest' image to show the relaxed area after defaecation and to visualise complete or incomplete emptying. This is the last in the series of images taken and is often the most useful in demonstrating pathology. An empty rectum gives the best chance to show prolapse, especially when using FDP, and incomplete emptying does affect accuracy in assessment for prolapse

If the practitioner is concerned that they may not have demonstrated pathology adequately they can, with the patient's consent, refill the rectum and acquire more images focused on the right area.[59]

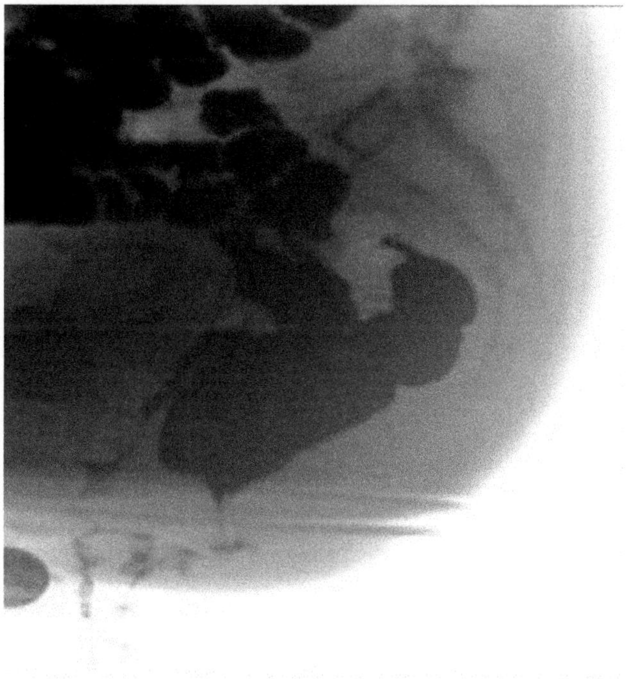

Fig. 21.25 Image taken at rest.

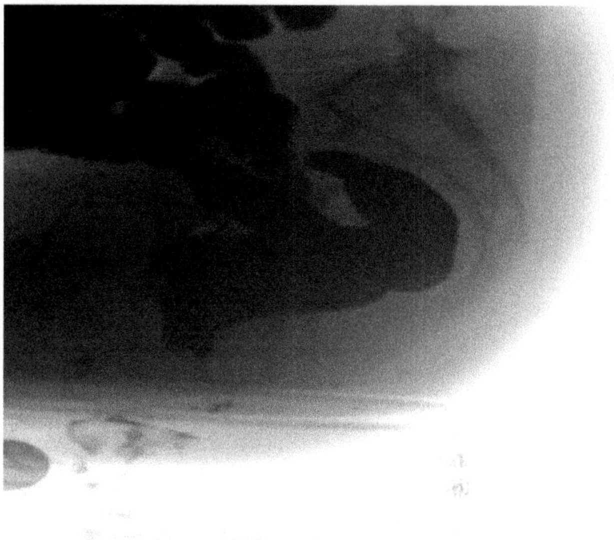

Fig. 21.26 Image captured at Kegel manoeuvre stage.

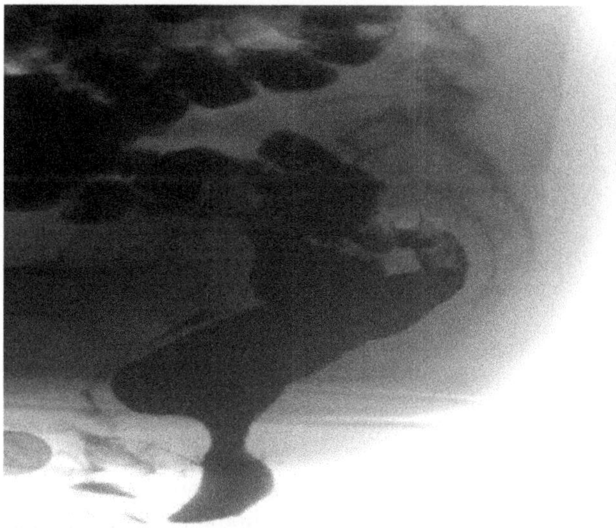

Fig. 21.27 Image captured at defaecation stage.

Potential Complications for the Procedure

Some patients can find the contrast medium hard to hold due to incontinence, this is why it is important to limit the movement between the examination and rectal insertion. The rectum needs to be adequately filled to ensure accurate diagnosis, and also to replicate the patient's symptoms.

It is important to note that some patients will have severe degrees of pelvic floor descent, therefore the images may have to be acquired lower than the sacral promontory; necessity for this can be determined during the dynamic images.[59]

In fluoroscopy, when vaginal contrast is often used during the examination, there is a potential that the vaginal contrast agent could be mistakenly positioned in the bladder (rare, but potentially very hazardous) or rectum. If placed in the rectum, the vagina will not be visualised properly.

Criteria for Assessing Image and Examination Quality

- The images should be free of artefacts, patients should be appropriately dressed for their scan reducing any artefacts from metal
- Superiorly the images should include the sacral promontory, medially and laterally the sacrum, coccyx and pubic symphysis. The images should include within them the rectum, bladder and, in females, the vagina and urethra (which helps in assessment of rectocoele). Inclusion of all required structures allows for accurate evaluation in order to lead to correct diagnosis, and means that the following assessments can be made:
  a. Measurement of the anorectal angle by connecting the longitudinal axis of the anal canal and the posterior rectal line, parallel to the longitudinal axis of the rectum. This angle is a way of measuring puborectal muscle activity. During pelvic floor contraction, this angle becomes more acute but during relaxation it is more obtuse and there are normal variants for these angles. It is this angle that is used to define whether the pelvic floor is normal or abnormal
  b. Diagnosis of a rectocoele (Fig. 21.28): the anterior wall of the rectum with a bulge that is wider than 2 cm anteriorly is considered clinically significant
  c. Diagnosis of intussusception (Fig. 21.28): there must be an infolding of the rectal wall greater than 3 mm thickness to be considered significant. This can present as a funnel shape during straining; less than 3 mm thickness represents mucosal prolapse but is usually not considered significant[60]

Images should show the rectum full and, by the end of the examination (where possible), empty

Post Procedure

The patient is allowed to return to the toilet and may wish to take a shower. It is good practice to offer products that may give comfort for the journey home: e.g., sanitary towel or absorbent pants.

Patients should be informed that their stools will be paler or white for a few days and they should be encouraged to take a high fibre diet and plenty of fluids over the next 48 hours to reduce the incidence of constipation.

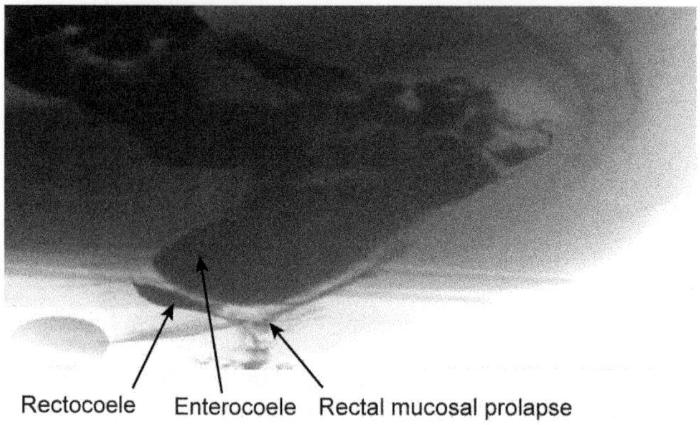

Fig. 21.28 Rectocoele, enterocoele and rectal mucosal prolapse intussuscepting the anal canal.

MAGNETIC RESONANCE DEFAECATING PROCTOGRAPHY

Preparation and Patient Care

Psychological and medicolegal preparation is outlined for MRDP under 'Patient preparation' at the start of this section of the chapter.

Contraindications for MRI should be checked with the patient; metallic artefacts should be excluded when the patient changes into an examination gown.

It is essential that during the examination the patient is given privacy and dignity at all times and also given the option that they can stop and withdraw their consent to continue at any point.

It is important that the radiographer keeps the environment secure by limiting the members of staff within the area, locking doors to prevent staff members walking in and placing no entry/do not disturb signs to bring awareness to that environment.

The radiographer should try to cover the patient as much as possible when performing intimate sections of the examination, for example placing a sheet over the patient when putting in the contrast media or putting a sheet over the lower half of the patient during the scan.

In addition to the MR scanner, the following equipment is required:

- Phosphate-based enema
- Incontinence pads
- Vinyl gloves
- Plastic apron
- 3 × 50 mL bladder tip syringes
- Ultrasound gel
- Commode or nearby toilet
- Lubricant
- Knee support pad
- Shower/warm water/cleansing wipes

Procedure

- A trained practitioner places a phosphate-based enema into the patient's anus. Once the patient feels ready, they

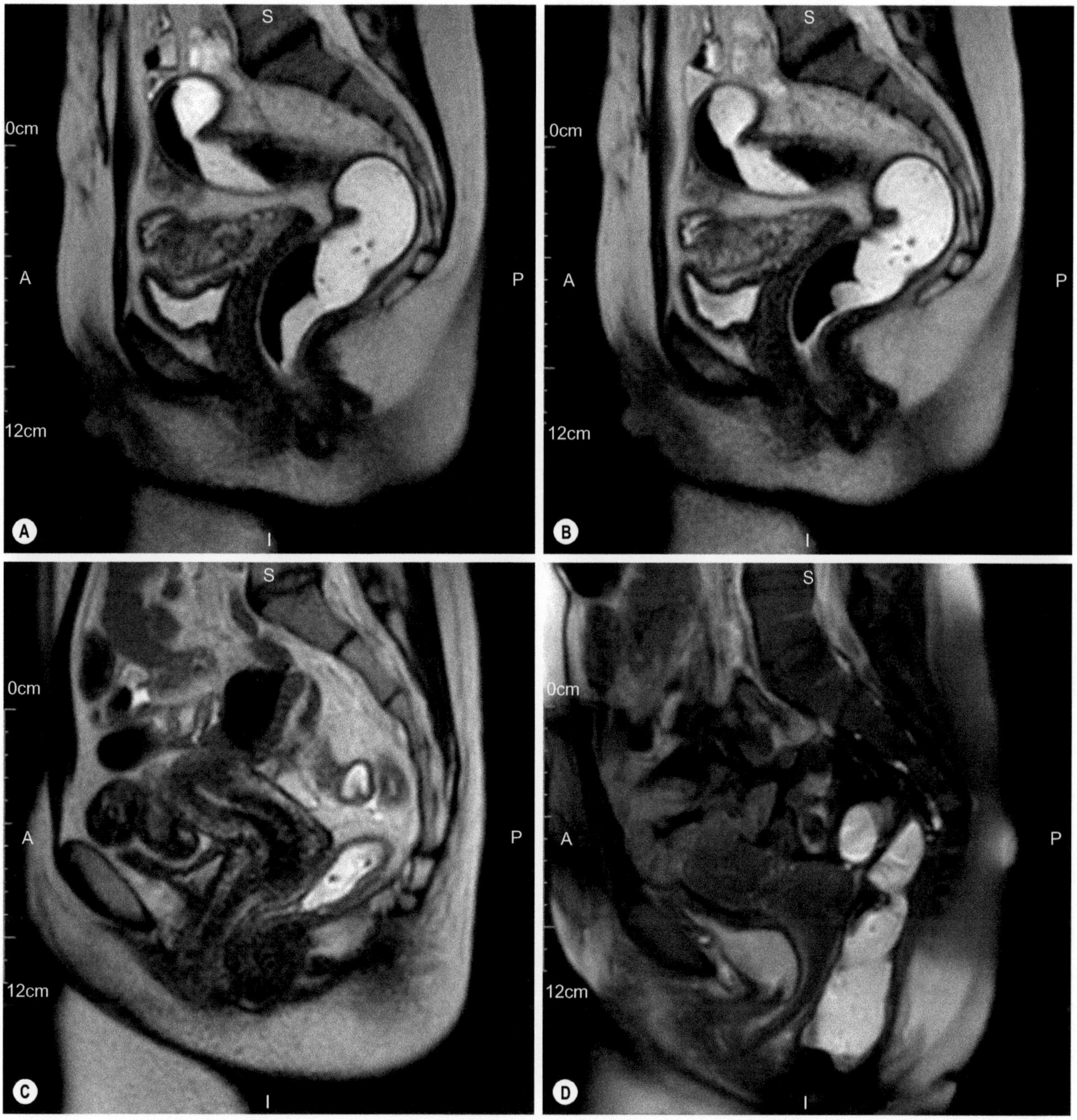

Fig. 21.29 (A–D) MRDP images: (A) image acquired 'at rest'; (B) squeezing (Kegel manoeuvre); (C) pushing down; (D) after defaecation.

are brought into the MRI suite. The radiographer then goes through the exercises again with the patient so that they understand the instructions fully

- A trained practitioner then administers the ultrasound gel into the patient's anus. This is usually approximately 150 mL. The patient is then asked to lie on their back with knees slightly bent with help from a foam pad. A pelvic torso coil is placed over the pelvis in order to obtain high-quality images
- Imaging is then performed using the following manoeuvres:
  a. At rest (Fig. 21.29A)
  b. Kegel manoeuvre (Fig. 21.29B)
  c. Valsalva manoeuvre (Fig. 21.29C)
  d. Defaecation (Fig. 21.29D)
- The radiographer then performs the dynamic scan. This is where the radiographer will be able to see the pelvic floor moving whilst it is being imaged. In this sequence the patient will perform:
  a. At rest
  b. Kegel manoeuvre
  c. Valsalva manoeuvre
  d. Defaecation, encouraging the patient to empty their rectum as much as possible (Fig. 21.29D). The dynamic sequence can be repeated several times to make sure that the patient empties their rectum
- After the dynamic sequence there are more images acquired at 'Kegel' and 'Valsalva'; this is to visualise how the pelvic floor is working without the weight of contrast within the rectum

- Then high-resolution images are taken at 'rest' in coronal plane and axial plane. This will visualise the levator ani in more detail
- Once all images are acquired, the patient is given an opportunity to clean up in the scanner room or offered a shower. It is good practice to offer products that may give comfort for the journey home, e.g., sanitary towel or absorbent pants

Accessory Organs of the Gastrointestinal Tract – Salivary Glands

Plain radiography imaging alone cannot be considered an accurate imaging method as only 50% of parotid gland and 20% of submandibular gland sialoliths are radio-opaque.[61] The first way that this issue was tackled was to use contrast-enhanced examinations (sialography), eventually supplemented by, or now superseded by, ultrasound CT, MRI, or RNI examinations. Since there are still some regions globally that do not have easy access to other imaging, contrast sialography is still covered at the end of this section

REFERRAL CRITERIA FOR IMAGING SALIVARY GLANDS

- Pain
- Swelling

Both symptoms are often noted on or after eating.
In addition to diagnosis, imaging is also a precursor to interventional techniques, such as basket removal of sialoliths.

ULTRASOUND

This has had an increasing role in assessing the salivary glands during the 21st century, particularly when using Doppler. All major pathologies exhibit classic signs of hypoechoic, anechoic or inhomogeneous areas that can be recognised and aid in differential diagnosis.[62] Owing to its non-invasive nature and capability in detecting numerous pathologies, ultrasound is considered to be the investigation of choice but it is known to be difficult to detect sialoliths with ultrasound, or in chronic cases where the gland does not function.[63]

It is particularly useful for assessing solid mass salivary gland pathology, and also effective in conjunction with fine needle aspiration because of the high resolution that can be attained. It has also been advocated as a quick and simple process to use in assisting fine needle aspiration of tumours.[63]

MAGNETIC RESONANCE SIALOGRAPHY

MRI has long been compared favourably to conventional techniques.[64] Its obvious advantage is that it uses hydrographic technique (relying on the presence of the patient's own saliva), so no cannulation is required, and of course no ionising radiation is used. However, to combat the spatial resolution difference a number of methods have been used: these include the use of a sialogogue for dynamic studies and also the use of small surface coils.[65,66] One showed that using a sialogogue and a passive occlusion device (a pad used to compress and occlude the opening of the duct) is comparable with interventional methods, particularly when assessing the parotid gland;[67] however it must be noted that the investigators had undertaken research on volunteers, recognising that further study on patients was required in order to assess diagnostic performance and the practicality of this technique.

When malignancy is identified via any imaging method, MRI is required to assess potential soft tissue invasion or perineural spread.[63]

COMPUTED TOMOGRAPHY

With duct cannulation and contrast enhancement, CT is also considered preferential to contrast radiography of the region. It is considered to be most useful in imaging (without contrast) for tumour enhancement or in patients who have a mass lesion. Radiation dose plays an important factor, especially compared to all other techniques; image quality is high and accuracy of the technique with or without contrast enhancement has been found to be of a comparable standard.[68] Cone beam CT can also be used to demonstrate the salivary glands.

RADIONUCLIDE IMAGING

RNI is particularly useful as a safe and reliable method to assess gland function and is known to have a role in diagnosis of Sjögren's syndrome and associated xerostomia.[69,70]

CONTRAST-ENHANCED X-RAY IMAGING OF THE SALIVARY GLANDS – SIALOGRAPHY

Usually only parotid and submandibular glands are imaged using contrast agents, as it is considered more difficult to cannulate the sublingual gland. Submental occlusal radiography can be used to assess the sublingual region but will only show radio-opaque calculi (see Dental Radiography, Chapter 14).

Contraindications

- Acute infection or inflammation[17,28]

Contrast Agent

- Water soluble contrast agent with an iodine content of 240–300 mg/mL *or* 480 mg/mL in an oily contrast agent. Neither contrast agent appears to be more advantageous than the other

Additional Equipment

- Small syringe (2 mL)
- Filling cannula
- Lacrimal dilator (sterile)
- 18G blunt needle with catheter (sterile)
- Sterile gloves
- Gauze swabs
- Sialogogue (used to stimulate salivation and help dilate the salivary duct for cannulation). This may be in the form of lemon juice, a citrus-flavoured sweet or sherbet

- Wooden spatula
- Mouthwash and disposable cup

Patient Preparation

- Removal of artefacts, including dentures
- After plain radiography has been undertaken, the sialogogue is administered to promote salivation and maximise visualisation of the salivary duct
- Explain to the patient that it will be necessary for them to indicate when the salivary duct feels full of contrast agent. Arrange for a distinctive sign to be given by the patient (e.g. raising a hand) when the relevant area feels tight or full. It is important that the patient understands the process *before* the procedure starts, as explanation while undergoing cannulation often proves ineffective
- Explain to the patient that it will be necessary for them to keep their lips closed gently over the cannula, to ensure it stays in place in the duct

For all areas, control images are taken prior to administration of the contrast agent; basic information on head positioning can be found in corresponding position descriptors in relevant chapters on radiography of the head or teeth (see Chapters 11 and 14), although centring and collimation differ for sialography. Some slight modifications from basic head positions will be outlined, if relevant.

PAROTID GLANDS

Control images for sialography can be taken prior to application of the sialogue, for preassessment of any radio-opaque calculi.

Image receptor (IR) position is dictated by patient position during the procedure, as patient or investigator preferences influence whether a supine or erect sitting position is used.

Control images required:

1. Anteroposterior (AP) (fronto-occipital (FO) position) projection with the head rotated 5° away from the side under investigation. Centre midway between the symphysis menti and the angle of the mandible on the side under examination. Collimate to include soft tissues of the neck and face, symphysis menti and zygoma on the side under examination. Figure 21.30 shows an AP projection (of the right submandibular gland) after contrast injection
2. Lateral, centred to the angle of mandible. Collimate to include soft tissues of the neck and under the chin, external auditory meatus, zygoma and to level with the ala of the nose anteriorly. Figure 21.31 shows a lateral projection (of the right parotid gland) after contrast injection
3. Lateral oblique with the patient's head (MSP) tilted 15° towards the side under investigation. Tube angle of 10–15° cranially, centre midway between the angles of mandible. Figure 21.32 shows a lateral oblique projection (of the right submandibular gland) after contrast injection

Technique

- If the gland is not visible, the sialogogue may be used to promote salivation
- Saliva is blotted away from the duct area using a gauze swab and the duct is dilated with a lacrimal dilator

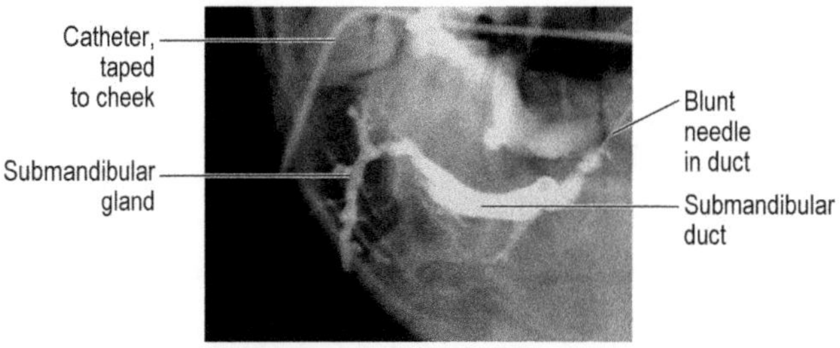

Fig. 21.30 AP – submandibular gland.

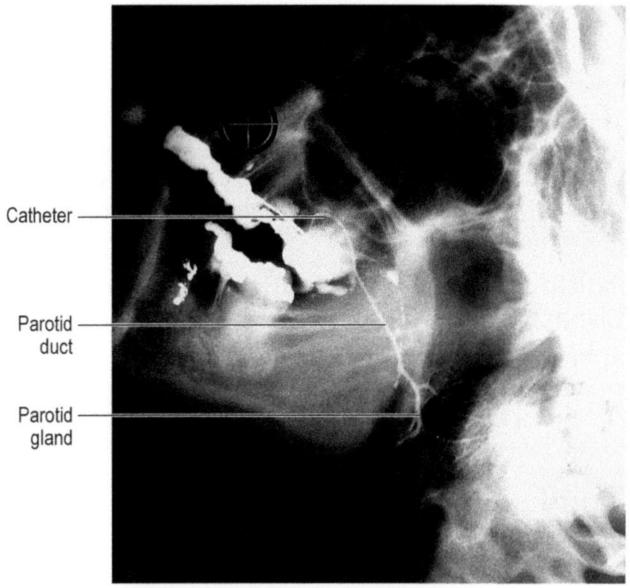

Fig. 21.31 Lateral – parotid gland. (Reproduced with permission from Ryan S, et al. *Anatomy for Diagnostic Imaging*. 2nd ed. London: Saunders; 2004.)

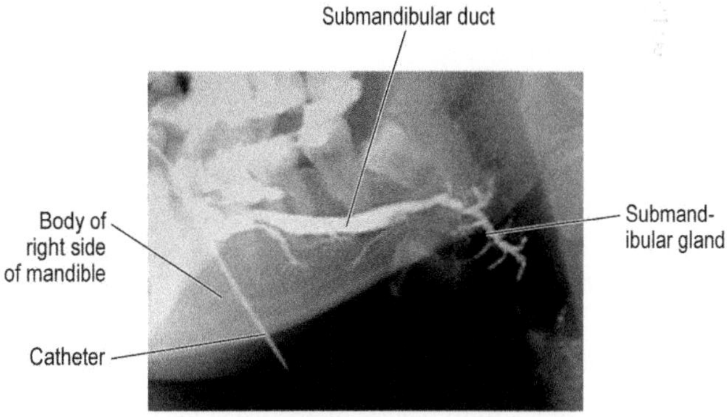

Fig. 21.32 Lateral oblique – submandibular gland.

- The duct is cannulated, using the blunt-ended sialographic needle/catheter apparatus
- Following cannulation, up to 2 mL of contrast are injected until the patient indicates that the gland feels 'full' (see the preparation section with regard to a signal for this)
- The catheter tubing is taped to the skin surface, away from the duct and gland area
- The precontrast images are repeated
- After the images have been taken the patient is given a mouthwash to promote saliva secretion and a lateral

view can then be taken to demonstrate drainage of the duct and any sialectasis, if present

SUBMANDIBULAR GLAND

Control images required:

1. A lower occlusal image, with the IR possibly displaced over to the side in question
2. Lateral, as for the parotid gland, centred to the angle of the mandible with the floor of the mouth depressed by a wooden spatula
3. Lateral oblique, as for the parotid gland

Technique

The procedure then follows that described for the parotid gland, but the occlusal film is not required after contrast introduction and it is not necessary to use a spatula in the lateral projection. A post-sialogogue lateral film is required.

Patient Aftercare: Parotid and Submandibular Glands

- Provide further mouthwash, if the patient requires it
- Advise the patient that they may experience an unusual taste (which may occur intermittently) until the contrast has fully drained

Potential Complications: Parotid and Submandibular Glands

- Infection
- Duct orifice damage
- Duct rupture

Accessory Organs of the Gastrointestinal Tract – Gallbladder and Biliary Tree

X-ray imaging with contrast has now been superseded by ultrasound and this has been the first imaging port of call for several decades, with other modalities playing their part in diagnostics.

ULTRASOUND

Ultrasound has a high degree of accuracy for the diagnosis of gallstones, similar to that of oral cholecystography, but with a number of significant advantages. It is also an excellent method of evaluating the common bile duct and common hepatic ducts without the use of contrast.

Advantages of ultrasound are:

- Patients fast for only 6 hours
- No contraindications
- Pain on scanning can be related to acute cholecystitis (Murphy's sign)
- No complications
- No use of ionising radiation
- Less time-consuming for the operator and patient
- Other structures can be imaged at the same time (e.g. bile duct, liver, pancreas)

RADIONUCLIDE IMAGING

Cholescintigraphy (or HIDA (hepatobiliary iminodiacetic acid) scan) is a useful adjunct to assess function, often after normal ultrasound has been performed for right upper quadrant pain, because a normal ^{99m}Tc-IDA scan excludes the diagnosis as it provides a direct assessment of cystic duct patency. This technique has high sensitivity and specificity, particularly for the diagnosis of acute cholecystitis (97% and 94%, respectively).[71]

COMPUTED TOMOGRAPHY

CT can be used to visualise the gallbladder but is not always as accurate as ultrasound in the diagnosis of gallstones, and has additional risks associated with the use of ionising radiation. CT can be useful in the very obese patient, as these patients prove difficult to image with ultrasound.

It has long been indicated that CT cholangiography has an increased role to play in the imaging of the biliary tree, providing precise and detailed evaluation of the system if the clinician has a comprehensive understanding of the technique.[72,73]

MAGNETIC RESONANCE IMAGING

This technique is constantly finding new applications as technology and expertise continue to grow in the field. The most common examination is the magnetic resonance cholangiopancreatogram (MRCP), which will be mentioned in more detail later in comparison with endoscopic retrograde cholangiopancreatography) (ERCP).

INTRAVENOUS CHOLANGIOGRAPHY (IVC)

This examination is almost never undertaken in the 21st century thanks to safer imaging via ultrasound, ERCP and MRCP.[28]

ORAL CHOLECYSTOGRAPHY

Ultrasound has almost exclusively replaced cholecystography in the UK but is still considered to be an option in other world regions with limited access to ultrasound.

The examination has three stages:

1. Control plain radiography
2. Contrast images
3. Gallbladder showing drainage of contrast after fatty meal (AFM)

Referral Criteria

- Suspected gallbladder pathology

Contraindications

- Hepatorenal disease
- Serum bilirubin levels in excess of 34 μmol/L
- Acute cholecystitis
- Dehydration
- Previous cholecystectomy

Contrast Agent

- There are a number of agents on the market, all producing the required result. The most common are sodium iopodate and iopanoic acid

FIRST STAGE: CONTROL IMAGE AND PATIENT PREPARATION

- Prior to the examination a *control image* is taken. Its use was advocated by Twomey et al.,[74] who estimated that it could aid in the diagnosis of up to 5% of calculi
- An information sheet and contrast agent are given to the patient to take home; this provides instructions on appointment time for the second stage of the examination, contrast agent and dietary preparation
- The patient is instructed to follow a light, fat-free diet on the day before the examination and to fast from 6 pm the night before their cholecystogram appointment.[28] They are encouraged to drink water to ensure hydration
- They are then instructed to take the contrast agent 12 hours prior to their appointment and are asked not to smoke

SECOND STAGE: EXAMINATION PROCEDURE AND POSITIONING TECHNIQUE

For prone and supine projections the IR is horizontal, employed with an antiscatter grid

Prone 20° LAO to Show the Fundus (Figs 21.33, 21.34)

Positioning

- From the prone position the right side is raised 20° and radiolucent pads are used to support the abdomen
- The right arm is placed on the pillow and the left knee flexed, to aid immobilisation

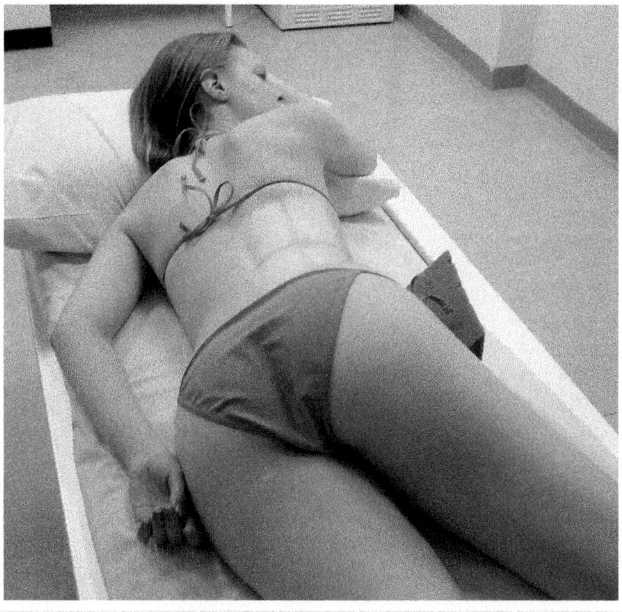

Fig. 21.33 LAO – gallbladder.

Central Ray and FRD

Vertical central ray
100 cm FRD

Centring

Level with the spinous process of L1, midway between the spine and the right flank

It is acknowledged that patient build will affect centring quite significantly. Slim patients will require centring to fall lower, closer to the spine, and well-built patients will require centring to lie higher and further from the midline (closer to the flank).[28]

Collimation

Collimate to include the soft tissue on the right of the abdomen, spine, 11th rib, iliac crest

Second 20° LAO After Ingestion of Contrast Agent

- Mark the posterior abdominal wall over the point used for centring, to aid positioning later in the examination. It will be necessary to explain the reason for this to the patient and gain consent. Document that consent has been given

Expose on arrested expiration

Exposing after full expiration will ensure that the gallbladder always lies in the same position in the abdomen for every exposure.

Supine 20° RPO to Show the Gallbladder Neck (Fig. 21.35)

The RPO projection may also clear appearances of faeces or bowel gas, which can obscure detail over the gallbladder.

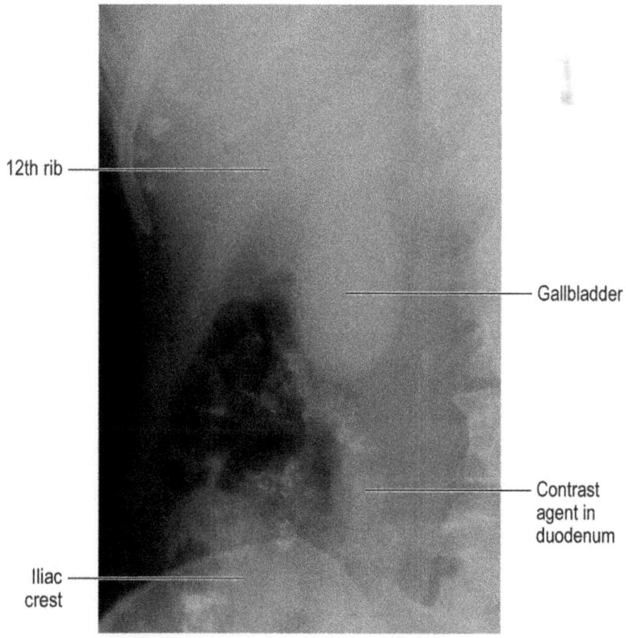

Fig. 21.34 LAO – gallbladder. The position and shape of the gallbladder will vary according to patient build. This example is of an 'average build' patient. In hypersthenic patients the gallbladder will be rounder and sit higher in the abdomen; it will also tend to lie more obliquely towards the lateral abdominal wall, or even horizontally. In asthenic patients the gallbladder will be longer and lie lower in the abdomen; it is also likely to lie closer to the spine. As a result, centring should be modified according to patient build.[8]

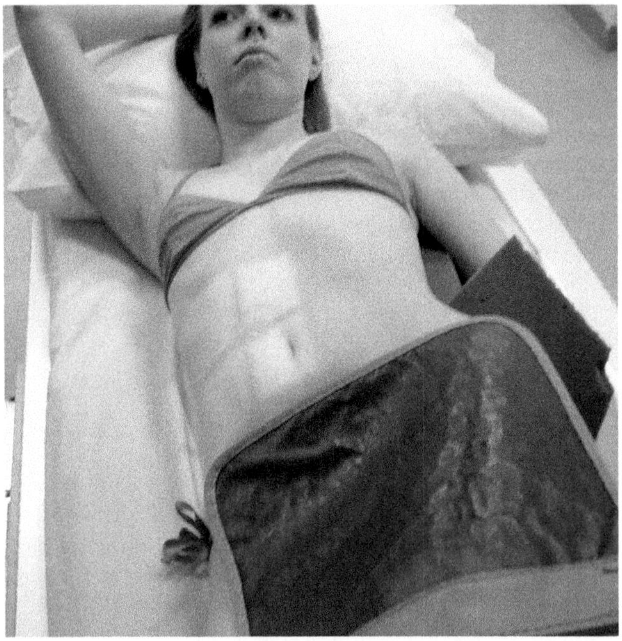

Fig. 21.35 Supine RPO – gallbladder.

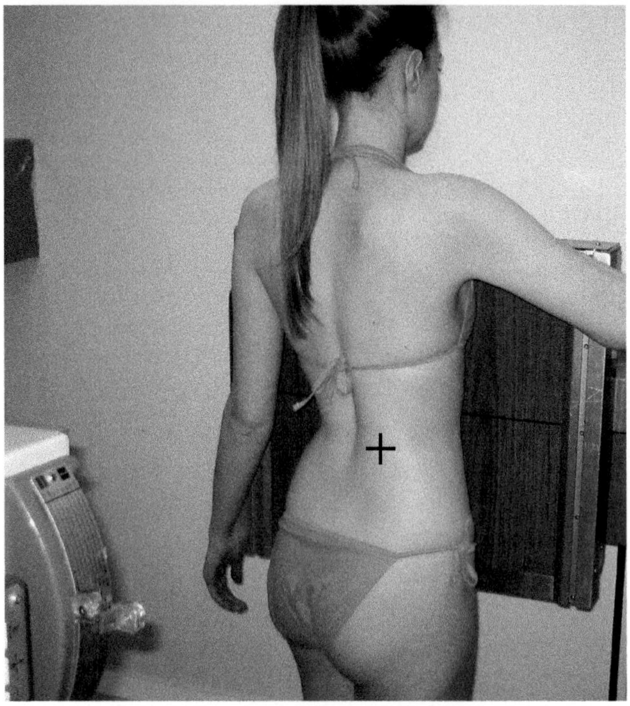

Fig. 21.36 LAO erect gallbladder.

Positioning

- From the supine abdomen position the patient is rotated 20° to their right
- The left side is supported on radiolucent pads

Central Ray and FRD

Vertical central ray
100 cm FRD

Centring

In the right midclavicular line, approximately 5 cm above the lower costal margin (but possibly varying with patient build)

> **For all projections:**
>
> Expose on arrested expiration; expiration ensures that the gallbladder lies in a more constant position for comparison of images

Collimation

Collimate to include the soft tissue on the right of the abdomen, spine, 11th rib, iliac crest

Erect 20° LAO (Figs 21.36, 21.37) for Possible Floating Gallstones

For erect projections the IR is vertical, used with an anti-scatter grid

Positioning

- From the erect posteroanterior (PA) position, the right side is turned 20° away from the IR
- The right arm is placed on top of the IR unit

Central Ray and FRD

Horizontal central ray
100 cm FRD

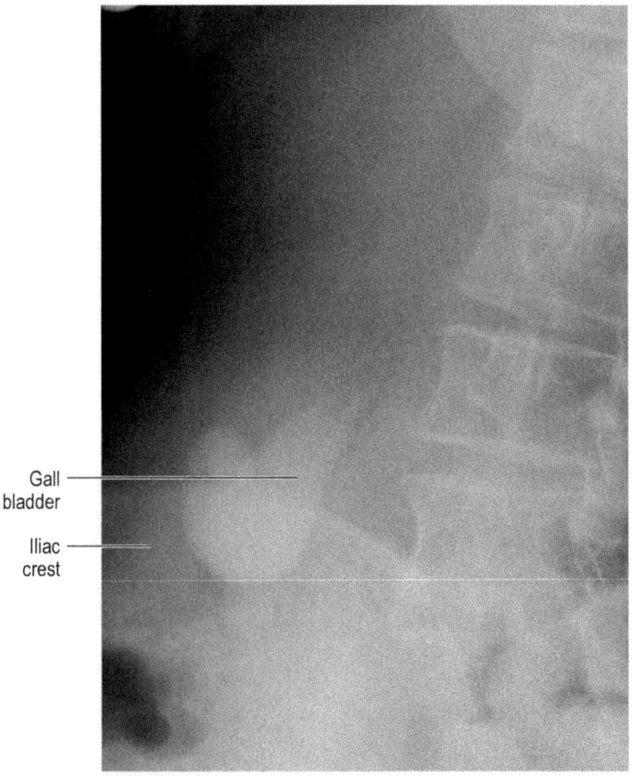

Fig. 21.37 LAO erect gallbladder. Note how much lower the gallbladder is in this position compared to the prone LAO image in Fig. 21.34.

Centring

Using the centring mark made after the prone 20° projection, centre 2–3 cm below and 2–3 cm medially to the mark. This allows for the change in gallbladder position that the erect position causes. Note that there may be no shift in gallbladder position for the hypersthenic patient.

Collimation

Collimate to include the soft tissue on the right of the abdomen, spine, 12th rib, iliac crest

If there are any overlying bowel shadows, fluoroscopic assessment may be made while the patient's trunk is rotated to clear the image of the gas from the gallbladder. If this method fails, conventional tomography may be required.

THIRD STAGE: AFM

The images for this stage should show that the gallbladder is emptying satisfactorily and is not obstructed by calculi. After satisfactory contrast images have shown the gallbladder, the patient is given a fatty meal (e.g. chocolate bar or a fat emulsion drink).

At this stage the images may be more strictly collimated, as the second-stage images can be studied to ascertain the exact gallbladder position; the radiographer uses the marks made over the second-stage centring points, adjusting the third-stage centring if the gallbladder has not been shown in the centre of the radiation field at the second phase. The gallbladder will also have contracted.

Thirty minutes after ingestion of the fatty food, a well-collimated prone 20° LAO image is taken (Fig. 21.38). It may be necessary to repeat the 20° erect LAO and/or the supine RPO.

Potential Complications[28]

- Nausea*
- Diarrhoea in up to 50% of patients
- Headache*
- Urticaria*

*These complications are rare.

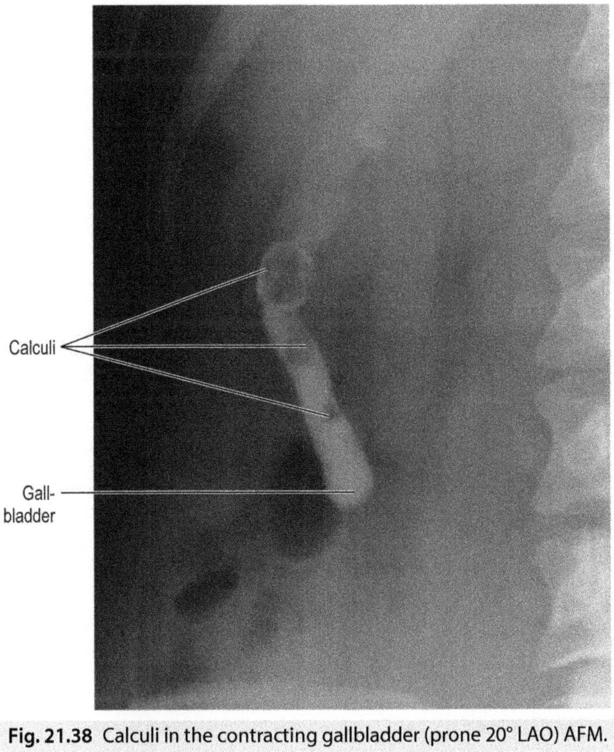

Fig. 21.38 Calculi in the contracting gallbladder (prone 20° LAO) AFM.

Other Diagnostic Techniques for the Gallbladder

OPERATIVE CHOLANGIOGRAPHY

The radiographer undertakes this examination under sterile conditions in the operating theatre.

Referral Criteria

- During cholecystectomy and/or bile duct surgery, if there is concern that calculi remain in the biliary tract

Contraindications

- There are no contraindications other than allergy to contrast agent

Contrast Agent

- Low iodine content, e.g. Niopam 150

Technique

This is a sterile procedure performed in the operating theatre. The surgeon will cannulate the cystic duct and introduce approximately 20 mL of the contrast agent. The aim is to show contrast flow into the duodenum and outline the length of the common bile duct (CBD) with minimal filling of the intrahepatic ducts (Fig. 21.39). Images of the area are taken using a mobile X-ray machine or, more frequently, using a mobile image intensifier (this can negate the need for further injections and reduces the risk of missing the information required by taking subsequent plain films). Sterile towels cover the abdomen and the surgeon generally indicates the region of interest by pointing or putting a spot of sterile water on the towel to aid correct centring. No radiographic positioning is necessary. The area is viewed and/or images are taken after 10 mL of contrast agent have been injected, and then exposure is repeated after a further 10 mL have been injected.

Potential Complications

- If the biliary tract is obstructed there is a risk that injection of contrast under pressure could cause septicaemia

POSTOPERATIVE (T-TUBE) CHOLANGIOGRAPHY

Referral Criteria

- To demonstrate or exclude calculi in the biliary tract if it is suspected that calculi remain in the tract after gallbladder surgery

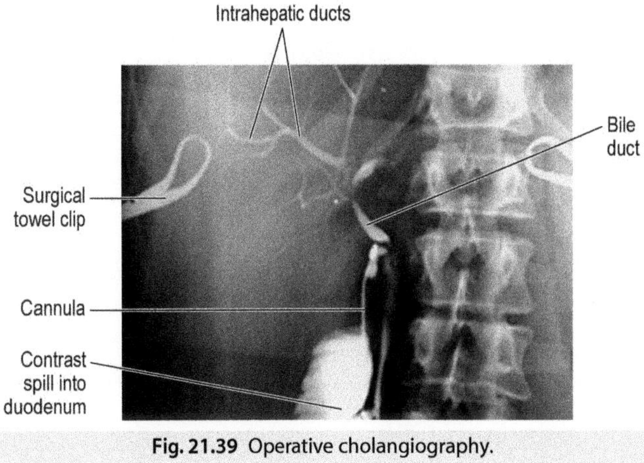

Fig. 21.39 Operative cholangiography.

Contraindications

- There are no contraindications other than allergy to contrast agent

Contrast Agent

- As for operative cholangiography

Additional Equipment

- Syringe and needle
- Filling cannula
- Antiseptic
- Gauze swabs
- Sterile gloves
- Clamp

Technique

- The examination is carried out using fluoroscopy, 7–10 days postoperatively
- The patient lies supine on the fluoroscopic couch and a fluoroscopic spot control film may be taken to show the position of the internal drain
- The external drainage tube is cleaned with antiseptic and clamped. A needle is inserted into the tube, between the clamp and the skin surface. Contrast agent is then injected until the ducts are demonstrated fluoroscopically
- Images are then taken, as required, after turning the patient until optimum visualisation of the area is achieved. Alternatively, if a C-arm intensifier is used, the tube may be rotated to achieve the same effect. It may be necessary to elevate the patient's head, shoulders and trunk (using table tilt) to assess duct drainage

Potential Complications

As for operative cholangiography.

PERCUTANEOUS TRANSHEPATIC CHOLANGIOGRAPHY (PTC)

This involves the introduction of contrast agent into the hepatobiliary system via a needle technique, through the lateral abdominal wall and into the liver. Needle insertion takes place using spot fluoroscopy for guidance.

Referral Criteria

- Jaundice: to check for hepatic bile duct obstruction
- Prior to interventional procedures, e.g. biliary drainage or stenting

Contraindications

- Tendency towards bleeding, platelets <100 000 or prothrombin time more than twice the control figure
- Infection of the biliary tract
- Hydatid disease

Contrast Agent

- Low osmolar contrast media with an iodine concentration of 150–300 mg/mL

Additional Equipment

- 22G flexible, long needle
- Small syringe and needle for administration of local anaesthetic
- Local anaesthetic
- Sterile gloves
- Antiseptic skin wash
- Gauze swabs
- Filling cannula
- Suturing equipment or skin sealant spray and skin dressing for after the procedure

Patient Preparation

- Results of blood tests must be available and checked to ensure they are within acceptable limits, because of the risks associated with bleeding
- The patient should also be given prophylactic antibiotics prior to the procedure (and also afterwards) to reduce the risk of infection
- Dietary preparation should include 'nil by mouth' to reduce the chance of nausea and/or vomiting
- It is recommended that the patient be given sedative premedication as the procedure can be uncomfortable
- As this is an invasive procedure and there are risks associated with it, written informed consent should be obtained

Technique

- The patient is positioned supine on the fluoroscopic couch. If a C-arm intensifier is being used, their right arm can be placed on an arm board and extended out to allow for the lateral C-arm movement and so that the lateral projection can be taken more easily. Using a C-arm intensifier means that the patient will not be required to turn during the procedure
- Initial screening of the region with the patient in full inspiration and expiration will allow the clinician to make a decision as to the best point to enter the liver
- Using aseptic technique, the area is cleansed and local anaesthesia given
- The flexible needle is inserted through the skin and into the liver with the patient in arrested respiration. The patient is then asked to breathe in a more shallow fashion to reduce needle movement and hence discomfort. The needle is advanced into the centre of the liver
- Contrast agent can then be injected into the liver as the needle is slowly withdrawn; this process can be repeated while moving the needle tip in any direction until the ducts begin to fill with contrast. The more dilated the ducts are, the easier cannulation will be. When the hepatic duct system is filled the needle can be withdrawn, unless access is still required for a therapeutic procedure
- Images taken may vary but often include:
  - supine
  - 45° lateromedial angle (from left and right); this will require 45° rotation of the patient in each direction if the C-arm is not available
  - right lateral
- Because contrast is heavier than bile it may be necessary to tilt the patient head down (Trendelenburg position) to ensure filling of the system. The patient can then be tilted more erect to check for obstruction or to see if contrast flows into the duodenum

Patient Aftercare

- After withdrawal of the needle, the area is sealed (or sutured) and a clean dressing is applied

- After the procedure, pulse and blood pressure should be taken every 15 minutes for the first hour and then half-hourly for 5 hours
- The wound site is monitored
- Abdomen size is monitored

Potential Complications

- (Morbidity is approximately 4%)
- Pyrexia
- Pancreatitis
- Perforation of the T-tube[28]

ENDOSCOPIC RETROGRADE CHOLANGIOPANCREATOGRAPHY (ERCP) (FIGS 21.40, 21.41)

Referral Criteria

- Extrahepatic biliary obstruction
- Jaundice
- Post-cholecystectomy patients who remain symptomatic
- Pancreatic disease
- Other diffuse biliary tract diseases

Contraindications

- HIV
- Australia antigen-positive
- Previous gastric surgery (affects the normal anatomy)
- Acute pancreatitis
- Severe cardiorespiratory disease

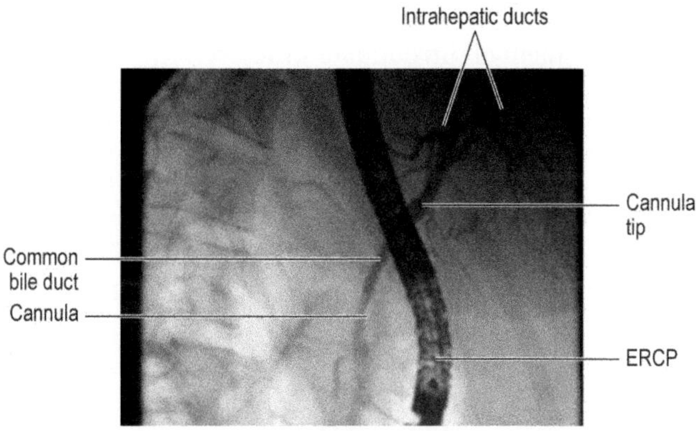

Fig. 21.40 ERCP.

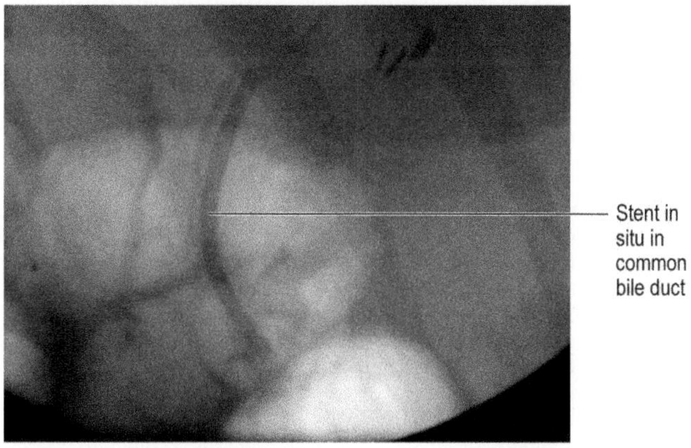

Fig. 21.41 ERCP – following stent insertion.

Contrast Agent

- Low osmolar contrast with an iodine concentration of 240–300 mg/mL is considered optimal. This is generally diluted to half strength with saline when cannulation has been confirmed to reduce the risk of obscuring any calculi and decrease the possibility of pancreatitis

Patient Preparation

- Nil by mouth for 4–6 hours prior to the procedure
- Antibiotic cover to reduce any infection risk
- As this is an invasive procedure which may need further therapeutic intervention, written informed consent must be obtained. Advance explanation is important as the patient will be sedated immediately before the examination

Technique

In the past, this procedure has generally been carried out by surgeons or gastroenterologists under fluoroscopic control, within a medical imaging department. Although this remains the more usual scenario, radiographers are increasingly carrying out this procedure.

- The patient's pharynx is anaesthetised using anaesthetic spray (to aid the passage of the endoscope); an intravenous sedative (e.g. diazepam or midazolam) is administered
- The patient is then asked to lie prone with their right side raised 30–45° and radiolucent pads are used to support the right side; the endoscope is then introduced
- During the procedure the patient is monitored for pulse and oxygen saturation to ensure their safety
- The endoscopist passes the scope into the duodenum and locates the ampulla of Vater (the bile duct orifice). Once located, a small catheter is positioned in the entrance and contrast agent introduced and viewed under fluoroscopic control. It is possible at this point for the endoscopist to cannulate the pancreas and obtain images, although repeated cannulation and introduction of contrast is to be avoided due to an increase in the risk of pancreatitis
- As contrast agent begins to fill the common bile duct, images can be taken which will demonstrate any calculi that might be present
- As for PTC, the patient may be tilted (a) into the Trendelenburg position to fill the intrahepatic ducts and (b) semi-erect to fill the distal end of the CBD and gallbladder
- If there is no need to progress to a therapeutic procedure, or a sphincterotomy has been performed (thereby aiding in the ease of recannulation of the duct), the scope may be removed; this will allow a better view of the duct, over which the scope may have been lying

Patient Aftercare

- The patient should continue to starve until sensation in their throat has returned
- The patient should have their pulse, temperature and blood pressure monitored half-hourly for 4–6 hours
- If pancreatitis is suspected, serum amylase tests should be undertaken

Potential Complications

- Damage caused by the endoscope (e.g. to the ampulla, distal ducts and the oesophagus)
- Acute pancreatitis 0.7–7.4%[28]

COMPARISON OF ERCP WITH PTC

ERCP has three main advantages over PTC:[28]

- ERCP enables visualisation of the ampulla, which can be the site of a tumour, and allows for biopsy during the procedure
- ERCP can demonstrate both the biliary tree and the pancreatic duct
- There are better therapeutic possibilities via ERCP, e.g. sphincterotomy, removal of stones via basket or balloon, drain or stent insertion

However, these do not negate PTC, which:

- Has a growing role as a precursor for interventional procedures that cannot be achieved via ERCP
- Generally shows the intrahepatic ducts better than ERCP, although the use of balloon catheters during ERCP means the endoscopist can improve their view of the area

Other Techniques for Assessing the Biliary Tree

ULTRASOUND

Whereas PTC may have been a primary investigation for obstructive jaundice in the past, ultrasound has now established itself in that role; it is non-invasive, involves no ionising radiation and has no complications. Ultrasound has become very accurate in assessing the level and cause of biliary obstruction; even early studies showed that the level of biliary obstruction was correctly noted in 95% of cases and the cause correctly noted in 88%,[75] and ultrasound equipment and techniques have improved significantly since that time.

COMPUTED TOMOGRAPHY

This has also proved itself an appropriate modality for the diagnosis of obstructive jaundice.[76] Studies have shown CT to be important in detection of early stage tumours and preoperative planning, along with MRI, MRCP and endoscopic ultrasound (EUS).[77,78]

MAGNETIC RESONANCE IMAGING

MRI has become increasingly useful for assessment of the biliary tree with MRCP (Fig. 21.42). Compared to endoscopy this is a non-invasive technique that negates the need for contrast injection. MRCP has long been known to have a high accuracy rate in evaluating common bile duct stones (choledocholithiasis).[79] However, it is advocated that patients with a high probability of disease should undergo ERCP, as some form of therapeutic procedure might be required. Since this investigation, other literature has concluded that MRCP has an extremely high sensitivity and

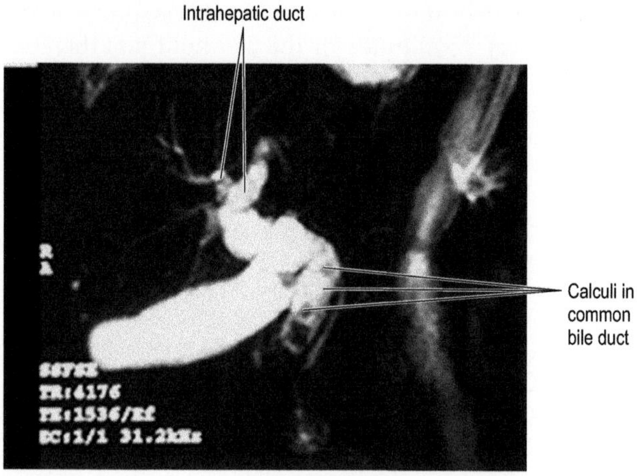

Fig. 21.42 MRCP.

specificity and is therefore an important imaging modality in this patient group, with more recent summaries indicating the value of MRCP as the single most useful modality for biliary malignancy.[80]

Assessment of the Pancreas

In X-radiography the pancreas is only visualised via ERCP with direct injection of contrast, but if a patient is suffering acute pancreatitis this is contraindicated. EUS, CT and MRI are the better methods for imaging the pancreas as they are non-invasive and also have the bonus of being able to show the involvement of surrounding structures.

Ultrasound has some limited value in overall evaluation of the area, due to difficulties created by gas in the colon and stomach, but may identify issues associated with pancreatitis such as biliary duct dilation in patients with a head of pancreas tumour. However, EUS is now more established as a medium that provides very high resolution images that are useful in both diagnosis and tissue sampling of pancreatic lesions via fine needle aspiration.[81]

References

1. Frøkjær JB, et al. Imaging of the gastrointestinal tract-novel technologies. *World J Gastroenterol*. 2009;15(2):160–168.
2. Maglinte D, et al. Advances in alimentary tract imaging. *World J Gastroenterol*. 2006;12(20):3139–3145.
3. Engin G. Computed tomography enteroclysis in the diagnosis of intestinal diseases. *J Computer Assist Tomogr*. 2008;32(1):9–16.
4. Moscandrew ME, Loftus Jr EV. Diagnostic advances in inflammatory bowel disease (imaging and laboratory). *Curr Gastroenterol Rep*. 2009;11(6):488–495.
5. Masselli G, et al. Small bowel neoplasms: prospective evaluation on MR enteroclysis. *Radiology*. 2009;1(3):743–750.
6. Swain P. The future of wireless capsule endoscopy. *World J Gastroenterol*. 2008;14(26):4142–4145.
7. NICE (National Institute for Health and Care Excellence). *Suspected Cancer: Recognition and Referral*. NICE guideline [NG12]; 2017. https://www.nice.org.uk/guidance/ng12.
8. European Society of Gastrointestinal Endoscopy. *Performance Measures for ERCP and Endoscopic Ultrasound: A European Society of Gastrointestinal Endoscopy (ESGE) Quality Improvement Initiative*. European Society of Gastrointestinal Endoscopy; 2018.
9. NICE (National Institute for Health and Care Excellence). *Pancreatic Cancer in Adults: Diagnosis and Management*. NICE guideline [NG85]; 2018. https://www.nice.org.uk/guidance/ng85.

10. Ponsaing LG, et al. Diagnostic procedures for submucosal tumors in the gastrointestinal tract. *World J Gastroenterol.* 2007;13(24):3301–3310.
11. NICE (National Institute for Health and Care Excellence). *Stroke and Transient Ischaemic Attack in over 16s: Diagnosis and Initial Management.* NICE guideline [NG128]; 2019. https://www.nice.org.uk/guidance/ng128.
12. *NICE (National Institute for Health and Care Excellence) (NICE) Gastro-Oesophageal Reflux Disease and Dyspepsia in Adults: Investigation and Management.* Clinical guideline [CG184]; 2014. https://www.nice.org.uk/guidance/cg184.
13. Chua TS, et al. Validation of 13C-urea breath test for the diagnosis of *Helicobacter pylori* infection in the Singapore population. *Singapore Med J.* 2002;43(8):55–57.
14. Moayyedi P, et al. New approaches to enhance the accuracy of the diagnosis of reflux disease. *Gut.* 2004;53:55–57.
15. Eckardt AJ, Eckardt VF. Current clinical approach to achalasia. *World J Gastroenterol.* 2009;15(32):3969–3975.
16. Chapman S, Nakielny R. *A Guide to Radiological Procedures.* 4th ed. Edinburgh: Saunders; 2001.
17. Whitley AS, et al. *Clark's Special Procedures in Diagnostic Imaging.* Oxford: Butterworth–Heinemann; 1999.
18. Ott DJ. In: Sutton D, Young WR, eds. *A Short Textbook of Clinical Imaging.* St Louis: Mosby; 1995.
19. Smith CM, et al. MicroRNAs, development of Barrett's esophagus, and progression to esophageal adenocarcinoma. *World J Gastroenterol.* 2010;16(5):531–537.
20. Varghese JC, Roy-Choudhury SH. Radiological imaging of the GI tract after bariatric surgery. *Gastrointest Endosc.* 2009;70(6):1176–1181.
21. Royal College of Radiologists. *iRefer: Making the Best Use of Clinical Radiology.* 8th ed. London: RCR; 2017. https://www.rcr.ac.uk/clinical-radiology/being-consultant/rcr-referral-guidelines/about-irefer.
22. Welbourn R, le Roux CW, Owen-Smith A, et al. Why the NHS should do more bariatric surgery; how much should we do? *Br Med J.* 2016;353(i):472.
23. Welbourn R, Hopkins J, Dixon JB, et al. Commissioning guidance for weight assessment and management in adults and children with severe complex obesity. *Obesity Rev.* 2018;19(1):14–27.
24. Bonilha HS, Humphries K, Blair J, et al. Radiation exposure time during MBSS: influence of swallowing impairment severity, medical diagnosis, clinician experience, and standardized protocol use. *Dysphagia.* 2013;28(1):77–85.
25. Logemann J. *Evaluation and Treatment of Swallowing Disorders.* 2nd ed. Austin, TX: Pro-Ed; 1998.
26. Logemann J. *Videofluoroscopy Conference.* Royal Preston Hospital; April 2008.
27. Miles A, McMillan J, Ward K, et al. Esophageal visualization as an adjunct to the videofluoroscopic study of swallowing. *Otolaryngol Head Neck Surg.* 2015;152(3):488–493.
28. Carver E, Carver B, eds. *Medical Imaging: Techniques, Reflection and Evaluation.* 2nd ed. Edinburgh: Churchill Livingstone; 2012.
29. Papp J. *Quality Management in the Imaging Sciences.* 6th ed. Elsevier; 2018:346.
30. British Society of Gastrointestinal and Abdominal Radiologists and the Royal College of Radiologists. *Guidance on the Use of CT Colonography for Suspected Colorectal Cancer.* London: The Royal College of Radiologists; September 2014. Report No.: BFCR(14)9.
31. Halligan S. CT colonography for investigation of patients with symptoms potentially suggestive of colorectal cancer: a review of the UK SIGGAR trials. *Br J Radiol.* 2013;86(1026):20130137.
32. Bryan G. *Diagnostic Radiography: A Concise Practical Manual.* 4th ed. Edinburgh: Churchill Livingstone; 1987.
33. Yucel C, et al. CT colonography for incomplete or contraindicated optical colonoscopy in older patients. *Am J Roentgenol.* 2008;190:145–150.
34. Bogoni L, et al. Computer-aided detection (CAD) for CT colonography: a tool to address growing need. *Br J Radiol.* 2005;78:S57–S62.
35. Winawer SJ, et al. A comparison of colonscopy and double-contrast barium enema for surveillance after polypectomy. *N Engl J Med.* 2000;342:1766–1772.
36. Steine S, et al. Double-contrast barium enema versus colonoscopy in the diagnosis of neoplastic disorders: aspects of decision-making in general practice. *Family Pract.* 1993;10:288–291.
37. Cancer Research UK. Bowel cancer incidence statistics. https://tinyurl.com/y5jr7wbb.
38. Office for National Statistics. *Cancer Survival in England: National Estimates for Patients Followed up to;* 2017. https://tinyurl.com/yyaqp8es.
39. Hodler J, et al. *Diseases of the Abdomen and Pelvis: Diagnostic Imaging and Interventional Techniques.* New York: Springer; 2006.
40. Neri E, et al. CT colonography versus double-contrast barium enema for screening of colorectal cancer: comparison of radiation burden. *Abdom Imaging.* 2010;35(5):596–601.
41. Burling D. CT colonography standards. *Clin Radiol.* 2010;65(6):474–480.
42. Keshav K, et al. Quality assessment for CT colonography: validation of automated measurement of colonic distention and residual fluid. *Am J Roentgenol.* 2007;189:1457–1463.
43. Tolan DJM, et al. Replacing barium enema with CT colonography in patients older than 70 years: the importance of detecting extra colonic abnormalities. *Am J Roentgenol.* 2007;189:1104–1111.
44. Barrett JF, et al. Artifacts in CT: recognition and avoidance. *Radiographics.* 2004;24:1679–1691.
45. S. Whipworm (Trichuris trichiura) | Parasites | Gastroenterology. [online] 2019. https://www.scribd.com/presentation/162674411/Whipworm-Trichuris-trichiura.
46. Gore RM, et al. *Textbook of Gastrointestinal Radiology.* Philadelphia: Saunders; 2007:890–904.
47. Saavedra Abril J. *MRI Defecography. Anatomic and Functional Cine-Based Evaluation of the Pelvic Floor Dysfunction.* European Society of Radiology [online]; 2015:1–27. C-2583. https://pdfs.semanticscholar.org/6737/5cbeda05a0924ba59113c75bbb93e6ab8d1d.pdf.
48. Rizal FE, Suliman I, Vessal S, et al. Investigating symptomatic evacuatory dysfunction. A comparative study between MRI and defecatory proctograms. *Colorectal Dis.* 2014;16:206.
49. Brown CG, Mohsen NS. Evaluation of pelvic floor dysfunction with dynamic MRI. *J Am Osteopath Coll Radiol.* 2017;6(3):13–18.
50. Pelvic Floor Center. Obstructive defecation. [online] 2019. http://www.pelvicfloorcenter.org/content/obstructive-defecation.
51. ASCRS. Rectocele. [online] 2019. https://www.fascrs.org/patients/disease-condition/rectocele-0.
52. Mayo Clinic. Intussusception. [online] 2019. https://www.mayoclinic.org/diseases-conditions/intussusception/symptoms-causes/syc-20351452.
53. Oxford GI. Enterocoele and sigmoidocoele. [online] 2011. https://www.oxfordgi.co.uk/enterocoele.
54. Ellis C, Essani R. Treatment of obstructed defecation. *Clin Colon Rectal Surg.* 2012;25(01):024–033.
55. Flusberg M, Sahni V, Erturk S, et al. Dynamic MR defecography: assessment of the usefulness of the defecation Phase. *AJR Am J Roentgenol.* 2011;196(4):W394–W399.
56. Guy's, St Thomas' NHS Foundation Trust. Having an MR proctogram. [online] 2019. https://www.guysandstthomas.nhs.uk/resources/patient-information/radiology/mr-proctogram.pdf.
57. Prasad R. The patient's experience of defaecating proctography: comparing magnetic resonance with conventional fluoroscopy techniques. *Radiography.* 2019;25:24–27.
58. Maglinte D. Functional imaging of the pelvic floor. *Radiology.* 2011;258(1):23–39.
59. Ayub G. Interpretation of defecating proctograms: getting to the bottom of it!. *Eur Soc Radiol.* 2014;C-1129:1–19.
60. Kim A. How to interpret a functional or motility test – defecography. *J Neurogastroenterol Motil.* 2019;17(4):416–420.
61. Greenberg MS, et al. *Burket's Oral Medicine.* 11th ed. Ontario: BC Decker Inc; 2008.
62. Bialek J, et al. US of the major salivary glands: anatomy and spatial relationships, pathologic conditions and pitfalls. *Radiography.* 2006;26:745–763.
63. Patel CM, et al. Imaging of salivary glands. *Imaging.* 2013;22:1.
64. Daneva S, et al. *Ultrasound and fine Needle Aspiration of the Salivary Glands.* ECR presentations; 1999:8. 008. lecture ref.
65. Takagi Y, et al. Fast and high resolution MR sialography using a small surface coil. *J Magn Reson Imaging.* 2005;22:29–37.
66. Wada H, et al. High resolution MR sialography of the parotid gland: comparison of microscopy coil and conventional small surface coil. *Proc Int Soc Magn Reson Med.* 2005;13:1078.
67. Hugill J, et al. MR sialography: the effect of a sialogogue and ductal occlusion in volunteers. *Br J Radiol.* 2008;81(967):583–586.
68. Purcell YM, et al. The diagnostic accuracy of contrast-enhanced CT of the neck for the investigation of sialolithiasis. *Am J Neuroradiol.* 2017;38(11):2161–2166.

69. Keyes J, et al. Best scintigraphic measures of parotid gland dysfunction in Sjögren's syndrome. *Arth Rheumatol.* 2010;62(suppl. 10):1887.
70. Aida M, et al. Value of salivary scintigraphy on Sjögren's syndrome. *J Nucl Med.* 2013;54(suppl 2):1934.
71. Zeisseman HA. Nuclear medicine hepatobiliary imaging. *Clin Gastroenterol Hepatol.* 2010;8(2):111–116.
72. Morosi C, et al. CT cholangiography: assessment of feasibility and diagnostic reliability. *Eur J Radiol.* 2009;72(1):114–117.
73. Hyodo MD, et al. CT and MR cholangiography: advantages and pitfalls in preoperative evaluation of biliary tree. *Br J Radiol.* 2012;85(1015): 887–896.
74. Twomey B, et al. The plain radiograph in oral cholecystography: should it be abandoned? *Br J Radiol.* 1983;56(662):99–100.
75. Gibson RN, et al. Bile duct obstruction radiologic evaluation of level cause and tumour respectability. *Radiology.* 1986;160:43–47.
76. Rishi P, et al. Value and accuracy of multi detector CT in obstructive jaundice. *Pol J Radiol.* 2016;81:303–309.
77. Hennedige TP, et al. Imaging of malignancies of the biliary tract – and update. *Canc Imag.* 2014;14(1):14.
78. Schima W. Biliary malignancies: multi-slice CT or MRI? *Canc Imag.* 2003;3(2):75–78.
79. Calvo MM, et al. Role of MRCP in patients with suspected choledocholithiasis. *Clin Proc.* 2002;77:422–428.
80. Hekimoglu K, et al. MRCP vs ERCP in the evaluation of biliary pathologies: review of current literature. *J Digest Dis.* 2008;9(3):162–169.
81. Quencer K, et al. Imaging of the pancreas: part 1. *Appl Radiol. September.* 2013;4. https://appliedradiology.com/articles/imaging-of-the-pancreas-part-1.

22 Genitourinary Contrast Imaging

KAREN KNAPP and ELIZABETH CARVER

As outlined in Chapter 20, contrast-enhanced imaging of the urinary tract was originally developed in the early 1920s, when suitable contrast agents were first used. For the most part of the 20th century contrast projection radiography was the only option for imaging of the tract, but all complementary imaging methods, and especially ultrasound, now offer a significant contribution to imaging the area. Throughout this chapter a suggested FRD is given for each examination description; however in practice a range of FRDs (typically from 100 cm to 120 cm), may be used, dependent on local protocol.

Ultrasound is an excellent imaging method that will show or estimate renal volume, parenchymal thickness, kidney shape and size, congenital development abnormalities, cysts, benign prostatic hypertrophy or carcinoma, hydronephrosis and tumours of the renal system. Use of colour Doppler will demonstrate the renal vascular system. The list is by no means exhaustive but does serve to show why ultrasound came to the forefront of imaging in this area.

Low radiation dose computed tomography (CT) of kidneys, ureters and bladder (KUB) has now moved towards extra-low dose CT KUB (equivalent dose to a projection radiography KUB exposure), making CT a suitable option in this area.[1] Comparison has been made between ultra-low dose (contrast-enhanced) CT and KUB (particularly relating to renal colic assessment), finding CT to be comparable in diagnostic yield to KUB.[2] Magnetic resonance imaging (MRI) also has a place in imaging the urinary system, thanks to its superior ability to demonstrate differences in soft tissue appearances.[3] Radionuclide imaging provides the opportunity for functional evaluation of the genitourinary system, including reflux assessment, along with assessment of renal scarring.[4] Further details on this are covered in Chapter 28. There is additional information on imaging methods for the urinary system at the end of the section on the urinary tract and within comments relating to common pathologies and clinical indications.

As a result of these developments in imaging, the use of intravenous urography (IVU) has slowly receded since the 1980s, mainly because of the increased availability and use of ultrasound. However, it may still be used globally, where there may still be difficulties using or accessing other imaging modalities (more specifically CT). The National Institute for Health and Care Excellence (NICE) states that CT should not be used for pregnant women because of the radiation exposure, and recommends ultrasound as the preferred imaging modality in this group. Children and young adults should also undergo an ultrasound scan and only have a CT scan if the former is inconclusive due to the radiation burden.[5]

Common Pathologies and Clinical Indications for Imaging of the Urinary System

This is not an exhaustive list and any suggested imaging methods are based on current UK guidelines.[5]

Calculus/Calculi

Renal calculi are formed in the urine and create problems for patients when they lodge in the urinary tract, causing severe pain (renal colic) and, potentially, ureteric obstruction, hydronephrosis and haematuria. Stones as small as 0.4 cm can cause renal colic, but pain scores are unrelated to stone size and location.[6] The constituents of calculi vary, but the most common are calcium oxalate and calcium phosphate; they are often radio-opaque (but can also be radiolucent and not visible via X-ray imaging) and can therefore be visualised on the projection radiographic image. However, owing to their (usually) small size they may not always be well visualised; this is also complicated by the surrounding (possible superimposition of) soft tissue structures of the abdominal viscera, and also mesenteric nodes and phleboliths. This obviously means that projection radiographic imaging of the abdomen, albeit a reasonable tool for imaging renal stones, is not as useful to determine ureteric stones and their position. Current UK guidelines recommend unenhanced low dose CT as the investigation of choice, with IVU indicated only when CT is unavailable.[5]

Large radio-opaque calculi may occupy the space within the pelvicalyceal system, filling it in almost exactly the same shape as the system; these are known as staghorn calculi (Fig. 22.1) and can mimic the appearance of a contrast-filled pelvicalyceal system. They can be an incidental finding seen on abdomen images.

Benign and Malignant Prostatic Disease

Although the prostate gland is not located within the urinary tract itself, prostatic disease affects urinary tract imaging by its extrinsic effects on the system. A large proportion of men from late middle age onwards will have an enlarged prostate due to benign prostatic hypertrophy/hyperplasia (BPH).[7] Symptoms of this include frequency of micturition, poor urine stream and dysuria. Extreme forms can cause bladder outlet obstruction. Although a benign condition, BPH will often require treatment in order to alleviate its symptoms, as they often significantly affect the patient's

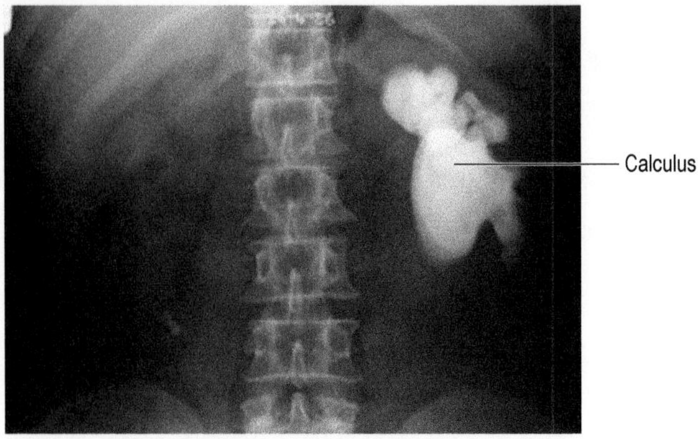

Fig. 22.1 Staghorn calculus on control image. The radio-opaque calculus has filled the pelvicalyceal system, almost mimicking a hydronephrotic kidney filled with contrast agent.

quality of life. It is important to differentiate between BPH and carcinoma of the prostate, which can cause similar symptoms.

If the urinary tract contains contrast agent and prostatic enlargement of any type is present, the bladder appears to have a depression at its base, in the shape of a mushroom. Bladder ultrasound with measurement of postvoid residual volume is the examination of choice when investigating BPH and the extent of its effect, and contrast radiography is not indicated for this condition.[8] Ultrasound will help differentiate between BPH and prostatic carcinoma and is usually used in conjunction with assessment of blood levels of prostate-specific antigen (PSA); an elevated PSA level may indicate malignancy. Multiparametric MRI is recommended in patients with persistent suspicion of prostate cancer.[9]

Commonly Encountered Malignant Tumours

The most common type affecting the intrinsic system is transitional cell carcinoma, and the most common location is the bladder. A common method of imaging assessment for bladder malignancy is ultrasound; however, cystoscopy is considered to be the optimum method. Epithelial cell tumours also affect the renal tract and are best demonstrated by contrast-enhanced CT. Computed tomography and MRI are useful for staging.[10]

Nephroblastoma (Wilms' tumour) is a malignant tumour affecting children: ultrasound is the first-line imaging test to identify the condition, with CT used to assess extent of the mass; MRI may also be useful and ^{18}F-fluorodeoxyglucose positron emission tomography fused with CT (PET-CT), provides information regarding the metabolic activity, which is accurately anatomically localized. This is potentially useful for staging as well as the assessment of treatment response.[11]

For the diagnosis of suspected renal cell adenocarcinoma or transitional cell carcinoma, the optimal methods of imaging have long been considered to be ultrasound, with an increasing use of contrast-enhanced ultrasound. Computed tomography, MRI and in particular multiparametric MRI, molecular imaging with ^{99m}technetium-sestamibi and single photon emission computed tomography (SPECT) have also been demonstrated to be useful.[12]

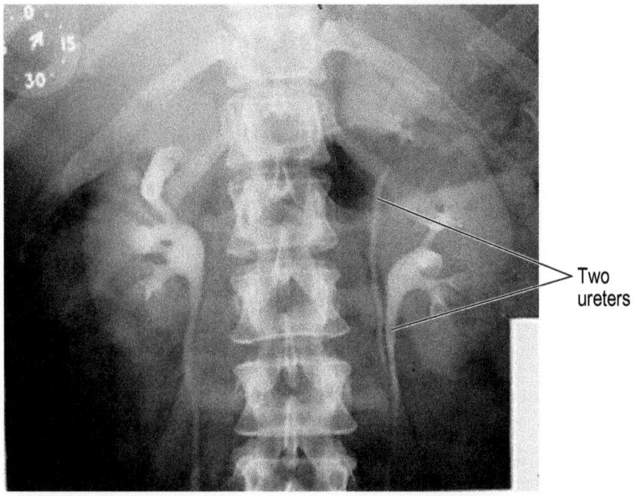

Fig. 22.2 Duplex system. In this case the pelvicalyceal systems are duplicated, but most duplex systems are not so extensive.

Duplex System

This is a duplication of part or parts of the urinary system involving the kidney and ureter. The most extensive form presents as a single kidney which has two sets of calyces, two renal pelvises and two ureters (Fig. 22.2); this may be unilateral or bilateral. Less extensive forms of the variant may show as two renal pelvises entering a single ureter, or two pelvises entering two ureters, which later fuse before entering the bladder. The variant is usually an incidental finding but is monitored in children because of its relationship to recurrent urinary tract infection (UTI).

Ectopic Kidney

The kidney is found in an area away from the usual site, sometimes on the opposite side to where it should lie (crossed ectopia).

Floating Kidney

The kidney may appear to be in a normal position or poses as a fixed ectopic kidney, which then moves as an examination progresses.

Horseshoe Kidney

A relatively rare variant. The two kidneys are joined at their upper or lower poles, the latter being by far the most common. Each kidney has its own ureter, and if the kidneys are joined at their lower pole X-ray contrast images show the calyces appearing similar to those in a 'normal' kidney which has been placed in an oblique position (Fig. 22.3). In these cases the ureters cannot leave the kidney pelvis and hilum medially as in the normal kidney, and travel forward and over the adjoined lower poles. Ultrasound, CT and MRI will also identify this variant.

'Reflux' and Pyelonephritis

More specifically known as ureteric or vesicoureteric reflux and reflux nephropathy; it commonly affects children. Urine flows backwards from the bladder owing to failure of the vesicoureteric valve. Reflux, in these cases, refers to backtracking of urine from the bladder into the

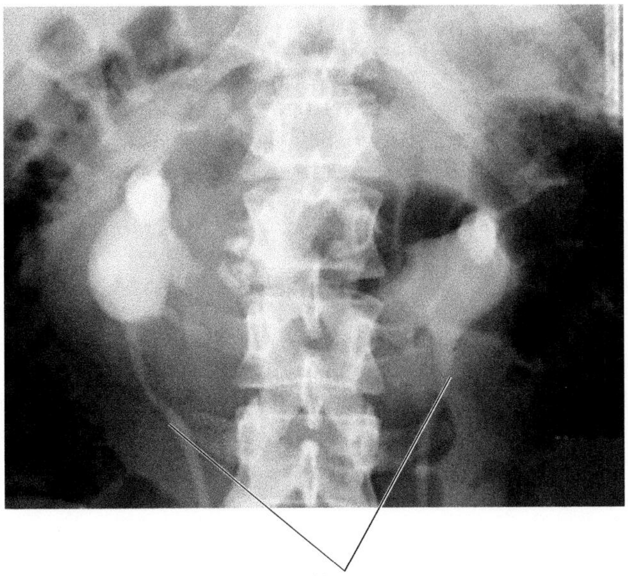

Fig. 22.3 Horseshoe kidney.

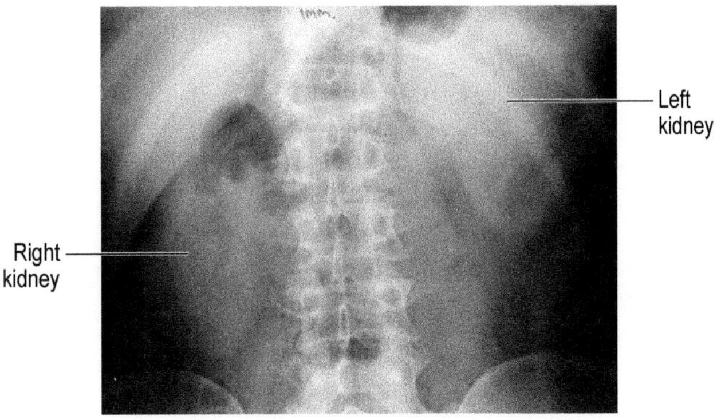

Fig. 22.4 Nephrogram.

ureter and upwards towards the kidney. This can lead to pyelonephritis, renal dysfunction and scarring, and in chronic cases, to renal failure. Vesicoureteric reflux can be assessed using micturating cystography and radionuclide imaging (RNI), which provides a non-invasive approach to diagnosis.[13,14]

Urinary Tract Obstruction

This can be due to a number of causes, either intrinsic or extrinsic. Obstruction affects the tract's ability to drain, potentially causing hydronephrosis, kidney enlargement and loss of renal cortex. If obstruction is caused by a calculus, unenhanced low dose CT is the imaging modality of choice. Contrast-enhanced CT (CT urogram), ultrasound, Doppler ultrasound, RNI and MRI all have a place if considering intrarenal blood flow, renal function, or assessment of patients who are not suitable for administration of intravenous contrast agent.[5]

Renal Transplant

Transplant patients will have one functioning kidney: the transplanted one, attached to a short ureter and placed in the right iliac fossa. The current recommendations for assessment of transplanted kidneys are for Doppler ultrasound with the use of RNI (can distinguish acute rejection) or MR/MR angiography (MRA) (if ultrasound is equivocal).[15,16]

Radiographic Examination of the Urinary System – Intravenous Urography (IVU)

Although the current UK guidelines no longer consider the intravenous urogram a front-line examination, a description of the technique follows as some centres still use it on occasion in an emergency situation if CT is unavailable. It must be envisaged that in the near future this examination may no longer be carried out.

The aim is to demonstrate the renal cortex, calyces, renal pelvis, pelviureteric junction, ureteric drainage and the bladder (although demonstration of the bladder may not be required). Contrast agent is administered intravenously and images of the system are obtained through various stages, from glomerular filtration to urine and contrast collection in calyces, and then on to ureteric drainage and bladder filling.

A range of projections are used for the IVU examination, in various combinations to demonstrate the system, and an appropriate selection of this combination will be discussed later in this section. Projections used are taken from the following list:

- Full-length KUB
- Prone KUB
- Cross-renal, collimated to the kidneys and upper ureters
- Oblique single kidney
- Bladder anteroposterior (AP) with caudal angle of approximately 15° to clear the bladder from the upper border of symphysis pubis
- Oblique bladder

Contrast agent can be seen almost immediately after injection, shown as a 'blush' in the renal cortex and known as a nephrogram (Fig. 22.4). This shows glomerular filtration of the contrast agent before it reaches the calyceal systems. It is important to see the renal outlines, as changes in the smooth outline may indicate the presence of tumours, cysts or cortical scarring. It also provides early information on renal size. It is possible to see appearances of renal blush for some time after injection and it is not always considered necessary to show the first blush immediately after injection of contrast agent, as renal outlines can be assessed along with the calyceal systems at later stages in the examination.

Around 5 minutes after injection the calyces should be seen to fill with contrast agent (Fig. 22.5), which then passes down the ureters to fill the bladder. In some cases the calyces empty quickly, preventing adequate demonstration of the calyces and renal pelvis. To counteract this, compression over the abdominal area level with the iliac crests is required, which restricts the flow of excreted contrast down the ureters. This therefore retains contrast agent in the kidney for a longer period to ensure adequate imaging of the collecting systems. Compression is usually left in place for around 5 minutes before an image of the kidneys is taken, but it must be noted that excessive and

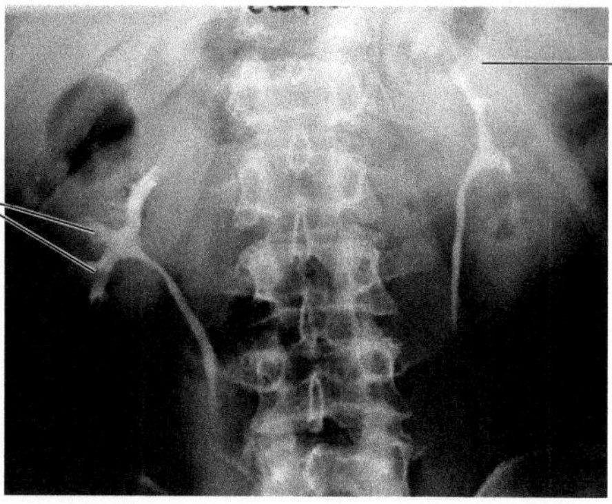

Fig. 22.5 Contrast agent in renal cortex and pelvicalyceal system.

prolonged compression may cause the calyces to appear slightly blunted and distended (imitating early hydronephrosis). It is recognised that compression is often applied routinely, often 5 minutes after injection, to ensure optimal contrast build-up in the calyces, but there are contraindications to the use of compression that must be considered. These include:

- Renal colic
- Known renal calculi
- Abdominal tenderness
- Recent abdominal surgery
- Recent pregnancy
- Renal transplant

In addition to fast drainage there may be other reasons for failure to demonstrate the cortex or calyces, and these are related to pathology or overlying bowel gas and faeces. Additional or supplementary projections/techniques may be necessary to improve visualisation in these situations. These include:

- Images in the opposite phase of suspended respiration to potentially change the position of overlying appearances such as bowel gas, faeces or radio-opacities
- Zonography to clear images of bowel gas and faeces
- Tomography to provide more detailed information after calyceal and renal pelvis images suggest or cannot exclude filling defects

Tomography (and zonography) should not be used routinely and most manufacturers now offer limited equipment with this capability, although digital tomosynthesis is now available on some equipment.[17]

Once the calyceal system has been demonstrated it is necessary to provide information on the ureters and bladder; evidence of ureteric drainage is especially important. A KUB projection (around 15–20 minutes after injection) will show most of the tract, including some early bladder information (Fig. 22.6). If the use of compression has been necessary it must be released before this KUB can be taken, in order to allow kidney drainage. Compression release usually allows for good visualisation of ureteric drainage, as the contrast-enhanced urine flows down the ureter. Some sections of the ureters may not be visible on the KUB, owing to the fact that urine is transported down these structures by peristalsis and portions of the ureters will be constricted; these portions will not be visible on the image. This in itself does not really pose a problem: if the ureter is obstructed then there should be other evidence to suggest this, including distended or blunted calyces, hydronephrosis (seen initially as delayed concentration of contrast agent and later as distended and club-shaped calyces), distended ureters (or even megaureter) and failure of contrast to pass the obstructed area on prone KUB or oblique bladder images. The prone KUB is particularly useful to show the ureteric obstruction site: the kidneys lie posteriorly in the retroperitoneal abdomen and the ureters extend from the kidneys anteriorly until they are approximately level with L4/L5 and then towards the bladder, which is situated anteriorly in the pelvis. Therefore, in the supine patient urine is moving in an upward direction for the first section of the ureter; turning the patient prone after sitting them upright for 5 minutes reverses this and allows the urine to drain towards the site of obstruction.

Series of Projections for the IVU

Texts describing excretion urography do vary on the suggested standard or routine 'protocol' for the examination,[18,19] but it must be accepted that owing to the decline in its use as a front-line examination a 'conventional' IVU series is no longer a valid concept. Providing a useful IVU series must be governed by the need to keep radiation dose to the patient as low as is reasonably practicable (ALARP), as stated in current regulations and guidelines,[20] and the need to use a series that will provide the best possible diagnostic images for each patient and their clinical history (or the appearances found as the examination progresses).

Considering the range of projections available, strategies to improve visualisation of key areas and effects of pathology on the appearances of the system, it is difficult to present a set of instructions that are guaranteed to work every time for every patient. The most important point is that, even if a set 'protocol' has been agreed, it is essential that radiographers carrying out IVU examinations must have a thorough understanding of the aims of the examination to ensure that those aims are met. An example of a 'full' IVU procedure is outlined as follows:

1. Control KUB on inspiration for assessment of gross anatomy and presence of obvious pathology, such as radio-opaque calculi
2. Position the patient for a cross-renal image
3. Injection of the contrast agent
4. Cross-renal 5 minutes after injection, to assess renal outlines and calyces and taken on arrested expiration. If calyces are not well demonstrated, apply compression if this is not contraindicated, and repeat the cross-renal 5 minutes later. If there is suspected pathology, or gas or faeces impair detail, undertake zonography or tomography of the renal area. Fulcrum heights selected for this will vary according to patient build, but three 'cuts' are usually taken from a range between 7 and 11 cm
5. If compression has not been applied, 15–20 minute KUB with contrast, taken on inspiration. If compression has been applied, release compression and undertake KUB after calyces have been adequately demonstrated
6. Collimated AP 15° caudal angle bladder image, taken after micturition

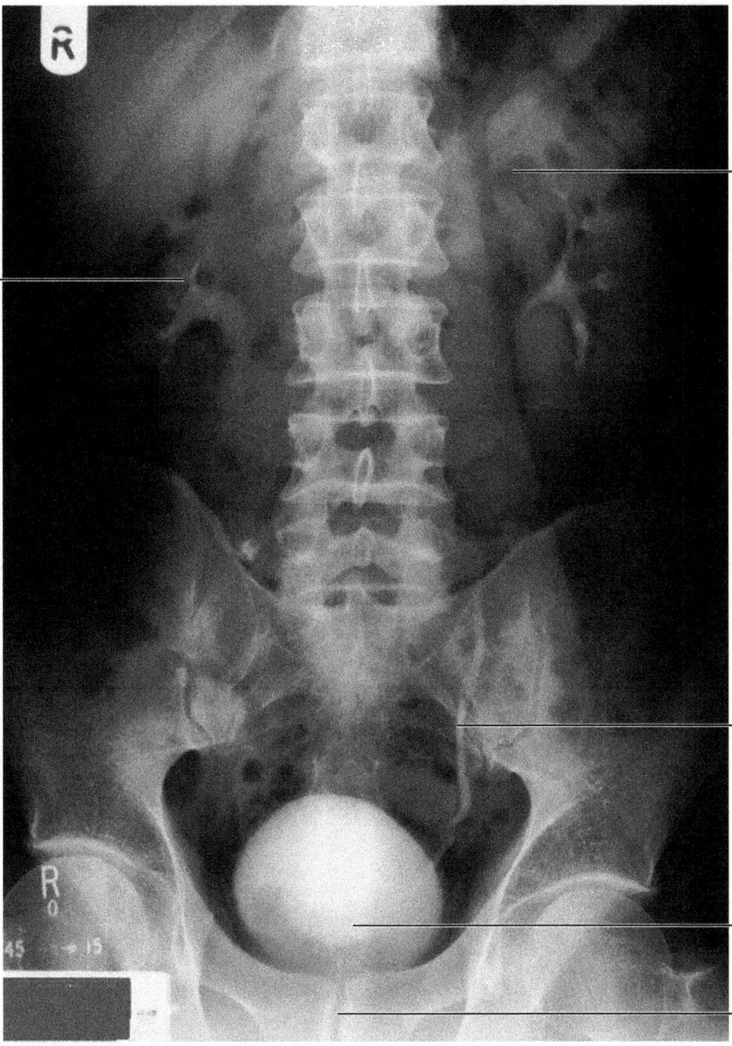

Fig. 22.6 KUB projection with contrast. The bladder appears to sit above the symphysis pubis, although its lower portion lies behind it in the pelvic cavity. The appearance is a result of oblique rays at the lower periphery of the beam, which project the symphysis clear of the bladder.

It is clear that this represents a significant number of exposures and it is increasingly rare to find that a full IVU series is undertaken in imaging departments. As the IVU is still undertaken in some centres, albeit with less frequency, it is necessary to outline how certain conditions may affect the IVU process.

Hydronephrosis (Fig. 22.7)

This may be known to pre-exist or may manifest itself during the examination as:

- Failure to demonstrate the calyces (especially easy to note when one kidney appears normal in comparison to a non-apparent kidney on the other side in the early stages of the examination). This is due to excessive urine, which dilutes the contrast agent, remaining in the kidney. Often there is concentration of the contrast agent later in the examination, but sometimes not for several hours. The cause of the hydronephrosis is impairment or obstruction of drainage at some point, from the pelviureteric junction down to the bladder, usually due to calculus or tumour. It can also be caused by bladder outlet obstruction
- Blunted and distended calyces
- Chronic hydronephrosis is likely to be accompanied by loss of renal cortex

Simple modification involves ensuring that there are delayed images of the affected kidney, initiated at around 20 minutes after injection, to allow for more contrast agent to mix with the urine and improve image contrast over the calyces and pelvis. If available, tomography may be useful, especially if gas and faeces make visualisation even more difficult. If the other kidney appears to be functioning the rest of the 'routine' aspect of the examination may continue, with further delayed images of the affected kidney being supplied at intervals (depending on how quickly concentration of contrast agent appears to be progressing). Micturition is delayed until adequate demonstration of both kidneys has been achieved, unless several hours pass and this is not possible.

Ureteric Obstruction

Hydronephrosis will manifest itself as a result of obstruction, and the radiographer will therefore initiate modification for

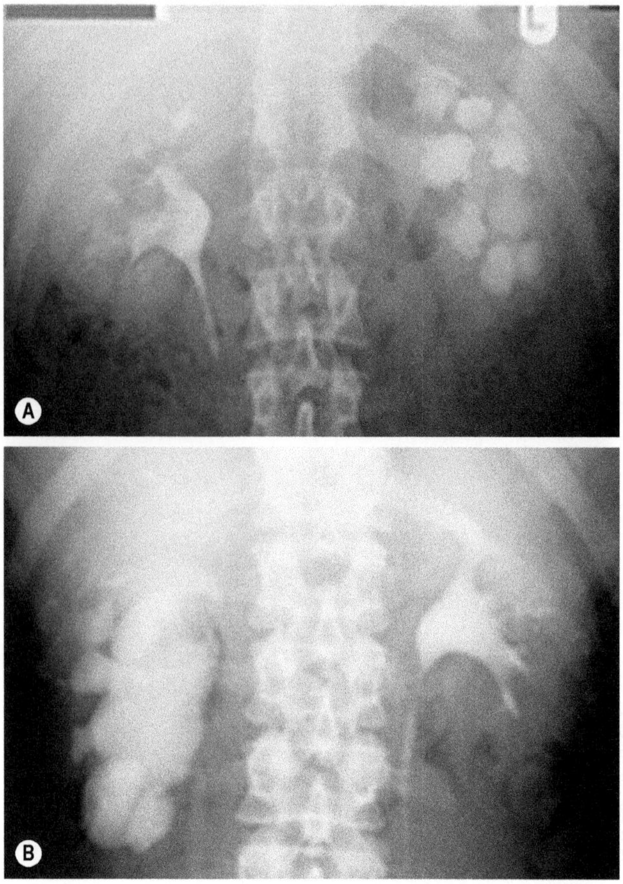

Fig. 22.7 Hydronephrosis. Two cases of hydronephrosis: (A) shows the left side with late concentration of contrast agent in the blunt calyces; (B) shows the affected right side, but in this case the distended renal pelvis is also seen. Compare the hydronephrotic kidney in both cases with the normal kidney on the opposite side.

hydronephrosis, followed by methods to show the site of obstruction. These include:

- Sitting the patient for 5 minutes (or 10–15 minutes if the hydronephrosis is severe) and then undertaking a prone KUB image
- Tilting the patient (if a tilt facility is available) with their head up for 5–15 minutes and undertaking a cross-renal image in this position
- When the suspected site of obstruction is at or near the vesicoureteric junction (where the lower ureter lies behind the contrast-filled bladder): oblique bladder, with affected side raised
- At post-micturition stage, undertaking a KUB image to show contrast and urine remaining in the ureter above the site of obstruction

Renal Colic as an Emergency

Exclusion of calculus is essential and a limited IVU series will offer this if the first choice of CT is unavailable. The acutely ill patient will present in the emergency situation. It is possible to keep radiation exposures to a minimum and a limited series is possible, suggested as:

1. Control KUB
2. Administration of contrast agent
3. KUB 15 minutes after injection

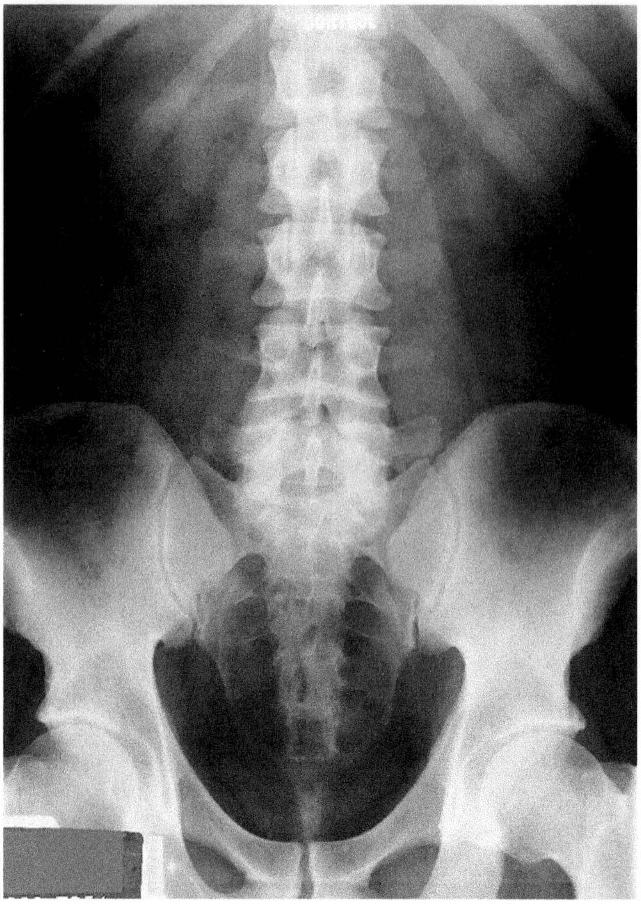

Fig. 22.8 KUB control.

Radiographic Projections for the IVU

For all IVU projections the image receptor (IR) is horizontal, using an antiscatter physical or virtual grid.

KIDNEYS, URETERS AND BLADDER (KUB) (FIG. 22.8)

This projection may be undertaken as a 'control' image for the IVU examination (Fig. 22.8) or as a standalone projection to assess the position of existing radio-opaque calculi. Discussion on the AP abdomen in Chapter 16 carries many points that are also relevant to the KUB projection.

Positioning

- The patient is initially positioned as for the supine abdomen (see Chapter 16, Fig. 16.1)

Beam Direction and FRD

Vertical
100–115 cm or higher in tall patients

Centring

In the midline at the level of the iliac crests

Collimation

Symphysis pubis, upper poles of kidneys

The lateral borders of collimation can be brought in to coincide with the ASISs (anterior superior iliac spines), as information on the whole of the abdomen will not be needed for the IVU unless additional general information on the abdomen is requested. This will avoid unnecessary irradiation of lateral portions of the abdomen.

Criteria for Assessing Image Quality

- Symphysis pubis and renal outlines are included on the image
- Spinous processes of the vertebrae are seen coincident with the midline of the image, and centralised and aligned down the middle of the vertebral bodies

> Expose on arrested respiration
> In the discussion on arrested respiration for the AP abdomen (Chapter 16) comments are made on the phase of arrested respiration during exposure. These are also relevant to the KUB projection, and exposure on suspended inspiration is recommended to ensure the whole of the system is included on this image.

- Symmetry of the iliac crests
- Sharp image demonstrating soft tissue of the kidneys in contrast with bowel gas and bony structures

Common Errors: KUB

Common Errors	Possible Reasons	Potential Impact on Interpretation
Symphysis pubis not included on the image	Inaccurate centring/positioning *or* tall patient? It may be necessary to undertake two projections to cover the area. It is suggested that these are (a) an image with symphysis pubis and as much upper tissue as possible is included, and (b) a cross-renal image. Excessive overlap of irradiated areas should be avoided	Bladder area cannot be fully assessed
Upper abdomen not included; symphysis pubis is well above the lower edge of the film	May have been centred using the lateral borders of iliac crest rather than the highest point of crests at the back	Upper poles of the kidneys may be missed and cannot be assessed
Vertebral column is not coincident with the midline of the film	Xiphisternum to symphysis line is inaccurately positioned, *or* scoliotic patient	Potential for missing part of a kidney on one side with a repeat required
Spinous processes are not demonstrated in the midline of vertebral bodies	MSP not perpendicular to table-top; palpate ASIS to ensure it is equidistant from the table *or* patient is scoliosed	Rotation may make comparison of renal outlines less accurate

PRONE KUB (FIG. 22.9A,B)

This projection is used to demonstrate the site of ureteric obstruction, draining the affected kidney so that contrast and urine lie at the lowest possible point (the site of obstruction). The patient should be asked to sit up for around 5 minutes to encourage kidney drainage, before turning prone for positioning. If the patient is unable to sit, their trunk can be propped up into a semi-recumbent position using pillows and sponges.

Positioning

- The patient is prone, head turned to the side and arms raised onto the pillow for stability and comfort. Care must be taken to ensure that any cannula in situ is not moved
- The median sagittal plane (MSP) is coincident with the long axis of the table
- For males, lead rubber or lead gonad protection is applied, below the buttocks, to protect the gonads
- ASISs are equidistant from the table-top

Beam Direction and FRD

Vertical
100–115 cm FRD or higher in large patients

Centring

Over the spine, level with the iliac crests

Collimation

- Symphysis pubis, renal outlines

> Expose on arrested inspiration

Criteria for Assessing Image Quality

- Symphysis pubis and renal outlines are included on the image. However, as this projection is intended to identify the location of ureteric obstruction, it may not be necessary to insist that all of the bladder and upper renal outlines are included
- Spinous processes of vertebrae seen coincident with the midline of the image, and centralised and aligned down the middle of the vertebral bodies
- Symmetry of iliac crests, which appear flattened out compared to their appearances on the supine AP image
- The symphysis pubis should appear to be deeper and the obturator foramina more open than in the AP projection
- Sharp image demonstrating contrast-filled structures in contrast with bowel gas and bony structures

Common Errors: Prone KUB

Common Error	Possible Reason	Potential Impact on Interpretation
Rotation, demonstrated by asymmetry of the iliac crests and spinous processes not seen in the midline of the vertebral column	Trunk has been turned to one side as the patient turns their head for comfort. Often this is addressed by simply turning the patient's head the opposite way	Rotation may make comparison of renal outlines less accurate

SUPINE ANTEROPOSTERIOR (AP) KIDNEYS ('CROSS-RENAL', 'CROSS-KIDNEY') (FIGS 22.4, 22.10)

Positioning

- The patient is positioned as for the supine AP abdomen

Beam direction and FRD

Vertical
100–115 cm FRD

Centring

In the midline, at a point between the xiphisternum and the level of the lower costal margins

COLLIMATION

Renal outlines

The lateral borders of collimation can be left as those used for the KUB projection, or modified after the KUB has been viewed.

Expose on arrested respiration

Exposure should be made on arrested expiration so that the renal shadows lie in a consistent position when exposures of the area are made at later stages in the examination.

Criteria for Assessing Image Quality

- Renal tissue outlines are shown on the image
- Spinous processes of vertebrae are seen coincident with the midline of the image, and centralised and aligned down the middle of the vertebral bodies
- Sharp image demonstrating renal outlines tissue in contrast with bowel gas and bony structures for this projection when undertaken without contrast enhancement. After injection of contrast agent, image contrast will be enhanced further and the renal outlines should still show in good contrast to other soft tissue; calyces and renal pelvis should also be seen in contrast with the renal cortex

Common Errors: Supine AP Kidneys

Common Errors	Possible Reasons	Potential Impact on Interpretation
Vertebral column not coincident with the midline of the film	Xiphisternum to symphysis line is inaccurately positioned, *or* scoliotic patient. Severe scoliosis may significantly alter the kidneys' positions and necessitate less stringent lateral collimation	Potential for missing part of a kidney on one side with a repeat required
Spinous processes not demonstrated in the midline of vertebral bodies	MSP is not perpendicular to the table-top; palpate ASIS to ensure it is equidistant from the table, *or* patient is scoliosed	Rotation may make comparison of renal outlines less accurate

OBLIQUE KIDNEY (FIG. 22.11A,B)

This projection is used at the control stage to ascertain the position of radio-opacities that appear to lie over the renal outline, or after injection of contrast to clear appearances of bowel gas or faecal matter from the renal image.

Positioning

- From the supine AP position the patient's trunk is rotated 30° *towards* the side under examination. Radiolucent pads are placed under the trunk to aid immobilisation and the arm on the lowered side is raised onto the pillow for comfort

Beam direction and FRD

Vertical
100 cm or 115 cm FRD

Centring

In the midline, midway between the xiphisternum and level of the lower costal margins

As the renal outlines generally lie with the left kidney slightly higher than the right, previous cross-renal images can be assessed to ascertain the exact kidney position before centring the beam for the oblique kidney projection. Note that centring is recommended as over the midline and not in the midclavicular line (sometimes erroneously quoted by students); this is due to the posterior position of the kidneys in the abdominal cavity – as the trunk rotates, the image of the kidney moves closer to the spine.

Collimation

Kidney under examination

Criteria for Assessing Image Quality

- Kidney under examination is seen on image
- If contrast agent has been injected the calyces and renal pelvis should appear shortened in a lateromedial direction

Common Error: Oblique Kidney

Common Error	Possible Reason	Potential Impact on Interpretation
Medial aspect of the kidney is omitted from the image	Centring over the midclavicular line rather than over the midline of the patient	The kidney cannot be fully assessed, necessitating a repeat.

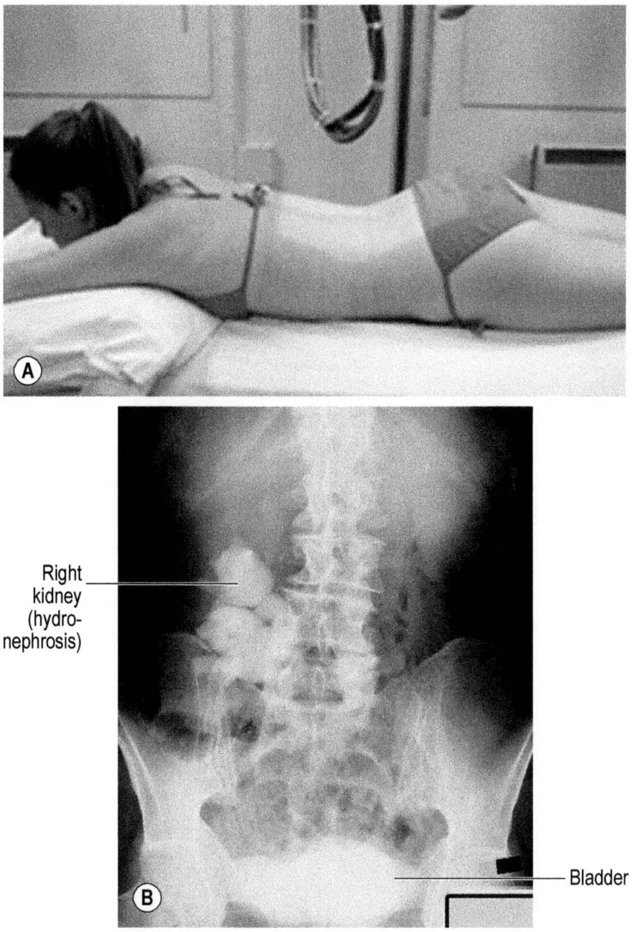

Fig. 22.9 Prone KUB. (B) is a prone image which shows hydronephrosis on the right side. Note how the position affects the appearances of the pelvis and bladder compared to the supine KUB in Fig. 22.7. The iliac crests appear flattened and much of the bladder now appears to lie behind the symphysis pubis (rather than above it as in the supine KUB). These differences are the result of the effects of oblique rays and change in position of the structures.

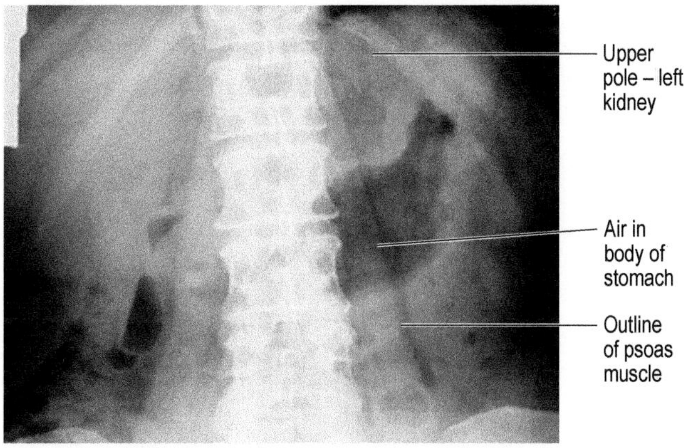

Fig. 22.10 Cross-renal control.

BLADDER: SUPINE AP 15° CAUDAL ANGLE (FIG. 22.12A,B)

Positioning

- The patient is positioned as for the supine abdomen (KUB)

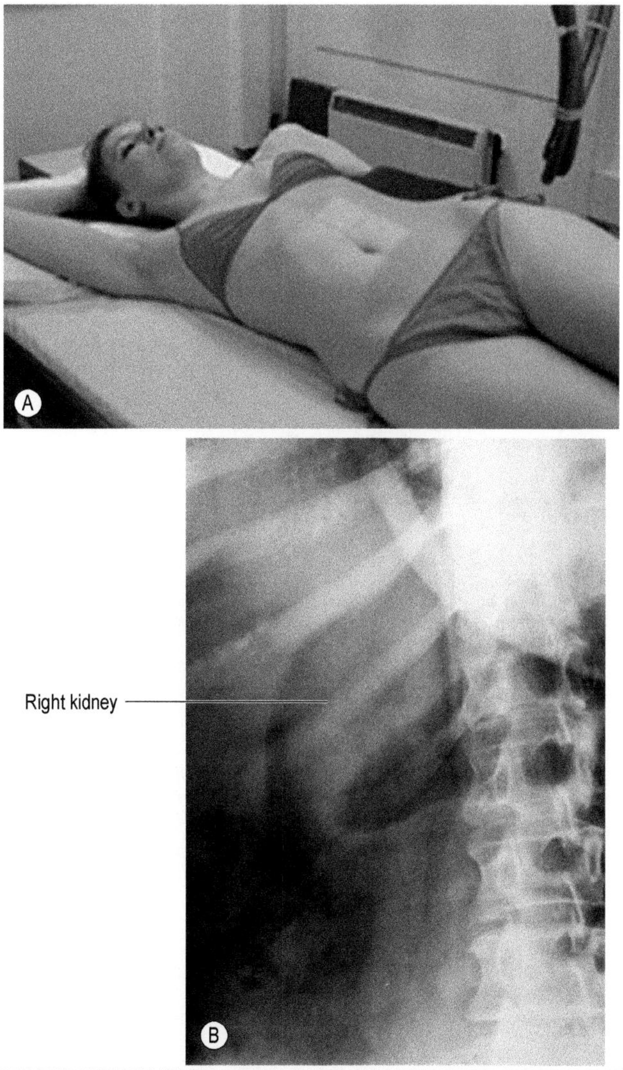

Fig. 22.11 Oblique kidney. (A) Note that the central ray is in the midline, not the midclavicular line (which is sometimes wrongly believed to be the centring plane for this projection); (B) the oblique kidney projection is often used before injection of contrast agent (as in this case) to provide further information on the position of opacities which overlie the kidney on supine images. It can also be used after injection of contrast agent, at any stage thereafter.

Beam Direction and FRD

Initially vertical, angled 15° caudally
100 cm or 115 cm FRD

Centring

In the midline, midway between the upper border of the symphysis pubis and the level of the ASIS

IR displacement may be necessary to ensure that the image lies within its boundaries.

Collimation

Symphysis pubis, bladder, lower ureters

Criteria for Assessing Image Quality

- Symphysis pubis, bladder and lower ureters are shown on the image
- Symphysis pubis is seen below and clear of the bladder

- Sharp image demonstrating the bladder in contrast with the surrounding soft tissue, if contrast has been used. This projection is less likely to be produced without contrast agent but is sometimes used as an additional control film if the lower abdomen has not been demonstrated on the KUB

Common Errors: Bladder – Supine AP 15° Caudal Angle

Common Errors	Possible Reasons	Potential Impact on Interpretation
Top of bladder is close to the top of the image, or outside collimation/boundaries of the film	Centring too low, often found to be over the symphysis pubis *or* IR was not placed correctly (too low)	Unable to fully visualise the bladder, necessitating a repeat image
Base of bladder is omitted from the boundaries of the film	Centring too high *or* IR was not displaced correctly (too high)	Unable to fully visualise the bladder, necessitating a repeat image

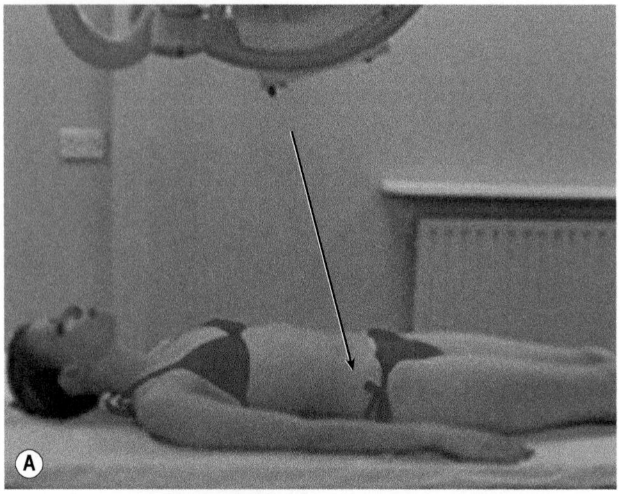

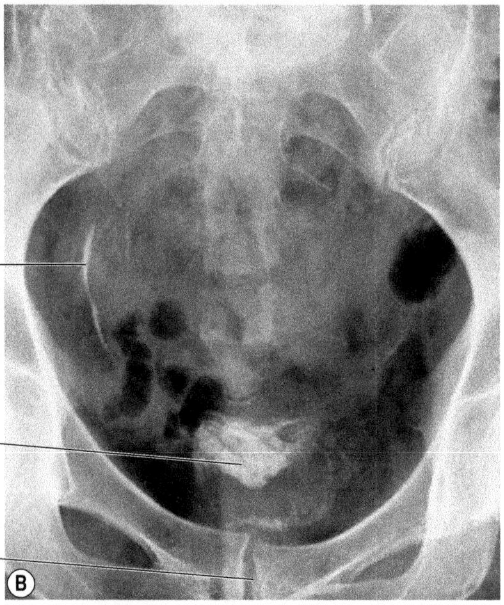

Fig. 22.12 15° bladder.

POSTERIOR OBLIQUE BLADDER (FIG. 22.13A,B)

This projection is usually used to demonstrate the lower end of the ureter as it enters the bladder posteriorly and inferiorly. To achieve this, the area is brought into profile by raising the side of interest; note that this is opposite obliquity to that required for the oblique kidney. Caudal angulation is not vital as the area of interest is the vesicoureteric junction, which is not superimposed over the pubis in an AP direction. However, angulation may reveal more information if it is required.

Positioning

- The patient is initially positioned as for the supine AP KUB
- The affected side is raised 30° and the trunk is supported and immobilised with radiolucent pads
- The arm on the lowered side is placed on the pillow for support

Beam Direction and FRD

Vertical or caudally angled 15°
100 cm or 115 cm FRD

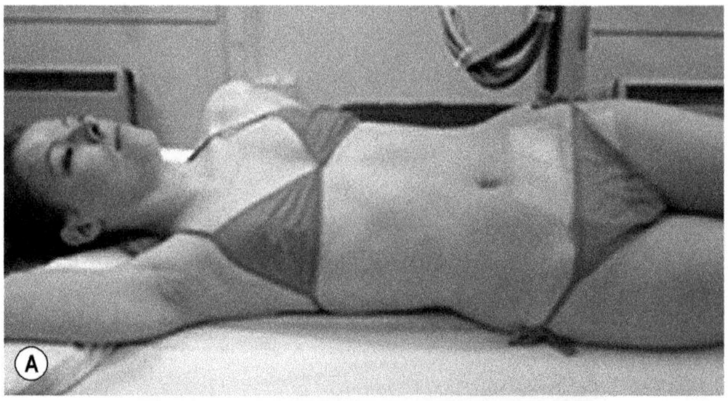

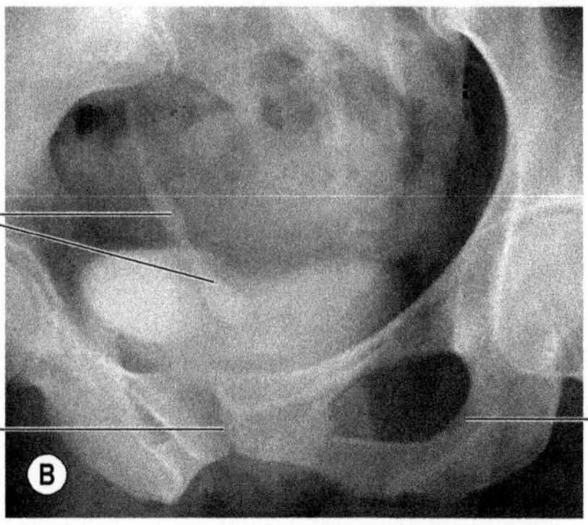

Fig. 22.13 Oblique bladder. The oblique projection aims to raise the lower end of the ureter in question to bring it from behind the bladder. In this case the intention was to show the lower end of the left ureter, which has failed to be demonstrated as there does not appear to be contrast agent in this lower portion (possibly because there is actually no obstruction at this point). The right ureter is seen, however, projected behind the contrast-filled bladder. There does appear to be some distension in this ureter, and an oblique with the right side raised will help confirm or exclude obstruction.

Centring

Midway between the middle of the upper border of the symphysis pubis and the ASIS on the raised side. IR displacement is required if an angle is used

Collimation

Symphysis pubis, bladder

Criteria for Assessing Image Quality

- Symphysis pubis and bladder are seen on the image
- Contrast-filled ureter on the raised side is seen at its site of entry into the bladder

Common Error: Bladder – Posterior Oblique

Common Error	Possible Reason	Potential Impact on Interpretation
Ischium of raised side is superimposed over lower ureter and bladder	Too much obliquity	Difficulty assessing the lower ureter and bladder due to superimposition of bony structures

Radiographic Examinations of the Bladder and Urethra – Cystography and Urethrography

It must be mentioned that ultrasound offers high-quality information on the bladder and prostate, especially due to its ability to differentiate between benign and malignant prostatic disease. It is also more efficient in its representation of disease affecting anterior and posterior bladder walls. It has largely replaced cystography in the adult, but cystography may still have a place in the assessment of vesicoureteric reflux, which is especially relevant in patients with recurrent UTI. This condition is most frequently assessed in children, but RNI provides a non-invasive and more acceptable method in this cohort.[21]

Cystography involves the administration of contrast agent via the urethra and into the bladder. Fluoroscopic investigation after surgery (e.g. radical cystoprostatectomy) is a quick and efficient method of identifying any possible leaks and is possibly the most common use for this particular examination. The examination is undertaken using fluoroscopic control, and bladder emptying and the urethra are also monitored while the patient micturates. This is termed *micturating cystourethrography* (MCU). The potential for embarrassment is clear, and the radiographer has the usual responsibility to respect the patient's privacy and dignity during the procedure. In addition, the radiographer must clearly convey that they know this is important for the patient. The opportunity for this lies in clear explanation of the procedure before the examination.

MICTURATING CYSTOURETHROGRAPHY (FIG. 22.14A,B)

Referral criteria

- Stress incontinence
- Suspected vesicoureteric reflux
- Assessment of the urethra in micturition

Contraindications

- Cystitis or other UTI infection
- Urethral stricture

Contrast Agent

- High or low osmolar contrast agent – up to 300 mL of 150 mg iodine (mgI) per mL

Additional Equipment

- Sterile towels
- Drip stand
- Saline
- Clamp
- Sterile gloves
- Gauze swabs
- Antiseptic skin wash and sterile receptacle
- Foley catheter
- Sterile anaesthetic jelly
- Incontinence pads
- Receptacle for receiving urine

Patient Preparation

- Explanation of the procedure, paying particular attention to the fact that patient privacy is taken most seriously. Requirement for micturition during the examination should also be explained and that it will be necessary for the patient to let staff know when their bladder feels full. The patient will also need to mimic the action of 'straining' without passing urine, and this must also be explained in advance
- Micturition immediately prior to the examination

Technique

- The area around the urethral opening is cleansed and the urethra is catheterised
- The bladder is drained of any remaining urine via the catheter
- After connecting the contrast agent to the catheter, the contrast agent vessel is hooked onto a drip stand and agent is allowed to run into the bladder; the flow should be controlled initially to allow early filling to be assessed fluoroscopically (to ensure that the catheter is positioned in the bladder and not in the vagina or ureter)
- Contrast agent is followed by saline, until the patient indicates that their bladder feels very full; it may be necessary to tilt the patient's head down slightly to ensure that the bladder fills completely
- Spot images are recorded in a variation of positions which include:
  - any position where vesicoureteric reflux is seen
  - AP
  - right posterior oblique (RPO) and left posterior oblique (LPO) (as shown in normal positioning descriptor outlined in Chapter 16) which will show distal ureters

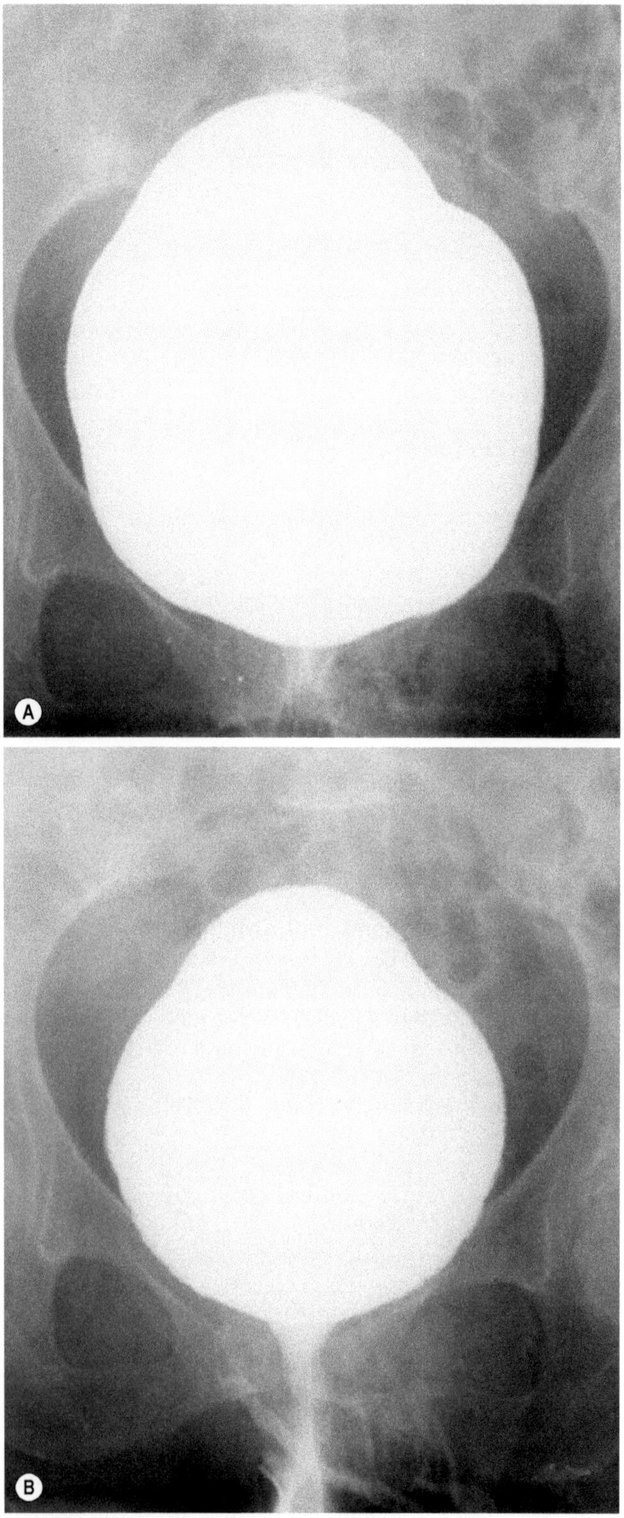

Fig. 22.14 (A) MCU – full bladder; (B) MCU – during micturition.

- lateral to demonstrate a fistula
- Additional images are taken with the patient 'straining'. The lateral is considered to be useful as well as an AP; male patients may be able to use a urine receptacle in the lateral decubitus position. For females, sitting erect will allow them to sit on a bedpan. This may require special equipment such as a high platform, which is placed against the erect fluoroscopy unit that has had the step removed
- The catheter is removed and further images are taken during micturition

Patient Aftercare

- The urethral area is wiped with a gauze swab
- The patient may wish to micturate further after the examination is complete
- The patient may wish to wash the genital area, and facilities should be available for this
- Antibiotic cover should be given to patients who have demonstrated vesicoureteric reflux

Possible Complications

- UTI
- (Rarely) reaction to contrast agent
- Perforation of the tract by the catheter

URETHROGRAPHY

Only the male urethra is examined by this method.

Referral Criteria

- Urethral fistula
- Congenital abnormality
- Urethral stricture

Contraindications

- UTI
- Recent cystoscopy or catheterisation
- Contrast agent
- 5–20 mL high osmolar contrast media (HOCM) or low osmolar contrast media (LOCM), 200–280 mgI/mL

Additional Equipment

- Sterile towels
- 20 mL syringe
- Filling tube for contrast agent
- Knuttson's (penile) clamp or urethral catheter with balloon
- Sterile water if a balloon catheter used
- 2 mL syringe for pushing water into the balloon
- Sterile gloves
- Gauze swabs
- Antiseptic skin wash and sterile receptacle
- Sterile anaesthetic jelly
- Incontinence pads
- Receptacle for receiving urine

Patient Preparation

- Explanation of the procedure
- Empty bladder

Technique

- The area is cleansed with antiseptic and anaesthetic jelly inserted into the urethra
- The penile clamp is applied to the tip of the urethra *or* the catheter inserted into the fossa navicularis. If the catheter is used it is also necessary to expand its balloon using 1 or 2 mL of water

- Approximately 5–10 mL of contrast agent is injected into the urethra and checked by fluoroscopic control. Further administration of contrast agent may be required to fill the long urethra or filling defects
- Spot images in RPO, LPO and AP positions are taken (following normal positioning descriptor as outlined in Chapter 16 and in Fig. 16.1), plus additional images if they provide useful information
- Further contrast filling may be necessary in order to allow the patient to micturate enough contrast agent to show the urethra during bladder voiding. Spot images may also be recorded during this action

Patient Aftercare

- Cleanse the area and allow the patient to micturate further if they wish

Possible Complications

- UTI
- Urethral tear

Other Methods for Imaging the Urinary System

ULTRASOUND

In many cases this has replaced contrast radiography as a first-line examination for the urinary system, but features such as the site of ureteric obstruction or calculus size may still require alternative imaging. Along with CT it is the front-line investigation for the assessment of a renal mass,[5] and is also an extremely useful tool for the assessment of renal transplant patients, particularly when using Doppler and contrast-enhanced ultrasound.[5,22]

COMPUTED TOMOGRAPHY

As a standalone investigation CT has certainly improved with the combination of low dose unenhanced and ultra-low dose techniques coming to the fore, especially in the acute situation.[5,23] Since the first edition of this book the need to discuss CT as a potential competitor in imaging the renal tract has diminished owing to its proven emergence as a main contributor to renal imaging, becoming the front-line recommendation for the detection of a renal mass.[12,23] An obvious advantage of CT is its ability to produce diagnostic images without contrast agent (unenhanced CT) and its associated risks. Another big attraction of CT urography is the 3D image reconstructions, which are now widely available. Advances in medical software mean that information obtained through coronal sectional imaging can be digitally reconfigured to produce accurate anatomy/pathology that can be viewed from any angle on a computer screen.

MAGNETIC RESONANCE IMAGING

The role of MRI should not be forgotten, particularly with regard to the question of risk of radiation dose to the patient. MRI can be used to demonstrate ureteric dilatation and obstruction.[12,24] It is not as accurate as other modalities in the diagnosis of small calculi, owing to the bright signal received from urine, which can obscure tiny stones. The place of MRI in this type of investigation is governed mainly by the patient and their suitability, or unsuitability, for other techniques. If the use of contrast agent or ionising radiation is contraindicated (e.g. in children or pregnant women), then MRI has proved its worth, especially as it compares favourably with contrast-enhanced CT when assessing renal masses.[25]

RADIONUCLIDE IMAGING

Renal function is effectively assessed by RNI, which is probably the most appropriate technique for this. It can differentiate between obstructive uropathy and non-obstructive dilatation of the renal pelvis, delineate areas of renal scarring due to infection, and localise ectopic kidneys after ultrasound fails to find their location. Its ability to assess function is also useful in the assessment of transplanted kidneys.[16] It can also assess vesicoureteric reflux, providing a less invasive and less traumatic diagnostic tool than cystography, as it does not involve urethral catheterization.[4]

Radiographic Examination of the Female Reproductive System

HYSTEROSALPINGOGRAPHY (HSG)

This is assessment of the anatomy of the uterus and uterine (fallopian) tubes, undertaken under fluoroscopic control. Spot images are recorded.

Referral Criteria

- Infertility – to check for patency of uterine (fallopian) tubes
- Recurrent spontaneous abortion (miscarriage)
- To assess patency of uterine tubes after reversal of female sterilisation
- It is possible that the procedure may have a therapeutic effect and clear obstructed uterine tubes

Contraindications

- Known or possible pregnancy
- Recent surgery
- Recent miscarriage
- Recent infection, such as pelvic inflammatory disease or salpingitis

Contrast Agent

- Approximately 20 mL HOCM or LOCM 280–300 mgI/mL

Additional Equipment

- Sterile towels
- 20 mL syringe
- Filling tube for contrast agent
- Sterile gloves
- Gauze swabs
- Antiseptic skin wash and sterile receptacle
- Vaginal speculum
- Vulsellum forceps
- Uterine cannula or Foley catheter
- Incontinence pads

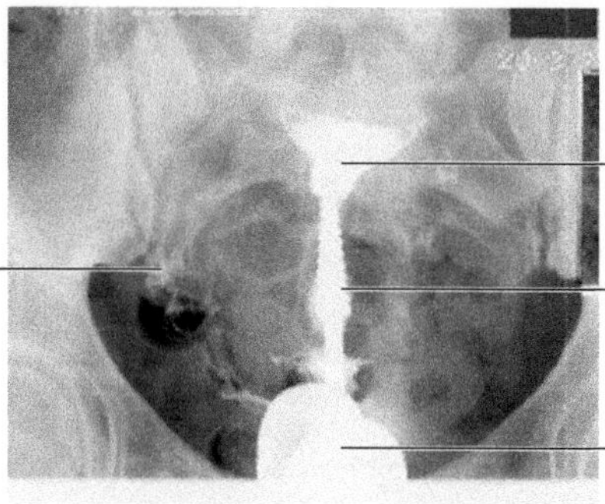

Fig. 22.15 Hysterosalpingogram.

- A portable Anglepoise light to help with visualisation of the cervix
- Sanitary pad

Patient Preparation

Prior to attending for the examination the patient is advised to use contraception from their last period and up to the examination, or abstain from sexual intercourse. Alternatively, the '10-day rule' is applied and the patient is only examined in this 10-day safe period after menstruation. However, some practitioners are reluctant to undertake the examination close to menstruation (i.e. within 4 days) to avoid the risk of extravasation or intravasation of contrast agent via the uterine endometrium.[26] If the 10-day rule is to be used in conjunction with this second rule, the patient can only be examined during days 5–10 of their menstrual cycle, providing a very narrow window of time. On the patient's arrival, the radiographer should ascertain that information on pregnancy status is correct.

- The patient may feel more comfortable if she micturates before the examination
- The procedure is explained, stressing that staff will observe the privacy rights of the patient. It will also be helpful to indicate that the procedure may be uncomfortable, rather than painful

Technique

- The area is cleansed and the speculum inserted to allow for location of the cervix
- The vagina and cervix are cleansed
- It may be necessary to stabilise the position of the cervix with the Vulsellum forceps before using the cannula. The cannula or catheter is inserted into the external os of the cervix and the contrast agent injected into the uterus. The speculum is removed, though sometimes it may be left in place if secure cannulisation of the cervix is at risk
- Filling of the uterine cavity is observed under pulsed or intermittent fluoroscopy
- Spot images are recorded in the AP position when the contrast agent is seen to reach the uterine cornua, when it starts to fill the fallopian (uterine) tubes, and then when the contrast agent has filled the tubes, spilling into the peritoneal cavity (Fig. 22.15)
- The cannula or catheter is removed and the area is wiped with gauze swabs

Patient Aftercare

- Give advice on using analgesia if the patient has low abdominal discomfort or slight cramps; advise that slight aching is not a matter for concern
- Provide the patient with a sanitary pad
- Explain that slight bleeding is possible and may last for a few days
- Advise that heavy bleeding or clotting is not normal and medical help should be sought if these occur

Possible Complications

- Trauma to the vagina or cervix
- Severe abdominal cramps
- Extravasation/intravasation of contrast agent via the endometrium to the uterine veins; this creates the risk of embolus
- Infection

Other Methods for Assessment of Fallopian Tubes and Uterine Abnormalities

MAGNETIC RESONANCE HSG

MRI is a viable alternative to the traditional HSG. However, as it does not use the traditional metal cannula but a plastic cannula with a balloon, it may be that this equipment aids in the result. MRI is the study of choice in infertile women owing to its high accuracy and detailed elaboration of uterovaginal anatomy.[27]

ULTRASOUND

Similar in principle to the HSG, but the hysterosonogram uses saline, ultrasonic contrast agent or ultrasound foam. Ultrasound foam contrast has been demonstrated to improve the diagnostic efficacy over saline for fallopian tube patency.[28] It is highly sensitive for identifying abnormalities in the uterus but cannot compete with the conventional method for assessing the fallopian tubes.[29]

References

1. Rodger F, Roditi G, Aboumarzouk OM. Diagnostic accuracy of low and ultra-low dose CT for identification of urinary tract stones: a systematic review. *Urol Int.* 2018;100(4):375–385.
2. Fowler J, Cutress M, Abubacker Z, et al. Clinical evaluation of ultra-low dose contrast-enhanced CT in patients presenting with acute ureteric colic. *Br J Med Surg Urol.* 2011;4(2):56–63.
3. Kalb B, Sharma P, Salman K, et al. Acute abdominal pain: is there a potential role for MRI in the setting of the emergency department in a patient with renal calculi? *J Magn Reson Imaging.* 2010;32(5):1012–1023.
4. Durand E, Chaumet-Riffaud P, Grenier N. Functional renal imaging: new trends in radiology and nuclear medicine. *Semin Nucl Med.* 2011;41(1):61–72.
5. NICE (National Institute f or Health and Care Excellence). *Renal and Ureteric Stones: Assessment and Management.* NICE guideline [NG118]; 2019. https://www.nice.org.uk/guidance/NG118.
6. Portis JL, Neises SM, Portis AJ. Pain is independent of stone burden and predicts surgical intervention in patients with ureteral stones. *J Urol.* 2018;200(3):597–603.
7. Ilo D, Raluy-Callado M, Graham-Clarke P, et al. Patient characteristics and treatment patterns for patients with benign prostatic hyperplasia, erectile dysfunction or co-occurring benign prostatic hyperplasia and erectile dysfunction in general practices

in the UK: a retrospective observational study. *Int J Clin Pract.* 2015;69(8):853–862.
8. Abdi H, Kazzazi A, Bazargani ST, et al. Imaging in benign prostatic hyperplasia: what is new? *Curr Opin Urol.* 2013;23(1):11–16.
9. Padhani AR, Allen C. Prostate tumours. In: Nicholson T, ed. *Recommendations for Cross-Sectional Imaging in Cancer Management.* 2nd ed. London: The Royal College of Radiologists; 2014:2. BFCR. 14.
10. Browne RF, Meehan CP, Colville J, et al. Transitional cell carcinoma of the upper urinary tract: spectrum of imaging findings. *Radiographics.* 2005;25(6):1609–1627.
11. Owens CM, Brisse HJ, Olsen ØE, et al. Bilateral disease and new trends in Wilms tumour. *Pediatr Radiol.* 2008;38(1):30–39.
12. Rossi SH, Prezzi D, Kelly-Morland C, et al. Imaging for the diagnosis and response assessment of renal tumours. *World J Urol.* 2018;36(12):1927–1942.
13. Fefferman NR, Sabach AS, Rivera R, et al. The efficacy of digital fluoroscopic image capture in the evaluation of vesicoureteral reflux in children. *Pediatr Radiol.* 2009;39(11):1179–1187.
14. Ziessman HA, Majd M. Importance of methodology on (99m)technetium dimercapto-succinic acid scintigraphic image quality: imaging pilot study for RIVUR (Randomized Intervention for Children with Vesicoureteral Reflux) multicenter investigation. *J Urol.* 2009;182(1):272–279.
15. Sugi MD, Joshi G, Maddu KK, et al. Imaging of renal transplant complications throughout the life of the allograft: comprehensive multimodality review. *Radiographics.* 2019;39(5):1327–1355.
16. Sharfuddin A. Renal relevant radiology: imaging in kidney transplantation. *Clin J Am Soc Nephrol.* 2014;9(2):416–429.
17. Neisius A, Astroza GM, Wang C, et al. Digital tomosynthesis: a new technique for imaging nephrolithiasis. Specific organ doses and effective doses compared with renal stone protocol noncontrast computed tomography. *Urology.* 2014;83(2):282–287.
18. Unett EM, Campling J, Royle AJ. *Radiographic Techniques and Image Evaluation.* London: Springer Science + Business Media; 2013.
19. Carver E, Wood D. Investigations of the genitourinary tract. In: Carver E, Carver B, eds. *Medical Imaging: Techniques, Reflection and Evaluation.* 2nd ed. Edinburgh: Churchill Livingstone; 2012:363.
20. *The Ionising Radiation (Medical Exposure) Regulations 2017 [IR(ME)R].* UK Statutory Instrument; 2017. No. 1322. https://www.legislation.gov.uk/uksi/2017/1322/contents/made.
21. Sükan A, Bayazit AK, Kibar M, et al. Comparison of direct radionuclide cystography and voiding direct cystography in the detection of vesicoureteral reflux. *Ann Nucl Med.* 2003;17(7):549–553.
22. Rimondini A, Denaro M, Bregant P, et al. Effective dose in X-ray examinations: comparison between unenhanced helical CT (UHCT) and intravenous urography (IVU) in the evaluation of renal colic. *Eur Radiol.* 2002;12(1, Suppl.):481.
23. Lee EY, Heiken JP, Huettner PC, et al. Renal cell carcinoma visible only during the corticomedullary phase of enhancement. *AJR Am J Roentgenol.* 2005;184(3 Suppl):S104–S106.
24. Chandarana H, Lee VS. Renal functional MRI: are we ready for clinical application? *AJR Am J Roentgenol.* 2009;192(6):1550–1557.
25. Ludwig DR, Ballard DH, Shetty AS, et al. Apparent diffusion coefficient distinguishes malignancy in T1-hyperintense small renal masses. *AJR Am J Roentgenol.* 2019;1–8.
26. Aitchison FA. *A Guide to Radiological Procedures.* 5th ed. London: Saunders; 2009.
27. Malek KA, Hassan M, Soliman A, et al. A prospective comparative study to assess the accuracy of MRI versus HSG in tubouterine causes of female infertility. *Middle East Fertility Soc J.* 2005;10:250–257.
28. Lim S L, Jung JJ, Yu SL, Rajeh H. A comparison of hysterosalpingo-foam sonography (HyFoSy) and hysterosalpingo-contrast sonography with saline medium (HyCoSy) in the assessment of tubal patency. *Eur J Obstet Gynecol Reprod Biol.* 2015;195:168–172.
29. Panchal S, Nagori C. A Imaging techniques for assessment of tubal status. *J Hum Reprod Sci.* 2014;7(1):2–12.

23 Vascular Imaging

MARK COWLING, COLIN MONAGHAN, BARRY CARVER, PATRICIA FOWLER AND ANDREW LAYT

There are now several non-invasive methods available for evaluation of the cardiovascular system, such as computed tomography angiography (CTA), magnetic resonance angiography (MRA) and ultrasound techniques, e.g. Doppler ultrasound. However, intra-arterial catheter angiography and venography remain important diagnostic tools and are likely to remain in clinical use for some years. Indeed, although it is invasive, intra-arterial catheter angiography has the benefit of being able to proceed directly to intervention should that be appropriate.

The vasculature of the head and neck is now most commonly imaged using techniques other than conventional catheter angiography, and is separately considered in the latter half of this chapter.

Imaging of the Cardiovascular System

EQUIPMENT

Digital subtraction angiography (DSA) has been available for over 40 years. It is noteworthy that in the 2000 NCEPOD (National Confidential Enquiry into Perioperative Deaths)[1] report on interventional vascular radiology it was stated that 8% of hospitals in the UK were still undertaking vascular work on barium screening systems. It seems likely, in the absence of more recent evidence, that this situation is now much improved, and certainly it should be considered unacceptable to be performing complex vascular imaging and intervention without access to DSA.

All dedicated DSA units have the X-ray tube and image intensifier mounted on a 'C-arm', allowing oblique views to be obtained easily without moving the patient. When angiographic images are acquired (often referred to as an angiographic run), a number of images are obtained before the intra-arterial injection of contrast; these are used as mask images. Contrast is then injected and the arteries are opacified. The mask image is then subtracted from the contrast images. All detail on the mask, such as bone, is thus removed from subsequent images, leaving only the contrast opacifying the vessels on the image; the finer detail is left unobscured by overlying structures. Digital acquisition of the image data means that the subtraction process is performed by computer, and the subtracted images are available in real time.

In general DSA is an excellent technique, but there can be problems with image quality, particularly due to patient movement. One method of dealing with this is to use a facility termed pixel shifting. This involves using the computer to move the mask and contrast images relative to one another such that they are properly aligned, thereby removing misregistration artefact (Fig. 23.1A,B). This method of image processing is most suited to movement in relatively simple anatomical structures such as a limb, and also in situations where movement has only been slight. More extreme movements can be very difficult, if not impossible, to correct by pixel shifting. This is because pixel shifting involves a simple translation of image data in two dimensions, whereas patient movement actually occurs in three dimensions, often involving a degree of rotation, rather than pure translation. Modern automated methods of pixel shifting can be of benefit where more extreme patient movement has occurred; however, there are still limitations to the technique, and attention to good patient positioning and explanation remains critical to obtaining good results.

Further degradation of image quality can be encountered owing to patient breathing and bowel peristalsis during an

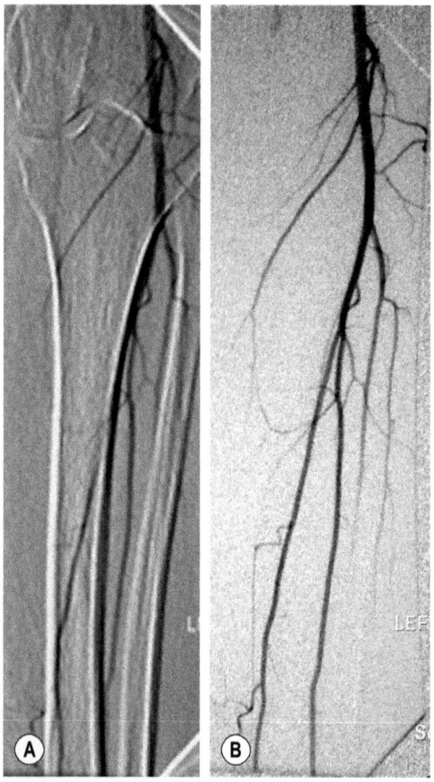

Fig. 23.1 (A) Digital subtraction arteriogram of distal calf showing misregistration artefact due to patient movement; (B) after pixel shifting the image quality is much improved.

acquisition. The former can be problematic in both the chest and the abdomen, and pixel shifting is of little value. It may prove necessary to perform the angiographic run again, but if a patient is very ill (the most common reason for being unable to suspend respiration adequately) it is often more helpful to acquire a larger number of masks than normal while the patient is breathing gently and 'remask' each image to improve the diagnostic quality. This involves changing to a different mask while looking at a single contrast image. The mask giving the least degree of misregistration artefact is chosen.

Misregistration due to bowel movement can cause marked degradation of images of the abdominal aorta and its branches, as well as the iliac arteries. In addition, it is nearly impossible to obtain images of diagnostic quality when undertaking mesenteric arteriography for gastrointestinal bleeding. Misregistration caused by gut peristalsis can be largely prevented by administering Buscopan (hyoscine-N-butylbromide) 20 mg, either intravenously or through the arteriography catheter. This abolishes peristalsis for about 15 minutes, thereby improving the quality of arteriographic images in the abdomen and pelvis. With regard to images obtained during mesenteric angiography for acute gastrointestinal bleeding, misregistration of bowel loops can give the impression of contrast extravasation into the lumen where there is none. Buscopan can be very helpful and should be administered, but it is also important to review the images without subtraction in order to avoid misdiagnosis.

Other techniques have been used to try to avoid problems with gut misregistration. For example, bowel loops can be displaced laterally by using a balloon between the patient and the image intensifier to compress the abdomen. However, such methods can often no longer be used because of the presence of proximity sensors in the equipment that prevent it from moving if it is in contact with the patient or any other object.

TECHNIQUE

Points of Access for Arteriography

Arteriography is most commonly performed by introducing a catheter through the common femoral artery in the groin. If this is not possible, the preferred route is to use the brachial artery at the level of the elbow joint. Alternatives include the radial artery, high brachial and axillary routes. Translumbar aortography, involving direct puncture of the abdominal aorta, is no longer practised in the UK.

The Transfemoral Approach

This involves the administration of local anaesthetic into the skin and deeper tissues, followed by the insertion of an arterial puncture needle. A suitable guide wire is introduced through the needle into the vessel. It is usual to observe the passage of the wire proximally through the iliac arteries into the abdominal aorta using fluoroscopy. This is helpful because it is possible for the wire to enter the inferior epigastric artery rather than the external iliac artery. This problem is immediately obvious if observed on fluoroscopy, and can be corrected. It should be noted, however, that as operators become more experienced and used to the 'feel' of the guide wire in the vessel, they may undertake little or no screening during this part of the procedure unless they encounter resistance to the passage of the wire.

The guide wire may fail to advance satisfactorily for a variety of reasons. Sometimes this can be resolved simply by repositioning the needle tip so that backflow of blood is improved, indicating that the needle tip has been positioned optimally within the vessel lumen. However, on other occasions it may be necessary to screen over the needle tip while the operator is manipulating the puncture needle, and possibly even injecting contrast. At such times the primary beam is very near the operator's hands. It is important that the screening radiographer remains vigilant and collimates as closely as possible to the needle tip to minimise the chances of the operator's hands entering the primary beam.

Once the guide wire has been correctly introduced into the aorta the needle is removed, leaving the wire in place, and a suitable catheter or sheath is introduced over it. The next stage in the procedure will depend very much on the examination to be performed, and will be dealt with below.

Complications of the transfemoral route are minimal during diagnostic arteriography; however, the recommended upper limit of complications for audit purposes is as high as 3%.[2]

The Transbrachial Route

This route is very useful if the femoral pulses are not palpable, but if a purely diagnostic study is required an alternative non-invasive method such as MRA or CTA should be considered. The complication rate associated with this route of access is in fact quite low, and in the past it would have been quite reasonable to use it routinely. It may even have had advantages for outpatient or day-case angiography. However, it is used much less frequently than the transfemoral route, probably because it is technically more demanding and therefore a little more time-consuming, and also because of concerns about placing a catheter across the origin of the left vertebral artery. The technique is very similar to that described above for the transfemoral route. However, a vascular sheath is used to facilitate the administration of antispasmodic and anticoagulant drugs during the procedure, as these are considered to reduce the incidence of brachial artery occlusion.

Most arterial territories can be examined using the transbrachial route, although the manipulations required are often more difficult because the catheters tend to be longer. In general, the left brachial approach will be used wherever possible, as this avoids placing the catheter across the origins of the great vessels as they arise from the aortic arch, with the associated potential for formation of pericatheter thrombus and consequent embolic stroke. Most frequently the femoral arteries will be examined, which involves placing the catheter inferiorly into the descending thoracic aorta and distally into the abdominal aorta. Although the initial brachial puncture and vascular sheath insertion can usually be achieved without fluoroscopy, when passing a pigtail catheter proximally into the brachial and subsequently axillary artery it is not at all uncommon for the catheter and guide wire to enter branches such as the circumflex humeral arteries. It is therefore necessary to use fluoroscopy to follow the passage of the catheter and guide wire.

It can be difficult to screen sufficiently laterally, and careful positioning of the patient before the start of the procedure is important. Modern angiographic tables are able to pivot laterally; moving the table in this way can be very helpful. Once the catheter and guide wire have reached the origin of the subclavian artery, the operator will manipulate the catheter into the descending aorta. Depending on the tortuosity of the vessels this may be relatively difficult. One of the issues is the proximity of aerated lung to the aortic arch, which can make the catheter very difficult to see. Use of filters, collimators and sometimes magnification can be very helpful in improving visibility. In addition, on modern angiographic units with pulsed fluoroscopy it can occasionally be helpful to raise the pulse rate, which will improve image quality.

Complications of brachial puncture for diagnostic arteriography are also said to be low, with a rate of up to 0.3% requiring surgery being reported.[3] Minor complications not requiring surgery and resolving spontaneously have been reported as 8–14% and major complications in 2.7%.[3,4]

Other Routes of Access

Other routes of access are now much less commonly used. The axillary and high brachial routes were associated with a relatively high incidence of haematoma formation and occasional consequent nerve damage (up to 2.4%),[5,6] owing to difficulty in achieving adequate compression. The translumbar route is no longer used in the UK because of the high incidence of retroperitoneal bleeding, the need for a general anaesthetic and lack of flexibility for performing selective arteriography. Of the other routes mentioned at the beginning of this section, the transradial approach has found favour with many cardiologists. However, although radiologists have used this approach for arteriography, it has not entered widespread use.[7]

ARTERIAL TERRITORIES EXAMINED

A variety of arterial territories can be examined, and the indications for each vary slightly. This section will discuss the approach to the examination of the various different territories, and, where relevant, will describe differences in technique according to the indication for the examination. Where projections are referred to, they are described using standard radiographic nomenclature. For example, with an under-couch tube, PA is a supine position, and anterior obliques are supine obliques with the named side of the oblique being that nearest the over-couch IR.

Femoral Arteriography

This describes examination of the abdominal aorta, iliac arteries and arteries of the lower limbs. Indications for femoral arteriography are:

- Intermittent claudication
- Critical limb ischaemia
- Acute limb ischaemia

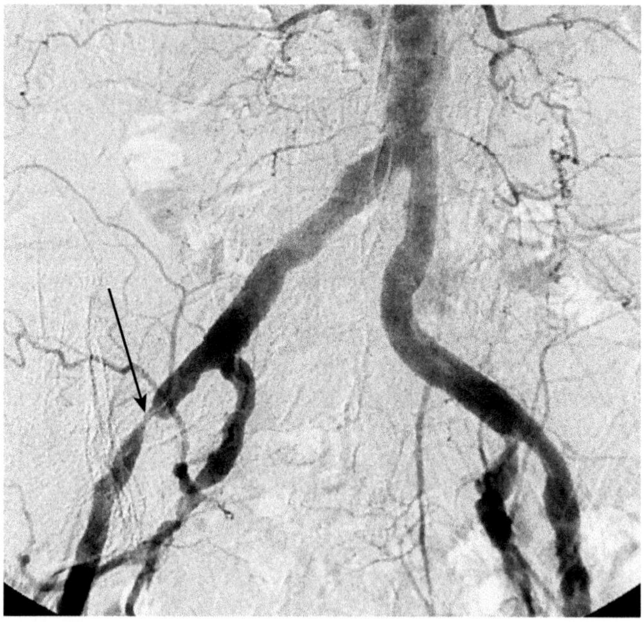

Fig. 23.2 Pelvic view from a digital subtraction arteriogram showing a severe focal stenosis of the right external iliac artery (*arrow*).

- Trauma
- Preoperative, e.g. prior to free flap skin grafting

The procedure is undertaken almost exclusively to demonstrate arterial stenoses and/or occlusions, and is the most commonly performed peripheral arteriogram at the time of writing (Fig. 23.2).

The patient lies supine on the angiographic table, legs placed as close together as possible, and supported to help keep them still during acquisitions.

Having gained arterial access, the catheter, typically a pigtail, is positioned within the abdominal aorta. Contrast is then introduced using a pressure injector. Exact protocols for injection vary. A typical protocol is to administer 25 mL of a non-ionic iodine-based contrast medium, 300 mgI/mL, at 10 mL per second. The pressure is set at 750 psi with a rise time of 0.5 seconds.

With many angiographic systems it is necessary to image the lower limb vessels in sections. Thus an abdominal aortogram will be performed, followed by a pelvic view to image the iliac vessels, and so on until the entire lower limb down to the foot has been imaged.

This is a disadvantage compared to the old film changer systems, where a bolus of contrast was administered, a series of views taken in one position, the table then automatically moved to the next position, another set of films exposed, and so on until the whole lower limb was imaged. This allowed only about 70 mL of contrast to be used, rather than up to 150 mL, for an equivalent DSA examination acquiring images at individual levels.

Of course, the traditional non-subtracted film-based systems did not allow imaging in real time, meaning that if there were a significant difference in flow rates down the two lower limbs, only the vessels in one of them might successfully be imaged. In addition, it is possible to dilute the contrast used in a DSA examination, making the contrast doses similar.

Modern systems have attempted to address this issue with 'bolus chasing'. Precise protocols vary between manufacturers, but the principle involves obtaining mask images along the entire length of both legs and then injecting a single bolus of contrast and following this as it flows distally along the lower limb vessels. The flow of contrast can be monitored in real time, meaning that the table movement can be slowed or hastened appropriately. Some systems also allow the speed of table movement to be set up automatically, depending on the time taken for a test bolus of contrast to reach the popliteal artery. Regardless of the method used, however, the system will provide subtracted images along the entire length of the lower limbs.

Although this facility is useful, the image quality is generally less good than that provided by static images, examining a single area at a time, because the signal-to-noise ratio is reduced. However, by using bolus chasing to perform an overall 'survey' of the lower limb vasculature, followed by static images over areas of concern, it is possible to reduce the overall contrast dose.

The C-arm allows appropriate oblique views to be performed. This can be most useful in the iliac arteries, where either the posteroanterior (PA) view has shown no abnormality when a lesion is suspected clinically, or where there is a suspicion of a stenosis on the PA view and confirmation of its location and severity is required. If the right iliac arteries are to be imaged then a left anterior oblique (LAO) projection is used, and if the left iliac arteries are to be examined a right anterior oblique (RAO) projection is used. An angulation of approximately 30° produces the best results.

Another area that is often shown poorly on the standard PA images is the origin of the profunda femoris artery. In this instance, LAO is used for the left side and RAO for the right side, with an angulation of 25–30%.

Renal Arteriography

The native renal arteries arise from the abdominal aorta. Their positions and number are variable, though they most frequently arise at the level of the L1/L2 vertebral bodies, and there is usually a single artery to each kidney. However, it is not at all unusual for a kidney to be supplied by two arteries, and they may be even more numerous than this. Furthermore, when the aorta is considered in cross-section, each artery may arise from either the anterior or the posterior quadrant. The most common arrangement is for the left renal artery to arise from the left posterior quadrant, and the right renal artery to originate from the right anterior quadrant. However, this is also very variable. Such anatomical variability requires scrupulous angiographic technique to ensure that every part of every renal artery is imaged.

Indications for renal arteriography include:

- Uncontrolled hypertension thought to be due to renal artery stenosis
- Rising serum creatinine thought to be due to renal artery stenosis or occlusion
- Bleeding after trauma, e.g. blunt trauma or renal biopsy

The commonest indication for renal arteriography is to search for possible renal artery stenosis. In the majority of patients the cause for this is atheroma, and such lesions are most frequently located at the origin of the renal artery. Therefore, flush aortography is used at least initially, and there may be no need to go on to selective arteriography for diagnosis.

The pigtail catheter is positioned in the abdominal aorta at about the level of the L1 vertebral body. The image is centred such that the entire abdominal aorta is imaged. Around 30 mL of a non-ionic iodine-based contrast medium, 300 mgI/mL, is administered at 15 mL/second, and images are acquired at two or three frames per second (Fig. 23.3). The first acquisition allows the number of renal arteries to be assessed, and may provide some information regarding the presence of stenoses. However, stenosis cannot be excluded until the renal artery origins have been satisfactorily visualised, and this almost always requires oblique views; magnification is also often helpful. Both LAO and RAO images centred on the renal arteries are obtained. Typically an angulation of 15° may be used, but sometimes different angulations are required.

If selective arteriography is required, for example if there is doubt about the presence of stenosis, especially if fibromuscular dysplasia is suspected, or because of bleeding from the kidney, a selective catheter will be introduced into the vessel origin, and having centred on the individual artery, contrast is injected by hand while images are acquired.

Occasionally arteriography is required for a renal transplant, for similar indications to those in native kidneys. The anatomy of transplant kidneys can produce some challenges for imaging. First, it is important to know whether the transplant is cadaveric or from a live donor. With the

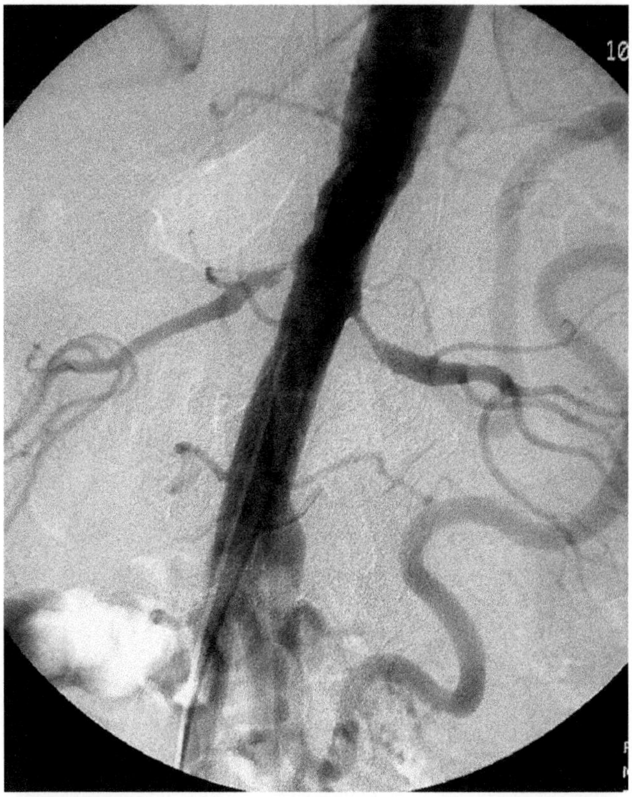

Fig. 23.3 Frontal view from a digital subtraction abdominal aortogram showing severe bilateral renal artery stenosis.

former, when the kidney is harvested it is possible to take a cuff of aorta so that the transplant kidney can be attached to the external iliac artery in one of the iliac fossae. It may require a number of obliques to profile the renal artery properly, as it may be quite tortuous. A kidney from a live donor will have a shorter artery, so will normally have been anastomosed to the internal iliac artery, but it will still lie in an iliac fossa.

In recent years non-invasive imaging of the renal arteries with MRA or CTA has been used much more frequently, and catheter angiography of the renal arteries purely for diagnosis is now unusual.

Mesenteric Arteriography

This examination is most commonly performed to identify a bleeding source, but may also be undertaken to identify stenoses or occlusions in the mesenteric vessels of patients suspected of suffering from bowel ischaemia (Fig. 23.4). In the latter case an abdominal aortogram is performed in the same way as for the renal arteries, but a lateral view is performed to profile the mesenteric vessel origins.

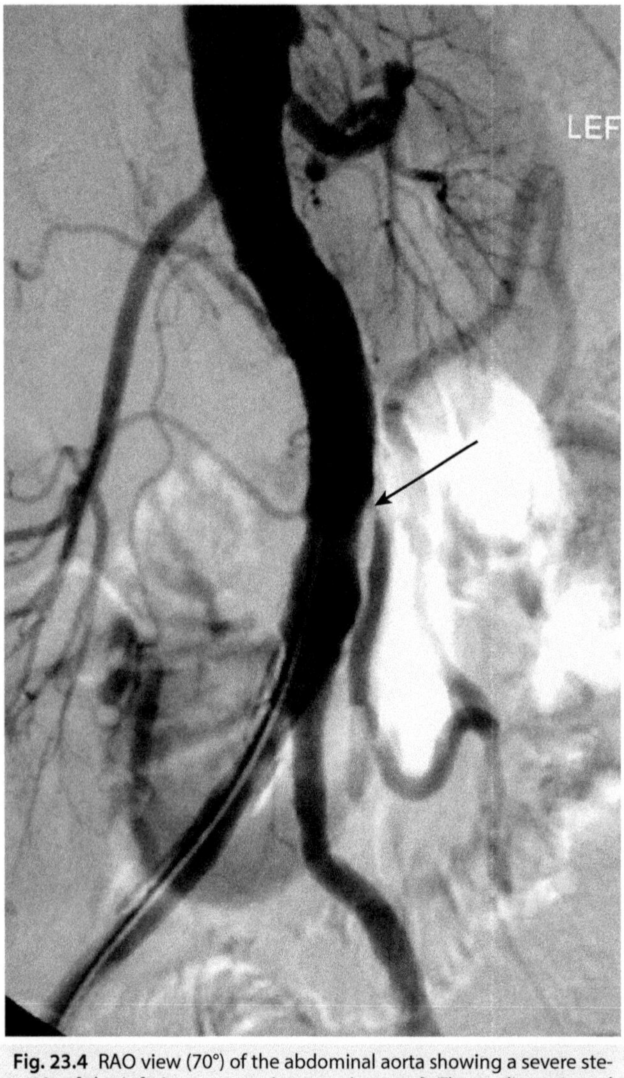

Fig. 23.4 RAO view (70°) of the abdominal aorta showing a severe stenosis of the inferior mesenteric artery (*arrowed*). The coeliac axis and superior mesenteric artery were occluded, and the patient was suffering from symptoms of mesenteric ischaemia.

In the case of mesenteric arteriography performed for gastrointestinal bleeding, selective arteriograms are performed on each individual vessel. Injection into the coeliac axis and the superior mesenteric artery is best performed with a pump, delivering around 20 mL of contrast medium at 6 mL per second. The inferior mesenteric artery is generally a smaller vessel, and is imaged using a hand injection. The operator may well advance the catheter more distally into the vessel to perform superselective injections. These will also be performed by hand, and will require magnified views.

Cardiac Arteriography

This is the radiological demonstration of not only the heart's structure but also its function. Whilst other modalities (CT and MRI) continue to make improvements in cardiac imaging, conventional catheter coronary angiography remains the gold standard for the investigation of coronary artery disease. Routinely only the left ventricle, ascending aorta and both left and right coronary arteries are studied. In order to reduce complications and risks, cardiac studies require constant monitoring of arterial pressures and electrocardiogram (ECG) waveforms.[8,9] This often requires the presence of ECG technicians, and it is quite common for these examinations to be performed by cardiologists.

High-quality fluoroscopic imaging equipment is essential, preferably using a biplanar system. Biplanar systems can reduce procedural times and the volume of contrast administered. However, single-plane dual-axis rotational angiographic techniques can also be effective.[10,11] High acquisition frame rates are essential, with all major equipment manufacturers offering cardiac units with exposure rates of between 7.5 and 50 frames per second. Arterial access was traditionally via the femoral approach, although the radial artery approach is gaining in popularity; this is due to easier access to the structures to the heart, less preparation for the patient, easier management of the puncture site and a faster recovery time.

Ventriculography

A pigtail catheter is guided across the aortic valve and positioned midchamber in the left ventricle. Correct positioning is essential to avoid complications (tachycardia or myocardial staining) or misleading results (forced mitral valve regurgitation).

Ventriculography is usually limited to two projections. RAO 30° and LAO 60° will demonstrate ventricular wall motion. A lateral projection is more useful in assessing mitral valve regurgitation.

A pressure injector should be used to deliver a bolus of contrast agent; 30 mL at 10 mL per second is usually sufficient to assess ventricular function.

Aortography

The same pigtail catheter can be withdrawn and positioned just above the aortic valve in order to perform an aortogram. Aortography is also usually limited to two projections. LAO 60° or lateral projections are useful for demonstrating ascending aortic dissections. Both projections offer an open view of the aortic arch and the position of the neck vessels. RAO 30° is also helpful in delineating aortic dissections and can also demonstrate more of the descending thoracic aorta.

Two projections will also allow assessment of any aneurysmal dilatations and the competency of the aortic valve.

A pressure injection of contrast agent should be used. Parameters of 40 mL of contrast at 20 mL per second are not uncommon.

Coronary Arteriography

The coronary arteries are cannulated using separate selective catheters. The positioning of the catheters is crucial to avoid occluding the artery or mimicking and/or camouflaging osteal diseases.[9]

The non-linear and oblique courses of the coronary arteries necessitate a number of different angiographic projections. The number of projections will vary from patient to patient. A combination of the following static projections is commonly used and will usually adequately demonstrate the coronary anatomy:

- Left coronary system: PA, lateral, RAO 30°, LAO 60°, RAO 30° with caudal 30°, LAO 60° with cranial 30°
- Right coronary artery: RAO 30°, LAO 60°, PA, lateral, LAO 60° with cranial 30°

Rotational angiographic projections often involve a dual axis rotation of the imaging system. The following swings should provide a comprehensive demonstration of the coronary tree:[12]

- Left coronary system: LAO 30° with cranial 30° via RAO 40° to LAO 40° with caudal 20°
- Right coronary artery: LAO 30° with cranial 30° via LAO 35° to RAO 30° with caudal 25°

Power injections of contrast can be used and are as safe as manual injections. However, manual injections offer advantages and flexibility for rapid repeat injections; 5–10 mL at 3–4 mL per second is commonly used for static acquisitions, and 3 mL per second can be used for rotational acquisitions.

Upper Limb Arteriography

This is required infrequently, as arterial pathology in the upper limb is much less common than in the lower limb. However, conditions such as subclavian steal (due to subclavian arterial occlusion), damage to the vessel because of trauma from cervical ribs or peripheral embolus may require arteriography. The examination will start with an arch aortogram, followed by selective catheterisation of the relevant subclavian artery, with views obtained along the length of the arm.

Venography

Until the 1990s venography was most commonly performed in the lower limb for diagnosis of deep vein thrombosis (DVT). DVT can now almost always be diagnosed or excluded on the basis of Doppler ultrasound, and venography is only rarely required. Once a vein on the dorsum of the foot has been cannulated, and tourniquets applied just above the ankle and just above the knee, contrast is injected and images of the calf are obtained in PA, RAO and LAO views. The knee tourniquet is then removed and views of the popliteal, femoral and iliac veins are obtained. It is also possible to perform arm venography and superior venacavography using similar techniques (Fig. 23.5).

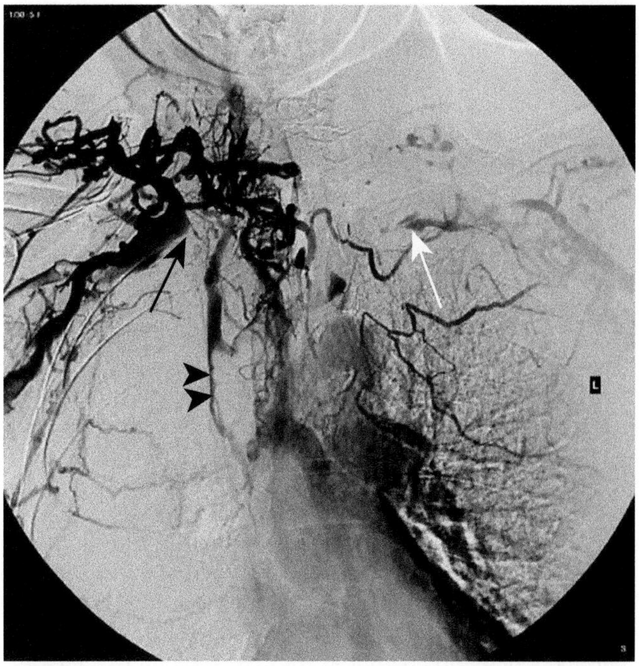

Fig. 23.5 Digital subtraction superior vena cavagram showing occlusion of the right (*black arrow*) and left (*white arrow*) brachiocephalic veins. The superior vena cava is narrow and contains thrombus (*double arrowheads*). The underlying diagnosis was bronchogenic carcinoma.

Vascular Imaging of the Head and Neck

EQUIPMENT

DSA remains the gold standard in the examination of the cerebral vasculature for many abnormalities. However, the less invasive alternatives are now adequate for many situations, and so its use is now confined to specialist applications such as prior to endovascular or neurosurgical treatment. It is advantageous to use a biplanar C-arm mounted fluoroscopic system rather than a single-plane system, to enable a reduction in examination time and the amount of radiological contrast medium administered. Biplanar is preferred for diagnostic use, and is considered essential for interventional use.

3D ROTATIONAL ANGIOGRAPHY

3D rotational angiography is useful to depict intracranial aneurysms, providing the facility to rotate the resultant angiographic image to display the vessels under examination to their best advantage. It is performed, using suitable equipment, by rotating the C-arm around the vessel of interest during contrast injection administered by injector pump. The catheter is positioned in the vessel as for a conventional angiogram. The vessel of interest is positioned at the isocentre under fluoroscopic control. The C-arm rotates to acquire a series of projections, typically over 5–10 seconds. Subtracted or non-subtracted images can be acquired. The resultant data set consists of a series of images taken at intervals around the vessel, which can be viewed and manipulated on a workstation. The images can be viewed as a multiplanar reformation, maximum intensity projection or volume-rendered.

Manipulating the 3D reformat of the images on a workstation allows the vessel to be viewed from any angle, without the need for further acquisitions. An appreciation of the morphology of the vessel, and any abnormality, can be gained, which can add significantly to the information obtained from conventional projections. It allows the operator to determine the optimum working projection (the C-arm position) at which to perform embolisation.

The ability to perform rotational angiography with 3D reformatting often removes the need for conventional supplementary oblique projections. The standard projections may be limited, depending on radiological preference, to frontal, lateral and rotational acquisitions for each vessel. Alternatively, the rotational acquisition may be used only where an abnormality is demonstrated conventionally.

Procedure

Fully informed consent must be obtained. Patients who are acutely ill may be unable to give consent, and may be treated as an emergency. Those undergoing diagnostic investigation may later undergo interventional treatment and will need to give their consent for this separately. Preparation is as for standard peripheral angiography, with the addition of a baseline neurological observation. Studies are routinely carried out with the patient awake, or with mild sedation. General anaesthesia may be used in the case of a patient who is unwell, or unable to cooperate, or where interventional treatment is undertaken.

Arterial access is normally gained via the femoral artery. The catheter and guide wire are advanced via the aorta and each cerebral vessel is selectively catheterised. Catheters for cerebral angiography have preshaped tips to facilitate vessel access. More than one catheter type may be used if vessels are tortuous or stenosed and a different shape is required. The catheter is often connected via a three-way tap to a pressurised saline flush, which is maintained throughout the procedure to minimise the risk of thrombus formation in the catheter.

Physiological monitoring is maintained throughout the procedure, with neurological observations at 15-minute intervals. Bed rest is necessary for 4 hours after the procedure, and during this time neurological and catheter site observations are made every 30 minutes.

Complications

- Stroke: risk of between about 0.1% and 1%. This may result from vessel dissection, arterial spasm or embolus
- Haematoma around the catheterisation site
- Allergy to local anaesthetic or contrast media

CEREBRAL ANGIOGRAPHY

The routine examination is the 'four-vessel angiogram' (right and left internal carotid arteries, right and left vertebral arteries). Both internal carotid arteries are selectively catheterised, with the tip of the catheter placed above the carotid bifurcation in the internal carotid artery. Often only one vertebral artery is selectively catheterised, as the termination of the contralateral vertebral artery may be filled by reflux, thereby demonstrating both posterior inferior cerebellar arteries with a single injection. Some centres include selective injections into both external carotids, particularly if a dural fistula is suspected.

It is prudent to first examine the vessel most suspected of having an abnormality, in case the procedure needs to be terminated before completion. Non-selective runs, for example with the catheter in the common carotid artery, may be performed if vascular access is difficult, but the quality of the study will be degraded by the superimposition of vessels.

Limited studies, e.g. of a single vessel, may be performed at follow-up.

A standard set of projections will be taken for each patient. This will vary slightly, depending on the radiologist's preference and the angiographic equipment used.

Internal Carotid Artery (Figs 23.6A,B–23.8A,B)

Typical standard projections are shown in the Table 23.1.

TABLE 23.1 Internal Carotid Artery Standard Projections

Projection	Positioning Guidelines	Field of View
Occipitofrontal (OF)	Petrous ridge viewed at the top of the orbit. Vertex at the top of the field of view	17 cm
Anterior oblique (AO)	From the OF position, oblique image intensifier to the side under examination 20–25°	17 cm
Lateral	Anterior of the skull at the top of the field, include from the skull base to the vertex, with as much of the rest of the cranium as possible	22 cm

Vertebral Artery (Figs 23.9A,B–23.11A,B)

Typical standard projections are shown in Table 23.2.

Final positioning adjustment is made under fluoroscopic control.

TABLE 23.2 Vertebral Artery Standard Projections

Projection	Positioning Guidelines	Field of View
FO 30° (Towne's)	Posterior clinoids viewed through foramen magnum. Foramen magnum positioned at the lower third of the field	17 cm
OF 20°	Petrous ridge at bottom of orbits. Include occiput in field of view	17 cm
Lateral	Include all of the occiput. Position with C2 at the bottom of the field of view	22 cm

Supplementary projections may be taken to exclude or demonstrate pathology (Table 23.3). These will depend on the patient's anatomy.

TABLE 23.3 Supplementary Projections

Supplementary Projection	Positioning Guidelines	Field of View
Orbital oblique	From the standard AO projection, angle caudally to project the petrous ridge at the bottom of the orbit	17 cm
Reverse oblique	AO 20–25° to the side opposite to the vessel under examination	17 cm
Submentovertical	Raise the patient's chin as much as possible (the head support may be removed) and angle cranially as much as the equipment will allow	17 cm

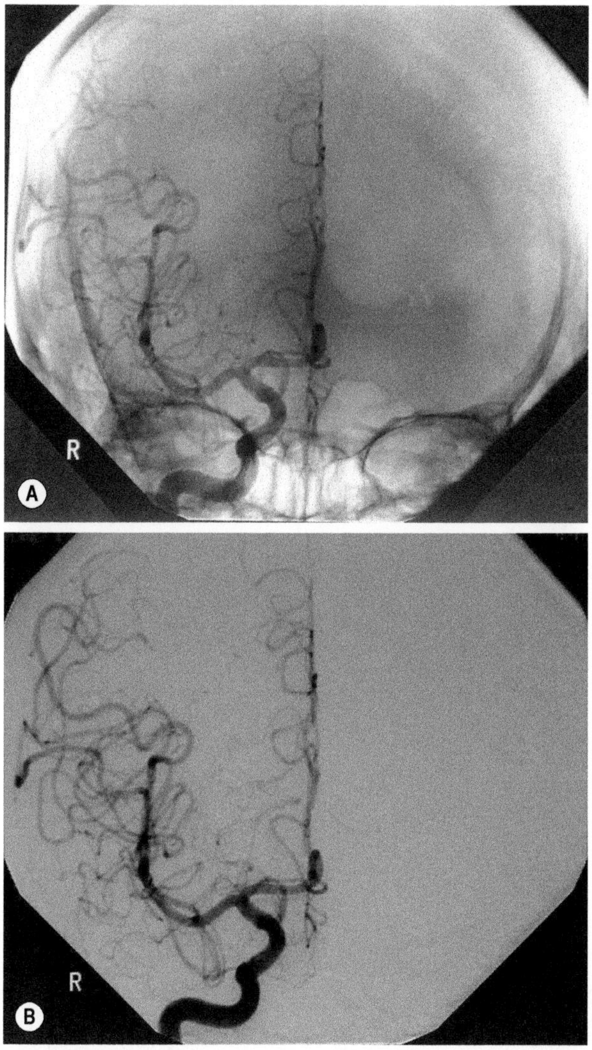

Fig. 23.6 OF projection following injection into the right internal carotid artery: (A) unsubtracted; (B) subtracted.

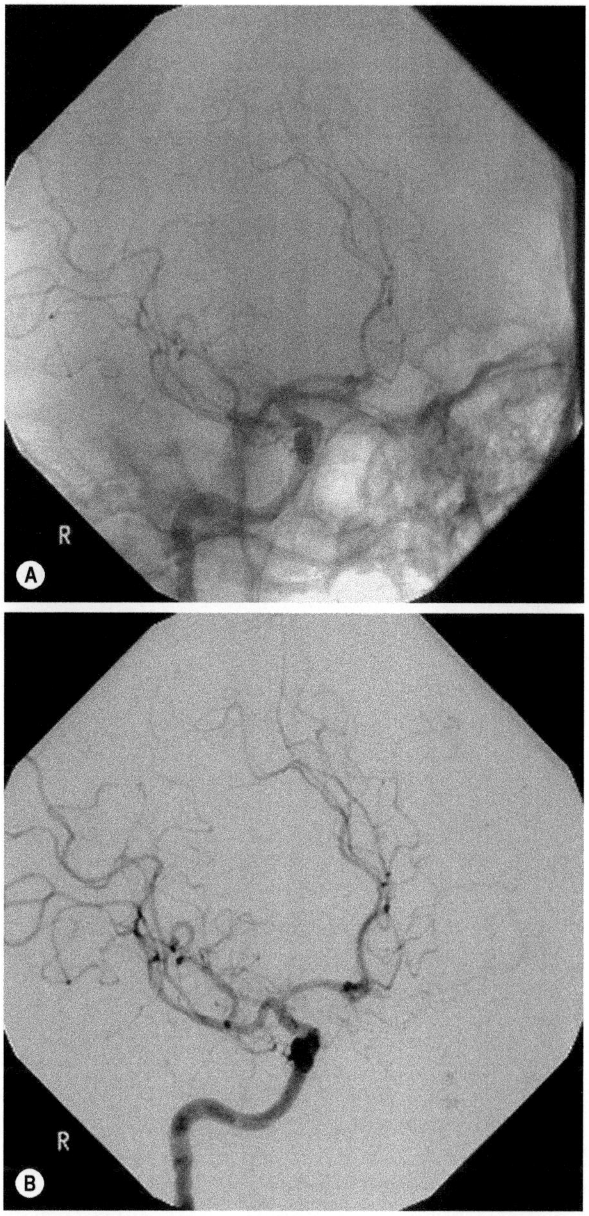

Fig. 23.7 AO projection following injection into the left internal carotid artery: (A) unsubtracted; (B) subtracted image.

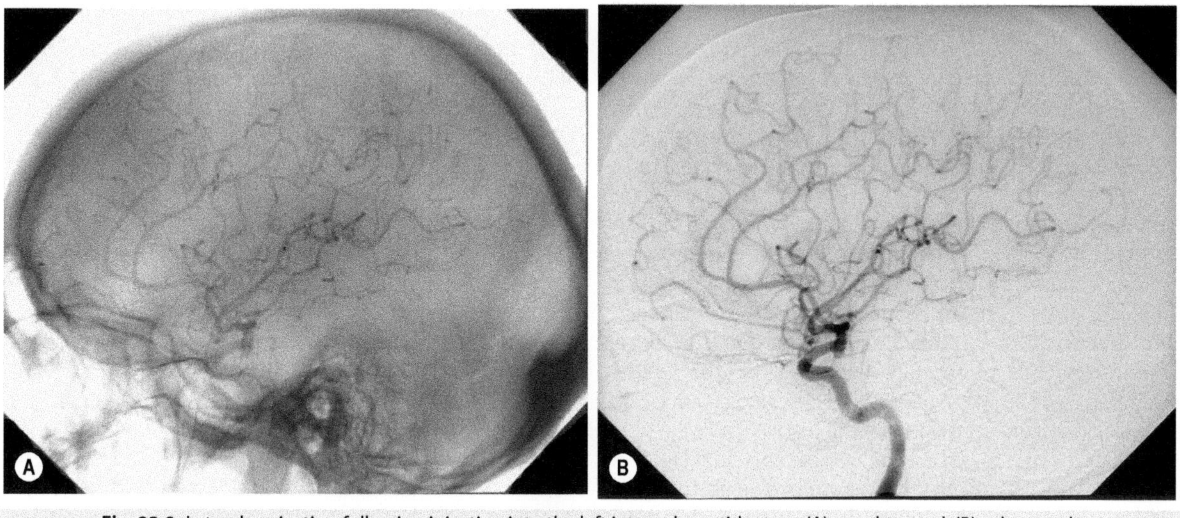

Fig. 23.8 Lateral projection following injection into the left internal carotid artery: (A) unsubtracted; (B) subtracted.

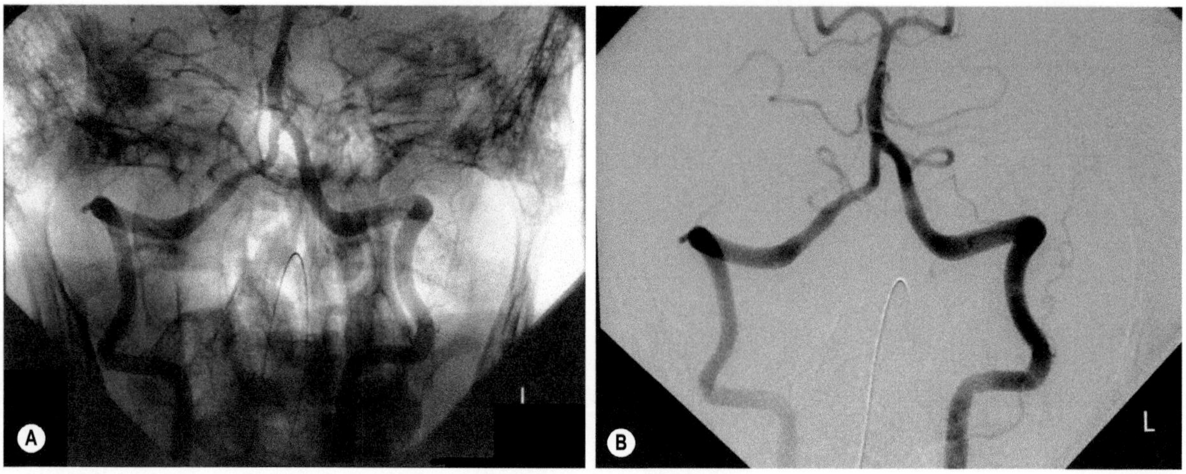

Fig. 23.9 FO 30° projection following injection into the left vertebral artery: (A) unsubtracted; (B) subtracted.

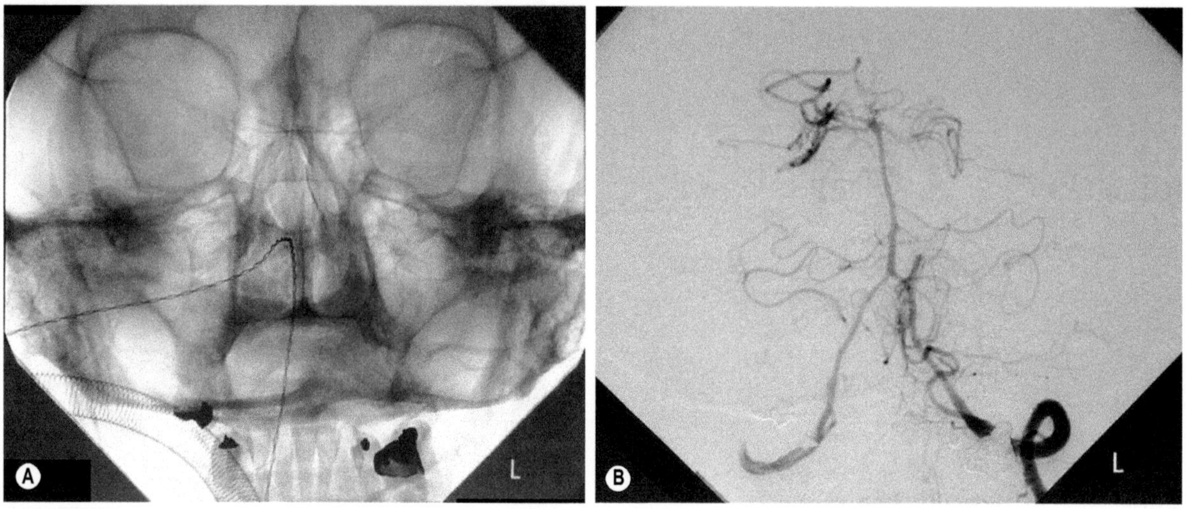

Fig. 23.10 OF 20° projection following injection into the left vertebral artery: (A) mask; (B) subtracted.

It is often difficult, with limited projections, to distinguish normal vessels from those with pathology, because the arteries are complex 3D structures. For example, a normal vascular loop may be superimposed over another vessel and mimic an aneurysm. Supplementary projections will allow a full understanding of the anatomy, including which vessels supply or drain any abnormality. It is important to demonstrate fully the morphology of aneurysms to determine the optimum treatment. Of particular interest is the ratio of diameter of the aneurysm body to the neck and the relationship of normal vessels to the aneurysm. The choice of projections, and the use of supplementary projections, is modified if 3D rotational angiography can be performed.

Neck Vessels. Examination of the extracranial portion of the arteries may be performed. The catheter is placed in the proximal vessel and injections are made as described above. A common indication is atheromatous stenosis of the carotid bifurcation. Standard projections for the common carotid artery are lateral and 20° AO.

CT ANGIOGRAPHY (CTA) (FIGS 23.12, 23.13)

CTA is acquired by obtaining CT images of a volume of tissue while a radiological contrast medium is flowing through it. The slice thickness used is dependent on the particular vessels of interest. A contrast medium is introduced intravenously via an automatic injector, the amount being dependent on the speed of flow and diameter of the vessels of interest, typically between 50 and 100 mL. The data obtained are reviewed as a maximum intensity projection or a 3D surface-rendered image. Post processing facilities enable extraction of surrounding data, and this, together with the ability to rotate the 3D image, enables optimum visualisation of the vessels under examination.

Although of lower resolution than conventional angiography, for most diagnostic purposes it is sufficient, and, although standard precautions for iodine-based contrast media must be observed, the advantage of being a less invasive technique means it is commonly used to image the cerebral and neck vessels.

As well as the arterial phase, delayed images can be used to image the cerebral venous system. Recent scanner developments mean that arterial and venous information can be easily obtained from a single acquisition, in conjunction with perfusion mapping.

The speed and simplicity of CTA means it is the method of choice to image vessels following trauma or other

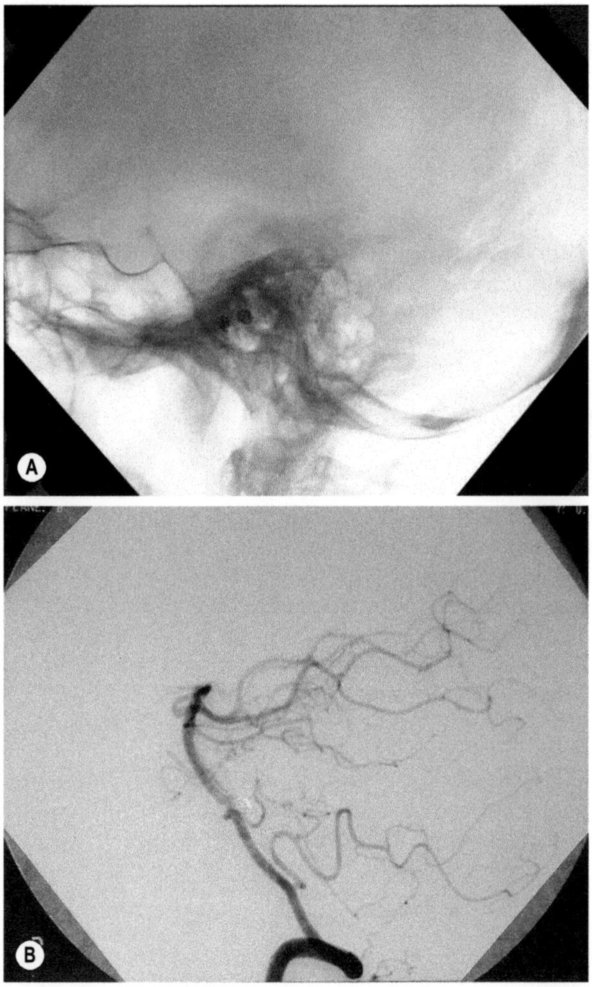

Fig. 23.11 Lateral projection following injection into the left vertebral artery: (A) unsubtracted; (B) subtracted.

emergency presentations, with DSA being performed only if the CTA is inconclusive.

MAGNETIC RESONANCE ANGIOGRAPHY (MRA) (FIG. 23.14)

Several imaging options are available using MRA. As described in Chapter 27, the most commonly used are time-of-flight (TOF) angiography, phase contrast angiography (PCA) and contrast-enhanced MRA (CEMRA). Each takes a different approach and has advantages and disadvantages in the investigation of the cerebral vessels. MRA techniques are still developing. MRA has the advantages of being minimally invasive with no radiation dose, and, with the exception of CEMRA, can be performed without exogenous contrast media. This makes its use suitable for screening studies, such as ruling out aneurysms in subjects with family history as a risk factor, or where regular follow-up studies are required, such as monitoring an unruptured aneurysm. MRA is useful in the evaluation of the neck vessels to look for stenosis or dissection.

The use of MRI is difficult in emergency situations where it may not be easy to establish whether the patient has factors that contraindicate MR, and also difficult for patients who are critically ill, because of limited access to the patient.

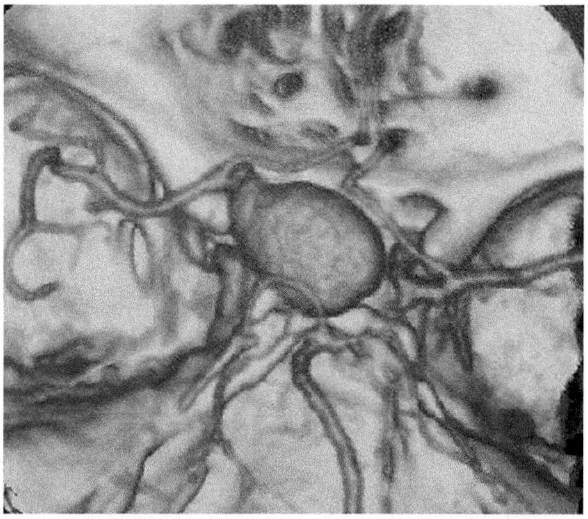

Fig. 23.12 Volume-rendered CTA demonstrating aneurysm.

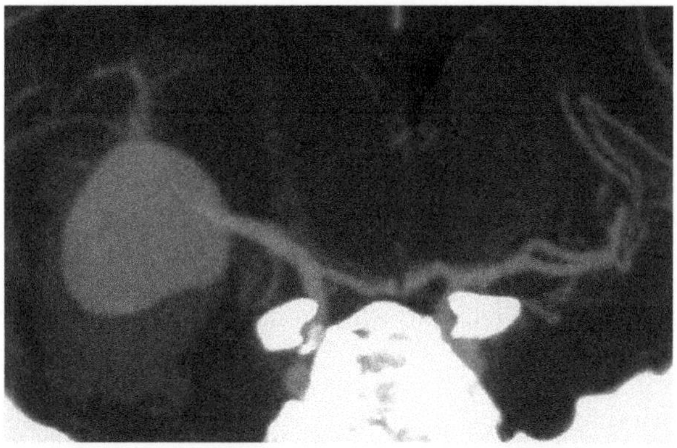

Fig. 23.13 CTA multiplanar reformat demonstrating aneurysm.

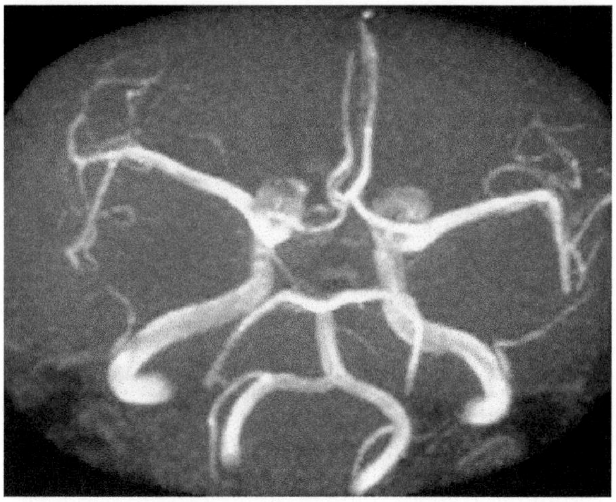

Fig. 23.14 MR TOF angiography.

DOPPLER ULTRASOUND

Doppler ultrasound is a well-established method of imaging the extracranial carotid arteries, particularly following transient ischaemic attacks (TIAs) or for those at risk of stroke. The aim of the investigation is to determine the presence or absence of atherosclerosis and the related degree of stenosis, prior to making decisions on appropriate treatment.[13]

A common place for the build-up of atherosclerosis is the carotid bifurcation, and this is a region of particular interest in Doppler ultrasound because it is an area of turbulence as the flow divides between the external and internal carotid arteries. The peak velocity and the relative changes in systole and diastole in different sections of the common, internal and external carotid arteries are indicators of the degree of stenosis. The vertebral arteries are also assessed to complete the examination. The degree of vessel stenosis will influence the selection of treatment method, which may include carotid endarterectomy or carotid stenting.[14] The urgency of imaging depends on the individual's risk of stroke.[15]

Doppler ultrasound also has a role in the follow-up of patients after carotid endarterectomy, and in the imaging of pulsatile masses and carotid dissection.[13] Doppler ultrasound examination of the extracranial vessels is dependent on a combination of grey-scale imaging, Doppler and colour flow analysis.[16] MRA and CTA may also be used in the imaging of these vessels.

Transcranial Doppler Ultrasound

Vessels in the cranium may be assessed by Doppler ultrasound using three possible approaches: transcranial, suboccipital or transorbital.[13] Transcranial Doppler ultrasound is widely used in perioperative carotid endarterectomy to determine the presence of emboli in the brain circulation, shown as high-intensity ultrasound signals.[17] It is also well established as a screening tool to determine the risk of stroke or TIA in those with sickle cell disease.[18–20] Other applications include the detection and assessment of vasopasm in patients with subarachnoid haemorrhage (SAH),[21,22] and the detection of circulating emboli in establishing the risk of stroke or TIA.[17] Clot lysis may be increased by combining transcranial Doppler ultrasound with thrombolytic drug therapy, particularly when combined with the use of microbubbles.[23–25] A newer development in clot lysis is the use of high-frequency ultrasound on a catheter tip to break up the clot.

COMMON EXAMINATIONS OF HEAD AND NECK

Cerebral Aneurysm

This is the most common indication for cerebral angiography. Aneurysmal rupture occurs in 6–12 patients per 100 000 population and the presence of asymptomatic aneurysms is thought to be in the region of 2% of the population.[26] A ruptured aneurysm presents the commonest cause of SAH in adults. The most common type is the saccular or berry aneurysm. Typically, defects develop due to the pressure of systolic waves causing herniation of the vessel wall.[27]

The average age of presentation is 40 years. Below this age presentation is more common in men than in women, but this reverses from 40 years upwards.[26] Over 90% of saccular aneurysms occur in the anterior circulation at branch points in the carotid supply,[28,29] the remaining 10% being in the posterior circulation.[26] In the anterior circulation approximately 25% are located in the middle cerebral artery distribution, 35% around the anterior cerebral artery and 30% associated with the internal carotid artery.[26,29,30] Cerebral aneurysms can range from 1–2 mm to 1–2 cm,[30] with the risk of bleeding generally increasing with size.[26,29,31]

The clinical presentation of rupture leading to SAH includes:

- Sudden severe headache[26,32,33]
- Rapid loss of consciousness[32,33]
- Vomiting[26,32]
- Photophobia[31]
- Nuchal rigidity[33]

Photophobia and nuchal rigidity result from meningeal irritation as a result of blood in the subarachnoid space.

Complications include:

- Rebleeding[29]
- Vasospasm with cerebral ischaemia[26]
- Hydrocephalus resulting from clot or obstruction of arachnoid villi by blood products[26,34]

The aim of imaging is to demonstrate the aneurysm neck and adjacent vessels to inform the choice of appropriate treatment methods: surgery or endovascular therapy.

Cerebral angiography supplemented with 3D rotational angiography enables a more exacting presentation of anatomical details than other approaches. DSA with 3D capabilities remains the gold standard, although CTA provides a non-invasive and cheaper alternative and is now the standard method of initial assessment. DSA is performed only if CTA is inconclusive.

Vasospasm may occur as a complication of SAH and will affect treatment decisions. It typically occurs 3–10 days after aneurysmal rupture.[31] In the imaging of vasospasm, CTA is more suited to the critically ill patient. CTA demonstrates anatomical configuration independent of the possible flow artefacts associated with MRA. Elevated velocities in transcranial Doppler ultrasound also have a role in confirming a clinical diagnosis.[35]

Arteriovenous Malformation (AVM)

AVMs are the second most common cause of SAH in adults. They result from developmental abnormalities of arterial and venous vessels leading to the formation of fragile vascular walls[27] as well as the lack of development of a capillary bed.[26] Typically they are made up of three parts: a core of dysplastic vessels known as a nidus, arterial feeding vessels and draining veins.[36] The associated vessels are hypertrophic and hyperplastic. AVMs are typically 3–4 cm in diameter[27] and are usually symptomatic by the age of 40 years.[26]

Clinical presentation:[26,34]

- Intracranial haemorrhage
- Seizure
- Headache
- Progressive neurological deficits

The aim of imaging is to obtain information on the layout of the vascular anatomy to inform treatment decisions. Information is required on the size and location of the nidus as well as the feeding and draining vessels. MRI and CT both have a role in providing information on the location of an AVM, with CTA providing additional information on the vascular anatomy. In preoperative assessment of AVMs there is a role for the range of imaging methods, but DSA remains the definitive procedure and provides optimum resolution for differentiation between vessels (Fig. 23.15).

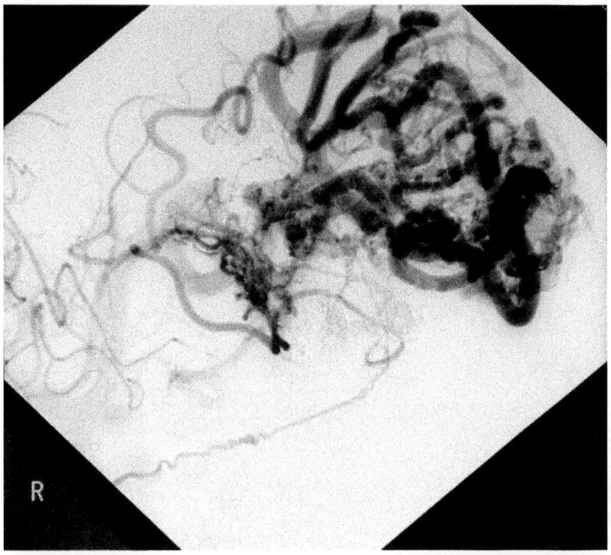

Fig. 23.15 Lateral projection following injection into the right common carotid artery. Subtracted image demonstrating an arteriovenous malformation.

Stroke

A first or recurrent stroke is experienced by over 100 000 people in England each year,[37] and stroke accounts for 11% of deaths worldwide.[38] Stroke may be divided into two main categories: *ischaemic*, accounting for around 85% of cases, and *haemorrhagic*, around 15%.[27,39]

Ischaemic Stroke. This type of stroke may lead to regional infarction or to small isolated areas known as lacunar infarcts. It occurs as a result of a regional lack of blood supply to the brain and can be due to occlusion of an artery by any mechanism, such as thrombosis, emboli or dissection. Thrombus may form intracranially or more commonly at the region of the carotid bifurcation, a common site for atheromatous disease and from where distal emboli frequently occur.

Haemodynamic ischaemic stroke may occur following: a reduction in perfusion for any reason; dissection of the vessels in the neck, particularly following trauma; vasospasm, a common complication of SAH; and can also be a complication of the use of some recreational drugs.

Haemorrhagic Stroke. Haemorrhagic stroke may result from bleeding into the brain tissue and may be the outcome of aneurysm rupture, AVM, or head injury. It can also be spontaneous, e.g. as a result of a hypertensive bleed. Cocaine and heroin abuse also increases the risk of cerebral haemorrhage and may lead to haemhorragic stroke.

The aim of imaging is to establish the diagnosis and to determine whether the event is purely ischaemic or has any haemorrhagic component. This can be established via CT examination as soon as possible after the event; urgent treatment has been shown to improve outcome in stroke.[15] Haemorrhage will contraindicate anticoagulant or thrombolytic treatment. Treatment of an ischaemic stroke is based on how much brain tissue has suffered irreversible damage and how much of the surrounding ischaemic tissue can be saved.

MR with diffusion and perfusion weighted imaging, or CT with perfusion imaging, can be used. MR has some advantages over CT in terms of radiation dose, sensitivity and specificity. The volume covered may be greater than is possible with CT perfusion techniques on some CT scanners, thereby allowing visualisation of, for example, small cortical lesions. However, MR may not be available in the emergency setting, is a difficult environment for patients requiring monitoring or ventilation, and is not suitable for patients with certain contraindications. The speed and wide accessibility of CT and an accuracy approaching that of MR makes it the most commonly used modality.

An unenhanced CT scan is first performed to rule out haemorrhage or other pathology. Perfusion CT can then be performed to evaluate an ischaemic stroke. A single bolus of contrast is injected while a volume of the brain is repeatedly scanned. The protocol will depend on the scanner configuration, with newer scanners offering wider coverage.

The change in attenuation caused as the contrast flows through the tissue is measured within each voxel and these data are used to produce different perfusion maps. Typically the mean transit time, the time the contrast takes to pass from the arterial to the venous phase (Fig. 23.16A), the time to peak, the time taken for the contrast to reach the maximum density, and the cerebral blood volume (CBV), volume of contrast within the blood vessels (Fig. 23.16B), are shown. From these measurements, cerebral blood flow (CBF) can be calculated (Fig. 23.16C). Comparison can be made between the affected and normal hemispheres, and the different maps viewed in combination to establish the degree of reversible damage. An area with reduction in CBF and increased or maintained CBV suggests tissue with reversible ischaemia, as the blood vessels dilate in an attempt to maintain cerebral perfusion. An area with matched reduction in CBF and CBV suggests infarcted tissue.

CTA can be used to demonstrate the site of the occlusion. The current generation of scanners allow CTA to be obtained from the perfusion data set without the additional injection of contrast.

Perfusion weighted MR can be used in a similar manner to CT perfusion. Diffusion weighted MR is very sensitive to early stroke changes, but the problems of imaging the acutely ill patient may limit its use compared to CT. The use of arterial spin labelling techniques allows perfusion imaging by magnetically 'labelling' blood during the scan. It therefore requires no injection of any contrast, so is completely non-invasive.

Transient Ischaemic Attack (TIA)

A transient ischaemic attack, sometimes described as a 'mini stroke', occurs when a cerebral artery is temporarily occluded, with the symptoms and signs resolving within 24 hours. Patients who have had a TIA are at high risk of stroke and should receive urgent assessment, including imaging. Diffusion weighted MRI is the best method of imaging the brain because of its

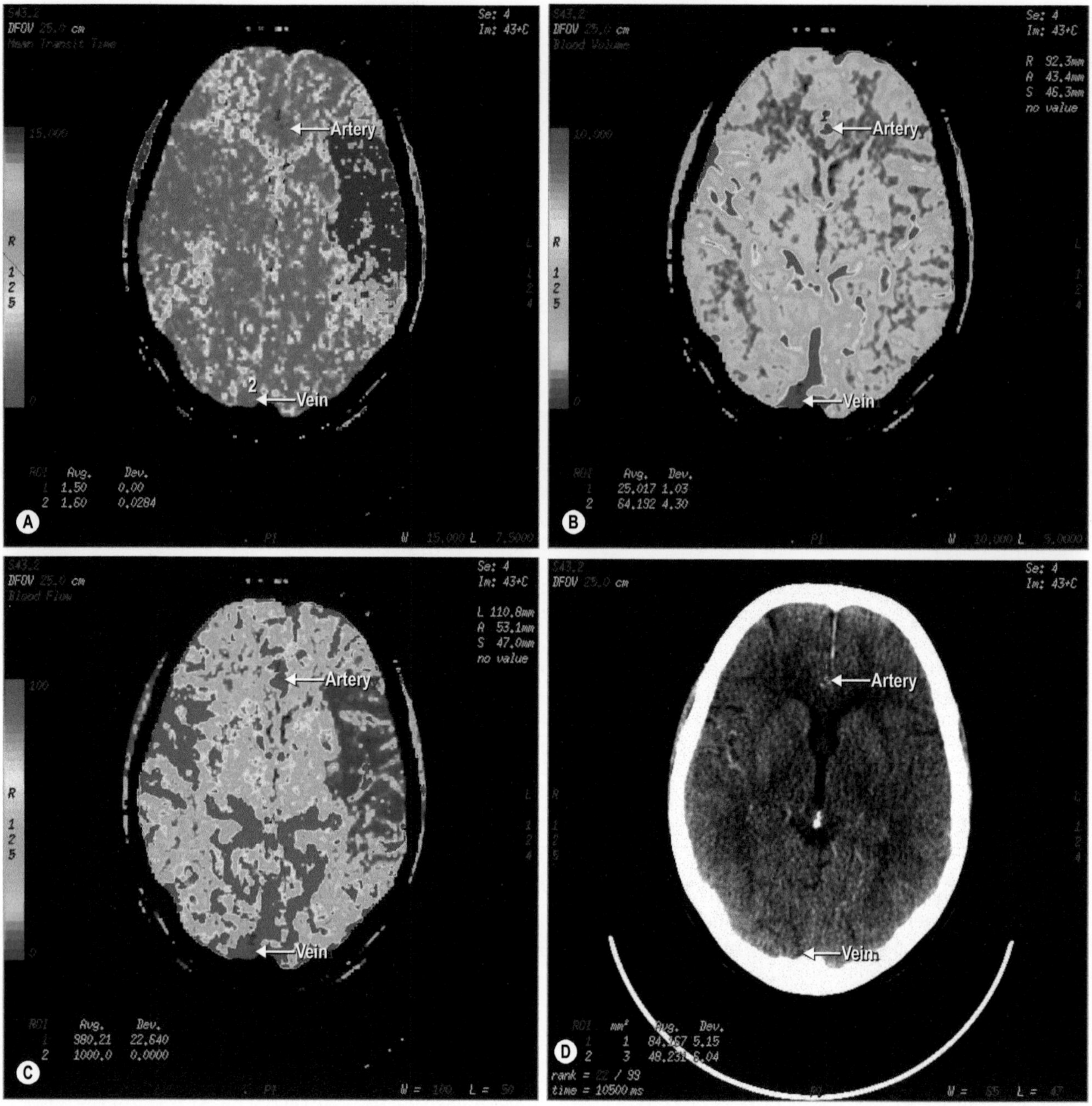

Fig. 23.16 A patient with an acute onset of right-sided weakness and dysphasia. The plain CT scan (D) shows small areas of hypodensity within the left cerebral hemisphere. The CT perfusion study demonstrates an extensive region of perfusion mismatch within the left middle cerebral artery.

sensitivity to subtle vascular changes, and is helpful in assessing which blood vessels may be involved. Imaging will help rule out other pathologies such as migraine or haemorrhage.[15] Carotid artery disease is a common cause of TIA, and imaging is important to determine whether carotid endarterectomy is required. Doppler ultrasound is the modality of choice, supplemented by MRA or CTA if inconclusive.

Tumour

Preoperative examination of the layout of the vascular supply to tumours is now more usually undertaken by magnetic resonance angiography (MRA). Preoperative devascularisation (embolisation) is used in some centres.

Conclusion

It has been said that the gold standard for the demonstration of vascular abnormalities remains conventional catheter angiography: this is a well-established and relatively safe technique for imaging the arterial tree. Where there has been evidence of substantial risk either locally, such as in the case of axillary artery puncture, or in the territory to be examined, such as the carotid arteries, other techniques or approaches have been used. However, many conditions can now be adequately demonstrated using alternative techniques that are less invasive and quicker.

The current mainstay of carotid artery imaging is Doppler ultrasound. Doppler ultrasound provides a non-invasive means of imaging the head and neck vessels, and is especially important in the management of patients presenting with TIA or stroke. However, this technique requires regular audit to ensure that there is minimal inter- and intra-observer variation. This approach has the benefit of removing the potential stroke risk associated with carotid angiography for an individual patient, but the hidden consequence is that if Doppler ultrasound results are inaccurate, some individuals may be treated inappropriately and some requiring treatment may not receive it. Furthermore, Doppler ultrasound does not produce an anatomical map for the surgeon or interventionist who will subsequently undertake treatment.

Continuing refinements in MRA mean that the use of this investigation will increase. With a range of different angiographic sequences available, this non-invasive non-ionising technique is ideal for imaging many vascular abnormalities. Acutely ill patients may be unable to cooperate with MRI scanning, and the restrictions of the MRI environment produce difficulties in imaging high-dependency patients.

Despite progress in non-invasive vascular imaging techniques such as MRA, a large number of invasive arteriograms are still carried out in the UK. This is at least on the surface undesirable, as the costs in terms of bed days of this strategy are relatively high. However, a significant number of patients will be unsuitable for MRI, for example due to having cardiac pacemakers, claustrophobia or other contraindications. Furthermore, MRA lends itself very much to planned outpatient-type work, such as may be undertaken in patients with intermittent claudication.

However, many such patients do not require imaging at all, as there is little evidence to support treatment in this group unless their exercise tolerance is less than 100 m. Patients with acute or chronic critical limb ischaemia require either urgent or, at the very least, prompt imaging and management to prevent limb loss. Owing to the pressure on MRI services and the consequent lack of availability of MRA in many places in the UK, most centres would find it difficult to provide such a non-invasive service on this basis. In addition, owing to its tendency to overestimate the severity of vascular lesions, there may be confusion between severe stenosis and occlusion in a vessel. Such a distinction can be critical in deciding whether to use open surgical or endovascular therapy. Using intra-arterial angiography in this clinical situation has the advantages of better distinction of stenosis versus occlusion, although it can still prove difficult to identify distal vessels, and of being able to proceed directly to endovascular therapy if that is appropriate.

CTA can be undertaken over large anatomical areas, such as the entire thorax, abdomen and pelvis, in a single breath-hold. It therefore has considerable advantages over DSA; such as being non-invasive, using a lower overall contrast dose when assessing large areas, and also demonstrating information about structures beyond the lumen of the vessel. Thus, in the assessment of aneurysmal disease the wall of the vessel and the true size of the aneurysm can be assessed. DSA can be misleading in this situation, as the presence of intramural thrombus can give a misleading impression of the size of the aneurysm. In addition, although CTA has the disadvantage over MRA of using ionising radiation, it has the advantage of being usable where MRI is contraindicated, e.g. if a patient has a pacemaker, and is less likely to cause claustrophobia. CTA also tends to be faster than MRA.

The widespread availability of modern CT scanners, with technology that continues to improve, means that CT has become the primary investigation for patients presenting with conditions such as SAH or stroke. Advances in hardware and processing software mean that diagnostic confidence in CTA compared to conventional DSA is high. Even relatively small vascular abnormalities, such as small aneurysms, can be demonstrated. This investigation can be performed on patients presenting from the Emergency Department, leading to rapid diagnosis, with demonstration of the morphology of vascular abnormalities, and subsequent expedition of effective treatment.

CTA is not suitable for all conditions: degradation due to metallic artefacts can make it unsuitable for patients with vascular clips or coils, and its demonstration of abnormalities such as small vessels in slow-flowing AVMs is inferior to that of conventional angiography. DSA will remain the investigation of choice for such conditions. DSA will continue to be performed where the results of other techniques are equivocal, but its use as a diagnostic tool has declined. The efficacy of interventional radiological treatment over conventional neurosurgery has long been accepted for many intracranial vascular abnormalities. The use of intra-arterial thrombolytic drugs, administered under DSA control, to treat acute stroke is another example of how the DSA room is now more dedicated to treatment than diagnosis.

References

1. Callum K, et al. Interventional vascular radiology and interventional neurovascular radiology. In: *A Report of the National Confidential Enquiry into Perioperative Deaths*. London: NCEPOD; 2000.
2. Royal College of Radiologists. *Standards in Vascular Radiology*. London: RCR; 1999. BFCR(99)9.
3. Treitl KM, König C, Reiser MF, Treitl M. Complications of transbrachial arterial access for peripheral endovascular interventions. *J Endovasc Ther*. 2015:22(1):63–70.
4. Heenan S, Grubnic S, Buckenham TM, et al. Transbrachial arteriography: indications and complications. *Clin Radiol*. 1996;51:205–209.
5. Chitwood R, Shepard AD, Shetty PC, et al. Surgical complications of transaxillary arteriography: a case control study. *J Vasc Surg*. 1996;23:844–849.
6. McIvor J, Rhymer J. 245 transaxillary arteriograms in arteriopathic patients: success rate and complications. *Clin Radiol*. 1992;45:390–394.
7. Cowling M, Buckenham TM, Belli AM. The role of transradial diagnostic angiography. *Cardiovasc Intervent Radiol*. 1997;20:103–106.
8. Noto T, Johnson L, Krone R, et al. Cardiac catheterization: a report of the Registry of the Society for cardiac angiography and interventions. *Catheterizat Cardiovasc Diagn*. 1991;24:75–83.
9. Kern M, Sorajja P, Lim M. *Cardiac Catheterization Handbook*. 6th ed. Philadelphia: Elsevier; 2015.
10. Grech M, Debono J, Xuereb RG, et al. A comparison between dual axis rotational angiography and conventional coronary angiography. *Catheterizat Cardiovasc Intervent*. 2012;80(4):576–580.
11. Klein AJ, Garcia JA. Rotational coronary angiography. *Cardiol Clin*. 2009;27(3):395–405.
12. Horisaki T, Iinuma K, Bakker N. Feasibility evaluation of dual axis rotational angiography in the diagnosis of coronary artery disease. *Med Mundi*. 2008;52(2):11–13.
13. Allan PL, Gallagher K. The carotid and vertebral arteries: transcranial colour Doppler. In: Allan PL, et al., ed. *Clinical Doppler Ultrasound*. 2nd ed. Edinburgh: Churchill Livingstone; 2006:41–72.

14. Zwolak RM, Siegel JI. Follow-up after carotid endarterectomy and stenting. In: Zierler RE, ed. *Strandness's Duplex Scanning in Vascular Disorders*. Philadelphia: Lippincott Williams & Wilkins; 2010.
15. NICE (National Institute for Health and Care Excellence). *Stroke and Transient Ischaemic Attack in over 16s: Diagnosis and Initial Management*. NICE guideline [NG128]; 2019. https://www.nice.org.uk/guidance/ng128.
16. Henningsen C. *Clinical Guide to Ultrasonography*. St Louis: Mosby; 2004.
17. King A, Markus HS. Doppler embolic signals in cerebrovascular disease and prediction of stroke risk: a systematic review and meta-analysis. *Stroke*. 2009;40:3711–3717.
18. Verduzco LA, Nathan DG. Sickle cell disease and stroke. *Blood*. 2009;114(25):5117–5125.
19. Pavlakis SG, et al. Transcranial Doppler ultrasonography (TCD) in infants with sickle cell anemia: baseline data from the BABY HUG trial. *Pediatr Blood Cancer*. 2010;54:256–259.
20. Roberts L, O'Driscoll S, Dick MC, et al. Stroke prevention in the young child with sickle cell anaemia. *Ann Hematol*. 2009;88(10):943–946.
21. American College of Radiology. *ACR Practice Guideline for the Performance of Transcranial Doppler Ultrasound for Adults and Children*. American College of Radiology; 2007.
22. Kinaid MS. Transcranial Doppler ultrasonography: a diagnostic tool of increasing utility. *Curr Opin Anaesthesiol*. 2008;21(5):552–559.
23. Csiba L. Ultrasound in acute ischaemic stroke. In: Brainin M, Heiss W-D, eds. *Textbook of Stroke Medicine*. Cambridge: Cambridge Medicine; 2010:58–76.
24. Rubiera M, Alexandrov AV. Sonothrombolysis in the management of cause ischaemic stroke. *Am J Cardiovasc Drug*. 2010;10(1):5–10.
25. Tsivgoulis G, Eggers J, Ribo M, et al. Safety and efficacy of ultrasound-enhanced thrombolysis: a comprehensive review and meta-analysis of randomized and nonrandomized studies. *Stroke*. 2010;41:280–287.
26. Lindsay K, Bone I. *Neurology and Neurosurgery Illustrated*. 4th ed. Edinburgh: Churchill Livingstone; 2004.
27. Stevens A, Lowe J. *Pathology*. 2nd ed. St Louis: Mosby; 2000.
28. Rubin R, Strayer DS. *Rubin's Pathology: Clinicopathologic Foundations of Medicine*. 5th ed. Philadelphia: Lippincott Williams & Wilkins; 2008.
29. Kumar V, Abbas AK, Mitchell R. *Robbins Basic Pathology*. 8th ed. Philadelphia: Saunders; 2008.
30. Reid R, Roberts F. *Pathology Illustrated*. 6th ed. Edinburgh: Churchill Livingstone; 2005.
31. Wiebers D, Whisnant JP, Huston J, et al. Unruptured intracranial aneurysms: natural history, clinical outcome, and risks of surgical and endovascular treatment. *Lancet*. 2003;362(9378):103–110.
32. Kumar P, Clark M. *Clinical Medicine*. 5th ed. Edinburgh: Churchill Livingstone; 2002.
33. Fitzgerald M, Folan-Curran J. *Clinical Neuroanatomy and Related Neuroscience*. 4th ed. Philadelphia: Saunders; 2002.
34. Porth C. *Pathophysiology*. 6th ed. New York: Lippincott–Raven; 2002.
35. Losseff N, et al. Stroke and cerebrovascular diseases. In: Clarke C, Howard R, Rossor M, et al., eds. *Neurology: A Queen Square Textbook*. Chichester: Wiley–Blackwell; 2009:109–154.
36. Lawton M, Spetzler R. Surgical management of acutely ruptured arteriovenous malformations. In: Welch K, et al., ed. *Primer on Cerebrovascular Diseases*. San Diego: Academic Press; 1997:511–519.
37. Royal College of Physicians Sentinel Stroke National Audit Programme (SSNAP). National clinical audit annual results portfolio March 2016–April 2017.
38. World Health Organization. *Top 10 causes of death*. www.who.int/news-room/fact-sheets/detail/the-top-10-causes-of-death. December 2020.
39. Rothwell PM, Coull AJ, Giles MF, et al. Change in stroke incidence, mortality, case-fatality, severity, and risk factors in Oxfordshire, UK from 1981 to 2004 (Oxford Vascular Study). *Lancet*. 2004;363(1004):1925–1933.

24 Interventional and Therapeutic Procedures

MARK COWLING

Interventional and therapeutic procedures undertaken in the medical imaging department locate body structures accurately before intervention and assess the progress of the procedure to follow. Interventional procedures often use a contrast radiology approach, but now almost equally often use computed tomography (CT), magnetic resonance imaging (MRI), or ultrasound (US). Interventional and therapeutic procedures include angioplasty, embolisation, dilatation, stent or filter insertion, stone removal and biopsy.

Peripheral angioplasty was first carried out in the femoral artery by Charles Dotter in the United States in 1964. He used coaxial catheters of progressively increasing sizes to widen the lumen of the vessel. Initial results were not as good as would be expected today; however, the equipment available has progressively developed such that results of angioplasty are now vastly improved and a number of other techniques are available for treatment of vascular lesions. These include embolisation in various arterial or venous territories and stent grafting for aneurysms.

Vascular Interventional Procedures

INDICATIONS

The most common indication for interventional vascular procedures is limb ischaemia, usually of the lower limb. This can present in a variety of ways, such as intermittent claudication (pain in the limb on exercise and relieved by rest), chronic critical limb ischaemia (e.g. causing rest pain, ulcers or gangrene) or acute limb ischaemia (causing pallor, coldness and numbness of the limb).

The common feature is the presence of stenoses or occlusions in the arteries supplying blood to the limb. In general, the greater the severity of the vascular disease, the greater the severity of the symptoms, although if quite severe vascular disease has developed slowly collaterals can form and prevent the symptoms from being as severe as might otherwise be the case. Limb ischaemia considered suitable for management by interventional radiological techniques can be treated in a variety of ways, such as angioplasty, stent insertion or thrombolysis. It is important to remember, however, that treatment is chosen on the basis of the symptoms, not simply the angiographic appearance.

Embolisation, on the other hand, may be undertaken for a variety of reasons. First, there may be uncontrolled bleeding: for example from the gastrointestinal tract, tumours in various sites and from the kidney, liver or other solid organs after trauma or biopsy. Embolisation is also useful in the treatment of some aneurysms. This is particularly true of aneurysms in the cerebral circulation, where coil embolisation may be used as an alternative to surgical aneurysm clipping to prevent recurrence of subarachnoid haemorrhage. Other indications include treatment of arteriovenous malformations and embolisation of the testicular vein for varicocoele. Uterine artery embolisation can be used for the treatment of uterine fibroids.

Stent grafting is used in the treatment of aneurysms. A true aneurysm describes a situation where the vessel is abnormally dilated because of expansion of all three layers of the vessel wall, making it prone to rupture. When such an aneurysm is present in the abdominal aorta, rupture causes bleeding and without emergency surgery is fatal. Therefore, if an abdominal aortic aneurysm measuring 5.5 cm or more in diameter is identified, it is usual for surgical aneurysm repair to be undertaken to remove the risk of rupture if the patient is sufficiently fit to undergo such major surgery. Since the 1990s stent grafts have been, and continue to be, developed; this can provide an alternative to open surgical repair, particularly in patients who might be at greater risk from open surgery. True aneurysms may also arise at other sites, such as the thoracic aorta and iliac arteries, and may also be amenable to treatment by stent grafting.

A false aneurysm is not surrounded by normal vessel wall. Instead, it represents the persistent leakage of blood into a cavity surrounded by haematoma. These are most commonly seen as a result of trauma to the vessel, often iatrogenic, but may also arise due to erosion by tumours, the presence of adjacent inflammation such as from acute pancreatitis, or the presence of infection in the vessel wall. Stent grafting may also be useful in the treatment of false aneurysms. However, if infection is thought likely to be present then a stent graft should be avoided if possible, as being of a foreign material its presence would make the infection impossible to eradicate. In deciding whether or not to use a stent graft the site of the false aneurysm should also be considered. For example, a false aneurysm arising from the common femoral artery (CFA) after arterial puncture is positioned directly over the hip joint: a stent graft implanted at this site would be subject to repeated stress and would eventually fail. False aneurysms at this site are therefore better treated with US-guided injection of thrombin, which thromboses the false aneurysm.

ANGIOPLASTY

The basic principles of angioplasty are the same in whichever vascular territory they are to be applied. These will be described first, followed by important caveats with respect to different arterial territories.

Once an arterial stenosis requiring treatment has been identified, it is traversed with a suitable guide wire and catheter combination. For very narrow stenoses, which can be very difficult to cross, it can be extremely helpful to use the 'roadmap' facility available on modern digital subtraction angiography (DSA) equipment. This allows contrast to be injected while screening, and the image of the vessels to be retained on the monitor. When the screening pedal is next depressed the image of the vessel remains superimposed over the real-time image of the catheter and guide wire as they are being manipulated. On newer angiography units it is also possible to superimpose an acquired angiographic run over the fluoroscopic image to aid guidewire and catheter manipulation.

Once the lesion has been crossed it is important that either a guide wire or a catheter should remain across it at all times until the procedure has been completed. When an angioplasty is undertaken, complications such as vessel dissection, occlusion due to acute thrombosis or distal embolisation, or even vessel rupture, may occur. If a guide wire has been left across the lesion it is a comparatively simple matter to go on to manage the complication appropriately. If the guide wire has been removed it may be possible to cross the lesion again, but this is often highly complex, is not always successful and may result in vessel dissection and irretrievable occlusion. At the very least, time will be taken up in crossing the lesion again, which in an acute situation is counterproductive.

Angioplasty itself is undertaken using a balloon catheter designed for the purpose. Balloons are available in a wide variety of diameters and lengths to suit the vessel and lesion being treated. The majority of balloons have radio-opaque markers at each end to facilitate the correct positioning of the device in relation to the stenosis (some have a marker in the middle). The balloon catheter is inserted through the vascular sheath over the guide wire and advanced into the correct position. This can be done using the roadmap, or bony landmarks may be chosen to facilitate positioning. The balloon is then inflated to the correct pressure (for that balloon) for 30 seconds in the first instance. It is then removed, leaving the guide wire in place, and an angiogram is performed to demonstrate the response. If the result of the angioplasty has been satisfactory, the guide wire can be safely removed. If the result is unsatisfactory, further balloon inflations may be undertaken, perhaps to a greater diameter or for a longer period of time. Depending on the site, a vascular stent may be inserted, or the use of a drug eluting balloon may be considered.

Drug eluting balloons work much in the same way as regular angioplasty balloons, however, as the name suggests, they are coated with a long-acting drug. The balloon is inflated and held at nominal pressure for 60 seconds, or two lots of 45 seconds. This allows time for the drug coating to be absorbed by the vessel wall and prevent the vessel re-stenosing. Drug-coated balloons will not be as effective in the long term as a stent, but are useful in areas where simply ballooning with a standard balloon is not enough.

Cutting balloons may also be used when a stenosis is too rigid to be ballooned alone. The balloon contains 2–4 tiny blades along the length of the balloon that cut through the first epithelial surface and allow the vessel to stretch when ballooning, without compromising the integrity of the vessel.

Iliac Angioplasty

The results of iliac angioplasty are generally very good, and for many years have experienced a low complication rate.[1,2] The procedure is safe and successful, and in many centres it is offered to patients who have intermittent claudication after 100 m walking or less. It may also be of great value as an adjunct to surgery.[3] For example, if a lower limb bypass graft is to be undertaken, iliac angioplasty to a stenosis above the proposed site of the proximal anastomosis will improve the inflow of blood, making a successful bypass more likely and reducing the extent of the surgery required.

When undertaking iliac angioplasty it is often possible to choose whether to approach the lesion ipsilaterally and retrogradely, or contralaterally and antegradely. An ipsilateral approach, puncturing the artery on the side to be treated followed by crossing the stenosis in a retrograde fashion, offers an advantage: should a vessel dissection occur it is unlikely to lead to vessel occlusion, as the blood flow distally along the vessel will tend to close the intimal flap. The alternative, which involves puncturing the contralateral femoral artery, crossing the aortic bifurcation and then traversing the lesion, is technically more demanding and, if a dissection occurs, the blood flow will tend to cause the intimal flap to extend distally, potentially causing vessel occlusion.

Superficial Femoral Artery (SFA) Angioplasty (Fig. 24.1A–D)

This procedure is most commonly undertaken for the management of critical lower limb ischaemia or short-distance intermittent claudication. Such ischaemia is most likely to be caused by SFA occlusion, rather than a simple stenosis; thus to perform an angioplasty the occlusion must first be crossed with a guide wire. This can be difficult, but the use of a hydrophilic guide wire will facilitate successful crossing in the vast majority of cases, with many operators electing to pass the guide wire subintimally. SFA angioplasty is less commonly performed for treatment of intermittent claudication, as generally the results are inferior to those of iliac angioplasty,[4,5] and two randomised studies have shown that the results are no better over the long term than those observed after a supervised exercise programme.[6,7]

As with iliac angioplasty, SFA lesions can be approached either contralaterally or ipsilaterally. The contralateral approach is the same in technical terms as that used for the iliac vessels. However, the ipsilateral approach to the SFA is technically more difficult, as an antegrade puncture of the CFA is required. To perform an antegrade puncture, the femoral head is first identified under fluoroscopy and its position marked on the skin surface with a metal marker. Local anaesthetic is infiltrated into the skin over the femoral pulse as it is palpated at this level. A puncture needle is introduced first and a guide wire is then introduced along the SFA. It is possible that the guide wire may pass into the profunda femoris,

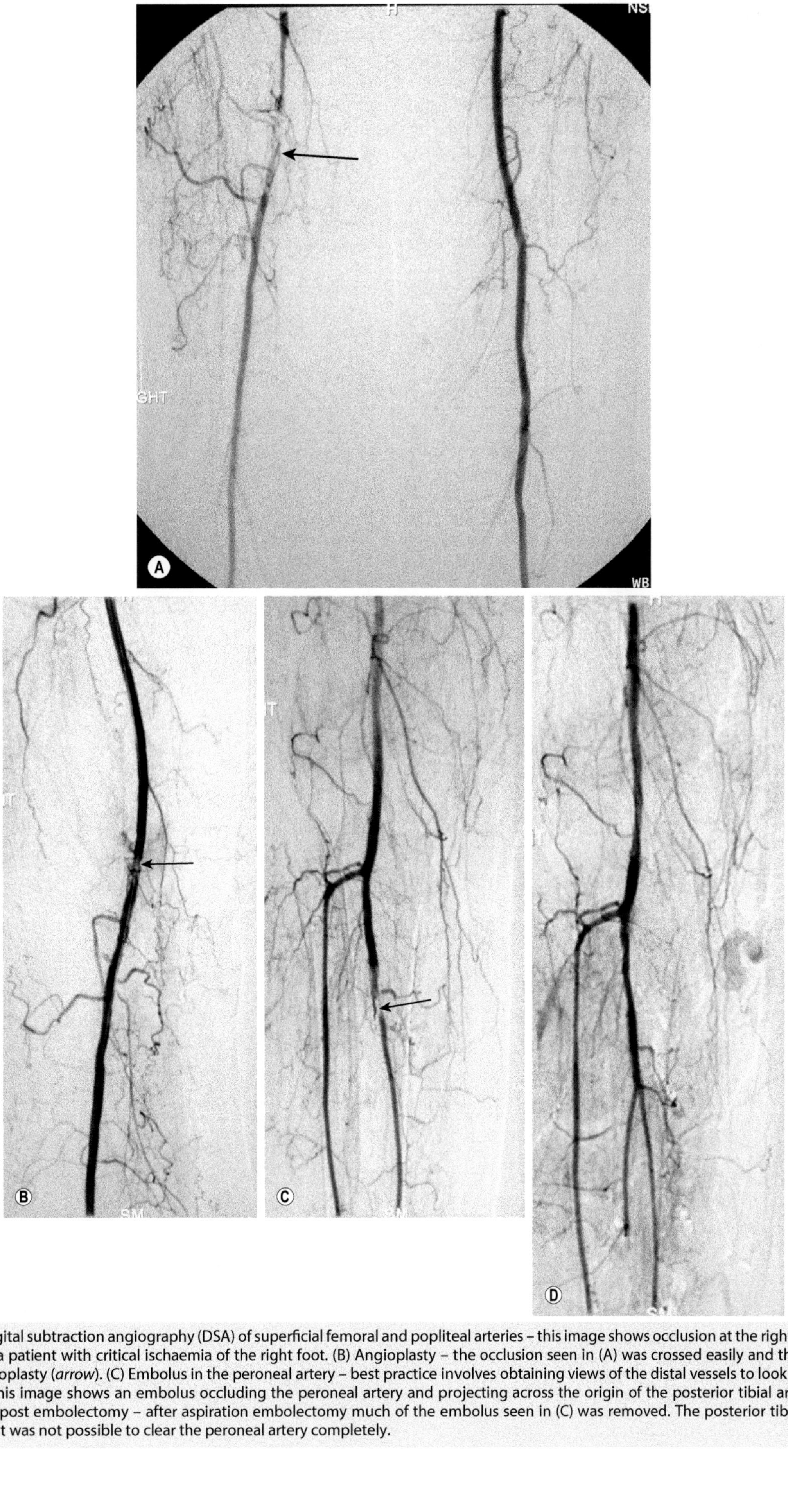

Fig. 24.1 (A) Digital subtraction angiography (DSA) of superficial femoral and popliteal arteries – this image shows occlusion at the right adductor canal level (*arrow*) in a patient with critical ischaemia of the right foot. (B) Angioplasty – the occlusion seen in (A) was crossed easily and there was a good result from angioplasty (*arrow*). (C) Embolus in the peroneal artery – best practice involves obtaining views of the distal vessels to look for any possible complication. This image shows an embolus occluding the peroneal artery and projecting across the origin of the posterior tibial artery (*arrow*). (D) Peroneal artery post embolectomy – after aspiration embolectomy much of the embolus seen in (C) was removed. The posterior tibial artery is now patent, though it was not possible to clear the peroneal artery completely.

and for this reason it is important to observe its progress under fluoroscopic control. If it proves difficult to enter the SFA, it may be necessary to screen over the needle tip while manipulating it into different positions to facilitate guide wire advancement. When doing this it is very easy for the operator to put their hands into the X-ray beam without realising. The radiographer can prevent or minimise this by centring only on the very tip of the needle, rather than its whole length, and using the collimators appropriately. Antegrade puncture is often used because the distance from the puncture site to the angioplasty site is short, avoiding the need to use very long guide wires. It also avoids any problems associated with catheter manipulation when dealing with tortuous iliac arteries or an acutely angled aortic bifurcation; in the event of a complication occurring, the subsequent management, e.g. aspiration embolectomy, is much more straightforward (Fig. 24.1C,D).

Popliteal Artery and the Tibial Vessels

Lesions in these vessels will only be treated with angioplasty in the presence of critical lower limb ischaemia or short-distance claudication (Fig. 24.2A,B). The

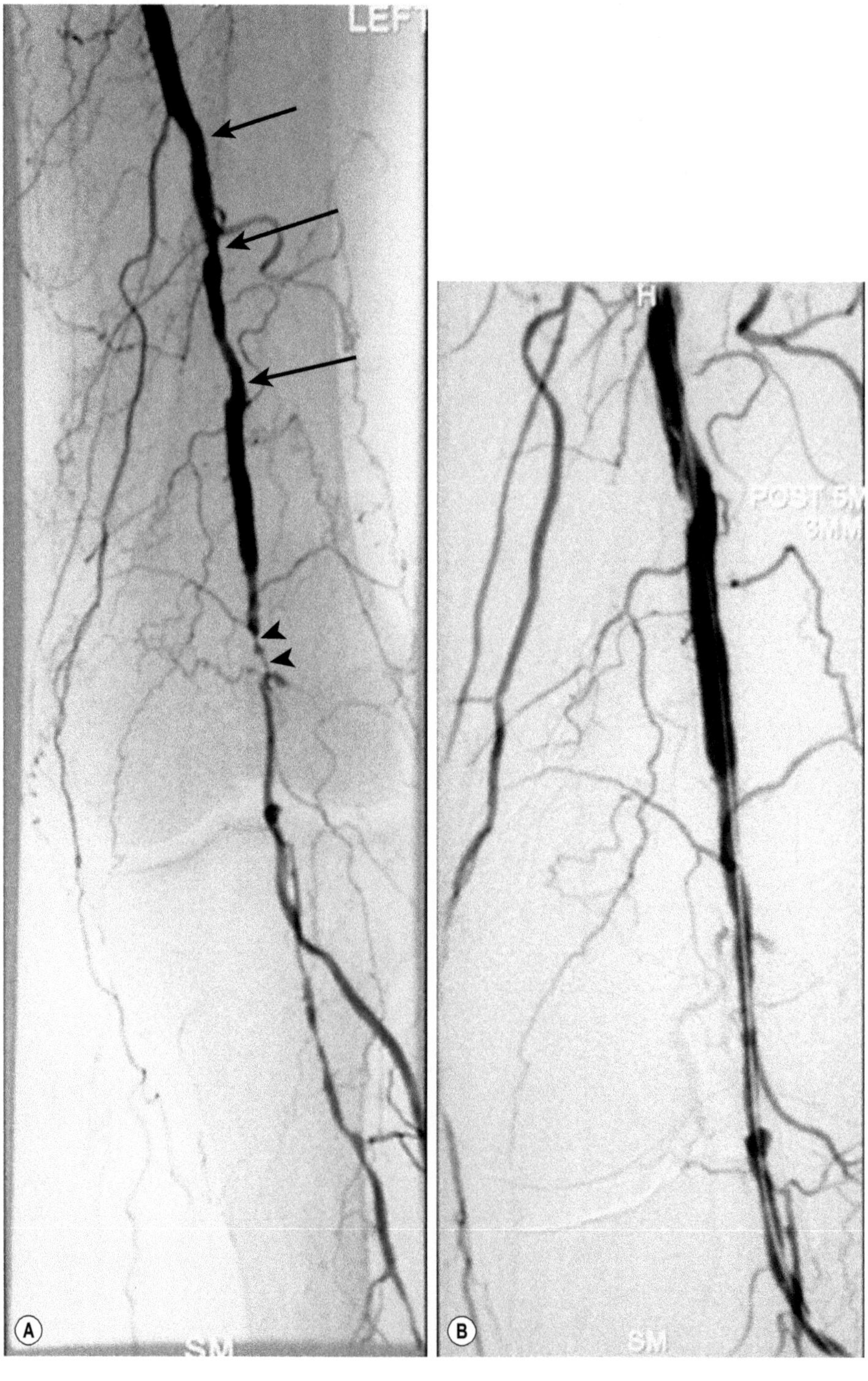

Fig. 24.2 (A) Stenosis of popliteal artery – arteriogram demonstrating a stenotic segment of above-knee popliteal artery (*arrows*) and a tight stenosis at the origin of the anterior tibial artery (*arrowheads*), which has an abnormally high take-off. (B) Arteriogram post angioplasty – a good technical result after angioplasty in the case shown in (A).

potential benefit of angioplasty at these sites in patients with uncomplicated intermittent claudication would be completely outweighed by the potential risk and the likelihood of future recurrence.[8] Technically there is very little difference between angioplasty performed here and elsewhere in the lower limb. Smaller diameter balloons are used, and many operators prefer to use finer guide wires.

VASCULAR STENT INSERTION

The term 'stent' describes a device designed to keep a passage or conduit open. Vascular stents have become accepted as extremely helpful both in maintaining patency where the result of angioplasty alone has been suboptimal, and in certain locations where they provide such markedly superior benefits compared to angioplasty alone that they are considered to be the first line of treatment.

Vascular stents are metallic, commonly made either of stainless steel or Nitinol. Nitinol is a nickel–titanium alloy which has great elasticity and 'shape memory', which allows it to return to its original state even after significant manipulation and bending. Stents may be self-expanding or balloon expandable. Prior to deployment, stents are compressed onto a delivery catheter; each end of the stent either has radio-opaque markers on the device itself or on the catheter, to facilitate correct positioning. The technique used for deployment of a stent is much the same as that described for angioplasty, with the obvious difference that instead of performing simple balloon dilatation, a stent is deployed instead. It will often prove necessary to perform angioplasty prior to stent deployment, and further angioplasty after deployment may be required to ensure that the stent is fully expanded.

Stents are used commonly in the iliac, renal and subclavian arteries, and are being used increasingly in the carotid arteries. Stents have previously been used only in the SFA as a 'bail-out' if angioplasty has resulted in vessel occlusion. However, evidence is starting to show, at least with more modern stent, e.g. Nitinol, designs, that for lesions >6 cm the use of stents may be the superior initial treatment.[9] Stents are not used routinely in the popliteal or tibial vessels, though devices are available to be used in the event of a suboptimal result.

Stenting the Iliac Artery (Fig. 24.3A,B)

It has been shown that if iliac angioplasty is technically successful there is no advantage in terms of clinical outcome in adding a stent.[10–11] However, in about 50% of cases the outcome from angioplasty is suboptimal, perhaps due, for example, to elastic recoil of the vessel wall or dissection causing flow limitation. Many professionals would add to this and include failure to reduce the intra-arterial pressure gradient across the lesion to less than 10 mmHg as an indication; although in practice this is not measured in many centres unless there is a perceived problem with the angiographic result.

The exception to this is the treatment of iliac artery occlusions where, if angioplasty alone is used, there is an incidence of peripheral embolisation of up to 50%.[10] For this reason, primary stenting is undertaken when treating iliac occlusions endovascularly. Thus, a self-expanding stent is first deployed across the occlusion and subsequently dilated using an angioplasty balloon.

Stenting the Renal Artery (Fig. 24.4A,B)

Renal artery stenosis is generally caused by one of two pathologies, either fibromuscular hyperplasia or atheroma. Fibromuscular hyperplasia is an uncommon cause of uncontrollable hypertension and responds well to angioplasty alone. Atheromatous renal artery stenosis (ARAS), when it requires treatment, responds very poorly to angioplasty alone, and it has clearly been demonstrated that primary stenting is superior in both the short and the longer term.[12] This happens because the vast majority of ARAS occurs at the origin of the vessel and is caused by aortic atheroma rather than true atheroma of the renal artery. Therefore, an expansile force applied to the stenosis causes shear stresses within the aortic plaque, rather than an expansile force within the renal artery lumen. Once the angioplasty balloon is removed the stenosis will frequently recur as the aortic plaque moves back into position.

Balloon-expandable stents are favoured for the treatment of ARAS. In order to avoid the stent being compressed by the aortic plaques, it is necessary to position the stent so that it projects 2–3 mm into the aortic lumen. Such precision is much easier to achieve with balloon-expandable stents, as they do not shorten when they are deployed. Although much improved over older designs, even modern self-expanding stents show some shortening.

Subclavian Stenting

Although stenoses or occlusions can occur in the subclavian arteries at any point, by far the commonest site of disease is the origin of the left subclavian artery. The majority of these lesions are asymptomatic. However, where there are symptoms of arm claudication or subclavian steal syndrome, intervention may be indicated. Stents are frequently used at this site, especially in the presence of arterial occlusion.

If there is occlusion at the origin of the left subclavian artery it is usually very difficult indeed to cross the lesion using a catheter inserted via the groin. It is therefore often helpful to use a transbrachial approach. Previously this often required a surgical cut-down onto the brachial artery for access, as 7Fr or 8Fr sheaths were required. Now sheaths of only 6Fr in diameter can be used, which allows for true percutaneous puncture.

VASCULAR STENT GRAFTS

As previously mentioned, stent grafts are used in the treatment of true or false aneurysms. The technology continues to evolve, and it is not possible to say at this point whether stent grafting will replace open surgery in the treatment of aneurysmal disease. However, as new stent graft designs become available the anatomical limitations to their use are gradually diminishing. There is also improving evidence to support the use of stent grafts in the treatment of thoracic aortic aneurysms, where the risks of surgery are considerably greater than those of open surgery for abdominal aneurysms.[13] Furthermore,

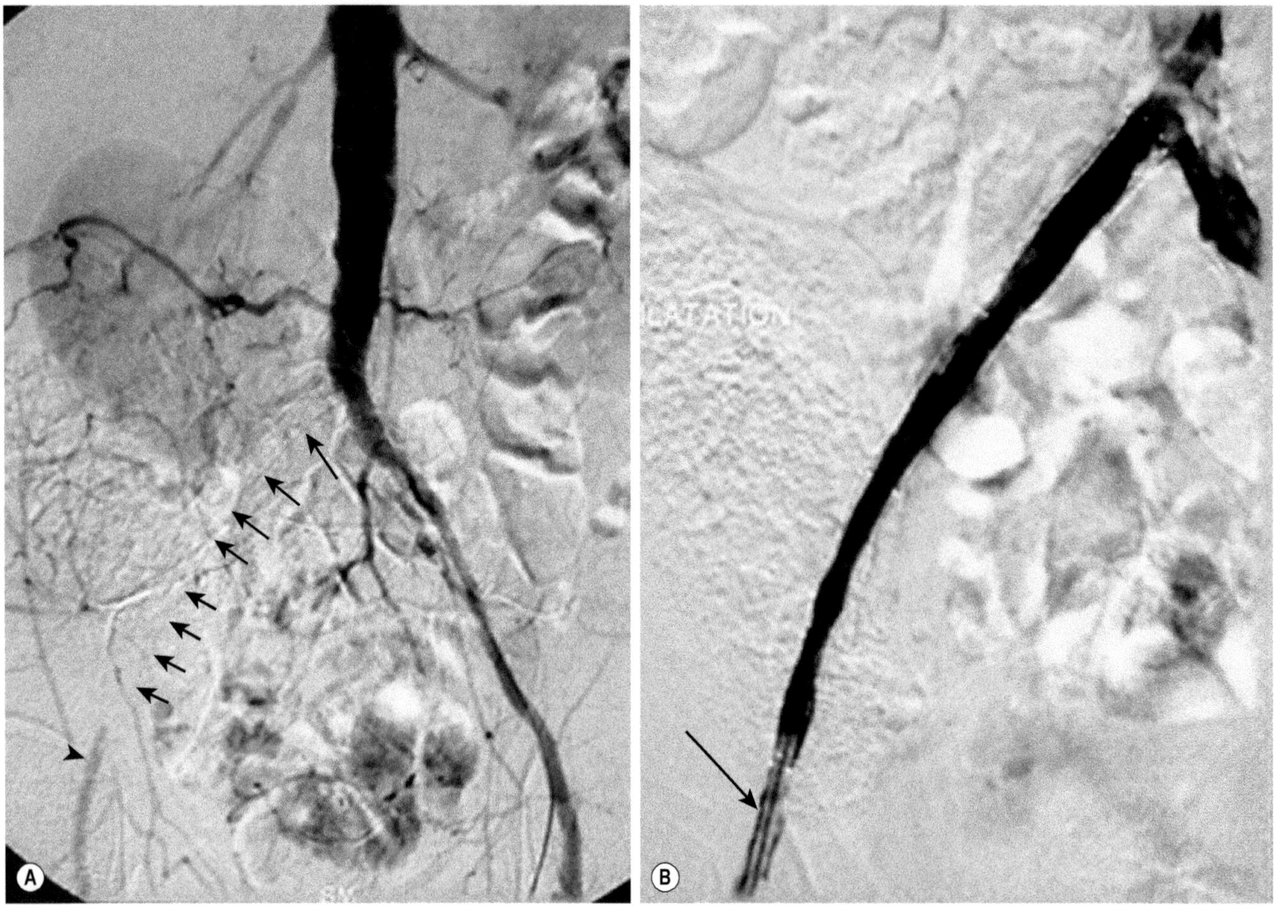

Fig. 24.3 (A) Occluded common iliac artery – patient with rest pain in the right foot. A previous right common iliac stent is now occluded, along with the external iliac artery (*arrows*). There is reconstitution of the common femoral artery distally (*arrowhead*). (B) Stenting the occlusion – the patient in (A) was considered a very poor risk for surgery, therefore the occlusion was successfully stented despite the fact that there was concern that the distal end of the stent would be very near the hip joint and might be damaged during hip flexion. There is a filling defect distally caused by the vascular sheath (*arrow*).

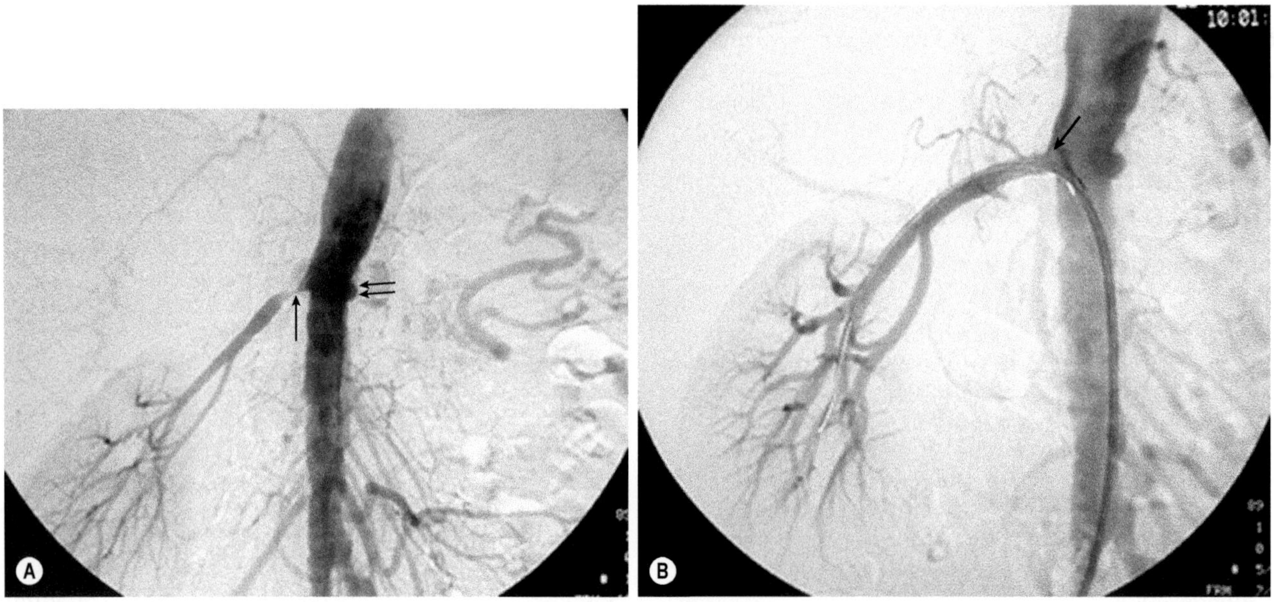

Fig. 24.4 (A) Renal artery stenosis – abdominal aortogram showing severe right renal artery stenosis (*arrow*) and an occluded left renal artery (*double arrow*). (B) Renal artery stent – the patient was experiencing episodes of flash pulmonary oedema and had deteriorating renal function; a right renal artery stent was inserted (*arrow*) with good technical and clinical results, with improvement in cardiac failure and greatly improved renal function.

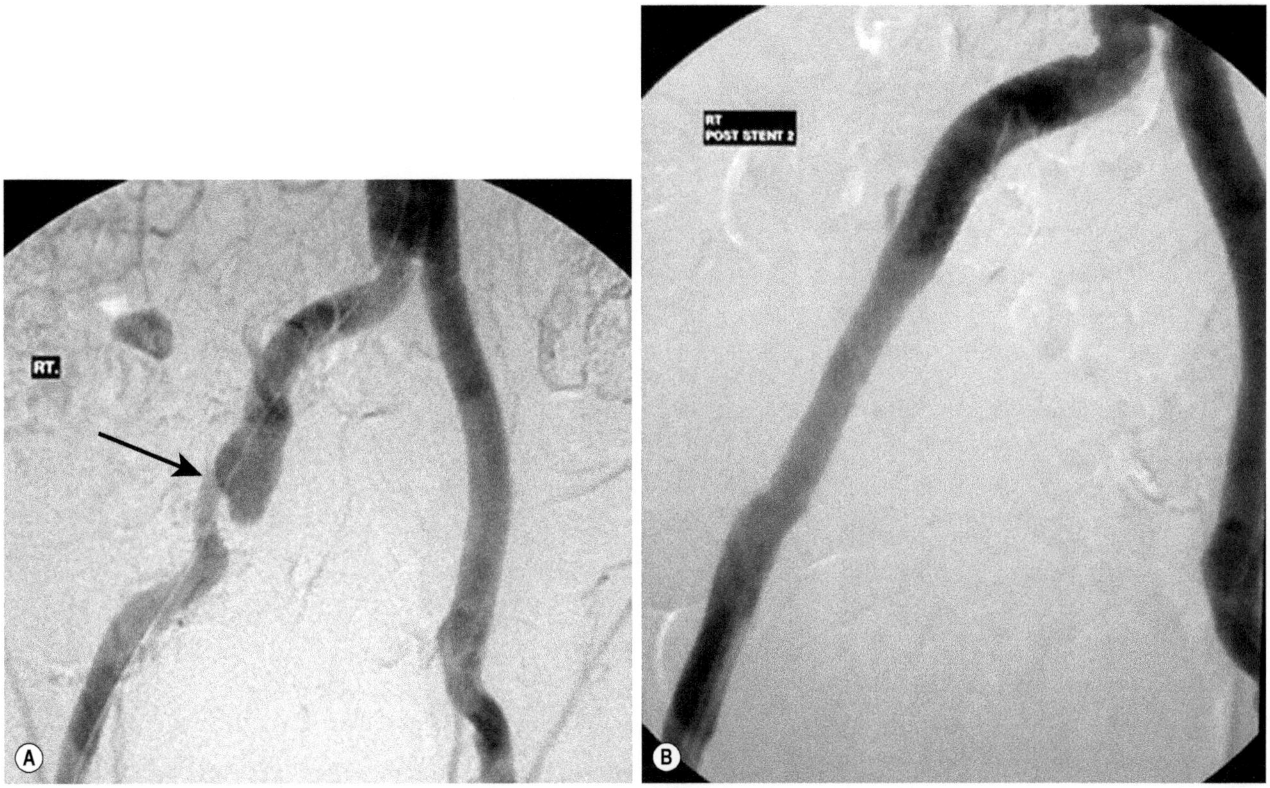

Fig. 24.5 (A) External iliac aneurysm – this arteriogram shows a 3 cm diameter external iliac aneurysm (*arrow*) arising at the distal end of an aorto-bi-iliac graft. (B) Treating the aneurysm with stent grafts – the aneurysm seen in (A) was successfully treated with two balloon expandable stent grafts.

there is some evidence to suggest that stent grafting may be of value in patients who would be at greater than average risk for abdominal surgery, for example if they have renal failure.[14–16] Randomised data have long shown a reduction in 30-day mortality when stent grafts are used for abdominal aortic aneurysm repair, compared to open surgery.[17,18]

When used for aortic aneurysms, stent graft delivery systems are large and require surgical exposure of one or both common femoral arteries. Smaller aneurysms, such as in the iliac arteries, can be treated without surgical exposure of vessels (Fig. 24.5A,B). Therefore, aortic stent graft procedures have frequently been performed in the operating theatre with a mobile image intensifier. A better alternative is to use an angiographic suite that has been constructed to operating theatre standards. This provides a sufficiently sterile environment with a high standard of imaging.

Prior to the stent graft procedure the aneurysm is assessed for the diameter of the proximal and distal landing zones, as well as the overall length of the device. A number of 'off the shelf' devices are available, and several manufacturers are able to supply custom-made stent grafts for more complex cases. The need for the latter has declined with time, although with the advent of branched devices there still may be a need for this.

Angiographic 'runs' are performed to ensure precise positioning of the device. For example, in stent grafting of abdominal aortic aneurysms it is clearly vital to avoid covering (and thereby occluding) the renal arteries with graft material. However, there are devices that have a bare stent at the proximal end which is designed to lie over the renal arteries. Once an image has been selected as the reference image for the deployment of the device it is vital that the C-arm is not moved. Even slight movement can cause errors due to parallax, which could cause misplacement of the stent graft.

EMBOLISATION

Commonly used embolisation agents include gelatin sponge (Fig. 24.6A–C) (for temporary embolisation), polyvinyl alcohol particles and coils (for permanent vessel occlusion). The full range of embolic materials available for clinical use is vast, complex and includes materials that would require a whole chapter to describe and explain in detail. Embolisation procedures are often complex and time-consuming, and may require the use of superselective coaxial catheter systems; multiple magnified views of the area are needed.

The basic principle of embolisation is to identify the target vessel and place the catheter tip in the correct location prior to introducing the embolic material. Generally one wishes to place the catheter as far distally as possible to avoid embolisation of normal tissue. In addition, when delivering particulate materials it is important to avoid reflux of emboli. It is important, therefore, to use continuous fluoroscopy when injecting such materials.

Some embolisation procedures are relatively simple, such as treatment of varicocoeles. Varicocoeles normally affect the left testis, and occur because the valve at the confluence of the left testicular and the renal vein is incompetent,

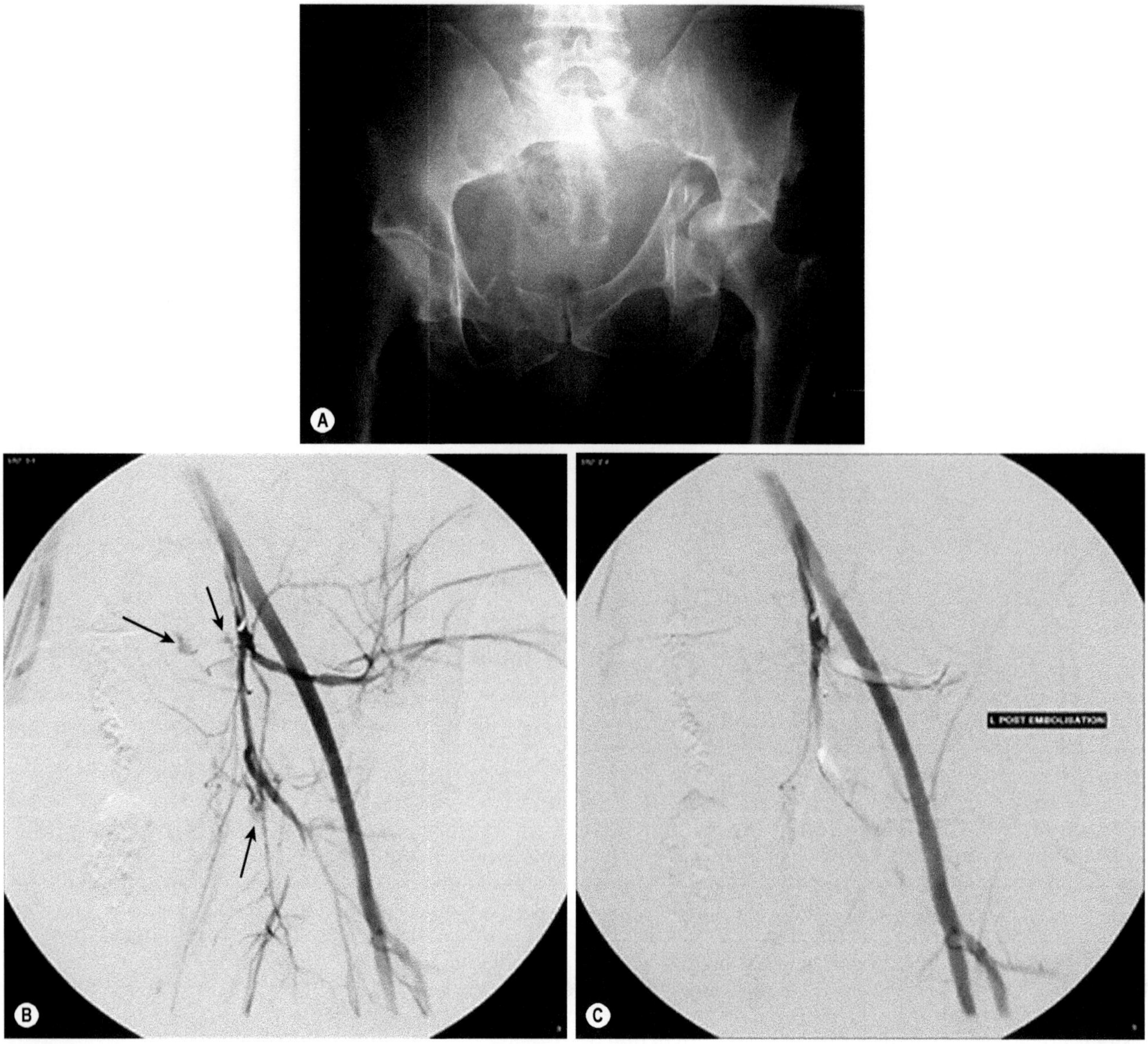

Fig. 24.6 (A) Plain radiographic image showing very obvious pelvic fracture involving the left acetabulum and the pubic rami on the right. Pelvic fractures can be associated with severe bleeding, as was the case here, and angiography with a view to embolisation was performed. (B) Iliac arteriogram after pelvic fracture – selective left internal iliac arteriogram showing at least three bleeding points (*arrows*) on the case seen in (A). Appearances were similar on the right side as well. (C) Embolisation after trauma to internal iliac artery – the case seen in (A) and (B) after embolisation with gelatin sponge; no further bleeding is seen.

allowing reflux of blood at systemic venous pressure into the venous drainage of the testis. Treatment involves embolisation of the left testicular vein. The procedure involves placing a catheter in the left renal vein and injecting contrast while screening, and also saving the fluoroscopic image. Once valve incompetence has been confirmed and the anatomy demonstrated, the testicular vein is entered and embolisation coils are placed along its length. Generally, patients requiring embolisation of the testicular vein are young, and it is clearly important to minimise radiation dose during this procedure.

Other procedures are more complex, such as embolisation for gastrointestinal bleeding (Fig. 24.7A–C), and require a more flexible approach to determine the precise anatomy and demonstrate the bleeding point accurately, followed by therapy. Highly complex situations, such as therapy for arteriovenous malformations, may be better referred to centres with a specialist interest in this area.

VENOUS INTERVENTIONS

Commonly undertaken venous interventions include placement of tunnelled venous lines and insertion of inferior vena cava (IVC) filters. Stents are also used in the venous system; however, the techniques used are very similar to those used in arteries, so it is not necessary to describe them in any greater detail.

Tunnelled Central Venous Lines

Tunnelled central venous lines are used for a variety of purposes, including administration of chemotherapy, total parenteral nutrition and temporary (and occasionally permanent) haemodialysis access. The line is tunnelled

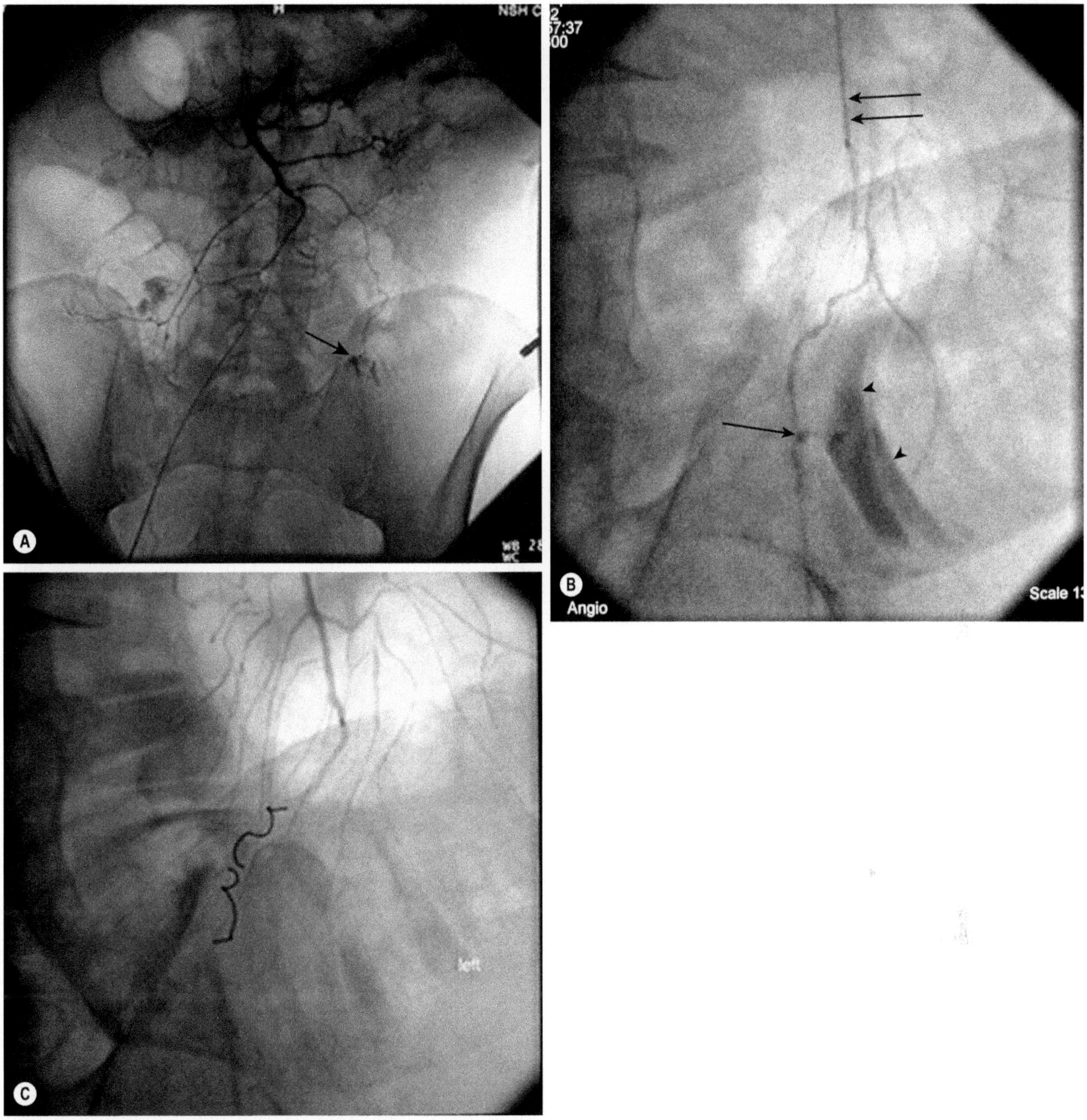

Fig. 24.7 (A) Mesenteric arteriogram – (without subtraction) showing a bleeding point in the distal ileum (*arrow*). There is also a calcified lymph node on the right side, which should not be confused with a bleeding point. (B) Superselective arteriogram – on the case seen in (A), using a microcatheter (*double arrow*) showing a bleeding point (*arrow*) which is allowing extravasation of contrast material into the bowel lumen (*arrowheads*). (C) Embolisation – the bleeding vessel seen in (A) and (B) was successfully embolised using two microcoils.

subcutaneously; near the point where the tunnel exits the skin the line has a Dacron cuff attached to it which becomes incorporated into the tissues, making accidental dislodgement much less likely than with non-tunnelled lines. There are also port systems available in which the entire device can be placed subcutaneously and be accessed percutaneously with a needle for drug administration.

The most commonly accessed vessels are probably the internal jugular veins, followed by the subclavian veins. On occasion, these vessels are occluded; this is particularly the case for patients who have had multiple central lines placed in the past, e.g. for haemodialysis. In these instances it may prove necessary to use alternative vessels, such as the external jugular vein, or even direct puncture of the IVC to provide venous access.

The best method of guiding the vessel puncture is US, which has the clear benefit of avoiding the use of ionising radiation and has been recommended by NICE for jugular vein puncture since 2002.[19] When performing subclavian vein puncture it is possible to opacify the target vein with contrast, and guide the puncture in this way. Fluoroscopy is used to identify the catheter tip when positioning it in the superior vena cava (SVC). The first choice of vein for puncture is the right internal jugular. This vein follows an almost straight course into the right brachiocephalic vein and subsequently the SVC, meaning that there is little potential for kinking of the introducer sheath during insertion. Use of the left internal jugular and subclavian veins is usually straightforward, whereas the use of the right subclavian vein can be difficult, as kinking of the introducer sheath can be a significant problem here.

The procedure is performed using local anaesthetic, often with light sedation. The target vein is punctured under imaging guidance, and the guide wire introduced; passage of the guide wire through the heart into the IVC confirms that a venous puncture has been achieved. A short incision is made at the puncture point, and a tunnel measuring approximately 6 cm long is formed on the anterior chest wall. A specific tunnelling device is used for the purpose, and the catheter is then drawn through the tunnel and inserted through a peel-away sheath into the vein (depending on the manufacturer there is some variation in the precise technique used, which is beyond the scope of this chapter). The catheter tip is visualised on fluoroscopy and positioned in the lower part of the SVC. By using image guidance for the insertion of tunnelled central venous catheters, complications should be minimised. For example, it has been known for many years that pneumothorax rates with image guided vein puncture are as low as 0%, compared to 5% with blind puncture.[20]

IVC Filters

IVC filters can be permanent or removable and are designed to prevent the passage of thrombus from the lower limbs into the pulmonary circulation, as prophylaxis against pulmonary embolism, which can be fatal. The standard treatment for deep vein thrombosis (DVT) is anticoagulation with heparin and subsequently oral anticoagulant therapy. IVC filters are therefore only used in certain situations, such as when anticoagulation is contraindicated, when pulmonary embolism has occurred despite adequate anticoagulation, and on occasion as prophylaxis against pulmonary embolism during surgery for pelvic trauma. However, the availability of removable filters in particular is changing practice; as clinicians become more familiar with these devices the indications for their use continue to evolve and expand.[21]

Many types of IVC filter are available, and insertion via the internal jugular or femoral routes is possible. A number of retrievable filters are available on the market. The principles of filter insertion are relatively simple. Access to the venous system is achieved and an inferior venacavagram is obtained to document the size of the IVC and the location of the renal veins. Assuming that the IVC is not of an abnormally large diameter, the filter is deployed below the level of the renal veins. Although it is occasionally necessary to deploy above the renal veins, this is to be avoided wherever possible so that in the event of IVC thrombosis the renal veins do not also become occluded.

IVC filters are effective at preventing pulmonary emboli[22] and have replaced the previous treatment of surgical ligation of the IVC. However, in the longer term IVC filters do not prevent recurrence of DVT. The complication rate of IVC filter insertion is low, but includes potential migration of the device, IVC thrombosis and IVC perforation. Therefore, wherever possible, removable IVC filters should be used and systems should be put in place to ensure that removal actually takes place if possible.

Future Developments and Current Impact of Interventional Vascular Procedures

These minimally invasive procedures have had a massive impact in the management of patients with vascular disease. For example, iliac angioplasty or stent insertion has now replaced surgery for many patients who require treatment for iliac artery disease. In addition, where open surgery is required, adjunctive angioplasty or stent insertion can be of great value in reducing the complexity of surgery undertaken. This chapter has necessarily concentrated on the better-established techniques or devices. However, there is constant development in the devices industry, and there is little doubt that solutions will be found for some of the problems encountered with current technology. Perhaps one of the best publicised examples is the continued development of drug eluting stents. The stent surface is coated with a drug that inhibits endothelial cell growth, preventing in-stent stenosis or occlusion by neointimal hyperplasia.[23,24]

Work is also progressing on the use of MRI for guidance when performing these procedures. Interventional MRI is becoming fairly well established in some areas, such as biopsy or image-guided surgery. However, the situation with vascular procedures is more complex, in that device movement needs to be monitored in real time. Work continues to be undertaken to allow catheter tracking to this end.[25]

Reflection on Endovascular Therapy

The evidence concerning the use of endovascular therapy in the management of intermittent claudication is fairly clear. However, in the management of critical limb ischaemia the issues are more complex. The argument that is frequently advanced is that attempting an endovascular procedure does not preclude the subsequent use of surgery, which is usually true. However, consumables for these procedures are relatively expensive and if, to take an extreme, they were rarely successful, endovascular therapy in this arena would be highly wasteful of resources. The evidence for their use is often conflicting. The patients being treated in the various studies are, of course, a heterogeneous group, and the endpoints used are often different, making direct comparisons between studies very difficult.

In the 'real world' endovascular therapy is used by many as the first line, with surgery being held in reserve. Surgery for critical limb ischaemia, which will usually involve some form of distal bypass, is complex and may not be possible if there is no good vein available for use as a graft. Furthermore, wounds from open surgery may become infected, which in an already compromised limb can be disastrous, especially if infection is due to a multiresistant organism. Surgery may also be relatively contraindicated if there is pre-existing infection in the limb secondary to ischaemia. If revascularisation fails, amputation will inevitably follow. Not only is this expensive in terms of resources for rehabilitation, but many patients never actually manage to use their prosthetic limb, and the mortality from amputation is also very high. Therefore, there is a need for pragmatism in this area. Even if patency rates from endovascular therapy for critical limb ischaemia are far from perfect, avoiding amputation can only be regarded as a good thing.

With regard to stent grafts, the picture is becoming clearer. There is no doubt that anatomically suitable thoracic aortic aneurysms should be treated by stent grafting, as the mortality and morbidity from open surgery is so high. With regard to the abdominal aorta, randomised trials showed reduced 30-day mortality compared to open surgery.[17] Confidence in the value of abdominal aortic stent grafts has increased, due to improved durability of devices which give better prospects for longer term outcomes.[18]

What of the future for conventional open vascular surgery? There has been much talk in the UK of the development of a single specialist with skills in both open and endovascular surgery. However, it has become apparent that the shortage of people wanting to enter both vascular surgery and interventional radiology requires that both groups of specialists remain at the present time. In addition, it is unlikely that there is sufficient time available in the training years to become competent in both. Elsewhere in Europe and the United States many vascular surgeons have adopted endovascular techniques. However, it is almost certainly true that individuals tend to concentrate on one or the other, as it is very difficult to remain highly skilled at both. For the foreseeable future there will be a continued need to use open surgical techniques, but as technology improves, endovascular therapy is likely to be used in ever-increasing numbers of patients.

Non-vascular Interventional Procedures or Therapies

This sphere of interventional radiology is often referred to as non-vascular interventional radiology and encompasses techniques in the gastrointestinal tract, liver and biliary system, the urogenital system, the musculoskeletal system and the airways. Before considering the interventional techniques used in specific systems, it is worth examining the subjects of biopsy and drainage, which are very commonly used techniques that do not fit within a systems categorisation as they are used in many organs and cavities.

IMAGE-GUIDED BIOPSY

This term refers to any procedure conducted under image guidance that yields tissue for histological or cytological examination. Although not strictly therapeutic, it is a common invasive procedure that is frequently a prerequisite to some form of therapy. Depending on the area biopsied the complications, although rare, can also be significant. The principles of fine needle aspiration (FNA), where cells are sampled with a narrow-gauge needle for cytological examination, and core biopsy, where a larger core of tissue is obtained for histological examination, are the same. However, if FNA is to be undertaken the diagnostic yield is greatly enhanced by a technician or cytologist being present at the time of biopsy to ensure that the sample is diagnostic. If that is not possible, experience shows that it is better, wherever feasible, to obtain a core of tissue for formal histological examination. This applies even in the lung, where one might imagine that a thinner needle would produce lower complication rates.

Biopsies are perhaps most commonly performed under either US or CT guidance. It is also possible, using non-ferromagnetic needles, to perform biopsies using interventional MRI scanners. The principles governing image-guided biopsies are very similar, with CT requiring additional considerations regarding the use of ionising radiation.

Having chosen the most suitable modality for performing a biopsy, and ensured that there are no contraindications such as abnormal blood clotting, the first decision concerns the position the patient should be placed in. This will be based on where the skin entry point needs to be, not only to allow the needle to follow the shortest path to the lesion, but also to avoid important structures such as vessels. Patient comfort and stability are important in ensuring safe execution of the procedure. Supine or prone positions are commonly used, having the advantage of being fairly stable, meaning that patient movement during the procedure is rarely a problem. Some older patients do have problems with lying prone for prolonged periods, especially if they have arthritis of their cervical spine, which may give neck pain during the procedure. Lying patients on their side may sometimes be necessary, and if so it is important that suitable support is provided to eliminate movement during the biopsy.

One must be cautious when performing a biopsy in a different position from that of the diagnostic imaging, as the relationships of various structures can be altered. A good example is when performing CT-guided adrenal gland biopsy. When a patient has a CT scan in the supine position the upper abdominal organs and diaphragm tend to fall backwards, obliterating much of the posterior costophrenic recess, giving an apparently straightforward path to the adrenal glands. However, the adrenal glands are in the retroperitoneum and it is necessary to perform a biopsy with the patient in the prone position. This causes the organs of the upper abdomen and the diaphragm to displace anteriorly, widening the posterior costophrenic recess and extending it caudally. In the majority of patients this means that aerated lung will now lie between the target adrenal gland and the nearest skin entry point. It is therefore necessary to insert the biopsy needle with a cranial angulation in order to travel upwards towards the adrenal gland while avoiding the lung. Use of CT fluoroscopy makes such manoeuvres more easily achievable as the needle can be viewed in real time.

In some situations there may be no immediately obvious path available. A good example is that of lesions in the chest positioned behind the heart. Clearly there is no path from the anterior chest wall, and trying to reach the lesion from a lateral approach would involve crossing a great deal of lung parenchyma, with the consequent risk of pneumothorax or even bleeding. It is possible to use a posterior approach by injecting normal saline paraspinally to produce a window through which the biopsy needle can pass. This avoids crossing lung parenchyma and any potential pneumothorax.

PERCUTANEOUS DRAINAGE PROCEDURES

A large number of drainage procedures are undertaken to treat abdominal or pelvic abscesses, as even in the antibiotic era, if pus is not drained from an abdominal or pelvic abscess cavity, the mortality rate remains high. Abdominal and pelvic abscesses may arise from a variety of causes, including as a complication of surgery, diverticular disease, Crohn's disease and pancreatitis. Pancreatitis may also cause pseudocysts in the pancreas itself, and abscesses may develop in the liver and occasionally the spleen. Drainage procedures are also increasingly being undertaken in the thorax, both for simple pleural effusions and for empyemas.

A variety of drains are available, varying from 6Fr (2 mm) to 16Fr (5.3 mm) in diameter. In general, the more viscous the material to be drained the wider the catheter required. If initial drainage with a catheter fails, it may be worth exchanging it for a larger one.

Drains can be inserted using US, CT, fluoroscopy or MRI for guidance. Clearly there are issues for MRI-guided procedures, related to the requirement to use non-ferrous materials.

The fluid collection or abscess is first identified via the chosen diagnostic imaging procedure and then the optimal position for intervention is decided upon in much the same way as for percutaneous biopsy. If a collection is relatively large and superficial it may be straightforward to insert a drain directly into it on a trocar, without the use of a guide wire. If this is to be done, it may be helpful to insert a narrow gauge Chiba needle first and check its position, to give an idea of the direction in which the larger drain needs to be inserted.

If the procedure is particularly complex it is often effective to insert an 18G Chiba needle under CT guidance and, having checked that the needle tip lies within the collection, insert a guide wire over which the drain can be inserted. There is less chance of kinking the guide wire if the procedure is visualised in real time, so CT fluoroscopy is again useful. If CT fluoroscopy is not available it may be advantageous, once the Chiba needle has been inserted, to move the patient into a fluoroscopy suite for guide wire insertion and drain introduction, but as long as the procedure is undertaken with extreme care, insertion of the guide wire and drain without fluoroscopy ought not to cause problems.

When draining pancreatic abscesses or pseudocysts, one must take particular care to prevent the formation of a fistula between the pancreas and the skin. This is best achieved by using a transgastric approach; thus if a fistula does form after drain removal, it will be between the pancreatic duct and the stomach, rather than the skin. Pancreatic secretions will therefore pass harmlessly into the stomach. Although it is possible to puncture the stomach under US guidance, the greater degree of confidence is given by using CT. Having entered the pseudocyst, a drain is inserted as for a normal collection. However, it should be noted that the fluid from pancreatic collections is often quite thick, and larger drains are often required.

Non-vascular Interventional Techniques: Gastrointestinal Tract

OESOPHAGUS

Interventional techniques in the oesophagus are most commonly used in the relief of obstruction which causes dysphagia, although treatment is sometimes required for oesophageal fistulae or perforations. Oesophageal obstruction may be due to benign causes such as peptic strictures caused by chronic reflux oesophagitis, achalasia, radiotherapy or ingestion of caustic substances. Alternatively, the cause may be malignancy, due to oesophageal carcinoma or extrinsic compression from malignant lymph nodes.

Oesophageal Dilatation

Oesophageal dilatation, when performed under fluoroscopy alone, is achieved using balloon dilators. It appears that many endoscopists are also switching to use balloons rather than bougies (a series of flexible dilators of increasing thickness). Dilatation alone is suitable only for treating benign lesions of the oesophagus (Fig. 24.8A,B), when dilatation is required owing to resection after surgery for malignancy, rather than due to the original malignancy; when used in an attempt to relieve malignant dysphagia the results are usually only very short-lived, and there is up to a 10% incidence of oesophageal perforation.

At the start of the procedure the patient is placed on the fluoroscopic table in the left lateral position. The throat is anaesthetised with xylocaine spray, and the patient is sedated. A suitable catheter and guide wire are used through a per oral approach to cross the stricture, and the catheter is exchanged for a balloon. The size of balloon used varies according to the type of lesion being treated. Thus fibrotic lesions such as those caused by radiotherapy or ingestion of caustic substances need to be treated initially with small angioplasty balloons, with diameters of 8–10 mm, as there is a high incidence of perforation. Over a number of treatments progressively larger balloons are used, with the aim of reaching a final diameter of 20 mm. Strictures resulting from chronic reflux oesophagitis can normally be treated with 20 mm balloons immediately, whereas in achalasia, where the aim is to tear muscle fibres, larger balloons of 30–40 mm in diameter are required.

It has long been recognised that technical success rates are around 95%.[26–28] These results are as good as if not better than those of bougienage, and avoid the morbidity and mortality associated with surgery. Stricture recurrence can be a problem, but up to 70% of patients remain asymptomatic at 2 years. Recurrent dysphagia can usually be successfully treated with repeat dilatation. The main potential complication of oesophageal dilatation is perforation. Overall, the perforation rate does appear to be very low, with some workers reporting no incidence of this; when taking consent from patients, quotation of a perforation rate of less than 1% can be supported.[25] However, there are important exceptions to this: for example, the perforation rate for dilatation of caustic strictures has been quoted as being as high as 25%. One would expect the situation to be similar for strictures induced by radiotherapy.

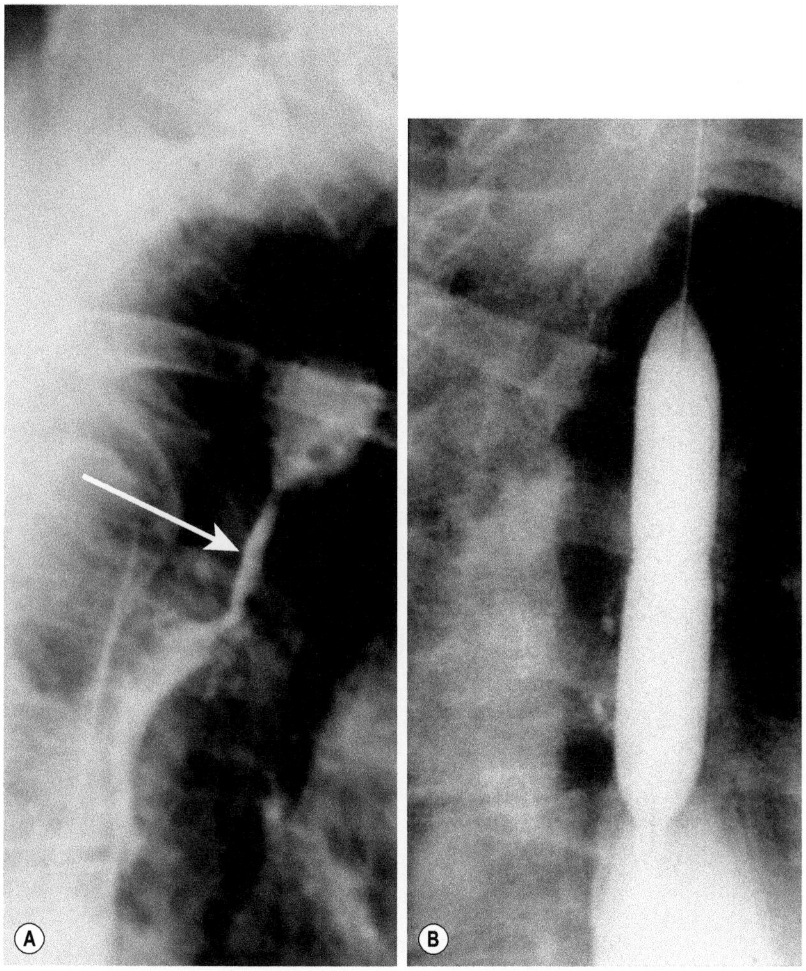

Fig. 24.8 (A) Stricture requiring oesophageal dilation – contrast swallow showing a tight stricture at the anastomosis between the upper oesophagus and a gastric pull-up after resection of an oesophageal carcinoma (*arrow*). (B) Oesophageal dilation – 20 mm oesophageal balloon fully inflated across the stricture.

Oesophageal Stent Insertion

At the time of presentation a significant proportion of patients with oesophageal carcinoma have lesions that are not amenable to surgical resection. However, they all have or will develop dysphagia that requires palliation. Available treatments include surgery, chemotherapy, radiotherapy, laser therapy, rigid plastic tubes and self-expanding metallic oesophageal stents. There is now wide experience in the use of oesophageal stents, and they form an important part of the palliation of malignant oesophageal obstruction.

The technique of insertion is very similar to that for oesophageal dilatation. However, once the stricture has been crossed with a guide wire it is pre-dilated to 15 mm in diameter. Using a balloon of a smaller diameter than the stent diminishes the risk of over-dilating the oesophagus, which would increase the risk of stent migration. Some practitioners do not dilate the oesophagus prior to deploying a stent; however, in some cases this may mean that the stent expands insufficiently to allow removal of the delivery system through it. Once the stent has been deployed the delivery system is removed and contrast medium injected to ensure patency and that there has been no perforation. After the patient has recovered from the sedation they are allowed initially to take sips of fluid, and over the next few hours to take increasing volumes.

The results of oesophageal stenting are generally good, improvement or complete relief of dysphagia in 83–100% of patients is well documented.[29–31] Complications include perforation, for which insertion of a covered stent is the treatment anyway; stent migration; pain; upper gastrointestinal haemorrhage; aspiration pneumonia and fistula formation. The results of stenting are known to be better than those reported for palliative surgery,[32] chemotherapy and radiotherapy,[33,34] in terms of both success in the relief of dysphagia and the complications encountered. Results of a randomised study have in addition shown stent insertion to be superior to the use of laser therapy.[35] Covered stents are also highly successful in sealing leaks and fistulae to the airways caused by malignant tumours[36] (Fig. 24.9A,B).

STOMACH AND DUODENUM

The two main interventional radiological procedures undertaken in this anatomical location are percutaneous gastrostomy and stent insertion. Balloon dilatation is occasionally undertaken for strictures involving surgical anastomoses or due to pyloric dysfunction after gastric pull-up operations performed for oesophageal carcinoma. However, such balloon dilatation differs little from that performed in the oesophagus, and will not be described in further detail here.

Percutaneous Gastrostomy

In many hospitals in the UK fluoroscopically guided gastrostomy insertion is only undertaken if the endoscopic

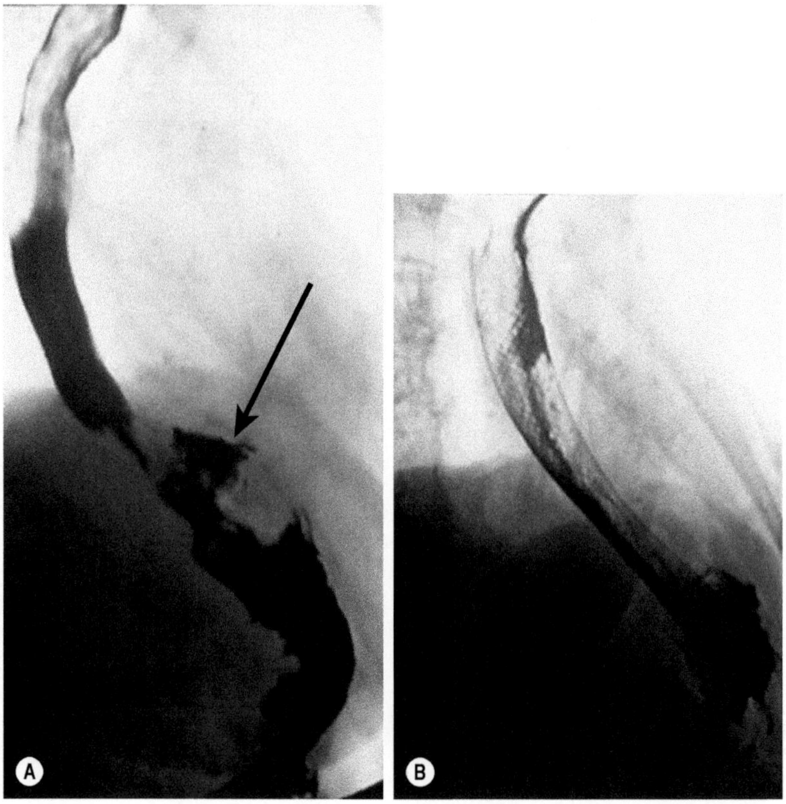

Fig. 24.9 (A) Oesophageal malignancy and endoscopic perforation – carcinoma of the oesophagogastric junction causing obstruction and associated with perforation after endoscopy (*arrow*). (B) Using a covered stent to treat a stricture and seal perforation – the stricture has been successfully treated and the perforation sealed with a covered oesophageal stent.

approach has failed. Gastrostomy is performed most commonly to provide enteral nutrition if there is an anatomical or functional difficulty in swallowing. It is also sometimes undertaken to decompress the stomach. Over the last few years fewer gastrostomies have been required in cases of oesophageal carcinoma because of the advent of oesophageal stents. One of the commonest reasons, if not the most common, for gastrostomy insertion is stroke causing swallowing difficulties.

Prior to gastrostomy a nasogastric tube needs to be inserted, preferably the day before, to drain gastric contents. A US scan is performed to identify the left lobe of the liver, and this is marked on the skin. In addition, some radiologists advocate the administration of barium the night before to opacify the transverse colon. Both of these are aimed at preventing inadvertent puncture of adjacent organs. The stomach is then fully inflated with air introduced via the nasogastric tube; this displaces the colon inferiorly and brings the anterior gastric wall as close as possible to the anterior abdominal wall. A suitable pathway to the stomach is identified under fluoroscopy and the skin is infiltrated with local anaesthetic. A needle is then passed into the stomach; either the stomach can be fixed to the anterior abdominal wall with 'T' fasteners, or a guide wire can be inserted, followed by proceeding directly to gastrostomy tube insertion.

Reports on the high technical success of the procedure (99–100%) are well established[37–39] Potential complications include reflux of the enteral feed into the oesophagus, with the risk of causing aspiration pneumonia. If such reflux occurs the gastrostomy can be converted to a gastrojejunostomy, which usually solves the problem. Further major complications of the procedure include severe bleeding, peritonitis and sepsis, and have been reported in 1.4–6.0% of cases. Minor complications include peritoneal irritation, local infection and tube migration or displacement.[37–39]

Gastric and Duodenal Stenting

In the stomach and duodenum stents are used in the management of strictures, which are usually caused by malignant tumours of the stomach or the pancreas. They are occasionally required for the treatment of pyloric dysfunction after gastric pull-up operations if balloon dilatation is unsuccessful.[40] Peptic strictures are becoming increasingly uncommon with improved treatment for peptic ulcer disease. Often insertion of gastric or duodenal stents for malignancy is only requested if patients are considered unfit for surgery. However, as experience grows, it would appear that stents are being used for these indications more commonly as an alternative to surgery in fit patients.

Stent procedures in the stomach and duodenum are technically more complex than those in the oesophagus. The reasons for this are that the large size and distensibility of the stomach allows space for loops of guide wire and catheter to form, and the fact that longer catheters and delivery systems are required, both making manipulation across strictures more difficult. For these reasons many workers advocate the use of endoscopy in conjunction with fluoroscopy; albeit not always required, endoscopic assistance can be very helpful in difficult cases.

Prior to the availability of dedicated stents, vascular wall stents were used (Fig. 24.10A,B), as the standard oesophageal stents were not available on a sufficiently long delivery system. However, there are now specific stents available for use in the stomach, duodenum and colon. The procedure is very similar to that for oesophageal stent insertion, apart from the different anatomical location, so it will not be described in any further detail. Success rates

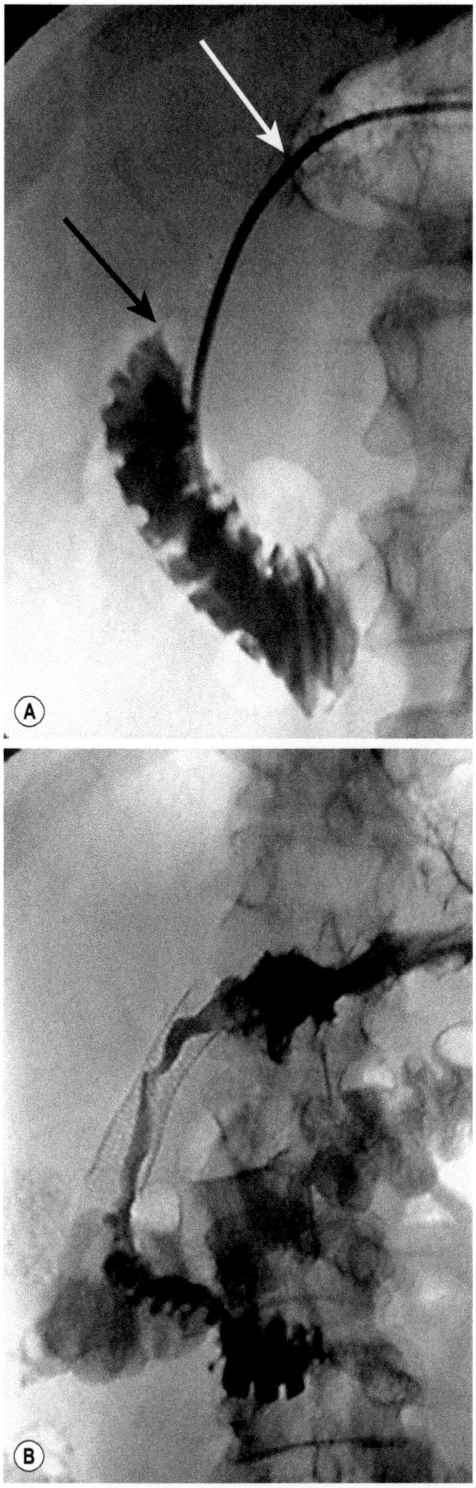

Fig. 24.10 (A) Gastric outlet obstruction – this patient had gastric outlet obstruction due to carcinoma of the pancreas. A catheter is positioned across the obstruction, the limits of which are defined by air in the stomach proximally and contrast in the duodenum distally (*arrows*). (B) Relieving gastric outlet obstruction – a contrast study performed on the day after stent deployment shows full stent expansion and complete relief of gastric outlet obstruction.

of 80–100% have been reported.[41–44] The only reported complication is aspiration of gastric contents into the airways, and this is infrequent. Although perforation of the stomach or the duodenum is a theoretical possibility it has not been reported.

COLON

Colonic Stents

Colonic stents were originally intended for temporary use in patients presenting with acute large bowel obstruction secondary to colonic carcinoma. This allows bowel preparation to be given and a primary bowel anastomosis to be formed at the time of tumour resection, rather than having to perform a defunctioning colostomy and return some weeks later to rejoin the bowel loops. However, more recently, colonic stents have been used as the sole treatment for obstruction for patients who will only receive palliative therapy. As such they are used not only in the management of unresectable colon tumours, but also in the management of other extensive pelvic tumours causing colonic obstruction.

A number of stents are available for use in the colon. The technique involves gaining access to the colon via a rectal approach and traversing the stricture with guide wire and catheter techniques (Fig. 24.11A,B). As the colon is tortuous and the haustra can make catheter and guide wire manipulation difficult, it may be helpful to use either a supporting sheath or a colonoscope to provide additional support. Once the stricture has been crossed the stent is deployed. Following deployment, balloon dilatation is occasionally required, though if possible this is to be avoided: rely instead on gradual stent expansion over 24 hours or so in order to minimise the risk of bowel perforation.

Around 70% of colonic carcinomas are on the left side of the large bowel. Clinical success rates of 64–100% are reported, with right-sided lesions being much more difficult to reach and treat.[45–47] In addition, cost reductions of around 28% were reported when using stents rather than the conventional approach of defunctioning colostomy. Complications of colonic perforation, stent displacement and obstruction have been reported. More minor complications include rectal bleeding, tenesmus, transient anorectal pain and fecal impaction.[45–47]

Non-vascular Interventional Techniques: The Biliary Tree

It should be noted that the majority of interventions in the biliary tree are undertaken at the time of endoscopic retrograde cholangiopancreatography (ERCP). However, if ERCP fails for any reason the percutaneous approach to the biliary tree is required. The most common procedure undertaken by interventionists in the biliary tree is stent insertion. Biliary drainage is also frequently carried out, usually prior to stenting, and there is occasionally a call to dilate benign biliary strictures. Biliary drainage will be described first, as access to the biliary tree is an essential component of all of these procedures.

Indications for intervention in the biliary tree include palliation of unresectable primary or metastatic malignancy, benign biliary strictures, sepsis accompanying biliary obstruction and preoperative decompression. ERCP is also frequently used in the treatment of calculi in the bile ducts, and percutaneous biliary intervention may be required where the bile ducts have been opacified at ERCP but it has not been possible to secure drainage with a stent; if obstructed bile ducts are left undrained in this situation there is a significant risk of cholangitis.

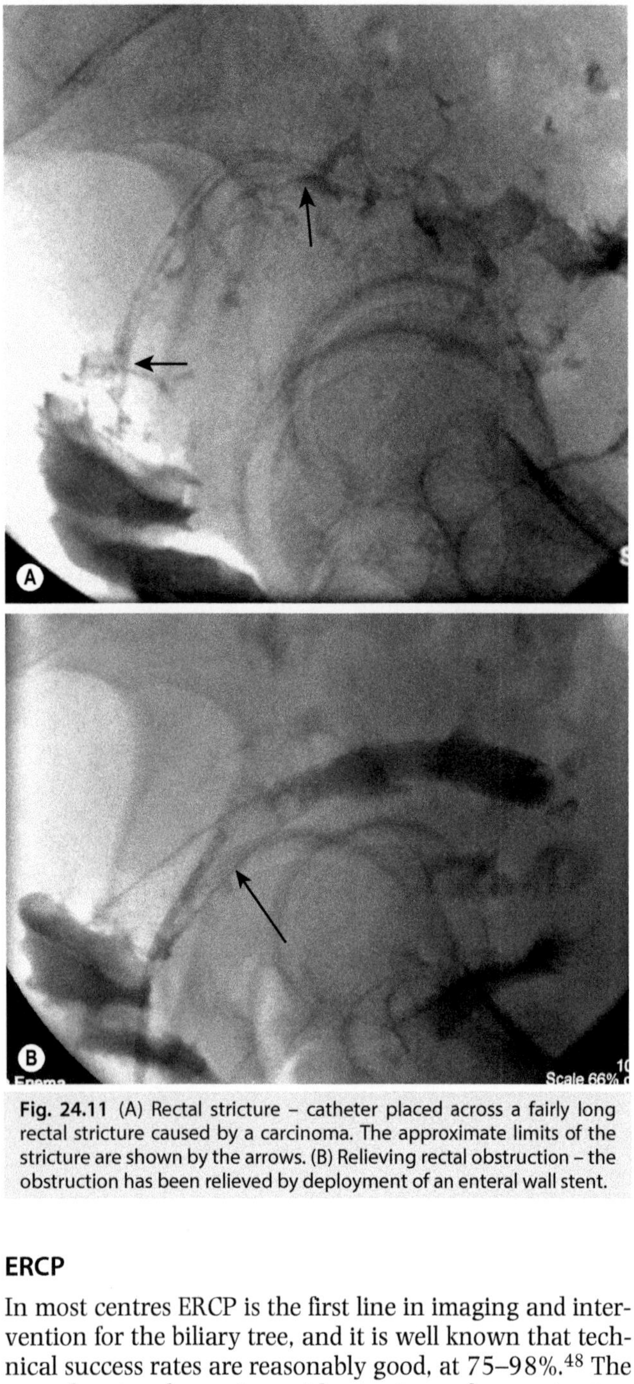

Fig. 24.11 (A) Rectal stricture – catheter placed across a fairly long rectal stricture caused by a carcinoma. The approximate limits of the stricture are shown by the arrows. (B) Relieving rectal obstruction – the obstruction has been relieved by deployment of an enteral wall stent.

ERCP

In most centres ERCP is the first line in imaging and intervention for the biliary tree, and it is well known that technical success rates are reasonably good, at 75–98%.[48] The procedure involves using a side-viewing endoscope to visualise and then cannulate the ampulla of Vater in the second part of the duodenum. Contrast is then injected through the cannula, and the biliary tree and pancreatic duct are opacified. Having made a diagnosis, appropriate therapy can often be delivered at the same sitting. Thus, in cases of obstruction a sphincterotomy is first performed; essentially this involves making a cut at the lower end of the common bile duct to allow instruments to pass. If obstruction is being caused by gallstones in the common bile duct, sphincterotomy alone occasionally allows a stone to drop out of the duct; more frequently it proves necessary to trawl the duct with baskets or balloons to extract the calculi. If there is a benign biliary stricture this can be balloon dilated, whereas malignant strictures require stent insertion.

ERCP is also of value if the biliary tree is not dilated. One example of this is in patients who have experienced bile duct trauma at the time of laparoscopic cholecystectomy and have a resultant biliary leak. Placement of a plastic biliary stent for around 6 weeks to divert the flow of bile away from the area of leakage into the duodenum will usually result in sealing of the leak. After 6 weeks the stent can be removed.

A further example is that of primary biliary sclerosis, where there is widespread narrowing of bile ducts. In this situation it is sometimes possible to identify a 'dominant stricture' that can be dilated, with the relief of some or all of the patient's symptoms.

Potential complications of ERCP include death, sepsis, haemorrhage and bile leak. If ERCP is not possible, for example due to previous partial gastrectomy or duodenal stenosis, or if it fails for some other reason, then percutaneous biliary intervention can be attempted. In addition, there are strong arguments for using percutaneous biliary intervention as the primary mode of palliation for malignant hilar strictures, i.e. proximal lesions that involve one or more of the common hepatic duct or right or left hepatic ducts.[49]

Percutaneous Biliary Drainage

The first step in any percutaneous biliary tract intervention is to gain access to the bile ducts. This is done by first performing a percutaneous transhepatic cholangiogram (PTC). Having ensured that the blood clotting is normal and prophylactic antibiotics have been administered, the patient is placed on the X-ray table in the supine position with their right arm raised above their head. The right upper quadrant is imaged by fluoroscopy and a suitable point for skin puncture is selected. Local anaesthetic is administered along with intravenous sedation and/or analgesia. A thin (22 or 21G) Chiba needle is advanced into the liver and then gradually withdrawn while contrast is gently injected. Several passes of the Chiba needle may be required in order to access a bile duct, although if the biliary tree is dilated it is rare to fail.

Once the bile ducts have been opacified a suitable guide wire is inserted through the Chiba needle. Occasionally it proves necessary to reposition the needle prior to guide wire insertion. The Chiba needle is exchanged for a coaxial dilator system, allowing insertion of a larger and stiffer guide wire. If biliary drainage alone is to be performed, it is possible at this stage to insert a pigtail drainage catheter over the guide wire into the bile duct, to provide external drainage of bile; this option may be chosen, for example, if there is cholangitis that requires treatment before definitive therapy.

If it is possible to pass the guide wire through the ampulla of Vater, it is possible to use an internal/external biliary drain. This device has drainage holes along a greater length than the standard external drainage catheter such that, when positioned with the pigtail in the duodenum, drainage holes lie above and below the papilla. This allows much of the bile to drain internally, while retaining access to the biliary tree for future intervention. Internal/external biliary drains tend to be more secure, and can be useful for providing internal drainage while making decisions regarding management.

Biliary Stenting

Both plastic and metallic stents are available for relief of biliary obstruction. At ERCP the vast majority of stents used are plastic, as they are relatively cheap. However, because they are much smaller in diameter than metallic stents they have a much greater tendency to block. There is evidence that, when stents are being used for the palliation of malignant biliary strictures, metallic stents are in fact more cost-effective than plastic devices because of the lower reintervention rate.[50,51]

When placing stents percutaneously, some consideration needs to be given to the size of the device being placed across the liver parenchyma. At 12Fr in diameter the plastic stents placed at ERCP are considered by many operators to be too large to be inserted through the liver, so many percutaneously placed stents are only 10Fr in diameter, with a consequent reduction in lumen size. It is advantageous to use self-expanding metallic stents percutaneously (Fig. 24.12A,B): these not only have the advantage of a small delivery system (6Fr), they also provide a much larger lumen (up to 10 mm, or the equivalent of 30Fr).

The other factor in deciding whether to use a metallic or plastic stent is the cause of the biliary stricture. If metallic stents are used in benign strictures, for example those caused by chronic pancreatitis, most will occlude over a period of months owing to the overgrowth of epithelial cells through the stent mesh. As a result, one can face great difficulties in management, and it is better where at all possible to manage such patients by ERCP and regular elective stent changes. In malignant biliary strictures the reduced reintervention rate and delivery system size associated with metallic stents makes a compelling case for their use.

Dilatation of Benign Biliary Strictures

There is a wide variety of potential causes for benign biliary strictures. However, in the Western world the majority are iatrogenic, either as a result of trauma to the bile ducts at the time of laparoscopic cholecystectomy or occurring at anastomoses formed between the small bowel and the biliary tree, either at the time of liver transplantation or at biliary bypass for the management of biliary strictures or surgery for pancreatic carcinoma. Benign biliary strictures may also be caused by chronic infection associated with bile duct calculi.

Decision-making and management in this patient group can be complex, and requires a multidisciplinary approach. Even relatively mild strictures can cause stone formation, cholangitis and cirrhosis. Surgery has traditionally been used, but ERCP is now much more important in the management of such patients, and good long-term results with plastic stents and repeated stent changes have been reported.[52,53] Where ERCP is not possible, perhaps because of previous surgery, percutaneous treatment may be required. Plastic stents are frequently used, and balloon dilatation of strictures is reported as being very successful. However, several treatments may be required in order to achieve a satisfactory result; if percutaneous therapy is to be used this will require long-term placement of a biliary drain, which is inconvenient for the patient.[54]

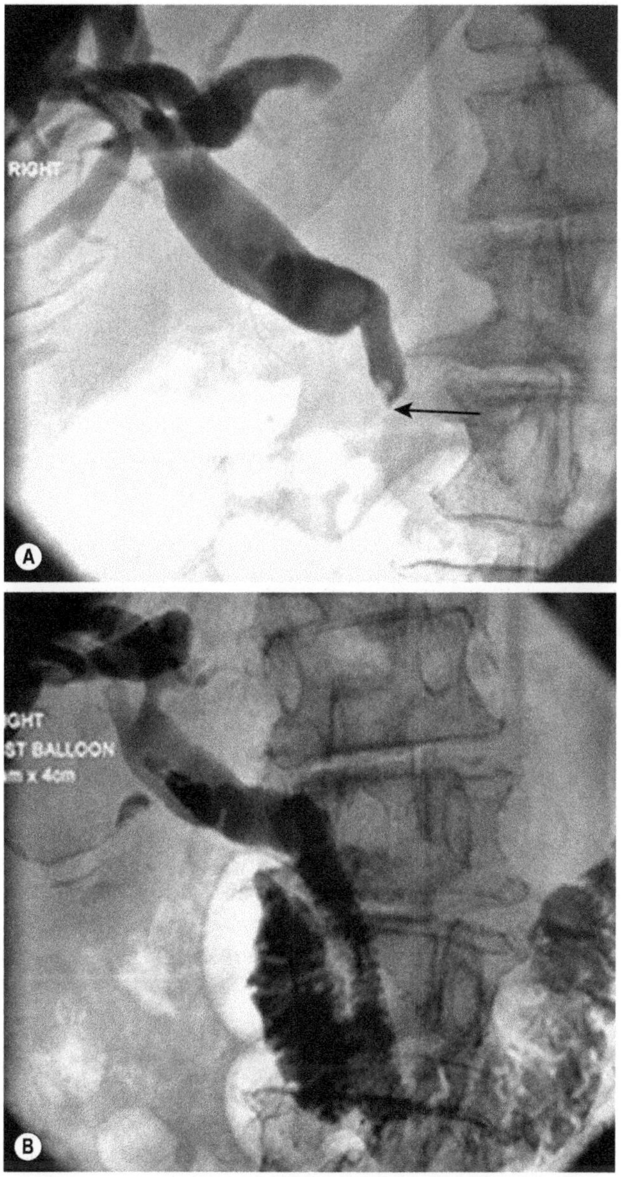

Fig. 24.12 (A) Obstructed common bile duct – cholangiogram performed via catheter positioned in the biliary tree. Complete obstruction of the distal common bile duct has been demonstrated (*arrow*). (B) Stenting bile duct obstruction – the obstruction has been relieved by the deployment of a 10 mm diameter self-expanding metallic stent.

Non-vascular Interventional Techniques: Urogenital Tract

The most widely undertaken procedure in the urogenital tract is percutaneous nephrostomy. Having gained access to the urinary tract it is also possible to introduce ureteric stents to relieve obstruction and use balloons to dilate strictures. Percutaneous nephrolithotomy (PCNL) is also used in the treatment of renal calculi. In recent years, increasing numbers of uterine artery embolisations (UAEs) have been performed for the treatment of uterine fibroids.

Percutaneous Nephrostomy

Percutaneous nephrostomy is usually performed to relieve urinary tract obstruction. An alternative approach is to place retrograde ureteric double 'J' stents cystoscopically. However, nephrostomy has advantages in certain situations, such as malignant obstruction and if infection is present (pyonephrosis).

The procedure itself can be carried out using either fluoroscopy or US alone or a combination of the two, which may ensure more confidence. The patient is placed prone on the fluoroscopy table with the side to be treated slightly elevated. A US scan is performed to identify the hydronephrotic kidney; it is usually possible to identify calyces and to select one for puncture. Wherever possible one aims to puncture a posterior lower pole calyx, as the arrangement of intrarenal vessels at this site means that the risk of bleeding complications is less with this approach. The skin and deep tissues are infiltrated with local anaesthetic and intravenous sedation and/or analgesia is administered. A suitable needle is then introduced into the collecting system under US guidance.

After the collecting system has been successfully punctured a stiff or superstiff guide wire is introduced; if at all possible the guide wire is directed down the ureter to give the most secure position. It is impossible to see this reliably on US and it is best visualised on fluoroscopy, hence the combined US and fluoroscopic method is most often preferred. Once the operator is satisfied with the guide wire position a suitable nephrostomy catheter (typically 8Fr in diameter) is introduced, fixed to the skin and attached to a drainage bag.

If the cause of the obstruction is self-limiting, such as a small ureteric calculus, the nephrostomy may only be required for a few days and then removed. Similarly, it may be removed after definitive treatment such as ureteroscopy and stone removal has been carried out. In other situations further intervention may be required, either at the same time as nephrostomy insertion or on another occasion. This will be discussed in the following sections.

Minor complications requiring no additional therapy are fairly common, and virtually every patient will develop transient mild haematuria. Severe bleeding necessitating transfusion or other intervention is reported as occurring in 1–3% of cases.[55]

Ureteric Stent Insertion

Ureteric obstruction may arise from a variety of causes. Antegrade stenting via a nephrostomy track is only rarely required for temporary causes such as calculi. However, causes such as strictures or obstruction caused by malignancy or radiotherapy can rarely be stented retrogradely, and antegrade ureteric stenting is of immense value in this patient group.[56,57]

The stents used have a pigtail shape at either end and are made of plastic. They need to be changed every few months, although this does not require repeat nephrostomy; once the obstruction has been crossed it is almost always possible to change stents retrogradely.

The principles behind antegrade ureteric stenting are relatively simple. Having gained access to the upper urinary tract by performing a nephrostomy, an angiographic catheter and guide wire are manipulated into the ureter and through the obstruction. The guide wire is exchanged for a stiff guide wire and a suitable size of stent is introduced over it. In order to achieve a suitable angle for stent insertion it may prove necessary to gain access via middle or even upper pole calyx, as attempting to push the stent forwards from a lower pole puncture can lead to a loop forming in the proximal guide wire, which is then pushed into the upper pole region. If stenting from a lower pole puncture, a peel-away sheath advanced into the proximal ureter will normally remedy this problem without having to resort to a further puncture.

Balloon Dilatation of Ureteric Strictures

Benign strictures in the native ureters may occur for a variety of reasons, including calculus disease, radiotherapy and surgical trauma. In renal transplants, ureteric strictures may be due to periureteric fibrosis, anastomotic fibrosis or ischaemia. Diffuse strictures caused by chronic rejection or necrosis cannot be successfully dilated with balloons.

The procedure is identical in many respects to that of ureteric stent insertion, except for the fact that a high-pressure balloon is placed across the stricture and dilated, followed by insertion of a stent. The stent is then removed some weeks later. Good long-term results can be anticipated in up to 50% of benign ureteric strictures.[58]

Percutaneous Nephrolithotomy (PCNL)

PCNL was developed in the mid-1970s and, as it became accepted, largely replaced open surgery for urinary tract stones. Despite the subsequent development of extracorporeal shockwave lithotripsy and ureteroscopic techniques, PCNL is still regularly used for the management of urinary tract stone disease.

PCNL may be carried out either in the operating theatre with a mobile image intensifier, or in the radiology department; in either instance the patient is placed under general anaesthesia. It is important to establish which calyces contain stones on preoperative imaging; the appropriate calyx for puncture is then selected. Initially the urologist performs a cystoscopy and passes a ureteric catheter into the proximal ureter. The patient is then turned prone, and the collecting system is opacified with contrast medium injected through the ureteric catheter. The chosen calyx is then punctured and a guide wire introduced and placed in the ureter.

A peel-away sheath is introduced over the guide wire, which allows the insertion of a second super-stiff guide wire. This provides two guide wires, one for dilating the track and the other as a safety guide to prevent access being lost. The track is dilated to 30Fr in diameter using either coaxial metal dilators or a balloon system, followed by insertion of a 30Fr working sheath. This allows the introduction of a nephroscope, baskets and mechanical lithotripters for the breaking up and removal of calculi. This part of the procedure is undertaken by urologists, so teamwork is very important.

After successful stone removal the working sheath is removed and a large nephrostomy tube left in situ for 1–2 days. Success rates for stone removal are high. The mortality rate for such large-bore access to the urinary tract is low (less than 0.3%).[59] Significant bleeding is more likely than with smaller-bore tubes, but can usually be managed by inserting a balloon dilatation catheter into the track to provide tamponade. If tamponade over a few days fails, angiography and embolisation may be needed.

Uterine Artery Embolisation (UAE) for Fibroids

Embolisation in general has been described earlier in this chapter. However, UAE for fibroids merits special consideration under genitourinary therapies.

The technique was first described in the mid-1990s and was taken up enthusiastically by many radiologists and patients alike. It is attractive as an alternative to hysterectomy as it is a day-case procedure, whereas hysterectomy is a major surgical procedure with a prolonged period of recovery often required. There are other clear resource benefits, such as a reduction in hospital bed and nursing care requirements compared to hysterectomy.

The technique involves selective catheterisation of both uterine arteries and embolisation is achieved using polyvinyl alcohol particles. A tightly collimated beam should be used, and where pulsed fluoroscopy is used the slowest pulse rate compatible with adequate visualisation should be employed. If at all possible, formal angiographic runs should be avoided, but where these are necessary they should be kept as short as possible. This is because the patients who undergo this examination are relatively young women, and one wishes to minimise the radiation dose to the pelvis.

Initial reports regarding UAE were very enthusiastic, claiming few if any complications and great success both for reducing the size of the fibroids themselves and in treating the associated symptoms. However, as experience with the technique has grown it has become apparent that it is not without complications. All patients experience pelvic pain of varying severity after the procedure, and many professionals advocate patient-controlled analgesia in the post procedure period to counter this. Perhaps the most worrying, though thankfully relatively uncommon, complication is sepsis. Although deaths are reported they are rare, and it should not be forgotten that hysterectomy has a significant morbidity and mortality. Randomised data indicated that the two treatments have similar outcomes,[60,61] so there is a strong case for patient choice, in the light of the available evidence, determining which treatment is used.

Reflection on Intervention and Therapies

This chapter illustrates the immense breadth of procedures undertaken by interventional radiologists today. Although there is much commonality between the techniques used, for example the use of catheter and guide wire manipulation, ever-increasing amounts of clinical knowledge are required for the safe application of these techniques. As a result, there has in many cases been a tendency for individuals to subspecialise further within interventional radiology, for example to concentrate on vascular radiology alone. In some cases organ specialists undertake the interventional procedures relevant to them. A good example of this is in musculoskeletal radiology, where specialists often undertake bone biopsy and even vertebroplasty; there is insufficient space to describe all of the available techniques in this chapter, hence their omission.

Another issue facing interventional radiologists is that as techniques become more complex, the clinicians looking after the patient will have less knowledge of them, making subsequent patient care more difficult. This is especially the case where junior staff care for a patient on the ward after the procedure.

There is thus a strong case for greater clinical involvement of interventional radiologists by performing ward rounds and maybe even outpatient clinics, both to assess patients prior to treatment and to follow them up afterwards. Such clinical involvement should also allow for improved quality of patient consent, given the direct communication with the expert in the interventional procedure, rather than a representative from a different specialist area. Although some might argue that this would be appropriate, the unique knowledge of imaging that is brought to these procedures by interventional radiologists should improve the quality of their conduct, although this would be difficult to measure.

References

1. Van Andel G, et al. Percutaneous transluminal dilatation of the iliac artery: long term results. *Radiology*. 1985;156:321–323.
2. Wolfe GL, et al. Surgery or PTA for peripheral vascular disease; a randomised controlled trial. *J Vasc Intervent Radiol*. 1993;4:639–648.
3. Ballard J. Aortoiliac stent deployment vs. surgical reconstruction. *J Vasc Surg*. 1998;28:94–103.
4. Lofberg A-M, et al. Percutaneous transluminal angioplasty of the femoropopliteal arteries in limbs with chronic critical lower limb ischaemia. *J Vasc Surg*. 2001;34:114–121.
5. Shaw M, et al. The results of subintimal angioplasty in a district general hospital. *Eur J Vasc Endovasc Surg*. 2002;24:524–527.
6. Perkins J, et al. Exercise training versus angioplasty for stable claudication: long and medium term results of a prospective, randomized trial. *Eur J Vasc Endovasc Surg*. 1996;11:409–413.
7. Whyman M, et al. Is intermittent claudication improved by percutaneous transluminal angioplasty? *J Vasc Surg*. 1997;26:551–557.
8. Brown K, et al. Infrapopliteal angioplasty: long term follow-up. *J Vasc Intervent Radiol*. 1993;4:139–144.
9. Tadros RO, Vouyouka AG, Ting W, Teodorescu V, Kim SY, et al. A Review of Superficial Femoral Artery Angioplasty and Stenting. *J Vasc Med Surg*. 2015;3:183.
10. Tetterooe E, et al. Randomised comparison of primary stent insertion versus primary angioplasty and selective stent insertion in iliac artery occlusive disease. *Lancet*. 1998;351:1153–1159.
11. Bosch J, Hunink M. Meta analysis of the results of PTA and stent placement in aortoiliac occlusive disease. *Radiology*. 1997;204:87–96.
12. Van de Ven P, et al. Arterial stenting and balloon angioplasty in ostial atherosclerotic renovascular disease: a randomised trial. *Lancet*. 1999;353(9149):282–286.
13. Reidy J, Taylor P. The use of stent grafts in thoracic aortic disease. *Cardiovasc Intervent Radiol*. 2000;23:249–251.
14. Faries P, et al. A multicentre experience with the Talent endovascular graft for the treatment of abdominal aortic aneurysms. *J Vasc Surg*. 2002;35:1123–1128.
15. The Vascular Surgical Society of Great Britain and Ireland and the British Society of Interventional Radiology. *Fifth Report on the Registry for Endovascular Treatment of Aneurysms*; 2001.
16. Katz D, et al. Operative mortality rates for intact and ruptured abdominal aortic aneurysms. An eleven year state wide experience. *J Vasc Surg*. 1994;19:804–817.
17. EVAR Trial Participants. Endovascular aneurysm repair versus open repair in patients with abdominal aortic aneurysm (EVAR trial 1): randomised controlled trial. *Lancet*. 2005;365:2179–2186.
18. Barleben A, Mathlouthi A, Mehta M, Nolte T, Valdes F, Malas MB. Ovation trial investigators, Long-term outcomes of the Ovation Stent Graft System investigational device exemption trial for endovascular abdominal aortic aneurysm repair. *J Vasc Surg*. 2020;72(5):1667–1673.
19. NICE (National Institute for Health and Clinical Excellence). *Guidance on the Use of Ultrasound Locating Devices for Placing central Venous Catheters*. Technology appraisal guidance [TA49]; 2002. https://www.nice.org.uk/guidance/TA49.
20. Lameris J, et al. Percutaneous placement of Hickman catheters: comparison of sonographic guided and blind techniques. *AJR Am J Roentgenol*. 1990;155:1097–1099.

21. DeYoung E, Minocha J. Inferior Vena Cava Filters: Guidelines, Best Practice, and Expanding Indications. *Semin Intervent Radiol.* 2016;33(2):65–70.
22. Decousus H, et al. A clinical trial of vena caval filters in the prevention of pulmonary embolism in patients with proximal deep vein thrombosis. *N Engl J Med.* 1998;338:409–416.
23. Senst B, et al. Drug Eluting Stent Compounds. 2020. Statpearls. https://pubmed.ncbi.nlm.nih.gov/30726034/.
24. Sousa J, et al. Two year angiographic and ultrasound follow-up after implantation of Sirolimus-eluting stents in human coronary arteries. *Circulation.* 2003;107:381–383.
25. Heidt T, et al. Real-time magnetic resonance imaging - guided coronary intervention in a porcine model. *Sci Rep.* 2019;9(1):18282.
26. McLean G, et al. Radiologically guided balloon dilatation of gastrointestinal strictures. *Radiology.* 1987;165:35–43.
27. Starcke E, et al. Esophageal stenosis: treatment with balloon catheters. *Radiology.* 1984;153:637–640.
28. Sabharwal T, et al. Balloon dilation for achalasia of the cardia: experience in 76 patients. *Radiology.* 2002;224:719–724.
29. Cowling M, et al. The use of self-expanding metallic stents in the management of malignant oesophageal strictures. *Br J Surg.* 1998;85:264–266.
30. Cwiekiel W, et al. Malignant esophageal strictures: treatment with a self expanding nitinol stent. *Radiology.* 1993;187:661–665.
31. Saxon R, et al. Treatment of malignant esophageal obstructions with covered metallic Z stents: long term results in 52 patients. *J Vasc Intervent Radiol.* 1995;6:747–754.
32. Earlam R, Chunha-Melo J. Oesophageal squamous cell carcinoma: 1. A critical review of surgery. *Br J Surg.* 1980;67:381–390.
33. Earlam R, Chunha-Melo J. Oesophageal squamous cell carcinoma: 2. A critical review of radiotherapy. *Br J Surg.* 1980;67:457–461.
34. Herskovic A, et al. Combined chemotherapy and radiotherapy compared to radiotherapy alone in patients with cancer of the oesophagus. *N Engl J Med.* 1992;326:1593–1598.
35. Adam A, et al. Palliation of inoperable esophageal carcinoma: a prospective randomized trial of laser therapy and stent placement. *Radiology.* 1997;202:344–348.
36. Morgan R, et al. Malignant esophageal fistulas and perforation: management with plastic-covered metallic endoprostheses. *Radiology.* 1997;204:527–532.
37. Hicks M, et al. Fluoroscopically guided percutaneous gastrostomy: analysis of 158 consecutive cases. *AJR Am J Roentgenol.* 1990;154:725–728.
38. Wills J. Percutaneous gastrostomy: applications in gastric carcinoma and gastroplasty stoma dilatation. *AJR Am J Roentgenol.* 1986;147:826–827.
39. De Baere T, et al. Percutaneous gastrostomy with fluoroscopic guidance: single centre experience in 500 consecutive cancer patients. *Radiology.* 1999;210:651–654.
40. Cowling M, et al. Self expanding metallic stents in the treatment of pyloric dysfunction after gastric pull-up operations. *Eur Radiol.* 1999;9:1123–1126.
41. Binkert C, et al. Benign and malignant stenoses of the stomach and duodenum: treatment with self-expanding metallic endoprostheses. *Radiology.* 1996;199:335–338.
42. Feretis C, et al. Palliation of malignant gastric outlet obstruction with self expanding metal stents. *Endoscopy.* 1996;28:225–228.
43. Wong Y, et al. Gastric outlet obstruction secondary to pancreatic cancer: surgical vs endoscopic palliation. *Surg Endosc.* 2002;16:310–312.
44. Yim H, et al. Clinical outcome of the use of enteral stents for palliation of patients with malignant upper GI obstruction. *Gastrointest Endosc.* 2001;53:329–332.
45. Mainar A, et al. Colorectal obstruction: treatment with metallic stents. *Radiology.* 1996;198:761–764.
46. Dauphine C, et al. Placement of self expanding metal stents for acute malignant large bowel obstruction: a collective review. *Ann Surg Oncol.* 2002;9:574–579.
47. Aviv R, et al. Radiological palliation of malignant colonic obstruction. *Clin Radiol.* 2002;57:347–351.
48. England R, Martin D. Endoscopic and percutaneous intervention in malignant obstructive jaundice. *Cardiovasc Intervent Radiol.* 1996;19:381–387.
49. Deviere J, et al. Long-term follow-up of patients with hilar malignant stricture treated by endoscopic internal biliary drainage. *Gastrointest Endosc.* 1988;34:95–101.
50. Prat F, et al. A randomised trial of endoscopic drainage methods for inoperable malignant strictures of the common bile duct. *Gastrointest Endosc.* 1998;47:1–7.
51. Davids P, et al. Randomised trial of self expanding metal stents versus polyethylene stents for distal malignant biliary obstruction. *Lancet.* 1992;340:1488–1492.
52. Draganov P, et al. Long term outcome in patients with benign biliary strictures treated endoscopically with multiple stents. *Gastrointest Endosc.* 2002;55:680–686.
53. Born P, et al. Long term results of endoscopic and percutaneous transhepatic treatment of benign biliary strictures. *Endoscopy.* 1999;31:725–731.
54. Gabelmann A, et al. Metallic stents in benign biliary strictures: long term effectiveness and interventional management of stent occlusion. *AJR Am J Roentgenol.* 2001;177:813–817.
55. Farrell T, Hicks M. A review of radiologically guided percutaneous nephrostomies in 303 patients. *J Vasc Intervent Radiol.* 1997;8:769–774.
56. Chitale S, et al. The management of ureteric obstruction secondary to malignant pelvic disease. *Clin Radiol.* 2002;57:1118–1121.
57. Sharma S, et al. A review of antegrade stenting in the management of the obstructed kidney. *Br J Urol.* 1996;78:511–515.
58. Lucey B, et al. Miscellaneous visceral renal intervention. *Semin Intervent Radiol.* 2000;17:367–372.
59. Segura J, et al. Percutaneous removal of kidney stones: review of 1000 cases. *J Urol.* 1985;134:1077–1081.
60. Dutton S, et al. A UK multicentre retrospective cohort study comparing hysterectomy and uterine artery embolisation for the treatment of symptomatic uterine fibroids (HOPEFUL study): main results and medium-term safety and efficacy. *Br J Obstet Gynecol.* 2007;114:1340–1351.
61. Hehenkamp WJ, et al. Symptomatic uterine fibroids: treatment with uterine artery embolisation or hysterectomy: results from the randomised clinical Embolisation versus Hysterectomy (EMMY) trial. *Radiology.* 2008;246:823–832.

25 *Breast Imaging*

JUDITH KELLY and RITA MARY BORGEN

Introduction and Rationale

Mammography is considered to be the most commonly implemented method of imaging the breast, and, definitively, it is *radiographic* imaging of the breast. The majority of mammograms are performed by women on women, and for the purposes of this chapter it is assumed that both client and mammographer are female (whilst acknowledging this is not always the case). It is not our intention to present a complete work on mammography and breast imaging – this is a brief introduction to a specialised field.

Although mammography is considered to be a major contributor to breast imaging, other imaging modalities are not ignored. A résumé of other methods is given in the chapter and ultrasound of the breast is given additional focus because of its complementary role alongside mammography.

Historically, mammography has always been performed by radiographers; however, in 2000 the Department of Health announced changes to be made to the Breast Screening Programme which meant a 40% increase in skilled staff was necessary.[1] To cope with the already critical shortage of radiographers and radiologists and the increase in demand a 'Skills Mix Project in Radiography'[2] was established and a four-tier structure was formed, the four tiers being:

- Consultant/lead practitioner
- Advanced practitioner
- Practitioner
- Assistant practitioner

Assistant practitioners work towards National Vocational Qualifications in the workplace, after which they are able to perform basic mammographic procedures under the supervision of a radiographer practitioner. Radiographers have the opportunity to undertake postgraduate training in order to advance their careers into clinical roles traditionally undertaken by radiologists, such as image reading, ultrasound scanning, magnetic resonance imaging (MRI) double reporting, and image-guided interventional procedures.[2]

Mammography is widely used in the investigation of symptomatic breast disease and is the modality used for breast screening. The Million Women Study calculated the sensitivity and specificity of mammography by following over 120 000 women after their screening mammogram, showing sensitivity to be 86.6% and specificity 96.8%.[3]

Symptomatic Mammography

Symptomatic women are usually referred by a clinician and present with a potentially significant breast problem, i.e. they have symptoms such as a palpable lump, nipple discharge and pain, or a visual change such as skin tethering or puckering.

Asymptomatic Mammography

The National Health Service Breast Screening Programme (NHSBSP) currently invites all women aged 50–70 years who are registered with a general practitioner (GP) to attend for a routine 3-yearly mammogram. Some regions in the UK have extended the age range for screening to 47–73 years as part of a trial to explore possible benefits of this. Results and conclusions are not available at the time of going to press and it is not clear when results and conclusions will be published. Asymptomatic women with a significant risk of breast cancer are offered yearly mammograms between the ages of 40 and 49.[4] High risk women are now included in the NHSBSP and undergo additional annual breast MRI until aged 50.

Whatever a woman's reason for attending, there will always be common anxieties. The most significant concern is likely to be the outcome or fear of positive results following the investigation, but for many women there are concerns about the procedure itself – is it painful, is it safe?

Communication with Women Undergoing Mammography

As for all interactions between patient and health professional, effective communication is vital during mammography and starts before the woman even attends for her mammogram. All women should receive suitable, accurate and helpful written information prior to their appointment. This could include information about the procedure itself and, for breast screening, details about the risks and benefits, thus enabling women to make an informed decision. Any other information that may help to reduce the potential for anxiety should be incorporated, such as instructions on how to find the unit, waiting times and other tests that may be undertaken during their visit.

The majority of women attending for a mammogram will be given a 'normal' result and therefore will be likely to meet only one member of the breast team: the mammographer. With this in mind, the mammographer has a vital role in ensuring that the client receives all the information she requires and needs, and that it is imparted in a compassionate and understandable manner. This is also important in encouraging women for future reattendance.

Essential communication stages:

- Before the mammogram, so that the woman knows what to expect and what is expected of her
- During the mammogram, to ensure that she knows what is currently happening and to enable her to voice any concerns or indicate any discomfort she may be experiencing
- After the mammogram, so that she knows when and how the results will be communicated.

Breast Screening

In 1957, the Commission of Chronic Illness in the United States defined screening as 'the presumptive identification of unrecognised disease ... by the application of tests, examinations or other procedures which can be applied rapidly'.[5]

No screening test can be considered perfect, but the World Health Organization's International Agency for Research on Cancer (IARC) concluded that there was sufficient evidence for the efficacy of breast screening of women between 50 and 69 years.[6] Some essential considerations for a screening programme include:

- Is the disease an important health problem for the population?
- Can the population at risk be readily identified?
- Does early treatment lead to a better outcome?
- Are the benefits of screening greater than the harm caused?
- Does the screening identify the disease at a preclinical stage?
- Is treatment of the preclinical disease widely available?
- Is the screening modality acceptable to the target population?
- Is the method to be used cost-effective?

In the UK mammography is currently offered every 3 years to women between the ages of 50 and 70. A pilot study currently under way may result in the age range being extended to 47–73 years.[7]

Mammography has been the screening modality used for every randomised trial that has shown a significant population reduction in breast cancer mortality.[8–11] It has a high sensitivity in the detection of breast cancers, particularly invasive carcinomas and ductal carcinoma in situ (DCIS).[3]

The use of a multidisciplinary approach when women are recalled following their initial mammogram ensures that the screening process is specific. The assessments used are further imaging, clinical examination and tissue sampling through biopsy.

Publication of the Forrest Report[5] on breast screening and the subsequent implementation of the NHSBSP revolutionised mammography in the UK. The report made numerous recommendations: projections that should be undertaken on each breast; the screening interval; interpretation of the mammograms; assessment and follow-up; and implementation of quality assurance and quality control procedures at every step of the programme. Recommendations regarding the setting up of an advisory committee and the Pritchard Report[12] then led to guidance on quality issues. Recommendations made in the Forrest and Pritchard Reports do not pertain only to screening mammography services, as they are pertinent wherever mammography is offered, thus ensuring equity of provision for all women.

Breast Disease Demonstrated with Mammography

BENIGN BREAST CONDITIONS

There are a number of benign breast conditions that may manifest on mammograms and approximately 90% of breast lumps are benign. Some examples are:

- *Benign breast change:* There is no evident disease process and changes are often brought about by hormonal variations. Conditions such as mastitis and fibroadenosis would come under this umbrella term.
- *Cysts:* Cystic changes in the breast are very common and, as with most benign breast conditions, tend to be bilateral.
- *Fibroadenoma:* These are often found incidentally as they are usually too small to feel. Larger lesions occur in younger women. Fibroadenomas in postmenopausal women do not grow (except in women on hormone replacement therapy) and new lesions seldom appear.

Mammographic Appearance of Benign Breast Conditions

Breast Condition	Mammographic Appearance
Cysts	Visualised as an increase in density, usually with well-defined, sharp edges
Fibroadenoma	Has no specific characteristic features but is usually well defined, often encapsulated and causes displacement of the surrounding tissues. When calcification occurs the lesion is said to have a 'popcorn' appearance

BREAST CANCER

United Kingdom breast cancer facts and statistics:[13]

- Breast cancer is the most common cancer in women
- The lifetime risk of developing cancer of the breast is 1 in 8
- 80% of breast cancers occur in postmenopausal women
- 5–10% of breast cancers are genetically related.
- Around 300 men are diagnosed in the UK each year
- Breast cancer can be divided into two main types:
  - In situ carcinoma: this is contained within the breast ducts or lobules, although it has the potential to become invasive
  - Invasive carcinoma: this has spread from the ducts or lobules into the surrounding breast tissue. It has the potential to metastasise, via the blood or lymphatic systems, to other parts of the body and may ultimately shorten the patient's life. Invasive cancers are graded histologically from 1 to 3, according to how similar the breast cancer cells are to normal cells of the same type. The higher the grade the more different the cancer cells are from normal cells and the more rapidly they reproduce[14]

Mammographic Appearance of Breast Cancer

Cancer Type	Mammographic Appearance
DCIS	Frequently microcalcifications (but not always)
Invasive ductal carcinoma	Usually spiculate mass, but often has calcification and parenchymal distortion
Invasive lobular carcinoma	Similar to ductal carcinoma but microcalcification is less common

Mammography is often not able to distinguish between benign and malignant masses, which is why breast imaging services do not stop at mammography but incorporate other imaging modalities such as ultrasound and MRI. However, it is possible to make some general observations from mammographic appearances:

- A spiculated mass with microcalcifications is highly suspicious and strongly indicates malignancy; any mass with distortion should be assumed to be malignant until proved otherwise
- Microcalcifications are difficult to evaluate but could represent DCIS
- Well-defined masses are frequently benign

Dose Implications for the Breast Undergoing Mammography

It is important to remember that mammography uses radiation and therefore has the potential to induce carcinoma by the biological effects of radiation. The risk is considered to be extremely low for the patient undergoing a single mammogram because the dose is well below the threshold for deterministic effects, and the reproductive cells are not exposed to primary radiation. Risks are highest in young women and are estimated to range from 9.1 fatal carcinomas induced per million per mGy in the 30–34-year age group, falling to 7.5 fatal carcinomas induced per million per mGy in the 45–49-year age group and 4.7 fatal carcinomas induced per million per mGy in the 60–64-year age group.[11]

For women of screening age in the UK the risk of radiation-induced breast cancer (including non-fatal tumours) is approximately 1 in 100 000 per mGy. Radiation dose for women attending the NHSBSP is taken to be on average 4.5 mGy per two-view screening examination. The risk of radiation-induced cancer for a woman attending mammographic screening (two projections) by the NHSBSP is about 1 in 20 000 per visit, and it is estimated that about 170 cancers are detected by the NHSBSP for every cancer induced.[15]

Digital Mammography

The NHSBSP approved the use of digital mammography for breast screening following the results of the Digital Mammographic Imaging Screening Trial (DMIST), which enrolled almost 50 000 women. Each woman in the trial underwent both film mammography and digital mammography and various factors were recorded, such as the age of the woman, density of the breast, thickness of the compressed breast, and radiation dose. Digital and film mammograms were reported separately before being compared, and it was determined that the sensitivity of film screen mammography was comparable to that of digital mammography in women with fatty breasts. However, in women with dense breasts the trial demonstrated significantly improved sensitivity of digital mammography over film screen mammography. Furthermore, the trial revealed that the radiation dose with digital mammography was 22% less than with film screen mammography.[16] In 2007 the Department of Health stated that all screening units should have at least one digital mammography set by 2010.[17]

Alternative and Complementary Imaging Techniques

MAGNETIC RESONANCE MAMMOGRAPHY (MRM)

MRM is increasingly used as an adjunct to mammography and ultrasound, although it currently has disadvantages such as high cost, limited availability and several contraindications (women with pacemakers, pregnant women, those with claustrophobia and women who are unable to lie in the required prone position, which is necessary when using a breast coil). It is, however, particularly useful for:[18]

- The assessment of implant leakages
- Imaging of dense, glandular breasts
- Evaluation of indeterminate breast lesions
- Evaluation of lesions with discordant size on clinical/conventional imaging assessment
- Imaging of suspected multicentric or multifocal lesions
- Differentiation of recurrent breast cancer from scar tissue
- Evaluation of the response of breast cancer to treatment
- Although MRI is of value in the scenarios outlined above, incorporating the resultant report findings into the future management of the patient should be taken into account otherwise the information gained from the MRI is of little value. It is therefore important that management plans based upon all the MRI findings are fully characterised and interpreted in context with the clinical situation.

NUCLEAR MEDICINE

There are three main uses of nuclear medicine in breast imaging:

1. *Sentinel node biopsy.* This involves the use of technetium-labelled colloid to label the first axillary lymph node to drain the breast – the sentinel node. If this node is metastasis free then axillary clearance can be avoided. Sentinel node status is able to accurately predict axillary lymph node status in over 95% of cases.[19]
2. *Scintimammography.* This involves the use of technetium-labelled sestamibi and, used as an adjunct to mammography, is comparable to MRM in both sensitivity and specificity in the demonstration of both palpable and impalpable tumours.[18]

3. *Preoperative image guided localisation of breast lesions with I^{125} seed.* This involves the placement of a titanium capsule contacting an I^{125} seed and gold marker into a tumour prior to surgery. This can be done in conjunction with either stereo or ultrasound guidance and can be combined with sentinel node biopsy.[20]

ULTRASOUND

Ultrasound of the breast has continued to increase in recent years, owing to advances in ultrasound technology and ultrasound-guided interventional techniques are fundamental in breast disease assessment but is not a standalone method for imaging the breast. It is, however, used more extensively than MRI, computed tomography (CT) and radionuclide imaging (RNI). As breast ultrasound is frequently used in conjunction with mammography, more detail on this imaging modality is included following descriptions of mammography technique.

DIGITAL BREAST TOMOSYNTHESIS

Many digital mammography sets now have this function. The woman is positioned as for a normal mammogram, but with reduced compression. The X ray tube then moves over the breast in an arc, taking a series of low-dose images as it moves. Once these images have been reconstructed (a matter of seconds) a three-dimensional image is produced which is displayed as slices throughout the breast, much like a CT scan. This is particularly useful for dense breasts as it eliminates the problem of overlapping tissue. The use of tomosynthesis as part of a breast screening programme has been trialled in the United States and early results suggested that, when performed as an adjunct to digital mammography, there was a 30–40% reduction in women being recalled for assessment.[21,22] When tomosynthesis was performed without digital mammography the recall rate was reduced by 10%.[21,22] Many breast units have implemented tomosynthesis within the NHS breast screening assessment context yet the discussions on tomosynthesis are by no means complete. Since the first papers were published, efficacy of tomosynthesis as part of breast screening has continued to be considered and clinical trials have been initiated in several locations globally; some are expected to take several years before results can be published and at least one trial is not expected to be completed until 2030.[23] In the meantime, published opinions vary regarding the efficacy of tomosynthesis as an adjunct to digital mammography, with some noting significant reduction in recall rates[24,25] and others advising caution when considering tomosynthesis as part of a screening programme until more data is available.[26] Use of tomosynthesis amongst recalled women has also been considered heterogeneous[25] and other research suggests that over-detection is a potential issue in a screening programme when using tomosynthesis; it does, however, acknowledge that it has benefits.[27] There is other suggestion that tomosynthesis as an adjunct to digital mammography does not lead to a reduction in recall rate amongst younger high-risk women, and that the effect of tomosynthesis on false-positive rate at prevalent screening remains uncertain.[28]

CONTRAST-ENHANCED MAMMOGRAPHY (CEM)

CEM is becoming a more widely available technique in symptomatic settings because of its ability to improve the diagnostic performance of mammography. It requires use of intravenous contrast agents in order to demonstrate uptake of breast cancers and is therefore able to compensate for some of the limitations of conventional mammography such as lack of contrast, overlapping structures and in dense breasts.

Mammography Technique

EQUIPMENT

The purchase, commissioning and quality control of suitable equipment are essential for the provision of a quality mammography service.[8] Equipment must be acceptable to both the operator and the client: it must be light and easy for the operator to use, and there must be no sharp edges in the sections of the unit that come into contact with the client. In addition, handles are necessary to help the client maintain the correct arm position for the oblique projection and for support, if necessary.

The machine consists simply of an X-ray tube connected to a breast support which houses the imaging detector on a C-shaped arm, with a moveable compression paddle between the two (Fig. 25.1).

FUNCTIONAL REQUIREMENTS

- *High-voltage generator.* The generator must supply a near DC high voltage with ripple less than 5%.

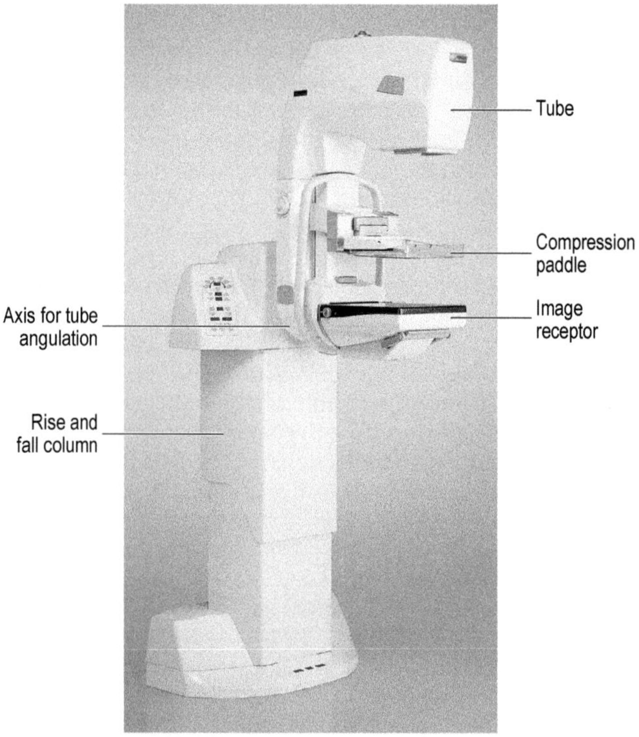

Fig. 25.1 Mammography unit. (Reproduced with permission from Xograph Imaging Systems.)

- *Kilovoltage (kVp) output.* Most modern mammography machines have automatic selection for kVp in order to optimise contrast. The generator provides a constant potential and the high voltage applied to the tube must be from 22 to 35 kVp in increments of 1 kVp.
- *Focal spot size.* The focal spot should be as small as possible to ensure adequate resolution, for example 0.3 mm for general mammography and 0.1 mm (small focus) for magnification views.
- *Tube current (mA).* In order to keep exposure times to a minimum (and thus reduce the likelihood of movement unsharpness) the tube current should be as high as possible. At 28 kVp the current should be at least 100 mA on large focus.
- *Grid.* A grid is essential to ensure optimum image quality; this may be incorporated within the detector on some digital systems.
- *AED.* An automatic exposure device is essential because of the wide variation in breast sizes and compositions. (As there is a need for high radiographic contrast and hence the system has low latitude, there is little scope for error in the selection of mAs.)[23]

IMAGE RECORDING

In line with other radiographic examinations, film/screen mammography has been replaced by digital mammography. The digital images are sent electronically to a computer workstation where they are post processed before being stored in the picture archiving and communication system (PACS). From here the images can be retrieved remotely on reporting workstations and monitors throughout the hospital. The images can also be viewed in other hospitals provided a suitable network link is in place.

DIGITAL MAMMOGRAPHY

This modality allows annotations to be applied digitally and images can be manipulated once produced. One of the main advantages of image manipulation is its ability to magnify the image more sharply than that associated with macro or magnification images, sometimes required to demonstrate suspicious areas already seen on mammograms. A further benefit of digital magnification is that it does not involve an additional exposure to radiation, unlike traditional magnification views.

VIEWING IMAGES

Digital mammography images can be viewed on any monitor linked to the network. However, for reporting purposes high-resolution 5 megapixel monitors are required.[29]

It is recommended that craniocaudal (CC) images are viewed 'back-to-back' with the posterior aspects of the breasts touching (Fig. 25.2A,B). Mediolateral obliques are viewed with the pectoral aspects touching (Fig. 25.3A,B). These strategies facilitate vital comparison of similar areas of each breast for each projection.

Mammographic Projections

Anatomical markers must be used on all projections undertaken and markers used in mammography usually incorporate legends, which identify the side under examination, the projection and, sometimes, the orientation of the axilla.

CRANIOCAUDAL (CC) (FIG. 25.4A,B)

Positioning

- The mammography unit is positioned with the image receptor (IR) holder horizontal and the height adjusted to slightly above the level of the inframammary angle
- The client faces the machine, standing approximately 5–6 cm back from it
- The client's arms hang loosely by her side and her head is turned away from the side to be examined
- The breast is lifted gently up and away from the chest wall (the mammographer will use the left hand to raise the right breast and the right hand to raise the left breast)
- With the mammographer supporting the breast, the height of the unit is adjusted so that the IR holder

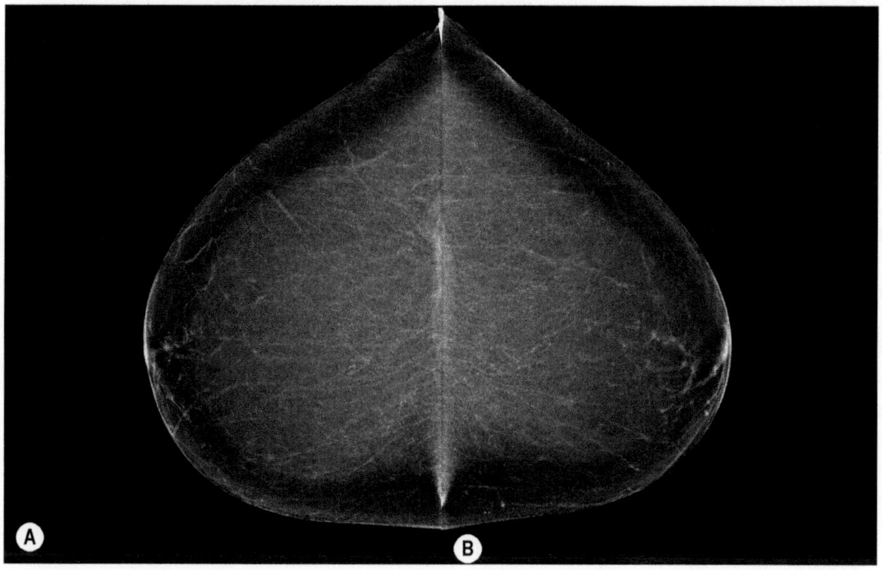

Fig. 25.2 Mounting craniocaudal images for viewing. (Images used courtesy IMS Italy.)

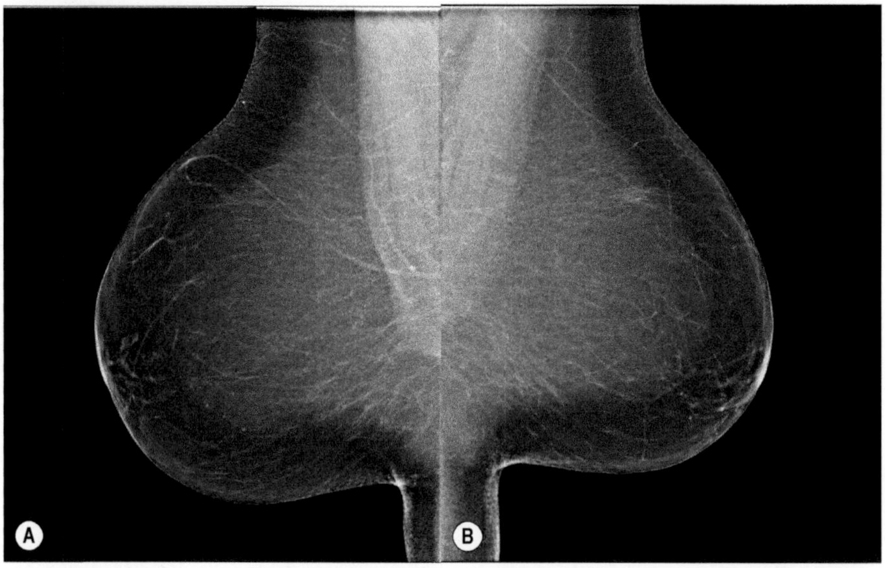

Fig. 25.3 Mounting mediolateral oblique images for viewing. (Images used courtesy IMS Italy.)

makes contact with the breast at the inframammary fold and the breast is at approximately 90° to the chest wall

- The client is asked to lean slightly forward until her rib cage is in contact with the machine. The breast is carefully placed onto the IR holder, ensuring that no skin folds are created underneath the breast
- The client is asked to lean slightly towards the side to be examined to bring the outer quadrant of the breast into contact with the IR holder. The mammographer gently pulls the lateral aspect of the breast onto the IR holder whilst making sure that the medial aspect of the breast remains in place. It may be necessary to adjust the unit height to ensure that the inferior aspect of the breast lies horizontally on the IR holder
- The mammographer places her thumb on the medial aspect of the breast and her fingers on the superior aspect; she then pulls gently forward towards the nipple to ensure no skin folds are created, while compression is applied slowly. During this process it is advisable that the mammographer maintains gentle pressure on the client's back, to ensure the maximum amount of breast tissue is included on the image
- The light beam diaphragm can be used while compression is applied, to check that:
  - the nipple is in profile
  - all the breast is within the main beam
  - both the medial and lateral margins are included
  - there are no skin folds
  - compression of the breast is adequate*
  - The client may need to hold their other breast laterally and against their body in order to avoid its inclusion on the image. Compression is a vital component in achieving good mammographic images. It is also a part of the examination that causes much concern for women. If the mammographer explains the need for compression at the start of the examination the client may be more able to tolerate any possible discomfort, knowing that better-quality images will be produced and the need for repeat examinations less likely.

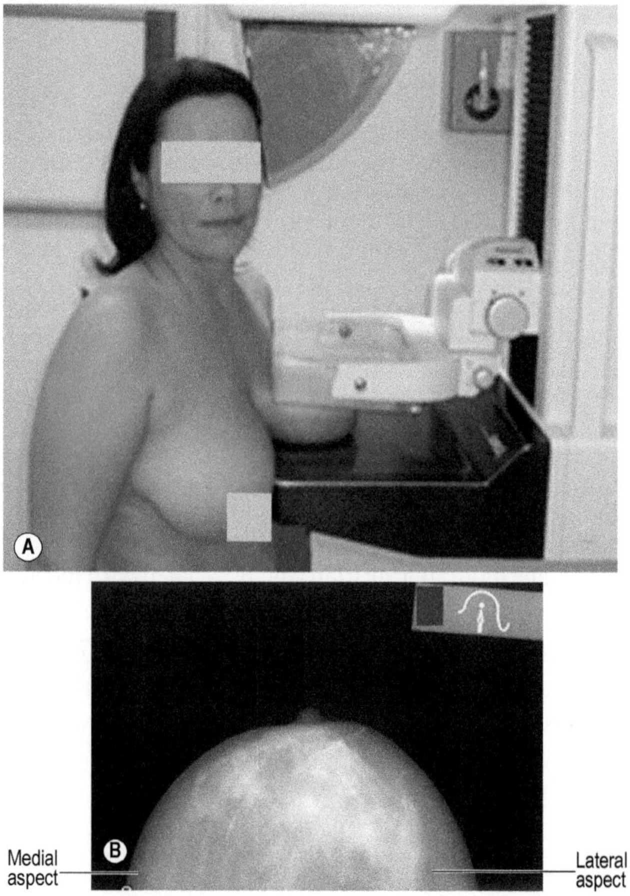

Fig. 25.4 (A) CC projection; (B) CC image.

*Compression of the breast greatly improves image quality by:

- reducing the thickness of breast tissue irradiated, thereby reducing the superimposition of breast tissues and reducing the radiation dose to the breast
- reducing geometric unsharpness
- reducing movement unsharpness

- improving contrast (by reducing internal X-ray beam scatter)

Application of the correct amount of compression comes with experience, although there are guidelines concerning the amount of pressure to be used. The maximum pressure allowed in the UK is 200 N,[1] although in practice this amount is not necessary and many manufacturers limit their equipment to 160 N.

Criteria for Assessing Image Quality

- The nipple is in profile
- The majority of the medial and lateral breast tissue (including some of the axillary tail) is included
- Pectoral muscle is at the centre of the edge of the image. However, this is seen in only approximately 30% of individuals
- An appropriate exposure has been used to provide optimum contrast between the different structures within the breast and adequate image density to demonstrate glandular tissue, muscle and fat
- Absence of artefact, including skin folds
- Absence of movement

Common Errors: CC Projection

Common Errors	Possible Reasons
Nipple is pointing downwards	IR holder may be too high – reduce height Skin on the underside of the breast may be caught at the proximal edge of the IR holder – reposition the breast by lifting it and gently pulling the underside of the breast forward Excess loose skin on the superior surface of the breast – apply tension to the skin surface, pulling it gently towards the thorax
Folds at the lateral aspect of the breast	There may be a pad of fat or skin above the upper outer quadrant – alter position of the arm The client may be leaning towards their medial aspect The breast may be twisted

MEDIOLATERAL OBLIQUE (MLO) (FIG. 25.5A,B)

Positioning

- The client faces the unit with feet apart
- From the position used for the CC projection, the unit is rotated through 40–50°, with the IR holder on the side of examination; the height is adjusted to bring the upper border of the IR holder level with the axilla. It may be necessary to further adjust the height during positioning
- The client raises the arm on the side under examination and also raises her chin (thus preventing superimposition of the mandible over the breast)
- The mammographer stands next to the side not under examination and holds the lateral aspect of the breast with one hand, whilst placing the other hand on the client's back
- The client is encouraged to lean forward into the machine and, with feet still facing forward, is asked to lean laterally towards the IR holder
- The mammographer slides her hand forward from between the lateral aspect of the breast and the IR holder, gently pulling the breast forward
- From the side under examination, the mammographer gently pulls the client's raised arm across and behind the IR holder, so that the corner of the receptor holder sits in the axilla. The client's hand is guided to the handle of the mammography unit for support and the elbow is positioned so it hangs down comfortably behind the IR holder
- The mammographer returns to the side not under examination and, with one hand holding the superior aspect and the other hand holding the inferior aspect of the breast, the mammographer gently lifts the breast and pulls it forward. The mammographer then uses the palm of one hand to hold the breast in place, whilst using the other hand to ensure there are no creases in the inframammary angle
- The thumb of the hand holding the breast is positioned under the breast while the fingers are spread across the breast. This maintains breast position in preparation for compression
- The light beam diaphragm is used to check that:
  - the nipple is in profile
  - the inframammary angle is clearly visible and included within the boundaries
  - there are no skin folds
  - the edge of the compression plate is adjacent to the thorax from immediately below the clavicle down to the inframammary angle
- Compression is applied slowly and evenly using the foot pedal while the mammographer maintains the breast in position, gradually moving her fingers forwards towards the nipple during compression. The thumb maintains the lift of the breast until compression is complete and the breast is held in place by the compression paddle
- When imaging large breasts it is advisable to use the fingers of the opposite hand to support the inferior aspect of the breast in order to avoid straining the thumb

Criteria for Asessing Image Quality

- The entire breast and skin surface are included
- The pectoral muscle lies at the level of the nipple and at an angle of 20–35° from the vertical
- The nipple is in profile
- The inframammary angle is clearly demonstrated
- There are no skin folds
- An appropriate exposure is used to provide optimum contrast between the different structures within the breast and adequate image density to demonstrate glandular tissue, muscle and fat
- There is absence of artefact
- There is absence of movement

Common Errors: MLO Projection

Common Errors	Possible Reasons
Skin folds at axilla	IR holder may be too high
Skin folds at inframammary angle	Overlap of the breast and abdominal wall – ask the client to stick their bottom out a little and ease out any creases
Nipple is not in profile	IR holder may be too high. The client may have rotated their hips – reposition
Pectoral muscle not across the image	IR holder may be too high – adjust and reposition the shoulder

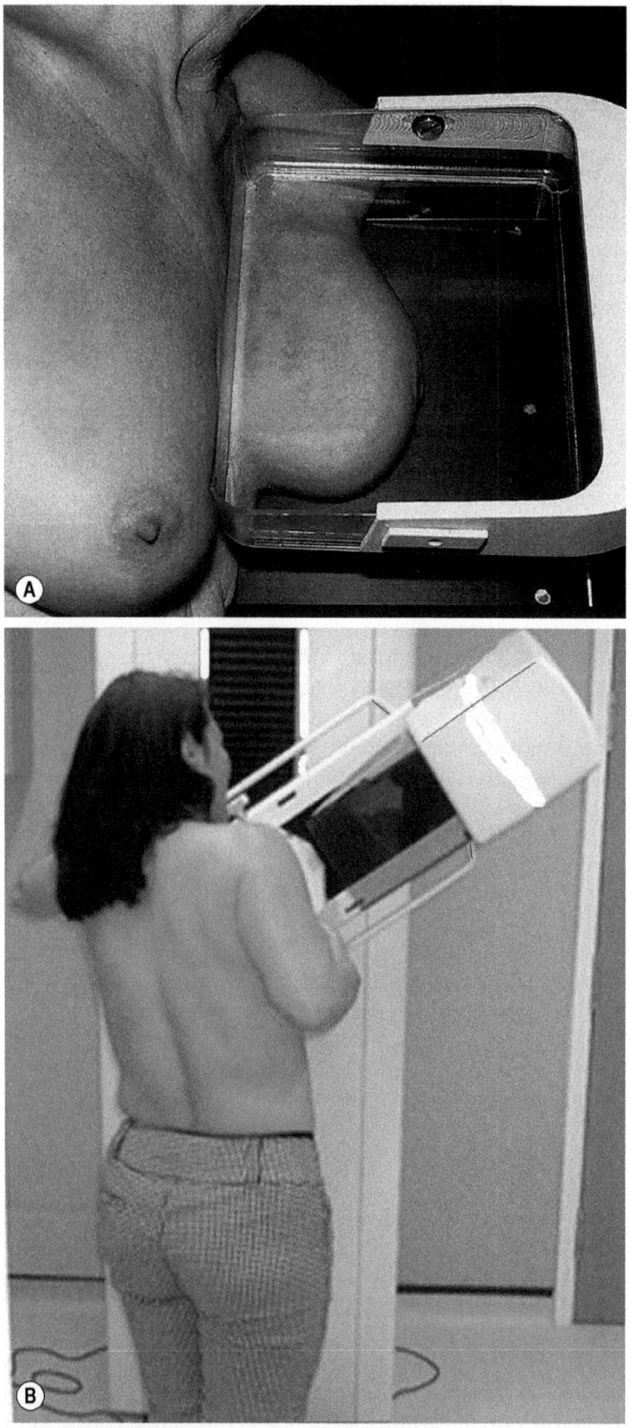

Fig. 25.5 (A) MLO projection; (B) MLO position demonstrating 45° angle of unit. (A, Reproduced with permission from Lee L, Stickland V, Wilson R, et al. *Fundamentals of Mammography*. 2nd ed. Edinburgh: Churchill Livingstone; 2003.)

PGMI (PERFECT, GOOD, MODERATE, INADEQUATE) SYSTEM

The PGMI system was introduced in the UK in the early 1990s as a grading system and guide to performance criteria in the classification of oblique mammograms. It is still used in training centres and mammography departments as a means of evaluating mammograms. It is important to remember, however, that CC films, though not assessed by the PGMI system, must not be forgotten in performance evaluation. Indeed, many breast screening units have modified the original PGMI forms to include the criteria necessary to evaluate CC films.

As the PGMI system is subjective, it is possible that individuals using it might grade the same images differently on separate occasions, and this is the main reason for questioning its validity. However, without a better system that uses both the MLO and the CC projections for training and continuing development, mammographers will continue to use PGMI.

The PGMI System: Summary[23]

P = Perfect. To be graded as a 'perfect' image, the following must apply:

1. Whole breast imaged thus:
   - Pectoral muscle to nipple level
   - Pectoral muscle at correct angle
   - Nipple in profile
   - Inframammary angle shown under the breast
2. Correct annotations:
   - Patient identification and examination date
   - Correct anatomical markers
   - Mammographer identification
3. Correct exposure
4. Adequate compression
5. No movement unsharpness
6. Absence of skin folds
7. Symmetrical images

G = Good. To be graded 'Good', both oblique images must meet criteria 1–5 from the list in the Perfect section. Inadequacy in 6 and 7 can be accepted if shown in a minor degree.

M = Moderate. 'Moderate' images are considered acceptable for diagnostic purposes. Acceptable errors are:

- Pectoral muscle not level with the nipple or not at the correct angle but the back of the breast is adequately shown
- Nipple not in profile but the retroareolar area is well defined

- Inframammary angle is not clearly demonstrated but the breast is adequately defined
- Artefacts are present but the image is not obscured
- More severe skin folds but the breast image is not obscured – when other criteria are adequately fulfilled

I = Inadequate

- If part of the breast is not imaged
- Inadequate compression: this may result in image unsharpness and reduce contrast
- Incorrect exposure
- Artefacts or skin folds that cover the image of the breast
- Inadequate or incorrect identification or annotation of anatomical markers

Supplementary Projections

There are a number of additional projections that can be used to supplement the basic CC and MLO projections. They are used to gain further information when a lesion or possible lesion has been seen on the original images, and are often all that is required to clarify any uncertainty. These additional projections can also be used in situations where the client has difficulty achieving the original position, leading to an inadequate examination, for example women who are disabled, wheelchair users, or those whose physical characteristics render positioning difficult and/or painful.

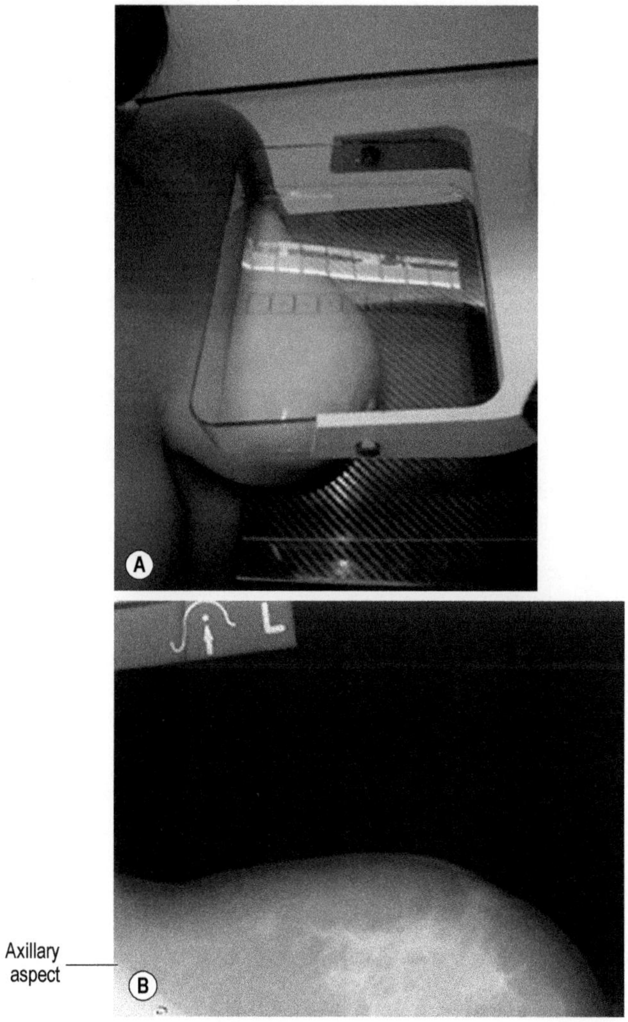

Fig. 25.6 Extended CC.

MEDIALLY ROTATED CRANIOCAUDAL PROJECTION (EXTENDED CC) (FIG. 25.6A,B)

This projection is useful to demonstrate more of the outer breast, towards the axillary tail. The equipment and the client are positioned as for the CC projection but the client then turns her feet 5–10° to the opposite side to that being examined, and is then turned further to include the lateral aspect of the breast. The medial portion of the breast will not be included on the image.

This projection will demonstrate lesions in the extreme lateral portion of the breast that are seen on the MLO but not on the CC image. It can also be used for women with large breasts who require more than one image in the CC position.

MEDIOLATERAL PROJECTION (FIG. 25.7A,B)

This projection is used to assess the depth of lesions for localisation and is particularly useful after localisation. The majority of the breast tissue is demonstrated, with the exception of the axillary tail.

Positioning (left breast described)

- The IR holder is vertical
- The client faces the machine with the lateral edge of the chest wall in line with the IR holder
- The left arm is raised and the client is encouraged to hold the support handle. The breast should be in line with the centre of the IR holder
- The mammographer uses her left hand to lift the client's humerus and her right hand to lift the breast up and away from the chest wall. The client is encouraged to lean into the machine, and while keeping the nipple in profile and the inframammary angle in view the right hand is used to ease the patient's axilla onto the corner of the IR holder by carefully pulling the upper portion of the pectoral muscle forward
- The client's arm is rested on top of the machine and, while supporting the breast with the right hand and maintaining the position of the left shoulder with the left hand, the mammographer applies compression ensuring that the nipple is in profile and the inframammary angle is clearly demonstrated prior to making the exposure

Criteria for Assessing Image Quality

- Inframammary angle is included
- Nipple is in profile
- Inferior portion of pectoral muscle is included

A *lateromedial* projection may also be undertaken if it is still necessary to demonstrate the inframammary angle. This essentially uses the opposite position of the mediolateral projection, with the client initially standing with the vertical IR holder between the breasts; the medial aspect of the breast under examination is placed against the IR holder's surface and the breast elevated, positioned and compressed similarly to the mediolateral projection (Fig. 25.8).

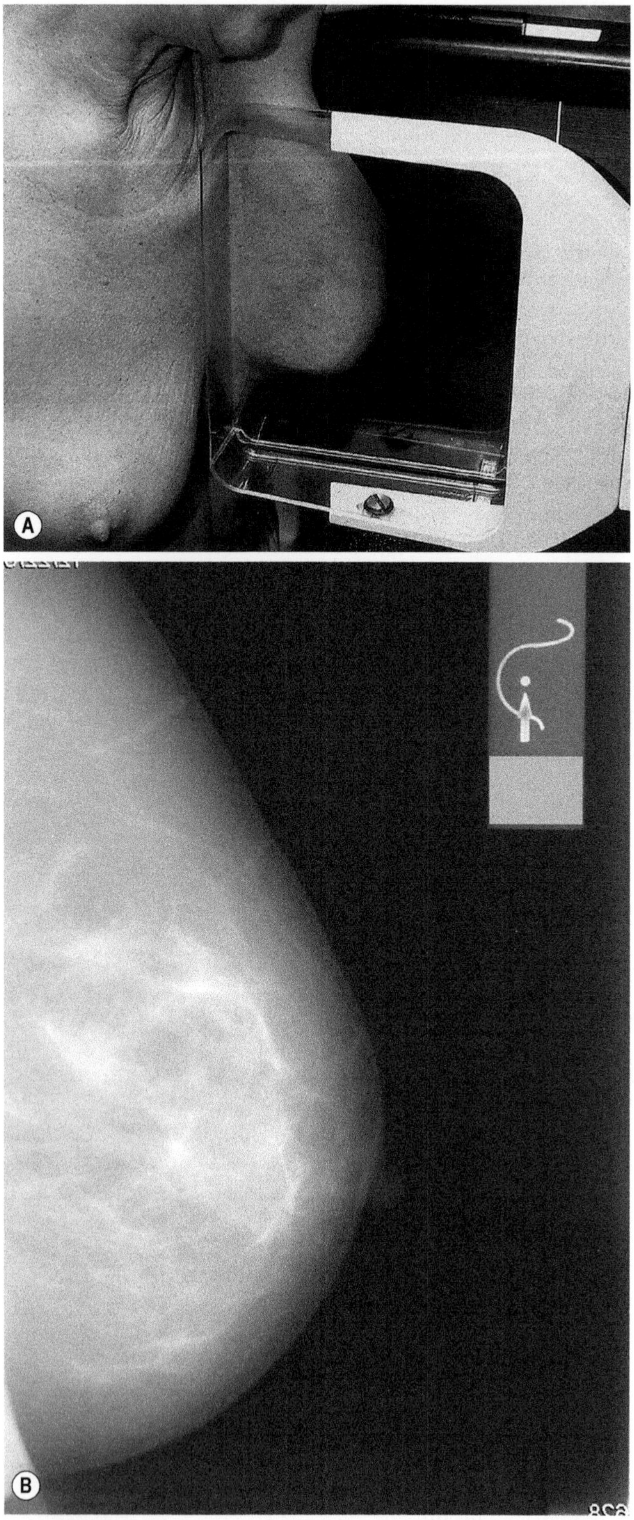

Fig. 25.7 Mediolateral. (A, Reproduced with permission from Lee L, Stickland V, Wilson R, et al. *Fundamentals of Mammography*. 2nd ed. Edinburgh: Churchill Livingstone; 2003.)

LOCALISED COMPRESSION VIEWS (PADDLE VIEWS)

These are used to demonstrate whether a lesion has clear or ill-defined borders and to demonstrate whether a lesion is merely a superimposition of tissues or indeed a genuine lesion. A small compression paddle is attached to the compression unit and this is applied over the area of the suspected lesion; it has the capacity to apply more effective and localised compression to a particular area of the breast.

Equipment requirements are:

- Fine focus
- Small localised compression paddle
- Moving grid
- Full field diaphragm

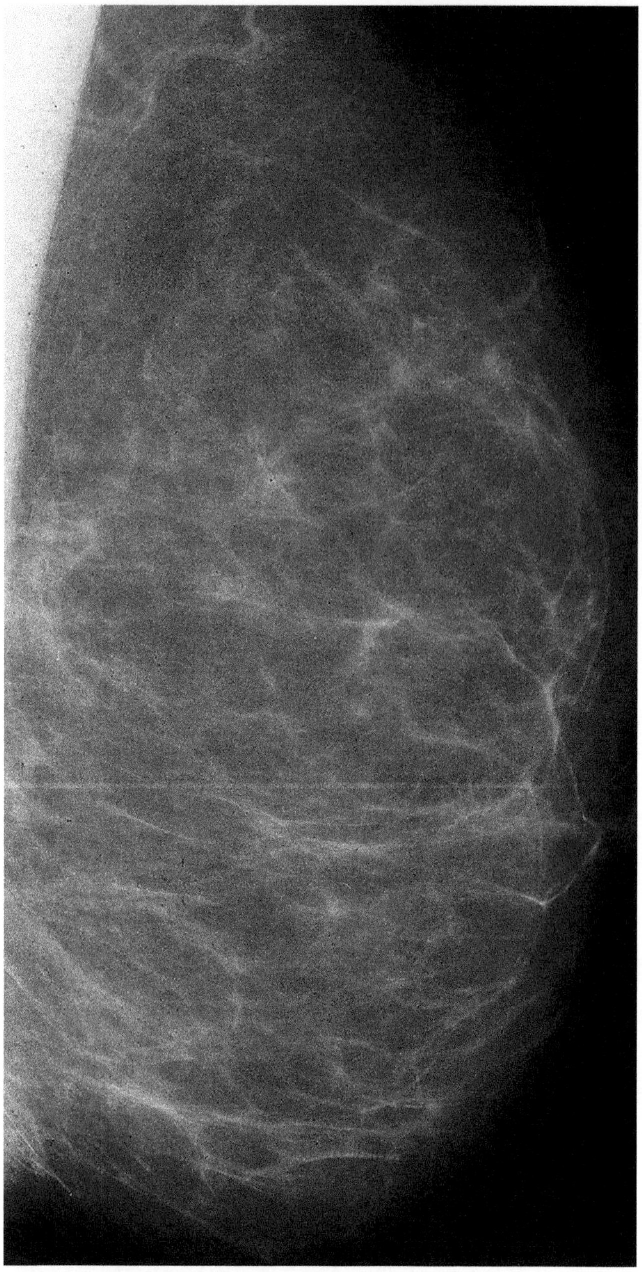

Fig. 25.8 Lateromedial. (Reproduced with permission from Lee L, Stickland V, Wilson R, et al. *Fundamentals of Mammography*. 2nd ed. Edinburgh: Churchill Livingstone; 2003.)

MAGNIFICATION (MACRO) VIEWS

These are used to magnify areas of suspicion seen on mammograms, usually areas of microcalcification, which may well demonstrate their characteristics more clearly when magnified. Additional magnification views frequently provide information regarding microcalcification extent and also further microcalcification not seen on the initial mammograms. This is vital for assessment of possible disease extent and informs further management where DCIS or invasive disease are diagnosed.

When undertaking magnification views, communication and explanation is important: if the client is aware of what is being done, why it is being done and what is required of her, she will be able to assist the mammographer more effectively.

Adaptations to equipment are required as follows:

- Fine focus
- Magnification platform
- Small localised compression paddle
- Full field diaphragm

Positioning is selected from existing images, using the projection most likely to demonstrate the suspicious appearance well; for calcifications these are CC and lateral. The breast is positioned in contact with the magnification platform rather than directly over the IR. The localised paddle is brought down over the area of suspicion.

Ultrasound

The use of ultrasound as an adjunct to X-ray mammography in the work-up of benign, indeterminate and suspicious breast lesions and as a first-line imaging investigation in women under 40 is now firmly embedded in breast diagnostic practice. Furthermore, ultrasound-guided interventional procedures have not only revolutionised the diagnostic management of impalpable and palpable breast lesions but have also resulted in very accurate preoperative diagnoses.

Ultrasound guided interventions include:

- Fine needle aspiration (FNA)
- Wide bore core biopsy
- Aspiration/drainage
- Vacuum-assisted biopsy
- Vacuum-assisted excision biopsy
- Guided localisation

Ultrasound-guided intervention is also recognised as preferable for sampling even clinically palpable lesions, as it is more accurate (thanks to real-time imaging) and considerably safer owing to the proximity of some breast lesions to the chest wall. Consequently, diagnostic excision (open) biopsies are now an infrequent procedure. Ultrasound is also used in initial staging of the axilla in patients with suspected breast cancer, and this facilitates the most appropriate surgical management for such cases. Any equivocal or suspicious nodes are sampled (either fine needle aspiration or core biopsy) preoperatively, and if found to contain metastatic disease an axillary clearance is performed. If no diseased nodes are found preoperatively the patient proceeds to sentinel node biopsy at the same time as surgery to remove the lesion.

As already mentioned in this chapter, MRI, ultrasound and RNI all have a role in identifying breast disease, but the technological developments in ultrasound have meant that this modality now offers high-quality images that are most suitable for demonstrating both breast anatomy and breast pathology. With regard to the dose implications of RNI and the range of contraindications and costs of MRI, the benefits of ultrasound are clear: availability, speed of examination and equipment cost.[25] Technologies are still evolving, with add-on software applications such as *elastography and contrast enhanced ultrasound* becoming increasingly available. These applications allow further lesion characterisation by providing information that assesses tissue stiffness and blood supply (tumours require additional vascularity in order to proliferate) leading to improved diagnostic confidence. However, the overall clinical benefits of such technologies are yet to be fully realised and integrated into routine practice.

The use of ultrasound in the diagnosis of breast disease, both independently and as an adjunct to mammography, is well documented and there are numerous texts and articles devoted to it. This chapter aims to provide an overview of breast ultrasound rather than exploring it in great depth.

NORMAL ULTRASONIC APPEARANCES OF THE BREAST

The breast comprises a mixture of tissue components which depend on age, hormonal status, structural changes (pathological, involutional, congenital) and particular individual characteristics. In young women breast tissue generally contains very little fat (i.e. is mainly breast parenchyma) but the ageing process causes glandular tissue to be replaced by fat and connective tissue. However, this does vary, and young women with large breasts may still have considerable volumes of fatty tissue.

Observing the breast in schematic sagittal section the following anatomy is seen:

- The skin surface: this is the superficial component of the breast and, when using high-resolution probes, demonstrates a homogeneous band that is more echogenic than the underlying fatty tissue
- Subcutaneous fat
- Cooper's ligaments (the septa of connective tissue surrounding and supporting the glans from the dermis to the pectoral fascia) appear as hyperechoic, oblique lines going into the parenchyma
- Breast parenchyma (ducts and lobules)
- Interlobular fibrofatty tissue
- The deep mammary fascia
- Pectoralis major and minor muscles
- Ribs and intercostal spaces
- Pleura and lung

A young, predominantly glandular breast is variably echogenic, whereas older breasts with more adipose tissue present as hypoechoic. Breast parenchyma is therefore not homogeneous. The parenchyma is seen to be triangular in shape with the apex towards the nipple, and is visualised as a well-defined, rounded nodule of medium echogenicity.

COMMON LESIONS SEEN WITH ULTRASOUND

Cysts

Cysts are such a common finding in women between the ages of 35 and 50 years that they are virtually considered a normal variant; however, they are rare in women under 25 and over 60 years.[25] Cysts can present as single or multiple and are often bilateral.

Simple cysts generally:

- Have well-defined margins
- Appear as rounded or ovoid in shape
- Are anechoic (no internal echoes)
- Are compressible
- Are seen to have a well-defined posterior wall with enhanced sound transmission
- Are seen to have thin shadows at the lesion edges
- Are completely encompassed by a thin echogenic capsule

Complex Cysts

A complex cyst can be defined as any cyst that does not meet the strict criteria for definition as a simple cyst (given above). They are also considered to be a common finding and the use of higher-resolution equipment probably contributes to this, owing to its ability to demonstrate small fluid particles and artefactual echoes within cysts. When characterising cystic breast lesions it is important that the operator excludes the presence of artefactual echoes within a simple cyst that can erroneously make them appear as solid lesions or complex cysts. Internal echoes can also often occur after incomplete aspiration of a simple cyst.

Benign Solid Lesions

The majority of benign breast tumours comprise a mixture of the three breast components: parenchyma, connective tissue and fat. The most common lesions are:

- *Fibroadenoma*: the most common benign breast tumour, affecting women between 20 and 40 years of age. They appear as a well-defined, solid lesion with smooth margins. Fibroadenomas are hypoechoic and internal echoes are usually present due to their macroscopic structure. They have an elongated shape and are not easily compressed.
- *Lipoma*: lipomas are less echogenic than fibroadenomas, being approximately isoechoic to intramammary fat. Lesion encapsulation differentiates them from normal fatty tissue and they are more compressible than fibroadenomas.

Malignant Lesions

Ultrasound is used in the diagnosis of breast cancer as an adjunct to mammography, which is the main initial diagnostic imaging tool. In this setting ultrasound is used to assess the internal structure, size, accurate location and the additional spread of any disease not seen mammographically. Carcinomas can exhibit a variety of ultrasonic characteristics and there is frequently an overlap between benign and malignant lesions (approximately 2% of carcinomas exhibit fibroadenoma-like features, i.e. smooth margins and homogeneous internal structure). However, in general, malignant lesions are very variable in shape; hypoechoic; cause posterior acoustic shadowing (as they are solid); have ill-defined/irregular margins and mixed internal echoes. If undiagnosed at an early stage the progression of disease is characterised ultrasonically by the appearance of alteration of the internal structure of the carcinoma in association with distortion of the surrounding stroma, possible skin infiltration and surrounding interstitial oedema.

LIMITATIONS OF ULTRASOUND IN BREAST DISEASE DIAGNOSIS

Like all imaging techniques, ultrasound is very examiner-dependent, and therefore experience and technique have a great effect on diagnostic accuracy. It is also equipment-dependent and, as already indicated, the quality of equipment used, appropriate transducers and settings are of paramount importance in achieving optimal images. Reproducibility can often be problematic, especially following any needle intervention (if haematoma has occurred), as this can alter ultrasonic appearances for some time afterwards.

Thorough, systematic examination can be very time-consuming in large, dense breasts and visualisation of microcalcification (often an indication of DCIS) is still unreliable, even with the most up-to-date equipment.

BREAST ULTRASOUND EQUIPMENT

Adequate ultrasound examination of any organ requires the use of appropriate equipment. Performing accurate high-quality breast ultrasound requires technical specifications at the very least equal to those for any other body part, demanding excellent spatial and contrast resolution. Only high-resolution instrumentation capable of producing high-quality images should be used.[30]

The breast is a superficial structure which requires the use of high-frequency near-field imaging using real-time hand-held transducers (7.5–15 mHz) with a linear array configuration and a 'footprint' of approximately 4–7 cm. When such equipment is used, many more normal structures in the breast tissue are seen, as well as appearances resulting from proliferative and fibrocystic change. A detailed knowledge of breast anatomy and pathology is therefore essential for accurate interpretation of such findings.

The 1998 Medical Devices Agency publication of guidance for ultrasound scanner used in breast imaging indicated that scanners should have the capability to:[31]

- Differentiate between solid and cystic lesions to 2 mm in diameter
- Display normal and abnormal breast tissue detail
- Image a 22G needle within the breast
- Measure the dimensions of breast lesions
- Penetrate breast thickness to 40 mm
- Demonstrate irregularities in lesion margins and surrounding breast tissue

The use of Doppler analysis during an examination provides the sonographer with an indication of blood flow to and from a lesion, thus helping further with the formation of a differential diagnosis. Doppler modes available include colour Doppler, power Doppler and pulsed Doppler with spectral analysis. As with conventional breast ultrasound, such applications require high-frequency transducers. There are a number of specific situations where there is a role for Doppler, including determination of the aggressiveness of suspicious or malignant lesions (high-grade lesions tend to have noticeably increased flow, whereas low-grade lesions have less tumour neovascularity); assessing response to tumour therapy; distinguishing fat necrosis and scarring from recurrent disease; distinguishing between inflammation and metastases where lymphadenopathy is seen.

THE ROLE OF ULTRASOUND WITH MAMMOGRAPHY

Breast ultrasound as a complementary imaging modality is most often used in the following situations:

- Evaluation of a mass already demonstrated mammographically; with an experienced sonographer ultrasound is highly sensitive in differentiating between solid and cystic lesions in the breast[32]
- To assist with needle guidance for localisation of lesions prior to surgery (see section on breast lesion localisation later in the chapter)
- To assist with needle guidance during breast interventional procedures, e.g. cyst aspirations or lesion biopsy
- Evaluation of dense breast tissue in symptomatic patients. Women most likely to have dense breasts are younger, premenopausal or on hormone replacement therapy. In the presence of dense breast tissue it is frequently difficult to distinguish mass lesions on mammograms

Wherever possible, mammograms for the patient under examination should be available to the sonographer to further aid the scan procedure, and to inform the differential diagnosis of breast problems.

SONOGRAPHY AS A STANDALONE DIAGNOSTIC TOOL

Ultrasound alone is not an appropriate means of screening women for breast cancer, and it is acknowledged that 'the use of ultrasound in population screening of asymptomatic women is associated with unacceptably high rates of both false positive and false negative outcomes'.[33] However, ultrasound is often used as the initial, and sometimes the only, imaging modality in the following situations:

- Determination of the nature of a palpable lump – solid or cystic
- Follow-up for patients with recurrent cysts
- Where the level of clinical suspicion at initial assessment is low and use of radiation may raise concern, e.g. in pregnant patients
- When the patient is under 40 years of age and presents with a clinical abnormality thought to be benign. Such a patient is likely to have dense breasts, greatly reducing the sensitivity and efficacy of mammography
- In extreme cases when a patient presenting with a clinical abnormality refuses mammographic assessment
- To ascertain the integrity of breast prostheses when rupture is clinically suspected
- In cases where compression used in mammography would be intolerable or inappropriate for the patient, e.g. in acute breast conditions such as abscess, recent trauma, and for assessment of the axilla only in cases of very advanced local disease

SUMMARY OF BREAST ULTRASOUND TECHNIQUE

- The patient is undressed from the waist up and is (usually) in the supine or supine oblique position, thereby reducing breast thickness, improving sound penetration and improving visualisation of deeper breast structures. Occasionally upper quadrant masses are better demonstrated in the erect position.
- The arm of the side under examination (ipsilateral) is extended above the head to stretch the pectoralis muscle, thereby enabling better fixation and immobilisation of the breast and ensuring good visualisation of the lower quadrants and the inframammary fold. This position also facilitates the reproducibility of clinically palpable findings.
- For optimal scanning the transducer should be held at the base, perpendicular to the skin surface, with gentle pressure applied to ensure complete contact. An angled transducer results in poor sound penetration. Compression is useful in reducing the thickness of the area to be examined and to assess changes in the shape of a lesion, e.g. flattening a cyst to confirm its nature. However, care must be taken that the pressure applied is just sufficient to maintain uniform contact with the skin surface but not so excessive that lesions are inadvertently pushed out of the scanning plane or structures are deformed within the parenchyma (the latter making them difficult to evaluate). Glandular tissue and fat are easily deformed but tumours are much firmer, exhibiting considerably less compressibility.
- The whole of the breast and its adjacent tissues are examined, from the inframammary fold to the peripheral areas of the upper quadrants, and from the anterior midaxillary line and the axillary tail to the lateral aspect of the sternum.
- Both sagittal and transverse scans are undertaken, involving overlap of scanning planes to ensure complete, systematic coverage of the breast, along with radial scanning around the areola complex. Because the lactiferous ducts converge radially toward the nipple areola from the periphery and terminate within the nipple, radial scans facilitate examination of the breast ductal structures.
- Any focal lesions demonstrated should be described along with a differential diagnosis, measured and documented in two planes. The position of any lesion within the breast should be provided as precisely as possible, for example in the left upper outer quadrant. Additionally, lesions/abnormalities may be described as represented on a clock face, e.g. 1 o'clock, 9 o'clock etc., and the distance from the nipple given.
- Mammographic and clinical findings should be correlated when appropriate.

STORING AND VIEWING ULTRASOUND IMAGES

It is now common practice for images of the examination to be produced and stored in radiology PACSs for ease of access. Some systems still facilitate printing of paper copies as well. The equipment used for PACS should be compatible with the ultrasound system.

Quality assurance (QA) and quality control are of paramount importance for any imaging modality; it is common practice for weekly and monthly QA checks to be undertaken on ultrasound units to ensure that ultrasound systems are operating consistently at their optimum level of performance.

Breast Lesion Localisation

Before the NHSBSP was introduced in 1988[1] most breast cancers were found only when a palpable lump had

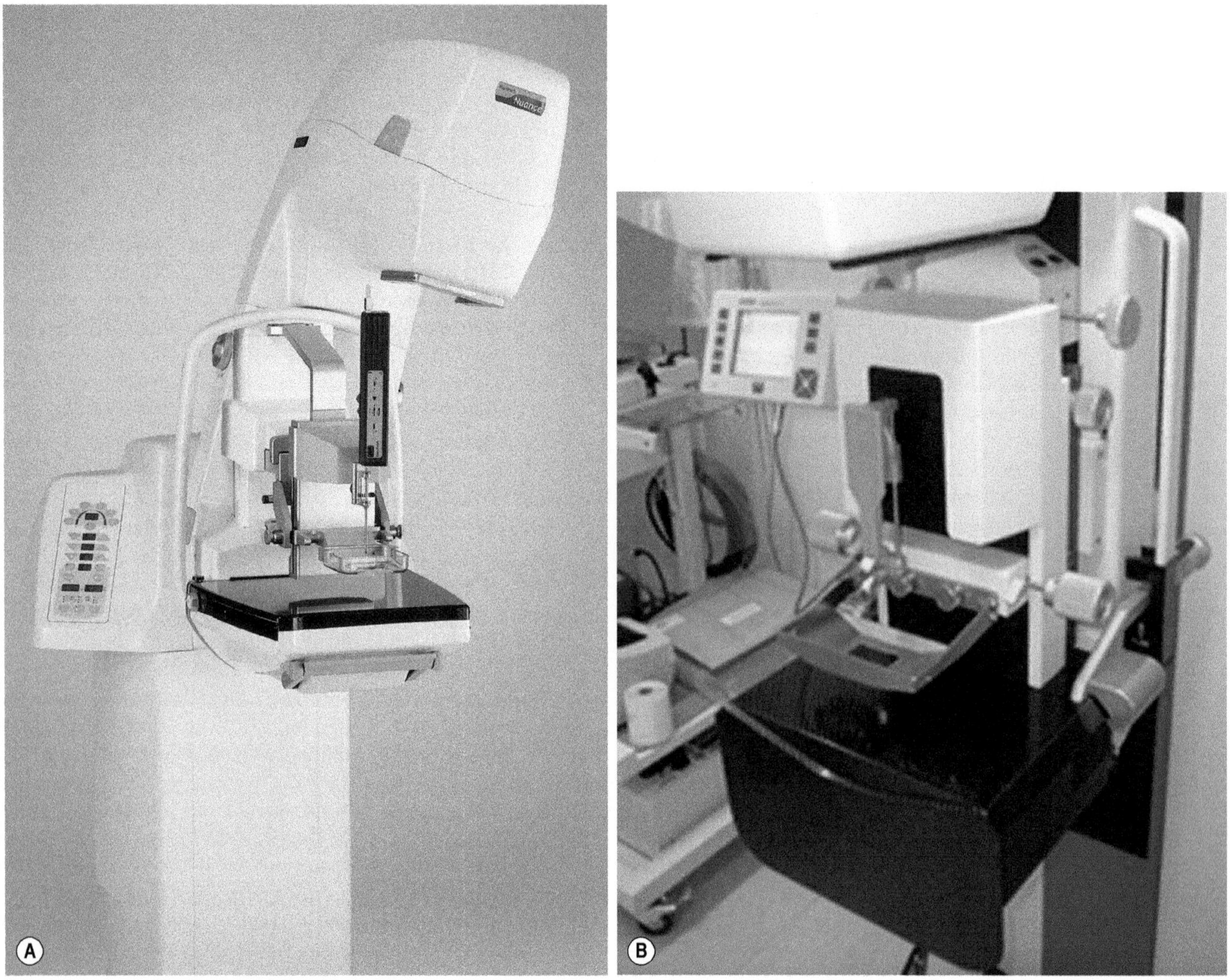

Fig. 25.9 **(A,B) Stereotactic units. Note the similarities between the two units.** (Reproduced with permission from Xograph Imaging Systems.)

formed, i.e. they were clinically detectable. The fact that the surgeons could feel these tumours meant that during breast-conserving surgery assistance was seldom necessary to locate the area to be excised; unfortunately, this also meant that tumours were more likely to be more advanced in their growth than those found via a screening mammogram.

Breast screening has increased the rate of diagnosis of breast cancers so small or so deep within the breast tissue that they are impalpable. In order for surgeons to remove these lesions accurately and achieve good cosmesis, the tumours need to be 'localised' under either X-ray or ultrasound guidance.

In most cases 'localisation' involves the insertion of a localisation needle into the breast under image guidance so that the tip is positioned just beyond and adjacent to the tumour. A flexible localisation wire is then passed through the needle and fixed in position with a hook or barb, depending on the type of localisation wire used (there are many different types). The wire remains in the breast with its tip acting as a landmark for the surgeon, who will surgically remove the lesion in question. In addition, the wire tip can often be seen ultrasonically; this can therefore be used to identify the lesion's area in relation to the skin surface to further improve surgical accuracy.

ULTRASOUND IN LOCALISATION

If a lesion is visible ultrasonically localisation is relatively straightforward; it is very accurate, as the 'real-time' imaging means the needle and its relationship to the lesion can be monitored as the needle is positioned and the wire deployed. Alternatively if the lesion is palpable and/or lying superficially within the breast, skin marking with semi-permanent ink is an alternative to wire localisation. This is performed with the patient in a position replicating that of the operating theatre, the skin is marked immediately above the lesion and the distance between the skin and the lesion measured and recorded. This is a totally non-invasive technique.

Ultrasound guidance should be the method of choice for localisation if possible; it is faster than X-ray guidance and adjustments for movement or incorrect needle placement can be made immediately. The patient is spared the discomfort of breast compression and is able to lie supine for the duration of the procedure. Moreover, further irradiation of the breast is avoided.

STEREOTAXIS IN LOCALISATION

If a lesion cannot be seen clearly under ultrasound, X-ray guidance using a stereotactic device is necessary. There are currently two types of stereotactic device available:

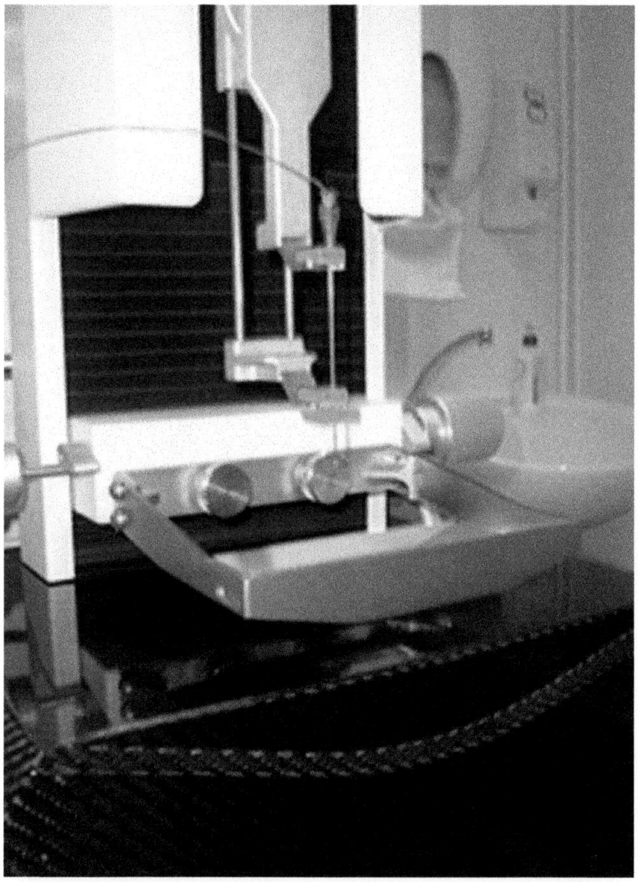

Fig. 25.10 Localisation needle and guidewire positioned in stereotactic unit.

one involves the patient lying prone on a biopsy table and the other is an attachment to an upright mammography unit. Figures 25.9A,B and 25.10 demonstrate the position of the localisation needle in the attached stereotactic unit. For the purposes of this chapter, the upright method will be described, as this is the type most commonly encountered in the UK.

The number of staff involved in the procedure should be kept to a minimum, but there should be sufficient to ensure a high-quality procedure and no compromise to patient safety, i.e. consideration must be given to the fact that the patient must never be left alone. An ideal number of staff is three: the mammographer, the practitioner performing the localisation and a second mammographer or nurse.

Before bringing the patient into the room it is important to ensure that everything is ready for the procedure to begin, thereby minimising any anxiety and distress the patient may feel. Ideally, the procedure should also be explained to the patient before she enters the room. She is then seated in front of the mammography unit and made as comfortable as possible; once positioned in the stereotactic device she will be required to stay still in order to reduce the margin of error when inserting the needle.

The breast position for localisation will have been determined by assessing the location of the lesion from previous mammograms. The patient is then appropriately positioned in the machine and the compression paddle is applied. Once positioned, the patient's comfort is ensured and maintained and the outline of the compression window is marked on her breast. If there is any subsequent movement of the breast this will be easily seen and repositioning can be performed if necessary. It is not easy for the patient to maintain her position as she may have to move her head to facilitate the swing of the X-ray tube. Two stereotactic images of the breast are required, with the tube being moved through an angle of 30° in between each exposure, and the patient position supported and maintained during the tube movement. The two images are displayed next to each other on the digital monitor. The images are checked to ensure that the abnormality is clearly demonstrated on both screens of the monitor. If necessary, the breast is repositioned and further images are taken. Once satisfactory stereotactic images have been obtained the abnormality is 'targeted' on each image and the coordinates of the target are then transmitted to the stereotactic device. The skin is cleansed and local anaesthetic administered before the needle is inserted into the breast through needle guides attached to the unit. The wire is then deployed so that the tip lies just beyond the lesion, and check images are taken in the craniocaudal and lateral positions to check its position. The wire tip must be positioned beyond the lesion so that the surgeon can follow the wire down to the area that needs to be removed. If the wire stops short of the abnormality, the surgeon may have difficulty in locating it.

Once the wire is deemed to be positioned satisfactorily the procedure is complete and sterile dry dressings are applied over the entry site and the wire itself. A detailed report is then written for the surgeon to inform them of the relation of the lesion to the wire tip and the length of wire within the breast. It can be helpful to include a diagram in the report demonstrating the position of the wire within the breast. The surgeon can also view the check images in the operating theatre. The patient is then escorted back to the ward to await surgery.

After surgery the excised tissue is returned for X-ray assessment. The tissue is imaged and, after comparison with the preoperative mammograms, the surgeon is informed by imaging department personnel about the presence of the abnormality within the excised tissue and the proximity of the abnormality to the borders of the tissue. PACS will also enable the surgeon to view images from theatre. This stereotactic procedure is also used to obtain core biopsies of the breast for histological assessment. Lesions biopsied usually include microcalcification clusters and isoechoic masses that may not be visible ultrasonically.

At the time of writing, new localisation techniques which do not involve the use of wires are being trialled in various centres. One such example is the Magseed, which is a metallic seed, smaller than a grain of rice, that can be accurately placed in the tumour up to 30 days before surgery.[34] Magseed is Food and Drug Administration (FDA) cleared in the United States and recently has become Conformité Européene (CE) marked for use across Europe – with the United Kingdom the first market to have access to it.

References

1. Department of Health. *The NHS Plan: A Plan for Investment, a Plan for Reform.* London: HMSO; 2000.
2. Department of Health. *Radiography Skills Mix: A Report on the Four-Tier Service Delivery Model.* London: HMSO; 2003.
3. Banks E, et al. Influence of personal characteristics of individual women on sensitivity and specificity of mammography in the Million Women Study: cohort study. *Br Med J.* 2004;329(7464):477.
4. NICE (National Institute for Health and Care Excellence). Familial breast cancer: classification, care and managing breast cancer and related risks in people with a family history of breast cancer. Clinical guideline [CG164]. www.nice.org.uk/guidance/CG164.
5. Forrest AP. Breast cancer: the decision to screen. *J Public Health Med.* 1991;13:2–12.
6. International Agency for Research on Cancer. *Mammography Screening Can Reduce Deaths from Breast Cancer.* Geneva: World Health Organization; 2002. Press release 139: 19 March.
7. Department of Health. *Cancer Reform Strategy.* London: HMSO; 2007.
8. Lee L, Strickland V, Wilson R, et al. *Fundamentals of Mammography.* 2nd ed. Edinburgh: Churchill Livingstone; 2003:143.
9. Bjurstram N, et al. The Gothenburg Breast Screening Trial. First results on mortality, incidence and mode of detection for women aged 39–49 years at randomisation. *Cancer.* 1997;80:2091–2099.
10. Nystrom L, Rutqvist LE, Wall S, et al. Breast cancer screening with mammography; overview of Swedish randomised trials. *Lancet.* 1993;341:973–978.
11. Shapiro S, Venet W, Strax P, et al. *Periodic Screening for Breast Cancer: The Health Insurance Plan Project and its Sequelae, 1963–1986.* London: Johns Hopkins University Press; 1988.
12. Pritchard J. *Quality Assurance Guidelines for Mammography. Report of a Sub-committee of the Radiology Advisory Committee of the Chief Medical Officer.* Oxford: NHSBSP Publications; 1990.
13. Breast Cancer Care. *Breast Cancer – the Facts*; 2019. [online] http://www.breastcancercare.org.uk/breast-cancer-breast-health/breast-awareness/breast-m8s/breast-cancer-the-facts/.
14. Cancer Research UK. *What Do 'grade' and 's-phase' Mean?*; 2019. [online] http://www.cancerhelp.org.uk/about-cancer/cancer-questions/what-do-grade-and-sphase-mean.
15. NHSBSP (National Health Service Breast Screening Programme). *Review of Radiation Risk in Breast Screening.* Publication No. 54; 2003.
16. Hendrick R, Pisano ED, Averbukh A, et al. Comparison of acquisition parameters and breast dose in digital mammography and screen-film mammography in the American College of radiology imaging network digital mammographic imaging screening trial. *AJR Am J Roentgenol.* 2010;194:362–369.
17. Department of Health. *Cancer Reform Strategy*; 2007. http://www.dh.gov.uk/en/Publicationsandstatistics/Publications/PublicationsPolicyAndGuidance/dh_081006.
18. Mann R, Kuhl CK, Kinkel K, et al. Breast MRI: guidelines from the European Society of breast imaging. *Eur Radiol.* 2008;18:1307–1318.
19. Pater J, Parulekar W. Sentinel lymph node biopsy in early breast cancer: has its time come? *J Natl Cancer Inst.* 2006;98(9):568–569.
20. Goudreau S, Joseph J, Seiler S. Preoperative radioactive seed localisation of non palpable breast lesions: technique, pitfalls and solutions. *Radiographics.* 2015;35:1319–1334.
21. Poplack S, Tosteson TD, Kogel CA, et al. Digital breast tomosynthesis: initial experience in 98 women with abnormal digital screening mammography. *AJR Am J Roentgenol.* 2007;189:616–623.
22. Gur D, Abrams GS, Chough DM, et al. Digital breast tomosynthesis: observer performance study. *AJR Am J Roentgenol.* 2009;193:586–591.
23. Weigel S, Gerss J, Hense H-W, et al. Digital breast tomosynthesis plus synthesised images versus standard full-field digital mammography in population-based screening (TOSYMA): protocol of a randomised controlled trial. *BMJ Open.* 2018;8(5). e020475.
24. Houssami N, Hunter K, Zackrisson S. Overview of tomosynthesis (3D mammography) for breast cancer screening. *Breast Cancer Management. Special Report.* 2017;6(1). https://www.futuremedicine.com/doi/full/10.2217/bmt-2016-0024.
25. Galati F, Marzocca F, Bassetti E, et al. Added value of digital breast tomosynthesis combined with digital mammography according to reader agreement: changes in BI-RADS rate and follow-up management. *Breast Care.* 2017;12:218–222.
26. Bernadi D, et al. Digital breast tomosynthesis (DBT): recommendations from the Italian College of breast radiologists (ICBR) by the Italian Society of medical radiology (SIRM) and the Italian group for mammography screening (GISMa). *Radiol Med.* 2017;122(10):723–730.
27. Bernadi D, et al. Effect of implementing digital breast tomosynthesis (DBT) instead of mammography on population screening outcomes including interval cancer rates: results of the Trento DBT pilot evaluation. *Breast.* 2020;50:135e–140.
28. Maxwell AJ, Michell M, Lim YY, et al. A randomised trial of screening with digital breast tomosynthesis plus conventional digital 2D mammography versus 2D mammography alone in younger higher risk women. *Eur J Radiol.* 2017;94:133–139.
29. NHS Cancer Screening Programmes. *Commissioning and Routine Testing of Full Field Digitial Mammography Systems*; 2019. NHSBSP equipment report 0604. Version 3; Available from: http://www.cancerscreening.nhs.uk/breastscreen/publications/nhsbsp-equipment-report-0604.pdf.
30. NHSBSP Ultrasound Working Group. *Review of the Use of Ultrasound Scanners in the UK Breast Screening Programme.* Publication 43 February; 1999.
31. MDA 1998 Further Revisions of Guidance Notes for Ultrasound Scanners Used in the Examination of the Breast, with Protocol for Quality Testing. Evaluation Report MDA/98/52. London: Medical Devices Agency, (Department of Health).
32. Ciatto S, Rosselli del Turco M, Catarzi S, et al. The contribution of ultrasonography to the differential diagnosis of breast cancer. *Neoplasma.* 1994;41(6):341–345.
33. Teh W, Wilson ARM. The role of ultrasound in breast cancer screening. A consensus statement by the European Group for Breast Cancer Screening. *Eur J Cancer.* 1998;34(4):449–450.
34. http://us.endomag.com.

Further Reading

Hogg P, Kelly J, Mercer C, eds. *Digital Mammography: A Holistic Approach.* New York: Springer; 2015.

Madjar H. *The Practice of Breast Ultrasound.* Stuttgart: Thieme; 2000.

Stavros AT. *Breast Ultrasound.* Philadelphia: Lippincott Williams & Wilkins; 2004.

26 Computed Tomography

BARRY CARVER and MARTINE HARRIS

Introduction

Radiography produces 2D images of 3D objects; it is important to remember that they are shadow projections ('Ex umbris eruditio'). This inevitably means that structures are superimposed and the structure that is the object of imaging may be obscured from view. To address this problem, focal plane tomography was developed shortly after the First World War, blurring out layers above and below the region of interest, to provide an image of the required structure, but again it is 2D and prone to equipment and operating problems. The ideal is a technique that allows for 3D rendition of images.

The advent of X-ray computed tomography (CT) has had a great impact on medical imaging, primarily because CT solves this fundamental limitation of radiography by eliminating the superimposition of imaged structures.

CT uses a rotating X-ray source coupled to a bank of detectors to produce diagnostic images of the body. The basic premise of CT is that the attenuation pattern of the X-rays can be measured during rotation and spatially located; the sum of attenuation at each point can then be calculated and displayed. Since its inception at the beginning of the 1970s CT has undergone significant technological evolution (or development) to become a major technique in the routine diagnosis (or exclusion) of disease, and scanners can be found in almost all hospitals in the UK.

Advantages

Advantages of CT include:

- Axial acquisition of cross-sectional images: with modern isotropic imaging, data can be post processed into multiple planes or rendered volumes, producing 2D or 3D images. Magnetic resonance (MR) is truly multiplanar as scans are acquired directly in different planes without the need for reconstruction; however the quality of CT isotropic reconstructions is high.
- Cross-sectional imaging has excellent low contrast resolution (LCR), which is superior to other imaging methods with the exception of MR, which matches and in some cases exceeds the LCR of CT.
- CT images also show good high contrast (spatial) resolution, and excellent bone detail. MR does not image bone directly due to the lack of free hydrogen within cortical bone.
- Digital imaging: this enables the manipulation of images, as well as post processing to other planes; the applied reconstruction algorithm and window settings can be adjusted to better visualise specific tissues. The application of filters and digital processing can enhance content, e.g. the use of edge enhancement for looking at bone or lung tissue.
- CT is generally well accepted by patients, certainly more so than MR, which is less well tolerated due to noise and claustrophobia. Contraindications for MR due to safety requirements do not apply to CT.
- CT is still more readily available than MRI and radionuclide imaging (RNI), being in situ in the vast majority of acute hospitals and imaging centres in the UK and supplied by a number of independent sector providers.

Disadvantages

Disadvantages of CT include:

- Due to its nature, CT is undeniably a high radiation dose technique and its increased use worldwide means that it contributes significantly to the total effective dose from medical imaging. Several dose reduction techniques have been introduced to optimise examinations, but radiation doses vary widely. Multiple examinations may approach the thresholds for deterministic radiation effects; for example cataract formation, as a result of the cumulative lens dose from a series of head CT scans, has been reported.[1]
- Metallic artefacts cause loss of image detail; this effect is much reduced by software corrections on many modern scanners.
- Soft tissue structures surrounded closely by bone can be difficult to image, e.g. in the posterior fossa, where the soft tissue contrast of MR is superior. This is again a problem largely overcome in the latest generation of scanners.
- Misregistration artefact can be caused by relative movement of the body structures from the acquisition of one single slice to the next, e.g. due to inconsistencies in the patient's respiratory pattern. If misregistration occurs then the reconstruction will be meaningless, as the same portion of anatomy could be portrayed at different positions in the reconstructed image. With the advent of single breath hold scanning this is now less of a consideration. Traditionally, when scanning two areas such as the chest and upper abdomen, many centres have overlapped the two acquisition blocks to ensure no loss of information due to breathing differences between the two acquisitions. There are, however, dose implications for this technique which are worthy of consideration. To solve problems of misregistration and unnecessary additional radiation exposure, most manufacturers now offer fast acquisition protocols that allow a single scan through the entire volume.

In some quarters there is an attitude that CT can be undertaken by anybody, including non-radiographically qualified staff, such as departmental assistants. It can be argued, however, that, along with every other branch of imaging, CT is operator-dependent. Image quality is dependent on factors that should be adjusted for each examination and, more important, for each patient. In addition, due to the high dose burden, all operators of CT equipment should be trained and skilled in optimising CT examinations.[2] Indeed, specific additional training requirements are mandatory in some countries, such as the United States[3]; unfortunately, the need for requirements such as this can be only too evident.[4]

Equipment Chronology

1874 Sir William Crookes constructs the cathode discharge tube. During his experiments over the next few years he discovers fogging of photographic plates stored near discharge tubes.

1895 Wilhelm Roentgen discovers X-rays whilst investigating gas discharge using a Crookes' tube.

1935 Grossman coins the term 'tomography' describing his apparatus for looking at detail in the lungs.[5]

1951 Godfrey Hounsfield starts work at EMI, initially working on early computers.

1956 Ronald Bracewell uses Fourier transforms to reconstruct solar images. At the same time Alan Cormack starts to work on solving 'line integrals'.

1958 Korenblyum and colleagues in Ukraine work on obtaining thin section X-ray images using mathematical reconstructions.

1961 William Oldendorf produces an image of the internal structure of a test object using a rotating object. He was unable to make further progress due to the lack of available equipment to provide the computation that would have been required.

1963 Cormack publishes a paper on mathematical reconstruction methods.

1965 David Kuhl, one of the pioneers of radionuclide imaging, produces a transmission image using a radioactive source coupled to a detector.[6]

1967 Bracewell produces a mathematical solution for reconstruction with fewer errors and artefact than found with Fourier.
Hounsfield and Ambrose come together to develop CT head scanning. Hounsfield uses an iterative algebraic technique rather than more complex mathematical formulae.

1971 The first clinical CT scanner is installed at Atkinson Morley Hospital (UK) under the supervision of James Ambrose. The first patient is scanned on 1 October. The first scanners were somewhat crude and took several minutes to produce each slice, which were of fairly poor quality. However, at the time, even these crude images were revolutionary, enabling a first non-invasive glimpse within the skull, at the soft tissue contents.

1972 Ambrose and Hounsfield discuss the clinical use of CT at the British Institute of Radiology annual conference.[7] Clinical images are shown at RSNA.

1973 Hounsfield and Ambrose publish papers describing the design and clinical applications of the CT system.[8,9]
EMI scanner becomes commercially available.
Hounsfield starts work on the second-generation scanner.

1974 Hounsfield produces abdominal images with a 20-second acquisition time.

1975 EMI CT 1010 second-generation scanner becomes available, soon to be followed by the CT 5005 – the first EMI body scanner.
In the next few years, third generation scanners become available but have problems with artefact; a problem solved by General Electric (GE). Fourth-generation scanners were later introduced to avoid the artefact problems initially suffered by the third-generation machines.

1979 Hounsfield and Cormack are awarded the Nobel prize for medicine.

1983 The first 2-second scanner introduced by GE (CT 9800).

1985 Electron beam CT developed.

1989 Siemens introduce spiral (helical) CT, using slip ring technology to enable the tube to rotate continuously without the need to go back to unwind its cables.

1992 Elscint Twin scans 2 slices simultaneously, which is a return to a method used by the original EMI scanners.

1998 Multislice CT initially incorporating 4 slices is introduced; GE, Picker, Siemens and Toshiba displayed systems at RSNA. Since then 8, 16, and on up to 320 … slice machines have become available. Sub-second scan times enable body areas to be scanned in a single breath hold. Advancements have in many cases had to wait on the development of computer systems robust enough to cope with the huge quantities of data generated, a problem initially encountered by Oldendorf.

2005 Siemens launch dual energy scanners, opening the potential for characterisation of chemical make up of materials via simultaneous imaging at different kV values.

2007 Toshiba launch Aquilion One 320 slice, ending the numbers game? Enables single rotation imaging of entire organs due to 16 cm coverage.
Further developments have built upon these foundations. As mentioned above, CT systems have been classified according to the motion of the X-ray tube and detectors during scanning. There have been several generations of CT scanner, which are described here in brief.

FIRST-GENERATION SCANNER (FIG. 26.1)

The first-generation CT scanner utilised a single pencil beam of X-rays being measured by a single detector. In order to cover the area of interest, the movement required is a combination of translation and rotation. In the initial position, the tube/detector assembly moves across the scan field of view (translation) and a series of measurements of transmitted intensity are made. It then rotates 1° to its next position before commencing another translation.

This is a very time-consuming method and typical scan times were of the order of 4 to 6 minutes per slice acquisition. The early scanners attempted to compensate by having two detectors to perform 2 slices at once, a technique now resurrected in the latest generation of spiral scanners that offer 'new' multislice acquisition.

- Advantages: It was the first of its kind and offered the first opportunity for axial imaging of the head.

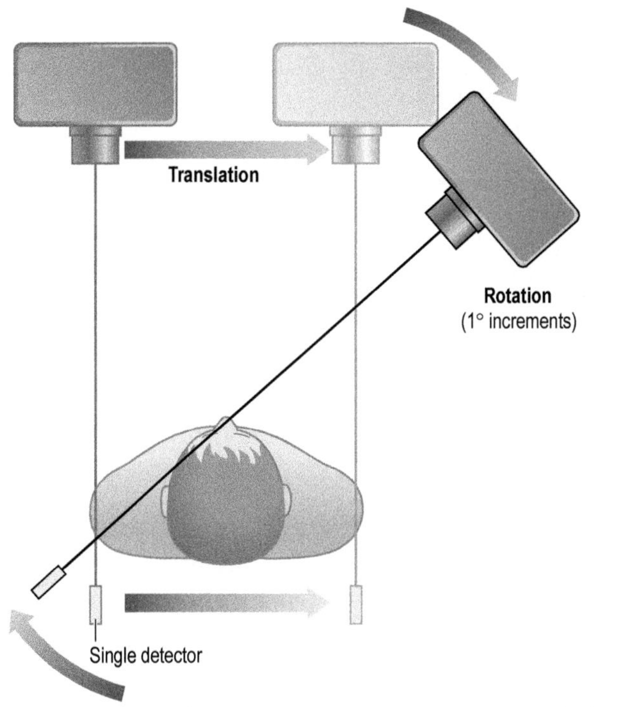

Fig. 26.1 Schematic of first-generation scanner.

- Disadvantages: Mechanically complex, slow scans, which were only practical for scanning the head of patients who could be adequately immobilised using a water bag. The water bag was used to reduce the range of information required as its density is closer than air to that of tissue.

SECOND-GENERATION SCANNER (FIG. 26.2)

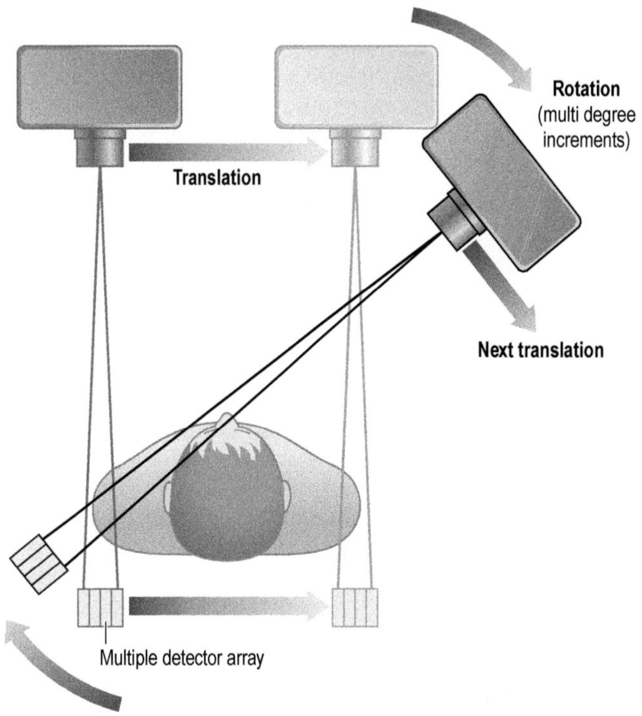

Fig. 26.2 Schematic of second-generation scanner.

The second generation used the same principles of movement as the first generation, i.e. a combination of translation and rotation, but utilised several innovations. Instead of a pencil beam, a narrow fan beam was now utilised, being measured by a bank of detectors. The fan beam is still not sufficient to cover the entire area of interest so translation and then rotation is still required, but because more information is being gathered at each position, multiple degree rotational incrementation is possible.

- Advantages: As several detectors were being utilised, scanning times were significantly reduced and quality was increased. Typical scan times of the order of 20–80 seconds per slice were achievable. Again 2 slices were acquired simultaneously on the EMI 1010 with a fixed slice thickness of 13 mm
- Disadvantages: The maintenance of the translate–rotate movement renders these scanners still mechanically complex.

THIRD-GENERATION SCANNER (FIG. 26.3)

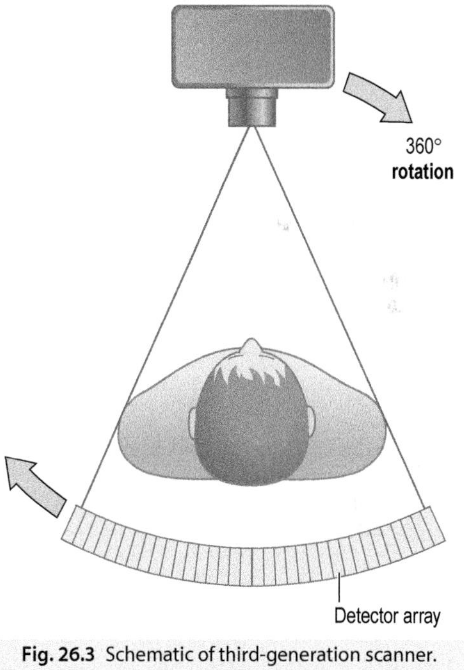

Fig. 26.3 Schematic of third-generation scanner.

Also known as a rotate–rotate scanner, this model was the first to do away with the requirement for translation across the patient by utilising a wide fan beam of X-rays. A large number of detectors (up to 1000) are used to allow for the increased beam width, and the tube and detectors are rigidly coupled and rotate jointly about the patient. Rotation only is required as the fan beam covers the entire body. It is this configuration that is still the most commonly used, even in the latest multislice and dual source equipment.

- Advantages: The greater number of detectors plus the rotation only movement allows shorter scan times, typically of the order of 2–8 seconds. The width of the fan beam can be adjusted (collimated) to limit the beam to the area under examination. Use of the rotation only

movement renders this type of unit mechanically simpler than its predecessors.
- Disadvantages: Detectors were expensive, therefore more detectors equals more cost. Also more processing power is required, as more information is gathered at one time. Initially problems were encountered with circular artefacts but this was overcome by adjusting the detectors.

FOURTH-GENERATION SCANNER (FIG. 26.4)

This scanner was similar to the third generation scanner; again using a wide fan beam, but with a complete circle of detectors around the patient. In this case only the tube rotates, with the detector ring being stationary.

- Advantages: Mechanically simpler due to having fewer moving parts. Scan times reduced and now taking 1–10 seconds.
- Disadvantages: The high number of detectors equals high cost. There were also greater calibration difficulties. As the tube is rotating within the detector ring, the detectors are further away from the patient leading to a greater penumbral effect.

ELECTRON BEAM COMPUTED TOMOGRAPHY (EBCT)

A completely different concept, the electron beam is directed to the anode rotating around the patient, and is again linked to a bank of detectors. As mechanical rotational movement is now not utilised, quick (50 ms) scans are possible. EBCT has been used for gated cardiac studies for some time. This was the only CT technology that could provide high-quality cardiac imaging for several years, but now commonly available multislice and dual source equipment can match EBCT in cardiac studies.

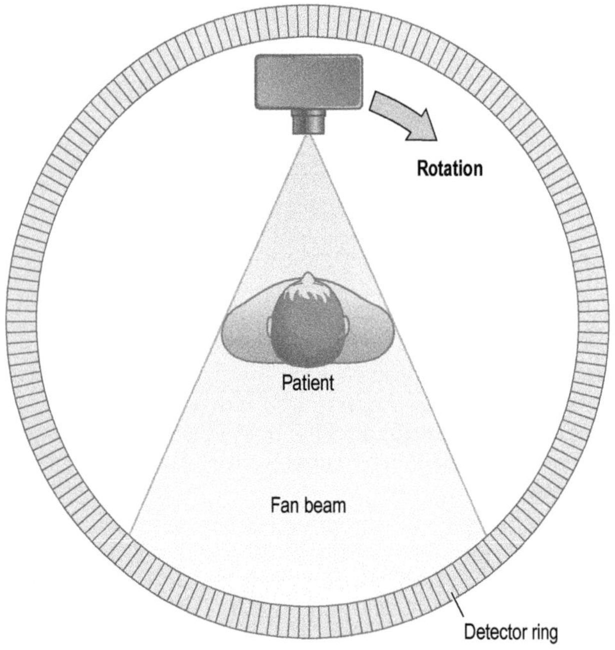

Fig. 26.4 Schematic of fourth-generation scanner.

SPIRAL/HELICAL CT

Helical scanners are also described as volume acquisition or spiral scanners. For clarity, the term helical will be used throughout this chapter.

In the 1990s, 'conventional' CT began to be replaced by helical scanners. Due to cost, availability and equipment replacement programmes, it was only in the late 1990s that these became the norm in the UK. Ironically, this occurred just as this technology itself was superseded with the introduction of multislice helical scanning.

Helical scanning differs from conventional CT in the method of data acquisition. Instead of a single 360° rotation that produces a single slice followed by an incremental table movement, in helical scanning, a volume of data is acquired.

One of the main advantages of this method of continuous data acquisition is its speed. As a large volume of data can be acquired very rapidly, a series of images that would take several minutes to acquire in conventional 'slice by slice' mode, can now be obtained in seconds.

This is due to both the use of slip ring technology, enabling continuous rotation of the X-ray tube around the gantry (without the cables which previously had to be 'unwound' by a return rotation prior to the next slice being obtained), and also improvements in the design of the tube and its drive motors enabling sub-second acquisition times.

This rapid data acquisition means that large areas of the patient can be imaged within a single breath hold, eliminating one of the major problems for image reconstruction and interpretation: misregistration. Respiratory misregistration can be completely eliminated, and the short scan times make it less likely that patient movement becomes a factor.

MULTISLICE CT

The greatest advance in scanner design was the multidetector volume acquisition scanner, ironically a return to one of the features of the original EMI scanner – multiple detector arrays. The difference is that the first EMI scanner had two rows of one detector, whereas the latest multislice scanners have tens of thousands of detector elements. The majority of scanners are of the third-generation type with rotating tube and detector array.

Large volumes can be rapidly imaged with thin slice widths enhancing the diagnostic capacity of CT. Large numbers of thin slices can be reconstructed to produce high quality volume-rendered images, with the elimination of 'stair step' artefacts, and the reduction of partial volume artefacts.

Advantages

Advantages of multislice CT include:

- Speed of acquisition – sub-second rotation speeds are now the norm.
- In comparison to single slice helical, multislice enables the same acquisition in a shorter time, or larger volumes to be scanned in the same time, or for thinner slices to be scanned.
- All manufacturers have sub-millimetre scan capabilities. Toshiba have detectors that are 0.5 mm, matching the

pixel size to produce a voxel that is the same size in each dimension, termed isotropic. Isotropic and near isotropic voxels enhance the 2D reformatting ability of the scanner, enabling high-quality multiplanar reconstructions from an axial data set. 3D reformats produced are also excellent, with none of the problems of possible misregistration and information loss inherent in MR due to its longer scan times.

- Modern multislice CT scanners have improved temporal resolution which allows sub-second high-quality imaging of dynamic anatomy, e.g. cardiac CT. However, functional analysis is better performed with MR.

WIDE DETECTOR CT

The next logical step after multislice CT was to develop wide area detector CT systems which allow expanded coverage of the body (up to 16 cm per tube rotation) in the z-axis and the opportunity to dynamically image visceral organs and bony joints. Wide detector CT eliminates the need to perform multiple acquisitions through a single organ such as the heart, which also improves motion and respiratory artefact. A reduction in the time taken to cover the area of interest potentially enables higher-quality imaging in patients who find it difficult to remain still for the duration of the scan, such as paediatric and trauma patients. Despite proven image quality and test accuracy benefits,[10] there are theoretical disadvantages to wide-detector imaging in terms of patient exposure and radiation dose efficiency. This is due to 'over- ranging' and changes to the shape of the X-ray beam aligned to the detector area. However, manufacturers have endeavoured to mitigate these issues and optimise the benefits.

DUAL SOURCE CT (FIG. 26.5)

An alternative strategy for increasing the speed of scan acquisition has been a new generation of dual source CT scanners. In these systems, a configuration of two X-ray tubes at an off-set of 90° on the CT gantry, and two corresponding adaptive array detector banks, rotate around the patient. Data is acquired twice as fast as single source scanners and there is greater flexibility in terms of modes of operation and the combination of two data sets acquired at the same anatomical level at the same time. This is particularly useful in cardiac imaging whereby each tube-detector coupling only needs to supply 90° of data to complete a 180° sinogram. Data from one cardiac cycle only is required to reconstruct an image and temporal resolution less than 100 milliseconds (ms) can be achieved regardless of heart rate.

These systems are also specifically designed to allow fast simultaneous scanning at low and high tube kilovoltage (kVp). The use of different X-ray spectra allows material decomposition of various chemical elements in the body based on absorption mechanisms.[11]

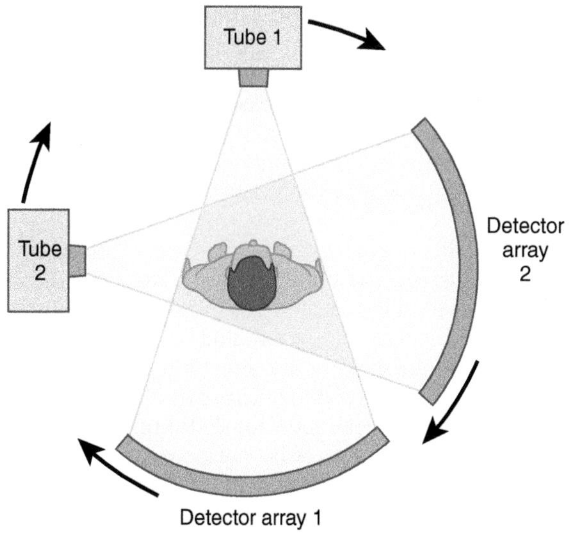

Fig. 26.5 Schematic of dual source scanner.

Equipment

THE X-RAY TUBE

Use of helical scanning, with its continuous rotation, means that huge demands are placed on the X-ray tube used in modern scanners. The tube needs to provide high output, whilst dealing effectively with dissipation of the heat produced. Air conditioning is generally required to maintain a comfortable temperature within the scan room and to assist with heat dissipation. Large anode discs in metal or ceramic tube envelopes are common, the anode usually being mostly graphite with a tungsten/rhenium target track.

BEAM SHAPING FILTER

In any CT scanner the X-ray beam produced is in fact heterogeneous, having a range of energies. Filters are applied to the beam on exiting the tube to reduce the range of energies. Filters also shape the beam to produce a more uniform result at the detectors in order to reduce the dynamic range required in the detector electronics.

COLLIMATORS

In a single slice system, a pre-patient collimator will limit the beam to the prescribed slice width at the centre of rotation; a post-patient collimator will then limit the beam incident on the detectors to the slice width. For example, pre-patient collimation to 4 mm will result in a 4 mm slice being produced.

In a multislice system, the beam is again collimated at the centre of rotation but the result will differ. For example, in a 4 slice system the 4 mm collimation given above will result in 4×1 mm slices being obtained.

TABLE

The table is an important element in CT. The table is usually of carbon fibre construction with rise and fall action; this gives strength without interfering with the resultant image, and facilitates patient handling. The table must be able to provide a wide range of movement at various speeds. Accuracy of movement is vital as any inconsistency would have detrimental effects on the image produced.

Table-tops are generally curved, except for those tables used in radiotherapy planning where a flat table-top is essential to allow CT simulation. Simulation needs to reproduce accurately the patient's position on the flat treatment table. Consequently, scanners used for both purposes will often have interchangeable table-tops for diagnostic and planning sessions.

DETECTORS (FIG. 26.6)

Modern detectors are of the solid-state type, mostly employing ultra-fast ceramic detector elements. An incident beam causes scintillation; the photon produced is then converted to an electrical signal by a photodiode and sent on to the electronics. The aim of any CT detector is to be accurate, stable and geometrically efficient. Image quality factors such as spatial resolution, artefacts and signal to noise ratio are influenced by the speed of detector response to X-ray excitation, low levels of afterglow after the X-ray source is turned off, cross-talk between detector elements and optimisation of light output and quantum detection efficiency.[12] The detector array is formed by a series of individual elements, as shown in Fig. 26.6.

Different manufacturers have differing approaches to the format of detector arrays, e.g. 16 slice, as can be seen in Fig. 26.7. The choice of array format affects the minimum slice width available, the number of slices available at minimum width, and the range of slice widths available.

DATA ACQUISITION SYSTEM (DAS)

The DAS 'reads' the measurements from the detector array, converts these analogue signals into digital format, and transmits the digital signal to the computer systems for reconstruction into the presented images.

The DAS needs to be able to deal rapidly with a vast amount of data being generated every second; development of these systems has been a limiting factor to the speed of development of larger and larger multislice arrays.

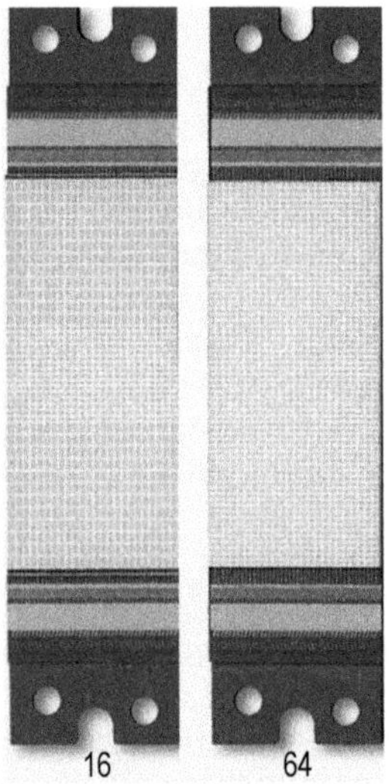

Fig. 26.6 Aquilion 16 and 64 detector arrays. Both provide up to 32 mm coverage per rotation. The 16 slice detector has 16×0.5 mm elements centrally, with 12×1 mm elements either side, enabling acquisition of 16×0.5 mm or 16×1 mm or 16×2 mm slices per rotation. The 64 slice detector provides 64×0.5 mm slices per rotation. (Reproduced with permission from Toshiba Medical.)

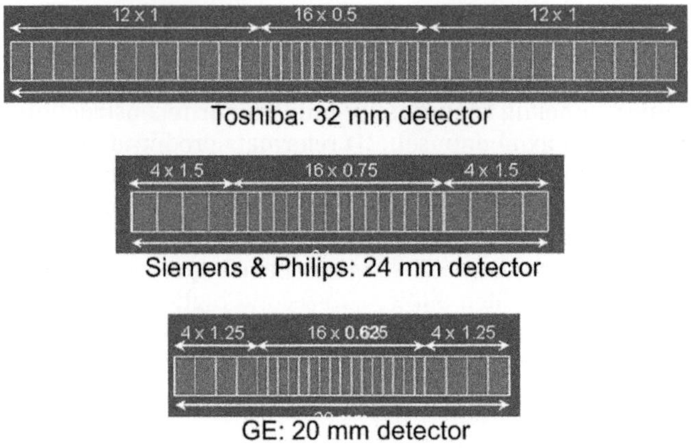

Fig. 26.7 Comparison of 16 slice detector arrays.

COMPUTER SYSTEM

The computer system processes operator input to set scanning parameters, patient information and archiving instructions. It also receives the information from the DAS which is then processed to form the image. A wide range of post processing options are available on modern scanners which again take place within this system, or alternatively on dedicated workstations. High-speed, high-capacity computers are required to perform these tasks at speeds that were unthought of until relatively recently, although for millennials these are part of everyday life.

Archiving requires some consideration; although archiving systems have greatly increased in capacity (and decreased in cost), the amount of data generated has also exploded. Only selected reconstructions are generally sent for storage and access on picture archiving and communication system (PACS); raw data, if stored, is often on high-capacity storage systems.

Physical Principles of Scanning

What happens to a homogeneous X-ray beam as it passes through an object? The X-ray photons interact with the material through which they pass and are attenuated by it. If the intensity of the emerging beam is measured, we know the initial intensity, hence the attenuation within the object can be measured.

With the X-ray tube of a CT scanner in one position, a narrow X-ray beam passes through the patient and the attenuation along the line taken by a particular beam through the patient can be calculated from the intensity of the emergent beam measured by a detector. The X-ray intensity transmitted through an object along a particular path contains information about all the material it has passed through, but does not allow the distribution of the material along the path to be discerned.

For the energies used in CT the attenuation of the beam is due to:

- Absorption: photoelectric
- Scattering: Compton (mainly)

Attenuation due to photoelectric absorption is strongly dependent on the atomic number of the material (αZ^3).

Attenuation due to Compton scattering does not depend upon atomic number, but on the number of free electrons present. The number of electrons per gram of an absorber is remarkably constant over a wide range of materials, however because their density varies considerably, the number of electrons per metre does show variation across a range of biological materials. It is this difference between attenuation processes which enables differentiation of chemical composition in dual energy equipment.

If we consider the simplistic case of a homogeneous beam passing through the medium, the attenuation within the tissues follows the Lambert–Beer law, which states:

$$I = I_0 e^{-\mu x}$$

where:

μ = linear attenuation coefficient
I_0 = original intensity
I = transmitted intensity
x = thickness of material

In CT we are interested in measuring the linear attenuation coefficient. Solving the Lambert–Beer equation for LAC, we get:

$$\mu = \frac{1}{x} . \ln\left(\frac{I_0}{I}\right)$$

I is measured by the detectors, I_0 and x are known, hence μ can be calculated.

As mentioned earlier, the X-ray beam produced is in fact heterogeneous, having a range of energies. Filters are applied to the beam on exiting the tube to reduce the range of energies incident on the detector array.

Traditionally a narrow beam was required for accurate localisation of the attenuating tissues. Readings are taken from multiple angles to give a series of values of linear attenuation of the beam along intersecting lines through the patient. For example, in Fig. 26.8, a bony object would have the same attenuating effect on 'beam 1' whether at position 'A' or 'B'. However, with the addition of 'beam 2' it is possible to localise the structure to position 'B'.

In general, then, the transmitted intensity depends on the sum of the attenuation coefficients for all points along the path of the beam. Thus, the log transmission measurement is sometimes referred to as a 'ray sum' or 'line integral' of the attenuation along the path.

A radiograph can be considered to be composed of many such ray sums, produced unidirectionally, hence superimposing all structures encountered by the beam. Because of the differences in transmitted intensity, interfaces between bone, tissue and air are well demonstrated. The differences between adjacent soft tissues are not sufficient for good differentiation and hence they are less well demonstrated.

To demonstrate soft tissues we need to eliminate superimposition by taking ray sums from multiple directions; these ray sum measurements can then be mathematically reconstructed to generate an axial image, formed by estimating the distribution of the linear attenuation coefficient within the irradiated volume. The image produced can then be digitally manipulated to maximise contrast, enabling adequate visualisation of subtle changes in tissue density.

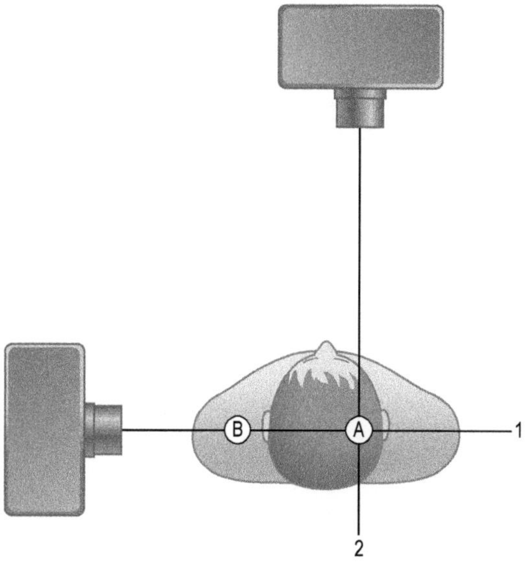

Fig. 26.8 Localisation of position.

The ability to produce such images is the main strength of CT as an imaging modality.

The information acquired by the detectors is passed to the computer. Once this data is committed to the computer memory it can be manipulated by the resident software to produce an image that is reconstructed on the screen of the viewing console. Reconstruction takes place via the application of a complex linear mathematical algorithm to the data obtained, traditionally this has been through a filtered back projection (FBP). Consideration of the detail of this mathematical process is beyond the scope of this chapter, but is well described in texts such as Seeram.[13]

Image reconstruction in its simplest form consists of recalling the digital information fed to the computer from the detectors via the DAS, and converting this information to an analogue voltage signal which controls the electron sweep within the display monitor.

Helical image reconstruction is more complex: because the table is continuously moving only one ray sum lies in the scan plane, the rest of the 'slice' information is interpolated from the acquired volume. 360° and 180° interpolations are used; a 360° interpolation requires data from two tube rotations for slice reconstruction, 180° interpolation allows smaller slice widths to be accurately reconstructed.

Multislice is more complex again, as it uses two or more data samples to produce each point within a projection, but the basic principles are the same. There is, however, an additional complication in that the more slices that are scanned, the wider the beam becomes in the *z* direction (along the patient length), meaning the beam ceases to be a narrow fan as seen in conventional and helical scanners; in multislice, the volume of data is the volume between two cones (Fig. 26.9). Each of the manufacturers has different mathematical methods for 'cone beam' correction; the complexity of the multislice reconstruction process is again beyond the scope of this chapter but is addressed in specialist texts.

The amount of movement within the data set is governed by the table movement, and is measured as the scan pitch. Helical pitch is defined as:

Pitch = 'table travel per rotation/nominal slice width'

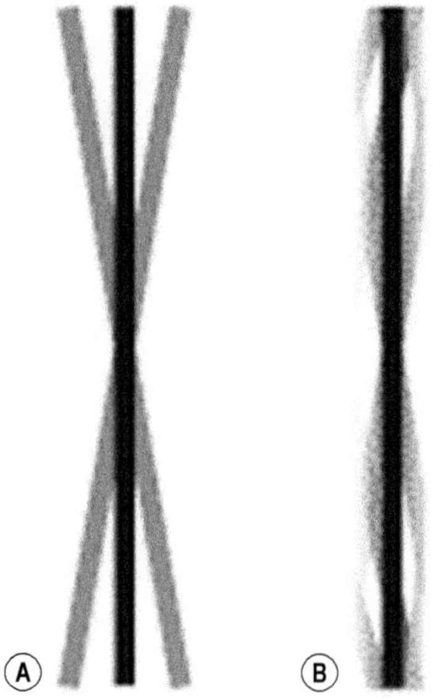

Fig. 26.9 Cone beam problem. (A) A wide X-ray beam is required to give full coverage of the detector elements. The beams produced at opposing angles form a cone; the slice profile is sharp at the centre but spatial resolution is lost at the edges due to 'cone beaming'. (B) For example, Toshiba's TCOT algorithm calculates these complex angles to provide a more accurate slice profile.

There are two definitions for pitch quoted in multislice, each of which provides a different number to represent pitch; it is therefore important to know which definition is in use when comparing techniques:

Pitch = 'table travel per rotation/X-ray beam width'

or

Pitch = 'table travel per rotation/detector width'

The data is stored within the computer as a matrix of intensities. The image produced consists of a matrix of cells with various brightness levels on the display monitor; the brightness of each cell is related to the intensity detected.

Each image square (or *pic*ture *el*ement) is called a pixel. The value of the number represented in each cell is relative, and is used to define image contrast. In CT the numeric information contained in each pixel is a CT number (or Hounsfield unit: HU) and is expressed relative to the density of water. The detector array is calibrated to give a zero value for water.

Each of these 2D picture elements represents a volume of patient data, the volume element, or voxel, and is equal to the pixel size × slice thickness (Fig. 26.10). If the voxel is the same size in each direction then it is called isotropic. This is the ideal for multiplanar reconstruction as the blocks are effectively the same when viewed from any direction, hence maximising the quality of reconstructions.

The size of image matrix used is determined by the characteristics of the equipment, and the storage capacity of the computer. The size of the image matrix is important as the more squares there are to form the image, the greater will be the image definition.

Measurement of the CT number of an object in an image can be useful for tissue characterisation, as by comparing it to known values such as those in Table 26.1 we can get a feel for the composition of the material (although a definitive tissue diagnosis cannot be made).

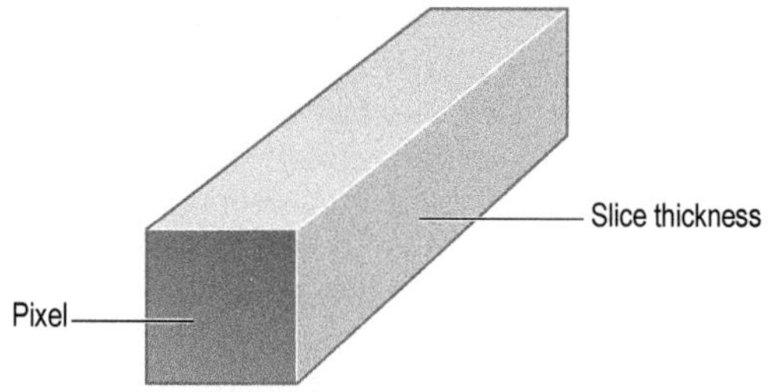

Fig. 26.10 Pixel and voxel.

TABLE 26.1 Hounsfield Unit Values for a Range of Tissues

Tissue Type	Hounsfield Unit
Air	−400+
Fat	−95
Water	0
CSF	10
Oedema	20–30
Clotted blood	30
White matter	30
Grey matter	35–55
Muscle	40–80
Kidney	50
Liver	60
Fresh blood	70
Calcification	~125
Cortical bone	1000

WINDOWING

The displayed image will comprise areas of high X-ray attenuation, shown in white; and low attenuation, shown in black. The intervening soft tissues will be shown in various shades of grey according to their individual attenuation properties.

As CT is sensitive to small changes in density, use can be made of the variation in shades of grey represented on the image to give better contrast discrimination. The image can be viewed on a variety of chosen settings to better view the particular structures of interest. This is termed 'windowing'.

The window level is set to the tissue of interest – this will place the tissue of interest in the midpoint of the grey scale. The window width is set to enable the required range of tissues to be viewed, and straddles the window level evenly. For example, a window width of 400 set with a window level of 40 will include tissues with HU values from −160 to 240. Anything below −160 will appear black, whilst anything above 240 will appear white. The shades of grey on the image will divide the 400 units to be demonstrated.

As window width is increased, each grey-scale shade represents a greater number of attenuation values, so more tissues are seen, but with a reduction in image contrast. Thus the image appears flat, i.e. it has an overall grey appearance. Lower window widths enable tissues of closer attenuation values to be discriminated so small changes in density may be seen. The image will be of high contrast, i.e. it has more black and white. Low widths make the noise inherent in the image appear more apparent.

Introduction of contrast media can raise the attenuation values of soft tissue structures. It is important to then adjust the window level accordingly to ensure the tissues of interest remain in the centre of the grey scale and that structures that need to be visualised remain within the range of the selected window width.

Thresholds can be set using specific HU values to produce a range of data sets to provide a variety of image types on modern scanners, e.g. maximum intensity projections (MIPs). Colourised images can also be produced on the workstation to delineate different structures, particularly in 3D, and surface-rendered images, for example.

Image Quality

It has previously been stated that CT can be considered to be an operator- or user-dependent modality; this is because the user has a direct influence on the quality of the images produced and, as will be discussed later, the radiation dose administered to the patient. Given the potential for the administration of high doses within CT, adequate training of appropriately qualified staff is essential.

The greatest influence on image quality results from the choice of scanning factors, which includes mA, scan time, slice thickness and kVp. These parameters essentially determine the number of photons emitted from the X-ray tube and registered on the detector, which in turn determines the noise level, which has a detrimental effect on image quality.

Noise is superimposed over the whole image as a uniform grainy appearance and is dependent on the number of photons reaching the detectors (signal to noise ratio). Several factors influence the noise level on the image, the primary ones being slice thickness, patient size and applied mAs. In order to obtain good-quality images, noise should be kept to a minimum. However, there is a trade-off to be made: images can be produced with almost no noise, but at the cost of increased dose as the noise level is related to the applied mAs. Noise varies as $(1/\text{dose})^{1/2}$, and consequently doubling the mAs applied (and therefore patient dose) only reduces noise by factor of about 1.4.

The influence of slice thickness has changed, particularly with the higher-end scanners (16 or more slices). Conventionally, thick slices would be used for general soft tissue use. More photons contribute to image quality so noise is lower, a larger area is covered more quickly, the dose is reduced and examination time is faster. Thinner slices were reserved for areas where high resolution was required; fewer photons contribute to the image, therefore noise level is higher, and to achieve a similar image quality to the thicker slice, the dose administered needs to be increased to improve the signal to noise ratio. More slices are also needed to cover the same area so dose is increased but resolution improves.

With more recent multislice units, the beam collimation is equivalent to a thick slice on a single slice unit (Fig. 26.11), so we have the benefits of a thick slice but can reconstruct very thin slices from this irradiation of the patient.

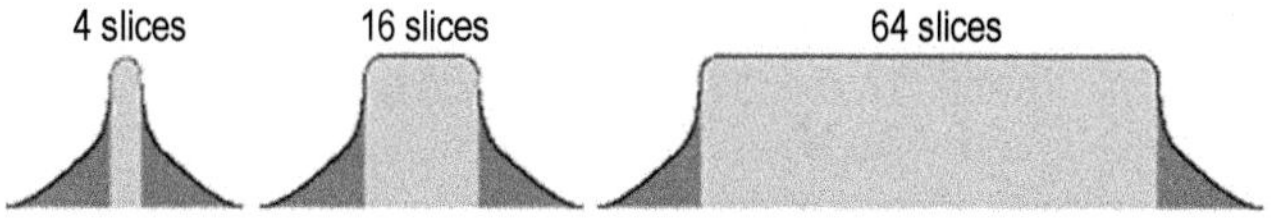

Fig. 26.11 Multislice *z* axis dose profiles. In single slice scanners the X-ray beam is a close match to the imaged width. 'Overbeaming' occurs in multislice scanners as there is a non-uniform beam distribution, but each detector requires equal beam intensity. The 'overbeamed' portion of the dose profile (generally a few mm – dark shading) can be seen for each scanner type. As the number of slices increases the proportion of excess radiation decreases with respect to the total profile, so the greater the number of slices the greater the 'overbeamed' dose efficiency.

For example, if we consider a 16 slice scanner with a detector array of 0.5 mm elements, an 8 mm collimation (thick slice on a standard helical scanner) can yield 16×0.5 mm images (very thin slice).

Reconstruction algorithms or filters are applied to the image reconstruction in conjunction with factors such as slice thickness, so that optimal image quality is obtained. They too affect the amount of noise and spatial resolution in the final image.

Increasing kVp provides greater penetration, hence this should be considered when scanning areas of higher attenuation; this can be utilised instead of, or as well as, increases in applied mA, depending on the patient habitus/anatomical area being examined.

Artefacts are patterns on an image that are not on the original object. There are many causes of CT artefact such as motion, metal, beam hardening and partial volume effect. Motion artefacts have been greatly reduced due to the rapid acquisitions available in multislice, in particular. The ability to scan whole body areas in a single breath hold has great advantages.

Some metals absorb X-rays producing radiation shadows; this results in a streak artefact in the reconstructed CT image. Where practicable, all metal objects such as jewellery, coins and clothing with metal fasteners should be removed in order to prevent this effect. This must, however, be balanced against the psychological needs of the patient. Only if the objects are likely to be situated within the scan field should they be removed. There is no need to change every patient into a hospital gown and indeed it is better for patient comfort and dignity if they can remain dressed wherever possible.

Beam hardening artefact appears as a streak artefact on the image. As the X-ray beam is heterogeneous on entering an object, particularly if it is high density, the lower energy photons are absorbed. This increases the effective energy of the beam, so adjacent soft tissues are more easily penetrated. This is also seen in non-circular areas such as the shoulder and pelvis where the attenuation is greater along the long axis, producing directional noise. This can be addressed by adaptive filters and correction software.

Partial volume artefact is caused by structures being partially included in the scan thickness. Each voxel represents an average attenuation value for the structures in that slice; if a high attenuation structure (e.g. bone) is partially included in a voxel, that voxel will have an average value higher than its surroundings, producing an error in reconstruction. This is avoided by the use of thinner slices (structures are then less often partially included) or volume artefact reduction software provided by several manufacturers. Truncation artefact occurs where parts of the anatomical area being imaged lies outside the FOV, e.g. with bariatric patients.

CT Safety: Dose

In a little over 40 years, CT has progressed from giving the first glimpse of imaging of cranial contents to the potential to replace planar radiography. However, with all CT examinations, the overriding concern is that of dose to the patient.

In 1989 in the UK it was reported that 20% of the dose from medical examinations was from CT, which at the time accounted for just 2% of examinations.[14] By 2018/19 this had grown to almost 70% of the dose and 13% of examinations.[15]

The introduction of multislice scanners produced an increase in patient dose as the first scanners of this type were less dose-efficient than single slice equipment due in large part to 'overbeaming' (see Fig. 26.11). With the production of more efficient detectors and increasing numbers of slices creating a greater effective slice width, this dose increase has been reduced.

Concern is warranted as tissue doses resulting from CT are amongst the highest used in diagnostic imaging. Repeat examinations can produce dose levels which approach and may exceed levels at which increased incidence of cancer has been observed,[2] hence the arguments put forward regarding hormesis and reduced risk from radiation exposure[16,17] do not apply to CT.

Effective dose equivalent (EDE) is, in many circumstances, the quantity used to describe patient dose, but due to the complex manner of its calculation it is difficult to assess for individual patients in CT. There is a requirement for recording of doses and those typically used in CT are the computed tomography dose index (CTDI), and dose length product (DLP), both of which can be used for approximation of EDE.

The first line of approach to dose reduction is to ensure appropriateness of the examination; CT must be the imaging modality best suited to answer the clinical question. In the UK there is a requirement for all complex examinations, such as CT, to be vetted and justified by a practitioner experienced in the imaging modality.[18] Given the greater capabilities of modern scanners, there is a wider variety of examinations and techniques available; multiphase contrast examinations should not be routine and should be used only for those clinical situations for which they are the most appropriate.

The operator can have a significant effect on administered dose through the principle of optimisation, with up to 50% reduction achievable by use of appropriate parameters, including automatic exposure control, reinforcing the case for appropriate training.[2] Auto exposure controls include kVp and mA modulation to match beam quality and quantity to patient body part. This can be achieved in a variety of ways. Two scout views can be used to assess the patient size, and then vary the mA slice by slice during the scan. Another alternative is using feedback from the previous rotation to determine the signal received by the detectors and alter the mA accordingly.

To appropriately manage radiation doses scanning techniques should be adopted that are not only tailored to the patient but also to the clinical task. This is of particular importance when implementing noise reduction techniques such as iterative reconstruction. The computational algorithms underlying these are considered proprietary although they share a common mechanism of dose and image quality optimisation through noise suppression and artefact reduction. The most sophisticated algorithms utilise artificial intelligence (AI) but all consider the physics of image acquisition, photon statistics (noise), properties of the object and geometry of the CT system. However, unlike traditional FBP algorithms, noise reduction techniques such as iterative reconstruction use non-linear operations that influence noise variance and image texture. Their use in low-contrast imaging and other specific clinical questions must be considered carefully through multidisciplinary experimentation.[19,20]

Despite the availability of these dose reduction measures, without proper training and awareness it has been reported that they often can be unused.[21]

Patient dose can be increased by failure to alter scan parameters to match the individual patient, especially in **children**, who **should not be scanned using adult protocols**.

Common Clinical Applications

CT is widely used in imaging virtually every anatomical region and the full range of clinical applications of CT is a text in itself. The following section therefore considers major areas for discussion; it is not intended to be a thorough evaluation of all CT applications. The use of CT in paediatrics is necessarily limited by the radiation burden, which is more significant due to the greater radiosensitivity of children's tissues. This is a specialist topic that will not be considered in detail within this chapter.

It would be inappropriate to attempt to be prescriptive regarding detailed protocols for examinations. In any case the differences in requirements of single slice compared to 16 slice and in turn both of these to 320 slice are such that this would not be possible.

As CT is a user-dependent modality, protocols vary widely and must take into account local preferences. In view of the high radiation burden associated with CT, any local variations should, however, fall within the framework of accepted best practice, with evidential support, rather than being simply an individual clinician's preference. It was previously reported that differing techniques for the same examination in different institutions have the potential to increase (or reduce) doses by a factor of greater than four;[22] this amount of variation is clearly unacceptable. The UK national dose survey in 2011 reported that dose reference levels remain broadly the same as for 1999, and there remain wide variations in technique for the same examination, and care needs to be taken regarding optimisation.[23]

The objective of the individual examination must always be considered, the objective being to provide the referring clinician with sufficient diagnostic information to enable the appropriate clinical management of the patient. Contrast enhancement is a good example of this; with modern scanning equipment it is possible to perform an initial unenhanced scan followed by multiphasic studies. Initial unenhanced images may not aid the answering of the clinical question and can therefore be omitted; the number of phases of contrast-enhanced scans should then be limited again to those that will address the clinical question for each individual patient, rather than blindly following a 'routine' protocol.

PREPARATION FOR THE EXAMINATION

Due to the association of CT with cancer (*CT – 'cancer test'*) it is important to remember that preparation is both mental and physical. A good explanation of the procedure can allay the patient's nervousness, which may be due not only to fear of the examination but also its result. Both European[24] and UK legislation[25,26] stipulate the need to provide 'adequate information' relating to the benefits and risks associated with radiation dose before exposure and the UK professional body has provided employers and staff with supporting guidance to fulfil these statutory requirements.[27]

The patient may be changed into a hospital gown, depending on departmental protocol, but if this is not necessary in order to remove artefacts from the scan field then consideration should be given to scanning the patient without having to undress to avoid depersonalisation.

As discussed in Chapter 20, any checks required for intravenous (IV) contrast administration should be made as appropriate. Here again there is a wide variety of local practice, particularly around administration to asthmatic patients, those with known renal insufficiency and to diabetic patients taking metformin. There will be a number of prophylactic measures taken by centres to ensure the safe use of iodinated IV contrast media both pre and post administration.[28,29]

For abdominal scanning the patient may be starved for several hours prior to the scan to avoid the appearances of food in the stomach, although starving may increase associated anxiety. An oral contrast medium is given at some centres to outline the bowel, which is typically administered at least an hour before scanning to allow transit. Increasingly, negative contrast is used, e.g. water, often for looking at the stomach, and this is finding increasing popularity in other abdominal examinations. Water has the advantages of being cheap, readily available and well tolerated by the patient.

'SCOUT'

For almost all examinations the first image taken is a scout (also called topogram, surview, scanogram). The X-ray beam and detectors are kept stationary as the patient moves through a thin, collimated beam of radiation. Dependent on anatomy and equipment, this projection may be performed as an AP, lateral, or both.

The scout is used for localisation and scan selection. Gross abnormalities may be demonstrated; also presence of metal or other artefacts may be seen. Dependent on the system, the single view or combination of two scouts will be used for calculation of mA modulation to reduce dose. This requires some thought on the part of the operator, for example when performing cranial CT and not utilising mA modulation: is it appropriate to perform two scouts? The reason for each aspect of every examination needs to be considered in order that the 'as low as reasonably practicable' (ALARP) principle is maintained.

USE OF IV CONTRAST

The high speed of modern equipment enables contrast enhancement to be viewed in multiple phases: arterial, portal venous, venous and delayed. As previously stated the selection of which phases are to be performed should be dictated by the clinical question to be answered.

Non-ionic iodinated contrast media delivered via a pressure injector is the norm; with the option to use a fixed timing delay related to the area of interest, use of test bolus to determine peak enhancement or bolus tracking of the contrast medium. When coupled with scanner software, accurate timing of contrast delivery is relatively straightforward. Again the dose implications of such methods must be considered; for example, if observing contrast build up in a region of interest, is it necessary to begin observation scans at the same time as starting the injection? Can the interscan delay be made longer to produce fewer of these scans but maintain an optimal start for the diagnostic scan?

Traditionally, contrast media volumes have been administered using a fixed-dose protocol that was related to the area of interest being scanned. However, in light of better scanner technology and knowledge of renal safety, many centres have now moved to a weight-based protocol, which means a reduced dosage of contrast media in the majority of cases. In a study looking at abdominal CT in 2016, George et al[30] were able to demonstrate that weight-based protocols (coupled with appropriate injection rates) could provide more consistent vessel and visceral enhancement and subjectively improve image quality.

CT angiography is made possible; multiplanar reconstruction, maximum intensity projections, 3D and surface-rendered images are easily created on the typical workstation. Large areas of anatomy can be demonstrated in a manner that is less invasive than conventional angiography, using less contrast and providing extra luminal information of the surrounding tissues and organs.

MAJOR TRAUMA

In the evaluation of major trauma, modern CT is invaluable, as it facilitates rapid and thorough evaluation of the head, neck, thorax, abdomen and pelvis. Imaging of patients who have suffered major trauma has changed radically following experience gained on the battlefield of recent conflicts, particularly Afghanistan.[31] NICE guidance[32] now advises that patients over the age of 16 who have suffered blunt major trauma, and suspected multiple injuries, should have whole body CT. They recommend a scout from vertex to toes, which together with clinical findings can be used to direct requirement of CT of the limbs, followed by a scan from vertex to mid thigh. There are many variations to this protocol in the literature and online: non-contrast coupled with contrast, biphasic/multiphasic etc. Example protocols are supplied within guidance from RCR;[33] typically patients are scanned head/neck + chest/abdomen/pelvis/and as far down the legs as possible.

It is recommended that this protocol should not be used for those aged under 16, where *'clinical judgement should inform the required areas for assessment'*.[32] Indeed it has been suggested that whilst whole body CT has been shown to improve mortality for adults, the benefit in children is 'unclear'.[34] Where contrast examinations of the abdomen are undertaken in children the 'Bastion protocol' for contrast administration should be used; this can be found in RCR guidelines,[35] and online, e.g. at the website of the British Society of Paediatric Radiology.[36]

BRAIN

CT is the investigation of choice in the trauma setting where bony injury and intracranial haemorrhage (ICH) are more readily demonstrated, and also for the investigation of acute stroke and paranasal sinus disease, although MR should be used for the staging of neoplasia prior to resection. Perfusion imaging is available for the demonstration of blood flow, particularly in the immediate investigation of stroke; as described in Chapter 23, the size of infarct and volume of ischaemic but viable brain tissue can be determined.

In head injury, CT is the investigation of choice where there is a suspicion of a clinically important brain injury. The Canadian Head CT rule[37] was adopted by both NICE[38] and the RCR[39] for their guidelines.

Patients presenting with acute stroke should be scanned as soon as possible (preferably within 1 hour), as per the national clinical guidelines for stroke.[40] The information required for appropriate treatment is whether or not the stroke is haemorrhagic, as this informs treatment options. In several centres radiographer reporting of cranial CT is utilised to assist with rapid diagnosis. Commonly, imaging will include non-contrast brain imaging and CT angiography for those where mechanical thrombectomy is an option ± perfusion where clinically available. This is designed to facilitate swift, appropriate treatment for this group of patients. Research has shown that rapid intervention can have significant results.

It *must* be remembered that:

'Stroke is a medical emergency. With active management in the initial hours after stroke onset ischaemic brain may be saved from infarction.'[41]

Common Indications

- Trauma
- Acute stroke
- Transient ischaemic attack (TIA)
- Space occupying lesion (SOL)
- Acute severe headache (suspected subarachnoid haemorrhage (SAH))
- Sinus disease

The use of CT for vascular studies of the head is covered in Chapter 23.

Typical Protocol

Lateral scan projection radiograph (SPR) from the skull base to vertex is commonly taken and used for planning axial slices/volume. In multiple trauma cases, the cervical vertebrae may be included.

In general, thinner slices are acquired through the posterior fossa which has often not been well visualised on CT. MR is superior if posterior fossa pathology is suspected. Whilst some centres still commonly performed cranial CT using sequential scans, there has been a move towards performing thin spiral scans to allow validated measurements to be reported for a number of clinical questions. Raw data is reformatted into the required slice thickness. Modern 64+ slice systems in particular demonstrate the posterior fossa well; thin slices are combined for viewing and provide good axial demonstration of this area. Isotropic or near isotropic multiplanar reconstructions are also readily produced.

Patient positioning for cranial CT has been the subject of debate. Many centres use a volume acquisition, typically planned parallel to the hard palate, enabling multiplanar reconstructions. The 'standard' approach has been to use the 'supraorbital baseline'; slices are planned parallel to a line running between the external auditory meatus (EAM) and the superior orbital ridge. The reasoning for this is to reduce the dose to the lens of the eye by not scanning through the globe. In practice, this is often badly performed as can be seen by the eyes being present on the lowermost images of many scans. This baseline exacerbates the problems of visualisation of the posterior fossa which is not optimally demonstrated.

The commonest alternative is the anthropological baseline, whilst irradiating the orbit, it does better demonstrate the posterior fossa, and the path of the optic nerve. This method is in use in some specialist neurocentres. The use of Bismuth shields has previously been suggested, but in common with other methods of contact shielding discussed in Chapter 3, is no longer recommended.[42]

Whichever baseline is to be used, and however the scan acquired, thought needs to be given to patient positioning in order to minimise the use of gantry angulation, which is to be avoided due to the potential to introduce artefacts in the posterior fossa and increase patient dose.[43]

Cranial CT is usually performed without the addition of contrast media. A second scan post administration of contrast is useful in some acute circumstances. The exception to this is in scanning for metastases when a single contrast-enhanced scan is usual; referral for MRI should also be considered subject to availability.

Cranial CT reporting by radiographers is a role development which has been demonstrated to be a feasible means for addressing radiologist shortages and of providing waiting list reduction. Studies have shown high accuracy rates are achievable after a suitable course of training,[44,45] and radiographers have taken on this role in some centres.

With multislice technology in particular, there is no longer any requirement for additional direct coronal scanning for e.g. paranasal sinuses, as high resolution reconstructions of ENT anatomy can be obtained in any plane (Figs 26.12 and 26.13). The effect of this when looking at fluid levels does, however, need to be considered.

SPINE

CT is of limited application other than in the case of trauma. Its use is mandatory in cases of cervical spine trauma and must be performed as soon as possible (preferably within 1 hour) where risk factors are identified and plain radiography findings are equivocal or have failed to demonstrate the cervicothoracic junction (see Chapter 9 for further discussion). CT is increasingly replacing plain radiographic imaging, particularly in cases of major trauma and/or when the patient is undergoing cranial CT. In the case of thoracic or lumbar trauma with neurological deficit, CT can be used to demonstrate bony detail.

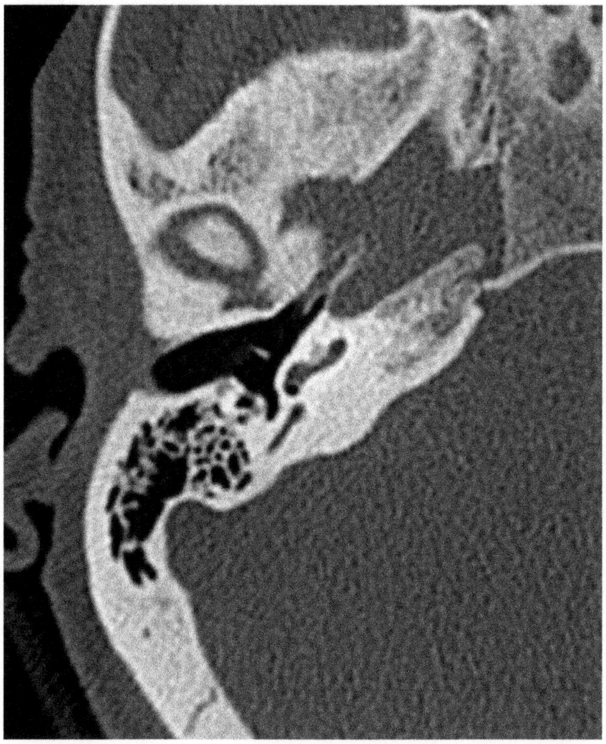

Fig. 26.12 **Cranial CT – high-resolution imaging of the temporal bone.** (Reproduced with permission from Toshiba Medical.)

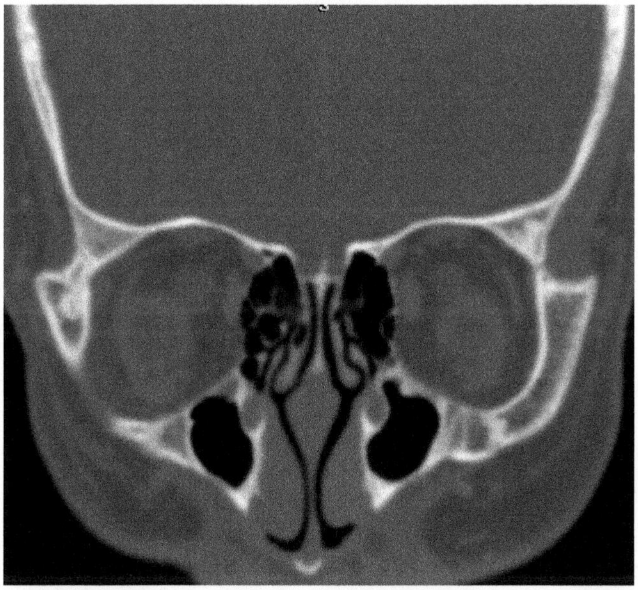

Fig. 26.13 **Cranial CT – coronal reconstruction used for viewing sinuses or facial bones.** (Reproduced with permission from Toshiba Medical.)

MRI is the investigation of choice for spinal pathology because of its greater soft tissue resolution and its ability for multiplanar imaging of the cord.

NECK

CT may be used for the staging of tumours in the neck and larynx; however, in the main, MR is better in this area and should be used where available. Protocols may exist

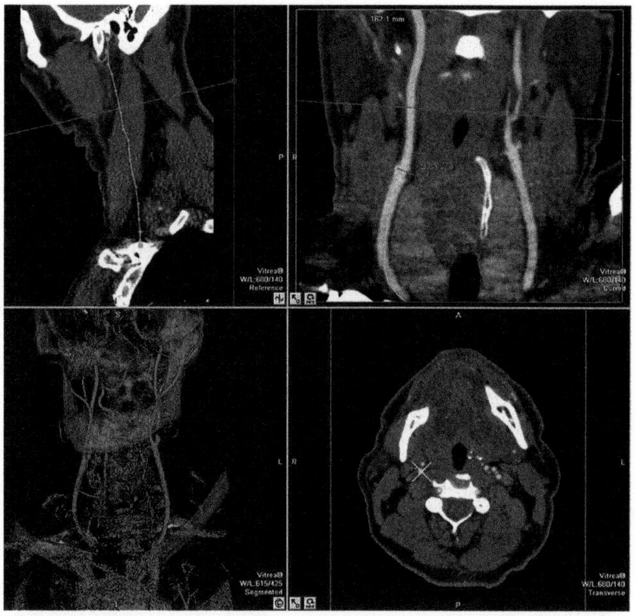

Fig. 26.14 **Neck CT – workstation images of carotid study.** (Reproduced with permission from Toshiba Medical.)

for salivary glands, vocal cord palsy, nodes and abscesses, although other investigations are generally used for the diagnosis of lesions in the neck. Carotid studies can be performed, as shown in Fig. 26.14.

CHEST

Justification for CT examination of young females should be particularly robust considering the potential for breast cancer induction.[46] It has previously been suggested that consideration should be given to the application of breast shielding, however this is not universally accepted and some advisory bodies do not recommend its use,[47] and techniques such as dose-modulation modes, which selectively limit the radiation exposure to sensitive organs, are more effective.

Staging of both chest primary lesions and metastatic spread from other primary sites in association with a chest radiograph, is a commonly seen utilisation of CT in this body area. Generally the thorax and upper abdomen are scanned; this is to enable assessment of upper abdominal lymphadenopathy and to view the adrenals and liver, particularly for metastatic spread. CT has high accuracy rates and can facilitate biopsy. Positron emission tomography (PET) is used in conjunction with CT within this context.

Nodal disease is well visualised. Specific sites in which nodes are often seen are the aortopulmonary window in the subcranial and perihilar regions and retrocrural area (Fig. 26.15). Multiplanar reconstructions can be helpful in interpretation, as can the use of varying window settings, and techniques such as the use of MIPs (Fig. 26.16).

High-resolution CT (HRCT) is used for detailed evaluation of the lung parenchyma. When scanning using thin slices on high end multislice equipment, utilising lung windows effectively provides 'free' HRCT imaging, which again can be reconstructed into any desired plane.

There has previously been debate on the use of 'low-dose' CT as a screening tool and several international projects are running to determine its impact[48] after Aberle et al[49] reported reductions in mortality from both lung cancer and all causes (20% and 6.7% respectively) in comparison to chest radiography.[50] Whilst CT may increase detection of early tumours, there is a high rate of detection of nodules which require follow-up with standard dose high resolution CT to classify them as benign, or otherwise, and prevent the requirement for unnecessary intervention[51] (approximately 23% of screened patients had nodules, and 2.7% had a malignancy in one large study).[52] The requirement for a second scan with 'normal' dose rates makes such screening costly, both financially and in terms of dose burden, particularly to asymptomatic patients. If patients with benign nodules are then followed up with interval scans the potential for extremely high dose burdens is clear.

It has been suggested that there is no difference in survival rate between patients with solitary lesions of 1 cm or 3 cm on diagnosis.[53] Further evaluation of the utility of CT screening is ongoing.

Rapid scan times enable visualisation of the entire thorax in a single breath hold, eliminating the previous problems associated with respiratory misregistration. Utilising software to optimise the timing of IV contrast injections, the area can be scanned in arterial phase, enabling demonstration of vascular structures in the thorax. CT is also the examination of choice for the investigation of pulmonary embolus. High accuracy rates are achieved even with lower doses of contrast media and the examination can, if required, be coupled with an examination of the upper legs for underlying deep vein thrombosis (Fig. 26.17). Dual energy scans enable accurate calculation of perfusion defects. Use of lower kV_p (80) has been shown to be effective for CT pulmonary angiography (CTPA), producing dose benefits without loss of image quality.[54]

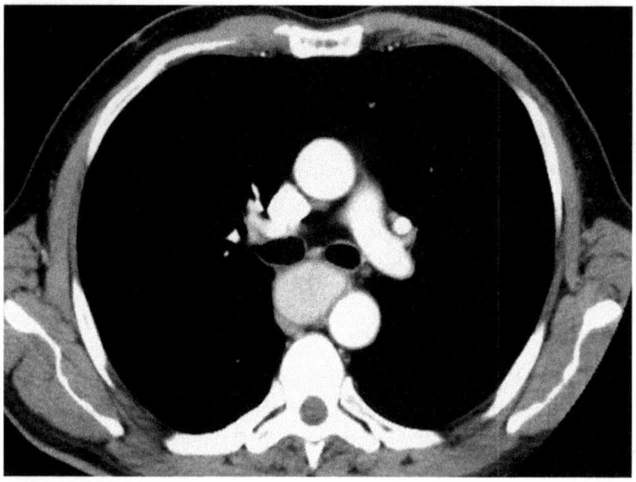

Fig. 26.15 CT thorax – axial slice through thorax. Excellent arterial contrast enhancement is seen on this image. (Reproduced with permission from Toshiba Medical.)

CARDIAC CT

Another use for fast scan times is in imaging of the heart. This has been described as the ultimate goal for multislice CT. Electrocardiogram (ECG) gating techniques enable high-quality imaging of the heart and associated vascular structures in as few as 3–5 cardiac cycles. Image quality now matches and in some cases exceeds that of EBCT, and availability of multislice scanners has certainly become more widespread than EBCT has been. Several indications exist for the use of cardiac CT, including chest pain, pre- or post-surgical intervention, coronary anomalies or failed catheter coronary angiography. The heart can be scanned via prospective or retrospective modes dependent on stability of heart rate; however, there are dose considerations with the latter. Dual source systems enable more rapid visualisation enabling temporal resolution to be reduced to 40–80 ms, comparable to that of EBCT (50 ms).[55]

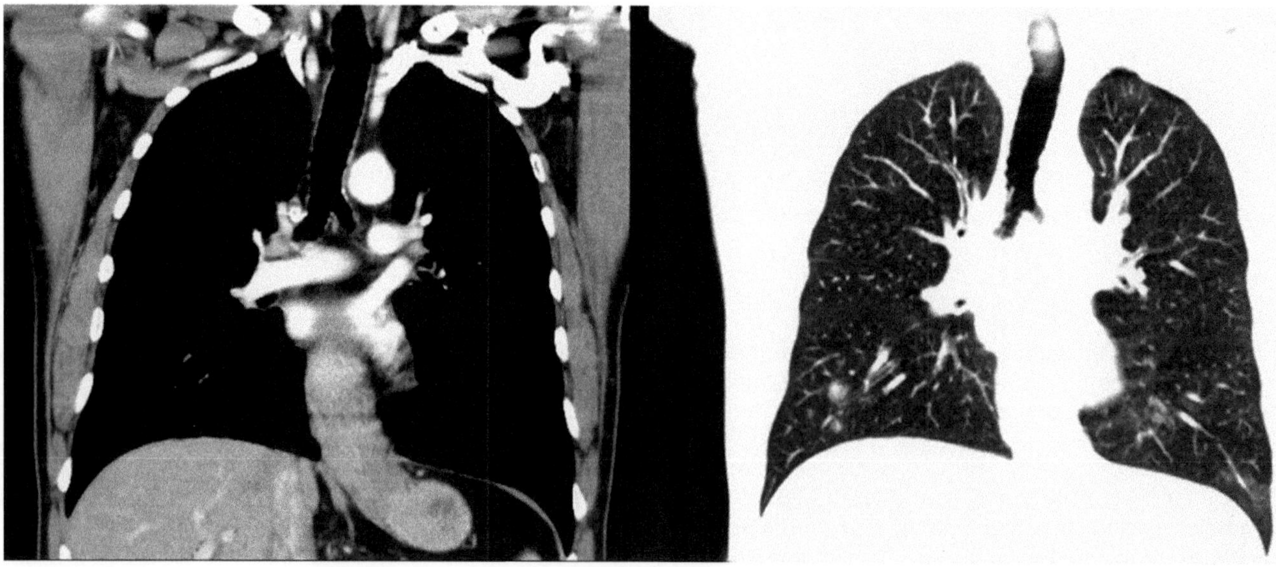

Fig. 26.16 CT thorax – coronal reconstructions viewed on 'soft tissue' and 'lung' windows. (Reproduced with permission from Toshiba Medical.)

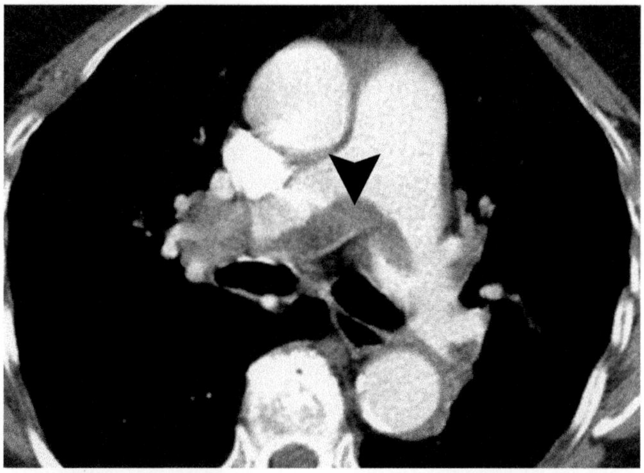

Fig. 26.17 CT thorax – PE scanning demonstrating saddle embolus (*arrowed*).

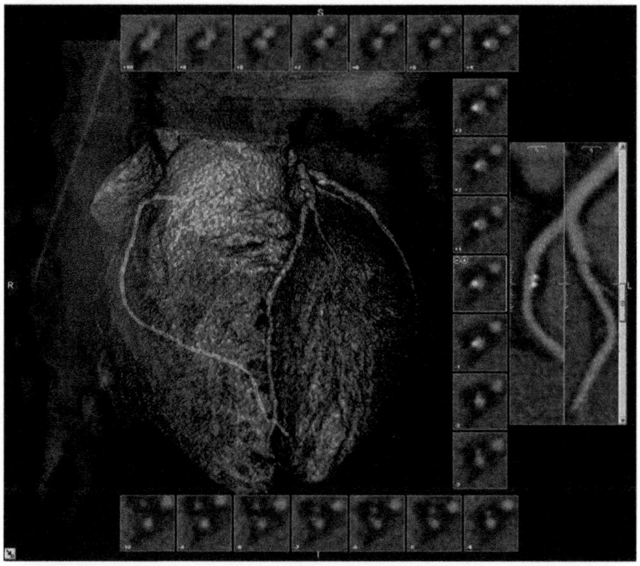

Fig. 26.18 Cardiac CT – CTA. High-quality 3D reconstruction from a 32 slice scanner. The sternum and great vessels can be seen semitransparent on this image. Curved reconstructions demonstrate the selected vessel which can be viewed 'sliced' in any direction. (Reproduced with permission from Toshiba Medical.)

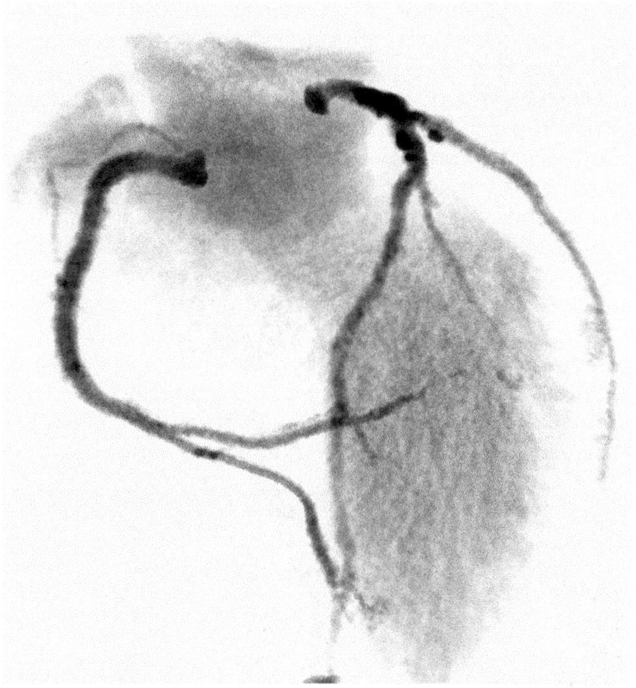

Fig. 26.19 Cardiac CT – CTA. The image here is manipulated to provide an 'angiographic' appearance. (Reproduced with permission from Toshiba Medical.)

Coronary artery calcium scoring has been in use for some time, and is used to provide an indication of the presence and amount of atherosclerotic plaque, enabling the detection of potential disease prior to the development of symptoms such as angina and dyspnoea. High-resolution, non-contrast scans are obtained and volumetric analysis used to produce a calcium score. This quantitative score can then be compared with a database of known scores adjusted for age and gender, and appropriate advice given on risk of coronary artery disease.

The information gained from calcium scoring does not give a direct measure of arterial narrowing, but has good correlation with the severity of underlying disease. It does not rule out the presence of soft non-calcified plaque. Whilst useful for patients with specific risk factors, screening remains impractical due to dose and cost.[56] Dissection, aneurysm and coarctation of the aorta can also be assessed, as well as the structure of the heart itself, often using the same gated techniques as cardiac CT to avoid misregistration (Figs 26.18 and 26.19). Such structural information can also be obtained using MRI, which should be considered as an alternative where available.

CTA is in widespread use and, with 320 slice machines now available, may even be used in some patients with atrial fibrillation, which has previously been a contraindication.[57]

ABDOMEN

Abdominal CT is a common examination that has a high diagnostic yield, but equally a high radiation dose burden. It is the examination of choice for nodal staging of many malignancies, including lymphoma. Whilst CT is generally thought to be the 'better' examination in cases of suspected abdominal mass, sepsis or pyrexia of unknown origin, ultrasound should be performed first. Ultrasound may yield the required information to answer the clinical question without the high radiation dose associated with abdominal CT, particularly in young adults. Both imaging methods may be used to facilitate image-guided biopsy, or drainage, or therapeutic radiofrequency ablation (RFA).

GASTROINTESTINAL TRACT

Oesophageal perforation may be demonstrated on a contrast barium swallow; however use of CT will enable the additional demonstration of complications in surrounding tissues. CT is also used for staging of oesophageal and stomach tumours; the primary tumour may be visualised and any local or nodal spread demonstrated. Water is useful as a negative oral contrast in this case as it enables visualisation of the stomach wall which may be partially obscured by the use of positive oral contrast media (Fig. 26.20).

In adults with acute abdominal pain, CT may be used to establish the cause and level of obstruction. Colonic lesions are well demonstrated by CT colonoscopy, with full and thorough bowel preparation results compare with direct colonoscopy. The use of reconstruction techniques such as virtual colonoscopy allows for comparable images but with the advantage of visualisation of involvement choice external to the lumen. CT is widely used as the investigation of choice as discussed in Chapter 21. CT colonoscopy forms an important part of the National Bowel Cancer Screening Programme (NBCSP) in England as CT also facilitates staging of lesions within the same examination (Figs 26.21–26.23).

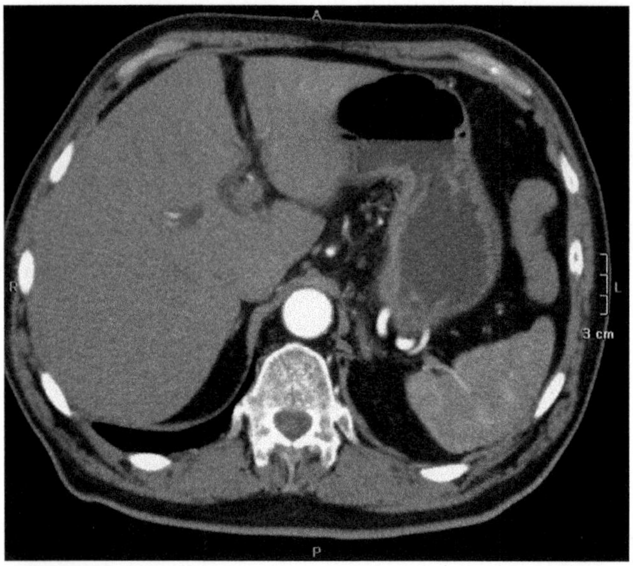

Fig. 26.20 CT of gastrointestinal tract (GIT). Use of water as negative contrast enables visualisation of the stomach wall. (Reproduced with permission from Toshiba Medical.)

LIVER (FIG. 26.24)

CT is far more sensitive than ultrasound (US) and is commonly used for staging prior to resection, although US is again usually the first-line investigation for diagnosis. The soft tissue contrast sensitivity of MR makes it the investigation of choice for staging of primary lesions, and if available, should be considered for the evaluation of metastases.

Although MR has become the most commonly used modality, where there are contraindications three-phase post-contrast techniques are useful for diagnosis and pre-surgical staging of liver metastases, which are the most frequently occurring malignant tumours of the liver. Many liver lesions look similar pre-contrast and can look similar at different timings following injection. The use of precontrast scans has been questioned for some time; both its utility and dose implications must be considered. CT can also be used in the investigation of cirrhosis, demonstrating fatty infiltration, and also to characterise possible haemangioma; the use of MRI should be considered in these cases.

KIDNEYS AND ADRENAL GLANDS

The adrenals are commonly scanned in association with the thorax for bronchial staging as they are a common site for metastatic spread from a lung primary (Fig. 26.25). Where further characterisation of adrenal lesions is required, MR is now often the examination of choice, particularly in young patients. Unenhanced CT of the kidneys, ureter and bladder (KUB) region has replaced the intravenous urogram (IVU), in the investigation of choice for renal colic and detection of calculi. It should be performed with reduced exposure factors as it has been shown that diagnostic accuracy can be maintained with a low dose protocol.[58] Following ultrasound and normal cystoscopy, the CT urogram is now often performed for visible haematuria and visualisation of upper renal tract pathophysiology, as well as follow-up of transitional cell and bladder tumours.

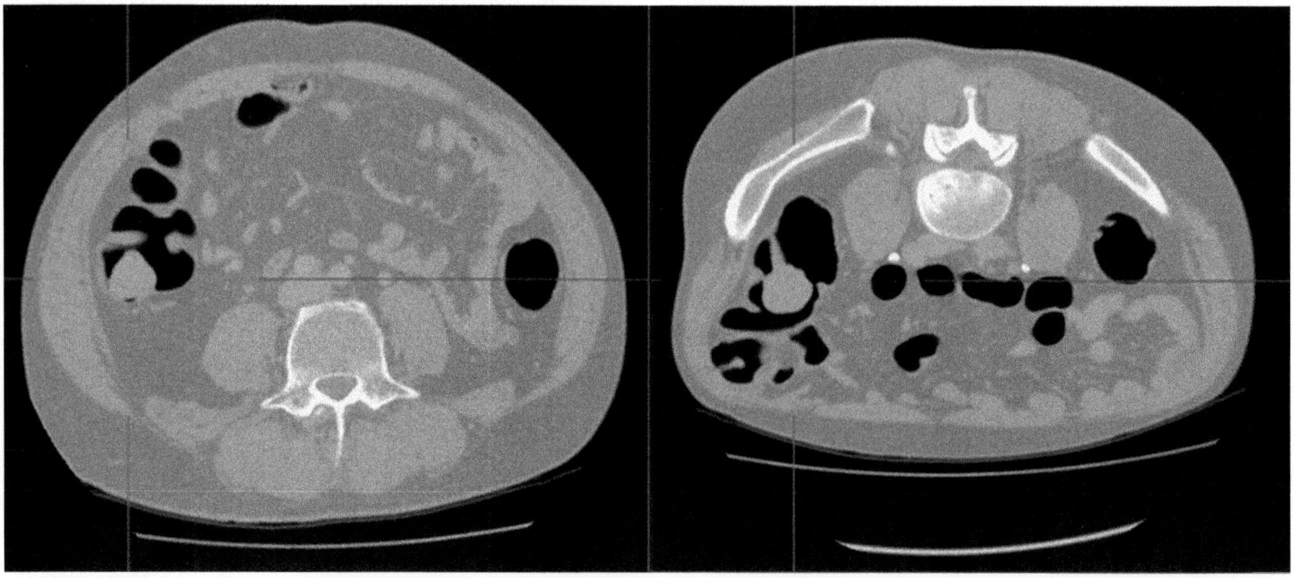

Fig. 26.21 CT of GIT – colon. Axial scans can visualise pathology external to the colon. A polyp is seen in the ascending colon. On the prone view the polyp has moved anteriorly under gravity and its stalk can be seen. (Reproduced with permission from Toshiba Medical.)

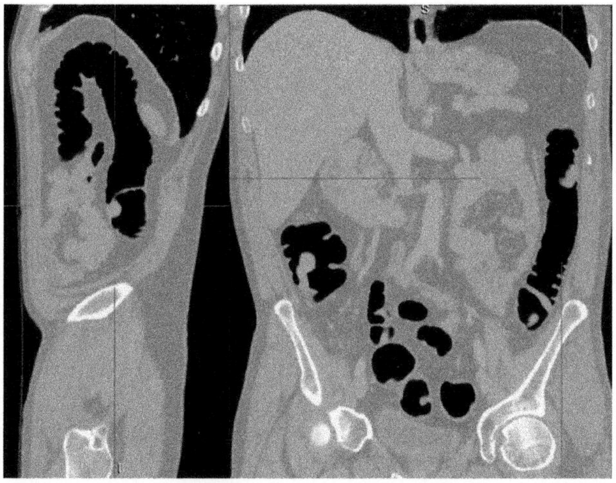

Fig. 26.22 CT of GIT – colon. Sagittal and coronal reconstructions from Fig. 26.21. (Reproduced with permission from Toshiba Medical.)

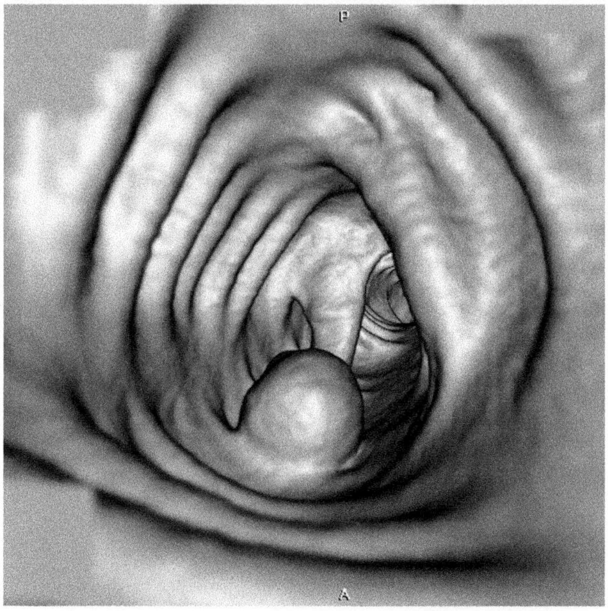

Fig. 26.23 CT of GIT – virtual colonoscopy. Prone reconstructions from patient in Fig. 26.21, demonstrating the polyp in the bowel, hanging from its stalk. (Reproduced with permission from Toshiba Medical.)

Contrast-enhanced CT is the investigation of choice for characterisation and follow-up of renal masses, again it is usual for US to be the first-line investigation, but CT can detect smaller lesions. MRI may be used in staging of advanced disease where it is superior to CT. CT is the examination of choice in renal trauma, in which case a non-contrast and post-contrast two-phase examination is indicated.

PANCREAS

US is better in thin patients and CT is better in larger individuals where the peripancreatic fat is useful for delineation. IV contrast enhancement is used to assess necrosis in the immediate post-acute phase of pancreatitis, and is better than US for follow up, but due to the dose implications, US should be used for monitoring chronic conditions. For pancreatic tumours, CT is required for staging, whilst both US and CT may be used to facilitate biopsy and drainage (Fig. 26.26).

MUSCULOSKELETAL SYSTEM

CT has an important place in musculoskeletal imaging due to its ability to demonstrate occult and complex fractures, and bone healing. For example, CT can be used to clarify a clinically suspected scaphoid fracture, but MRI is better where it is available. Conventional radiography is still the first-line technique for the detection of fractures and dislocations. RNI is sensitive though not specific for the detection of occult or stress fractures and metastatic disease. US and MRI are the investigations of choice for associated soft tissue injuries. Extremity cone beam computed tomography (CBCT) might also have a place in the diagnosis and management of musculoskeletal injuries and chronic conditions as it offers the same high resolution, 3D images as conventional CT, with potentially lower radiation dose.

Currently, CT is used for orthopaedic surgical planning, clarification of complex fractures and demonstration of developmental deformities. Areas of particular value are the tibial plateau, ankle, calcaneus, and pelvic fractures (Figs 26.27 and 26.28). CT can also be utilised for leg length measurement,

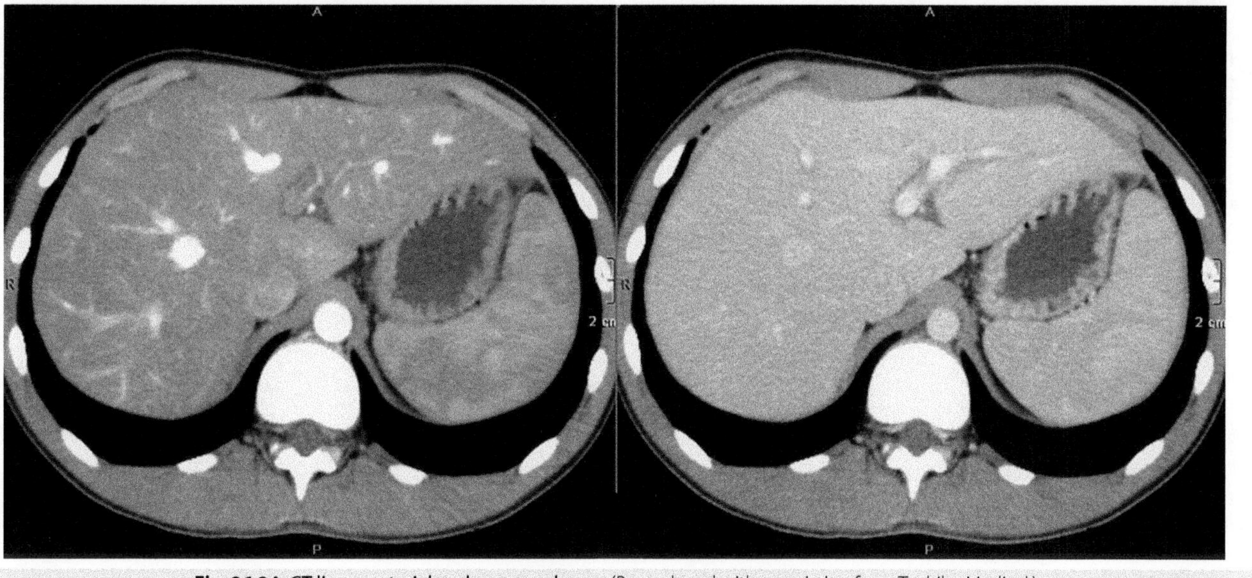

Fig. 26.24 CT liver – arterial and venous phases. (Reproduced with permission from Toshiba Medical.)

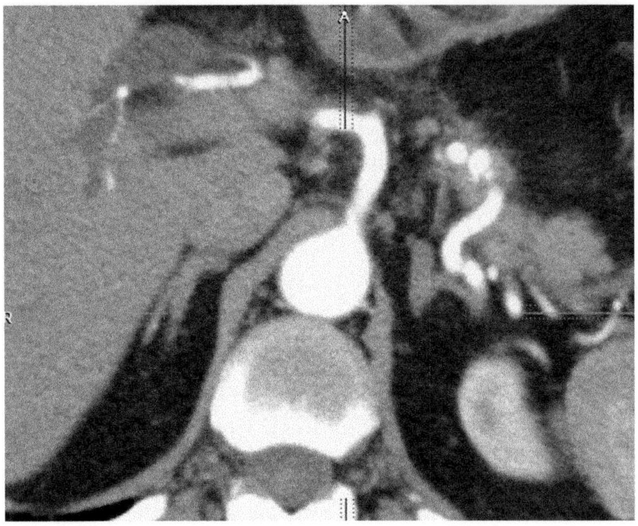

Fig. 26.25 CT adrenals. (Reproduced with permission from Toshiba Medical.)

assessment of scoliosis and prosthetic planning. If scout views are used for measurement they have the advantage of being obtained using a non-divergent beam, rendering measurement more accurate. High-end scans can produce 4D cine-like images, useful to assess musculoskeletal function.

CT ANGIOGRAPHY

CT has long been used to image vascular structures, but multislice technology opened up a new range of examinations, which are now achievable due to increased speed, coverage and reconstruction techniques. The aorta is commonly scanned for dissection and aneurysmal disease; coronal reconstructions, MIPs or 3D images can clearly resolve questions, for example, regarding renal artery involvement (Fig. 26.29). Where vascular surgery is planned angiography is often performed prior as a way of measuring disease (and thus the prosthetic required), and post surgery to rule out endovascular leaks.

Peripheral angiography can be performed in a far less invasive manner than traditional angiography (Figs 26.30 and 26.31); the dose advantages of magnetic resonance angiography (MRA) should be considered where this technique is available. This is an area where the ability to scan faster with more slices may be disadvantageous, as it is possible to scan faster than the travel of the contrast bolus.

Future Developments

New technology is being launched on a regular basis and such developments have made CT the most rapidly evolving imaging technology. No sooner was spiral CT replaced by quad multislice, than it in turn has been replaced by 8 slice and now 320 slice machines offering 4D CT applications, and additionally the multiple possibilities of the application of dual source, dual energy scanning. Already it is possible to scan 16 cm volumes in a single rotation, this may be extended by the development of flat plate digital detector systems raising the possibility of single rotation scanning of a larger body area. This could produce a data set of an anatomical area, e.g. the chest, from which could be reconstructed a chest image plus lateral and obliques as required, as well as slices in any plane, 3D and MIP reconstructions – all from a single rotation. This would have a similar acquisition time to standard chest X-ray. Dose and noise reduction technologies will continue to expand in line with these developments as the medical community strives to optimise CT examinations.

C-arm CT systems have been developed for use in operating theatres, and interventional suites. These systems can be used as a standard image intensifier; the CT function is selected and a series of images taken at fixed angles as the intensifier C-arm rotates around a preselected isocentre (Fig. 26.32).

These advances in medical imaging technology are being driven by the rapid advances in computing and associated technologies, such as machine learning algorithms, and AI systems. Already we can look to the

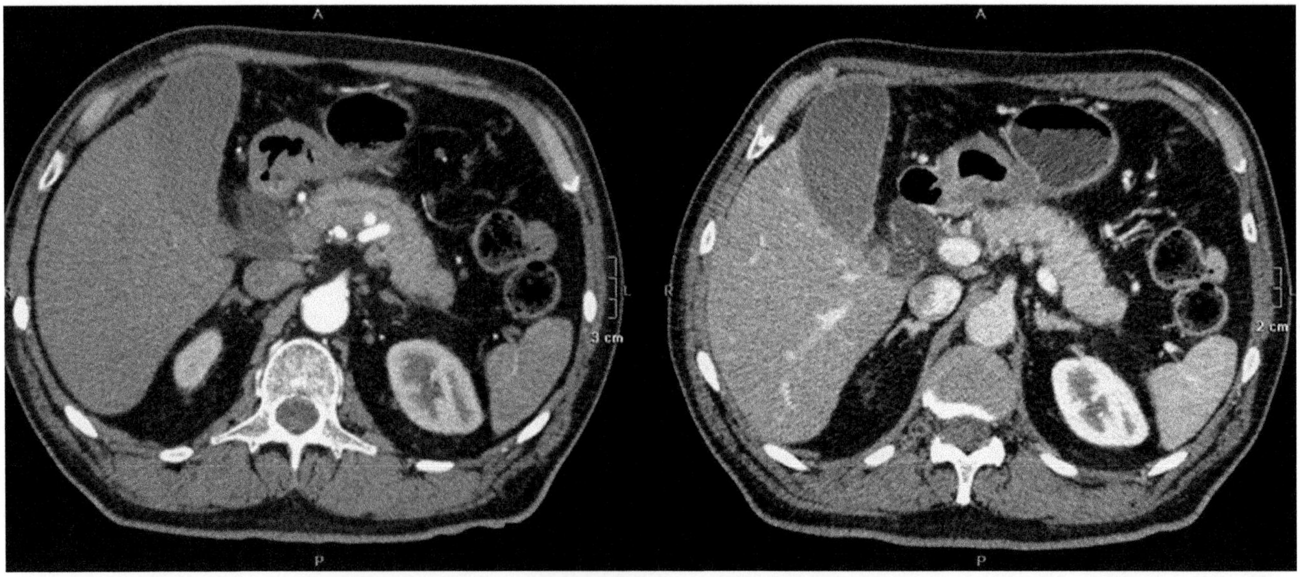

Fig. 26.26 CT pancreas – arterial and venous phases. (Reproduced with permission from Toshiba Medical.)

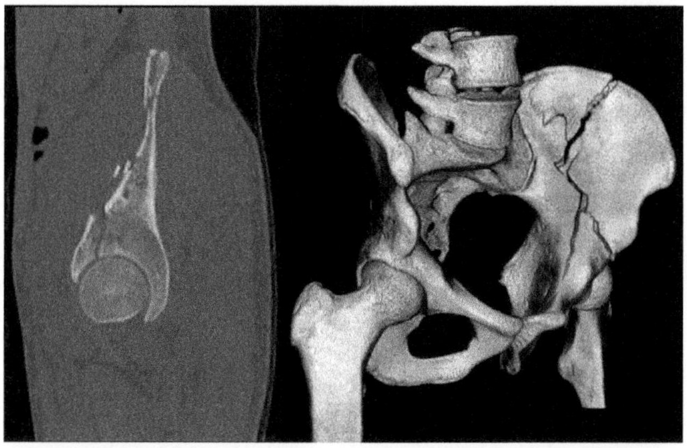

Fig. 26.27 CT pelvis. A combination of oblique reconstructions and surface rendered images are used here to clarify a complex fracture. (Reproduced with permission from Toshiba Medical.)

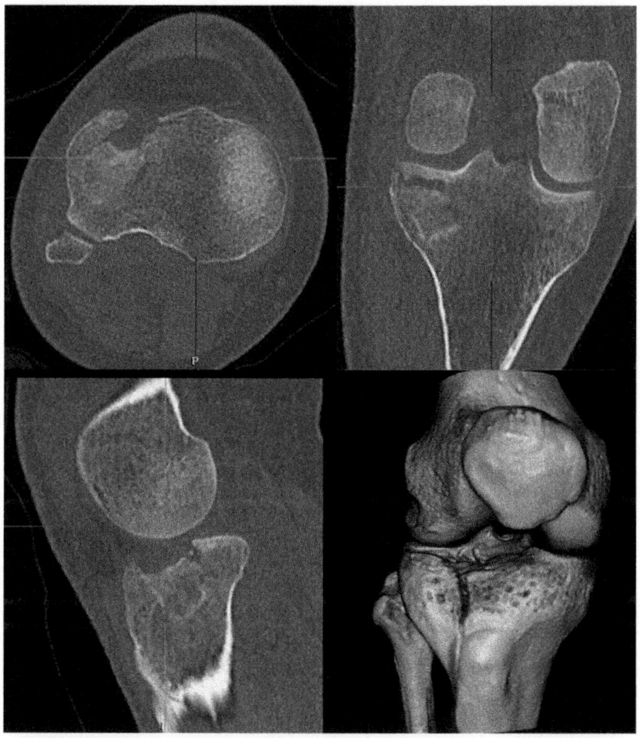

Fig. 26.28 CT knee. Tibial plateau fracture, well demonstrated by axial scan, coronal and sagittal reformats, and surface rendered 3D image. (Reproduced with permission from Toshiba Medical.)

image registration of various cross-sectional studies, for example the registration of CT and MRI images may enable bony and soft tissue structures and their relationships to be better demonstrated than is possible with each individual modality.[59] CT and PET images can be combined to provide anatomical and functional information simultaneously.

It continues to be an exciting and challenging time to be working with this dynamic imaging modality.

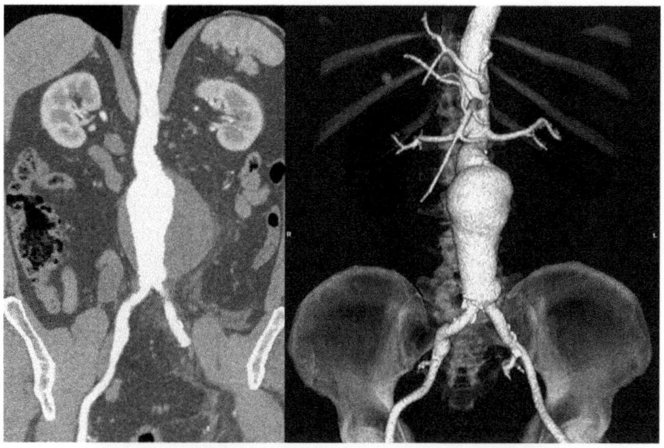

Fig. 26.29 CTA – abdominal aortic aneurysm. Curved MIP demonstrating extent and location of aneurysm. 3D image demonstrates non-involvement of renal arteries. (Reproduced with permission from Toshiba Medical.)

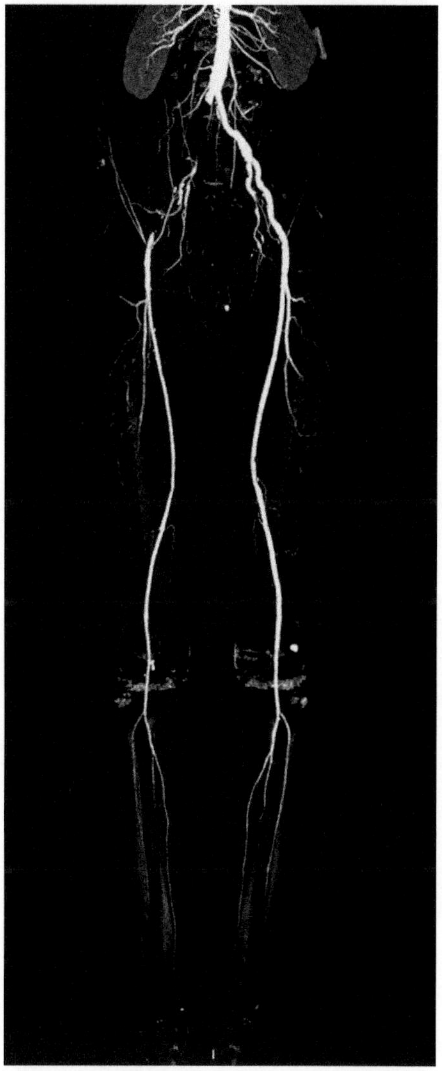

Fig. 26.30 CTA – peripheral angiography. Coverage from renal arteries to ankles shown on this MIP. (Reproduced with permission from Toshiba Medical.)

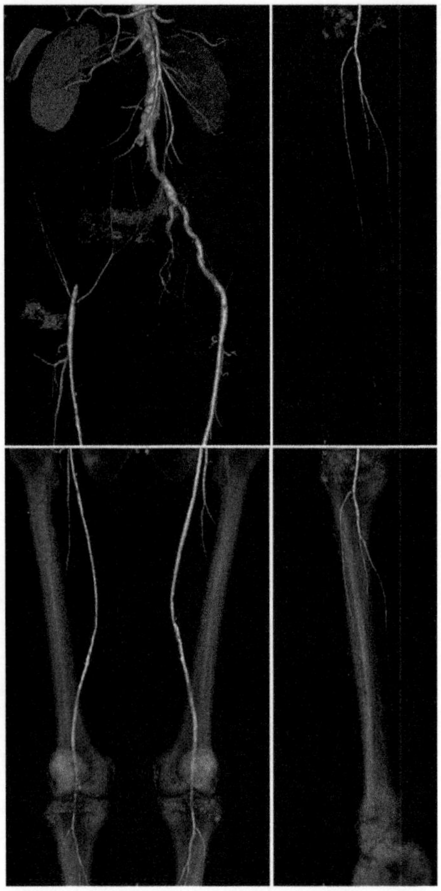

Fig. 26.31 CTA – peripheral angiography. Using image reformatting, a single volumetric acquisition can be used to view key areas from different planes/angles, and with or without semi-transparent bone for positional reference. (Reproduced with permission from Toshiba Medical.)

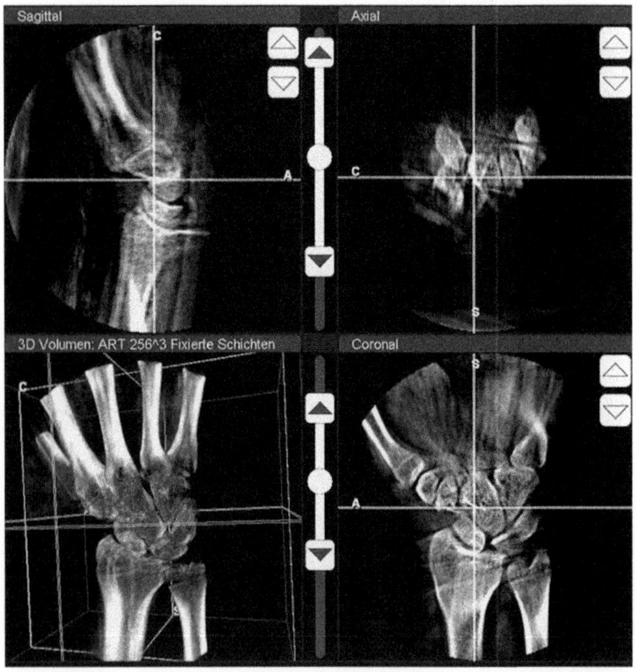

Fig. 26.32 Vario 3D. Multiplanar and 3D images reconstructed from images taken during rotation of the C-arm. (Reproduced with permission from Xograph.)

References

1. Yuan M-K, Tsai D-C, Chang S-C, et al. The risk of cataract associated with repeated head and neck studies: a nationwide population based study. *AJR Am J Roentgenol*. 2013;201:626–630.
2. ICRP (International Commission for Radiological Protection). *Managing Patient Dose in Computed Tomography*. Elsevier; 2000. ICRP Publication No. 87.
3. American College of Radiology. *ACR Practice Guideline for Performing and Interpreting Diagnostic Computed Tomography (CT)*. ACR; 2002.
4. Bogdanich W. Radiation Overdoses point up Dangers of CT Scans. New York Times, October 16. http://www.nytimes.com/2009/10/16/us/16radiation.html.
5. Grossmann G. Lung tomography. *Br J Radiol*. 1935;8:733.
6. Kuhl D. Transmission scanning. *Radiology*. 1966;87:278–284.
7. Ambrose J, Hounsfield G. Computerised transverse axial tomography. *Br J Radiol*. 1972;46:148.
8. Hounsfield G. Computerised transverse axial scanning (tomography), Part 1: description of system. *Br J Radiol*. 1973;46:1016.
9. Ambrose J, Hounsfield G. Computerised transverse axial scanning (tomography), Part 2: clinical applications. *Br J Radiol*. 1973;46:1023.
10. Kitagawa K, Lardo AC, Lima JAC, et al. Prospective ECG-gated 320 row detector computed tomography: implications for CT angiography and perfusion imaging. *Int J Cardiovasc Imag*. 2009;25:201.
11. Petersilka M, Brider H, Krauss B, et al. Technical principles of dual source CT. *Eur J Radiol*. 2008;68:362–368.
12. Shefer E, Altman A, Behling R, et al. State of the art of CT detectors and sources: a literature review. *Curr Radiol Rep*. 2013;1:76–91.
13. Seeram E. *Computed Tomography: Physical Principles, Clinical Applications, and Quality Control*. 4th ed. Philadelphia: Saunders; 2015.
14. Shrimpton P, et al. *Survey of CT Practice in the UK. Part 2: Dosimetric Aspects*. London: HMSO; 1991. NRPB-R249.
15. NHS England Diagnostic Imaging Dataset statistical release19 December 2019 (NHS England and NHS Improvement). https://www.england.nhs.uk/statistics/wp-content/uploads/sites/2/2019/12/Annual-Statistical-Release-2018-19-PDF-1.9MB.pdf.
16. Cameron J. UKRC 2004 debate: moderate dose rate ionising radiation increases longevity. *Br J Radiol*. 2005;78:11–13.
17. Feinendegen L. UKRC 2004 debate: evidence for beneficial low level radiation effects and radiation hormesis. *Br J Radiol*. 2005;78:3–7.
18. *The Ionising Radiation (Medical Exposure) Regulations*. UK Statutory Instrument 2000 No. 1059; 2000. https://www.legislation.gov.uk/uksi/2000/1059/contents/made.
19. Harris MA, Huckle J, Anthony D, et al. The acceptability of iterative reconstruction algorithms in head CT: an assessment of Sinogram Affirmed Iterative Reconstruction (SAFIRE) vs. Filtered Back Projection (FBP) using phantoms. *J Med Imaging Radiat Sci*. 2017;48:259–269.
20. Mileto A, Guimares LS, McCullough CH, et al. State of the art in abdominal CT: the limits of iterative reconstruction algorithms. *Radiology*. 2019;00:1–13.
21. Freiherr G. Dose-saving technologies proliferate throughout CT. *Diagn Imaging*. 2010;32. http://www.diagnosticimaging.com/view/dose-saving-technologies-proliferate-throughout-ct.
22. Shrimpton P, Jessen KA, Geleijns J, et al. Reference doses in computed tomography. *Radiat Protect Dosim*. 1998;80:55–59.
23. Shrimpton P, Hillier MC, Meeson C, et al. *Doses from CT Examinations in the UK – 2011 Review*. Public Health England; 2014.
24. European Commission. Council directive 2013/59/Euratom. *Official Journal of the European Union*. 2013. Available at: http://eur-lex.europa.eu/LexUriServ/LexUriServ.do?uri=OJ:L:2014:013:0001:0073:EN:PDF.
25. *The Ionising Radiation (Medical Exposure) Regulations*. UK Statutory Instrument 2017 No. 1322; 2017. [IR(ME)R]. https://www.legislation.gov.uk/uksi/2017/1322/contents/made.
26. *The Ionising Radiation (Medical Exposure) Regulations (Northern Ireland)*. Statutory Instrument 2018 No. 17; 2018. https://www.legislation.gov.uk/nisr/2018/17/contents/made.
27. Society and College of Radiographers. *Communicating Radiation Benefit and Risk Information to Individuals under the Ionising Radiation (Medical Exposure) Regulations IR(ME)R*. London: Society and College of Radiographers; 2018.
28. Harris MA, Snaith B, Clarke R. Strategies for assessing renal function prior to outpatient contrast-enhanced CT: a UK survey. *Br J Radiol*. 2016;89:20160077.

29. Williams K, Probst H. Use of IV contrast media in radiotherapy planning CT scans: a UK audit. *Radiography*. 2016;22:S28–S32.
30. George AJ. Comparison between a fixed-dose contrast protocol and a weight-based contrast dosing protocol in abdominal CT. *Clin Radiol.* 2016;71:1314.
31. Graham R. Battlefield radiology. *Br J Radiol.* 2012;85(1020): 1556–1565.
32. NICE (National Institute for Health and Care Excellence). *Major Trauma: Assessment and Initial Management.* NICE guideline [NG39]; 2016. https://www.nice.org.uk/guidance/ng39.
33. Royal College of Radiologists. *Standards of Practice and Guidance for Trauma Radiology in Severely Injured Patients.* 2nd ed. London: RCR; 2015.
34. Meltzer J, Stone Jr ME, Reddy SH, et al. Association of whole-body CT with mortality risk in children with blunt trauma. *JAMA Pediatrics.* 2018;172(6):542–549.
35. Royal College of Radiologists. *Paediatric Trauma Protocols.* London: RCR; 2014.
36. British Society of Paediatric Radiology. Camp Bastion Contrast Calculator. https://www.mybspr.org/contrastwheel.htm.
37. Steill I, Wells GA, Vandemheen K, et al. The Canadian CT head rule for patients with minor head injury. *Lancet.* 2001;357:1391–1396.
38. NICE (National Institute for Health and Care Excellence). *Head Injury: Assessment and Early Management.* Clinical guideline [CG176]; 2019. https://www.nice.org.uk/guidance/cg176.
39. Royal College of Radiologists Working Party. *Making the Best Use of a Department of Clinical Radiology: Guidelines for Doctors.* 6th ed. London: RCR; 2007.
40. Intercollegiate Stroke Working Party. *National Clinical Guidelines for Stroke.* 5th ed. London: Royal College of Physicians; 2016.
41. Intercollegiate Stroke Working Party. *National Clinical Guidelines for Stroke.* 2nd ed. London: Royal College of Physicians; 2004.
42. AAPM position statement PP26-B 2017 (PP26-A 2012) AAPM position statement on the use of bismuth shielding for the purpose of dose reduction in CT scanning. https://www.aapm.org/publicgeneral/bismuthshielding.pdf.
43. Murphy U. Dose implications of gantry tilt in cranial computerised tomography. Radiography Ireland. 6(3):137–139.
44. Carver B. Meeting service needs: cranial CT reporting by radiographers. In: *Proceedings of UKRC 2004.* BIR Congress Series; 2004:10.
45. Carver B. Is cranial CT reporting by radiographers a feasible option to assist radiologist workload and provide a route for radiographer role extension?. In: *RSNA Scientific Assembly and Annual Meeting Program.* Oak Brook, IL: RSNA; 2004:553.
46. Jansen-van der Weide M, Greuter MJW, Jansen L, et al. Exposure to low-dose radiation and the risk of breast cancer among women with a familial or genetic predisposition: a meta-analysis. *Eur Radiol.* 2010;20:2547–2556.
47. AAPM position statement on the use of patient gonadal and fetal shielding 2019; PP32-A; 4/2/2019. https://www.aapm.org/org/policies/details.asp?id=468&type=PP.
48. Wise J. Mobile lung cancer testing in supermarket car parks is to be expanded. *BMJ.* 2017;359:j5450.
49. Aberle DR. National lung screening trial research team. Reduced lung cancer mortality with low-dose computed tomographic screening. *N Engl J Med.* 2011;365:395–409.
50. Baldwin DR, et al. Low dose CT screening for lung cancer. *BMJ.* 2017;359:j5742.
51. Bach P, Jett JR, Pastorino U, et al. Computed tomography screening and lung cancer outcomes. *J Am Med Assoc.* 2007;297(9):953–961.
52. Henschke C, McCauley DI, Yankelevitz DF, et al. Early lung cancer action project: a summary of the findings on baseline screening. *Oncol.* 2001;6:147–152.
53. Patz E, Rossi S, Harpole DH, et al. Correlation of tumour size and survival in patients with Stage 1A non-small cell lung cancer. *Chest.* 2000;117:1568–1571.
54. Zamboni G, Guariglia S, Bonfante A, et al. Low voltage CTPA for patients with suspected pulmonary embolism. *Eur J Radiol.* 2012;81(4):e580–584.
55. Flohr T, McCullough CH, Bruder H, et al. First performance evaluation of a dual-source CT system. *Eur Radiol.* 2006;16:256–268.
56. Blankstein R, Budoff MJ, Shaw LJ, et al. Predictors of coronary heart disease events among asymptomatic persons with low low-density lipoprotein cholesterol. *J Am Coll Cardiol.* 2011;58:364–374.
57. Xu L, Fan Z, Yu W, et al. Diagnostic performance of 320-detector CT coronary angiography in patients with atrial fibrillation: preliminary results 2011. *Eur Radiol.* 2011;21:936–943.
58. Meagher T, Sukumar VP, Collingwood J, et al. Low dose computed tomography in suspected acute renal colic. *Clin Radiol.* 2001;56:873–876.
59. Panigraphy A, Caruthers SD, Krejza J, et al. Registration of three-dimensional MR and CT studies of the cervical spine. *Am J Neuroradiol.* 2000;21:282–289.

27 *Magnetic Resonance Imaging*

JOHN TALBOT

Introduction

Nuclear magnetic resonance (NMR) is a process whereby atomic nuclei are placed into a powerful external magnetic field and perturbed by an electromagnetic field which is applied at a particular frequency. The technique was developed at the end of the 1940s and became a popular method for analysing samples of chemical compounds using spectroscopy over the following three decades. NMR was first conceptualised as a potential imaging modality in 1969, shortly after the initial development of computed tomography (CT) in 1967. The first image was created in 1973 by Professor Paul Lauterbur in the United States and the first human image was made in 1976 by Professor Sir Peter Mansfield and colleagues in the UK.

Magnetic resonance imaging (MRI) uses a combination of spatially varying magnetic fields, temporally varying magnetic field gradients and low-energy electromagnetic radiation to produce diagnostic images of the body. The basic premise of MRI is that a radiofrequency pulse is applied to the hydrogen nuclei within the patient's tissues which causes them to change their energy state and net magnetic alignment to an external magnetic field. As the nuclei return to equilibrium, their emitted energy can be received by a radio antenna (coil), measured and spatially located.

MRI is a first-line technique in the routine diagnosis of disease, and scanners can be found in all major hospitals. MRI is not only used in routine imaging scenarios, but also in specialties such as cardiac imaging, neurological imaging and radiotherapy.

Like CT, MRI is a cross-sectional imaging modality acquiring user-definable slices having variable size (field of view, FOV) and thickness. MRI does, however, have certain advantages over CT:

- MRI uses non-ionising radiation rather than X-rays. To be precise, MRI uses electromagnetic radiation in the radiofrequency range – between 6 and 340 MHz, depending on the magnetic field strength of the scanner. This portion of the electromagnetic spectrum has a longer wavelength than that of X-rays and is correspondingly less energetic and less damaging to tissues.
- MRI has excellent soft tissue contrast. MRI is unique among diagnostic modalities in that the signal that forms the image is generated by the body tissue itself. Radiographs and CT rely on X-rays passing through, and being attenuated by, the area under investigation. Although the user has control over the penetrating power and intensity of the beam, the resulting image is still essentially a shadow of the anatomy. MRI, on the other hand, has multiple user-definable parameters which exploit the molecular behaviour of the tissues and can significantly modify the contrast-to-noise ratio of such.
- MRI acquires images in any geometric plane without having to modify the position of the patient. Although CT data can be post processed into many different planes and rendered volumes, the acquisition plane is still essentially axial.
- MRI can obtain both structural (morphological) information and *functional* information. Functional MRI (fMRI) exploits the fact that MRI can detect minute changes in the chemical composition of body tissues, such as the amount of haemoglobin versus deoxyhaemoglobin. The principle of fMRI imaging is to rapidly acquire a series of images of the brain and to statistically analyse the images for differences between them. This is usually done after a baseline scan, and the patient is asked to perform a physical or mental task during acquisition.

There is a developing trend for more powerful scanners, operating at higher magnetic field strengths (up to 10 tesla for human research), which can investigate metabolic function[1] and have microscopic resolution.

Equipment Chronology

1938 In the 1930s American physicist Isidor Rabi researched methods of observing atomic spectra. During his work he demonstrated that the spin state in a molecular beam can be reoriented in a magnetic field. In 1944 he received the Nobel Prize in physics 'for his resonance method for recording the magnetic properties of atomic nuclei'.[2]

1946 The process of NMR was discovered by the independently operating research teams of Felix Bloch (Stanford University) and Edwin Purcell (Harvard University).

1948 Nicolaas Bloembergen presented his theory of relaxation times, based on experiments in Purcell's laboratory.

1950 Irwin Hahn 'accidentally' discovered spin echoes while working on relaxation experiments. He originally cursed the symmetrical oscilloscope reading as an 'annoying glitch'.

1950s NMR was used in the field of analytical chemistry.

1960s NMR spectroscopy revolutionised the non-destructive analysis of the composition of chemical compounds. These techniques tested very small samples that were placed inside high-field magnets having a very narrow bore only a few centimetres wide. Paramagnetic reagents were used in NMR spectroscopy and can be thought of as the forerunners of modern MRI contrast media.

1966 Richard Ernst showed that Fourier transform increases the sensitivity of magnetic resonance (MR) spectroscopy.

1969 Dr Raymond Damadian (SUNY Downstate Medical Centre) used NMR spectroscopy in research into sodium and potassium in living cells. This led him to his first experiments with NMR and caused him to first propose the possibility of an NMR body scanner.[3]

1971 Following animal studies on rats, Damadian discovered noticeable differences in the NMR signals emitted by healthy tissues and tumours. He authored a paper entitled 'Tumor detection by nuclear magnetic resonance',[4] and although this work was met with scepticism from many quarters Damadian maintained his idea of the MR body scanner.

1972 Damadian filed the first of his patents for an MRI body scanner. The patent described how liquid helium could be used to create a supercooled electromagnet housed within a cylindrical cryostat. The patent also described how the nuclei of hydrogen atoms in the body would react to the resultant magnetic field, and how a 3D spatial localisation method could encode the signals into an image.

1973 The journal *Nature* published an article written by Professor Paul Lauterbur, Professor of Chemistry at SUNY, entitled 'Image formation by induced local interaction: examples employing magnetic resonance'.[5] Lauterbur described a new imaging technique for which he coined the term *zeugmatography* (from the Greek meaning 'to join together'). This alluded to the principle of his technique, which involved the joining of two magnetic fields in the spatial localisation of two test tubes filled with water sitting in a bath of deuterium oxide (heavy water). Lauterbur used a static main magnetic field over which he applied an additional gradient magnetic field. He then used a back-projection method (similar to that used in CT) to produce an image of the two test tubes (Fig. 27.1).

This landmark imaging experiment was of great importance for two reasons. Firstly, it was the first time that NMR had given spatial information rather than just spectroscopic information. Secondly, it was the first time frequency had been used as a spatial encoding mechanism. This was achieved by the use of the gradient magnetic fields and forms the basis for all modern frequency encoding still used today. Professor Lauterbur received a Nobel Prize for this and other work in the field of MRI in 2003.

1973 In the same year Professor Peter Mansfield was beginning his studies into NMR at the University of Nottingham in the UK. He initially worked on studies of solid objects, such as crystals. However, one year later, Mansfield and collaborator Alan Garroway filed a patent and published a paper on image formation by NMR.[6]

1975 Richard Ernst proposed the Fourier transform as an image reconstruction method in MRI. Mansfield and another colleague, Andrew Maudsley, who were also working in the field of spatial encoding, proposed a technique that could produce in vivo imaging.

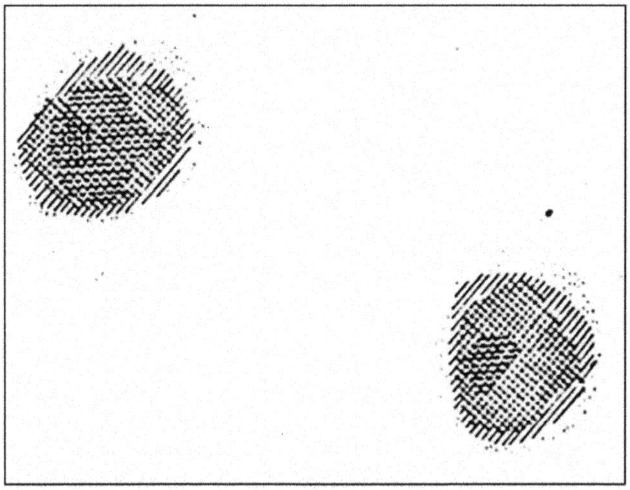

Fig. 27.1 The first use of spatial encoding with NMR by Professor Paul Lauterbur. The shaded areas represent the spatial position of two tubes filled with water.[5] (Image reproduced by kind permission of Professor Paul Lauterbur and *Nature*.)

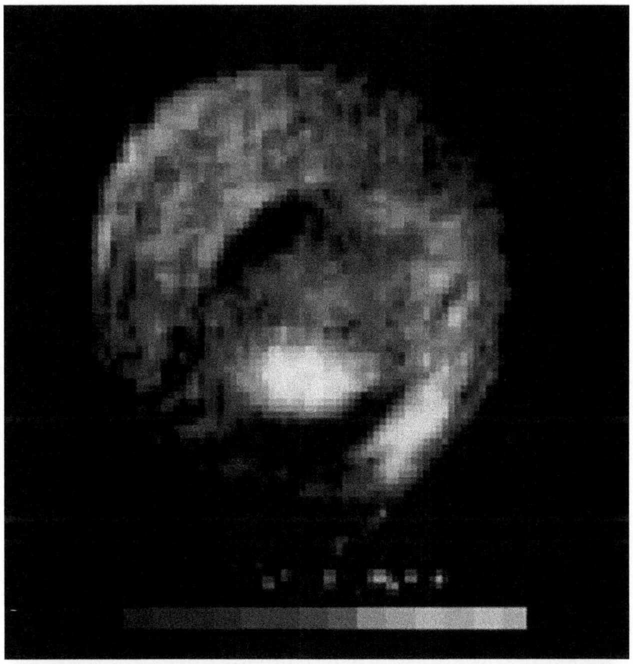

Fig. 27.2 First human MRI scan by Mansfield and Maudsley.[7] Axial cross-section through a finger. (Image reproduced by kind permission of Professor Mansfield. Mansfield P, Maudsley A. Medical imaging by NMR. *Br J Radiol.* 1977;50:188.)

1976 Mansfield et al began to study ways of fast imaging using NMR and an improved picture display. They produced the first in vivo image of human anatomy, a cross-section through a finger (Fig. 27.2).[7]

1977 Damadian, aided by graduate students, built a prototype NMR body scanner consisting of a homemade superconducting magnet. The magnet itself was made of nearly 50 km of niobium–titanium wire spun onto a cylinder. The magnet bore itself was 134 cm in diameter, large enough to allow the positioning of a human body. To ensure superconductivity the magnet was supercooled using liquid helium.

The receive coil was constructed from cardboard and copper wire and designed to be worn around the body like a corset, very much like modern phased-array wrap-around body coils. Research assistant Laurence Minkoff was placed into the scanner. The receive coil was positioned around his thorax and signal readings taken in a procedure that lasted nearly 5 hours. The result was a rudimentary image, plotted by hand from the data acquired using crayons. It showed a 2D view of Minkoff's chest, including his heart and lungs.[8] Meanwhile, in the UK, Mansfield et al published two papers on imaging using NMR and a paper on multiplanar image formation.[9–11]

1978 Following on from earlier images of small body parts, Mansfield presented his first image through the abdomen. He also published animal studies showing how NMR could be used in the diagnosis of tumours. Mansfield invented echo-planar imaging, a technique that made MRI image acquisition much faster. Scan times were now short enough to make MRI imaging a practicable technique for human diagnostics.
Professor Paul Lauterbur began work on finding a suitable MRI contrast agent in this year using paramagnetic reagents in an animal study.[12]

1979 The Mansfield team continued their studies into the NMR imaging of tumours, specifically carcinoma of the breast.

1980 In the late 1970s and early 1980s many groups took up the challenge to produce a commercially viable MRI system. This needed to be large enough to scan a human but also to have sufficiently good field homogeneity to produce diagnostic images. These pioneers included the group from the Hammersmith Hospital (Professor R. Steiner and Professor G. Bydder) working in conjunction with Picker Ltd at Wembley (Dr I. Young), two independent groups in Nottingham (Professor P. Mansfield and Dr W. Moore), and in Aberdeen (Professor J. Mallard and Dr J. Hutchinson).

1981 Mansfield and his team introduced the concept of real-time moving images by NMR and presented a paper critically evaluating NMR imaging techniques.[13]
Philips Medical Systems produced their first scanner.
Schering applied for a patent for an MRI contrast agent, gadolinium diethylenetriamine penta-acetic acid (DTPA).

1983 The first commercial MR scanner in Europe (from Picker Ltd) was installed at the Department of Diagnostic Radiology at the University of Manchester Medical School (Professor I. Isherwood and Professor B. Pullen).

1984 MRI contrast agent gadolinium DTPA (Magnevist, Schering) was tested on humans.

1985–1990 In the latter half of the 1980s NMR applications and refinements began to evolve rapidly and included dynamic imaging, cardiac applications, more efficient shimming methods, active magnetic shielding and surface coil improvements.
Gadolinium DTPA was licensed for use in brain and spine imaging. Approval for use in other body areas followed.

1990–present Since the advent of commercial scanning, MRI equipment has been constantly modified and improved. These improvements have not just been in the physical construction but also in the design of the software used to produce the pulse sequences used in scanning.

Instrumentation and pulse sequence design will be discussed more fully in the following sections, but still in the historical context of MRI it is worth mentioning here some of the advances that have been made in the design of MRI scanners over recent years.

In the field of medical imaging the word 'nuclear' has been dropped from the term 'nuclear magnetic resonance imaging'. A commonly cited reason for this is that the word 'nuclear' has connotations with nuclear power, nuclear war and radioactivity in general – which may be unnecessarily off-putting in the context of a scan that does not use ionising radiation. A more likely explanation is that the name change was a result of a radiological turf-war, and was used to identify the fact that the modality did not belong in the same domain as nuclear medicine.

Although there are variations, such as 'open' magnets and Fonar's Erect system,[14] most modern scanners still have the same basic design featuring a closed-bore superconducting magnet orientated horizontally, allowing the patient to be positioned supine within the field. There have been many modifications and improvements to the original design since the advent of clinical scanning, and some of these are outlined in the next section.

Science and Instrumentation

MRI scanners can be categorised in terms of flux density (field strength). The unit used to measure magnetic flux density is the tesla (T): 1 T equals 10 000 gauss.[15] The empirical gauss unit was replaced by the tesla under the International System, but is still often used to describe magnetic fields having a low flux density; for example, the Earth's magnetic field varies from 0.2 to 0.7 gauss. For high flux densities, the tesla is a more appropriate unit. Clinical scanners are generally described as ultra-high-field, high-field, mid-field, or low-field systems:

- Ultra-high-field (3.0 T and above)
- High-field (1.0 T and above)
- Mid-field (0.5 T)
- Low-field (<0.15 to 0.5 T)

3T scanners were originally developed for research purposes, but are now used fairly commonly in the clinical setting for the benefits that high-field imaging brings.

Modern research scanners are often of considerably higher field strength than clinical scanners and can employ flux-densities as high as 10.0T for human research. These machines are typically used for applications such as fMRI and spectroscopy. At the time of writing, the most powerful research MRI scanner in the world is the 21 T magnet at the National High Magnetic Field Laboratory, Tallahassee, Florida. The scanner has a vertical bore just 10 cm wide, which is just large enough to perform studies on rats and mice.

MRI scanner design falls into two main categories: closed-bore and so-called open systems.

OPEN MAGNET SYSTEMS

Open systems are configured with either a vertical or horizontal magnetic field. The patient is positioned between the poles of the magnet, usually in a supine position, although some systems allow the patient to sit or stand. Open systems do not completely encircle the patient and therefore allow better access for biopsy etc. They are more patient-friendly in terms of claustrophobia, and allow nervous patients or children to stay close to their parent or carer throughout the entire procedure. Their other major advantage is in permitting access for patients with an increased BMI (body mass index), who would not fit in a closed-bore scanner. The main trade-off is that open systems tend to have slightly poorer geometric accuracy than closed-bore systems.

Open systems may use permanent magnets, resistive electromagnets and superconducting electromagnets in their design. The highest field strength found in open systems is currently 1.2 T.

Permanent Magnets

Permanent magnet systems generally have two opposing magnetic plates (shoes) constructed from a highly magnetic alloy of metals such as iron, nickel and neodymium. The patient lies on a couch inside the imaging volume between these plates.

From a cost point of view, these scanners are relatively cheap to run and maintain as they do not require expensive cryogen fills.

The disadvantages of permanent magnet design include the fact that it is difficult to achieve flux densities above 0.7 T and the scanners tend to be very heavy. Weighing up to 15 tons, they may be difficult to site, requiring deep structural foundations for the magnet room. They are also permanently magnetised and the field cannot be quenched in an emergency.

Resistive Magnets

These machines use an electromagnet to generate a magnetic field. An electromagnet is typically constructed from a coil of wire through which current is passed. Resistive systems are usually of the open configuration, but lighter and smaller in design than permanent magnet systems. They also have the advantage that they may be switched off when not in use.

Because the coil is not supercooled, there are cost implications in having to supply power when in use. This is offset by the fact that they do not require cryogen refills.

The main disadvantage of these systems is that the field strength is limited by the amount of current that can be applied to the coil without causing overheating due to resistivity in the windings. To achieve a high field, the number of windings would have to be increased significantly, which would result in an oversized and heavy system.

Superconducting Magnets

Superconducting systems use electromagnets that are supercooled by cryogens. The conductor used in the windings of a superconductive system is made from an alloy of niobium and titanium insulated with copper. This material is superconductive, which means that at extremely low temperatures the resistance to electrical current drops to virtually zero. The advantage is that a very high current can be applied to the windings without any associated heating, which results in the production of a very powerful magnetic field. The current will also continue to flow indefinitely while the coils are maintained at a low temperature. To achieve this low temperature, the coils are immersed in liquid helium. At such a low temperature the resistive copper becomes an insulator rather than a conductor because the current takes the path of least resistance through the niobium/titanium core. Copper is used because in the event that the magnetic solenoids should become resistive (such as during a magnet quench) the resulting heat can be conducted away efficiently. This reduces the risk of damage to the solenoids due to overheating.

To generate the main magnetic field, an electrical current is applied to the windings, gradually increasing until the magnet is ramped up to the desired field strength. The supply can then be disconnected and the current will continue to flow through the windings for as long as the low temperature is maintained.

CLOSED-BORE MAGNET SYSTEMS

The modern closed-bore scanner design resembles a CT scanner, but with the patient aperture having a depth of 70–100 cm. This is a great improvement over early systems, where the patient was totally enclosed by the bore. The MRI scanner itself consists of a large cylindrical supercooled electromagnet mounted inside a cryostat with various room temperature components arranged inside the warm bore of the cryostat.

The major system components, when viewed in transverse cross-section, form concentric circles, as shown in Fig. 27.3.

Working from the outermost structure inwards, the important components are the outer cover, cryostat, active shielding, main magnet, shim system, gradient system, radiofrequency (RF) transmitter/receiver and receive coils. These are discussed in more detail below.

Outer Cover

This is a plastic or fibreglass shell protecting the scan components from damage and dust.

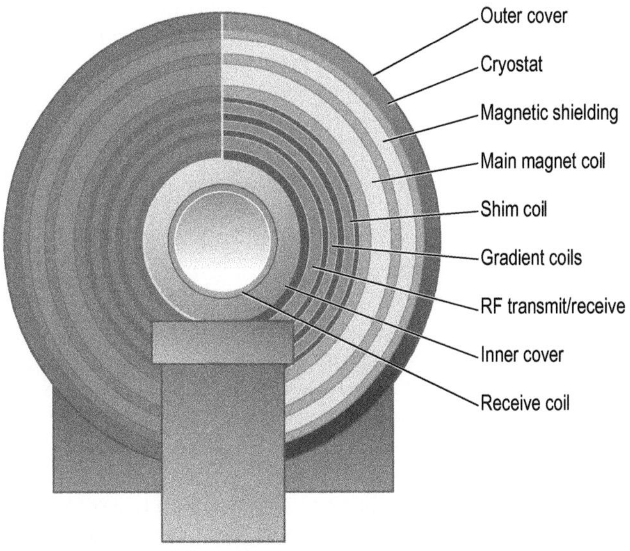

Fig. 27.3 The components of a closed-bore MRI scanner in transverse cross-section.

Cryostat

The cryostat is essentially a large Dewar flask having an outer steel casing and an internal aluminium cryogen chamber which also houses the main magnet solenoids and active shielding coils. Its main function is to maintain up to 1600 litres of the cryogen used to maintain the superconductivity of the solenoid electromagnets. The cryogen of choice in modern MRI systems is liquid helium; with a boiling point of −269°C (4°K), liquid helium creates the ideal environment for superconductivity. Helium is extracted from natural gas, and is therefore an increasingly rare and finite resource, with only a handful of extraction sites worldwide. At room temperature this expensive resource would boil off to the atmosphere, so the cryostat has the primary goal of reducing or eliminating helium boil-off. Firstly, the entire cryostat is cooled by a cold-head or chiller to reduce heat transfer by conduction. One of the main sources of heat inside the MRI scanner is the gradient coil (described in a later section). The chiller is important in offsetting the heat produced by this room-temperature solenoid. Secondly, the cryostat is evacuated to prevent heat-transfer by convection. Finally, the inner cryogen chamber is swathed in a reflective aluminised-mylar heat-shield which is very effective in reflecting the absorption of radiant heat. A combination of these factors, coupled with sophisticated helium re-condensing features, provides a highly efficient device that typically contains and preserves the cryogen for the expected service-life of the scanner. Recent technological advances by one of the major manufacturers has created a very efficient cryogen system requiring less than 8 litres of liquid helium to maintain superconductivity. This has two major advantages in that the running costs are reduced and the need for a cryogen vent is eliminated. This provides more flexibility in siting the equipment.

The cryostat is equipped with a wide-bore cryogen vent, colloquially known as the quench pipe, to allow the expulsion of helium gas in the event of a quench. The term *quench* refers to the suppression or stifling of the main magnetic field, achieved by causing the liquid helium to boil off rapidly to the atmosphere. A quench can be manually activated in the event of an emergency, but can also occur spontaneously. Spontaneous quenches are usually due to contaminants such as ice particles being inadvertently drawn into the cryostat. One litre of liquid helium produces approximately 730 litres of gas,[16] and a full cryostat can liberate around 1 million litres of gas in a fairly short explosive burst. This gas must be safely vented away from the patient and other personnel because, although non-toxic, it can quickly displace oxygen in the magnet room and other areas. There has been at least one reported case where suffocation has occurred as a result of cryogen leakage. There is usually a button in the magnet room that can be activated to quench the system in the event of an emergency. It should be noted from a safety viewpoint that the magnetic field can take from several seconds, to several minutes to reduce.

Magnetic Shielding

Early MRI scanners were not shielded and the main magnetic field was therefore not confined to the magnet room. The fringe field, as it is known, could extend beyond the boundaries of the building. This was a safety concern, because certain implanted medical devices, particularly cardiac pacemakers, may be adversely affected by a strong magnetic field. To maintain the magnetic field within a reasonable area (or footprint), magnetic shielding was originally achieved by bolting large metal plates around the body of the scanner or within the walls of the magnet room. Modern scanners feature an *active shielding* system that uses electromagnetic bucking coils positioned around each end of the main magnet generating an equal but opposite field. This provides for a much smaller and (for the patient) less intimidating equipment design. It also permits the MRI scanner to be sited in the imaging department without interfering with the operation of other nearby modalities such as the CT scanner. Passive shielding has been largely discontinued in favour of the more cost-effective active shielding which can now also be used on ultra-high-field scanners.

Magnet

Inside the cryostat is the main electromagnet. This is a solenoid magnet, constructed in separate segments. Superconductive wire is wound around a reel-shaped structure known as a bobbin. These segmented solenoids are formed by continuous strips of niobium–titanium alloy wire, many kilometres in length. The wire is wound onto the reel evenly and carefully under the control of a technician. The magnetic field thus generated is known as B_0, is of very high flux density and the segmented design provides a high degree of homogeneity over a 40–50 cm imaging volume.

Shim System

Moving further towards the centre of the scanner, the next component is known as the shim system.

As stated, MRI demands a homogeneous magnetic field. Homogeneity can be described in terms of parts per million (ppm). Perfect homogeneity is difficult to achieve. On delivery the raw magnetic field of the scanner is homogeneous to approximately 100 ppm. This can be further improved by a process known as shimming. Shimming can be either active, passive, or dynamic.

Passive shimming is performed by placing metal plates (or shims) at strategic positions inside the scanner assembly. This is facilitated by the use of sliding plastic shim trays arranged around the circumference of the magnet bore. Each tray can be removed in turn and typically has a number of hollow sections along its length designed to house small ferromagnetic shims. The placement of the shims is calculated by software after scanning a moveable test-sample inside a device known as a plotting-rig. It is usually only performed once, when the system is first commissioned for use.

Active shimming serves a similar function to passive shimming, but employs electromagnets.

Dynamic shimming uses the gradient coil, a resistive electromagnet that is activated every time a pulse sequence is performed. The primary function of the gradient coil is to create slopes along the main magnetic field, but modern systems also allow this coil to create offsets to spatial magnetic field variations. This technique can correct for any field inhomogeneity caused (for example) by the introduction of differently sized patients into the magnet bore.

After shimming, the homogeneity of the magnetic field should be better than 4 ppm, which equates to a difference in precessional frequency of <4 Hz over a 22 cm spherical volume. A full explanation of precessional frequency can be found later.

The homogeneous volume of the magnet bore in closed-bore scanners can be described as an imaginary sphere approximately 40–50 cm diameter, centred at the very mid-point of the bore in all three directions – the point known as the magnetic isocentre.

Gradient System

The main difference between MRI and NMR spectroscopy is the ability to determine the spatial origin of the signal returned by a sample. Spatial encoding is performed by the application of gradients to the main magnetic field. The gradient coil forms the next layer in the construction of the MRI scanner and consists of another set of electromagnetic windings orientated inside a cylindrical structure encircling the bore. These coils are very sophisticated on modern scanners and the conductive elements are not wound, but typically etched into copper sheet. The resulting winding pattern resembles the whirls of a fingerprint – giving the name 'fingerprint coil'.

Each element of the gradient set can be individually activated by the application of an electrical current sent from three gradient amplifiers. This results in the generation of a secondary field superimposed onto the main magnetic field on either side of the isocentre and producing a linear slope in magnetic field strength. The orientation of the elements in the gradient coil allows the gradient to be applied in any plane.

In convention with the modern 3D cartesian coordinate system, the three orthogonal planes are given the labels X, Y and Z. There are differences between manufacturers in the way gradient directions are interpreted, but for a majority of closed-bore scanners, with a patient lying in the magnet in the head-first supine position, the X, Y and Z directions are as follows:

- X direction: left to right (horizontal)
- Y direction: posterior to anterior (vertical)
- Z direction: inferior to superior (end-to-end)

Open systems have a vertical magnetic field, and therefore the Z direction is anterior to posterior and the Y direction inferior to superior. Activating the gradient coils in isolation allows the selection of sagittal, coronal and axial slices. Activation of the different gradient elements in tandem can produce imaging planes with any degree of obliquity, i.e. para-sagittal, para-coronal or para-axial.

When purchasing a scanner, it is worth investigating the various specifications of gradient system offered by the manufacturer. The speed and power of gradients vary, and there is usually a cost implication when purchasing high-speed power gradients because they require better gradient amplification and may require water-cooling owing to resistivity effects. This cost is often justified because the decreased acquisition time will allow higher throughput and increased temporal resolution for dynamic studies. Increased gradient strength will also provide higher spatial resolution, thinner slices and a smaller, minimum FOV. For applications such as fMRI, spectroscopy, perfusion and diffusion imaging, power gradients are strongly recommended.

Gradient amplitude is usually measured in milliTesla (mT) per metre, describing a change in magnetic flux-density over a distance in metres. At the time of writing, power gradients for clinical use deliver around 80 mT/m. In terms of acquisition time it is more meaningful to describe the speed at which gradients can be applied. This factor is known as the slew-rate and is measured in mT/m per millisecond. It describes not only the change in flux-density over distance, but also the time taken to achieve that gradient application. The limiting factor for gradient applications in patient scanning is the point at which physical side effects occur. Volunteers undergoing research scans at high gradient amplitude/speed have reported unpleasant temporary bioeffects, such as flashing visual disturbances known as magnetophosphenes and peripheral nerve stimulation causing tingling sensations in the extremities. These effects are caused by electromagnetic induction in nerve fibres and stop when the acquisition ceases.

Another important point to mention about the gradient system is that it is responsible for the acoustic noises made during scanning. MRI scans can be very loud, reaching over 100 decibels for some pulse sequences.[17] The reason for this noise is that the gradient coils carry current and are situated in the main magnetic field. Faraday's Law of Electromagnetic Induction states that a conductor lying in a magnetic field will move if unrestricted. The MRI gradient system is subject to a current of rapidly changing polarity and the resulting Lorentz forces will cause the structure to vibrate vigorously against its mountings. The higher the amplitude and speed of the gradient system, the louder and more unpleasant the noise becomes. This acoustic noise problem has been tackled by the use of ear defenders, music systems and special noise-cancelling headphones. There have also been recent developments in pulse-sequence design that can greatly decrease the sound levels of MRI acquisitions using relatively low amplitude gradient steps.[18]

Radiofrequency (RF) Transmitter/Receiver

The innermost component consists of an RF transceiver, another electromagnetic coil designed to transmit and receive RF pulses. The primary purpose of this transmitter is to produce a secondary electromagnetic field (known as B_1) at 90° to the main magnetic field. This is achieved by the use of an RF synthesizer, which generates a sine cardinal waveform which is then amplified and used to generate an alternating electric current to the transmitter coil. The frequency of this alternating current is matched to the precessional frequency of hydrogen nuclei within the patient, allowing a transfer of energy from the secondary field to the oscillating nuclei by the process of NMR. Modern scanners may employ a multi-element transmit coil, permitting a more homogeneous distribution of RF throughout the imaging volume. This is a particularly desirable feature at high field strengths, where standing wave effects can spoil image quality in the form of a shading artifact.[19] A secondary advantage is a reduction in RF deposition to the patient during image acquisition.

Receive Coils

Having transmitted an electromagnetic pulse into the patient, the system then has the task of receiving the returning signal; the mechanism behind this is covered in the next section. Although the body coil is capable of receiving RF, it has inherent image quality problems, primarily a poor signal-to-noise ratio (SNR). The efficiency of a receiver coil is determined by what is known as its filling-factor and this is maximised when the coil conforms closely to the shape and volume of the anatomy under investigation. The integral body-coil is situated a significant distance away from the area under investigation, and when imaging a small region of interest such as the knee, the body coil tends to receive a comparatively high level of random electrical noise compared to useful signal. For this reason, manufacturers provide a wide range of purpose-built receiver coils designed to be positioned in close proximity to the area under investigation, and sized to match the FOV required.

The three main types of receive coils are as follows.

Surface Coils. Surface coils are falling out of use in favour of phased-array volume coils, however they are still useful for imaging small structures such as finger joints or wrists. These coils are typically circular or elliptical in shape and consist of a wire antenna encased in a padded protective jacket. Generic surface coils are positioned close to the skin surface over the region of interest, such as the temporomandibular joint or wrist.

Surface coils receive less electrical noise than large volume coils such as the body coil, and because of this, and because of their close proximity to the patient, surface coils have a good inherent SNR. Their main disadvantage is the fact that they can only receive signal from a depth approximately equal to the coil diameter ×0.5. A 12 cm diameter coil will, therefore, only image structures to a depth of 6 cm below the surface of the skin. Signal falls off significantly with further distance from the coil. For uniform signal reception, a volume coil is required.

Volume Coils. Volume coils are designed to enclose the entire region of interest, usually the body, head, elbow, wrist, knee, ankle or foot. Their design often resembles a cylinder or birdcage, and the head coil often incorporates a mirror or prism allowing the patient to see an unrestricted view down the magnet bore. Some coils are very flexible and can be wrapped around the area under investigation. Volume coils detect signal uniformly across the region of interest without the loss of penetration associated with surface coils. The SNR is usually high because the coil size is matched to the region of interest resulting in a high filling factor. Some receive coils are also capable of transmitting RF.

Phased-Array Coils. A phased array refers to a number of receive coils ganged together. The signal detected by each element of the array is incorporated into one large FOV. Phased-array coils offer the coverage of the body coil but with the high SNR of a surface coil. The elements themselves can be selected or deselected depending upon the anatomical coverage sought. For example, a phased-array spine coil might have five elements, only one of which would be switched on for a cervical study. A cervicothoracic study may require three elements to be activated, and a scan for the whole spinal cord may employ all five elements simultaneously. Currently there are phased-array versions of coils used for most anatomical areas.

Modern phased-array coils have multiple elements, typically up to 32 or more, each detecting signal which may be routed through its own channel. This makes for a high SNR, as the noise collected by each element is random and tends to average out in the reconstructed image. Recent developments in coil technology have further improved SNR by digitising the data in the coil assembly rather than in a separate computer. This allows the acquired data to be transmitted back to the host computer via a fibre-optic cable which is unaffected by external interference or losses found in traditional wired connections. Phased-array coils can also be used for parallel imaging, whereby each element contributes to the collection of data for the image and shortens acquisition time accordingly.

PATIENT TRANSPORT SYSTEM

The patient couch has evolved over the years into a fairly sophisticated mechanism that allows accurate positioning of the region of interest using laser positioning devices.

Table movement and positioning are controlled by the scan computer, ensuring that the region under examination is always positioned optimally at the homogeneous isocentre of the magnet for every acquisition. Recent advances also permit acquisitions to be made during continuous table-movement permitting a larger, seamless FOV. With the advent of phased-array coils it is now possible to position the patient for one examination area and then perform imaging of multiple regions without physically disturbing the patient. An example of this is contrast-enhanced magnetic resonance angiography (CEMRA), where a single injection of contrast agent is imaged in stages as it passes in a bolus through the arterial system from the abdomen to the lower extremities. This kind of scan requires fast acquisition times and also very rapid (or continuous) table movement between areas of interest.

When purchasing a scanner it is well worth investigating the option of a detachable patient table. Detachable tables offer the advantage of a non-ferrous (safe) patient trolley that can quickly remove the patient from the scan room in an emergency, such as a magnet quench or in the event of a cardiac arrest. Having a second detachable table can improve patient throughput by allowing the positioning of non-ambulant patients in readiness for their procedure while the previous patient is still being scanned on the other table.

MRI Safety

The scope of MRI safety considerations is very wide and there are books and websites devoted to this complicated topic.[20] This section provides a brief overview, not a complete safety strategy, and practitioners working (or intending to work) in the field of MRI should seek further information before entering the MRI environment. The Medicine and Healthcare products Regulatory Agency (MHRA) offers safety guidelines for the use of MRI; local unit guidelines and hospital health and safety procedures should also be consulted.

RF PULSES

From a radiation protection viewpoint, MRI can be said to be a relatively safe modality. The electromagnetic radiation used is non-ionising and therefore does not present the risk of radiation-induced cancers associated with X-ray exposure. RF applications do, however, deploy energy into the body tissues, measured in watts per kilogram (W/kg), and this causes a heating effect, particularly at high field strengths. Many of the body systems can be adversely affected by overheating, so the scanner requires information about patient weight to ensure that safe levels are not exceeded.[21]

Burns associated with RF-induced heating of the patient or any attached leads or devices account for a majority of adverse incidents associated with this modality.

MAGNETIC FIELDS

The magnetic fields used in MRI can pose a significant safety risk to staff and patients owing to:

- Projectiles attracted to the main magnetic field
- Damage to implanted devices by the main magnetic field
- Torque applied to implanted devices and foreign bodies by the main magnetic field
- Nerve stimulation due to gradient magnetic fields
- Damage to implanted devices due to RF magnetic fields
- Heating of tissues or implanted devices due to RF magnetic fields

Projectiles

Projectiles due to translational or attractive displacement have caused a number of deaths and injuries to patients since 1980. Ferromagnetic objects such as wheelchairs, stretcher poles, floor polishers, oxygen cylinders and ancillary equipment have a strong attraction to the main magnetic field and may be dragged from the floor into the magnet bore. Experimentation by one equipment manufacturer has demonstrated that ferromagnetic objects may reach a speed of up to 60 kilometres per hour and follow a complex trajectory through the scanner causing serious trauma to a patient (and damage to the equipment, costing hundreds of thousands of pounds to repair).[22]

Implanted Devices

Implanted devices such as pacemakers and aneurysm clips may be adversely affected by a strong magnetic field. This may cause torque (twisting) of the device or may cause it to cease functioning correctly. There have been a number of deaths caused by patients entering the proximity of an MRI scanner with a pacemaker in situ. Other implanted devices deemed unsafe and therefore contraindicated include cochlear implants, breast implants with magnetic ports and some types of stents. Recent developments have allowed the production of conditionally safe devices such as pacemakers that can be programmed into an MRI-safe operating mode. A comprehensive research-based list of tested devices and implants can be found on Dr Frank Shellock's resource at https://www.mrisafety.com.[20]

The application of rapidly fluctuating gradient magnetic fields and RF pulses can induce voltages in conductive elements of a device, causing damage. Electromagnetic induction can occur in any looped conductor. For this reason cables must be insulated and not in direct contact with the patient's skin and the patient must not lie in a position where skin surfaces are in direct contact, for example the hands must not be linked or arms and legs crossed.[21]

Foreign Bodies

Items such as shrapnel and other metal fragments may experience a torque or attraction to the main magnetic field. This may lead to haemorrhage or damage to internal organs. Deflection of intraocular foreign bodies can also cause damage to the interior of the eye.[23]

To prevent patients with contraindications from entering the scan environment it is common policy to administer a screening form on attendance. In addition to the MHRA, the British Association of MR Radiographers offers the following advice:

The MR safety questionnaire should be designed to determine if there is any reason that the patient or individual would undergo an adverse reaction if they were to undergo an MRI investigation.[24]

They suggest that the questionnaire should be designed to obtain information concerning:

- Relevant previous surgery
- Prior injury from metallic foreign bodies
- Pregnancy
- Electrically, magnetically or mechanically activated devices

Further consideration should be given to:

- Permanent colouring techniques
- Body piercing
- Previous reaction to contrast agent
- Breastfeeding
- Last menstrual period

A set of example questions is also available from their website.[24]

It is good practice to inform patients of contraindications at the time of their appointment letter. This will prevent inconvenience to the patient and gaps in workflow if an individual cannot be scanned.

The Physical Principles of MRI

As already stated, the basic mechanism of MRI is that a radiofrequency is applied to the hydrogen nuclei in the patient's tissues which causes them to change their energy state and net magnetic alignment to an external magnetic field. As the nuclei lose this energy their magnetic moments realign with the field and their transmitted energy can be measured and spatially located. This technique uses a series of electromagnetic pulses and magnetic field gradient applications, collectively known as a pulse sequence. The timing of the pulse sequence components determines image contrast by exploiting the different molecular behaviours of the various body tissues such as collagen, fat, muscle and free water.

RESONANCE

Resonance can be defined as *the transfer of energy from one oscillating body to another*. In NMR this refers to the transfer of energy from an electromagnetic wave (radio wave) to the nucleus of an atom. To understand how this process works, the properties of electromagnetic waves and atomic nuclei must first be considered.

Electromagnetic Waves

Electromagnetic waves form a broad spectrum comprising different kinds of radiation. They travel at the speed of light, but have different wavelengths and therefore exhibit different frequencies. This means that if the waveforms are plotted on a graph or oscilloscope, some would have more cycles per second than others. Frequency is measured in hertz: 1 Hz = 1 cycle per second. The electromagnetic spectrum encompasses waves with a wide range of frequencies for example 10^2 Hz (radio waves) through microwaves and visible light to high-energy waves of the frequency 10^{24} Hz (X-rays and gamma rays). High-energy ionising radiation will damage biological tissue, whereas the lower-energy components of the spectrum such as radio waves are comparatively unlikely to cause permanent harm.

Atomic Nuclei

In the traditional Bohr model of the atom (proposed by Niels Bohr in 1913)[25] there is an arrangement of subatomic particles called protons, neutrons and electrons. Protons and neutrons (collectively called nucleons) are bound together to form a nucleus, with the electrons existing in discrete orbits around the nucleus like satellites around a planet. Modern science had modified this model slightly to describe the electron 'cloud' – a roughly spherical area surrounding the nucleus where there is a statistical probability of finding electrons.

In the classical model, all of the subatomic particles can be described in terms of mass, electric charge and movement:

- Electrons have negligible mass, are negatively charged, spin on their own axes in either direction and orbit the nucleus
- Protons have measurable mass, are positively charged and spin on their own axis in either direction
- Neutrons also have mass, have no electrical charge and spin on their own axes in either direction

Nuclei can contain differing numbers of protons and neutrons. Elements are assigned a mass number referring to the number of nucleons present and an atomic number that reflects the number of protons present.

If a nucleus has an even number of nucleons (such as helium, which has two protons and two neutrons) the nucleus will exhibit a positive electrical charge (due to the protons), but because the nucleons can spin in either direction the 'clockwise' spins will cancel out the 'anticlockwise' spins. The nucleus will therefore have a net positive charge but no net spin.

If a nucleus has an odd number of nucleons (as in lithium, which has three protons and four neutrons) there will be a net positive charge and a net spin. This is because there will be an unpaired spinning proton in the nucleus. Whenever there is an electrically charged spinning particle, a magnetic field will be generated by that particle. Nuclei having an odd mass number therefore have an induced magnetic field.

THE HYDROGEN NUCLEUS

The nucleus used in anatomical MRI imaging is the hydrogen atom. Hydrogen is chosen because its nucleus is a solitary proton with spin, charge and hence a magnetic moment. Hydrogen is by far the most common element in the universe, accounting for 75% of everything that is known to exist,[26] and accounts for approximately 60% of the atoms in the human body.

Quantum theory states that different atomic nuclei exist in one of several possible energy states. The number of possible energy states of an individual nucleus varies depending upon the element in question. The single hydrogen proton can only spin in one of two possible directions; its magnetic field can therefore only be generated in one of two possible orientations, and it exists in one of two energy states.

Normally the orientation of these tiny magnetic vectors is distributed randomly, but when subjected to an external magnetic field, such as that found inside an MRI scanner, the magnetic vectors of the nuclei will all align with the external field B_0. Approximately half of the nuclei will align with their magnetic vector pointing in the same direction as the main magnetic field (called spin-up) and the other half will align with their magnetic vectors in the opposite direction (spin-down). The nuclei can absorb energy from, and emit energy to, the main magnetic field and therefore flip between the two energy states constantly. However, as it requires less energy to align *with* the external field rather than *against* it, the ratio between spin-up and spin-down nuclei will change, and after a few seconds there will be slightly more spins in the low-energy/spin-up orientation than in the high-energy/spin-down orientation (Figs 27.4 and 27.5).

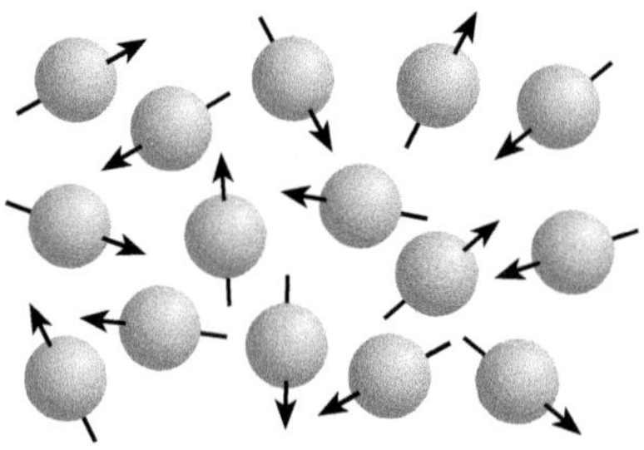

Fig. 27.4 Magnetic vectors of hydrogen nuclei in random alignment.

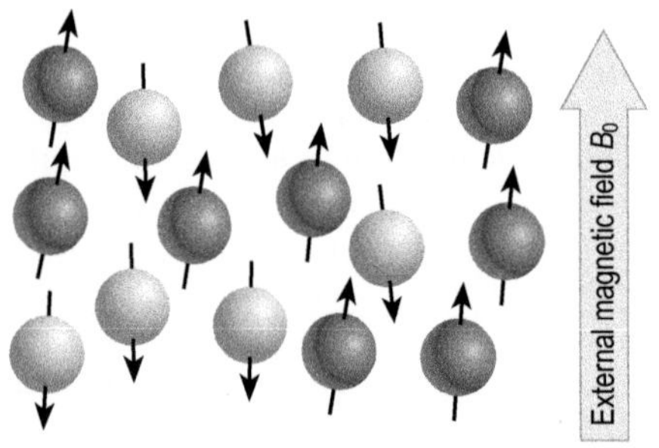

Fig. 27.5 Magnetic vectors of hydrogen nuclei in an external magnetic field.

THE NET MAGNETIC VECTOR (NMV)

In MRI it is the behaviour of the combined magnetism of all the hydrogen nuclei within a sample of tissue that is important. This bulk magnetic vector is also known as the net magnetic vector (NMV). As more of the hydrogen nuclei shift their magnetic vector into the parallel orientation, the NMV becomes aligned with B_0. This is because, at the outset, the populations of spin-up and spin-down nuclei are equal and their magnetic fields cancel out. Over time, more spins attain the spin-up orientation and the NMV becomes aligned accordingly. The resulting magnetisation is said to be 'longitudinal' or in the +Z direction. The time taken for the NMV to make this shift is known as T1[27] and is an important factor in image contrast (to be absolutely precise, T1 is defined as the time taken for 63% of the longitudinal magnetisation to orientate into the +Z direction).

The actual ratio between spin-up and spin-down nuclei is very small: in approximately every million spins there are only three extra spin-up nuclei. This does not sound like many, but when you remember that there are some 7×10^{27} atoms in the human body, this equates to billions of extra spin-up nuclei in a tissue sample, and it is these nuclei that provide the signal and contrast on an MRI scan. For the rest of this chapter, the magnetic vectors of these surplus nuclei will simply be referred to as the 'spins'.

One final important point to note is that the surfeit of spin-up nuclei increases with flux density (field strength). This is because more energy is required to oppose a strong field than a weaker field, and the spin-up and spin-down populations will reflect this. High-field scanners therefore have an inherently better SNR than low-field systems.

PRECESSION

When describing motion in the atom earlier, the terms *spinning* and *orbiting* were mentioned. There is also another important kind of motion involved in NMR, known as precession. When the nuclei are subjected to an external magnetic field they not only spin on their axes but they also wobble slightly. This is often described as being analogous to a spinning top. Consider a gyroscope spinning on a tabletop: it will spin at hundreds of revolutions per minute but will also be seen to wobble at a much slower rate. Imagine a line drawn through the vertical axis of the gyroscope: as the gyroscope wobbles this imaginary line will prescribe a cone shape. This movement is known as precession and is due to gravity. The *speed* at which the gyroscope wobbles is also related to gravity: on the moon, with less gravity, the gyroscope would precess more slowly (fewer wobbles per minute) than on the Earth.

The spinning hydrogen nuclei also precess, not because of gravity but owing to the presence of the external magnetic field. If the field strength is increased, the nuclei will precess at a faster rate; if the external field is reduced they will precess more slowly.

Phase and Frequency

The precessional speed and orientation of a spinning nucleus can be described in terms of frequency and phase.

The frequency of precession (i.e. how many wobbles per second) can be calculated by an equation first published by mathematician Joseph Larmor (1857–1942), and it is the only equation used in this chapter.

The Larmor equation states that:

$$\omega = \gamma B_0$$

where:

ω is the angular precessional frequency of the proton
γ is the gyromagnetic ratio of the nucleus
B_0 is the external field strength

Every nucleus has its own fixed gyromagnetic ratio expressed in hertz/tesla. For hydrogen this is 42.6 MHz/T, so at a field strength of 1 T the hydrogen nuclei will be precessing at a frequency of 42.6 MHz (at 1.5 T it will be 63.9 MHz and so on).

Knowledge of the precessional frequency for hydrogen at a particular field strength is important because in order to resonate the nuclei it is necessary to apply an electromagnetic wave at a matching frequency, and this will differ depending upon the field strength of the scanner being used.

Phase is a term that can be used to describe the angular orientation of the magnetic vector of a nucleus compared to other nuclei nearby. The gyroscope analogy can be expanded to explain phase. It was stated earlier that the vertical axis of a precessing gyroscope (or nucleus) prescribes a cone shape. If the gyroscope is viewed from above, the top of the gyroscope can be seen to move in a circular path as it wobbles about its axis. That is to say, its orientation goes from a 12 o'clock position round to 3 o'clock, 6 o'clock, 9 o'clock and finally ends up back at 12 o'clock. If a number of gyroscopes were set spinning at the same time, it is unlikely that they would all precess in synchrony. Even though they might be spinning at the same speed (frequency), one gyroscope might be at the 12 o'clock position while its neighbour is at 6 o'clock. This is analogous to the spins being out of phase with each other.

At equilibrium the nuclei are all precessing at the same frequency because they are all in the same magnetic field strength, but they are out of synchrony when it comes to the orientation of their vectors. The orientation of a single vector around its cone-shaped path is known as its phase position, and at equilibrium the spins can be said to be out of phase (Figs 27.6 and 27.7).

SIGNAL

To construct an image it is necessary to receive signal from the region of interest and spatially encode it. MRI signal is in the form of a weak electromagnetic wave created by the oscillating net magnetic vector of the spins following excitation by an RF pulse.

Faraday's law of electromagnetic induction states that:

The induced electromotive force or EMF in any closed circuit is equal to the time rate of change of the magnetic flux through the circuit.[28]

In the case of the MRI signal, the NMV is a moving magnetic field that will induce a voltage in an antenna (or conductive loop) placed in proximity to the region of interest. The maximum signal is generated when the NMV is 90° to B_0 and the contributing individual vectors are in phase.

At equilibrium the NMV is aligned in the same direction as B_0 and the spins are out of phase. There is no coherent

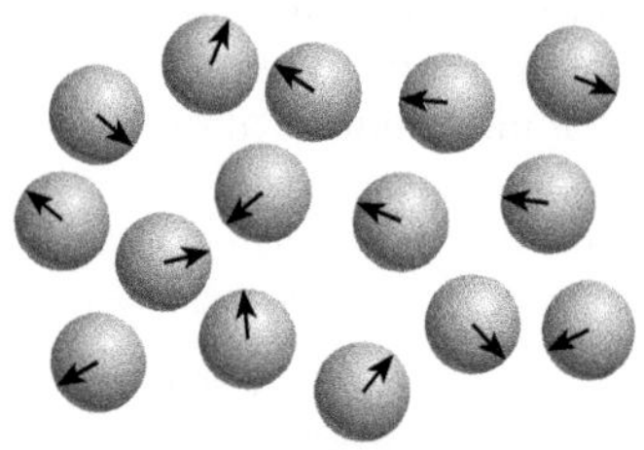

Fig. 27.6 The magnetic vectors of hydrogen nuclei, out of phase. (These spins are depicted as being viewed from 'above', i.e. we are looking from a direction parallel to the main magnetic field.) Dephased magnetic vectors cancel out, resulting in a loss of signal.

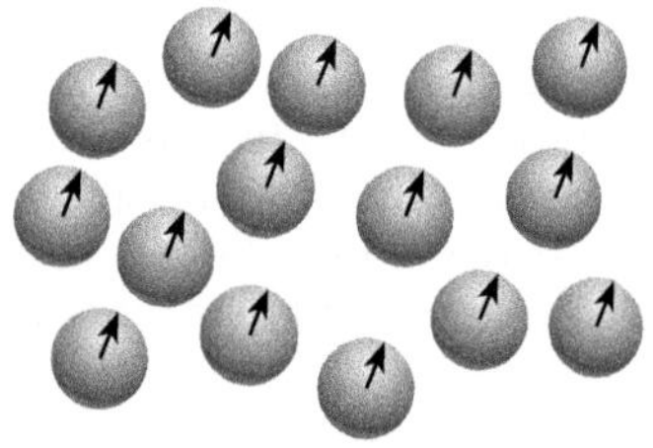

Fig. 27.7 The magnetic vectors of hydrogen nuclei, in phase. The combined magnetic effect of all these spins is known as the net magnetic vector (NMV).

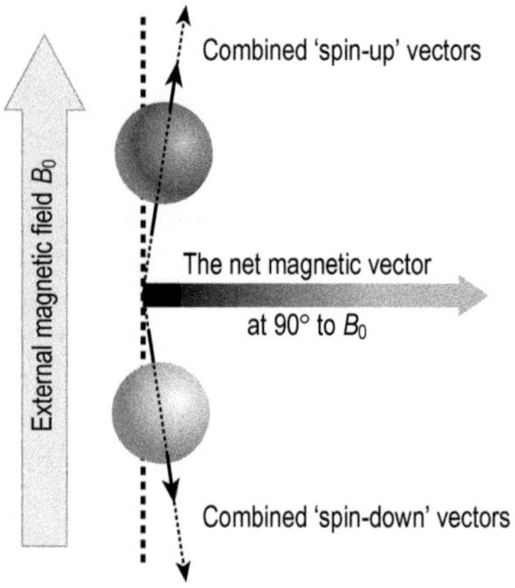

Fig. 27.8 The NMV following a 90° RF pulse.

transverse magnetisation to be detected by the receiver coil. To generate signal an RF pulse at the Larmor frequency transfers energy to the nuclei in the sample. This process of resonance has two important effects:

1. First, the surfeit of nuclei in the low-energy spin-up direction will absorb energy and become high-energy spin-down nuclei. If the right amount of RF is used the populations of spin-up and spin-down nuclei will become equal; the scanner determines the critical amount of RF required to do this during the prescan. The effect of having equal populations of spin-up and spin-down nuclei is that the NMV will change orientation. Instead of being aligned with the main magnetic field, the NMV will rotate (or more accurately nutate) to precess at 90° to B_0. This reflects the sum of all the spin-up vectors and all of the spin-down vectors as they transcribe their cone-shaped precessional path. In this orientation the vector may be detected using a suitable antenna (receive coil). This magnetisation is said to be in the transverse plane, i.e. the RF pulse has converted longitudinal magnetisation into transverse magnetisation. Because it has changed the angle of the NMV by 90° the pulse used is known as a 90° RF pulse (Fig. 27.8).
2. The second effect of the RF pulse is that it forces the magnetic vectors of the spins to precess in phase. This is important, as the signal from out-of-phase spins cancels out and cannot be detected by the receive coil. In-phase spins result in an NMV that precesses at the Larmor frequency at 90° to B_0 and produces maximum signal in the receive coil.

The spins do not stay in phase for very long, for two reasons. The main cause of dephasing is field inhomogeneity, even with a field homogeneous to 4 ppm there will be a fluctuation in field strength across the imaging volume. The secondary cause of dephasing is the fact that the nuclei have their own microscopic magnetic fields, and these fields interact over time, attracting and repelling each other, a process known as spin–spin interaction. The important point to note here is that dephasing due to inhomogeneity is undesirable, as it causes signal loss indiscriminately, whereas spin–spin interactions are desirable because they provide a powerful contrast mechanism. Fortunately the dephasing caused by inhomogeneity can be reversed by the use of a 180° RF pulse. The signal that would otherwise be lost reappears briefly as the spins come back into phase; this is known as a spin echo.

The time taken for the spins to lose (63% of) their phase coherence due to spin–spin interactions is known as T2, and it is this that can be exploited as a contrast mechanism.

CONTRAST

So far it has been stated that signal from hydrogen nuclei can be generated in a tissue sample and detected by a receive coil. In order to make a diagnostic image, however, it is necessary to create contrast between different structures/tissues/pathologies.

There are various factors affecting contrast on an MRI image, but the three most important are:

- T1 recovery
- T2 decay
- Proton density (PD)

T1

It was mentioned earlier that when a 90° RF pulse is applied to the sample, any longitudinal magnetisation is converted into transverse magnetisation. It is also true to say that any (residual) transverse magnetisation will be tipped into the longitudinal plane. The reason that this factor can be used to produce contrast on the image is that different tissues have different rates of T1 recovery.

As an example, there is a marked difference between the recovery rates of fat and pure water. Following a 90° RF pulse, fat recovers its longitudinal magnetisation quickly (200 ms). This is because it has large molecules with relatively slow brownian motion that can dissipate energy fairly readily. This means that, in fat, the spin population loses the absorbed energy quickly and the fat vector regains its low-energy spin-up orientation.

Pure water, on the other hand, has high-energy molecules with rapid brownian motion that cannot dissipate energy readily. Pure water nuclei therefore retain the absorbed energy and the magnetic vector associated with pure water remains in the transverse plane for longer than that of fat. The NMV from water can take up to 4 seconds to recover its longitudinal magnetisation.

If a second 90° RF pulse is rapidly applied to the sample, the fully recovered NMV from fat will once again be flipped into the transverse plane, giving maximum signal, but the partially recovered water vector will be flipped back into the longitudinal plane in the −Z direction. With little transverse magnetisation to be detected by the coil, water will subsequently return only a limited signal (Fig. 27.9).

If more time were allowed between RF pulses, fat and water vectors would each have time to recover their longitudinal magnetisation and would both be flipped 90° by successive RF pulses, reducing T1 contrast.

The time between RF applications is known as the TR (time to repetition); a T1-weighted image uses a short TR (e.g. 300 ms) and will exhibit relatively hyperintense (bright) fat and relatively hypointense (dark) fluid.

A T1-weighted sequence tends to demonstrate morphology clearly because it has a short echo time that yields a high SNR.

T1 weighting is the contrast of choice when using gadolinium enhancement, as gadolinium is a T1-shortening agent. Such scans are usually performed before and after administration of contrast agent to ensure that any hyperintensity on the image is due to enhancement rather than being an inherently T1-bright structure, such as fat or haemorrhage.

The fact that fat exhibits a high signal on T1 weighting makes this sequence sensitive to changes in bone marrow, including metastasis and avascular necrosis. If the fat content of bone marrow is replaced, the signal level will fall and the affected area will appear relatively hypointense on T1 weighting.

T2

Following the removal of the 90° RF pulse, the spins dephase rapidly.

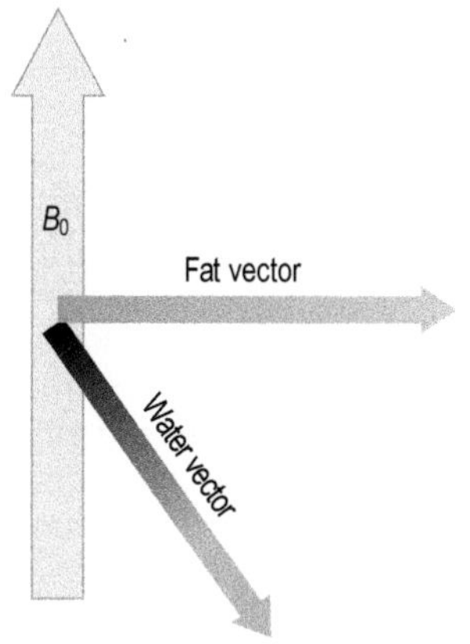

Fig. 27.9 Fat and water vectors during rapid TR. Fat vector is repeatedly flipped to 90° but water is flipped to beyond 90° and the signal becomes saturated.

The reason that T2 dephasing provides an image contrast mechanism is that different tissues lose phase coherence at different rates. The most marked difference here is between solids and pure water molecules. Following the removal of the 90° RF pulse, the magnetic vectors of slow-tumbling tightly packed nuclei in solid structures such as collagen have a marked effect upon each other and dephase readily and quickly. Although a somewhat counter-intuitive concept, in water molecules the comparatively rapid tumbling rate causes local magnetic field fluctuations to average out over time. In other words, the molecules are affected by the north and south poles of neighbouring dipoles in equal measure. This averaging-out causes their magnetic vectors to stay in phase for longer.

Contrast is therefore obtained by waiting for a certain time after the application of the 90° RF pulse before sampling the returning signal. Any tissues that have lost phase coherence (e.g. fat or collagen) will appear less intense than tissues whose spins are still in phase (e.g. water).

The time between the 90° RF pulse and the collection of the signal is known as the TE (time to echo); a T2-weighted image uses a long TE (e.g. 100 ms or above) and will exhibit high signal from water, but very reduced signal from solids.

Proton Density (PD)

The term proton density (PD) refers to the number of hydrogen nuclei present in a given volume of tissue. To compare extremes, think of air and water. There are more hydrogen nuclei in the fluid-filled ventricles of the brain than in the nearby air-filled paranasal sinuses. A PD-weighted image will therefore have varying degrees of signal from different tissues. A PD image is obtained by using parameters that reduce T1 and T2 contrast, i.e. a long TR to reduce T1 effects and a short TE to reduce T2 effects. When the influence of these contrast mechanisms is so diminished, an image is returned whereby the signal intensity of the various anatomical structures is determined principally by the concentration of hydrogen within those tissues. PD images could be said to be the most anatomically accurate, in some cases looking very much like monochrome postmortem photographs.

Weighting

When describing the contrast of an MRI image the term 'weighting' is used to indicate that the contrast is weighted or heavily influenced by one of the above parameters. Image contrast never results purely from one of these parameters alone, as all images are affected to some degree by T1, T2 and PD. For example, the air-filled sinuses may appear as hypointense as a melanoma metastasis on a T2-weighted scan. However, the lack of signal from the sinuses does not relate to T2 contrast but rather, a low proton density. Conversely, a melanoma metastasis contains plenty of hydrogen protons, but rapid dephasing creates the low-intensity T2 contrast.

SPATIAL ENCODING

Having generated signal and determined the contrast required, the final stage of the procedure is to spatially encode the signal so that it can be reconstructed into a diagnostic image. Spatial encoding using gradient magnetic fields was first proposed by Lauterbur in 1973,[5] further developed by Mansfield, and a variation of his technique is still used in scanning today. The principle relies on the fact that spins across the imaging volume can be assigned a particular spatial location depending on their frequency of precession or changing phase position measured over a certain timeframe. Spatial encoding for a 2D slice is achieved by the use of three gradients that perform the following functions:

- Determining the slice position
- Encoding the position of the spins in the horizontal axis of the image
- Encoding the position of the spins in the vertical axis of the image

Slice Position

Determining the slice position is the first part of spatial encoding. As mentioned in an earlier section, resonance can only occur if the energy source exhibits the resonant frequency as the target. An example of this would be to obtain two tuning-forks both tuned to the same note, place one of them in a stand and strike the second against an object to start it vibrating. If the vibrating fork is held in close proximity to the silent fork the transfer of energy between the two will induce vibration in the silent fork, even though there has been no physical contact. The critical factor is that they must be tuned to exactly the same note (frequency). This experiment would not work if a tuning fork playing the note A was held close to a tuning fork tuned to the note B.

The aim of slice selection is to resonate a thin section of tissue rather than the entire patient: consider a single slice through an abdomen on a patient who is lying supine and head first in the scanner.

The resonant frequency of the hydrogen nuclei can be calculated using the Larmor equation, and similarly if a gradient is applied at a known strength, the precessional frequencies of the spins along the length of the gradient can also be calculated. If a gradient is applied over a certain volume (centred at the magnetic isocentre), the mid-part of the gradient will remain at the centre frequency while spins at the ends of the gradient will exhibit either a slightly lower or a slightly higher frequency. If an RF pulse were applied at the centre frequency it would only resonate the spins at the isocentre. The spins elsewhere along the slope would not be affected, as their induced frequencies would not match the transmitted frequency. If an RF pulse was applied at a slightly higher frequency it would only resonate spins at a spatial allocation towards the higher frequency end of the gradient (Fig. 27.10). To achieve an axial slice it is therefore necessary to apply a gradient in the Z direction during transmission of the 90° RF pulse.

In reality, it is not quite that simple, because slices must have a finite thickness, so a range of frequencies must be applied to excite a narrow band of spins along the corresponding part of the gradient. This range of frequencies is known as the *transmit bandwidth*.

Phase Encoding

Having selected the slice position, it is now necessary to locate the signal returning from within that FOV. First, consider the signal originating from the horizontal axis of the image (left to right on a supine patient). To encode this signal, another magnetic field gradient application is performed. This time the gradient coils are used to apply a slope in the X direction across the magnet bore from right to left. This causes the precession of the spins to speed up or slow down depending on their location. Importantly, the gradient is then turned off. In the absence of the gradient the spins return to the centre frequency, but because of the time spent inside the gradient their *phase* positions will have shifted along this axis. Spins at the isocentre were still at the centre frequency during the gradient application, so their phase position will be unchanged – say at 12 o'clock (or 0°). Spins that were briefly precessing more rapidly than those at the isocentre might have an advanced phase position of 5 o'clock (or 150°). Spins that were situated at the lower-than-centre frequency portion of the slope might have a phase position of 7 o'clock (−150°) (Fig. 27.11).

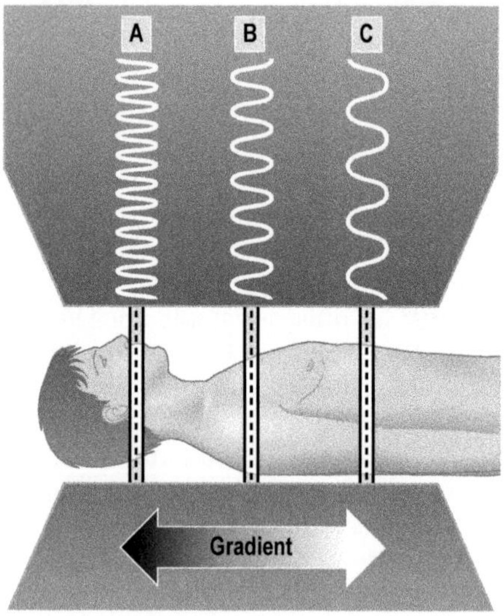

Fig. 27.10 Applied RF pulses at different frequencies resonate different slice positions along a magnetic field gradient. Radiofrequency A only resonates spins having the precessional frequency corresponding to the position of the topmost slice. Radiofrequency B is at the centre frequency and only resonates spins at the isocentre. Radiofrequency C only resonates spins having the precessional frequency corresponding to the position of the lowermost slice.

This *phase encoding* gradient is applied many times during the pulse sequence at gradually changing amplitudes, causing a different amount of phase shift across the FOV each time (repetition). The key point to note is that the phase position of the signal from a discrete point along the phase encoding axis will change its phase position incrementally each TR (e.g. TR 01 – 0°, TR 01 – 10°, TR 01 – 20°, TR 01 – 30°, and so forth). Mapped over time this gives the appearance of a frequency, i.e. a waveform having cycles. The spatial resolution in the phase direction is determined by the number of phase encodings performed, typically 128, 256, 512, 1024 or 2048 pixels. A 512 matrix will therefore require 512 RF applications (512 repetitions), and because the TR is of fixed length, a scan having a matrix of 512 will take twice as long to perform as a scan having a matrix of 256.

Frequency Encoding

Having applied the previous two gradients, the slice position has been determined and data collected enabling

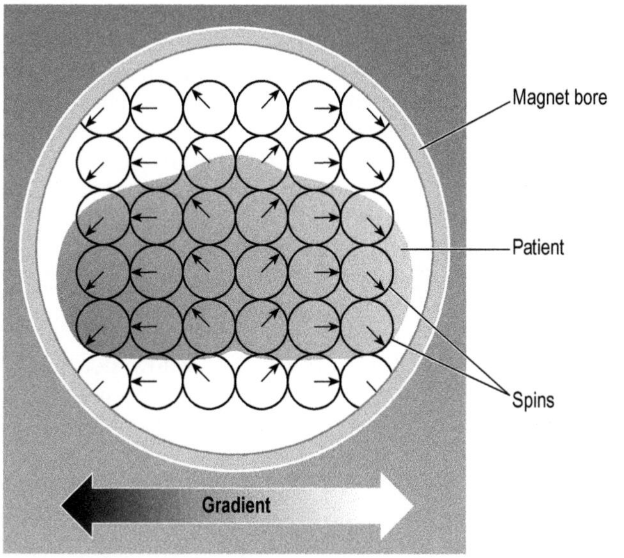

Fig. 27.11 The application of a secondary gradient across the field of view changes the precessional frequencies of the spins. When it is turned off, the phase positions of some columns of spins will be advanced or retarded compared to the spins that remained at the centre frequency (isocentre).

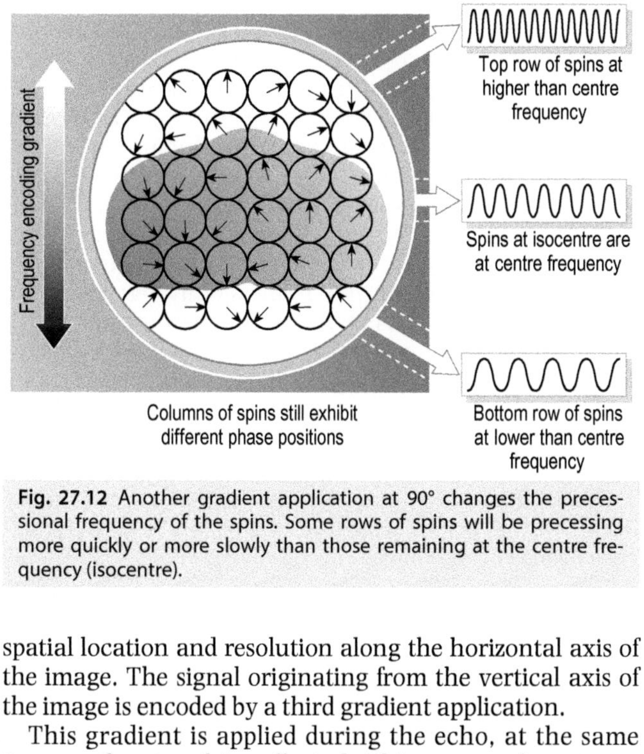

Fig. 27.12 Another gradient application at 90° changes the precessional frequency of the spins. Some rows of spins will be precessing more quickly or more slowly than those remaining at the centre frequency (isocentre).

spatial location and resolution along the horizontal axis of the image. The signal originating from the vertical axis of the image is encoded by a third gradient application.

This gradient is applied during the echo, at the same time as the signal is collected. This causes the returning signal to exhibit a range of different precessional frequencies from the spins along the horizontal axis of the region of interest. The gradient is therefore known as either the *frequency encoding* gradient or the *readout* gradient. Once again the spins at isocentre will remain at the centre frequency, but the spins at each end of the gradient will either precess more quickly or more slowly depending on the magnetic field slope. The net effect of this is that the receive coil detects a range of frequencies at time TE (Fig. 27.12).

Having acquired the signal, the system computer uses a mathematical calculation on the collected data known as the Fourier transform (devised by Jean Baptiste Joseph Fourier, 1768–1830), which essentially isolates the individual frequencies and their intensities. Because the applied gradient is linear in nature, each intensity measured will be in a linear arrangement corresponding to its spatial position of origin.

A useful analogy is to imagine playing the note 'middle C' on a piano and asking a concert pianist to name the note. Middle C is the central note on the keyboard, and on hearing the sound they would likely be able to identify it as such. They have 'received' a frequency (261.63 Hz) and have assigned it a spatial location (the middle). Middle C can be thought of as the central frequency in MRI, with all of the other white notes representing the range of frequencies along the gradient axis. If a pianist were to play a chord by pressing down on several piano keys at once, the Fourier transform would be able to identify the separate notes (frequencies) – and how hard each key had been pressed (signal intensities). To further develop this analogy, imagine looking at a graphic equaliser such as might be found on a mobile phone music player. The equaliser often displays a bouncing spectrum-analysis of the music being played. This is essentially a histogram of the frequencies present in the digital waveform of the music file at any given moment in time. The bass notes to the left, the high pitched frequencies to the right and middle C being in the centre. The height of the bars represents the amount of signal being returned at each frequency. In an MRI image these would be equivalent to the amount of signal being returned from each column of voxels in the frequency direction.

In terms of spatial encoding, the principle behind the phase and frequency encoding gradients is more or less identical, the difference being the sampling rate. All of the frequencies in a single spin echo are collected (sampled) in 20 ms or less; the data used to reconstruct an equivalent waveform in the phase direction are sampled each repetition and, therefore, take the entire duration of the scan to acquire. Either way, the result is a waveform created from the samples collected and this can be Fourier transformed to present the amplitude of each sample in space.

PULSE SEQUENCES

The succession of RF pulses and gradient applications used in spatial encoding is known as a pulse sequence. Pulse sequences can be divided into two main categories, known as spin echo and gradient echo (GE). The main difference between the two is that spin echo pulse sequences use a 180° RF pulse to rephase the signal that would otherwise be lost due to field inhomogeneity. GE uses a magnetic field gradient to produce an echo but does not correct for field inhomogeneity dephasing. GE is typically faster than spin echo but is prone to artefactual appearances such as susceptibility effects seen when patients have metallic implants. Figure 27.13 shows the order of events in a typical spin echo and GE pulse sequence.

These basic pulse sequences have been enhanced and developed to include new contrast mechanisms and methods of rapid acquisition; these include inversion recovery sequences, fast spin echo (FSE), driven equilibrium,

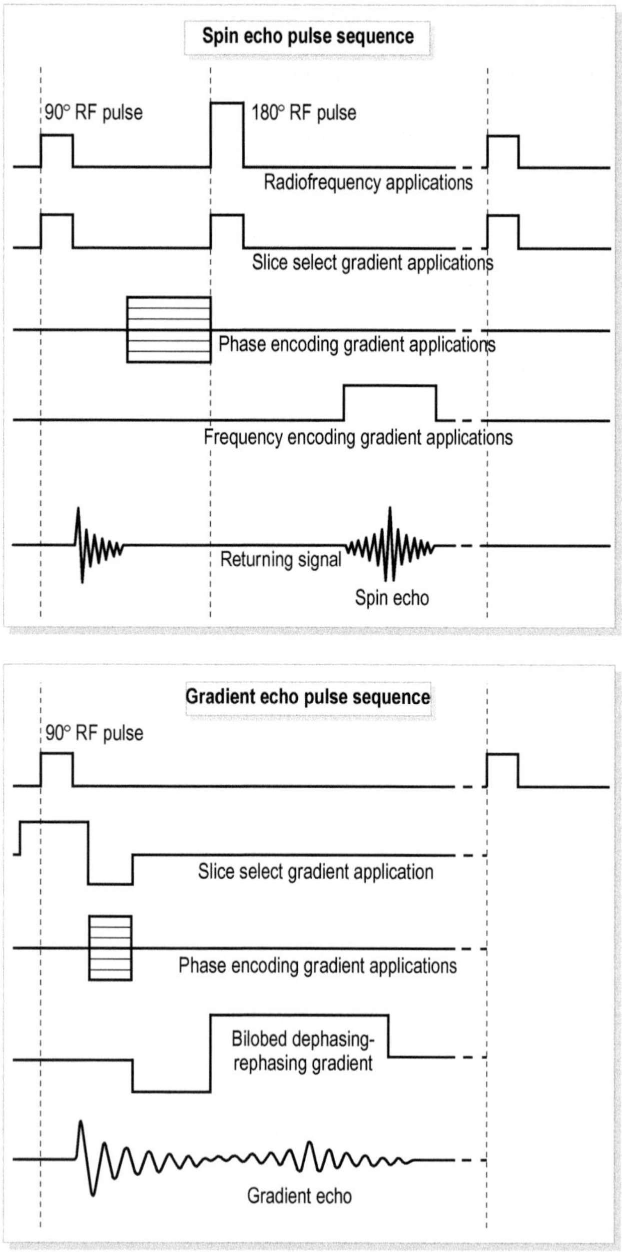

Fig. 27.13 Simplified spin echo and gradient echo (GE) pulse sequence diagrams. Note that the GE uses another magnetic field gradient application to produce an echo of signal rather than a 180° RF pulse.

single-shot imaging and echo-planar imaging. Further description of MRI pulse sequences can be found in the clinical applications section of this chapter.

CONTRAST MEDIA

Despite the excellent soft tissue capabilities of MRI and its inherently high contrast-to-noise ratio, the development of contrast media for MRI began in tandem with the first scans in 1978. MRI contrast media can be broadly classified into two main categories, positive and negative.

Positive Contrast Media – T1 Agents

Positive contrast agents produce an increase in signal intensity in affected tissues. In MRI the principal positive agents contain gadolinium as their active ingredient. In its native state gadolinium is a silver metal named after a Finnish chemist, Johan Gadolin. Like many other metals, gadolinium is mined for use in industry and its medical application forms only a small percentage of its global use. It is a lanthanide element at number 64 in the periodic table. At room temperature gadolinium is paramagnetic. This is to say that it aligns to and adds to an external magnetic field. Gadolinium is toxic and therefore is attached to a chelate or ligand to produce a contrast agent.

Its mechanism as a contrast agent relies on the fact that it causes T1 shortening at fairly low doses. This ability is due to the presence of seven unpaired electrons that form dipolar bonds with hydrogen nuclei in the tissues (blood). The result of this is that the molecular tumbling rate of water is reduced, allowing a more efficient energy exchange. With a rapid TR, water is able to recover much of its longitudinal magnetisation between RF pulses; this results in more magnetisation available to be flipped into the transverse plane. In simple terms, water combined with gadolinium chelate behaves more like fat, and is therefore hyperintense on a T1-weighted image.

Negative Contrast Media – T2 Agents

Negative contrast agents have now largely fallen from favour, but their action produces a decrease in signal intensity in affected tissues. In MRI the principal negative agents typically contain iron oxide as their active ingredient. These compounds consist of microcrystalline magnetite cores coated with dextranes or siloxanes. This impervious coating prevents the iron from binding with the body tissues.

The mechanism of a negative contrast agent relies on the fact that it causes T2 shortening at fairly low doses. The signal loss seen in areas of uptake is due to magnetic susceptibility effects. Spins in cells containing the superparamagnetic iron oxide will have a slightly higher precessional frequency than those surrounding them. This results in dephasing at the boundaries of these microscopic areas and a net loss of signal. This is because transverse magnetisation must be coherent (i.e. in phase) to produce maximum signal, and effects that cause dephasing will reduce the signal intensity.

USE OF MRI CONTRAST MEDIA

Although MRI has the inherent ability to distinguish between types of soft tissue, there are times when the use of contrast media is unavoidable.

Lesion Conspicuity

The use of contrast media can greatly increase the conspicuity of certain lesions. This is of particular importance where the presence of lesions would radically alter the treatment plan. As an example, a patient diagnosed with a single cerebral metastasis might be considered a candidate for surgery. If, by increasing conspicuity, gadolinium enhancement demonstrated the presence of multiple smaller lesions, it is less likely that surgery would be considered.[29]

Lesion Characterisation

Certain lesions are difficult to characterise using the inherent contrast parameters of MRI. For example, a neurofibroma returns a high signal on T2 weighting and a low to intermediate signal on T1. Other lesions, such as proteinaceous cysts, would also have similar contrast characteristics. Cystic lesions, however, do not tend to enhance, whereas a neurofibroma does.

Lesion Extent

On unenhanced T1-weighted images the boundaries of some lesions are not clearly defined. T2 weighting demonstrates pathology very well, but there is often a lot of associated oedema affecting the surrounding tissues that can distort the appearance of a lesion. The true size, shape and position of a lesion are usually better appreciated on a T1-weighted contrast-enhanced image.

Contrast-Enhanced MRA (CEMRA)

Blood vessels can be imaged by MRI using flow-dependent techniques that do not require the use of an exogenous contrast agent. Such studies produce contrast that relies on the flow of spins relative to their surroundings. These techniques suffer from certain shortcomings, such as artefactual over-estimation of stenoses, the ability to image flow only in a particular direction and small fields of view.

The use of gadolinium has reduced most of these problems. CEMRA allows a larger FOV, gives a more anatomical picture of the anatomy, more accurately reproduces the size of stenoses and shortens acquisition time to a matter of seconds.

Other considerations when deciding whether to use contrast include:

- *Throughput:* on low-field systems having longer acquisition times or only having conventional spin echo (CSE) rather than FSE, it may be quicker to make a diagnosis using contrast where the alternative would be to perform a number of more time-consuming sequences to make the same diagnosis. An example is acoustic neuroma, T1 pre and post gadolinium (10 minutes) vs a high-resolution T2-weighted scan (20 minutes)
- *Dynamic studies:* in some body areas such as the liver and breast, where different kinds of lesion may exhibit different rates of contrast uptake, a diagnosis is more readily ascertained by dynamic contrast-enhanced scanning (DCE MRI). This technique uses a series of short sequences performed after injection of gadolinium chelate and calculates the uptake curve and appearance of lesions in the arterial, venous and delayed stages post injection. This can give more information than a simple pre and post contrast scan

Common Clinical Applications

MRI is now used in imaging virtually every anatomical region, and the full range of clinical applications of MRI is therefore well beyond the scope of this chapter. The following section will cover only the most commonly requested examinations, and it is intended that the protocols suggested will act as a basic guide. MRI protocols vary widely and must take into account the preferences of the reporting radiologist/radiographer, the time available, the compliance of the patient, and the field strength and capabilities of the scanner hardware/software. Do not alter scan protocols without consulting other users or backing up the originals! The recommended pulse sequences are generic and are commonly found on equipment from all manufacturers.

PULSE SEQUENCES

The pulse sequences referred to in the protocols in the next section of this chapter are described in more detail here.

Spin Echo and Fast (Turbo) Spin Echo Sequences

Conventional spin echo (CSE) sequences use a 180° RF pulse to help eliminate undesirable dephasing due to field inhomogeneity. The result is a sequence that offers high-quality images which are relatively artefact free. The main trade-off is that the scan time can be relatively long compared to FSE or GE techniques. Attempts to reduce scan time, for example by reducing the phase matrix, the TR and the number of signal averages, typically result in a deterioration of image quality in terms of resolution, weighting and SNR, respectively.

It is possible to use more than one 180° pulse in a spin echo repetition, and therefore collect multiple echoes each having different TE values during the same acquisition. Multiple echo sequences result in more than one set of images, each set of slices having identical anatomical locations but different contrast characteristics. A common example is a dual echo sequence providing one set of T2-weighted images and a second set of PD-weighted images. A Dixon technique gradient echo sequence is also dual echo, but uses gradients to produce the echoes without a 180° pulse.

Dual (multiple) echo can also be used in a technique known as T2 relaxometry, where there are a number of echoes at different TE values, allowing regions of interest to be drawn and T2 relaxation curves produced for various tissues.

For T1 weighting CSE is a perfectly acceptable sequence choice because T1 contrast relies on a short repetition time, which inherently shortens scan time.

T1-weighted FSE sequences are also available but have some associated trade-offs in terms of weighting and maximum available slice number without offering a significant time saving over CSE T1-weighted images.

FSE sequences, introduced in 1990, shorten scan time by collecting more data per repetition. This is facilitated by the use of numerous 180° RF pulses within each TR period which, in turn, yield a whole train of echoes rather than just one echo per repetition. The echo train length is a user-definable parameter and shortens the scan time proportionally, so an echo train of 8 would reduce an 8 minute scan to a 1 minute scan. The longest echo train at the time of writing is 728, allowing the acquisition of an entire high-resolution image in a single shot.

FSE is usually the sequence of choice for T2-weighted studies because scan factors would make a CSE T2-weighted sequence impracticably slow (the TR must be long to reduce T1 effects). Historically, CSE T2-weighted sequences could take up to 30 minutes to acquire, compared to just a couple of minutes (or less) for FSE.

The trade-offs with FSE include a higher RF deposition to the patient (heating) and a slight change in weighting (higher fat signal on T2-weighted images compared to CSE). If it is thought that hyperintense fat might reduce the conspicuity of fluid-filled lesions, it is possible to select a fat saturation pulse as an additional imaging option. This technique applies an additional RF pulse to the region of interest every repetition. The frequency of the additional pulse is finely tuned to match only the resonant frequency of fat nuclei. Because fat receives more RF than the other tissues, the signal is saturated, essentially removed from the resulting images.

Single Shot (SSFSE)

Single-shot techniques have greatly shortened acquisition times in MRI. These sequences take FSE to the extreme, in that they apply numerous 180° pulses allowing collection of all of the signal for a slice after a single excitation pulse. This allows imaging while the patient is free-breathing. The snapshot effect of the scan typically freezes motion in areas of the body where movement can otherwise cause artefactual problems. Uses therefore include abdominal imaging and imaging on non-compliant children. Note that the images are taken one slice at a time, and although motion is frozen on each slice, the anatomy may appear at very different positions on each slice if the patient has moved significantly between each slice acquisition. For the same reason, an abdominal data set may not be perfectly contiguous if the patient is asked to hold their breath for each slice.

Inversion Recovery

The term 'inversion recovery' refers to the fact that an additional RF pulse is applied at the beginning of the pulse sequence that tips the NMV by 180° into the −Z direction. Following the application of a 180° pulse, the magnetic vectors of the tissues recover their longitudinal magnetisation to a certain degree before the application of a 90° RF pulse. The time interval between the 180° and the 90° pulses provides a powerful contrast parameter, known as the tau or 'time from inversion'. Different tissues recover their longitudinal magnetisation at different rates and by changing the timing of the 90° RF pulse, the image contrast can be altered significantly. Signal can even be nulled (eliminated) from selected tissues if required. The mechanism depends entirely upon the manipulation of the longitudinal and transverse components of magnetisation in various tissues, each having their own rate of recovery. The timing of the 90° pulse is chosen to occur at a time when signal from the desired tissue has recovered to be exactly at 90° to the main magnetic field and is therefore flipped back into complete inversion (90° + 90° = 180°).

Inversion recovery sequences can be very valuable when imaging at very low or very high field strengths. T1-weighted spin echo sequences suffer from poor contrast at these extremes, but inversion recovery provides a method of achieving images having high fat signal and hypointense fluid.

Like spin-echo, inversion recovery sequences can also be speeded up with the addition of an echo train.

STIR (Short Tau Inversion Recovery)

In STIR the timing of the 90° RF pulse is set to eliminate any signal from fat. Because the mechanism of STIR relies on longitudinal magnetisation changes rather than precessional frequency, STIR is a robust method of fat suppression that is effective even in the presence of poor field homogeneity. Field inhomogeneity causes a drift in precessional frequency across the imaging volume, and this is a factor that can often spoil spectral fat saturation methods. STIR sequences are very sensitive to pathology and are starting to be used in whole body MRI screening protocols. STIR is also sensitive to bone marrow changes and trabecular microfracture (bone bruising).

FLAIR (Fluid-Attenuated Inversion Recovery)

FLAIR is a commonly used inversion recovery technique whereby the timing is chosen to remove any signal from fluid such as cerebrospinal fluid (CSF). Proteinaceous fluid such as that found in pathology will still appear bright, making this an ideal technique for assessing periventricular disease in the brain or increasing the conspicuity of the cranial nerves.

Gradient Echo (GE)

GE sequences were developed primarily to reduce acquisition times. A gradient application is used to dephase and rephase the spins, rather than a 180° RF pulse. Contrast is achieved by the use of variable flip angles (i.e. not just 90°) combined with the TR, the TE, and whether or not residual transverse magnetisation is allowed to contribute to image contrast. Shortened TR and TE makes for a faster sequence, but with some trade-offs.

GE sequences are more affected by susceptibility artefact than spin echo, a fact that is exploited in the diagnosis of haemorrhage. The iron content of haemoglobin causes susceptibility artefact and is therefore more readily demonstrated on GE sequences than with on spin echo. Susceptibility artefact can be a problem, however, when there is metal close to the region of interest, such as dental fixings. In these areas spin echo or FSE may be required to reduce the artefact.

T2*-weighted GE is also sensitive to flow, causing flowing spins to appear hyperintense on the images (NB: * indicates that field inhomogeneity effects have contributed to the dephasing time of the spins; in GE this is because there has been no 180° pulse used). This feature, coupled with a short minimum TE and TR, is exploited in flow-dependent MRA sequences. The use of flow compensation makes GE the sequence of choice where flow may cause image degradation. This includes the spine (CSF flow) and the joints (blood flow in the region of interest).

Another feature of GE is the ability to use echo times that exploit the precessional frequency difference of fat and water. At 1.5 T the magnetic vectors of fat nuclei precess 220 Hz more slowly than those of water. This means that they will drift in and out of phase with each other over time. Fat and water nuclei will be in phase approximately every 4.2 ms at 1.5 T. If the TE is set at a multiple of this factor, signal will be generated from voxels containing fat and water components. If a TE is chosen when fat and water vectors are out of phase there will be a corresponding loss of signal. This is useful in characterising disease where there is a change in the fat to water ratio (such as fatty infiltration of the liver), or lesions where there is a known fat/water content (such as adenoma). Modern developments have resulted in gradient echo sequences that can obtain signal at different TE values in the same acquisition. These may include in and out of phase data that can be post processed to give fat-only or water-only images. This is known as the Dixon technique.

3D Volume Scans

Volume imaging typically uses GE sequences with an additional phase encoding gradient applied in the slice selection plane. This allows the acquisition of very thin contiguous sections. 2D techniques require a gap between slices of 10–20% of the slice thickness to avoid an artefact known as cross-excitation. Volume imaging does not require a slice gap and is therefore recommended in 3D reconstruction and volume measurement techniques, where a gap between slices would cause distortion and inaccuracy. Because the slice (partition) thickness can be reduced in comparison to a 2D scan it is possible to achieve isotropic voxels (having the same dimensions of width, depth and height). This is also useful in image reconstruction, as the resolution will be the same in every plane (including the slice select direction). This is also one of the reasons why 3D sequences are used in flow-dependent MRA.

Inflow Angiography (also called Time-of-Flight)

Inflow angiography is a flow-dependent method of imaging the vasculature. It relies on the use of GE sequences having a rapid TR causing saturation of signal from tissues within the imaging volume, but allowing spins entering the imaging volume to emit signal briefly before becoming saturated themselves. This is known as the *entry slice phenomenon*. The term *time-of-flight* (TOF) is not a particularly apt name for this technique, as TOF can also cause flow to *lack* signal if the flowing nuclei are moving at high speed.

This *high-velocity signal loss* – whereby spins inside an imaging volume flow out of the slice before rephasing occurs – is kept to a minimum by the use of a short time to echo (TE). The base data therefore demonstrate high-signal flow against a saturated, hypointense background. Anatomical images may be reconstructed from the base-data using a post processing technique called maximum intensity projection (MIP). This process reconstructs the data from different virtual points of view and constructs an anatomical-looking representation of the vasculature. The reconstructed images can over-exaggerate the size of stenoses and underestimate the true lumen size of vessels, and in reporting inflow MRA procedures it is recommended that the base data are also taken into consideration.

Another shortcoming of this sequence is that it is sensitive to tissues having high signal on T1 weighting. This includes fat and some stages of haemorrhage (methaemoglobin) that may obscure the vessels on an MIP.

Phase Contrast Angiography (PCA)

PCA uses a subtraction method to differentiate between flowing and stationary spins. The pulse sequence used is GE with an additional gradient application known as the velocity encoding gradient or VENC. The steepness of this additional gradient is a user-definable parameter used to differentiate between differing flow velocities (e.g. between arterial and venous flow). The principle of this technique is that two acquisitions are performed to encode flow along a particular direction.

The first acquisition uses a VENC that results in the flowing nuclei acquiring an advanced phase position compared to the stationary background spins. The second acquisition uses a flow compensating gradient such as that used in artefact reduction techniques. This gradient causes both stationary and moving spins to retain the *same* phase position. When the data from the two acquisitions are digitally subtracted the resulting images show only the difference, i.e. the flowing spins. This technique can be time-consuming, as the VENC may need to be applied in all three orthogonal planes (X, Y and Z) if flow is tortuous. The advantages are in the excellent background suppression and the fact that phase images can be created in which flow can be shown as black or white, depending on direction. The subtraction technique means that, unlike TOF images, phase contrast images are not obscured by tissues having short T1 times.

Contrast-Enhanced MRA (CEMRA)

As outlined above, phase contrast and inflow angiograms have certain image quality and artefact issues. Most of these problems can be resolved by the use of positive contrast media. In CEMRA, a bolus of gadolinium-based contrast media is injected into a vein, usually in the antecubital fossa. When the bolus reaches the region of interest, a T1-weighted 3D volume GE sequence is performed while the patient holds their breath/keeps perfectly still. This technique has the following advantages:

- Shorter RF pulses may be used
- Shorter TR and thinner sections may be obtained under 1 mm
- Large 3D data volumes may be collected in a 6–20 second breath hold
- Larger fields of view are possible than with inflow MRA and PCA because in-plane flow may be imaged; as an example, the aorta can be imaged with coronal slices rather than axial

The rationale behind the technique is that paramagnetic contrast agents shorten the T1 time of blood. This makes it possible to acquire an MRA in which image contrast is due to the differences in the T1 relaxation times between blood and surrounding tissues. This is an advantage because it results in a more anatomical image. Flow-dependent methods such as inflow MRA and PCA only yield signal from moving blood. Vessels containing very slow flow or stationary flow cannot be visualised. Using CEMRA it is (theoretically) possible to image vessels containing stationary blood, provided there is contrast agent present. This means that CEMRA does not tend to suffer from flow-related artefacts such as over-estimation of stenosis, incorrect representation of lumen diameter and saturation signal loss due to in-plane flow.

Ideally, the dose of contrast agent used must be sufficient to shorten the T1 time of blood compared to the background tissues. A short TR can then be used which saturates signal from all structures apart from blood. The background tissue having the shortest T1 is fat, 270 ms at 1.5 T, so enough gadolinium must be injected per bolus to shorten the blood T1 to under 270 ms.

It is of vital importance in CEMRA that the acquisition is timed so that data are collected during the short time in which the bolus of contrast is present within the imaging volume.

To simplify the procedure and reduce the likelihood of human error, modern scanners have protocols that feature sequences of such high temporal resolution that the operator can inject the entire contrast bolus using a syringe pump and witness its arrival in the vessel of interest in real time. This permits the user to initiate the main data acquisition when the contrast is in exactly the required area.

Moving table-top studies allow the bolus to be chased into the extremities in much the same way as in early iodine-enhanced radiographic arteriography.[30]

To sum up the main advantages of this technique:

- CEMRA is capable of imaging in-plane flow (i.e. it is not restricted to perpendicular flow like inflow MRA).
- Because CEMRA can image in-plane flow, a wider FOV can be achieved in a short timeframe. This is because, for example, the aorta can be imaged using relatively few coronal slices, whereas with in-flow techniques it would require many axial slices.
- Signal is not dependent upon flow (i.e. flow of any speed will yield high signal).

Despite these advantages, the use of CEMRA is declining slightly in favour of CT angiography, particularly in light of recent concerns around the use of gadolinium. In patients where gadolinium is contraindicated there are other non-contrast methods of blood-vessel imaging, such as so-called 'fresh-blood' imaging where data are collected in systolic and asystolic phases of the cardiac cycle and digitally subtracted to leave the vessels on the image.

Diffusion Techniques

MRI scanners are capable of differentiating between moving and relatively stationary spins. The mechanism behind this was covered in an earlier section on phase contrast angiography. Modern systems with very powerful gradients can take this principle to a microscopic level and can differentiate between the molecular diffusion rates in different tissue environments. This is facilitated by the fact that the random thermal motion of water molecules causes a net flow along an unrestricted pathway, resulting in a loss of signal. Any adjacent area where flow is restricted due to pathology (such as stroke) will not experience as much signal loss and will appear comparatively hyperintense.

Perfusion Imaging

Perfusion studies use dynamic contrast enhancement combined with a high temporal resolution scan technique. As the contrast perfuses through the region of interest it will cause either an increase in signal intensity on T1-weighted sequences or a drop in signal intensity when T2* weighting is employed. The high temporal resolution allows rapid re-acquisition of the same slice or block of slices over time. The T2* technique is often used as part of a stroke protocol, where the healthy tissue experiences a signal drop due to susceptibility effects of the gadolinium leaving the poorly perfusing pathology comparatively hyperintense.

Suggested MRI Protocols by Body Area

BRAIN

MRI of the brain can be used to assess structure, pathology and brain function.

MRI has surpassed CT for imaging of the brain owing to its superior sensitivity and soft tissue contrast; for example, MRI can detect demyelination even in early inflammatory lesions where CT studies have shown no abnormality.

The posterior fossa is well demonstrated on MRI images as MRI does not suffer from the beam-hardening artefacts associated with CT scans of this region. Aneurysms and vascular anomalies may be demonstrated using flow-dependent imaging techniques that can demonstrate vasculature without the need for iodinated contrast media. These techniques have additional advantages in that they are comparatively cheap, very quick to perform, have no risk of contrast agent-related side effects, use no ionising radiation and are more comfortable for the patient than a catheter study.

The multiplanar capabilities of MRI mean that slices can be acquired in non-orthogonal angles. This allows imaging along structures such as the trigeminal nerve and optic nerve as well as sagittal imaging of the pituitary fossa and coronal imaging of the hippocampus.

The functional capabilities of MRI are still being investigated and developed; fMRI is a technique that uses MR imaging to measure the metabolic changes that take place in the cortex of the brain during activation. The areas of the brain responsible for speech, sight, hearing and motor function can vary slightly between individuals. fMRI can be used to assess these areas prior to surgery, allowing the resection of tumours without damaging nearby structures that are critical to the patient. fMRI research is currently looking at applications in the fields of stroke, pain and the seat of language and memory.

MRI does have some disadvantages in comparison with CT in that it may have poorer geometric accuracy, particularly in open scanners, and is less able to assess bone structure. MRI is not ideal for the trauma patient because of projectile hazards due to incomplete safety screening and attached monitors, etc. CT provides a more immediate solution and can assess bony head injury more readily.

Common Indications

- Haemorrhage
- Infection
- Inflammatory processes/multiple sclerosis
- Ischaemia
- Acute ischaemic stroke
- Neurodegenerative disease
- Seizures
- Tumours
- Vascular abnormalities

Equipment Needed

Quadrature volume head coil or quadrature phased-array head coil

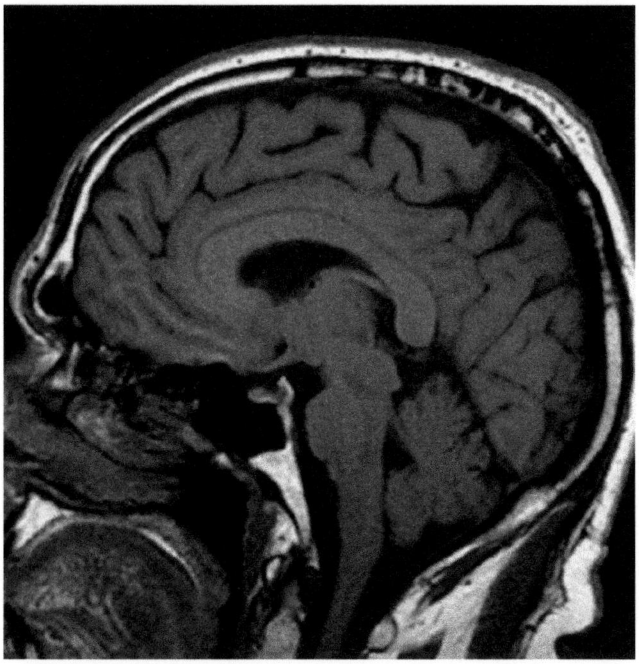

Fig. 27.14 T1-weighted, sagittal brain. (Reproduced with permission from Philips Medical Systems.)

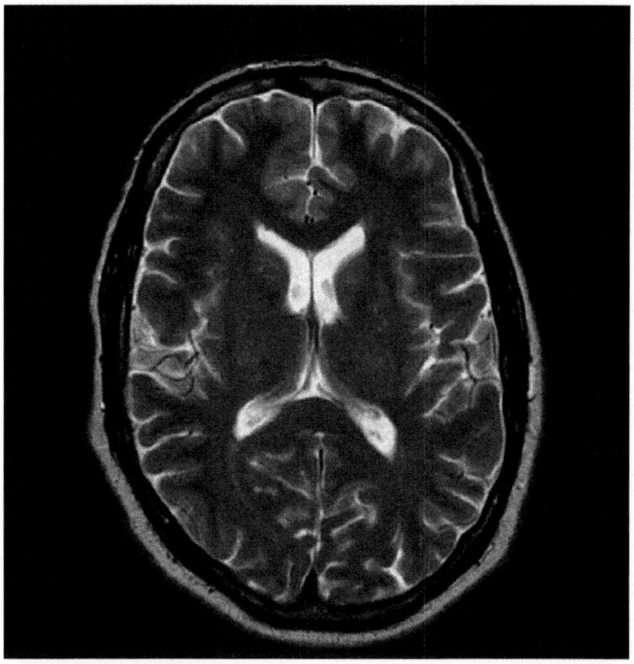

Fig. 27.15 T2-weighted, FSE, axial brain. (Reproduced with permission from Philips Medical Systems.)

Routine Protocol

The routine protocol may include the sequences shown in the following table and in Figs 27.14–27.16.

Routine MRI Protocol: Brain

	Weighting	Orientation	Pulse Sequence
1	T1	Three planes	GE (localiser)
2	T1	Sagittal	CSE/FSE
3	T2 or T2/PD	Axial or coronal	FSE (TSE)
4	T2	Axial/coronal/sagittal	FLAIR

It is important to standardise the imaging planes used for every patient. This is because each individual will lie with the head tilted to a different extent (chin up or chin down). The sagittal localiser will allow the operator to use a common landmark for the prescription of all axial images. This can be along the hard palate or the line joining the anterior to posterior commissures. Slices should be positioned to cover the foramen magnum to vertex.

Additional sequences may be added to the protocol as follows:

Tumour or Infection (Fig. 27.17)

	Weighting	Orientation	Pulse Sequence
1	T1 (± gadolinium)	Axial/sagittal/ coronal	CSE/FSE

T1-weighted images are used with positive contrast enhancement. Positive extracellular contrast media are able to cross any disruption of the blood–brain barrier. This results in the positive enhancement of brain tumours, infection and other lesions, such as active multiple sclerosis plaques.

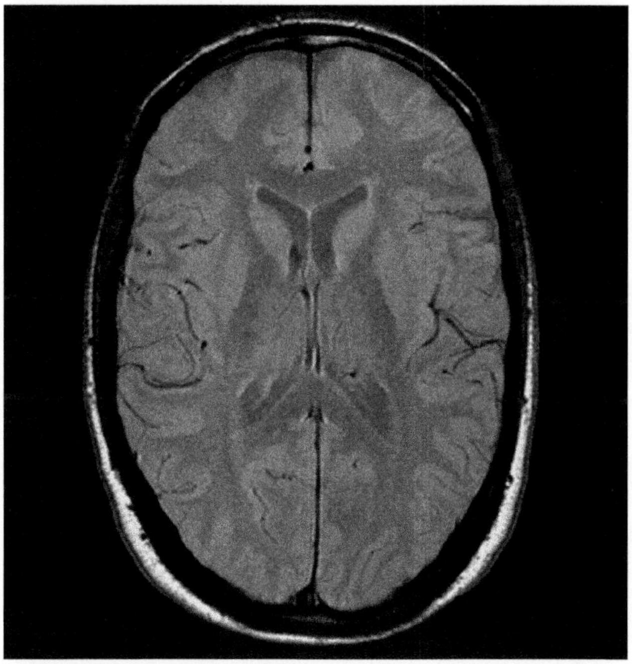

Fig. 27.16 PD-weighted spin echo, axial brain. (Reproduced with permission from Philips Medical Systems.)

Multiple Sclerosis

	Weighting	Orientation	Pulse Sequence
1	T2	Axial/coronal/sagittal	FLAIR

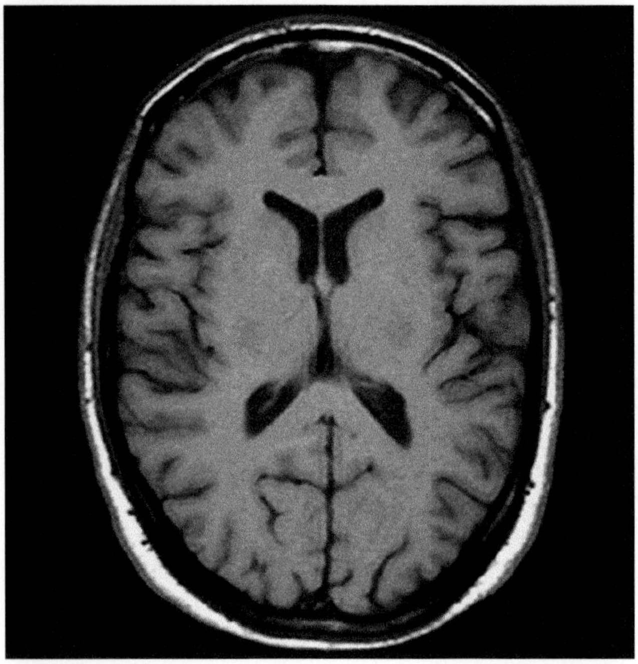

Fig. 27.17 T1-weighted, spin echo, axial brain. (Reproduced with permission from Philips Medical Systems.)

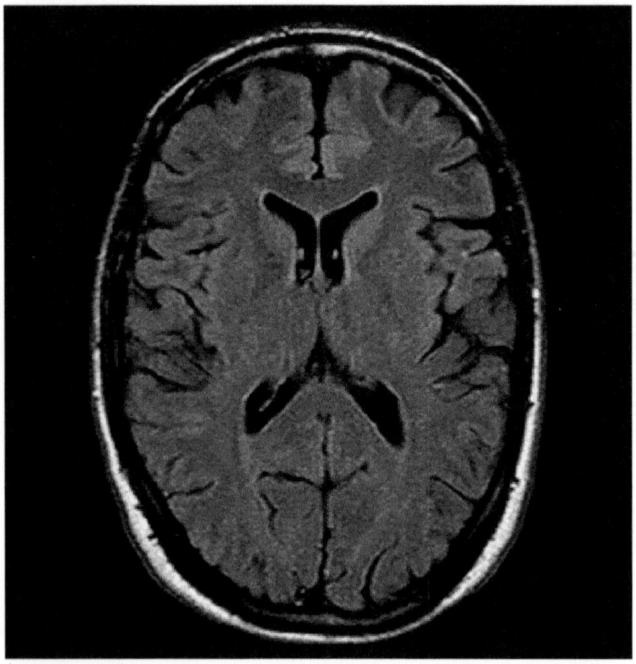

Fig. 27.18 Fluid-attenuated inversion recovery T2-weighted, axial brain. Note that an inversion time has been selected to null signal from water so the ventricles appear hypointense despite the T2 weighting. (Reproduced with permission from Philips Medical Systems.)

FLAIR uses inversion recovery to suppress signal from the CSF in the ventricles, but not the signal from proteinaceous fluid in areas of demyelination. This is useful in defining the extent of periventricular disease (Fig. 27.18).

Epilepsy (Figs 27.19, 27.20).
The protocol may include some of the sequences shown in the following table.

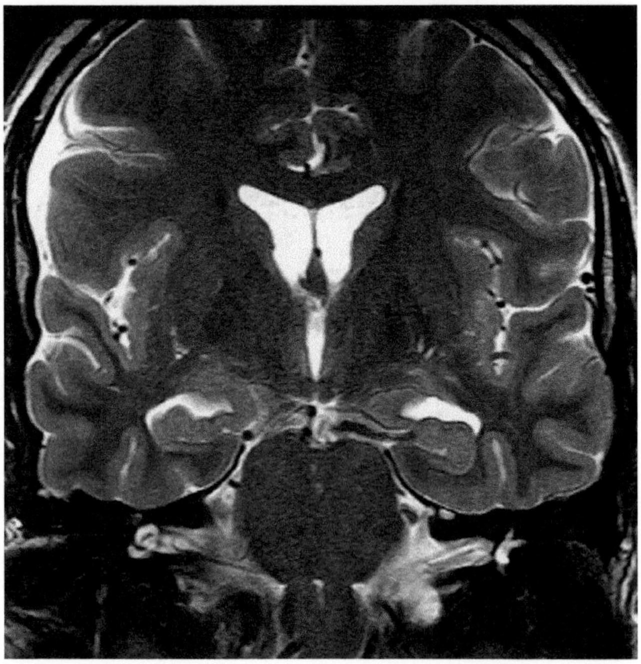

Fig. 27.19 High-resolution T2-weighted, FSE, coronal – brain. (Reproduced with permission from Philips Medical Systems.)

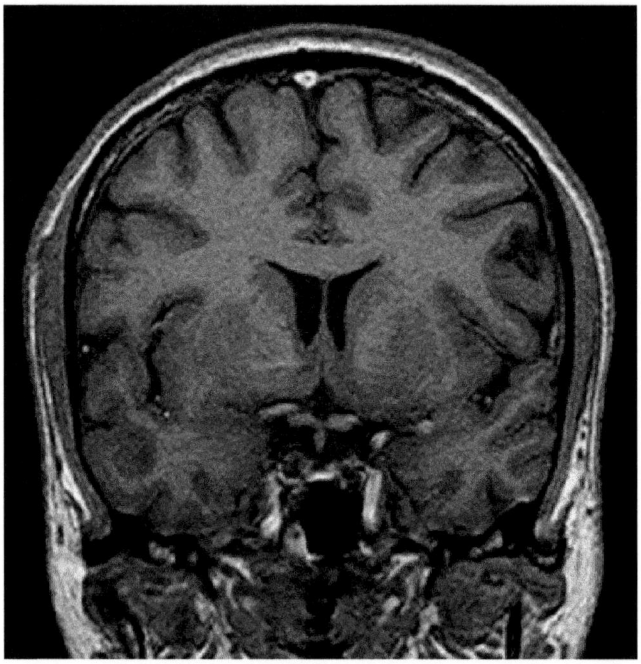

Fig. 27.20 T1-weighted incoherent GE, 3D volume – brain. (Reproduced with permission from Philips Medical Systems.)

	Weighting	Orientation	Pulse Sequence
1	T2	Axial	FSE (TSE)
2	T1	Sagittal	CSE/FSE
3	T1	Coronal (thin slices)	Fast inversion recovery
4	T2	Coronal (thin slices)	FSE (TSE)
5	T1	Coronal 3D volume	GE
6	T2	Coronal 3D volume	FLAIR

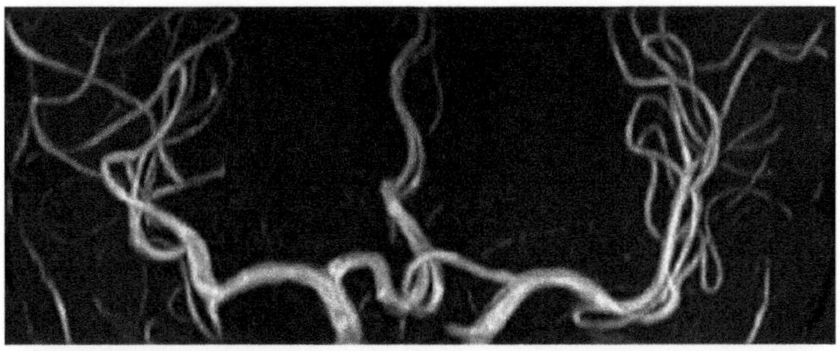

Fig. 27.21 3D TOF (post maximum intensity projection) – cerebral angiogram. (Reproduced with permission from Philips Medical Systems.)

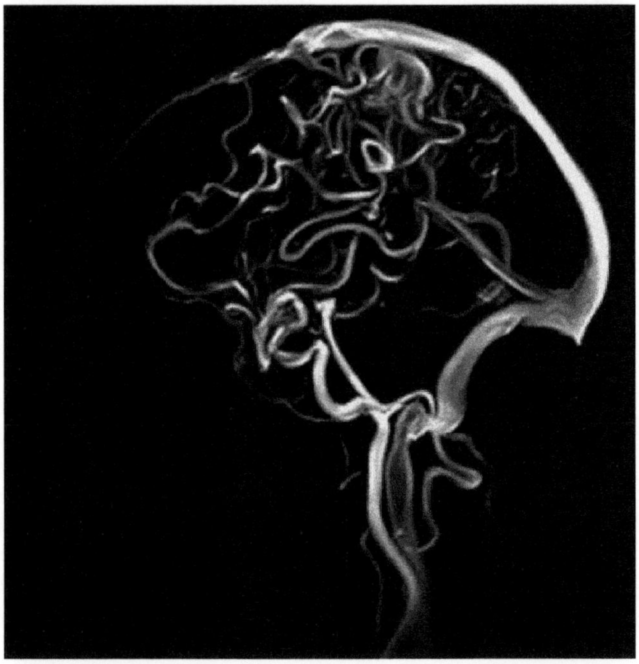

Fig. 27.22 PCA – cranial vessels. (Reproduced with permission from Philips Medical Systems.)

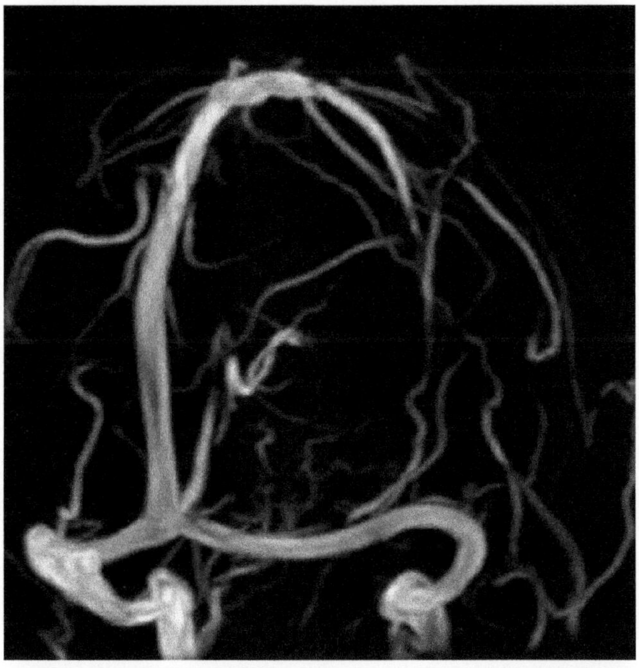

Fig. 27.23 Phase contrast venography of the brain. (Reproduced with permission from Philips Medical Systems.)

High-resolution T2-weighted scans orientated at 90° to the long axis of the temporal lobe can be useful in assessing hippocampal disease (sclerosis) and structure.

A *3D volume* acquisition will allow the measurement of hippocampal or frontal lobe volumes, as there is no slice gap.

Vascular Abnormalities and Presence of Flow (Fig. 27.21)

	Vessels	Orientation	Pulse Sequence
1	Arteries/aneurysms	Axial	3D inflow MRA
2	Veins	Sagittal oblique	2D inflow MRA
3	Veins	Axial	3D phase contrast MRA

3D TOF gives a high-resolution image having isotropic (i.e. cubic) voxels. This allows MIPs having the same resolution along every axis. The FOV (slab thickness) is limited owing to saturation effects.

2D TOF can be acquired one slice at a time and therefore allows wider coverage than 3D acquisition. Individual 2D slices are not thick enough to cause saturation of slow-moving inflowing spins and therefore can be used for venography. Non-isotropic voxels result in lower resolution of the MIP images.

Phase contrast studies allow the encoding of flow in any direction, not just perpendicular flow. The VENC can be selected for arterial or venous flow (Figs 27.22 and 27.23).

Assessment of the Internal Auditory Meati or Trigeminal Nerves (Fig. 27.24)

	Weighting	Orientation	Pulse Sequence
1	T2/T2*	Axial (thin slices)/3D volume	FSE (TSE)/balanced GE

Or

	Weighting	Orientation	Pulse Sequence
1	T1 (pre/post gadolinium)	Axial/coronal (thin slices)	CSE/FSE

Thin slices 2–3 mm give high-resolution images of the acoustic nerves to exclude acoustic neuroma or other pathology. A *3D volume* acquisition has the additional advantage of requiring no slice gap. T1-weighted pre and post contrast studies can demonstrate lesions within the trigeminal nerve and reveal vascular abnormalities in adjacent vessels which may be causing symptoms due to compression and pulsatile irritation.

Note that balanced GE can be used as an alternative to T2-weighted FSE, as it has the advantage of reducing CSF flow motion artefacts.

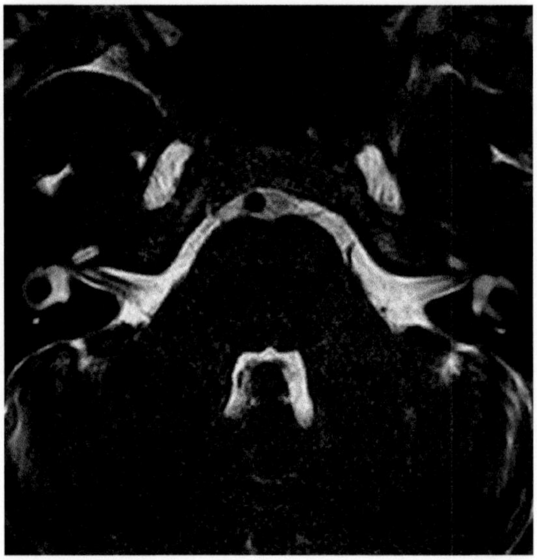

Fig. 27.24 High-resolution T2-weighted FSE, axial – internal auditory meati. (Reproduced with permission from Philips Medical Systems.)

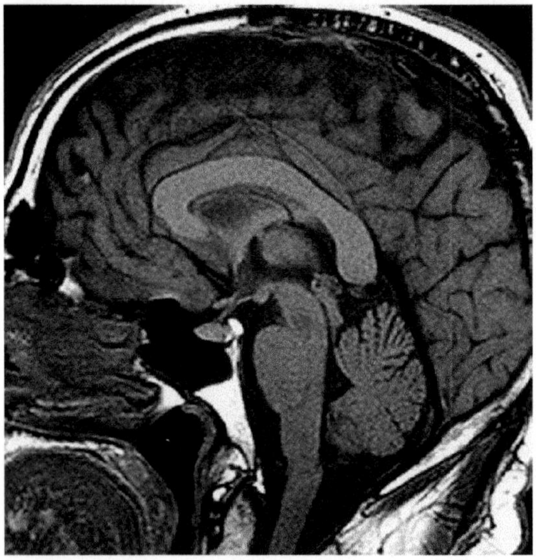

Fig. 27.25 High-resolution T1-weighted spin echo, sagittal – pituitary fossa. (Reproduced with permission from Philips Medical Systems.)

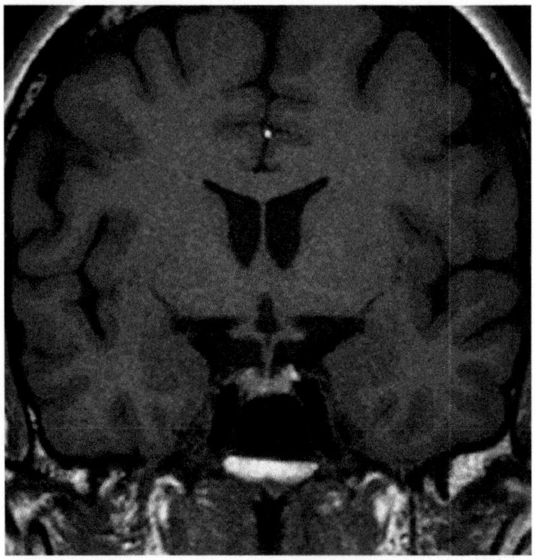

Fig. 27.26 High-resolution T1-weighted spin echo, coronal – pituitary fossa. (Reproduced with permission from Philips Medical Systems.)

Pituitary Fossa (Figs 27.25, 27.26)

	Weighting	Orientation	Pulse Sequence
1	T1 (pre/post gadolinium)	Sagittal/coronal (thin slices)	CSE/FSE

The absence of a blood–brain barrier in the pituitary gland and stalk results in homogeneous enhancement after gadolinium chelate injection. A focal hypointense area within the gland immediately after Gd-DTPA is abnormal and is the most common appearance of an adenoma.

Orbits (Figs 27.27, 27.28)

	Weighting	Orientation	Pulse Sequence
1	T2 (fat suppression)	Axial/coronal (thin slices)	STIR/FSE (TSE)
2	T1 (pre/post gadolinium)	Axial/coronal/sagittal (thin slices)	CSE/FSE

STIR and T2 fat-suppressed sequences reduce the signal from retro-orbital fat, improving contrast in assessing the optic nerves. If fat suppression is required on the T1-weighted images chemical fat saturation may be used. Appropriately angled parasagittal projections can be used to demonstrate the optic nerve along its full length to the optic chiasm. Note that this protocol may also be used in imaging the other cranial nerves.

SPINE

The spine is an anatomical area that is inherently suited to MRI. The area is relatively immobile, has good PD and excellent contrast-to-noise ratio. Artefactual appearances can occur due to the movement of nearby structures such as the throat, anterior body wall, heart and bowel, but these can usually be reduced by using a pre-saturation pulse. A pre-saturation pulse is a user-defined region that is subjected to additional RF pulses to suppress all signal. If a region is not emitting signal then it cannot cause artefactual appearances on the image.

In many cases MRI is replacing conventional radiography of the spine because of the wealth of additional information it provides and because of its non-ionising nature.

Common Indications

- Congenital abnormalities
- Cord atrophy
- Cord compression
- Degenerative disease
- Demyelination
- Disc disease (new and recurrent following surgery)

- Epidural fibrosis (following surgery)
- Haemorrhage
- Infarction
- Infection
- Metastatic disease
- Tumour
- Vascular malformations

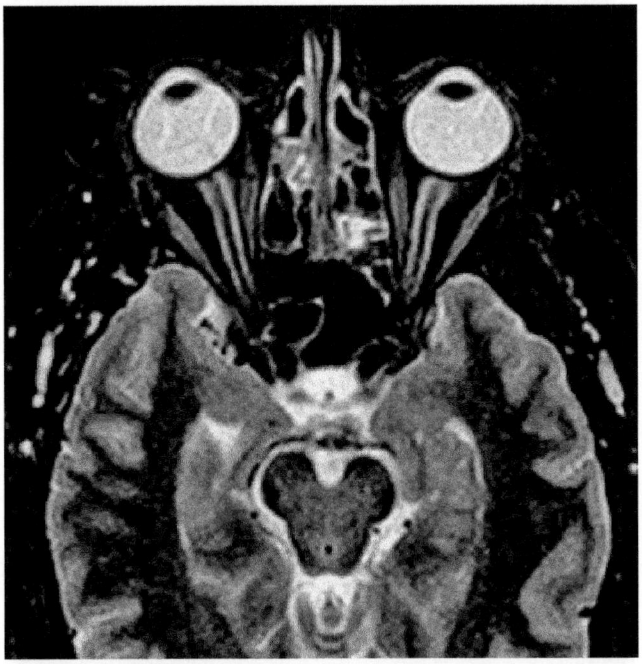

Fig. 27.27 **STIR, axial – orbits.** (Reproduced with permission from Philips Medical Systems.)

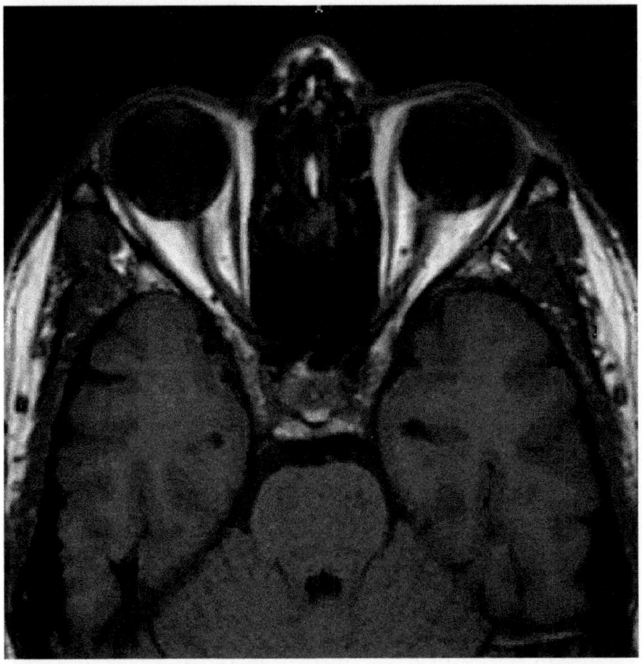

Fig. 27.28 **T1-weighted spin echo, axial – orbits.** (Reproduced with permission from Philips Medical Systems.)

The soft tissue capabilities of MRI make it particularly suited to the demonstration of congenital abnormalities such as Chiari malformation, spina bifida, cord tethering, dysraphisms and diastematomyelia.

Changes in bone marrow are also well demonstrated and make MRI a useful tool in the assessment of metastatic disease. Bone marrow is usually of intermediate signal on T1 weighting because of its fat content. Metastatic infiltration has a higher water content and therefore reduces the signal in affected areas.

MRI has a unique sensitivity to demyelinating conditions; T2-weighted sagittal images of the cord are therefore valuable in demonstrating lesions of multiple sclerosis. CT rarely shows such lesions, although areas may enhance on delayed scanning after a double dose of iodinated contrast medium in advanced cases of disease.

Tumours are well demonstrated on MRI, usually causing a widening of the cord, high signal on T2 weighting and possible enhancement on T1-weighted images. There are several classifications of cord tumour that can be differentiated by close inspection of MRI images in many cases.

The contrast-to-noise ratio generated on T2 weighting between CSF and cord allows MRI to replace conventional myelography in most cases. Disc disease, cord compression and spinal stenosis will cause indentation of the theca.

Haemorrhage can be detected using GE sequences owing to increased susceptibility effects.

CERVICAL SPINE

Equipment Needed

Volume neck coil, quadrature phased-array neurovascular coil, quadrature spine coil or quadrature phased-array spine coil

Routine Protocol

The routine protocol may include the sequences shown in the following table and in Figs 27.29–27.33.

Routine MRI Protocol: Cervical Spine

	Weighting	Orientation	Pulse Sequence
1	T1	Three planes	GE (localiser)
2	T2	Sagittal	FSE (TSE)
3	T1	Sagittal	CSE/FSE
4	T2/T2*	Axial/3D volume	FSE (TSE)/GE
5	T1	Axial	CSE/FSE

The coronal localiser will allow the operator to orientate the sagittal sections. The FOV should include the posterior fossa to the second thoracic vertebra. The sagittal localiser allows the operator to prescribe the axial slices. Axial slices should cover the intervertebral discs.

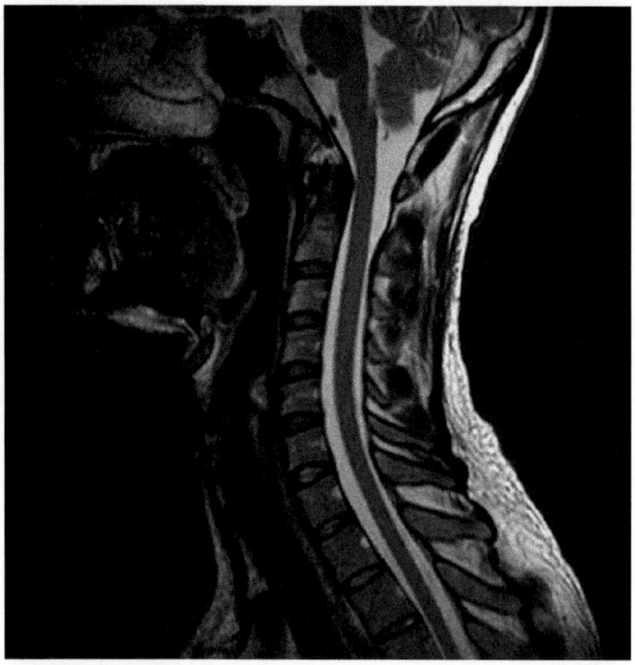

Fig. 27.29 T2-weighted FSE, sagittal – cervical spine. (Reproduced with permission from Philips Medical Systems.)

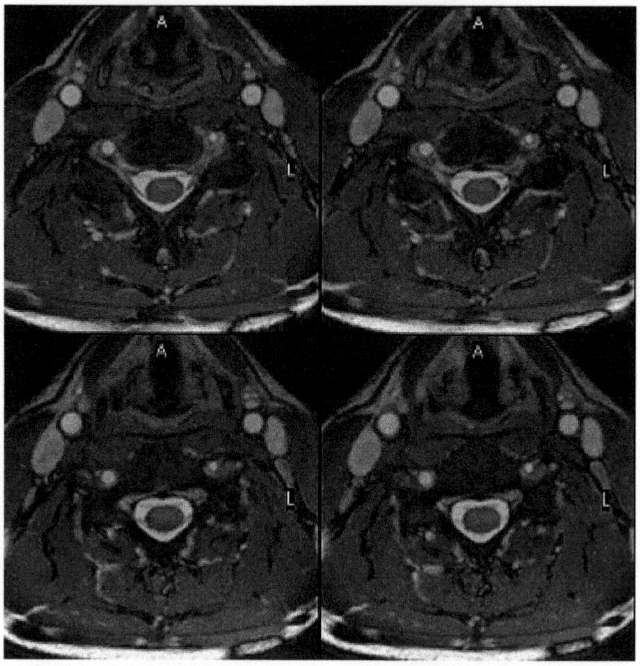

Fig. 27.31 T2*-weighted GE, axial – cervical spine. (Reproduced with permission from Philips Medical Systems.)

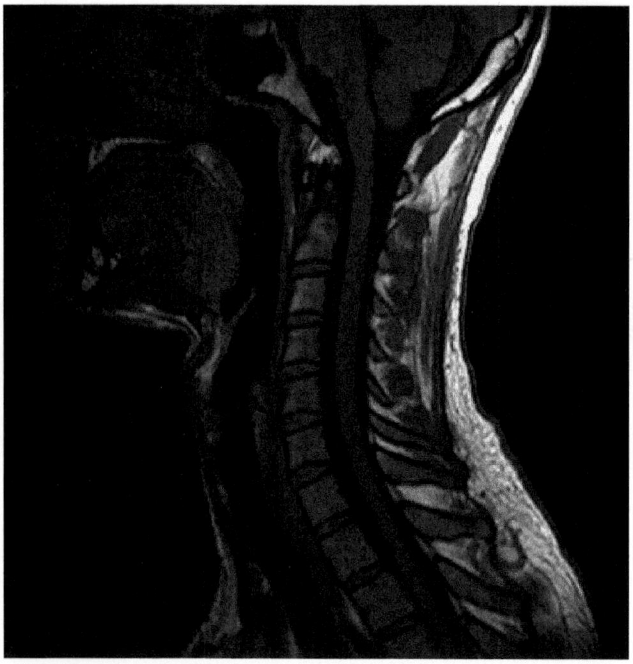

Fig. 27.30 T1-weighted spin echo, sagittal – cervical spine. (Reproduced with permission from Philips Medical Systems.)

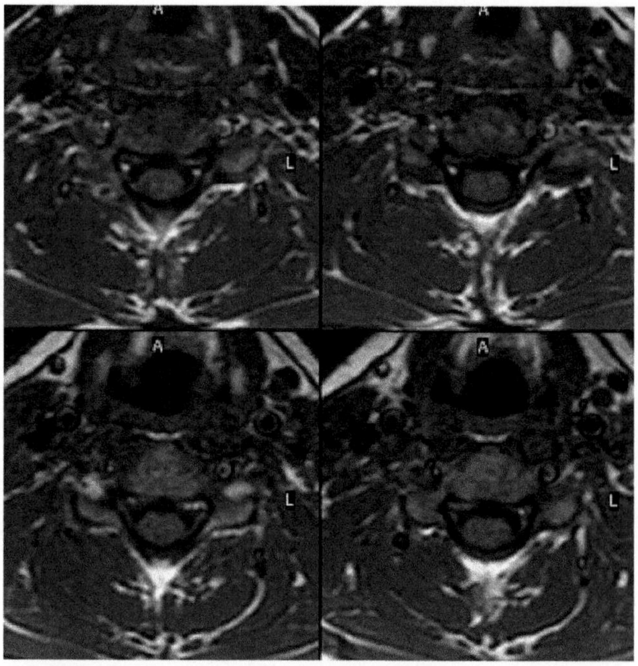

Fig. 27.32 T1-weighted spin echo, axial – cervical spine. (Reproduced with permission from Philips Medical Systems.)

Additional sequences may be added to the protocol as follows.

Syringomyelia or Tumour (Fig. 27.34)

	Weighting	Orientation	Pulse Sequence
1	T2	Sagittal	STIR
2	T1 (pre/post gadolinium)	Sagittal/axial	CSE/FSE

T1 weighting is used with positive contrast enhancement. STIR images are useful to demonstrate intrinsic signal change within the cord and bone marrow. If fat suppression is required on the T1-weighted images, chemical fat saturation may be used. In cases of syringomyelia, the full length of the lesion must be demonstrated. This may include separate scans of the thoracic and lumbar regions.

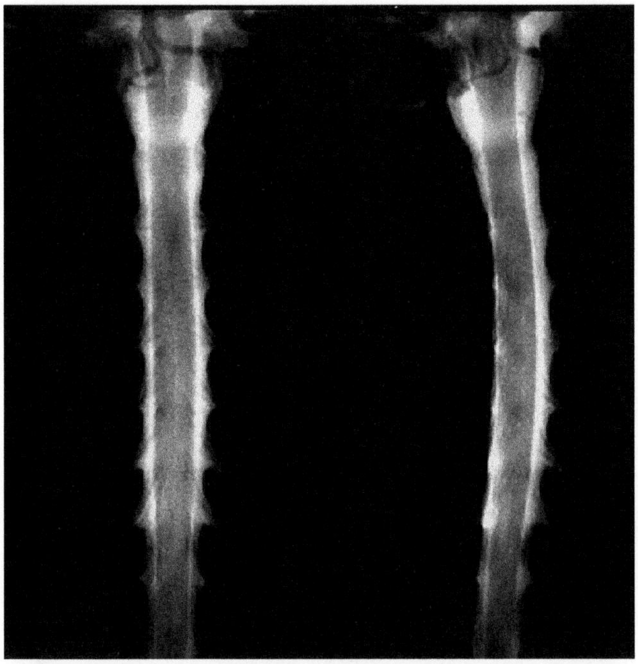

Fig. 27.33 Long T2-weighted 'myelographic' maximum intensity projection – cervical spine. (Reproduced with permission from Philips Medical Systems.)

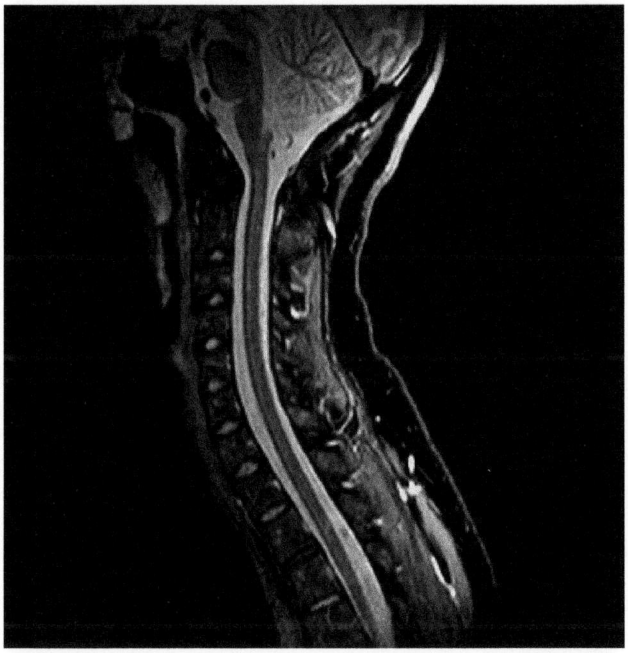

Fig. 27.34 Short tau inversion recovery, sagittal – cervical spine. (Reproduced with permission from Philips Medical Systems.)

Brachial Plexus

	Weighting	Orientation	Pulse Sequence
1	T2	Coronal	FSE (TSE)/STIR
2	T1	Coronal/axial	CSE/FSE
3	T2	Axial	FSE (TSE)

Slices prescribed from the angle of the mandible to the lung apices. Coronal sections are not usually very useful in routine spine imaging but are very useful when looking for lesions such as neurofibroma. The coronal plane demonstrates the classic dumbbell shape of the lesion which may not be appreciated on sagittal views. If fat suppression is required, STIR may be used.

THORACIC SPINE

Equipment Needed

Quadrature spine coil or quadrature phased-array spine coil

Routine Protocol

The routine protocol may include the sequences shown in the following table and in Figs 27.35 and 27.36.

Routine MRI Protocol: Thoracic Spine

	Weighting	Orientation	Pulse Sequence
1	T1	Three planes	GE (localiser)
2	T2	Sagittal	FSE (TSE)
3	T1	Sagittal	CSE/FSE
4	T2/T2*	Axial/3D volume	FSE (TSE)/GE
5	T1	Axial	CSE/FSE

The coronal localiser will allow the operator to orientate the sagittal sections. The FOV should include the seventh cervical vertebra to the first lumbar vertebra. Identification of vertebral level can be facilitated by including the second cervical vertebra on at least one sequence (such as the localiser). The sagittal localiser allows the operator to prescribe the axial slices. Axial slices should cover any relevant intervertebral discs.

Additional sequences may be added to the protocol as follows.

Syringomyelia or Tumour

	Weighting	Orientation	Pulse Sequence
1	T2	Sagittal	STIR
2	T1 (pre/post gadolinium)	Sagittal	CSE/FSE
3	T1 (pre/post gadolinium)	Axial	CSE/FSE

T1 weighting is used with positive contrast enhancement. STIR images are useful to demonstrate intrinsic signal change within the cord and bone marrow. If fat suppression is required on the T1-weighted images chemical fat saturation may be used. In cases of syringomyelia, the full length of the lesion must be demonstrated. This may include separate scans of the cervical and lumbar regions.

Scoliosis

	Weighting	Orientation	Pulse Sequence
1	T1 or T2	Coronal	CSE/FSE

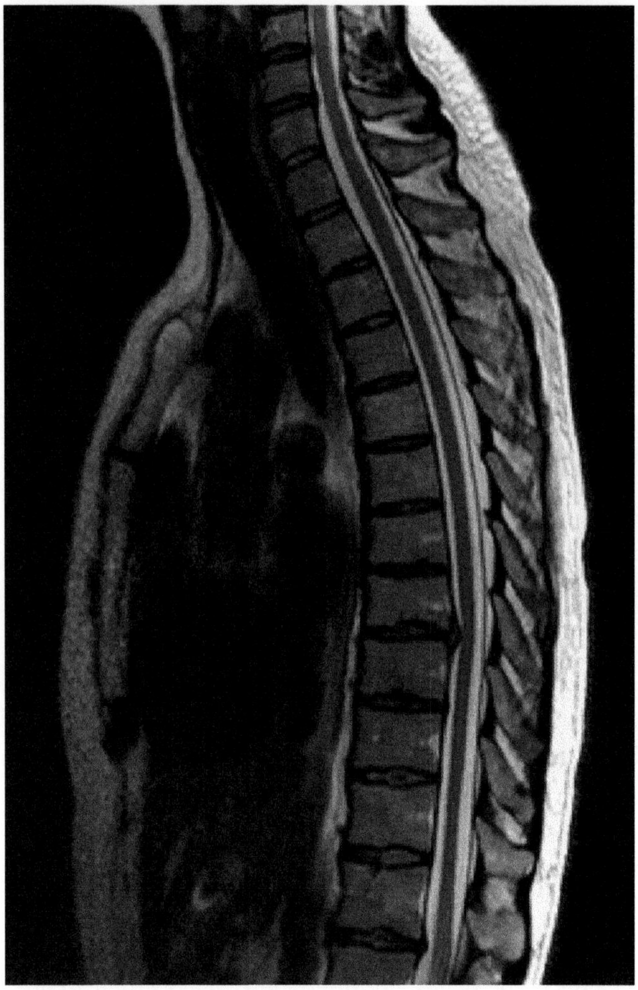

Fig. 27.35 T2-weighted FSE, sagittal – thoracic spine. (Reproduced with permission from Philips Medical Systems.)

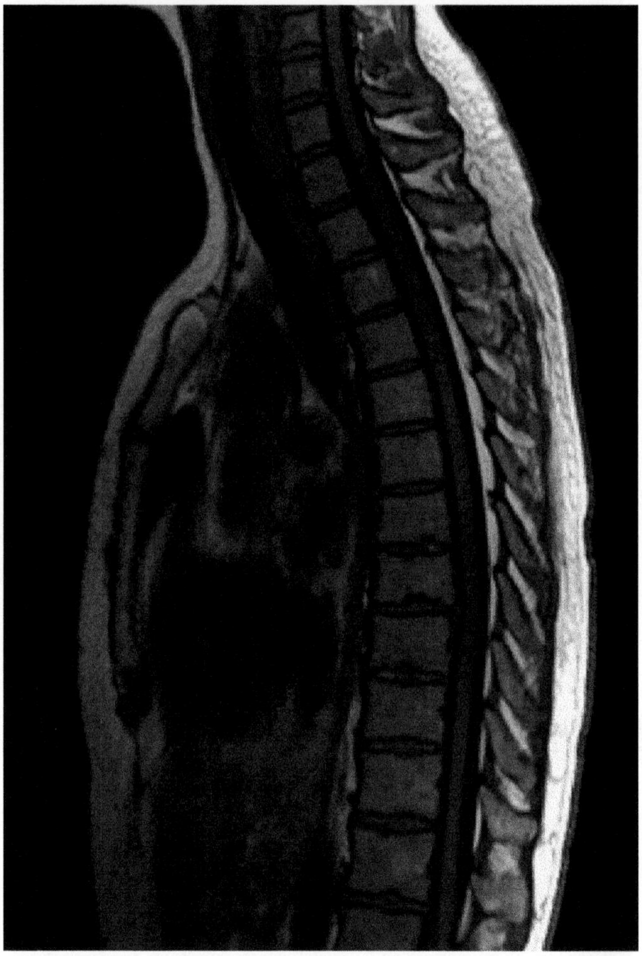

Fig. 27.36 T1-weighted spin echo, sagittal – thoracic spine. (Reproduced with permission from Philips Medical Systems.)

Scoliosis causes the spine to curve out of the sagittal plane and therefore a coronal data set will provide better coverage and more readily understandable anatomical information.

LUMBAR–SACRAL SPINE

Equipment Needed

Quadrature spine coil or quadrature phased-array spine coil

Routine Protocol

The routine protocol may include the sequences shown in the following table and in Figs 27.37–27.39.

Routine MRI Protocol: Lumbar–Sacral Spine

	Weighting	Orientation	Pulse Sequence
1	T1	Three planes	GE (localiser)
2	T2	Sagittal	FSE (TSE) or STIR
3	T1	Sagittal	CSE/FSE
4	T2	Axial	FSE (TSE)
5	T1	Axial	CSE/FSE

The coronal localiser will allow the operator to orientate the sagittal sections. The FOV should include the 12th thoracic vertebra to the tip of the coccyx. The sagittal localiser allows the operator to prescribe the axial slices. Axial slices should cover any relevant intervertebral discs.

STIR may be used instead of T2 sagittal images, particularly if the examination is a limited replacement for radiographic evaluation. STIR is sometimes described as a 'search and destroy' sequence due to its sensitivity to pathology.

Additional sequences may be added to the protocol as follows.

Syringomyelia or Tumour

	Weighting	Orientation	Pulse Sequence
1	T2	Sagittal	STIR
2	T1 (pre/post gadolinium)	Sagittal	CSE/FSE
3	T1 (pre/post gadolinium)	Axial	CSE/FSE

T1 weighting is used with positive contrast enhancement. STIR images are useful to demonstrate intrinsic signal change within the cord and bone marrow. If fat suppression is required on the T1-weighted images chemical fat saturation may be used. In cases of syringomyelia,

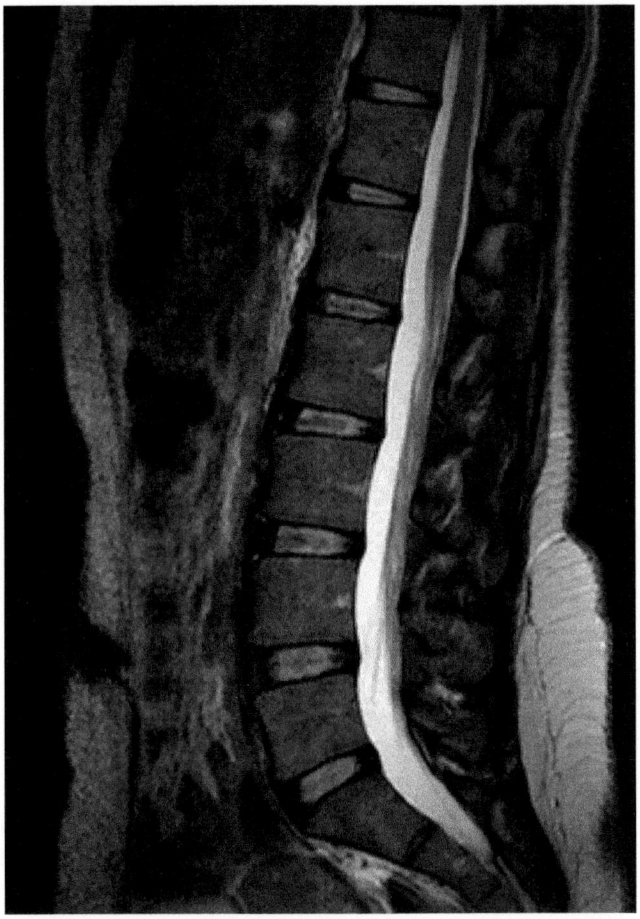

Fig. 27.37 T2-weighted FSE, sagittal – lumbar sacral spine. (Reproduced with permission from Philips Medical Systems.)

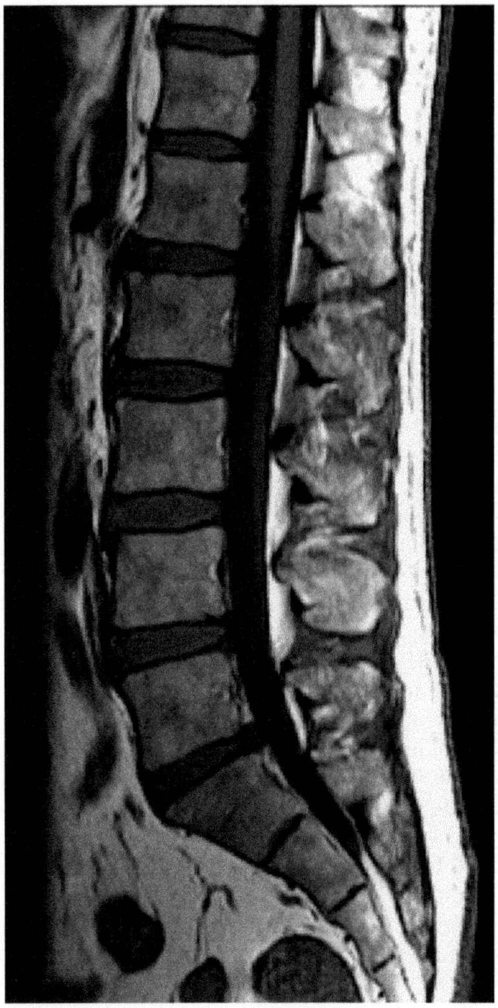

Fig. 27.38 T1-weighted spin echo, sagittal – lumbar sacral spine. (Reproduced with permission from Philips Medical Systems.)

the full length of the lesion must be demonstrated. This may include separate scans of the cervical and thoracic regions.

Some MR systems have moving-table techniques and software capabilities that enable image fusion from separately acquired data sets so that a reconstructed whole spine can be visualised. This both speeds up the acquisition of data as re-centering/patient re-positioning for each area becomes unnecessary, and is useful in ascertaining the correct vertebral level of any lesions demonstrated.

MUSCULOSKELETAL SYSTEM

MRI has an important role in the diagnosis and treatment of musculoskeletal disorders. MRI accurately depicts soft tissue injuries such as muscle, ligament and meniscal tears as well as cartilage and bone injuries. Muscle has an intermediate to slightly long T1 relaxation time and a short T2 relaxation time. It appears relatively hypointense on both T1- and T2-weighted sequences, particularly FSE T2.

The fat planes allow identification of individual muscles owing to fat's hyperintensity on T1 weighting. Injured muscles have associated oedema and haemorrhage, which prolong the T1 and T2 relaxation times of the injured tissue, so T2-weighted images with fat

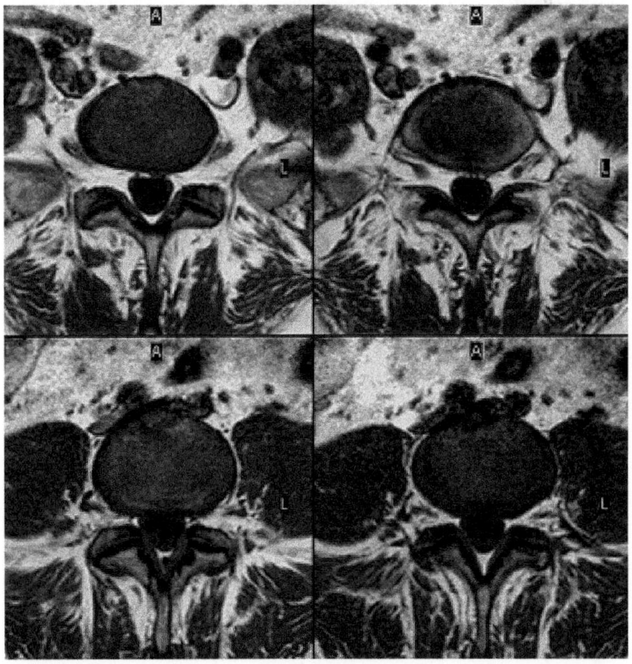

Fig. 27.39 T1-weighted spin echo, axial – lumbar spine. (Reproduced with permission from Philips Medical Systems.)

suppression (or STIR images) demonstrate tears. Water-bearing oedematous tissue is hyperintense compared to the relatively hypointense muscle and saturated signal of fat.

T1-weighted imaging may be useful in providing information about haemorrhage, which has changing intensity with time owing to the altering state of the haemoglobin component (oxyhaemoglobin, deoxyhaemoglobin, intracellular methaemoglobin, extracellular methaemoglobin and haemosiderin).

PD-weighted images have an inherently high SNR and have been found to be well suited to the visualisation of the internal structures of joints such as the knee. Fat-saturated PD-weighted images have increased water sensitivity and are useful in the detection of bone marrow oedema, and in demonstrating hyaline cartilage surface injuries or irregularities.[31]

This knowledge is invaluable in formulating the optimum treatment plan for a patient. The sensitivity of MRI is such that it can detect injuries such as rotator cuff tendonitis and bone bruising. These injuries are ideally treated conservatively, so an MRI scan can spare the patient unnecessary surgery. MRI is also an ideal modality to diagnose bone and soft tissue tumours, infection and avascular necrosis of bone.

MRI studies may now also include MR arthrography. This technique involves the injection of a dilute solution of gadolinium chelate (1 in 100 dilution) into the joint capsule followed by T1 fat-saturated images. The joint capsule is distended by the high-signal gadolinium and allows better visualisation of the intra-articular structures. The dilution is required because in an undiluted state the gadolinium would cause T2 shortening and reduce signal intensity rather than increase it.

SHOULDER

The shoulder joint allows a wide range of movement at the cost of having a shallow socket. It is therefore susceptible to a range of soft tissue injury involving the ligaments and tendons of the rotator cuff.

Common Indications

- Rotator cuff disease
- Labral injury
- Biceps tendon disruption

Equipment Needed

Dedicated phased-array shoulder coil, phased-array flex coil, surface coil or wrap-around coil

Routine Protocol

The routine protocol may include the sequences shown in the following table and in Figs 27.40–27.42.

Routine MRI Protocol: Shoulder

	Weighting	Orientation	Pulse Sequence
1	T1	Three planes	GE (localiser)
2	T1/T2/PD (fat suppression)	Sagittal	CSE/FSE
3	T1	Coronal	CSE/FSE
4	T2/PD (fat suppression)	Coronal	FSE (TSE)
5	T2*/PD (fat suppression)	Axial	GE/FSE (TSE)
6	T1	Axial	FSE/CSE

The axial localiser will allow the operator to orientate the coronal sections parallel to the tendon of the supraspinatus muscle. The FOV should include the entire joint and rotator cuff.

The parasagittal sections may be prescribed from the paracoronal data to ensure perpendicular orientation. MR arthrography may be performed in examinations of the shoulder joint.

ELBOW

The elbow is a very stable joint but elbow dislocations and fractures are common.

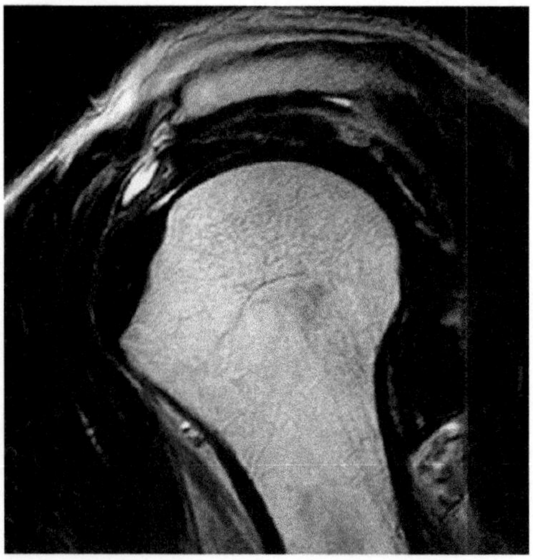

Fig. 27.40 T2-weighted FSE, sagittal – shoulder joint. (Reproduced with permission from Philips Medical Systems.)

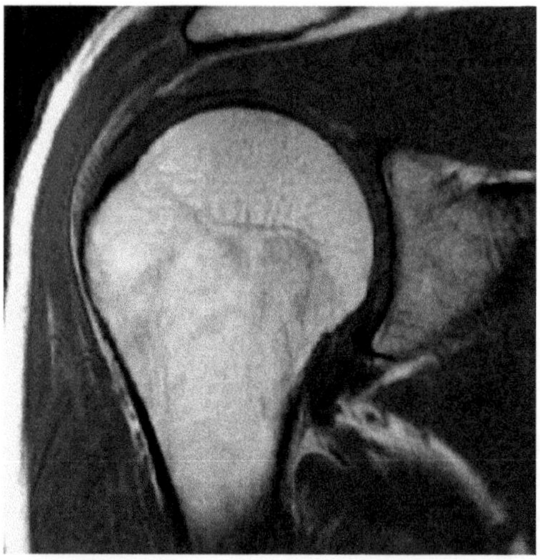

Fig. 27.41 T1-weighted spin echo, coronal – shoulder joint. (Reproduced with permission from Philips Medical Systems.)

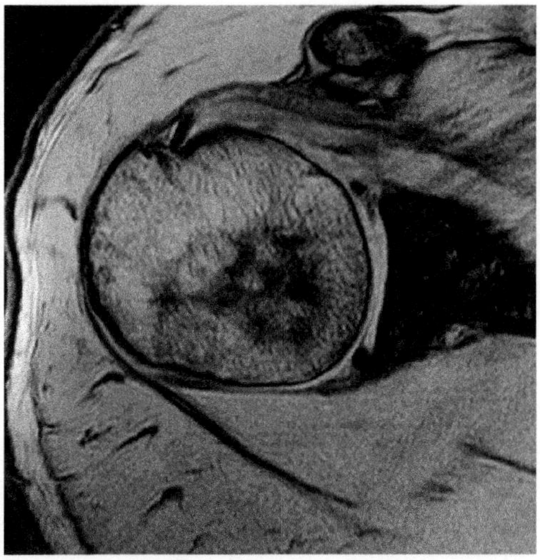

Fig. 27.42 T2*-weighted GE, axial – shoulder joint. (Reproduced with permission from Philips Medical Systems.)

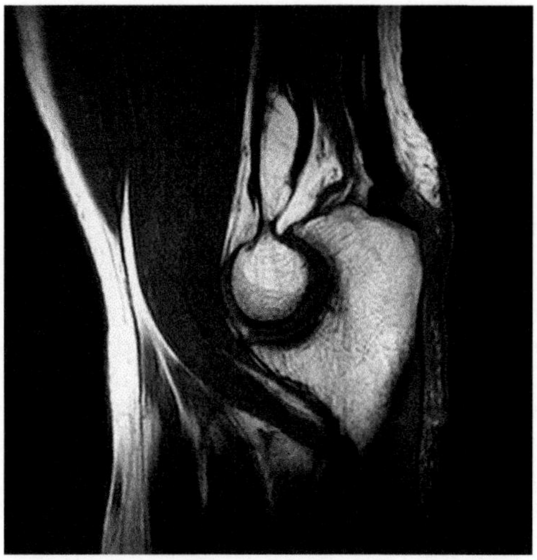

Fig. 27.43 T1-weighted spin echo, sagittal – elbow joint. (Reproduced with permission from Philips Medical Systems.)

Complex elbow injuries involve related fractures and/or neurovascular injuries. MRI is not particularly useful in acute trauma where conventional radiography can be used to assess bony injury. In the subacute setting, however, MRI is invaluable in assessing soft tissue damage.

From a practical viewpoint the elbow can be difficult to image owing to its location lateral to the trunk. Comfortable patient positioning is therefore of great importance.

Common Indications

- Ligament and tendon injury
- Articular cartilage injury
- Occult fractures
- Assessment of neurovascular structures

Equipment Needed

Dedicated phased-array elbow (extremity) coil, phased-array flex coil, surface coil or wrap-around coil

Routine Protocol

The routine protocol may include the sequences shown in the following table and in Figs 27.43–27.45.

Routine MRI Protocol: Elbow

	Weighting	Orientation	Pulse Sequence
1	T1	Three planes	GE (localiser)
2	T1	Sagittal (thin slices)	CSE/FSE
3	T1	Coronal (thin slices)	CSE/FSE
4	T1	Axial (thin slices)	CSE/FSE
5	PD or T2 (fat suppression)	Axial (thin slices)	FSE (TSE)
6	PD or T2 (fat suppression)	Coronal (thin slices)	FSE (TSE)
7	T2*	Sagittal 3D volume	GE

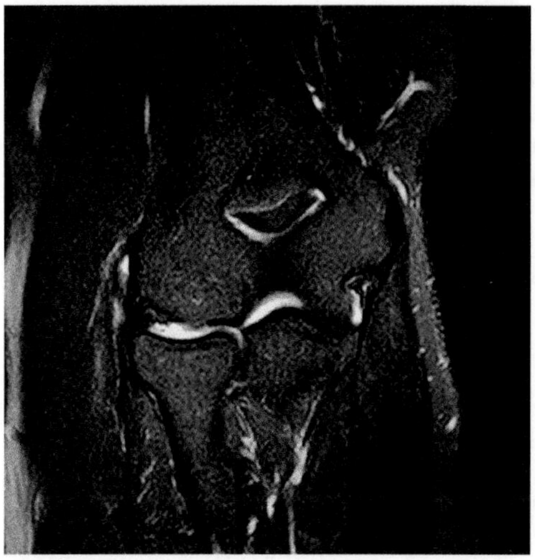

Fig. 27.44 T2-weighted FSE with fat saturation, coronal – elbow joint. (Reproduced with permission from Philips Medical Systems.)

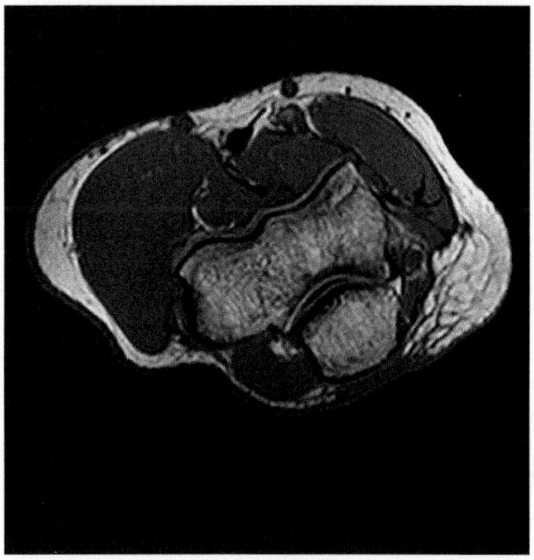

Fig. 27.45 T1-weighted incoherent GE, axial – elbow joint. (Reproduced with permission from Philips Medical Systems.)

The axial localiser will allow the operator to orientate the sagittal and coronal sections. The FOV should include the entire joint, the distal humerus and the proximal radius and ulna, including the biceps tendon distal insertion at the radial tuberosity.

MR arthrography may be performed for examination of the elbow joint.

WRIST

In the wrist, dislocations and fractures are common.

MRI is not particularly useful in acute trauma, where conventional radiography can be used to assess bony injury. In the subacute setting, however, MRI is invaluable in assessing occult fractures, avascular necrosis, soft tissue damage and instability due to ligament damage. As an anatomical area, the wrist is not particularly amenable to MRI. Bone and ligaments have low PD and there is a degree of flow from veins and arteries.

Common Indications

- Ganglia
- Carpal tunnel syndrome
- Occult fractures/scaphoid injury
- Assessment of ligaments
- General pain/repetitive strain injury
- Avascular necrosis
- Synovitis
- Rheumatoid disease

Equipment Needed

Dedicated phased-array wrist (extremity) coil, phased-array flex coil, surface coil or wrap-around coil

Routine Protocol

The routine protocol may include the sequences shown in the following table and in Figs 27.46–27.48.

Routine MRI Protocol: Wrist

	Weighting	Orientation	Pulse Sequence
1	T1	Three planes	GE (localiser)
2	T1	Axial/coronal (thin slices)	CSE/FSE
3	T2*	Coronal 3D volume	GE
4	PD (fat suppression)	Coronal/sagittal (thin slices)	FSE (TSE)
5	T2 or PD (fat suppression)	Axial (thin slices)	FSE (TSE)
6	T2	Coronal (thin slices)	STIR

The sagittal localiser will allow the operator to orientate the coronal and axial sections. The FOV should include the entire joint, carpal bones and distal ulna and radius. Sagittal imaging is occasionally used as it can help demonstrate carpal dislocations.

MR arthrography may be performed for examination of the wrist joint to demonstrate ligament injury.

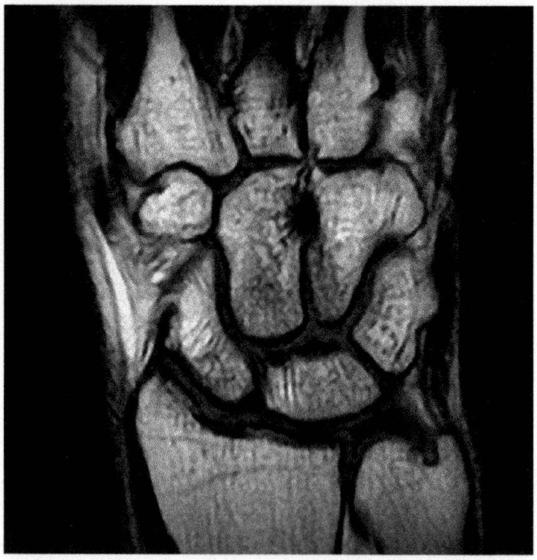

Fig. 27.46 T1-weighted spin echo, coronal – wrist joint. (Reproduced with permission from Philips Medical Systems.)

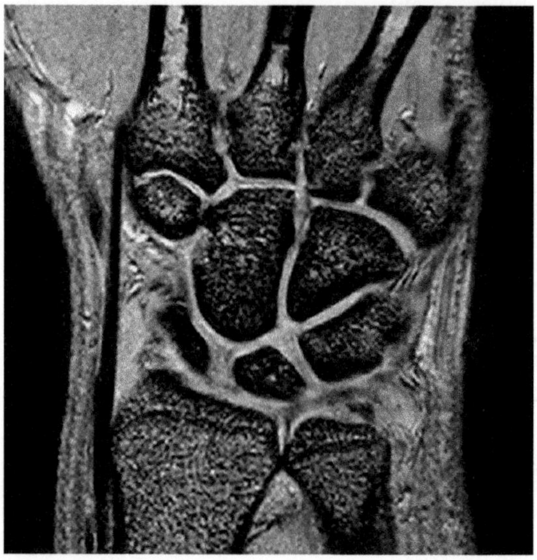

Fig. 27.47 T2*-weighted coherent GE, coronal – wrist joint. (Reproduced with permission from Philips Medical Systems.)

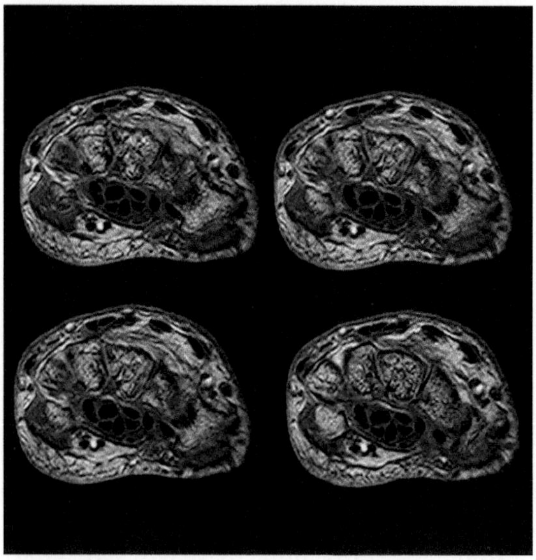

Fig. 27.48 T2*-weighted coherent GE 3D volume – wrist joint. (Reproduced with permission from Philips Medical Systems.)

HIP

Hip pain is a very common clinical problem and can have a wide number of causes, some musculoskeletal and some not related to the joint itself (e.g. sciatica, hernia or aneurysm).

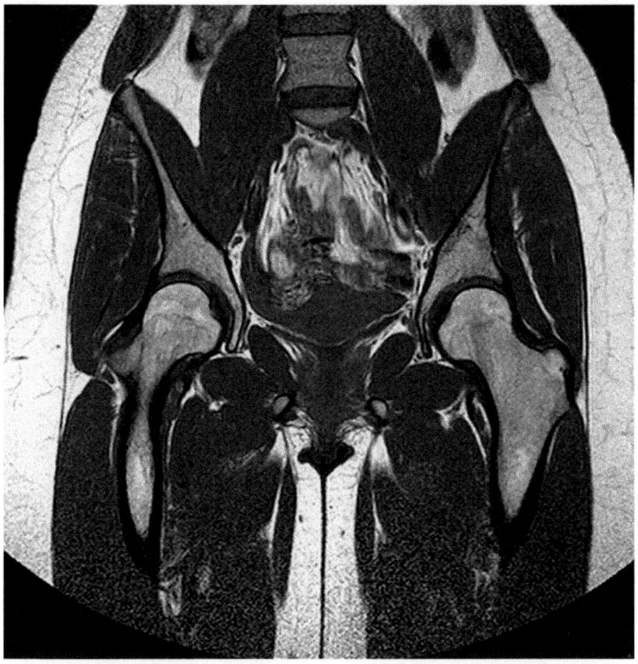

Fig. 27.49 T1-weighted coronal – hip joints. (Reproduced with permission from Philips Medical Systems.)

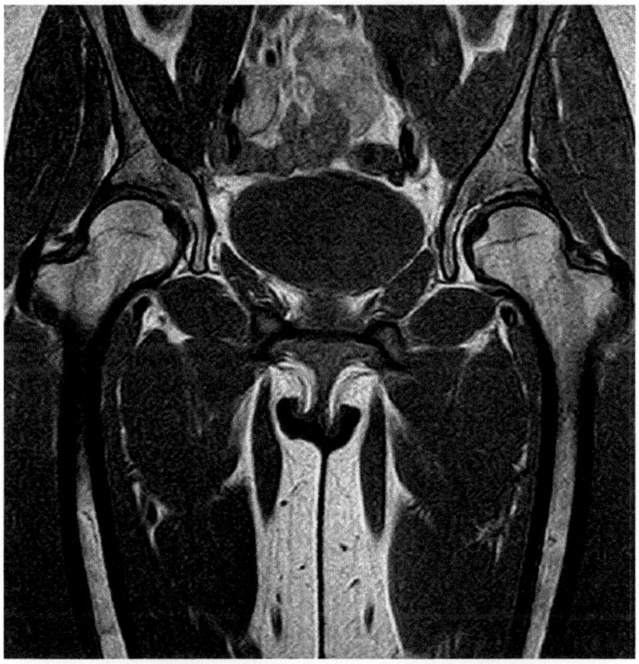

Fig. 27.50 PD-weighted, coronal – hip joints. (Reproduced with permission from Philips Medical Systems.)

As an anatomical area, the hip is very amenable to MRI as it has a high PD and is easily immobilised.

Common Indications

- Avascular necrosis
- Bone marrow disorders
- Occult fractures
- Neoplasm
- Osteomyelitis
- Labral injury

Equipment Needed

Phased-array torso coil

Routine Protocol

The routine protocol may be bilateral or unilateral (having a reduced FOV). It may include the sequences shown in the following table and in Figs 27.49 and 27.50.

Routine MRI Protocol: Hip

	Weighting	Orientation	Pulse Sequence
1	T1	Three planes	GE (localiser)
2	T1	Coronal	CSE/FSE
3	T2 or PD (fat suppression)	Coronal	STIR/FSE (TSE)
4	T1/T2 (fat suppression)	Axial	CSE/FSE

The FOV should cover the area from above the acetabulum to below the lesser trochanter. MR arthrography may be performed in examinations of the hip joint to demonstrate labral cartilage injuries.

KNEE

Plain radiography of the knee is of little value unless there has been a direct trauma to the joint causing bone fracture. MRI can accurately demonstrate the soft tissue structures of the knee and detect quite subtle damage to these components.

Common Indications

- Arthritis
- Bone bruising (trabecular microfracture)
- Cartilage injury chondromalacia
- Cruciate ligament damage
- Evaluation of knee pain
- Infection (osteomyelitis)
- Neoplasm
- Patellar disorders/maltracking

Equipment Needed

Dedicated quadrature volume knee coil (may be transmit/receive), or phased-array knee coil

Routine Protocol

The routine protocol may include the sequences shown in the following table and in Figs 27.51–27.56.

Routine MRI Protocol: Knee

	Weighting	Orientation	Pulse Sequence
1	T1	Three planes	GE (localiser)
2	PD (± fat suppression)	Sagittal	FSE (TSE)
3	T1	Sagittal	CSE/FSE
4	T2/PD (fat suppression)	Coronal	FSE (TSE)
5	T1	Coronal	CSE/FSE
6	T2/PD (fat suppression)	Axial	FSE (TSE)
7	T2*	Sagittal/volume	GE

The FOV should cover the entire joint and should include the skin surfaces laterally and medially.

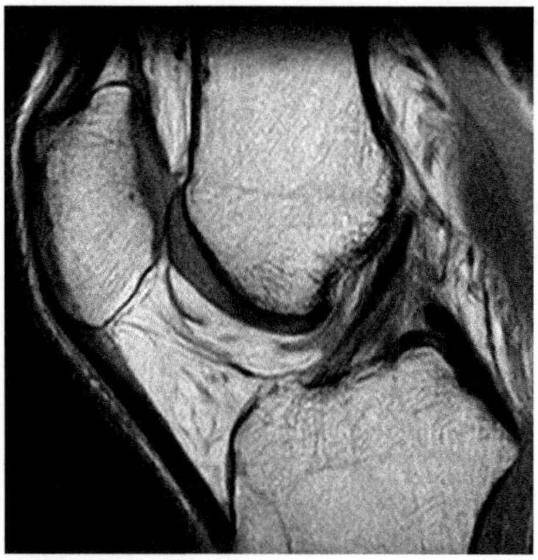

Fig. 27.51 PD-weighted, sagittal – knee joint. (Reproduced with permission from Philips Medical Systems.)

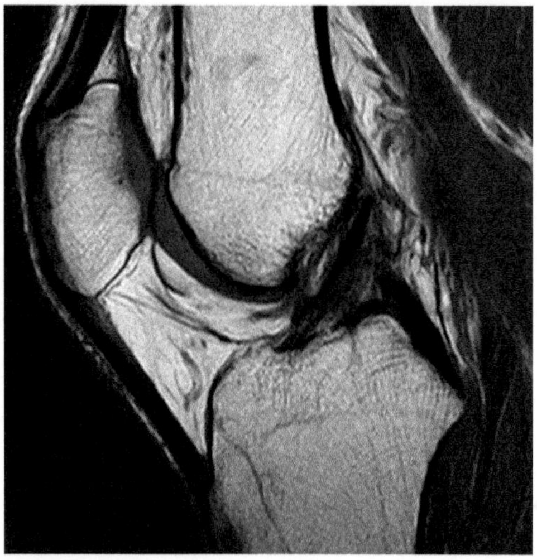

Fig. 27.52 T1-weighted sagittal – knee joint. (Reproduced with permission from Philips Medical Systems.)

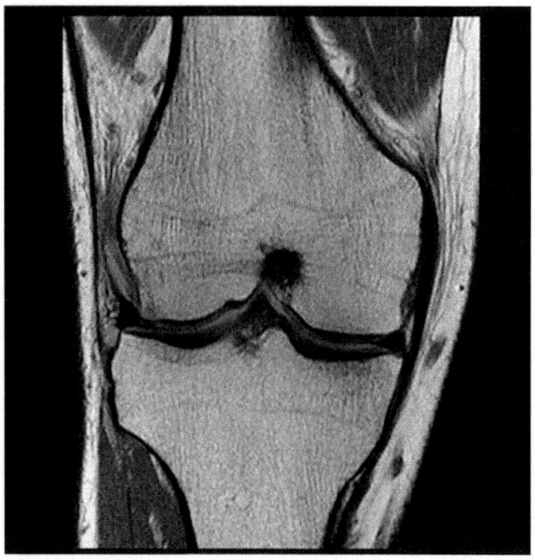

Fig. 27.53 PD-weighted, coronal – knee joint. (Reproduced with permission from Philips Medical Systems.)

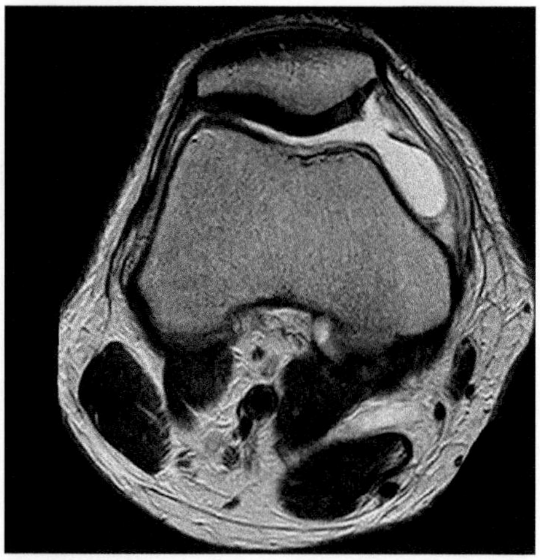

Fig. 27.54 T2-weighted FSE, axial – knee joint. (Reproduced with permission from Philips Medical Systems.)

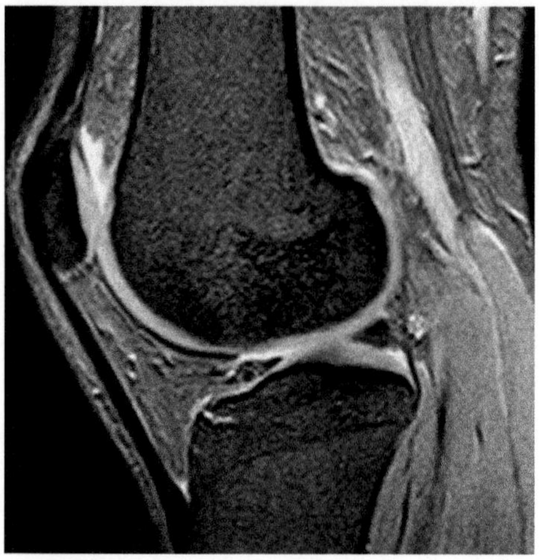

Fig. 27.55 T2*-weighted coherent GE, sagittal – knee joint. (Reproduced with permission from Philips Medical Systems.)

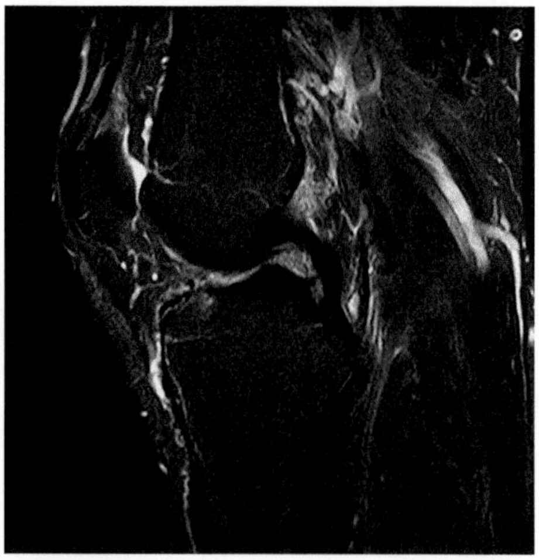

Fig. 27.56 STIR, sagittal – knee joint. (Reproduced with permission from Philips Medical Systems.)

ANKLE

Plain X-rays of the ankle are of use when ruling out fracture or joint instability.

MRI can demonstrate the soft tissue components of the joint. MR arthrography can be performed in the ankle joint to demonstrate ligament tears and intra-articular lesions.

Common Indications

- Arthritis
- Bone bruising (trabecular microfracture)
- Cartilage injury chondromalacia
- Ligament damage
- Infection
- Neoplasm

Equipment Needed

Phased-array extremity coil or quadrature volume knee coil

Routine Protocol

The routine protocol may include the sequences shown in the following table and in Figs 27.57 and 27.58.

Routine MRI Protocol: Ankle

	Weighting	Orientation	Pulse Sequence
1	T1	Three planes	GE (localiser)
2	T1	Coronal	CSE/FSE
3	T2/PD (fat suppression)	Coronal	STIR/FSE (TSE)
4	T1	Sagittal	CSE/FSE
5	T2	Sagittal	FSE (TSE)
6	T2/PD (fat suppression)	Sagittal	STIR/FSE (TSE)
7	T2 (fat suppression)	Axial	FSE (TSE)
8	T1	Axial	CSE/FSE

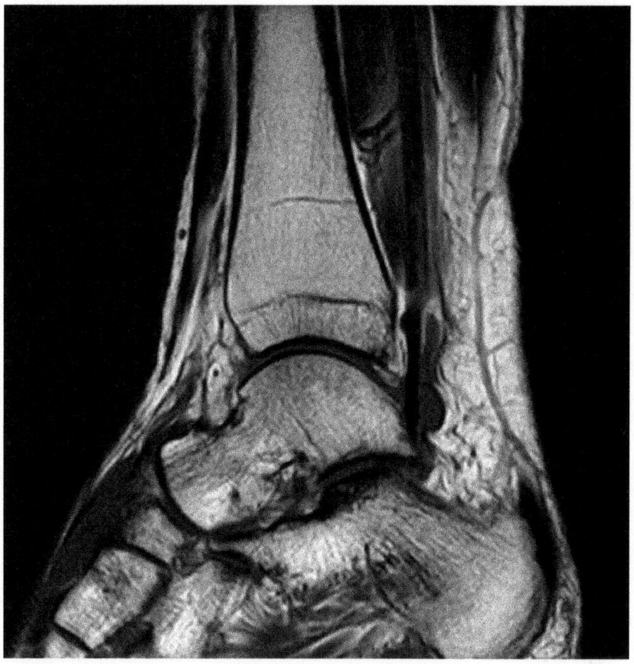

Fig. 27.57 **T1-weighted sagittal – ankle joint.** (Reproduced with permission from Philips Medical Systems.)

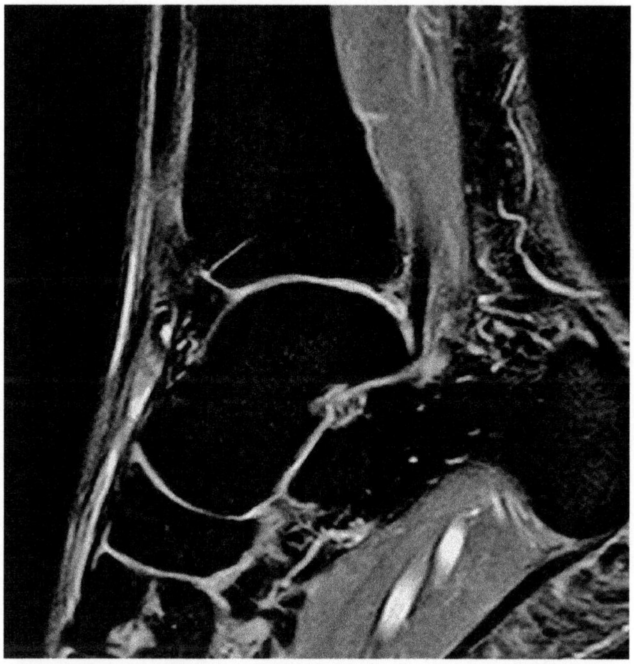

Fig. 27.58 **STIR, sagittal – ankle joint.** (Reproduced with permission from Philips Medical Systems.)

BREAST

MRI is very sensitive at detecting breast lesions and unlike mammography is not limited by dense tissue. Specificity is variable, however, and MRI is therefore used in combination with clinical examination, mammography, ultrasound and biopsy to obtain an accurate diagnosis.

Focal lesions within the breast usually enhance after the administration of gadolinium contrast, and T1-weighted 3D volume imaging data with or without fat suppression are collected dynamically (DCE MRI). The technique should feature both high spatial and temporal resolution for accurate analysis. Enhancement curves are produced for regions of interest. Lesions can then be characterised by the pattern and rate of enhancement, malignant lesions tending to have rapid bright enhancement with rapid wash-out.[32]

Diffusion weighted imaging (DWI) is a technique that is gaining popularity performed in conjunction with DCE MRI. Information can be acquired from DWI sequences to demonstrate the random motion of water molecules in the body and the free or restricted motion of such molecules. Post processing software allows the generation of apparent diffusion coefficient (ADC) maps for assessment of a lesion's diffusion and ADC values assisting in breast tumour characterisation. Many malignant lesions exhibit restricted diffusion and appear hypointense on ADC but hyperintense on DWI.[33,34]

Common Indications

- Screening high-risk groups
- Guided biopsy
- Staging extent of known disease
- Diagnosing recurrent disease
- Lesion characterisation after equivocal ultrasound/mammography results
- Neoadjuvant radiotherapy response
- Implant integrity/rupture

Equipment Needed

Dedicated phased-array breast coil or phased-array torso coil with breast support

Routine Protocol

The routine protocol may include the sequences shown in the following table.

Routine MRI Protocol: Breast

	Weighting	Orientation	Pulse Sequence
1	T1	Three planes	GE (localiser)
2	T2	Coronal	SSFSE[a]
3	T2 (± fat suppression)	Axial (± 3D volume)	SSFSE/STIR
4	T1 (dynamic) (+ gadolinium) (± fat suppression)	Axial/sagittal/coronal volume	GE, may use Dixon technique if available
5	T1 (post gadolinium)	Sagittal of each breast	FSE (TSE)/GE
6	T2 (± water suppression)	Axial/sagittal	STIR, FLAIR
7	DWI (± multiple B_0 values)	Axial	EPI

[a]If single-shot is not available/preferred, FSE may be used. T1 3D dynamic volume with fat suppression negates the need for subtraction images. It is desirable for the 3D acquisition to have isotropic (i.e. cubic) voxels. This allows reconstruction in orthogonal and oblique planes with the same resolution along every axis. This may negate the need for other acquisitions post contrast.

ABDOMEN

The commonly imaged areas in abdominal MRI include the liver, the pancreas, the kidneys and adrenal glands, and the reproductive system. With the advent of new hardware and pulse sequences the trend seems to be towards breath-hold and free breathing scans. T2 weighting can be achieved using SSFSE, T1 weighting by GE. Conventional spin echo may also be used in conjunction with motion reduction techniques such as diaphragm tracking (navigators). This involves locating a region of interest over the diaphragm and using the resulting periodic read-out to control data collection as the patient breathes.

LIVER

Liver MRI is commonly used for the detection and characterisation of focal liver lesions, especially tumours. On a T1-weighted sequence the signal intensity of normal liver is greater than that of muscle or spleen, less than that of subcutaneous fat and approximately the same as that of the pancreas. On T2-weighted sequences normal liver tissue is of relatively low signal owing to short T2 relaxation time, and is less intense than spleen. Focal lesions in the liver generally enhance after the administration of Gd-DTPA.

The liver is a common site for metastatic disease, and so imaging of metastases is a very common indication for liver MRI. Metastases generally appear at a lower signal intensity than normal liver tissue on T1-weighted images, but owing to the presence of oedema they are usually hyperintense on T2-weighted sequences. They can also have haemorrhagic components, which appear as inhomogeneous areas at varying intensities depending upon the age of the haemorrhage and the weighting used.

Imaging usually involves DCE studies, where diagnosis is based on the rate and pattern of enhancement of any lesions present.

Several manufacturers also offer hepatobiliary gadolinium-based agents. Healthy liver cells enhance and their contrast enhancement accumulates over time. The focal lesions remain low in signal on post-contrast T1-weighted fat-suppressed images owing to nil or poor uptake of contrast by abnormal cells.

Common Indications

- Characterisation of benign/malignant lesions
- Assessment of diffuse liver disease, e.g. fatty liver, haemochromatosis
- Visualisation of biliary tree in obstructive jaundice

Equipment Needed

Phased-array torso coil
Respiratory compensation/triggering

Routine Protocol

The routine protocol may include the sequences shown in the following table and in Figs 27.59–27.61.

Routine MRI Protocol: Liver

	Weighting	Orientation	Pulse Sequence
1	T1	Three planes	GE (localiser)
2	T1 (pre gadolinium) (±fat suppression)	Axial/3D volume (breath hold)	GE, may use Dixon technique if available
3	T1 (dynamic) (+ gadolinium) (fat suppression)	Axial/3D volume (breath hold)	GE
4	T2 (fat suppression)	Axial (breath hold)	SSFSE[a]
5	T1	Axial/coronal (breath hold)	GE
6	T2/T2*	Axial/coronal (free breathing)	SSFSE[a] (triggered)/balanced GE
7	T1	Axial (breath hold)	GE, fat and water in phase (may be a dual echo)
8	T1	Axial (breath hold)	GE, fat and water out of phase (may be a dual echo)

[a]If single shot is not available/preferred, FSE with respiratory gating may be used.

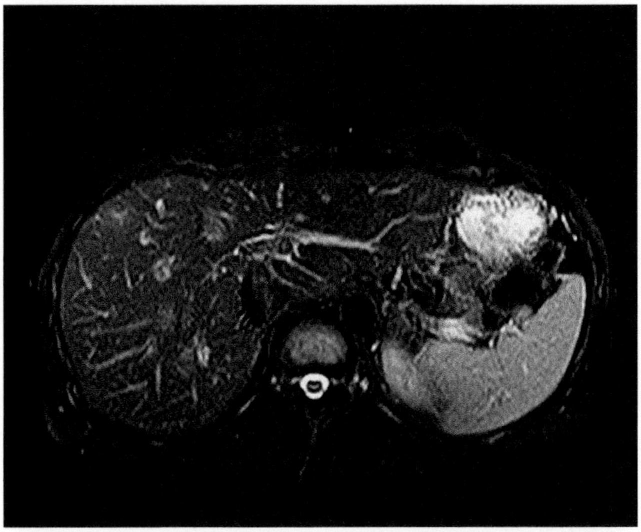

Fig. 27.59 T2-weighted single-shot – liver (patient free breathing). (Reproduced with permission from Philips Medical Systems.)

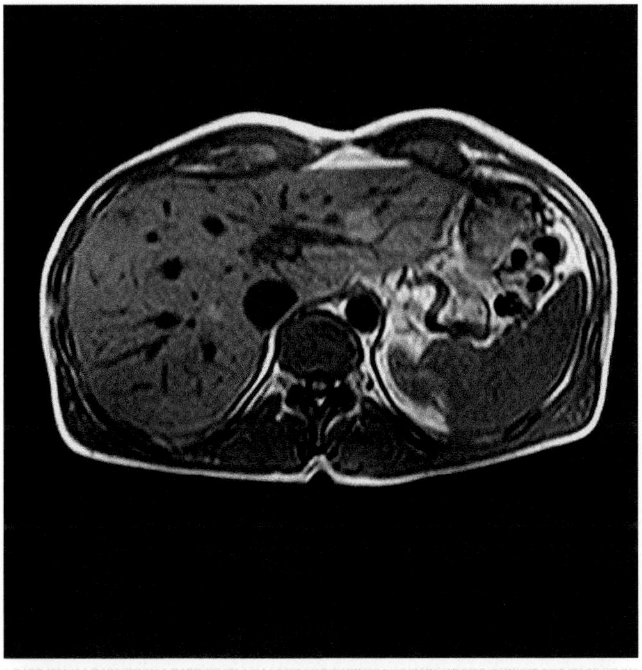

Fig. 27.60 T1-weighted GE – liver (breath holding). (Reproduced with permission from Philips Medical Systems.)

Free-breathing SSFSE is usually performed with respiratory gating to ensure that each slice is acquired at the same point in the respiratory cycle.

Balanced gradient sequences can be used as an alternative to T2-weighted FSE as they also reduce circulatory/biliary flow artefacts.

In- and out-of-phase imaging (either run separately or as one dual acquisition) can help to diagnose fatty liver, as voxels containing fat and water will decrease in signal intensity on the out-of-phase image (Fig. 27.61).

Dynamic scanning can help to differentiate between enhancing liver lesions. These studies are performed after

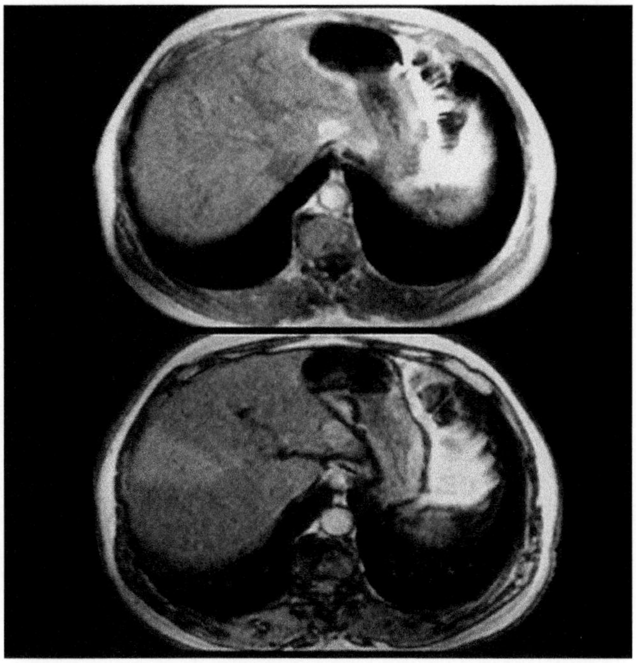

Fig. 27.61 In- and out-of-phase imaging in the liver. (Reproduced with permission from Philips Medical Systems.)

positive contrast agent injection, typically in the arterial, portal, venous and delayed phases. Fat suppression may be used following contrast injection to help improve the contrast-to-noise ratio.

Multiple echo T2-weighted sequences may be useful in characterising haemangiomas as these lesions remain hyperintense on late echoes.

The biliary tree may be imaged using T2-weighted sequences having very long echo times (Fig. 27.62). This provides an image resembling an endoscopic retrograde cholangiopancreatogram, but without the need for any intervention or contrast media. This technique is often referred to as a magnetic resonance cholangiopancreatogram (MRCP). A very long echo time (perhaps up to 600 ms) results in an image where only water spins are still in phase. If a 3D volume technique is used the data can also be post processed using MIP to give multiprojectional images.

PANCREAS

The pancreas can be seen on a Tl-weighted image as a medium signal intensity structure with an intensity similar to that of the liver, surrounded by hyperintense fat. With increased age the homogeneity of the pancreas decreases due to parenchymal atrophy. The margins of the gland may be smooth or lobulated, and the pancreatic duct is shown as a low signal intensity structure on Tl-weighted images. Narrow slice thickness is required to show the duct as it is less than 2 mm across. Fat-suppression imaging leaves the pancreas as a homogenous high-signal structure which has a greater signal intensity than any of the surrounding structures. The pancreatic duct may also be demonstrated on MRCP.

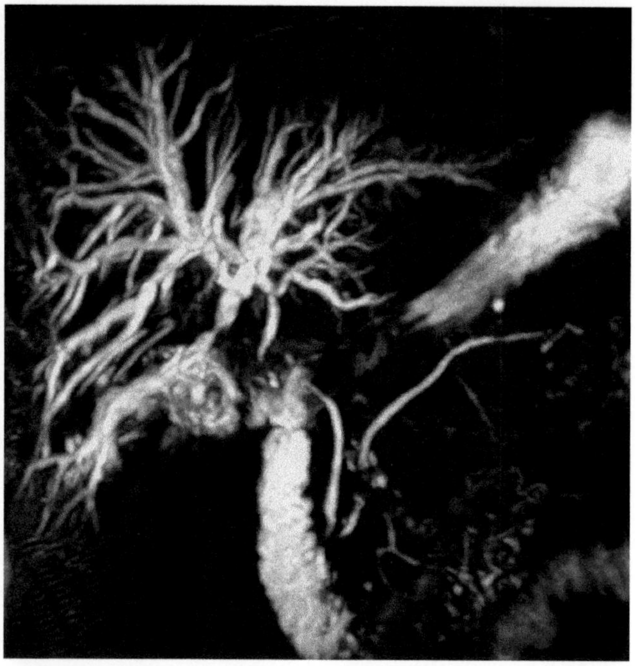

Fig. 27.62 Heavy T2 weighting and maximum intensity projection – biliary tree. (Reproduced with permission from Philips Medical Systems.)

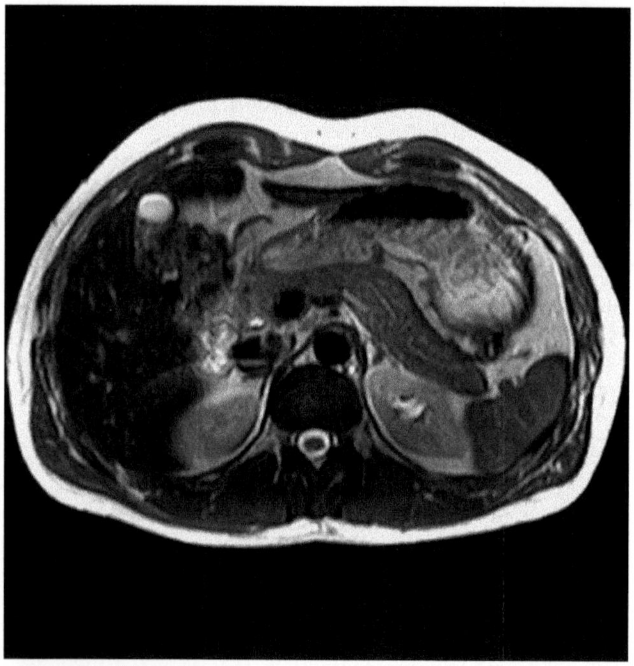

Fig. 27.63 T2-weighted axial – pancreas. (Reproduced with permission from Philips Medical Systems.)

Common Indications

- Evaluation of pancreatitis
- Neoplasms
- Trauma

Equipment Needed

Phased-array torso coil
Respiratory compensation/triggering

Routine Protocol

The routine protocol may include the sequences shown in the following table and in Fig. 27.63.

Routine MRI Protocol: Pancreas

	Weighting	Orientation	Pulse Sequence
1	T1	Three planes	GE (localiser)
2	T1 (± fat suppression)	Axial (thin slices) or 3D volume (breath-hold)	GE
3	T1	Axial (breath-hold) respiratory compensation	FSE (TSE)/GE
4	T2/T2*	Axial (breath-hold)	SSFSE[a]/balanced GE
5	T1	Axial (breath-hold)	GE fat and water in phase
6	T1	Axial (breath-hold)	GE fat and water out of phase

[a]If single shot is not available/preferred, FSE with respiratory gating may be used.

On T1-weighted images the normal pancreas has higher signal intensity than any other abdominal organ.

Fat-saturated T1-weighted sequences are useful for distinguishing normal from abnormal pancreatic parenchyma because distracting high signal from intra-abdominal fat is removed. For patients unable to hold their breath, respiratory compensated spin echo sequences may be performed.

Breath-holding, in- and out-of-phase, T1-weighted GE images display similar anatomical information as spin echo sequences but with the additional bonus of signal suppression due to fat and water phase opposition. This technique, which is also used in the liver, can help in distinguishing between some common lesions and tumours in this anatomical area. These include adenoma (in the adrenal area), focal fatty change in the pancreas and renal cell carcinoma metastasis in the pancreas.[35–40]

KIDNEYS

The diagnosis of malignant renal masses requires visualisation of the mass and usually positive enhancement with gadolinium-based contrast media. Typically, T1-weighted GE sequences are used.

For renal transplant assessment, T2-weighted sequences and contrast-enhanced 3D GE sequences give anatomical information about causes of graft dysfunction. These may be supplemented by dynamic contrast renography and MRA. MRA is also frequently used for renal artery stenosis as a non-ionising radiation alternative to CT.

MR urography is a technique that has gained popularity, as information can be acquired from either *static-fluid* imaging using T2-weighted images with long echo times or *excretory* imaging using delayed, contrast-enhanced, T1-weighted fat-suppressed 3D GE sequences to assess kidney function. These can be performed pre and post contrast to provide subtraction data.[41]

Common Indications

- Adrenal gland assessment
- Neoplasms
- Renal transplant

Equipment Needed

- Phased-array torso coil
- Respiratory compensation/gating

Routine Protocol

The routine protocol may include the sequences shown in the following table and in Figs 27.64–27.66.

Routine MRI Protocol: Kidneys

	Weighting	Orientation	Pulse Sequence
1	T1	Three planes	GE (localiser)
2	T1	Coronal	CSE/FSE/GE
3	T1	Axial	CSE/FSE/GE
4	T2 (± fat suppression)/ T2*	Coronal/axial (breath-hold)	SSFSE[a]/balanced GE
5	T1	Axial (breath-hold)	GE fat and water in phase
6	T1	Axial (breath-hold)	GE fat and water out of phase

[a]If single shot is not available/preferred, FSE with respiratory gating may be utilised.

If renal angiography is needed (Fig. 27.67)

	Weighting	Orientation	Pulse Sequence
1	T1	Coronal 3D volume	GE

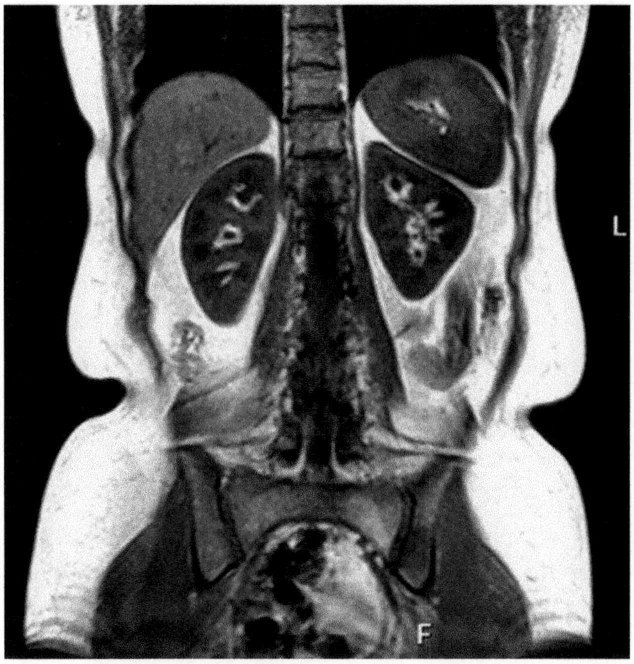

Fig. 27.64 **T1-weighted coronal – kidneys.** (Reproduced with permission from Philips Medical Systems.)

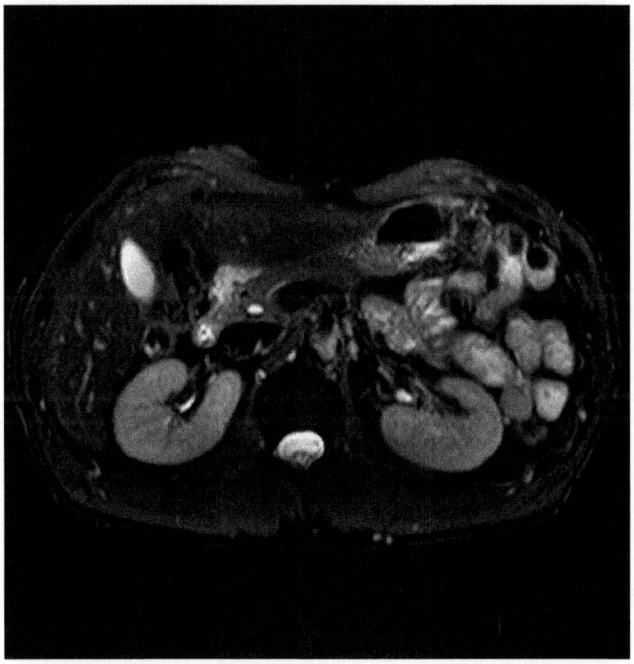

Fig. 27.65 **T2-weighted (fat suppression), axial – kidneys.** (Reproduced with permission from Philips Medical Systems.)

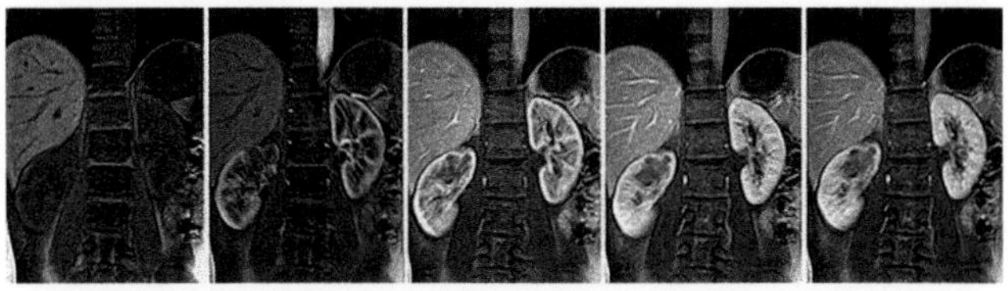

Fig. 27.66 **T1-weighted dynamic study, coronal – kidneys.** (Reproduced with permission from Philips Medical Systems.)

PELVIS

The pelvis presents an ideal area for MRI imaging. It has a high PD, good inherent contrast-to-noise ratio, and is easily immobilised using compression.

Common Indications

- Anal fistulae
- Assessment of prostate gland (male)
- Fibroids (female)
- Location of undescended testis (male)
- Neoplasms (prostate, cervix, uterus, ovaries, bladder, rectum)

Equipment Needed

Phased-array torso coil, compression band

Routine Protocol

The routine protocol may include the sequences shown in the following table and in Figs 27.68–27.70.

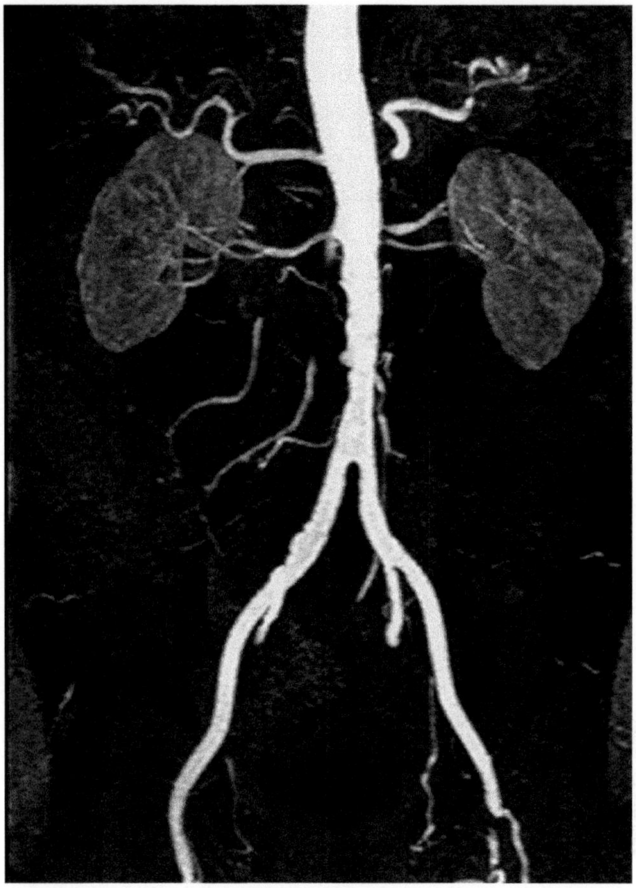

Fig. 27.67 Renal contrast-enhanced MRA. (Reproduced with permission from Philips Medical Systems.)

Routine MRI Protocol: Pelvis

	Weighting	Orientation	Pulse Sequence
1	T1	Three planes	GE (localiser)
2	T1	Axial	FSE (TSE)
3	T2	Axial	FSE/SSFSE[a]
4	T2	Coronal	FSE/SSFSE[a]
5	T2	Sagittal	FSE/SSFSE[a]

[a]If single shot is not available/preferred, FSE with respiratory gating may be utilised.

For anal fistulae

	Weighting	Orientation	Pulse Sequence
1	PD/T2 (fat suppression)	Coronal	FSE (TSE)
2	T2 (± fat suppression)	Sagittal	FSE (TSE)
3	T2 (± fat suppression)	Axial	FSE (TSE)
4	T1	Axial	FSE (TSE)

STIR may be used instead of FSE.

PROSTATE

MRI is becoming more popular as the imaging choice for prostate cancer detection and guiding management. MRI is used in combination with clinical examination, ultrasound and biopsy to obtain an accurate diagnosis.

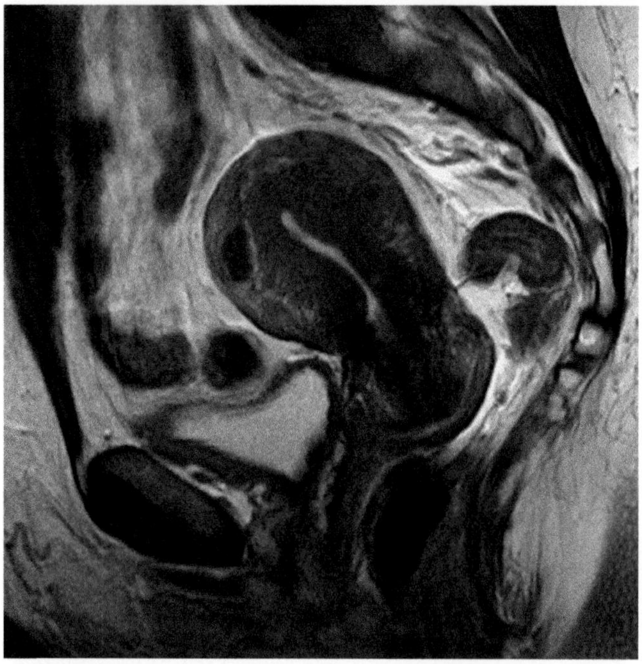

Fig. 27.68 T2-weighted sagittal – female pelvis. (Reproduced with permission from Philips Medical Systems.)

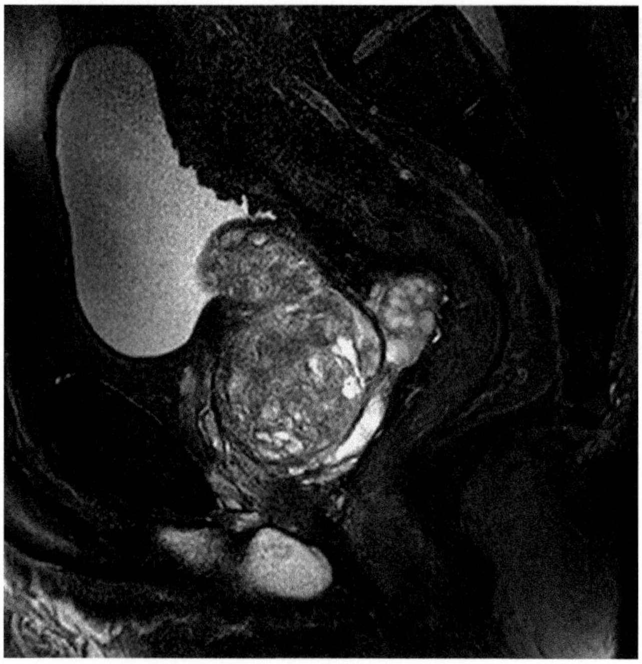

Fig. 27.69 T2-weighted (fat suppression), sagittal – male pelvis. (Reproduced with permission from Philips Medical Systems.)

Focal lesions within the prostate usually enhance after the administration of gadolinium contrast. T1-weighted, 3D volume imaging data with or without fat suppression are acquired dynamically (DCE MRI). The technique should feature both high spatial and temporal resolution for accurate analysis. Enhancement curves are produced for regions of interest. Lesions

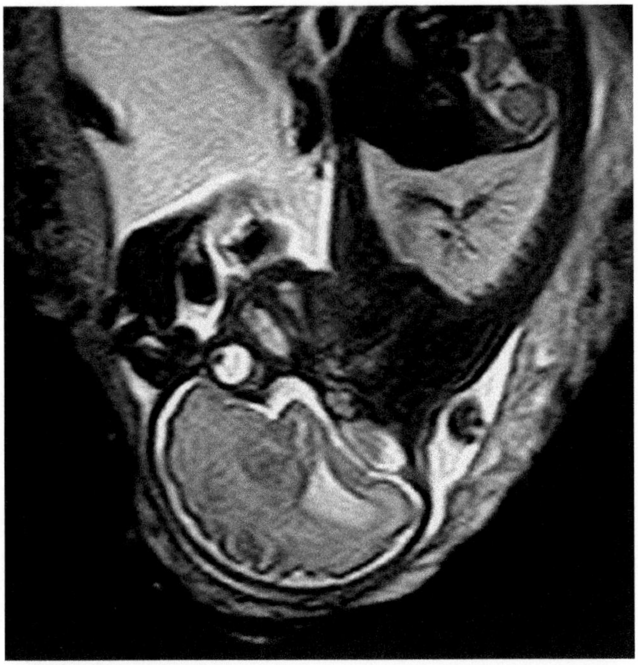

Fig. 27.70 T2-weighted sagittal – fetus. (Reproduced with permission from Philips Medical Systems.)

can then be characterised by the pattern and rate of enhancement, malignant lesions tending to have rapid bright enhancement with rapid wash-out or persistent enhancement.[42]

DWI may be used in the assessment of a lesion's diffusion and ADC values assisting in prostate tumour characterisation. Malignant lesions in the prostate generally have restricted diffusion and appear hypointense on ADC but hyperintense on DWI.[42]

Common Indications

- Screening high-risk groups
- Guided biopsy
- Evaluation after negative biopsy with elevated PSA
- Surgical planning or post surgical assessment
- Staging extent of known disease, extracapsular extension
- Diagnosing recurrent disease
- Active surveillance
- Radiation planning

Equipment Needed

Dedicated phased-array torso coil or phased-array torso coil; intra-cavitary endo-rectal coils are used dependent on local procedures

Routine Protocol

The routine protocol may include the sequences shown in the following table.

Routine MRI Protocol: Prostate

	Weighting	Orientation	Pulse Sequence
1	T1	Three planes	GE (localiser)
2	T2	Sagittal (small FOV, thin slices)	FSE (TSE)
3	T2	Coronal (small FOV, thin slices)	FSE (TSE)
4	T2	Axial (small FOV, thin slices)	FSE (TSE)
5	T1 (dynamic) (+ gadolinium) (± fat suppression)	Axial 3D volume	GE
6	T1	Axial whole pelvis	FSE (TSE)/GE
7	T1	Coronal whole pelvis	FSE (TSE)/GE
8	DWI (± multiple B_0 values may be required)	Axial	EPI

If single shot is not available/preferred, FSE may be used. T1 3D dynamic volume with fat suppression negates the need for subtraction images.

References

1. Chang G, Wang L, Schweitzer ME, et al. 3D Na MRI of human skeletal muscle at 7 Tesla: initial experience. *Eur Radiol.* 2010;20(8):2039–2046.
2. https://www.nobelprize.org/prizes/physics/1944/rabi/facts/.
3. Wakefield J. *The 'indomitable' MRI.* Smithsonian magazine; 2000. https://www.smithsonianmag.com/science-nature/the-indomitable-mri-29126670/.
4. Damadian R. Tumor detection by nuclear magnetic resonance. *Science.* 1971;171(976):1151–1153.
5. Lauterbur P. Image formation by induced local interaction; examples employing magnetic resonance. *Nature.* 1973;242(5394):190–191.
6. Garroway P, Grannell PK, Mansfield P. Image formation in NMR by a selective irradiative process. *J Phys C (Solid State Physics).* 1974;7:457.
7. Mansfield P, Maudsley A. Medical imaging by NMR. *Br J Radiol.* 1977;50:188.
8. Damadian R, Goldsmith M, Minkoff L. NMR in Cancer: XVI. FONAR image of the live human body. *Physiol Chem Phys.* 1977;9:97–100.
9. Mansfield P, Maudsley A. Planar spin imaging by NMR. *J Phys C (Solid State Physics).* 1976;9:L409–L411.
10. Mansfield P, Maudsley A. Line scan proton spin imaging in biological structures by NMR. *Phys Med Biol.* 1976;21:847–852.
11. Mansfield P. Multi-planar image formation using NMR spin echoes. *J Phys C (Solid State Physics).* 1977;10(3):L55–L58.
12. Lauterbur P, Dias M, Rudin A. Augmentation of tissue water proton spin-lattice relaxation rates by in vivo addition of paramagnetic ions. In: Dutton P, et al., ed. *Frontiers of Biological Energetics.* New York: Academic Press; 1978:752–759.
13. Ordidge R, Mansfield P, Coupland RE. Rapid biomedical imaging by NMR. *Br J Radiol.* 1981;54:850–855.
14. http://www.fonar.com/standup.htm.
15. Philips. Basic principles of MR imaging. Philips Medical Systems.
16. Baker G. *The Science and Technology Facilities Council.* Safety in the Handling and Use of Cryogenic Liquids; 2008.
17. Ezzeddine B. Active noise cancellation system for magnetic resonance imaging. Neuroscience Directions. 1(1), p3. Wallace-Kettering Neuroscience Institute.
18. Alibek S, Vogel M, Sun W, et al. Acoustic noise reduction in MRI using Silent Scan: an initial experience. *Diagn Intervent Radiol.* 2014;20(4):360–363.
19. Imai Y. New MultiTransmit technology advances 3T imaging. *Fieldstrength Magazine.* 2009;(38). Best, Philips Medical Systems.
20. http://www.mrisafety.com.
21. Shellock F. *Reference Manual for MRI Safety, Implants and Devices.* Los Angeles: Biomedical Research Publishing Group; 2007.

22. Chaljub G, Kramer LA, Johnson 3rd RF, et al. Projectile cylinder accidents resulting from the presence of ferromagnetic nitrous oxide or oxygen tanks in the MR suite. *AJR Am J Roentgenol.* 2001;177:27–30.
23. Vote B, Simpson AJ. X-ray turns a blind eye to ferrous metal. *Clin Exper Ophthalmol.* 2001;29:262–264.
24. http://www.bamrr.org.
25. Graham D, Cloke P, Vosper M, et al. *Principles of Radiological Physics.* 5th ed. Edinburgh: Elsevier; 2007.
26. Singh S. *Big Bang.* London: Harper Collins; 2005.
27. Hashemi R, Bradley W. *The Basics of MRI.* Baltimore, MD: Williams and Wilkins; 1997.
28. Sadiku MNO. *Elements of Electromagnetics.* 4th ed. Oxford: Oxford University Press; 2007.
29. Anslow P, Talbot J, et al. *Somerset MRI Course CD ROM.* Vol. 2. MRI Education Company; 2001.
30. Meaney J. Magnetic resonance angiography of the peripheral arteries: current status. *Eur Radiol.* 2003;13(4):836–852.
31. Lal NR, Jamadar DA, Doi K, et al. Evaluation of bone contusions with fat-saturated fast spin-echo proton-density magnetic resonance imaging. *Canad Assoc Radiol J.* 2000;51:182–185.
32. Shinil K, Shah SK, Greatrex KV. Current role of magnetic resonance imaging in breast imaging: a primer for the primary care physician. *J Am Board Fam Med.* 2005;18:6.
33. Korteweg MA, Veldhuis WB, Visser F, et al. Feasibility of 7 Tesla breast magnetic resonance imaging determination of intrinsic sensitivity and high-resolution magnetic resonance imaging, diffusion-weighted imaging, and (1)H-magnetic resonance spectroscopy of breast cancer patients receiving neoadjuvant therapy. *Invest Radiol.* 2011;46:370–376.
34. Rahbar H, Partridge S. Multiparametric breast MRI of breast cancer. *Magn Reson Imaging Clin North Am.* 2016;24(1):223–238.
35. Mitchell D, Crovello M, Matteucci T, et al. Benign adrenocortical masses: diagnosis with chemical shift MR imaging. *Radiology.* 1992;185:345–351.
36. Outwater E, Siegelman ES, Radecki PD, et al. Distinction between benign and malignant adrenal masses: value of T1-weighted chemical-shift MR imaging. *Am J Roentgenol.* 1995;165:579–583.
37. Jacobs J, Coleman BG, Arger PH, et al. Pancreatic sparing of focal fatty infiltration. *Radiology.* 1994;190:437–439.
38. Isserow J, Siegelman ES, Mammone J. Focal fatty infiltration of the pancreas: MR characterization with chemical shift imaging. *Am J Roentgenol.* 1999;173:1263–1265.
39. Outwater E, Bhatia M, Siegelman ES, et al. Lipid in renal clear cell carcinoma: detection on opposed-phase gradient-echo MR images. *Radiology.* 1997;205:103–107.
40. Carucci L, Siegelman ES, Feldman MS, et al. Pancreatic metastasis from clear cell renal carcinoma: diagnosis with chemical shift MRI. *J Comput Assist Tomogr.* 1999;23:934–936.
41. Leyendecker J, Barnes CE, Zagoria RA. MR urography: techniques and clinical applications. *Radiographics.* 2008;28:1.
42. Hegde J, Mulkern RV, Panych LP, et al. Multiparametric MRI of prostate cancer: an update on state-of-the-art techniques and their performance in detecting and localizing prostate cancer. *J Magn Reson Imaging.* 2013;37:1035–1054.

28 Radionuclide Imaging

ROBERT GORDON

Introduction

Nuclear medicine has three distinct practice areas: diagnostic radionuclide imaging incorporating positron emission tomography (PET), in vitro laboratory-based diagnostics and unsealed source radionuclide therapy. In all three areas the power of nuclear medicine is its ability to diagnose and/or treat disease at a physiological or molecular level.

When radioactive substances are administered to patients, whether for diagnostic or therapeutic purposes, they are collectively referred to as radiopharmaceuticals. For diagnostic imaging these radiopharmaceuticals provide a way of visualising patterns of biological activity in the organs of interest. This is achieved by imaging the distribution of radiopharmaceuticals which are selected based on their ability to be taken up by the organ or pathology of interest. Abnormalities including trauma or the effects of pathogenic invasion can be identified using carefully targeted radiopharmaceuticals. The great advantage of nuclear medicine imaging is that, except in the case of trauma, physiological changes usually precede anatomical changes.[1]

In vitro nuclear medicine utilises radioactive substances on human tissue and/or fluid samples to diagnose a wide range of pathologies. The most common in vitro test performed in nuclear medicine departments' laboratories is the glomerular filtration rate test (GFR) used to calculate precise renal function. There are several approved techniques to ascertain accurate GFR values in nuclear medicine using either technetium 99m (^{99m}Tc)-labelled DTPA or chromium 51 (^{51}Cr)-labelled EDTA.

Unsealed source therapy is used in the clinical management of both benign and malignant disease. The intention is to deliver an appropriate radiation dose to the pathological tissue in order to cause cell death. Consequently, radioactive substances that emit beta particles are commonly used. Radionuclide therapy for malignant disease is generally performed in oncology units, not least because the radiation protection restrictions are stringent and expensive to implement. A wide range of malignant diseases can be treated in this fashion, for example, thyroid cancer using iodine (^{131}I). In addition to emitting beta particles, ^{131}I decay also produces gamma photons with an energy of 364 keV, which can be imaged using a standard gamma camera to provide information regarding disease progression. Although these high-energy photons are sub-optimal for imaging when compared to using ^{123}I for the same purpose, the choice to image with ^{131}I does not result in an additional radioactive dose to the patient and can present an efficient and cost-effective option for diagnosis. The most common benign disease to be treated using ^{131}I is thyrotoxicosis, but at a much lower dosage. Iodine 131 should be discouraged for standalone scintigraphy, however, due to the large radiation burden to the radiosensitive thyroid gland.

Nuclear medicine is highly reliant on the skills of a multidisciplinary team to match a suspected clinical condition to an appropriate nuclear medicine investigation. The selection process must be considerate of multiple factors including the availability and appropriateness of the pharmaceutical and radioisotope, dosimetry and scanning technique in addition to applying the principles of 'as low as reasonably practicable' (ALARP). Any decision to proceed must be balanced in terms of net benefit resulting from the radiation dose.

Equipment Chronology

1896 Henri Becquerel discovers radioactivity.

1930s Cyclotron invented, providing means to produce usable quantities of radionuclides. Technetium 99m (^{99m}Tc) first produced in the late 1930s.

1940s Radionuclides become available for medical use.

Early 1950 Cassen et al produced a scintillation detector mounted in an automatic scanning gantry, which was probably the first incarnation of the rectilinear scanner.[2]

1953 First study involving the imaging positron emitters published.[3] As cyclotrons became more available, development accelerated due to the availability of positron-emitting radionuclides that could be labelled as clinically useful molecules. Even so, PET remained only a research tool until the late 1970s.

Late 1950s Commercial machines available: these devices allowed the acquisition of an image by tracing a collimated scintillation detector in a rectilinear pattern over the area of interest. Rectilinear scanners, however, were very slow and could not produce images of dynamic processes.

Hal Anger developed a scintillation detector, which has since become known as the gamma camera.[4] This device is kept stationary and collects gamma rays over the field of view, resulting in much more rapid image acquisition than the rectilinear scanner and allowing dynamic imaging.

1960 Developed at the Brookhaven National Laboratory the molybdenum/technetium (^{99}Mo/^{99m}Tc) generator became commercially available. One of the earliest reported uses of ^{99m}Tc was for brain scanning.[5]

1963 First single photon emission tomography study published.[6]

This technique acquired data at a series of angular positions around the patient allowing the production of multiplanar images. By 1964 commercial Anger gamma camera systems available.

1967 Hounsfield develops computer algorithms for image production. These algorithms accounted for attenuation and scatter and converted the emission tomography technique to single photon emission computed tomography (SPECT). At this time reconstruction of data took several hours; however, owing to advances in computing, the same processes today take a few seconds.

1970s Radiopharmaceuticals developed allowing imaging of most organs in the body.

Mid 1970s Rotating gantries developed to allow automatic SPECT acquisitions.

Late 1970s Clinical PET systems started to become commercially available.

1980s Cardiac radiopharmaceuticals became available.

Since the 1980s, systems for planar, dynamic and SPECT acquisition, have been commercially available and have been further developed and refined.

1990s Rectangular camera heads replaced circular ones to allow imaging of greater areas.

Late 1990s PET started to become routinely used as a clinical tool in the United States. A proliferation of literature started to appear to indicate that PET had a value in the diagnosis and management of certain malignant conditions, and it was not long before it was realised that PET imaging was an essential component in the management of certain cancers. The American healthcare economy then drove the PET market, and as a consequence PET scanning systems and cyclotrons became more available and at a lower cost. The increased clinical use of PET encouraged more research to be conducted into its potential applications and presently a large number of dedicated PET centres exist purely for research purposes.

2000 PET-CT named *Time* magazine medical invention of the year.

Early 2000s First clinical PET-CT systems installed in the UK.

Late 2000s Increased proliferation of PET-CT services throughout the UK increasing the availability of clinical PET-CT.

Mid 2010s More than 30 hospitals now offering PET-CT facilities in the UK; an ever-expanding network of centres means PET-CT is now more available than at any other time.

Science and Instrumentation

RADIOACTIVITY

The atoms of some substances are unstable owing to an imbalance in the number of protons and neutrons in the nucleus. Such substances emit radiation spontaneously and are said to be radioactive. Radiation is emitted from a radioactive atom when it undergoes disintegration, i.e. a transformation or decay to another atom. The radioactivity of a substance is defined as the number of disintegrations per second. The unit of radioactivity is the Becquerel (Bq): 1 Bq = 1 disintegration per second.

TABLE 28.1 Ideal Radionuclide Requirements for Use in Nuclear Medicine Imaging

Property	Ideal Requirements
Radiation emitted	Detection relies on radiation being emitted from the body and thus requires a penetrating form of radiation, i.e. gamma rays
Energy	The gamma rays must possess sufficient energy to escape the body but, conversely, their energy must be low enough to allow them to be efficiently stopped within the detector
Half-life	The radioactivity must be sufficient to allow good image quality throughout the duration of the imaging period. The half-life must therefore be long enough to allow this. Conversely, if the half-life is much longer than the period of imaging, this may result in a higher exposure to the patient than is necessary
Cost and availability	The ideal radiopharmaceutical will be cheap and readily available

As atoms decay over time, the amount of radioactivity of a substance reduces. The time taken for the level of radioactivity to reduce to a half of its original value is called the half-life of the radionuclide. The radiation emitted by a radioactive substance can be of several types, e.g. alpha particles, beta particles, positrons or gamma rays. For imaging purposes, only penetrating radiation, such as gamma radiation, is of use.

RADIONUCLIDES

Table 28.1 gives the ideal radionuclide requirements for use in nuclear medicine imaging.

Technetium 99m (^{99m}Tc) is the most common radionuclide used in nuclear medicine and the physical characteristics of ^{99m}Tc (half-life and gamma-ray emission) are ideal for gamma camera imaging, not only because the gamma-ray energy is well suited to gamma camera detection, but also there is no particulate emission (reducing potential patient dose and harm). Although its short half-life (approximately 6 hours) could be considered self-limiting in terms of geographical availability, the invention of the molybdenum (^{99}Mo) generator allowed for a ready supply of ^{99m}Tc in most hospital locations. To handle this, on-site 'radiopharmacies' have developed which conform to pharmacy grade standards set out by the Medicines and Healthcare products Regulation Agency (MHRA) in the UK and are optimised for the handling of radioactive products to produce radiopharmaceuticals suitable for patient administration. In the radiopharmacy, the ^{99}Mo generator can be eluted multiple times a day to allow for a ready supply of ^{99m}Tc (elution is a method of washing ^{99m}Tc from ^{99}Mo into a sterile saline solution).

^{99m}Tc can be chemically bound to an extensive range of non-radioactive chemical compounds, which can remain chemically stable for substantial periods of time after introduction into the patient, allowing imaging to take place. Examples of uses of ^{99m}Tc include phosphate labelled to ^{99m}Tc, which permits bone imaging, and ^{99m}Tc labelled to a chelate (e.g. diethylenediaminetetra-acetic acid) for renal imaging. Other commonly used

TABLE 28.2 Other Commonly Used Radionuclides

Radionuclide	Production Method	Principal Photon Energy (keV)	Used to Image
^{99m}Tc	Generator (parent: reactor)	140.5	Skeleton, heart, lung perfusion, kidneys, brain, thyroid
^{201}Tl	Cyclotron	78	Heart, parathyroid
^{123}I	Cyclotron	160	Phaeochromocytoma, thyroid, brain
^{67}Ga	Cyclotron	93{185}300	Inflammation and infection
^{131}I	Reactor	364	Thyroid
^{81m}Kr	Generator (parent: cyclotron)	191	Lung ventilation

radionuclides, and their uses in nuclear medicine imaging, are given in Table 28.2.

All radiopharmaceuticals for PET imaging are positron emitters. Positrons annihilate with atomic electrons within a short distance to produce two 511 keV gamma-ray photons (travelling 180° apart). Only coincidence events are registered and contribute to image formation with single events being disregarded. PET radionuclides or their parent isotopes are cyclotron produced. If the cyclotron is offsite, the half-life of the radionuclide must be sufficiently long to allow it to be transported to the imaging centre while enough activity remains. The most common PET radionuclides currently in clinical use are the cyclotron-produced fluorine 18 (^{18}F) ($T1/2 = 110$ minutes) and generator-produced gallium 68 (^{68}Ga) ($T1/2 = 68$ minutes),[7] although additional tracers including carbon 11 (^{11}C), ammonia 13 (13N) and rubidium 82 (^{82}Rb) are also available.[8]

CHEMICAL COMPONENT

The chemical component attached to the radionuclide determines where the radiopharmaceutical travels in the body. There are several ways in which a desirable distribution can be achieved, including:

- Using a chemical found physiologically in the organ of interest, e.g. iodine for imaging the thyroid.
- Using an analogue. This is a chemical that simulates one found physiologically, for instance thallium is a potassium analogue and thus can be used to image muscle. Similarly, fluorodeoxyglucose (FDG) is a glucose analogue and can be labelled with ^{18}F for PET imaging to illustrate areas of high glucose metabolism, which has several clinical uses.
- Labelling cells that fight disease, thereby targeting the areas of disease, e.g. white blood cells or antibodies.

Radiopharmaceuticals are normally administered intravenously but are occasionally given subcutaneously, orally or via inhalation. Once incorporated, the radiopharmaceutical remains in the body for a period determined by the chemical form, the half-life of the radionuclide and the physiology of the patient. The patient will receive a radiation dose that will depend on the radioactivity administered and the residence time (i.e. the time during which the radionuclide is present in the body). The effective dose, which allows comparison with other imaging modalities using ionising radiation, is determined from the weighted sum of the absorbed doses to each organ. The weighting factors are organ-dependent owing to their different radiosensitivities.

THE GAMMA CAMERA

Until the introduction of the gamma camera, imaging was performed on rectilinear scanners using a limited range of radiopharmaceuticals. These scanners tended to produce poor-quality low-resolution images. The gamma camera changed this, resulting in massively improved image quality, thereby increasing the diagnostic value of this modality. The basic principles of operation of the gamma camera have remained largely unchanged from its inception until today, although more recent developments, including the advent of hybrid imaging have greatly increased the clinical usefulness of the gamma camera and, as a result, it continues to be used extensively.

The critical component of the gamma camera is the detector itself. A gamma camera detector consists of several components which work in tandem to create an image from the gamma rays emitted by the patient, primarily a scintillation crystal and an array of photo-multiplier tubes (Fig. 28.1).

There are a number of scintillation materials available although the most commonly used material in a gamma camera is sodium iodide, which contains a small amount of thallium impurity [NaI(Tl)]. The thallium impurity significantly increases the amount of light produced. Solid-state cadmium zinc telluride (CZT) crystals are also used clinically although largely in the form of dedicated cardiac scanners for myocardial perfusion imaging. CZT-based detectors have been shown to be superior to NaI(Tl) detectors in terms of sensitivity and spatial resolution and therefore offer the potential benefit of being able to reduce either patient doses or acquisition times, or potentially both, when compared to NaI(Tl) detectors. CZT require fixed collimators making them unsuitable for the imaging of high-energy isotopes such as ^{131}I and indium 111 (^{111}In) and the comparatively high cost of CZT detectors is likely to be a restrictive factor in financially constrained hospitals for at least the short term.

The properties of the detector affect many aspects of the image, as detailed below:

- *Light output*: This can be split into two distinct areas:
  - scintillate in response to a high proportion of the gamma rays that are incident upon it (this is dependent upon the density and the effective atomic number of the material which should be relatively high in both cases).

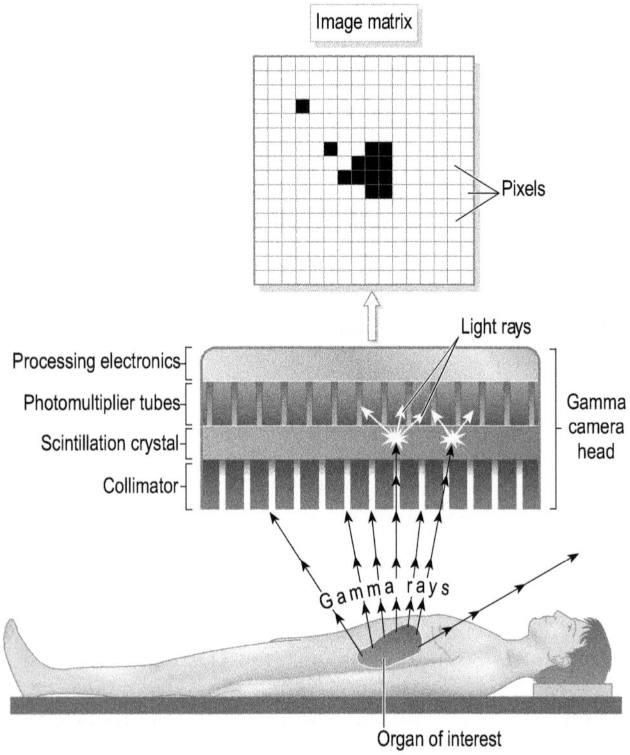

Fig. 28.1 Schematic diagram of a gamma camera showing the gamma rays emitted by the patient, the collimator allowing only those aligned with the collimator holes to pass through to the scintillation crystal. Light rays produced by the crystal are detected and quantified to obtain energy and positional information used to assign a count to the correct pixel location in the image matrix.

- produce short duration scintillations, the intensity of which should be proportional to the energy of the radiation absorbed but equally of high enough energy to be detected. This proportionality relationship allows for energy discrimination, enabling gamma rays outside a certain energy range to be disregarded, a feature which reduces the impact of scattered photons on the resultant image. The time duration of the scintillation is important because a long-lasting scintillation will adversely impact the detection of the next scintillation, reducing the efficiency of detection by the photomultiplier tube. The time delay between detected scintillations is known as the *dead-time* and ideally should be as low as possible.
- *Transparency*: All scintillations produced will need to travel through the crystal to reach the photomultiplier tube. A lack of crystal transparency is detrimental to the number of scintillations detected.
- *Thickness*: If the crystal is too thin, the gamma rays will pass through undetected. Conversely, increasing the thickness of the crystal will increase the distance between scintillations and the photomultiplier tubes detecting them, the impact of which is increased uncertainty in the point of origin and a resultant poorer-quality image.

Packed into the space behind the scintillator crystal are many PMTs, the role of which is to convert the scintillation detected into an electronic pulse. Those PMTs positioned around the point of a scintillation will detect some amount of light, at a level proportional to their distance from the scintillation. Those closest will detect more light and, in turn, produce a greater electronic pulse, whereas those further away will produce proportionally smaller pulses. The relative magnitude of these pulses can then be used to determine the point of light emission. The pixel count value in a corresponding location in a digital matrix can then be allocated, allowing the accumulation of an image (Fig. 28.2).

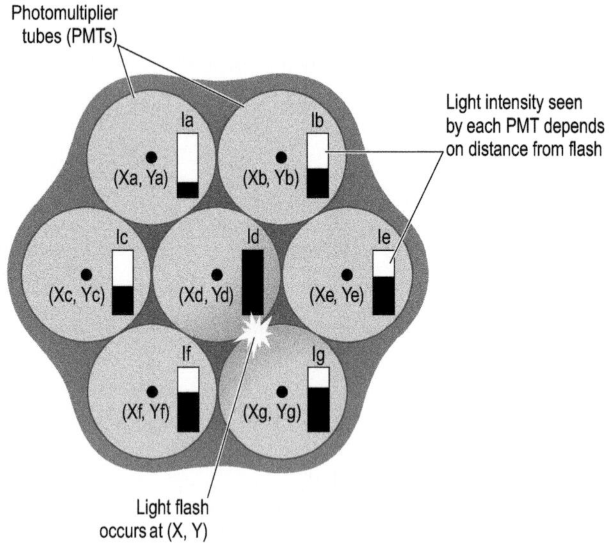

Fig. 28.2 The intensity of light detected depends on the distance of the PMT from the position within the crystal where the gamma ray was absorbed and the light flash occurred. These relative intensities are used to reduce a weighted average of the PMT positions (Xa, Ya), (Xb, Yb) etc. to determine the origin of the light flash.

However, the system so far described does not provide a method of tracing the point of light emission in the detector back to the point of origin of the gamma ray within the patient, which is critical to producing a meaningful image. This is the function of the collimator.

A collimator is essentially a block of attenuating material with a network of holes and is attached to the gamma camera between the detector crystal and the patient. Collimators vary with regard to their thickness and the number, direction and diameter of the holes but in the case of the most common type of collimator, the parallel-hole collimator, the holes act as a filter to allow only gamma rays travelling perpendicular to the face of the collimator to pass through to the crystal and be detected with non-perpendicular gamma rays being attenuated. In this way there is a direct one-to-one mapping between the origin of the gamma ray and the position of the pixel within the image matrix. A flow diagram illustrating the process of nuclear medicine image formation is shown in Fig. 28.3.

A trade-off exists between resolution and sensitivity within collimators such that a collimator used to produce a high-resolution image will have lower sensitivity and therefore take longer to obtain the same number of counts than a high-sensitivity collimator, and vice versa. Parallel-hole collimators can be sub-categorised based on their physical properties:

- *Low Energy High Resolution (LEHR)* – a relatively thin collimator designed for low-energy isotopes including

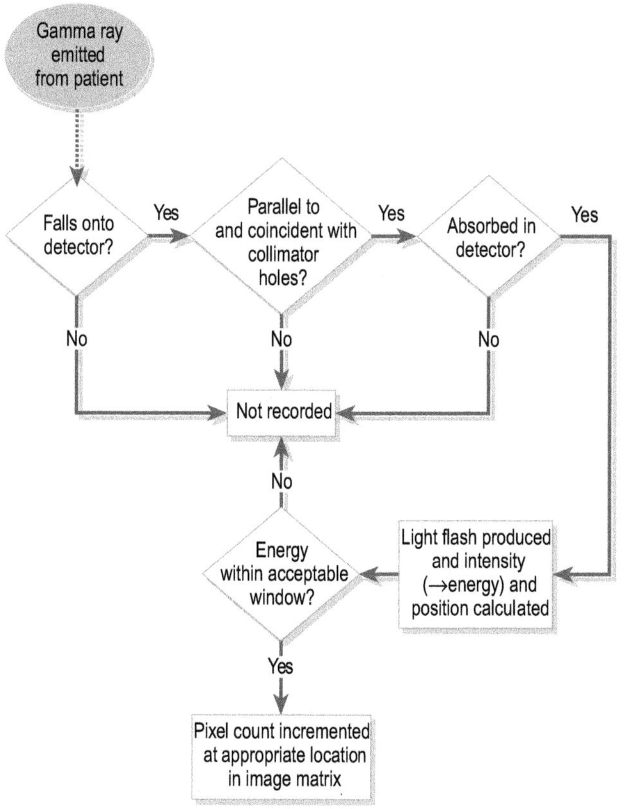

Fig. 28.3 The imaging process.

technetium. LEHR collimators have proportionally smaller diameter holes allowing for a better ability to distinguish between two points close together resulting in a higher-resolution image and might be used in, for example, delayed phase bone scans. The adverse effect of this higher resolution is poorer sensitivity.

- *Low Energy All Purpose (LEAP)/Low Energy High Sensitivity* – similar to LEHR, these are thin, low-energy optimised collimators. The holes are of larger diameter allowing more gamma photons through with a compromise on the resolution of the image produced. The benefit of these collimators is in the higher sensitivity resulting from a greater proportion of gamma photons passing through. These collimators are ideal for imaging techniques where a high count rate is desired, such as dynamic renal imaging, for example.
- *Medium Energy* – these collimators are generally thicker than the low-energy group of collimators and have thicker septa (the thickness of the attenuating material between holes) to reduce septal penetration, a situation where a high-energy photon is energetic enough to pass through the attenuating material between holes on route to the crystal. Septal penetration degrades the quality of image produced as photons travelling in a direction non-perpendicular to the collimator face may pass through and be detected, blurring the resultant image. Medium Energy collimators are commonly used to image isotopes such as ^{111}In and ^{67}Ga, both of which emit photons with energies in excess of 200 keV.
- *High Energy* – the thickest collimators of all. These are most commonly used to image ^{131}I which emits photons of 364 keV. The high levels of attenuating material significantly impact on the number of photons that pass through the collimator resulting in a relatively poor quality image when compared to the low energy range of collimators but this is offset by the fact that a patient can be imaged following a single administration of a therapeutic dose of ^{131}I negating the need for additional radiation exposures to the patient.

Other geometric arrangements of holes are also available. The holes of a diverging-hole collimator fan outwards and allow demagnification of the object, which is useful for large objects. Converging-hole or fan beam collimators fan inwards, providing magnification of the object, and are commonly used in brain imaging. Pinhole collimators have a single aperture at the end of a conical-shaped lead shield that allows magnification of objects near to the aperture and demagnification further away. The magnitude of the collimating effect of all these collimators depends on the distance from the collimator, and distortions in the image will occur with increased distance. This is particularly the case with the pinhole collimator, which can only be used effectively with thin objects. Despite this, the pinhole collimator is a very useful way of providing magnified images of, for example, the thyroid gland or small bone joints in children.

MULTIHEADED GAMMA CAMERAS

Gamma cameras can be purchased with one, two or three detector heads, each consisting of scintillation crystal, collimator and associated electronics. In most common use are the dual-headed systems, and many of the available systems can offer flexibility in the position and orientation of the heads. The advantage of multihead gamma cameras is basically that of speed. Dual-headed cameras can be used for whole-body scanning systems: one head can acquire data anteriorly and the other posteriorly simultaneously. For SPECT imaging, multiheaded cameras allow each head to acquire data from part of the complete revolution, thereby speeding up acquisition by a factor equal to the number of detector heads. Three-headed systems are most commonly used for dedicated brain SPECT imaging.

SINGLE PHOTON EMISSION COMPUTED TOMOGRAPHY (SPECT)

Static or dynamic planar nuclear medicine images are acquired with the gamma camera in a fixed position relative to the patient for the duration of imaging. SPECT imaging, on the other hand, acquires a series of images as the gamma camera rotates around the patient. These images, or *projections*, can then be mathematically reconstructed to form a 3D dataset from which slices through the body or 3D visualisations can be formed, in a similar way to X-ray CT.

This imaging technique allows much greater contrast owing to the effective removal of overlying structures present in planar imaging. Some common applications are in assessing myocardial perfusion, brain functionality and bone lesions.

SPECT-CT SYSTEMS

It is becoming increasingly common for gamma cameras and CT scanners to be housed on the same system to give what are termed SPECT-CT or hybrid systems. The CT scanners for this purpose range from low-dose non-diagnostic CT to fully fledged multislice diagnostic CT systems, depending on their intended use.

The CT component provides two advantages:

- *Attenuation correction*: Gamma rays emitted from within the patient are attenuated by various anatomical structures before they leave the patient and are detected by the gamma camera. The amount of attenuation varies depending on the path the gamma ray travels along from its point of origin, i.e. which anatomical structures the rays have to pass through, and this will vary with the orientation of the camera during a SPECT acquisition.

  The number of gamma rays detected may not actually represent the distribution of the radiopharmaceutical in the body: for example, during myocardial perfusion imaging on large-breasted female patients there may be more attenuation from the front than from the side, giving rise to artificially low counts in the anterior wall of the heart when the data are reconstructed.

  To obtain an accurate image of the actual distribution, it is necessary to know the attenuation of the various anatomical structures so that the attenuation differences at different angles can be corrected for. This is achieved by acquiring a transmission image via CT. If X-rays of similar energy as the gamma rays are used, the resulting CT image will effectively be an attenuation map and can be used as a correction in the reconstruction process. The resolution of the CT images for this purpose need not be particularly high, and it is therefore possible to use a low-dose CT protocol. Some systems acquire the CT over a relatively long time period compared to conventional CT examinations, which are normally performed during a breath-hold. This has the advantage that the CT images are more consistent with the relatively long SPECT acquisition, making the attenuation map a better match than one obtained from a breath-hold.
- *Image fusion*: The limited spatial resolution of nuclear medicine imaging, together with the efficient targeting of some radiopharmaceuticals, can result in specific uptake which is difficult to localise. On the other hand, a CT image provides good anatomical detail without the functional information. By overlaying the nuclear medicine SPECT images onto the corresponding CT image, the best of both modalities can be obtained. It is possible, for example, to see exactly which bone is affected by infection or trauma of complex areas such as the hand or foot or to pinpoint the precise location of a tumour. Hybrid systems are calibrated such that the CT and SPECT images can be accurately and consistently co-registered, and this must be checked as part of routine quality control.

POSITRON EMISSION TOMOGRAPHY (PET)

PET scanning is rapidly gaining popularity in the UK and is fast becoming part of a routine nuclear medicine service. The numbers of PET-CT scans increased both in terms of the total number of scans performed and the diversity of scans performed. Approximately 71 000 in 2012/13 to approximately 98 000 in 2015/16.[9] These included:

- ^{18}F-fluorodeoxyglucose (FDG) used for a range of investigations, including oncological, neurological and in the diagnosis of infection.[8]
- Gallium 68 (^{68}Ga)-labelled prostate-specific membrane antigen (PSMA) in the detection of recurrent or metastatic prostate cancer[10]
- Carbon 11 (^{11}C) choline used in the diagnosis of prostate cancer[11]
- Rubidium 82 (^{82}Rb) chloride utilised in the assessment of myocardial perfusion as an alternative to the traditional nuclear medicine myocardial perfusion study[12,13]

PET imaging is desirable because positron emitting radionuclides are relatively simple to label to biologically active organic molecules, although the comparative poor quality of images produced by a standalone PET scanner limited its clinical effectiveness. The widespread addition of a CT scanner to the system resulting in the creation of the hybrid PET-CT (positron emission tomography-computed tomography) system has greatly improved the quality of images and as a result the diagnostic usefulness of the modality has increased. By far the most common PET radiopharmaceutical is ^{18}F-FDG, which provides an image of glucose metabolism that is useful in oncology, cardiology and neurology.

The technologies and techniques employed in PET imaging are adaptations from conventional nuclear medicine with a number of differences designed to optimise the coincidence detection of single energy gamma rays following an annihilation event. There are three significant areas of difference between a gamma camera and a PET scanner:

- *Scintillation crystal*: Where gamma cameras are required to detect a range of energies depending on the isotope of choice, all PET tracers result in the production of mono-energetic gamma rays with an energy of 511 keV. For this reason, the properties of the crystal can be selected to maximise the detection of such high-energy photons.
- *Gantry*: The PET scanner gantry is designed differently to a gamma camera. The detector heads configuration of a gamma camera, consisting of multiple PM tubes to a large single crystal, has been revised so that in a PET scanner, a number of much smaller crystals are connected to each PM tube. Several PM tubes are then bound together to form a detector 'block'. The blocks are formed into a circular configuration inside the gantry creating a detector ring. Modern scanners consist of a number of detector rings to aid more rapid scanning and the production of higher-quality images. Furthermore, each detector block within the ring is electronically linked to several blocks on the opposite side of the gantry facilitating the detection of coincidence gamma rays.
- *Collimator*: There is no requirement for a conventional collimator in PET scanning. The physical collimator is replaced by an electronic collimator which selectively disregards any non-coincidence event and any photons that fall outside the 511 keV energy window.

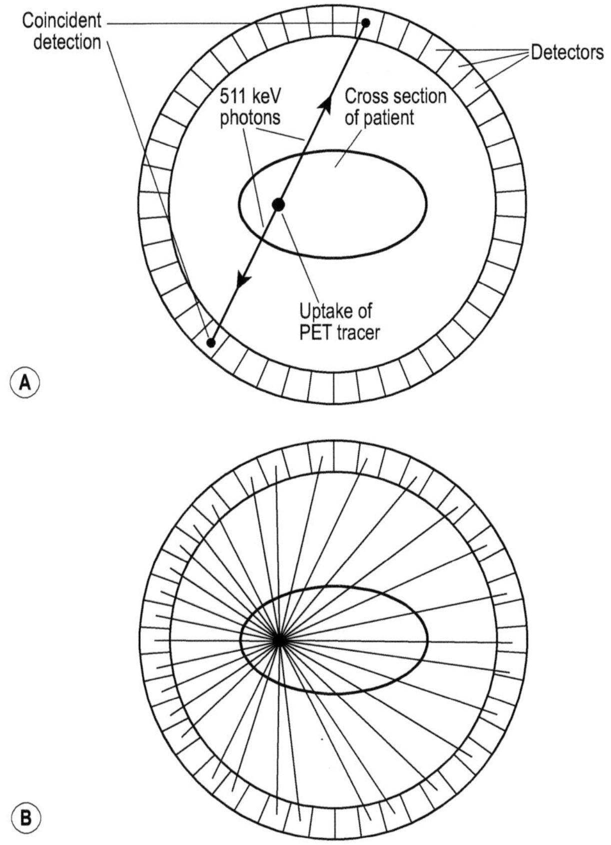

Fig. 28.4 The principle of operation of a PET scanner.

The basic principle of PET imaging is shown in Fig. 28.4A,B. PET tracers emit positrons that annihilate with electrons to form two 511 keV energy photons which are emitted in approximately opposite directions. Where this annihilation event occurs in the centre of the gantry, the two photons will travel and strike detectors at opposite sides of the PET gantry simultaneously and will therefore register as a coincidence event. The point of origin of the photons must then be somewhere along a line between the two detection events called the line of response. When sufficient coincident events have been accumulated, the distribution in the body is indicated by a superimposition of these lines. Reconstruction of the data is similar to that discussed for SPECT and produces a 3D dataset, which can be used to obtain slices through the area of interest.

Attenuation causes a particular problem in PET imaging due to the nature of coincidence detection. In order for a decay event to be recorded, both emitted photons resulting from the annihilation event must detected. Full or partial attenuation of either photon will result in both being discarded. For this reason, the addition of a CT scanner to a PET scanner offers significant benefit. The CT attenuation map allows for a correction map to be created to artificially boost the numbers of counts in areas adversely affected by attenuation. This correction factor has significantly improved the quality of a PET scanner, the result of which is that standalone PET scanners are no longer purchased for diagnostic imaging, instead replaced by the hybrid PET-CT scanners.

Image Acquisition and Quality

The image information leaving the gamma camera head(s) in the form of the X, Y and Z signal is stored in digital form and can be manipulated later to provide image and quantitative data. The final data output is highly dependent on radiographic technique. Once the patient has been correctly prepared and the radiopharmaceutical administered, the appropriate imaging acquisition factors need to be selected and the patient correctly positioned at the predetermined time.

Gamma cameras acquire images using different techniques depending on the nature of the physiological process involved. Some of these operator-dependent parameters are described below.

- *Planar imaging*
  - *Static*: The most basic acquisition is a static planar image. In this mode of operation the gamma camera head is simply positioned over the area of interest and an image acquired for a specified period of time or a number of counts (detected photons). High resolution is generally optimised for this imaging technique with scans taking, in the main, 3–5 minutes per view.
  - *Dynamic*: Dynamic planar imaging allows a succession of images (frames) to be acquired over a specified time-period. The operator will have control over the time duration of each frame, and most systems allow several phases to be acquired either simultaneously or in succession, e.g. a rapid succession of frames initially, followed by a series of longer duration frames. This mode of operation is commonly used to image initial blood flow to an area or the excretion of an organ over time. Subsequent processing of such studies can yield curves showing variations in uptake over time (time–activity curves). For dynamic imaging, short frame times are often required (e.g. 10 seconds per frame) in order to accurately capture what can be relatively rapid functional changes.
- *Whole body scanning*: This allows data to be acquired over an area greater than the field of view of the detector head. This is achieved by patient movement relative to the detector, similar to the motion of the patient couch through a CT scanner. The process is significantly slower than a CT scan due to the need to acquire sufficient count statistics (noise against resolution) and a typical whole body scan can take around 20 minutes. There are two distinct methods of achieving this motion:
  - *'Step and shoot' mode* – several automatically programmed distinct detector positions are used to acquire individual images, which are subsequently 'knitted' together.
  - *Continuous scanning mode* – either the gamma camera gantry or the patient couch is moved slowly during acquisition to build up the whole body image.
- *Dual energy acquisition*: The ability of the gamma camera to discriminate incident energies is exploited to produce two simultaneous frames of separate data representing differing images of the distribution of more than one administered radionuclide. An example would be with 190 keV gamma rays of ^{81m}Kr gas during a lung ventilation scan being stored in one frame and the 140 keV

gamma rays from the ^{99m}Tc lung perfusion image being simultaneously stored in another frame. This capability can also be exploited when imaging isotopes with multiple energy peaks, such as ^{111}In which has energy peaks at approximately 173 keV and 247 keV to improve the quality of images produced.

- *Gated acquisition*: A technique used to subdivide data into individual frames is controlled by a physiological 'switching' process, for example by connecting electrocardiograph (ECG) electrodes to the patient and using 'R' wave pulses to initiate and terminate a sequence of frames: e.g. 'gated' SPECT in myocardial perfusion imaging. In this example, the data can be used for motion studies of the heart and calculating physiological information.
- *Single photon emission computed tomography (SPECT)*: Multiple frames of data are acquired at predefined locations around a central axis within the patient. This can be in a 'step and shoot' mode, where the camera head(s) rotates a fixed number of degrees, stops, acquires a frame of image data for a predefined period, and then moves on to acquire the next frame. A 'continuous' mode allows the head(s) to rotate continually while acquiring data at the required angles. The final data can be reconstructed into three orthogonal planes.
- *Body contouring*: Spatial resolution is related to the distance between the detector and the patient. The closer the detector is to the patient, the sharper the images are. For static imaging, it is fairly straightforward for the operator to position the gamma camera heads as close to the patient as possible. However, for whole-body scanning or SPECT acquisition the detectors are constantly moving relative to the patient, making it difficult for the operator to optimise the position manually during the scan. To overcome this, some systems have methods of achieving this optimisation automatically. There are two basic methods:
  - *'Learn mode'* – the operator programs the position of the camera heads at certain positions of the scan individually to fit the patient; the system will then move the camera heads during the scan to those predefined positions.
  - *Body surface detector* – an infra-red beam, or capacitive sensors, mounted on the surface of the camera head, determines how far to move the camera head towards the patient during the scan.

  The latter method has the advantage that it can adjust in real time, e.g. if the patient has moved during the course of the scan.
- *Image matrix*: The image acquired by a gamma camera is divided into pixels to form an image matrix, examples of which include 64×64, 128×128 and 256×256 matrix sizes. The matrix size affects the spatial resolution of the image; larger pixel sizes acquire a higher number of counts per pixel than smaller pixel sizes, useful in dynamic imaging. Smaller pixel sizes, however, produce higher resolution images but require more counts per pixel to achieve data of sufficient quality due to the effect of statistical noise.

Statistical noise arises from uncertainties in the number of counts in each pixel of the image. As radioactive decay is a random process, acquired counts follow a Poisson distribution. This means that the uncertainty, measured as the standard deviation of the mean, is equal to the square root of the number of counts. For a pixel with 100 counts the standard deviation is 10, which is 10% of the mean. Similarly, a pixel count of 10000 has a standard deviation of 1%, the result of which is a more statistically sound image. The higher the number of counts, the lower the relative uncertainty or noise. Doubling the number of counts improves the noise by a factor of the square root of 2 (1.4). The pixel size has an important impact on this, as larger pixels will collect more counts and thus will inherently have less noise.

SCATTER

Scatter adversely affects the quality of the image. It occurs both within the patient and in the detector. Scatter of gamma rays in the patient causes them to change direction. In some cases a gamma ray may be scattered towards the gamma camera and, if detected, would result in a count being assigned to a wrong pixel within the image matrix, thereby adding to the noise. In many cases the collimator would filter out such scattered gamma rays but, if the new direction of the gamma ray was parallel to the collimator holes, it would reach the crystal and be detected. This is where the energy discrimination is applied. The gamma ray will have lost some energy as a result of the scatter interaction. Because the light intensity produced by the scintillator detector is proportional to the energy absorbed, the system can distinguish such scattered gamma rays and disregard them. Unfortunately, however, the various processes involved in the detection of photons carry their own uncertainties, which means that even unscattered gamma rays may appear to have energies slightly above or below the expected energy (photopeak). This means that there has to be a range (energy window) of acceptable energies applied, which in turn results in some scatter being included. In modern systems, with improved and more stable components, the detection uncertainties have reduced, allowing the window of acceptable energies to be narrowed and hence more noise to be eliminated, with a consequent improvement in image quality. As discussed above, scatter has a significant detrimental impact on PET imaging due to the nature of coincidence detection.

ANNOTATION AND ORIENTATION FOR VIEWING

Nuclear medicine images need to be correctly orientated for viewing and marked with the appropriate anatomical side. It is common practice to use a cobalt (^{57}Co) marker to identify the correct orientation during imaging, and for later viewing. Another point of note is that, contrary to the practice in radiography of denoting a projection by the 'entry' and 'exit' route of the incident radiation (anteroposterior, AP; posteroanterior, PA), it is correct in nuclear medicine practice to denote the body part directly adjacent to the surface of the collimator, e.g. anterior image or posterior image – not AP or PA. Also, images at 90°, e.g. 'lateral knee', would be correctly annotated as being 'lateral aspect' if the lateral aspect of the knee were adjacent to the collimator. Finally, a study should always have the radiopharmaceutical used, delay time to imaging and acquisition time/number of counts acquired marked on the images. Correct annotation is vital for effective image evaluation.

QUALITY CONTROL

As with any other imaging system, regular assessment of equipment performance is essential. Some of the parameters assessed routinely for a gamma camera are given below.

- *Uniformity*: The gamma camera has a large field of view and the count-rate observed over its surface for a uniform source should be constant. This is tested either by placing a large uniform source of radioactivity on the collimated camera or by using a small volume source at a distance from the uncollimated detector. An image is acquired in each case and assessed visually and quantitatively for non-uniformity.
- *Energy resolution*: The range of apparent energies erroneously assigned to unscattered gamma rays due to the uncertainties involved in the detection process has been mentioned previously. Energy resolution is essentially a measure of this. A uniform source of radiation is used and data are acquired in the form of a plot of 'the number of gamma rays being assigned a particular energy' against 'energy'. The result is a gaussian curve centered on the photopeak, and the energy resolution is defined as the full-width half maximum (FWHM) of that curve. The smaller the value the better, as this means that the energy acceptance window can be narrowed, thereby reducing image noise.
- *Spatial resolution*: The test consists of imaging a narrow line source and then producing a curve profile through the resulting image. The profile will be a gaussian curve and the spatial resolution is defined as the FWHM of the curve. The smaller the value the better, as this means that the camera can resolve objects that are closer together.
- *Centre of rotation (COR)*: This involves the acquisition of SPECT data of a single or multiple point source phantom to ensure rotational alignment is within accepted tolerance. The greater the COR offset, the poorer the spatial resolution of the gamma camera. Correction of a COR offset may be either electronic or mechanical and the importance of routinely performing the quality control check cannot be overstated, particularly on systems with a heavy SPECT workload as it can identify potential mechanical safety issues at an early stage.
- *Radiochemical purity*: In addition to the quality control checks required to ensure that all radiation detecting equipment is operating safely and effectively, the utilisation of radiopharmaceuticals in nuclear medicine mandates the implementation and application of a robust quality assurance program as part of the overall quality control regimen. Radiochemical purity can be defined as the proportion of total radioactivity in the sample associated with the desired labelled species and is important for a number of reasons. Unbound radioactivity within a radiopharmaceutical will result both in undesirable uptake and increased radioactive exposure to non-target areas. A common example of this in nuclear medicine is unbound pertechnetate in a technetium-based radiopharmaceutical which results in the visualisation of non-desirous gastric, thyroid and salivary gland uptake on the scan and increased radioactive exposure to those areas. This is of particular significance in relation to the thyroid gland, which has a high level of radiosensitivity. There are several methods of assessing radiochemical purity but all are based on the principle of separating different radioactive complexes from within a sample and comparing their distribution to accepted limits supplied by the manufacturer.[6] The process can be challenging as radiochemical purity relies on a sufficient level of radioactivity in the sample to determine distribution patterns and this can be difficult to achieve, particularly for short-lived isotopes.

Safety

Radiation protection in nuclear medicine has always been complex and highly regulated. The use of unsealed radioactive sources is highly hazardous because they can lead to contamination, from which people may receive internal and external radiation doses. The scenario became more complex when X-ray machines were attached to radionuclide scanners, creating PET-CT and SPECT-CT systems. Such hybrid systems have associated X-ray energies (continuous spectra) together with single photon gamma radionuclides and positron radionuclides.

The use of radioisotopes demands particular working practices which minimise the exposure time to the source and maximise both the distance from the source and the shielding of the source.

- *Time*: Minimising the amount of time spent in close proximity to a radioactive source is vital to reducing exposure levels to staff. There is a linear relationship between exposure time and radioactive dose – halving the time exposed to the source will halve the dose received, although this is no excuse for sloppy practice. It does, however, present a unique challenge in a nuclear medicine environment due to the fact that the source of radioactivity is often the patient.
- *Distance*: Unlike the linear relationship between time and dose, the relationship between distance and dose obeys the inverse square law, i.e. increasing distance by a factor of 2 reduces the dose received by a factor of 4. Whilst patient care should never be compromised, it is of paramount importance that working practices are adopted to reduce the exposure of staff to radioactivity. Simple measures such as taking a step back from the patient when communicating can be a highly effective measure.
- *Shielding*: High activity tasks such as dispensing and injecting patient doses and disposing of clinical waste carry significant associated doses to staff. As a result, nuclear medicine staff utilise a number of pieces of paraphernalia designed to reduce this dose. Tungsten or lead syringe shields, injection boxes and attenuating sharps box containers in addition to lead glass and lead bricks are all commonly found within the department to shield the staff from radioactive sources. The thickness of shielding is dependent on the nature of the workload, e.g. PET departments require thicker shielding due to position decay producing higher energy and more penetrating photons than single photon-emitting isotopes.

There are also a number of specific design characteristics highly evident in laboratory and clinical areas in which radionuclides are prepared and given to patients to enhance protection further. Examples include the need for non-absorbent surfaces and splash guards. Also, because patient urine can be radioactive, designated toilets have to be provided. At regular intervals, and in a systematic fashion, the nuclear imaging department should be monitored for contamination, using a calibrated contamination meter.

In relation to radionuclide and X-ray exposures, the patient should be afforded the least amount of radiation consistent with attaining a diagnosis. This philosophy is articulated in international guidance and national regulations. In many countries specific upper levels are set for particular diagnostic procedures, and these should be adhered to. The radiation exposure of those professionals who work in nuclear medicine imaging departments should be monitored, in accordance with legal requirements.

SUPPLY OF UNSEALED SOURCES FOR IMAGING

It is necessary to have a radiopharmacy facility 'on site' or within a relatively short distance of the gamma camera suite, in order to provide an effective nuclear medicine imaging service. Those without 'on-site' radiopharmacy facilities usually have a radiopharmaceutical dispensary to which daily deliveries can be made.

The radiopharmacy is sited in a 'clean' room where the air is 'ultrafiltered' and has a positive pressure. This, together with protective laminar flow cabinets and clothing, ensures the microbial sterility of the manufactured radiopharmaceuticals. Quality tests are undertaken on the eluate from the ^{99m}Tc generator to check for microbial sterility, and purity (in that it is free of the parent nuclide, ^{99}Mo) and structural alumina from within the generator. Dispensed radiopharmaceuticals are measured according to volume and radioactivity required at a reference time. Calculations are made to account for the physical half-life of the particular radionuclide used and a larger volume is dispensed, to allow for the decay time until administration later in the day at the required activity. Clearly this indicates that the patient's actual attendance time must be in concordance with the allocated appointment and administration time, and this, again, underlines the importance of good advance preparation. In addition to patient explanation, this should include careful explanation to ward personnel if the patient is attending from a ward area rather than from home.

The radioactivity administered to the patient is checked in a calibrator (ionisation chamber) before leaving the radiopharmacy, and it is good practice to double-check the intended activity directly before patient administration. Any patient administration must be within agreed tolerance of the diagnostic reference levels to give results consistent with the minimum amount of radioactivity necessary. It is obligatory to scale down adult activities for administration to children. Schemes for fractional reduction usually try to maintain similar image acquisition times as that of the equivalent adult scan. The converse is also occasionally necessary where increased doses are administered in order to achieve diagnostic quality results in obese patients. Most departments follow their national professional and regulatory bodies' advice in terms of administered activity, but there is usually scope for local variation.

Fundamentals of Nuclear Medicine Technique

The basic principles of nuclear medicine instrumentation necessitate careful radiographic technique to ensure optimal image quality. Conventional radiographic positioning principles lend themselves to being applied in a nuclear medicine setting. Care must be taken to avoid simulating or masking disease by poor positioning of the patient in relation to the gamma camera, misuse of radioactive anatomical markers or incorrect use of imaging equipment and technical parameters.

Optimal patient preparation is paramount for a successful outcome from nuclear medicine investigations. Many procedures can be ruined by incorrect advice or poor patient compliance prior to the investigation. This can partly be remedied by having clear written protocols for each investigation type and by providing the patient with unambiguous written instructions on how to prepare for the investigation. The advice can include the cessation of certain drugs, avoidance of particular foods, or avoiding food intake altogether for certain procedures. This sometimes involves dialogue with the referring clinician regarding interactions, and carefully relaying advice to the patient. An example of a failed procedure would be the patient who has consumed caffeine on the day of a pharmacological myocardial perfusion stress study. Caffeine has a deleterious action on the effectiveness of some pharmacological stressing agents, giving a dubious result when using dipyridamole or adenosine. The examination might need to be repeated in this scenario, clearly with associated additional risks from the repeated test. For this reason, an in-depth patient interview should be carried out prior to performing the procedure to ensure that the patient is caffeine-free.

It is necessary to have a thorough knowledge of human physiology and anatomy to fully understand the complexities of nuclear medicine imaging investigations. An understanding of how various radiopharmaceuticals are 'handled' by the body (pharmacokinetics) is necessary in order to undertake the appropriate investigation for the clinical question being asked, and to interpret the image appearance correctly. Some image appearances can also represent technical defects in terms of radiopharmaceutical quality or equipment failure.

Common Nuclear Medicine Investigations

Nuclear medicine has many techniques for imaging organs and systems of the human body. The focus here is on some common investigations, to illustrate the rationale involved for imaging, and to suggest their usefulness in the clinical setting.

SKELETAL SCINTIGRAPHY

The bone scan still represents a significant part of the workload of most nuclear medicine departments. This examination is highly sensitive: it can image bone pathology and trauma at a cellular level. More recently the increasing

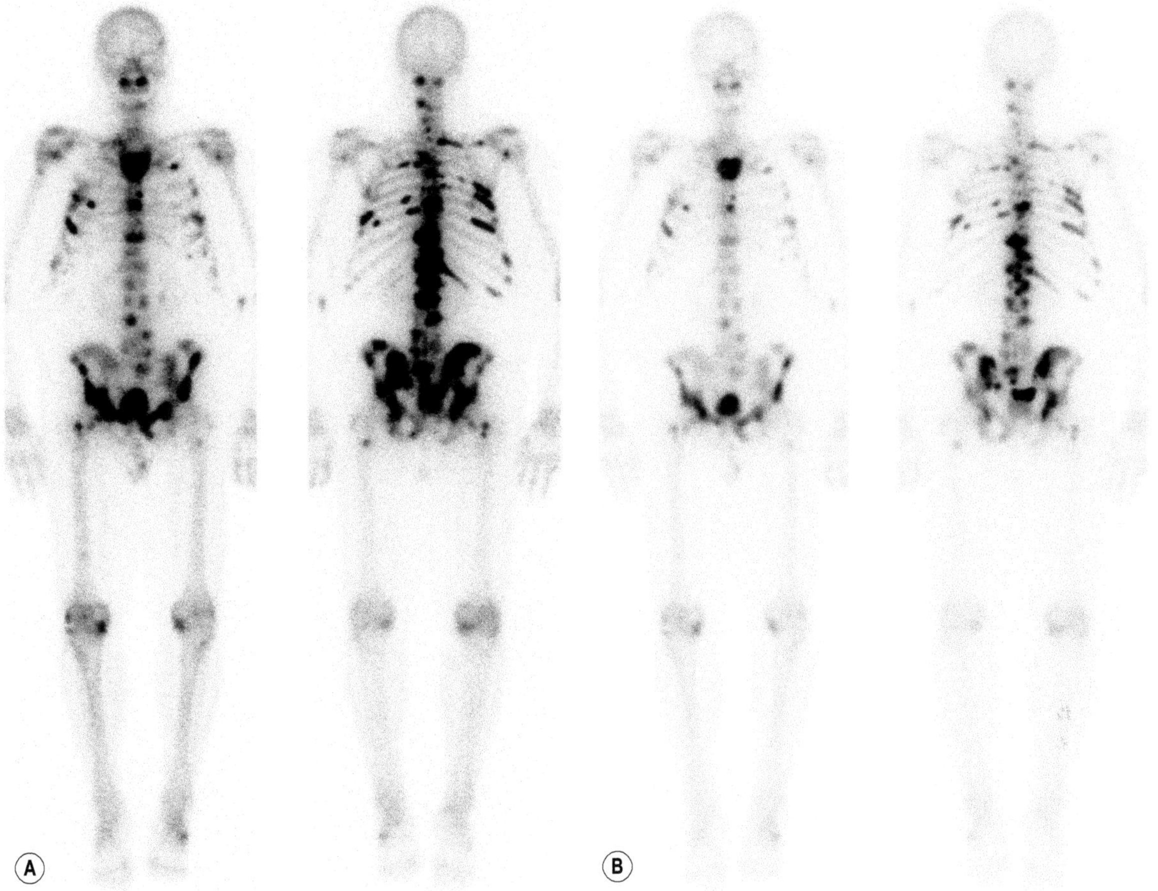

Fig. 28.5 Metastatic deposits. This bone scan shows multiple areas of increased uptake of ^{99m}Tc-HDP at 3 hours, indicating multiple metastatic deposits in the skeleton. The pattern of uptake suggests a definitive diagnosis.

capability of magnetic resonance scanners to image the whole skeleton has shown promising results and, subject to cost and availability, it could become a suitable alternative for some traditional skeletal scintigraphy indications in the future.

Isotope bone scanning has been shown to be a highly sensitive method of imaging bone disease, and it can show abnormal areas with a high level of sensitivity and specificity. Widespread implementation of SPECT-CT imaging in bone scintigraphy has further improved the diagnostic usefulness of the test with sensitivity and specificity quoted at 92% and 82% respectively in the identification of bone lesions.[14] Furthermore, Alazraki et al[15] reported that over 95% of bones scintigraphy investigations were abnormal where a projection radiograph demonstrated an abnormality, again demonstrating a high degree of sensitivity.

Common indications would include screening for metastatic bone disease; isolating primary bone tumours; confirming occult fractures; identifying potential areas of bone infection or osteomyelitis; differentiating infection from loosening orthopaedic hardware; and investigating metabolic bone diseases, e.g. Paget's disease or microfractures in cases of osteoporosis.

Limitations include its lack of specificity in characterising disease of bone. In many instances there is a need for scan results to be interpreted with clinical history and relevant radiographs in order to make a definitive diagnosis. However, the recognition of particular radiopharmaceutical distribution patterns can allow for a more accurate provisional diagnosis, by understanding the characteristic patterns of uptake of ^{99m}Tc-MDP (methylene diphosphonate), for example:[16]

- *Metastases*: often with multiple lesions with random distribution in the skeleton (Fig. 28.5)
- *Superscan*: high skeletal metabolic activity in conjunction with low or absent urinary tract and soft tissue uptake (Fig. 28.6)
- *Osteomyelitis*: with intense increased uptake on a three-phase bone scan

Given that there are some instances where a bone scan can be interpreted fairly safely on its own, Sharp et al confirm the general non-specificity of the technique by quoting some examples of non-specific abnormal uptake, which need further investigation to clarify their aetiology.[17]

Examples of appearances with *non-specific* interpretation:

- *Osteomalacia with associated pseudo fractures*: can be mistaken for multiple metastases in the skeleton or vice versa
- Simple collapsed vertebrae showing linear increase uptake in spine: can be mistaken for discitis or vice versa
- *A solitary spinal lesion can be interpreted as a metastasis*: could alternatively be due to fracture of the pars interarticularis; osteoid osteoma; active arthropathy, or primary tumour such as chondrosarcoma

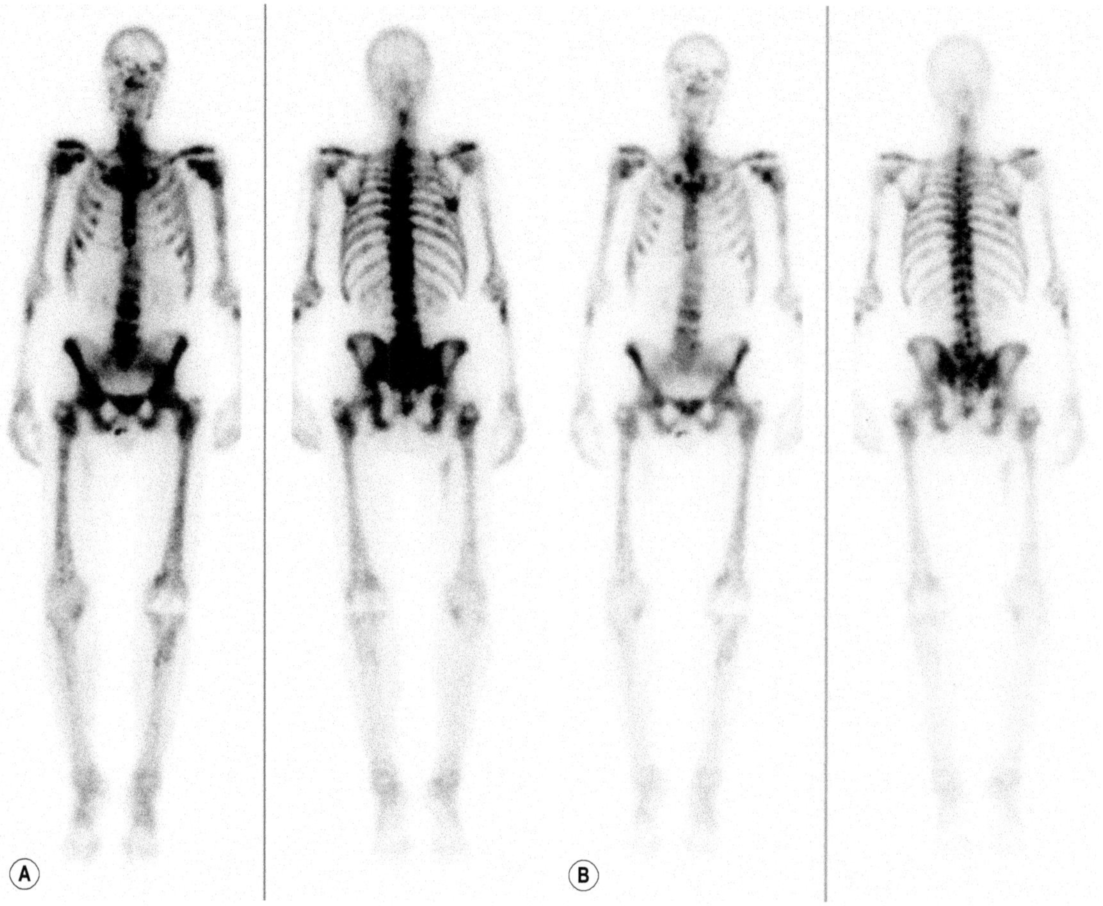

Fig. 28.6 Superscan. This bone scan demonstrates an example of a superscan with high skeletal metabolic activity and resultant uptake and low or absent urinary tract and soft tissue uptake.

Symmetry is of prime importance in the determination of a normal whole-body bone scan, and it is important that the two halves of the skeleton should be mirror images of each other. There should be uniform uptake of the radiotracer in the skeleton, and uptake in organs such as the kidneys and bladder is to be expected. Uptake in the soft tissues of the body can also be an indicator of disease, and should be considered to be a normal area of concern during the interpretation of such an investigation; care needs to be exercised when 'windowing' these areas (Fig. 28.7).[16]

It is important not only to recognise increased uptake of radiopharmaceutical due to abnormal malignant osteoblastic activity, but also to be aware of a false-negative scan, as in the case of multiple myeloma or renal cell carcinoma.[16] Here the characteristic interpretative sign is that of a 'cold' lesion where there is little or no radio-emission from bone. This is of prime importance when justifying the examination, and, once undertaken, must be considered in relation to the clinical history provided.

In cases where systemic disease is concerned the whole skeleton should be imaged. Localised disease present on planar images can sometimes be related to a systemic problem, and so a whole-body bone scan can help to characterise the disease. An example of this would be the multifocal appearance seen with many arthropathies.[17] Given that the nature of this examination only requires one radiopharmaceutical injection, then additional imaging carries no increased radiation burden.

Practical Considerations

^{99m}Tc-MDP and ^{99m}Tc-HDP (hydroxymethylene diphosphonate) are both commonly used. They are adsorbed onto the surface of bone by incorporation into the hydroxyapatite crystal formed by osteoblastic activity. Radiopharmaceutical uptake in bone is related to blood flow and osteoblastic activity. There is no appreciable difference in image quality between the two radiopharmaceuticals, although it has been suggested that there is higher skeletal uptake with HDP.[18] Peak uptake in bone is shown to be at approximately 1 hour[19] and the usual delay to imaging of 3 hours is related to soft tissue clearance by the kidneys of background activity resulting from non-adsorbed phosphonate. Less than 10% of administered activity is present in the blood compartment at 1 hour, and this drops to 2% at 4 hours.[20] It is normal to visualise renal drainage of the tracer and bladder filling, which needs to be emptied prior to imaging. Increased hydration has been conventionally used to improve the object-to-background ratio of radiotracer to improve image quality; however, Klemenz et al[21] showed that increased hydration had little effect on image quality, and that quality is more related to time delay to imaging and deteriorates with increasing patient age. Increased hydration is, however, recommended to reduce the radiation burden to the bladder wall.[21]

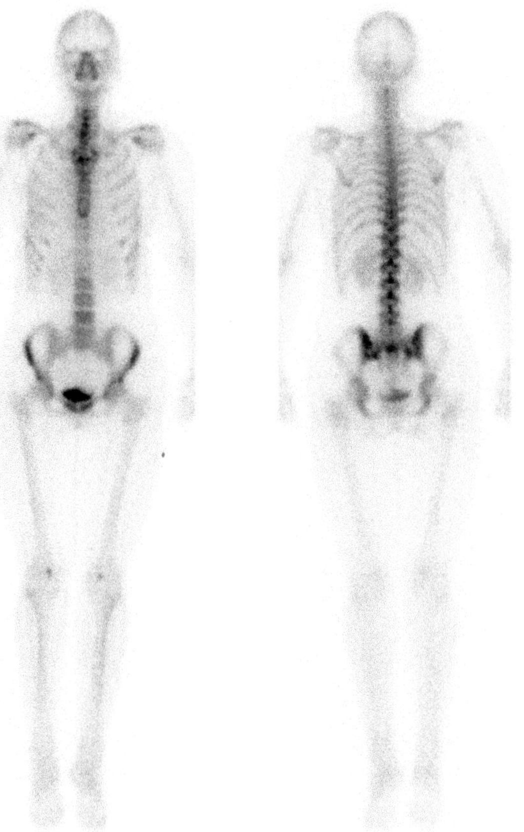

Fig. 28.7 Normal bone scan showing symmetrical uptake throughout the skeleton, with soft tissue visible, and the expected activity in the kidneys, ureters and bladder.

NUCLEAR CARDIOLOGY

Conventional coronary angiography and CT angiography (CTA) are used to image the patency and location of coronary vessels. Nuclear medicine imaging has the ability to demonstrate functioning and non-functioning areas of the myocardium. Radiopharmaceuticals can be used to perfuse the left ventricular wall: under-perfusion of a region of the left ventricle under exercise conditions will be indicative of a narrowing of the related diseased coronary artery or suggest previous damage from ischaemic events. A repeat examination at rest will indicate whether the diseased area has perfused normally when not under stress conditions and is hence more likely to respond to revascularisation surgery; or if it remains unperfused, suggesting irreversible disease best managed medically (Fig. 28.8).

The stress test is now usually done pharmacologically, as it allows for better patient compliance and is more reproducible than dynamic exercise using a treadmill. Adenosine and dipyridamole are potent coronary artery vasodilators that increase coronary blood flow to levels similar to those achieved with maximal physical exercise. The relative ventricular perfusion between 'stress' and 'rest' is useful in differentiating reversible from non-reversible ischaemia in this scenario. Pharmacological stressing techniques allow the cardiac vessels to be imaged at maximum dilatation, highlighting decreased perfusion due to narrowing caused by arteriosclerosis, or indeed lack of myocardial uptake indicative of permanent damage.

Until recently some false-positive results were inevitable owing to the attenuation of gamma rays during SPECT data acquisition. Modern SPECT-CT systems create an attenuation map of the patient which is then used to correct the original gamma ray image, to minimise error and improve diagnostic reliability (Fig. 28.9).

During the imaging procedure it is possible to also use the electrical signal from the beating heart to electronically 'gate' the SPECT acquisition. This allows the myocardium to be viewed as a beating entity to illustrate ventricular motion; left ventricular ejection fraction can also be estimated using this technique.

^{99m}Tc-MIBI (2-methoxyisobutylisonitrile) or ^{99m}Tc-tetrofosmin injected intravenously at peak stress, and at rest (on another occasion), will be trapped in the myocardium and will be representative of myocardial perfusion, with minimal redistribution prior to imaging. SPECT imaging then allows tomographic reconstruction in three planes, delineating areas of decreased perfusion due to ischaemia or infarction.

Ischaemic myocardium is sometimes stunned into inactivity functionally, which can seem to be non-viable on a stress and rest study. Evidence shows that stunned (or 'hibernating') myocardium can be successfully reperfused surgically, with a subsequent improvement in myocardial function in some cases.

In addition to ^{99m}Tc-based agents, thallium 201 (^{201}Tl) may also be used for myocardial perfusion imaging (MPI) studies. Thallium is advantageous in that it redistributes in the myocardium after a short period of time and so can be used to represent stress perfusion immediately following the stress procedure followed by delayed imaging performed to represent resting perfusion. This technique can be useful in identifying hibernating myocardium, although the poorer imaging properties of thallium photons (80 keV) restrict the clinical effectiveness compared to technetium-based agents.

PULMONARY EMBOLI

Ventilation–perfusion (V/Q) lung scanning remains a useful method of diagnosing pulmonary embolism (PE), although CT pulmonary angiography (CTPA) continues to be the imaging method of choice. CTPA elicits controversy when imaging young or pregnant women owing to the relatively high absorbed dose of X-rays in the breast tissue. Fetal dose remains low enough with V/Q scanning to justify the technique in this scenario. Also, as CT scanners are usually in high demand it might be that patients could be stratified according to presentation and risk of PE. The V/Q scan is recommended, and remains sensitive to PE, when the chest X-ray is normal and the patient's symptoms are consistent with PE. V/Q scanning also has value in evaluating lung function prior to surgery, with its ability to quantify uptake and give functional ratios.

An injection of ^{99m}Tc-MAA (macro-aggregated albumin) is trapped in the capillaries of the lungs with homogenous distribution indicating patent perfusion. The presence of a PE in the lungs generally results in a characteristic wedge-shaped defect which may be sub-segmental, segmental or lobular depending on the location and size of the PE.

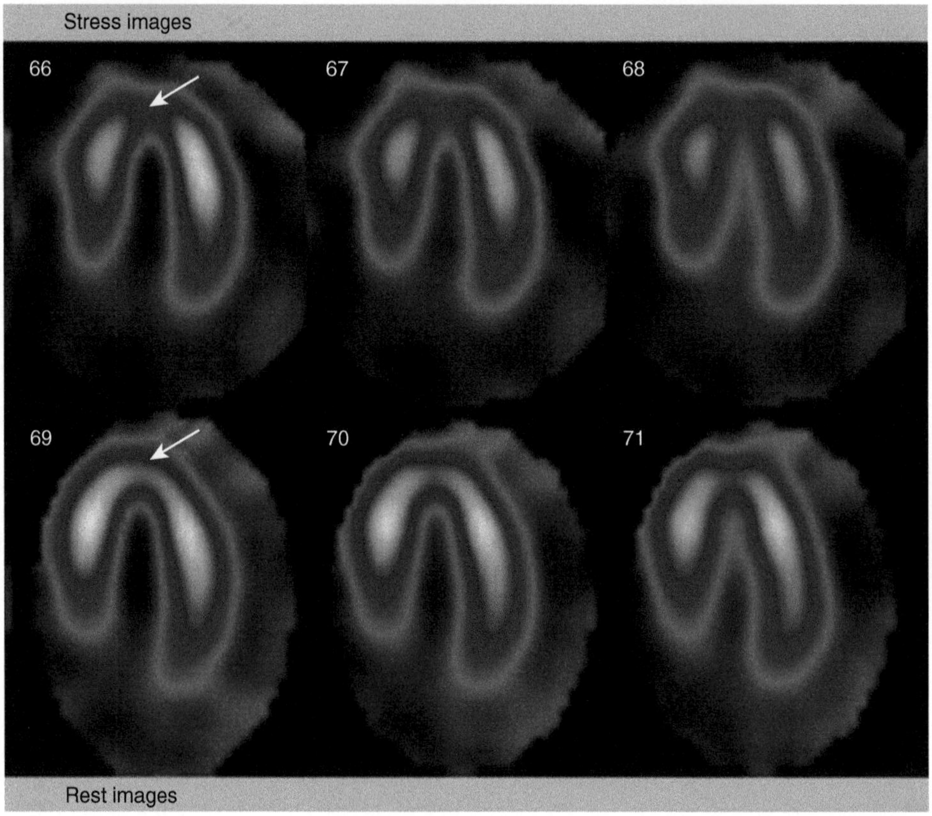

Fig. 28.8 Horizontal long axial (HLA) slice of left ventricle with perfusion defect at 'stress' (top row) which perfuses normally on the 'rest' scan (bottom row), confirming exercise-induced ischaemia.

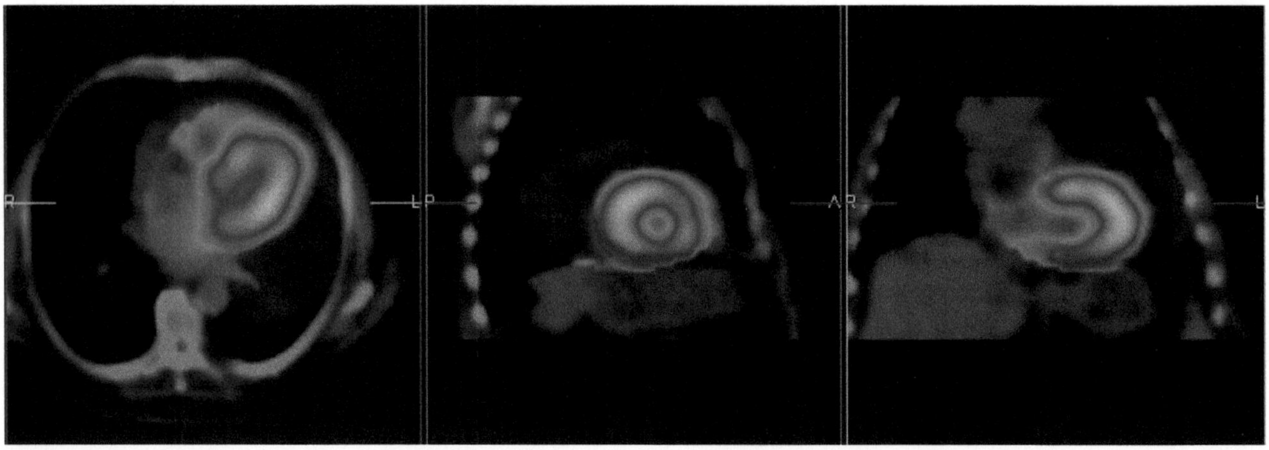

Fig. 28.9 CT attenuation correction map is applied to the acquired data creating an attenuation corrected dataset. This can be compared to the non-corrected data to minimise the impact of attenuating structures in the chest, thus reducing the likelihood of false-positive results.

Increased diagnostic accuracy can be achieved with the addition of a ventilation scan as affected areas of the lung generally demonstrate normal ventilation in the short term and therefore a scan representing abnormal perfusion with normal ventilation (a mismatch) is highly indicative of acute PE (Fig. 28.10A,B). Several methods of ventilation are available including the inhalation of a radioactive gas (^{81m}Kr) or aerosol (^{99m}Tc-labelled DTPA or Technegas) to visualise the patent airways. Gaseous ventilation can be both methodologically advantageous and superior in terms of image quality as the different energies of ^{81m}Kr and ^{99m}Tc allow for dual-isotope acquisition, where the patient inhales the gas in real time allowing the gamma camera to simultaneously acquire both ^{81m}Kr ventilation and ^{99m}Tc perfusion data.

Ventilation using either ^{99m}Tc-DTPA or Technegas must be performed sequentially with the ventilation phase being acquired before an administration of a saturation dose of ^{99m}Tc-MAA is administered to allow the visualisation of lung perfusion.[22]

ENDOCRINOLOGY

Sodium pertechnetate (^{99m}Tc-NaTcO$_4^-$), the raw eluate of the molybdenum/technetium generator, is readily available and can be used to image the thyroid gland. A delay

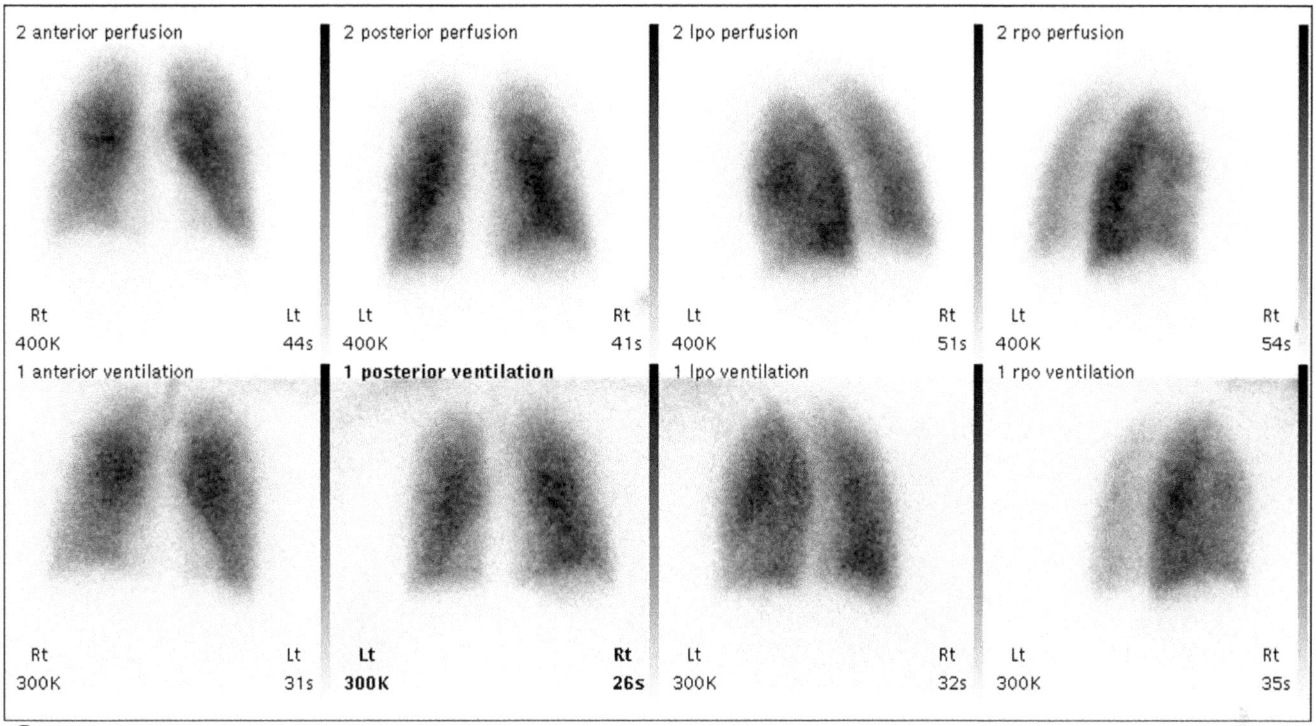

(A)

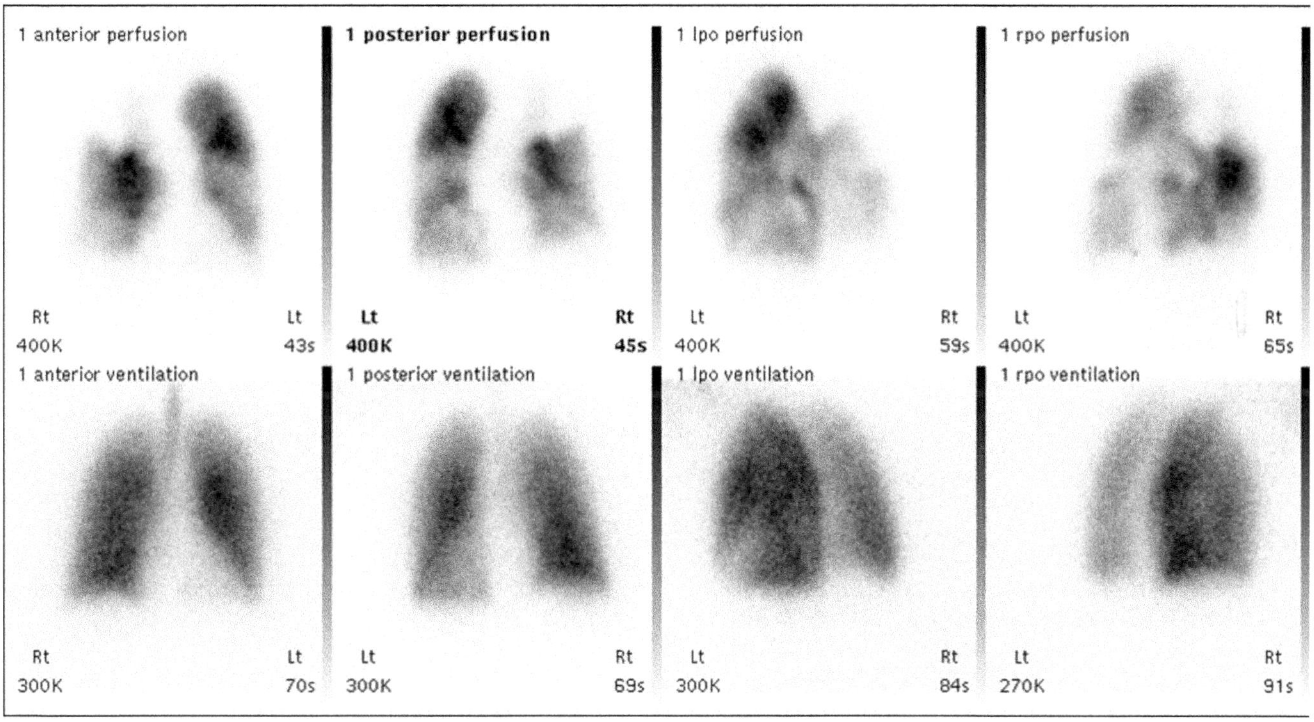

(B)

Fig. 28.10 (A) A normal ventilation and perfusion scan where the radioactive gas and MAA particles are free to flow around the normal lung. (B) Multiple areas of photopenia. The MAA has not been able to circulate freely around the lung when impeded by pulmonary emboli; however, the lung ventilation with radioactive gas is free to fill the lung unimpeded, as emboli affect the blood circulation and not the aeration. This is a classic mismatch, giving a high confidence of pulmonary emboli.

of 20 minutes after intravenous administration shows trapping of the pertechnetate ions in the gland. Abnormal tissue can be highlighted as cold hypofunctioning nodules, or hot hyperfunctioning nodules. Iodine 123 is also used for imaging the thyroid gland but gives a higher radiation burden,[23] as it is trapped and taken up by the gland. Iodine 123 has an advantage in imaging metastatic thyroid deposits in the skeleton, and the theoretical improved detection of retrosternal extension of the thyroid gland, owing to its higher emissive energy and lower background activity.

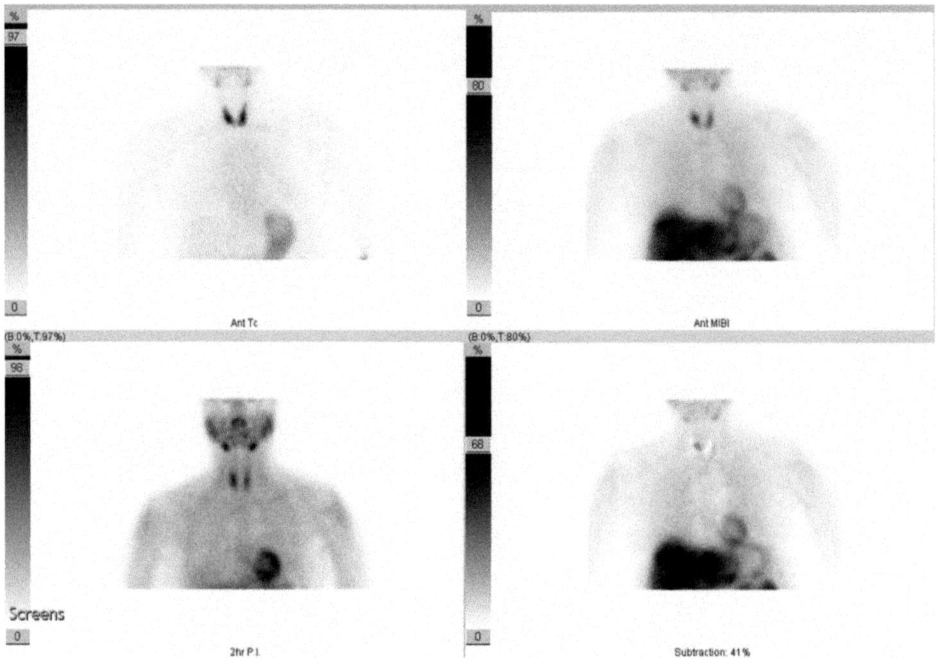

Fig. 28.11 Technetium 99m-sestamibi parathyroid scan. Showing ^{99m}Tc pertechnetate only, early ^{99m}Tc-sestamibi 'wash-in', delayed ^{99m}Tc-sestamibi 'wash-out' and post subtraction images (99mTc-sestamibi image with ^{99m}Tc pertechnetate uptake subtracted to demonstrate abnormal uptake of ^{99m}Tc-sestamibi by the parathyroid adenoma).

MR, CT and ultrasound are all useful in the anatomical evaluation of the thyroid gland, but nuclear medicine imaging provides the necessary functional information together with characteristic uptake in various tumours.[24] Although ultrasound can determine whether a nodule is solid or cystic, the value of nuclear medicine imaging is that of characterisation of the function of the nodule. It has been shown that 99% of 'hot' nodules are benign, whereas 10–20% of palpable cold nodules are malignant.[24]

Thyroid scintigraphy is also useful in the evaluation of thyroiditis in its various forms, and the characteristic uptake of radiopharmaceutical can help evaluate the stages of the disease. Thyroid uptake measurements are possible in nuclear medicine imaging, where a figure can be quoted of the percentage uptake in the gland at a certain time after administration. This is then useful for comparison with the norm, and helps differentiate Graves' disease from other causes of hyperthyroidism, e.g. subacute thyroiditis; and it has a role in the estimation of radioiodine required in thyroid ablation therapy.[24]

Congenital hypothyroidism in neonates can have a devastating effect on mental development if left undiagnosed. Most centres now screen for this condition soon after birth. Should blood tests show an abnormally low level of thyroid hormones then a technetium thyroid scan is urgently indicated to show the location and function of any thyroid tissue.

In the case of hyperparathyroidism, conventional practice was to image abnormal parathyroid glands with $^{99m}Tc/^{201}Tl$ subtraction techniques. Normal thyroid tissue would be highlighted by technetium and thallium is used to label both the thyroid and parathyroid glands. Digital subtraction of the normal ^{99m}Tc uptake from the ^{201}Tl would leave abnormal thallium activity in the parathyroid gland displayed on the resultant image. This is a useful technique but difficult to perform, requiring the use of expensive and poorly available thallium, not to mention absolute patient compliance, and results in a high radiation dose (>18 mSv).[23]

Technetium-sestamibi has more recently been successfully used in highlighting abnormal parathyroid tissue in place of thallium. Sestamibi is localised in parathyroid adenomas by concentration in the mitochondria-rich tumour, which is related to blood flow.[24] Images are acquired at 15 minutes and 2 hours following administration, as it has been shown that some tumours are more apparent at an early stage (Fig. 28.11). Theory dictates that sestamibi concentrates in the adenoma within 2 hours by which time any normal uptake will have 'washed out'.[24]

Parathyroid glands can be ectopic in the neck or mediastinum and are difficult to localise surgically.[25] The radionuclide technique has advantages over other imaging modalities with respect to imaging ectopic tissue, as it can image the whole area concerned, giving high sensitivity in the detection of adenomas. Sensitivity has been quoted from as high as 86% for planar studies to 90.5% with SPECT.[26] By performing SPECT/CT fusion, anatomical information is readily available for the surgeon to limit the incision size necessary and minimise the operating time (Fig. 28.12).

RENAL TRACT

There are many radiopharmaceuticals available for imaging the renal parenchyma and drainage system; the two most commonly used are discussed here.

Technetium 99m-MAG3 (mercaptoacetyl triglycine) is routinely used to image the kidneys, collecting system and bladder. Following intravenous administration it is rapidly removed from the blood circulation, primarily by tubular secretion. Renal function can thus be imaged with rapid dynamic frames over 30 minutes' duration, and a diuretic can be used to differentiate between true obstructive uropathy or non-obstructed dilatation of the

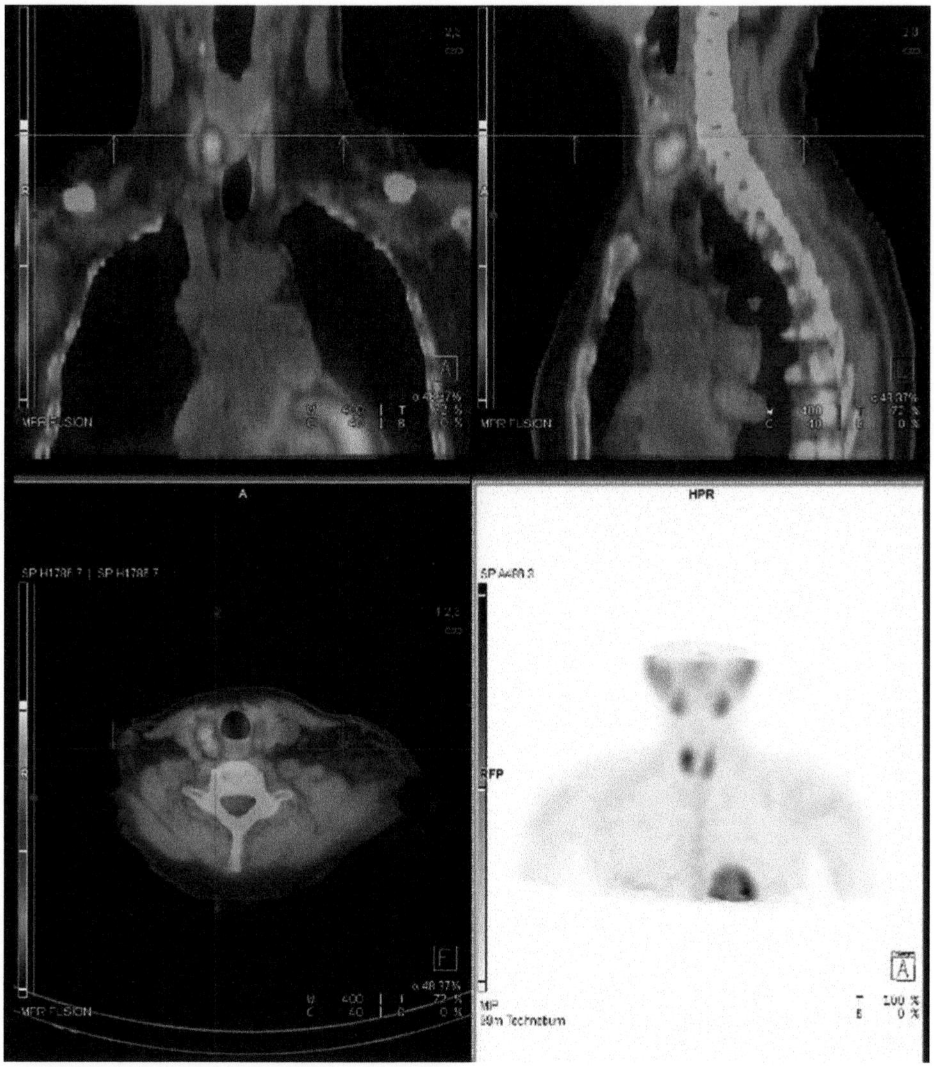

Fig. 28.12 The adenoma is accurately localised using SPECT-CT.

renal pelvis.[27] Data analysis can produce time–activity curves, which have diagnostic value in themselves, and a figure is usually quoted for relative renal uptake (Fig. 28.13). Patients with suspected vesicoureteric reflux can have further imaging while voiding, which will show as an activity peak in the ureter. This technique is less traumatic for paediatric patients as direct catheterisation is not necessary as in the conventional radiological method.

In contrast, ^{99m}Tc-DMSA (dimercaptosuccinic acid) is used to image the renal parenchyma, where the radiopharmaceutical is absorbed in the proximal convoluted tubules, thus being highly representative of functioning tissue. Its value is in being able to delineate areas of scarring (non-function) caused by infection, and localising ectopic kidneys which may have been absent on an ultrasound scan. Owing to its complete binding to the tubules there is no pelvirenal activity to denigrate the images, and it is especially useful in providing quantisation of relative renal function (Fig. 28.14).[27]

GASTROINTESTINAL (GI) IMAGING

There are a number of clinically effective nuclear medicine investigations in relation to the GI system. For a gastric emptying study radiolabelled food is used to image gastric motility. Technetium is used as a recipe ingredient for scrambled eggs or porridge, enabling the gamma camera to visualise stomach and intestinal food transit. This procedure can be used to assess excessively fast or slow transit times by exploiting the quantitative abilities of nuclear medicine, with a 'half-time' quoted for emptying gastric contents. The approximate normal half-time is quoted at 40 minutes for a solid meal[28] (Fig. 28.15).

A GI bleed study is useful in the identification and diagnosis of gastrointestinal bleeding utilising labelled red cells which will pool in the abdomen as a result of a bleed. This study requires early phase dynamic imaging but may require several hours of sequential imaging in order to detect slow bleeds. Needless to say, the patient must be actively bleeding at the point of commencing the study for the procedure to be successful.

Another useful imaging technique is a Meckel's diverticulum study. Damage to the bowel wall from acid secreting gastric mucosa, known as a Meckel's diverticulum, can result in peri-rectal (PR) bleeding. Sodium pertechnetate is naturally taken up by gastric mucosa, and this phenomenon can be used to advantage by highlighting suspect areas of ectopic gastric tissue within the whole abdomen. The patient is imaged dynamically immediately post injection and a positive

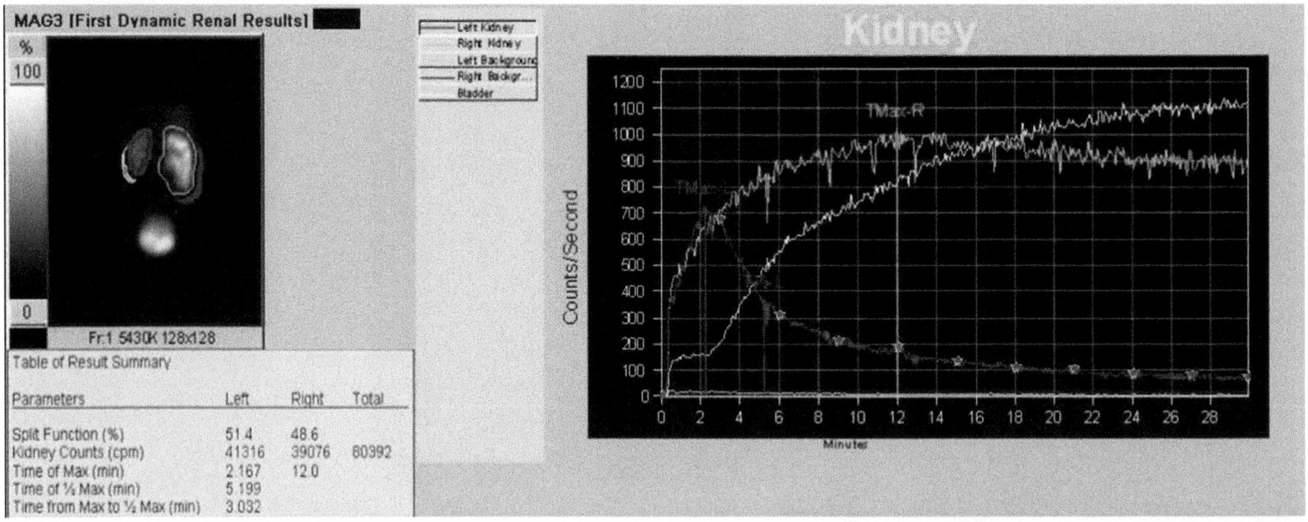

Fig. 28.13 Technetium 99m-MAG3 dynamic renogram showing the processed data from the dynamic frames of a 30-minute scan. Normal uptake and excretion can be seen on the curve for the left kidney, compared to the poor uptake and drainage of the right kidney. Furosemide was administered at T = −15.

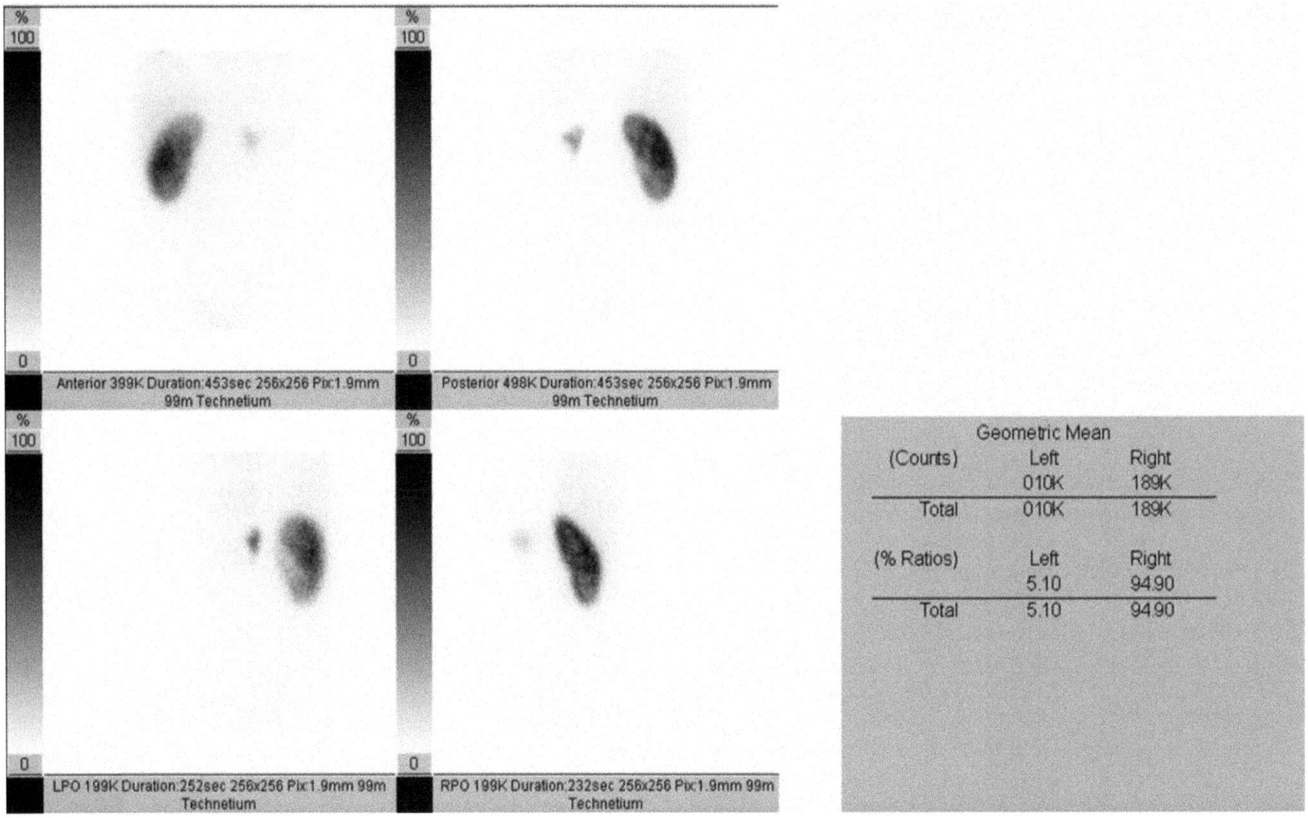

Fig. 28.14 Technetium 99m-DMSA static renal scan. These images represent a poorly functioning left kidney with a split renal function of 95% right kidney and only 5% left kidney.

scan is indicated by a characteristic blushing in the abdomen on the scan. This study is an ideal candidate for SPECT-CT imaging as any areas of suspicious uptake can be accurately localised to aid subsequent surgical intervention.[29]

INFECTION IMAGING

Radiolabelled white cells, mouse antibodies, ^{99m}Tc-HIG (human immunoglobulin) and ^{67}Ga can be used for imaging infection. The choice of radiopharmaceutical is usually made in the light of the medical history, and each has its own merit. The basic principle, however, is that the injected radiopharmaceutical will pool in an area of infection, and is especially useful in imaging infected orthopaedic hardware and pyrexia of unknown origin, where the whole body may be imaged.

It should be noted here that a radiolabelled white cell study cannot be performed in the absence of an on-site radiopharmacy as the labelling process involves the manipulation of

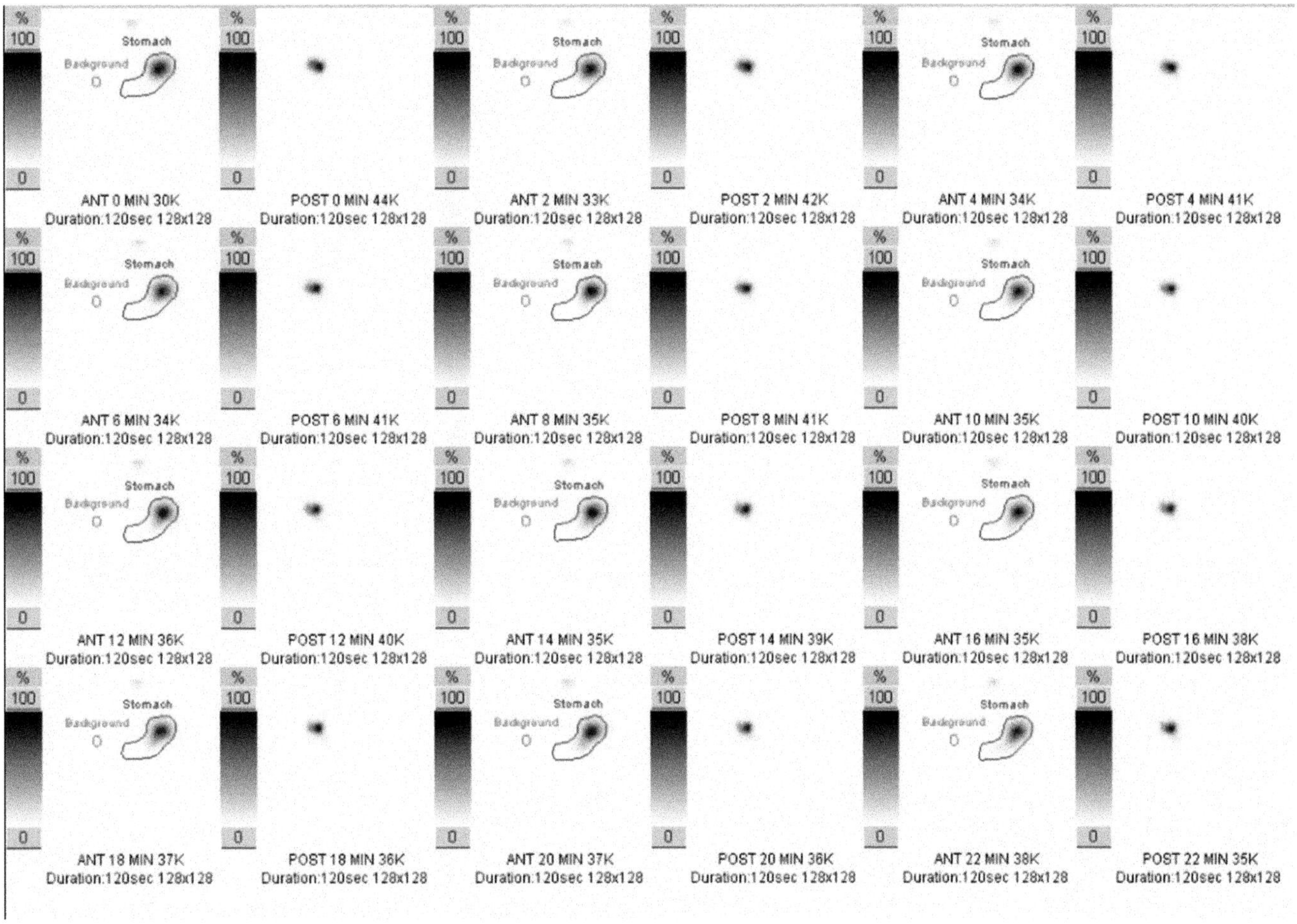

(A)

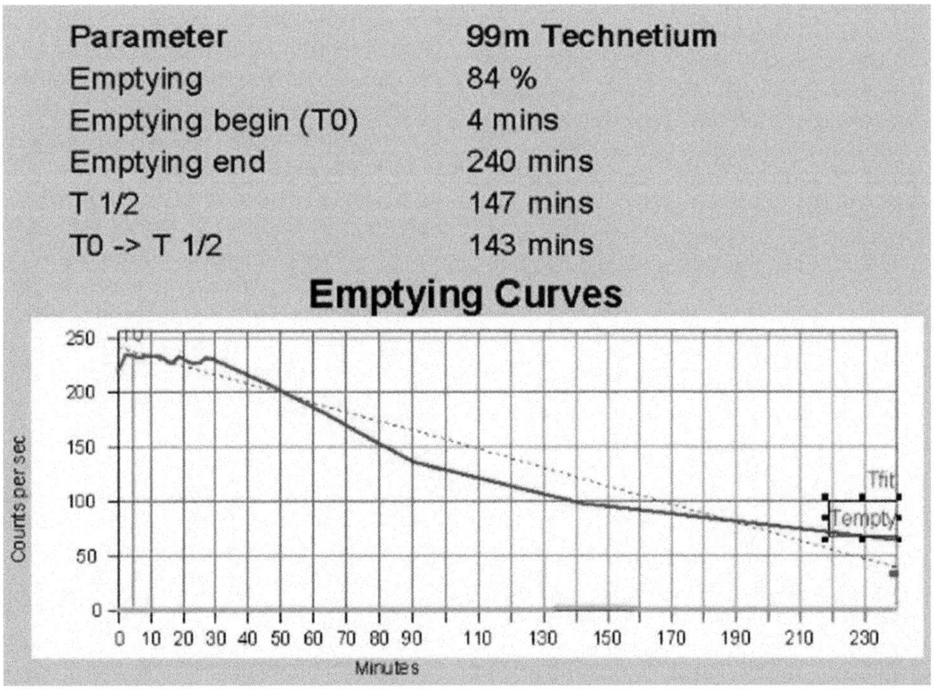

(B)

Fig. 28.15 Demonstrating gastroparesis: food remains in the stomach for an extended period, causing chronic nausea and vomiting. The estimated half-time in this case is 147 minutes.

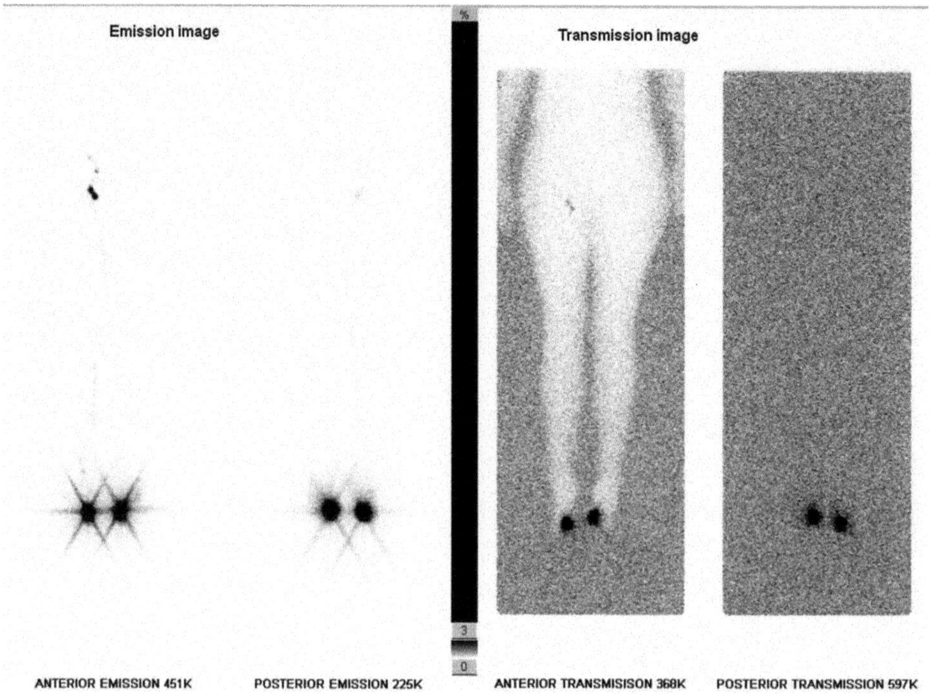

Fig. 28.16 An example of a abnormal lymphangiogram demonstrating normal lymphatic drainage on the right with delayed or obstructed drainage on the left. Anatomical localisation is obtained using a ^{57}Co flood source.

a patient's blood *in vitro* prior to re-administering into the patient. Clearly this will have an impact on the study technique and radiopharmaceutical used for the procedure.

BILIARY SYSTEM

Ultrasound and CT have largely taken over the role of imaging the liver, but ^{99m}Tc-HIDA (hepatobiliary iminodiacetic acid) continues to be the method of choice for imaging the biliary tree with suspected cholecystitis or biliary leakages postoperatively. Ultrasound is used for imaging calculi in the biliary system, but is not as consistent and specific as HIDA in the diagnosis of acute cholecystitis. The radiographic cholecystogram in this respect should be considered obsolete.[29] HIDA is also useful in imaging biliary reflux, and in the confirmation of biliary leakage following surgery.

LYMPHATICS

Technetium-labelled colloids can be used to image the lymphatic drainage. The technique is much easier to perform than a conventional lymphangiogram, and satisfactorily delineates areas of stasis (Fig. 28.16).

Another widely used lymphatic imaging method is in the localisation of the sentinel lymph node, the first node in the lymphatic chain, which drains fluid away from breast tumours and skin melanoma. A subcutaneous injection forming a radioactive bleb in the area of interest (either areola or close to the site of a melanoma) will drain via the lymphatics. During this process, the sentinel node is labelled and can be identified during surgery using a gamma probe and removed (Fig. 28.17). If the sentinel node is localised and shown to be disease free, then clinicians can be reasonably confident that the tumour has not spread via the lymphatics.

NEUROLOGY

Iodine 123-labelled DATSCAN is used in the diagnosis of Parkinson's disease to differentiate between true Parkinson's disease and an essential tremor. DATSCAN has an affinity for dopamine transporters in the brain and presents with a characteristic 'comma' shape in normal subjects representing the caudate nucleus and putamen. A significant reduction in uptake in this region of the brain can be symptomatic of one of a number of Parkinsonian syndromes which require further investigation. The most common positive presentation is of a 'full-stop' pattern (Fig. 28.18A,B).

In addition to DATSCAN, ^{99m}Tc-labelled HMPAO (hexamethylpropylene amine oxime) crosses the blood–brain barrier and becomes fixed in the brain. It can be used to visualise the vascular supply to the brain in the assessment of cerebrovascular disease. Disease-specific patterns of radiopharmaceutical uptake can be indicative of a transient ischaemic attack (TIA), complete stroke or Alzheimer's disease.

A nuclear medicine cerebrospinal fluid (CSF) study can be used to identify and localise the presence of a CSF leak or to assess the patency of an intracranial shunt. Referrals are commonly split into two categories – patients presenting with abnormally high CSF pressures (in the case of an occluded intracranial shunt) and patients presenting with abnormally low CSF pressures (in the case of suspected CSF leakage). A lumbar puncture is used to penetrate the 'closed' CSF system to administer ^{111}In-labelled DTPA and images are often acquired over several days.

A patent, and therefore normally operating shunt should result in rapid drainage of the isotope into the abdominal cavity (Figs 28.19A and B demonstrate a normally functioning shunt compared to a non-functioning shunt). Occlusion of any part of the drain will result in high pressure and often debilitating headaches.

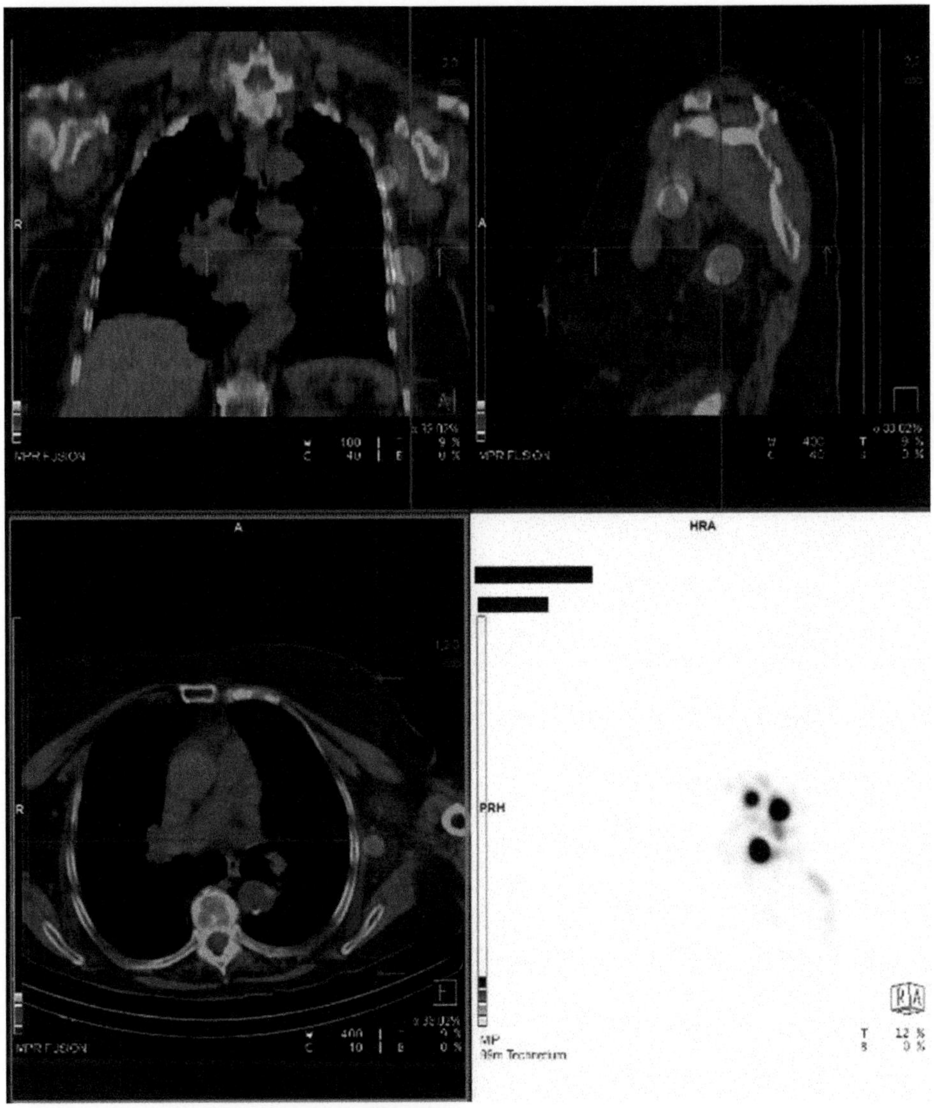

Fig. 28.17 Sentinel lymph node studies are an increasingly utilised investigation to identify the primary drainage lymph nodes prior to surgery. These investigations are commonly performed for breast cancer patients and patients with malignant melanomas.

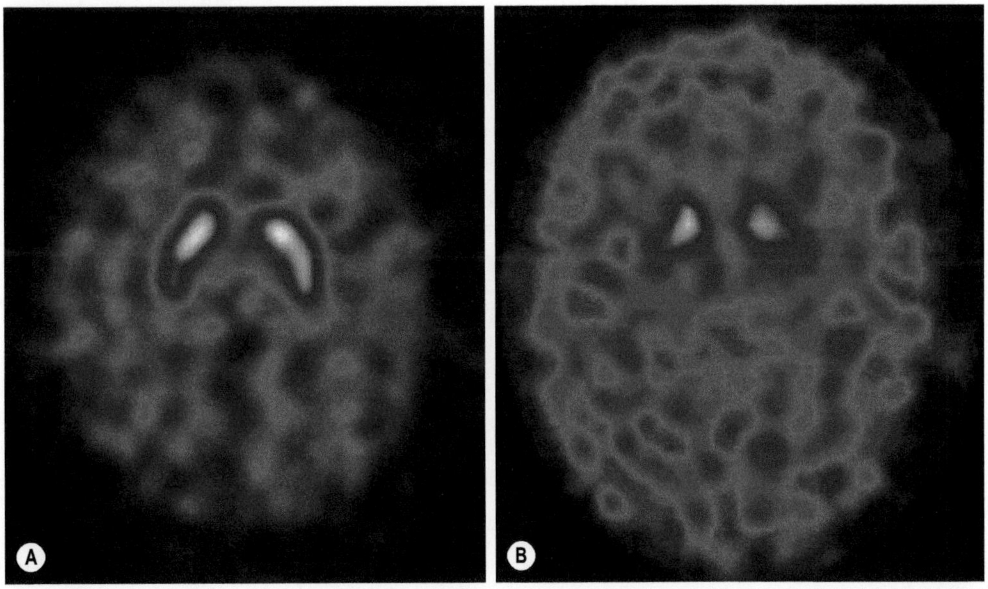

Fig. 28.18 (A) Normal uptake of DATSCAN in the brain in an area associated with dopamine transporters; (B) reduced uptake associated with Parkinson's disease.

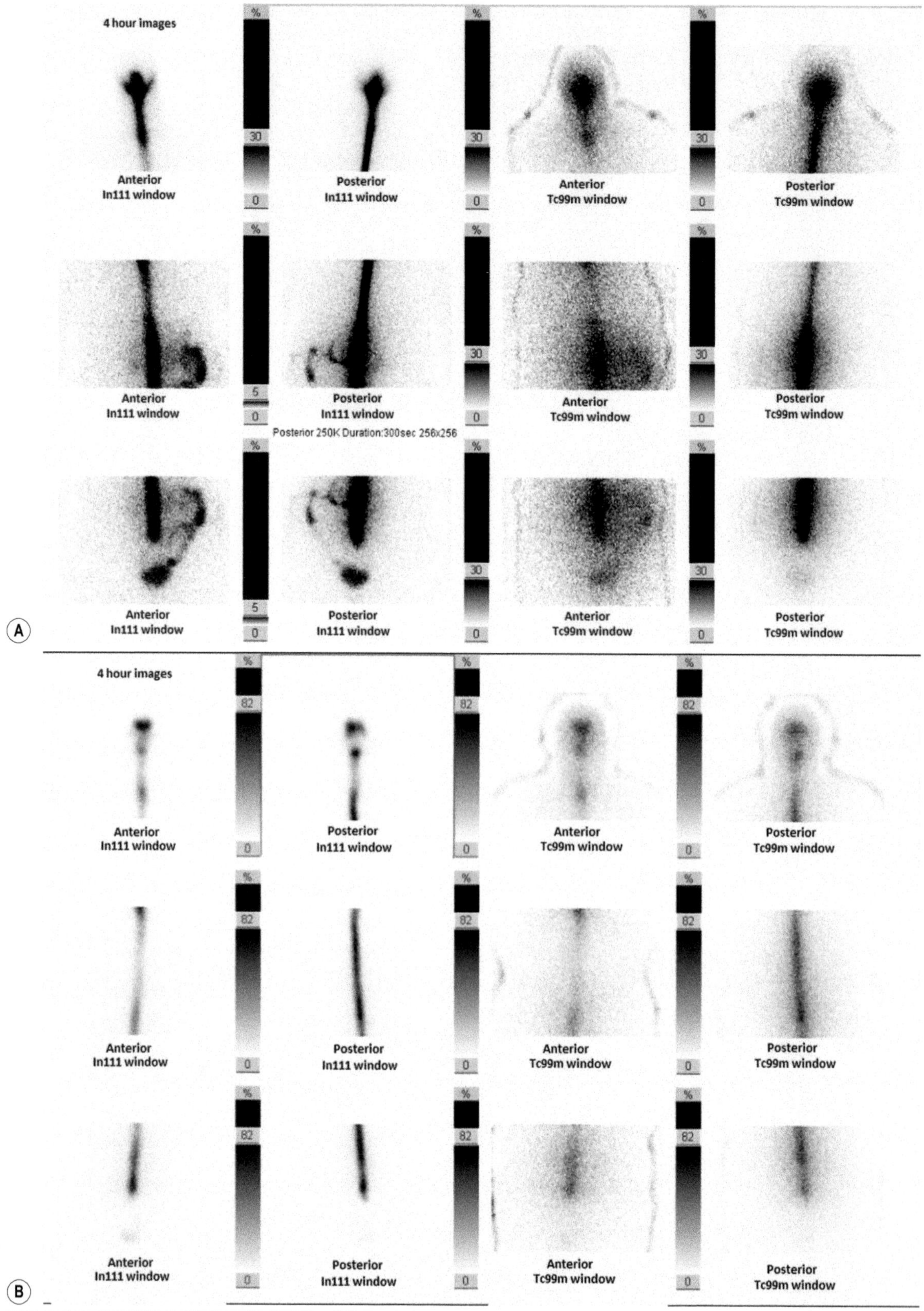

Fig. 28.19 A cerebrospinal fluid (CSF) study demonstrating the different presentations of a patent intracranial shunt (A) compared to a non-patent shunt (B).

The detection of a CSF leak can be identified visually although this is difficult unless the leak is large enough to result in rapid CSF leakage. Where an intracranial leak is suspected, nasal pledgets can be applied to absorb leaking CSF through the nasal cavity. These can then be measured using a radioactive well counter to determine abnormally high concentrations of CSF, indicating an intracranial CSF leak.

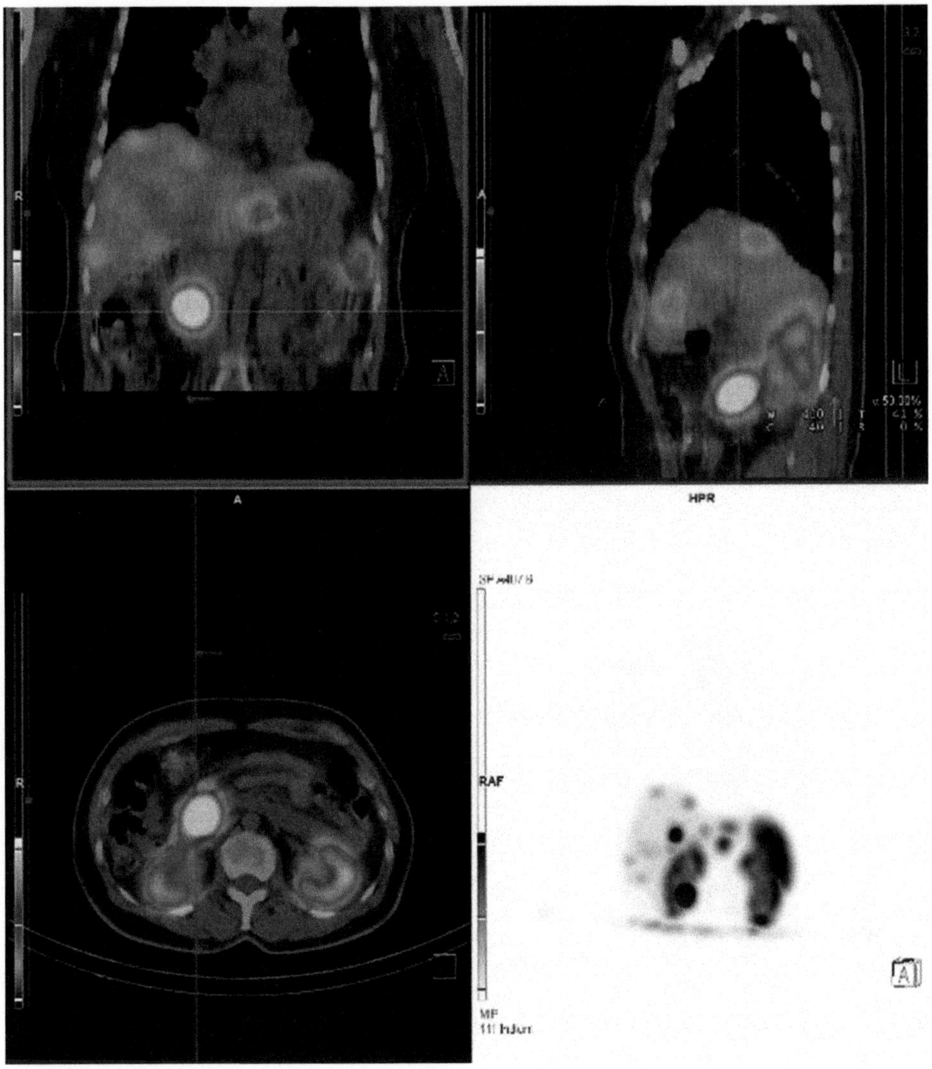

Fig. 28.20 A SPECT-CT reconstruction demonstrating multiple areas of increased ^{111}In octreotide uptake, in this instance suggestive of neuroendocrine tumour metastases.

TUMOUR STUDIES

Neuroendocrine tumour-labelling studies, such as ^{111}In-labelled octreotide and ^{123}I-labelled metaiodobenzylguanidine (mIBG) studies, are used to target and identify neuroendocrine tumours, which can occupy numerous sites in the body and are difficult to characterise with other standalone imaging modalities such as CT or MR. Octreotide studies have long been a useful method of characterising such tumours although in the past the technique was restricted by the limitations in localising the precise position of the tumour. SPECT-CT imaging in this instance has dramatically improved the clinical usefulness of these studies, as labelled tumours can be localised to within millimeters (Fig. 28.20).

PET-CT

Positron emission tomography (PET) imaging started several decades ago, using expensive dedicated imaging technology and requiring a nearby supply of specialist radiopharmaceuticals from a particle accelerator (cyclotron). Because positron-emitting radiopharmaceuticals have relatively short half-lives, the close proximity of a cyclotron to the PET centre was essential, and this often added to the cost of establishing a PET service. Cost restrictions and failure to show a clear value of PET imaging to the clinical routine meant its development was inhibited for many years.

In recent years, PET has begun to establish itself at the forefront of diagnostic imaging, particularly in the assessment of tumour metabolic activity and infection using ^{18}F-FDG. As already mentioned, this has in part been facilitated by the widespread installation of high-quality hybrid systems combining high-quality PET scanners with diagnostic quality CT scanners. The subsequent improvement in the study quality has led to a situation where standalone PET scanners are rapidly becoming obsolete and PET-CT is standard.

The value and use of PET-CT imaging is evolving at a tremendous rate and there has been a proliferation of articles in the literature attesting to its value. More recent literature surrounds its use in molecular imaging. There is the potential to detect preclinical disease (i.e. the patient has no signs or symptoms); when this is combined with molecular therapy (which might be radionuclide-based) it presents as a powerful mechanism for the detection and treatment of disease.

In the UK, as a direct consequence of a government initiative there has been steady growth in PET-CT imaging facilities. Dictated by cost and the requirement for geographical accessibility for patients, in the first instance a high proportion of these clinical PET-CT services were provided on mobile scanners. Clinical value, clinical demand and finance will no doubt determine whether fixed rather than mobile PET-CT sites will increase in number.

CLINICAL PET-CT

The most widespread PET-CT studies utilise ^{18}F-FDG as the radiopharmaceutical of choice and for this reason ^{18}F-FDG will be discussed for the majority of this section.

An analogue of glucose, ^{18}F-FDG is metabolised by the body to give an indication of the metabolic rate of a tumour with a higher metabolic rate resulting in a higher proportion of uptake to the area. A Standardised Uptake Value (SUV) is reported for focal areas of increased uptake. The SUV is not an absolute value but represents a measurement of the level of uptake compared to amount of activity administered either per bodyweight or body surface area.

Patient Preparation

The proportion of tracer uptake is affected by a number of factors for which the preparation of the patient prior to the administration of the dose is of paramount importance:

- *Diet*: The patient should be fasted for several hours prior to the study – this is generally accepted as 6 hours for non-diabetic or non-insulin-dependent diabetic patients and 4 hours for insulin-dependent diabetic patients. A high level of blood glucose resulting from recent food intake will result in high levels of muscular uptake of ^{18}F-FDG which in turn will reduce the levels of uptake in any specific areas of interest, e.g. tumour uptake.
- *Medication*: Some medications can have a detrimental impact on the quality of the scan. Oramorph, for example, may contain glucose and therefore should be avoided. Also, metformin can cause high concentrations of ^{18}F-FDG uptake which has a significantly adverse impact on the quality of the scan and also the ability of the radiologist to detect smaller lesions in the abdominal area.
- *Medical interventions*: Chemotherapy, radiotherapy, biopsies and surgery cause abnormal uptake patterns on a PET scan and a full patient history should be taken prior to booking a scan to ensure an optimum time delay is implemented prior to scanning. Radiotherapy, for example, has been shown to result in non-specific inflammation which presents as an area of increased uptake of ^{18}F-FDG. A minimum of 12 weeks is usually required to allow this inflammation to subside and to ensure that the PET-CT scan is of optimum diagnostic usefulness.[30]
- *Medical conditions*: Recent injuries and infections can result in focal uptake of ^{18}F-FDG and part of the pre-test interview should include investigating the general well-being of the patient.
- *Environmental conditions*: ^{18}F-FDG distribution can be affected by a number of environmental factors. Brown adipose fat or tissue (BAT) is involved in the generation of heat through glucose metabolism to maintain core body temperature. If the patient is cold during the uptake period, it can result in significant areas of uptake on the PET-CT scan which may be mistaken for malignancy, may mask small lesions and ultimately will reduce the confidence in the scan. It is important to ensure that patients are kept warm following the administration of ^{18}F-FDG as this will suppress the requirement for heat generation by BAT and ensure optimum image quality.[31]
- *Exercise and movement*: Vigorous exercise should be avoided for at least 24 hours before the scan as this can lead to muscular uptake which can degrade the quality of the scan. Post injection movement should also be kept to a minimum as this can also result in high levels of muscular uptake.[32]

^{18}F-FDG PET-CT PROCEDURE

The technique used to perform a PET-CT scan is site-specific and can be influenced by the technical specifications of the scanner or the capacity demands of the department. The amount of radioactivity administered to the patient is variable and can be both weight scaled or fixed dose, although a standard 60-minute patient 'resting' duration between the injection and scan is commonly applied. During this rest period, the patient should be discouraged from moving vigorously to avoid unwanted muscular uptake of radiopharmaceutical.

Scanning protocols can also vary between sites but generally consist of one of three common scan regimens for oncological ^{18}F-FDG work, which is dictated by the clinical history of the patient:

- Total-body – the whole of the patient
- Half-body – skull base to proximal third of femur (Fig. 28.21)
- Half-body plus head and neck – vertex to proximal third of femur

When compared to conventional nuclear medicine, whereby 2D and 3D scan types can be selected, all scanning in PET-CT is 3D, which reduces the requirement for variety of technique.

The scanning parameters also vary between sites. Traditionally, PET scans are performed in bed positions where each bed position represents a single scanner field of view with sufficient overlap to create a continuous whole-body scan, utilising a step-and-shoot technique. Each bed position, analogous to a 3D gamma camera static image, must be acquired for a sufficient time-period to produce an adequate number of counts in the image to reduce the impact of statistical noise. This is dependent on the dose administered to the patient and the time delay between injection and scan but is generally between 2 and 4 minutes per bed position, resulting in a standard 'half-body' scan duration of 20–30 minutes.

One limitation of the step-and-shoot method of imaging is that total scan lengths are constrained by bed positions. Therefore, a patient whose optimal scan length falls somewhere between five and six bed positions will either have a scan that is shorter than required, or, more likely longer than required and results in a higher than necessary CT dose. More recently, manufacturers have introduced a continuous whole-body facility which replaces step-and-shoot

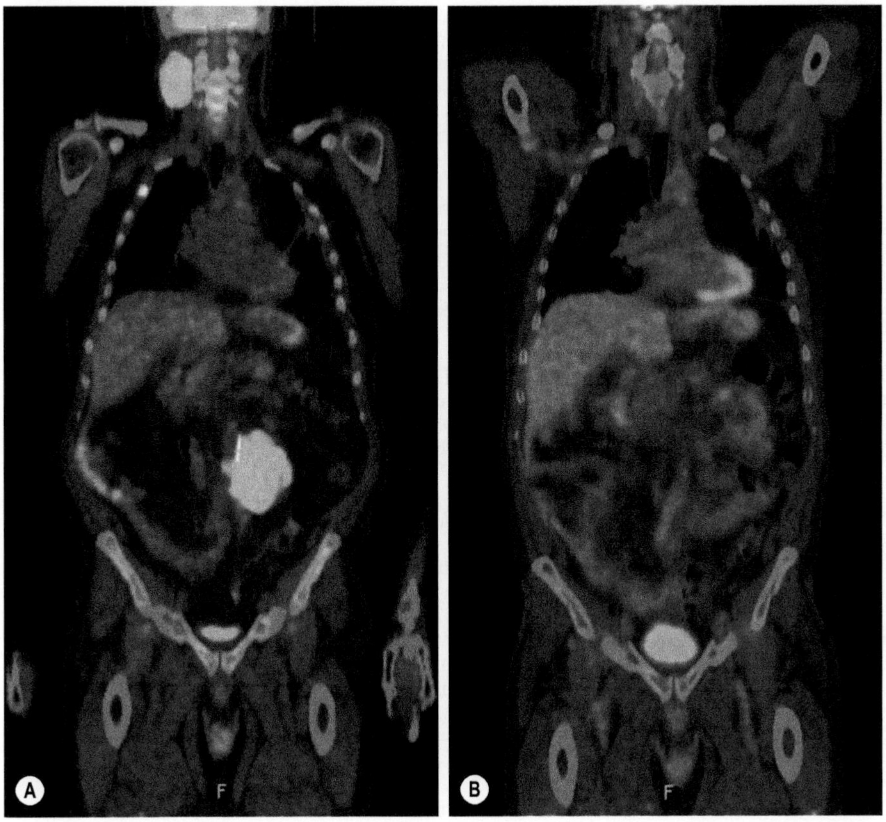

Fig. 28.21 A comparison between a pre-treatment ^{18}FDG PET-CT scan for lymphoma and a post-treatment scan. The scan demonstrates a significant reduction in FDG uptake indicating a positive response to treatment.

imaging with continuous bed motion. This can be a useful tool in optimising PET scanning for the patient and offering a more flexible approach to scanning. Figures 28.21A and B demonstrate pre- and post-treatment PET-CT scans for lymphoma.

Summary

At present, nuclear medicine imaging comprises a complex mixture of imaging systems, radiopharmaceuticals and protocols. Imaging systems, in particular, have evolved significantly since the initial development of the gamma camera. Advances in camera technology and associated software have resulted in improved resolution (image quality), and in some instances a reduction in imaging time. Overall, this has facilitated an improvement in diagnostic accuracy, clinical usefulness and patient throughput. To counterbalance the increasing complexity and diversity of modern nuclear medicine there has been a proliferation of multicamera departments. Generally speaking, year on year, there has been a steady increase in gamma camera studies, albeit with the introduction of complementary imaging modalities there has been a reduction in some specific imaging procedures at various junctures. A notable example of this is that gamma camera brain imaging went into decline when the CT scanner became a standard X-ray department feature.

In recent years the notion of using CT technology integrally with SPECT gamma camera technology has become universally accepted. This was a direct consequence of the advances and discoveries made in PET-CT. SPECT gamma cameras can now be purchased with or without CT systems, and can be low dose (for attenuation correction) or diagnostic quality.

The final advancement in nuclear medicine technology worthy of note is PET-MR – this represents the latest evolution in hybrid technology. Simultaneous acquisition of MR and PET data is achievable, and the ability to be used as a standalone MR scanner removes issues concerning productivity.[33] This hybrid technology is currently in its infancy, but commercial systems are already on the market. Although is it primarily used for research at the moment, it is likely that, as with PET-CT and SPECT-CT, there could be a growth in these scanners as robust research evidence emerges and as finances permit.

Significant advances continue to be made in radiopharmaceutical design, for both therapy and diagnosis. A major challenge is presented to the nuclear medicine imaging community, and beyond, as to how to make effective use of the imaging tools. It has become evident that the personnel who operate the technology and interpret the images need to evolve too. In the recent past, imaging technologies tended to be discrete and isolated although the introduction of PACS (picture archiving and communication systems) facilitated better proximity of different modalities in terms of image viewing and manipulation. This trend is being further advanced with the growth of hybrid imaging and there is a growing requirement for healthcare workers to have broader competencies, or at the very least to work in multi-skilled interdependent clinical teams. Strong consideration needs to be given to ensure that nuclear medicine clinical professionals are supported in the development of their skill base to ensure that the demands of these developing technologies can continue to be met. In this manner nuclear medicine can continue to grow and develop and maintain its relevance to clinical practice.

References

1. Bailey D, Adamson K. Nuclear medicine: from photons to physiology. *Curr Pharm Design*. 2003;9:903–916.
2. Cassen B, Curits L, Reed C, et al. Instrumentation for I-131 use in medical studies. *Nucleonics*. 1951;9:46–50.
3. Brownell GL, Sweet WL. Localization of brain tumors with positron emitters. *Nucleonics*. 1953;11:40–45.
4. Anger HO. Scintillation camera. *Rev Sci Instrument*. 1958;29:27–33.
5. Kuhl DE, Edwards RQ. Cylindrical and section radioisotope scanning of the liver and brain. *Radiology*. 1964;83:926–935.
6. Kuhl DE, Edwards RQ. Image separation radioisotope scanning. *Radiology*. 1963;80:653–661.
7. Duncan K. Radiopharmaceuticals in PET imaging. *J Nucl Med Technol*. 1998;26:228–234.
8. https://www.rcr.ac.uk/system/files/publication/field_publication_files/bfcr163_pet-ct.pdf.
9. https://www.england.nhs.uk/statistics/wp-content/uploads/sites/2/2018/03/Provisional-Monthly-Diagnostic-Imaging-Dataset-Statistics-2018-03-22.pdf.
10. Rousseau E, Wilson D, Lacroix-Poisson F, et al. A prospective study on 18F-DCFPyL PSMA PET/ct imaging in biochemical recurrence of prostate cancer. *J Nucl Med*. 2019;60(6).
11. Schwartzenbock S, Souvatzoglou M, Krause BJ. Choline PET and PET/CT in the primary diagnosis and staging of prostate cancer. *Theranostics*. 2012;2(3):318–330.
12. Ghotbi AA, Kjaer A, Hasbak P. Review: comparison of PET rubidium-82 with conventional. *SPECT Myocard Perfus Imaging*. 2014;34(3):163–170.
13. Theobald T. *Sampson's Textbook of Radiopharmacy*. 4th ed. London: Pharmaceutical Press; 2011.
14. Even-Sapir E, Metser U, Mishani E, et al. The detection of bone metastases in patients with high-risk prostate cancer: 99mTc-MDP planar bone scintigraphy, single- and multi-field-of-view SPECT, 18F-fluoride PET, and 18F-fluoride PET/CT. *J Nucl Med*. 2006;47:287–297.
15. Alazraki NA. In: Resnick WB, ed. *Bone and Joint Imaging – Radionuclide Techniques*. 2nd ed. London: Saunders; 1996.
16. Ryan PJ, Fogelman I. Musculoskeletal section. In: Britton KE, Collier D, Maisey M, Siraj QH, eds. *Clinical Nuclear Medicine*. 3rd ed. London: Chapman and Hall; 1998.
17. Sharp PF, Gemmell HG, Murray AD, eds. *Practical Nuclear Medicine*. 3rd ed. London: Springer; 2005.
18. Brown M, O'Connor MK, Hung JC, et al. Technical aspects of bone scintigraphy. *Radiol Clin North Am*. 1993;31(4):721–730.
19. Mallinckrodt Medical BV. *Summary of Product Characteristics*; 1996.
20. McKillop J, Fogelman I. *Benign and Malignant Bone Disease. Clinician's Guide to Nuclear Medicine Series (British Nuclear Medicine Society)*. Edinburgh: Churchill Livingstone; 1991.
21. Klemenz B, Katzwinkel J, Kaiser KP, et al. The influence of differences in hydration on bone-to-soft tissue ratios and image quality in bone scintigraphy. *Clin Nucl Med*. 1999;24(7):483–487.
22. Bajc M, Neilly JB, Minaiti M, et al. EANM guidelines for ventilation/perfusion scintigraphy – Part 1. Pulmonary imaging with ventilation/perfusion single photon emission tomography. *Eur J Nucl Med Mol Imaging*. 2009;36:1356–1370.
23. Administration of Radioactive Substances Advisory Committee. *Notes for Guidance on the Clinical Administration of Radiopharmaceuticals and Use of Sealed Radioactive Sources*; 2006.
24. Martin WH, Sandler MP, and Gross MD In: Sharp PF, Gemmell HG, Murray AD, eds. *Practical Nuclear Medicine*. London: Springer; 2005.
25. Coakley A, Wells C. In: Britton KE, Collier D, Maisey M, Siraj QH, eds. *Clinical Nuclear Medicine*. 3rd ed. London: Chapman & Hall; 1998:331–381.
26. Billotey C, Sarfati E, Aurengo A, et al. Advantages of SPECT in technetium-99-m-sestamibi parathyroid scintigraphy. *J Nucl Med*. 1996;37:1773–1778.
27. Testa H, Prescott M. *A Clinician's Guide to Nuclear Medicine – Nephrourology*. Amersham: British Nuclear Medicine Society; 1996.
28. Harding L, Notghi A. In: Sharp PF, Gemmell HG, Murray AD, eds. *Practical Nuclear Medicine*. London: Springer; 2005.
29. Harding L, Robinson P. *Clinician's Guide to Nuclear Medicine – Gastroenterology*. London: British Nuclear Medicine Society; 1990:20160764.
30. Cliffe H, Patel C, Prestwich R, et al. Radiotherapy response evaluation using FDG PET-CT – established and emerging applications. Br J Radiol. 201;90.
31. Steinberg JD, Vogel W, Vegt E. Factors influencing brown fat activation in FDG PET/CT: a retrospective analysis of 15,0001 cases. *Br J Radiol*. 2017;90:20170093.
32. Jackson RS, Schlarman TC, Hubble WL, et al. Prevalence and patterns of physiologic muscle uptake detected with whole-body 18F-FDG PET. *J Nucl Med Technol*. 2006;34:29–33.

29 Ultrasound

JULIE BURNAGE and BARRY CARVER

Introduction

Since the introduction of ultrasound (US) to medical imaging in the 1960s, its popularity has grown and applications widened into numerous subspecialties of medicine. Excluding plain radiography, ultrasound scans are the most commonly undertaken diagnostic imaging examinations in the UK. There are few people in the UK who will not have heard of ultrasound or seen images of 'baby scans'. The use of ultrasound in obstetric care is well recognised, although its importance is overlooked by many and the critical role it plays in antenatal care is often reduced to that of 'gender determination', yet the role diagnostic ultrasound plays in many other subspecialties of medicine is not widely understood.

Ultrasound is widely used because:

- It is safe: it does not involve the use of ionising radiation (although there are biological effects discussed later in this chapter).
- It is 'patient friendly' and well tolerated.
- Measurements are reliable, accurate and reproducible.
- Ultrasound scanning is dynamic and so disease processes can be detected or excluded quickly which means that patients can be put on the right pathway sooner than might otherwise happen.
- The cost of an ultrasound scan is considerably less than modalities such as CT or MR.
- The equipment comes in many formats from traditional large machines via laptop to pocket sized; as such it can be used in a variety of locations, including at the bedside.

Historically, the use of ultrasound was confined to the imaging department and in the main scans were performed by radiologists and radiographers; but advances in technology and the relatively low cost of machines mean that an ever-increasing and diverse range of healthcare professionals now use ultrasound in their own departments on a daily basis.

As well as sonographers, whose primary role is ultrasound scanning, there are dedicated practitioners performing specific ultrasound examinations; for example clinical vascular scientists undertaking vascular studies, cardiac physiologists carrying out echocardiography, abdominal aortic aneurysm (AAA) screening technicians working on national screening programmes, and healthcare assistants (HCA) working in termination of pregnancy clinics and using ultrasound to date a pregnancy. Additionally there are several groups of healthcare professionals using ultrasound as a 'tool': physiotherapists, midwives, anaesthetists, urologists, Obs/Gynae and Emergency Department consultants among others; for them, ultrasound is an adjunct to, rather than the main part of their work. Acronyms such as PoCUS (Point-of-Care Ultrasound) and FAST (Focused Assessment (or Abdominal) Sonography in Trauma) are recognised worldwide.

In order to support colleagues across medicine in the safe and competent use of ultrasound, the Royal College of Radiologists (RCR) produced 'Ultrasound training recommendations for medical and surgical specialties'; in 2017 the 3rd edition was published, emphasising that:

The medical use of ultrasound remains highly operator-dependent in spite of advances in technology, and the interests of the patient are best served by the provision of an ultrasound service which offers the maximum clinical benefit and optimum use of resources; that is, with appropriately trained personnel using equipment of appropriate quality.[1]

The Consortium for the Accreditation of Sonographic Education (CASE) publishes its list of accredited formal post-graduate and focused short courses to facilitate the training of all professionals in the UK.[2]

No matter who is performing an ultrasound scan and no matter what their profession or background they must be properly trained and competent, and work within a robust governance framework, which includes best practice protocols and policies, and which include regular competency assessments and audit.

Equipment Chronology

1790 Spallanzani found that bats manoeuvre using hearing rather than sight.

1801 Young's work on light shows that waves can be combined to become stronger or cancel each other out.

1826 Colladon determines the speed of sound through water.

1843 Physicist Christian Doppler describes an effect which explains a change in the perceived frequency of sound emitted by a moving source.

1880 The Curie brothers discover the piezoelectric effect in crystalline materials.

1917 Langevin invents the hydrophone. The device was able to send and receive low-frequency sound waves through water, and was used to detect submarines in World War I.

1936 Siemens launch the Sonostat, a therapeutic ultrasound machine that used the heating effects on tissue.

Early 1940s Growth of use of A-mode ultrasound materials testing.
1942 Dussik publishes his work on transmission ultrasound of the brain; the first medical ultrasound publication?
Late 1940s Ludwig studies the difference in sound waves as they travel through various tissues in animals, later applying these findings to human subjects.
1949 Wild assesses the thickness of bowel tissue and pioneers early developments in ultrasound.
1951 Professor Ian Donald, Dr John McVicar, and engineer Tom Brown produce static, black and white 2D scanning.
1954 Edler and Hertz publish their work on measuring cardiac movement.[3]
1958 Donald's equipment now able to demonstrate pathology in live volunteers. Publishes 'Investigation of abdominal masses by pulsed ultrasound'.[4]
1962 First contact 2D scanner developed, commercially launched in 1963.
1965 Advances in materials technology enable improvements in equipment and the development of real-time images. 'Diasonograph' designed – the first commercially produced ultrasound machine.
1972 First linear array scanners available.
1973 Grey-scale 2D available; developing computer technologies make ultrasound faster, with improving images.
1974 Duplex pulsed Doppler.
1980s Fast real-time scanners become widespread, enabling wider range of hospital-based clinical applications.
1984 First 3D fetal ultrasound.
1985 Real-time colour flow Doppler.[5]
1990s Digital processing enables high-resolution imaging using broadband transducers. Image quality and improvements in accuracy further increase the role of ultrasound, particularly in breast imaging and cancer detection. Contrast-enhanced ultrasound introduced.
2000s 3D and 4D fetal imaging becomes widespread. 3D scans are used in other applications, e.g. gynaecology and cardiac scanning. Laptop and handheld machines become available.

Developments in ultrasound are ongoing, for example the recent and ongoing development of strain/compression and shearwave sono-elastography.

Physical Principles of Ultrasound

Sound is a form of mechanical energy travelling from a vibrating source through a medium (sound cannot travel through a vacuum because there are no molecules for the vibrations to move through). It is transmitted as series of longitudinal waves, i.e. the energy travels along in the same direction as the particles of the medium vibrate. As a sound wave travels through a medium it undergoes compression (where the particles are closest together) and rarefaction (where the particles are furthest apart). Ultrasound has a high pitch (frequency) typically greater than 1 MHz, which is above the human audible hearing range of around 20 Hz to 20 000 Hz.

As with sound and other wave propagation, the properties of an ultrasound wave are governed by the equation

$$\nu = f\lambda$$

where:

v is the speed of sound which is dependent upon the transmitting medium: in ultrasound the medium is soft tissue and v has a relatively constant value of 1540 m/s, so even though the sound wave may travel through fat, bone, muscle fluid etc., machines are calibrated to assume the constant velocity of 1540 m/s.

f is the frequency (number of waves that pass a point per unit of time) or 'pitch'. In ultrasound, the frequency used is determined by the choice of transducer and equipment 'presets'.

λ is the wavelength (the distance between adjacent identical parts of a wave, e.g. between adjacent compressions). In ultrasound, penetration is proportional to wavelength, so given that v is constant, it is clear that to increase the penetrative ability of the ultrasound (i.e. to assess deeper structures), then λ must be increased and f must be reduced and likewise, if assessing structures which are closer to the surface, then f must be increased and λ reduced.

PRODUCTION OF AN ULTRASOUND WAVE (FIG. 29.1)

In 1880, Pierre and Jacques Curie, discovered that by applying pressure on certain substances, e.g. crystals, they could produce electricity. This they called the piezoelectric effect, the name derived from the Greek word for squeeze, *piezein*. Applying a voltage (electrical energy) to a piezoelectric material (crystals in the transducer) causes the crystal to expand and contract and the vibrations produced (mechanical energy) generate a sound wave.

This also applies in reverse: when a returning wave arrives at the crystal the resulting contraction and expansion generates an electric current, which can be read as a signal used to generate an image and the stronger the force coming back to the crystal, the greater the amplitude of the electrical signal generated. The amplitude of the signal is converted into signal *b*rightness on the screen and this is why it is called *B*-mode scanning. The crystal in an ultrasound transducer is therefore both a transmitter and receiver of sound waves.

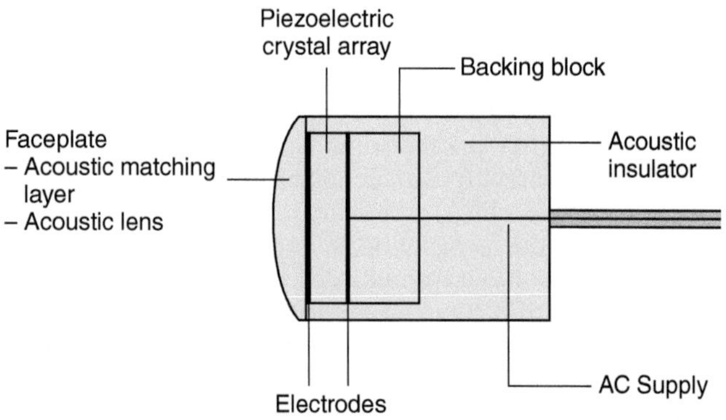

Fig. 29.1 Schematic of 'basic' transducer structure.

Originally transducers had a fixed, single crystal but modern transducers have multiple elements which can be 'fired' independently (or in groups) which enables the ultrasound beam to be focused, shaped and steered for optimum image quality.

The quality of the image determines the ability to diagnose; it is important that much of the ultrasound wave is able to penetrate through and return from tissues and structures. To this end the transducer is constructed such that it has a 'coating' similar to skin and, coupled with the use of ultrasound gel, the reflective interface between the transducer and the skin is minimised (see acoustic impedance mismatch below).

ULTRASOUND WAVE INTERACTIONS

As an ultrasound wave travels through the patient it will interact with layers between different tissues. These interactions will cause the wave to be attenuated, i.e. energy is lost as the generated wave traverses the patient. There are several mechanisms by which the wave is attenuated:

- *Absorption*: As the wave passes through the patient some of its energy is lost in the tissues through which it passes. The rate of absorption is dependent upon the tissue type and the frequency of the wave. As the wave passes through tissue, it generates heat. This is useful in therapeutic applications of ultrasound but is a potential hazard in diagnostic use.
- *Reflection*: Each tissue type has an 'acoustic impedance' (the resistance of the tissue to the propagation of the wave), when the ultrasound beam strikes a boundary between different tissue types, reflection occurs with some of the echoes going back to the transducer. The degree of reflection depends not on individual acoustic impedance of tissue but on the difference in the acoustic impedance of the tissues either side of the boundary – the acoustic impedance mismatch.
- *Acoustic impedance mismatch*: The acoustic impedance, Z, is the resistance of tissue to wave propagation and is the product of the density, ρ, of the tissue and speed of sound, ν, in the tissue.

$$Z = \nu\rho$$

A large mismatch creates a lot of reflection with little transmission; the mismatch between soft tissue and air is such that this interface is almost impenetrable by the wave, hence the necessity of ultrasound gel.

- *Refraction*: If the sound wave hits a tissue boundary at an angle that is not perpendicular to the interface, it may undergo a change of direction – refraction. The system does not know that the echoes are not coming back in a straight line and so a structure will appear on the screen in a different place to where it actually is in the body. This can lead to misregistration and measurement artefacts.
- *Scatter*: Scattering occurs when ultrasound interacts with very small targets (rather than strong boundaries) whose dimensions are similar to or smaller than the wavelength. The ultrasound is reflected in multiple directions and the echoes received back are much weaker than those from different tissue interfaces. Scattering is what gives the liver parenchyma or uterine myometrium their appearance on ultrasound, for example.
- *Diffraction*: This is the spreading or 'diverging' of the ultrasound beam as it travels from the transducer face through the tissue. The further the beam is from the source, the less intense it becomes.

IMAGE FORMATION

Crystals in the transducer are 'fired' in turn (often in groups) and as the pulses pass through the patient and after the processes of attenuation, echoes are reflected back to the transducer and are turned into electrical signals which are then manipulated and processed by the ultrasound machine to produce an image. The time taken for the echo to arrive back at the transducer indicates the depth of the tissue interface, and the size of the signal indicates the amount of reflection at the interface.

When the signal is processed, many of the processing functions can be controlled by the sonographer to produce the required image. The quality of the image on screen is dependent on a competent practitioner manipulating the equipment controls and adapting technique to account for the patient being scanned. The basic controls include:

- *Power*: Increasing the power increases the intensity of the ultrasound beam and therefore the overall 'brightness' of the image. Because power has a direct effect on the thermal and mechanical indices (see 'ultrasound safety' later in this chapter), it is important that the sonographer follows the ALARP (as low as reasonably practicable) principle.
- *Transducer selection* (Fig. 29.2): A variety of transducers are available and they are 'multi-frequency'. The higher the frequency of a transducer, the better the resolution but at the expense of the depth of penetration. For superficial structures, e.g. testes, soft tissue lumps or the thyroid gland, a higher frequency probe should be used. In very slim patients, using a high-frequency probe will often demonstrate the abdominal organs or liver edge more clearly than an abdominal (lower frequency) probe.

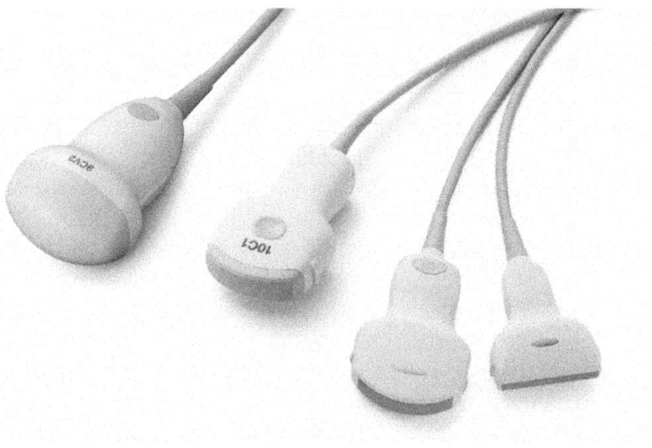

Fig. 29.2 Selection of transducers. (Reproduced with permission from Canon Medical Systems.)

There are a plethora of probes available and when a machine is purchased thought should be given to the case mix for the equipment so that appropriate probe packages can be chosen. A hockey stick probe used for musculoskeletal applications is of no use in a busy obstetric department, likewise a high-frequency endocavity probe will not be needed in a cardiac scanning department.

- *Time gain compensation (TGC)*: Because of the attenuation of the ultrasound beam as it passes through and returns from tissues, signals that take longer to return from deep interfaces are weaker than those from shallower interfaces which return faster; the correct use of TGC 'balances out' these signals. The TGC control does this by amplifying the echoes returning from deeper structures. The TGC control is a number of sliders, each of which corresponds to a different depth in the tissue. Moving one of the sliders to the right increases the brightness of the image at that specific depth. Moving all of the sliders to the right increases the brightness of the whole image.
- *Overall gain*: When echoes return to the transducer they are converted into small voltages. In order to produce an image, these voltages must be amplified before they can be processed. The overall gain is usually a rotating dial that amplifies or reduces all the signals received. Increasing the overall gain will make the overall image brighter and vice versa.
- *Focus*: The image quality is best when the region of interest is in the narrowest part of the ultrasound beam; the focus control enables the operator to adjust where the beam narrows. Beyond the focal zone, the beam starts to diverge and the resolution of the image is poorer. When assessing small structures, for example an ovary, it is better to use one focal zone but if looking at large structure such as the liver, it can be useful to have multiple focal zones so that the beam is narrower for a greater depth of tissue.
- *Depth*: The depth control does not change how far the ultrasound beam penetrates into the body but it does change the maximum depth of the tissue displayed on the screen. It is important that the region of interest fills most of the screen so that regions deeper than the area of interest are not visible. For optimum visualisation, the depth should be adjusted before zoom is used.
- *Zoom/Magnification*: The zoom function enables small regions of interest to be enlarged so that they can be examined more easily. In addition, by 'zooming' an area, other things that are not of interest are removed from the image, which facilitates visual acuity. On application of the zoom function a box appears which the operator moves using the trackball to encompass the region of interest (ROI). There are two types of zoom, read and write. Write zoom is used during 'live' scanning and has the advantage of improving the image quality because it magnifies the image in real time. Read zoom magnifies an area of a frozen image and because each pixel will be magnified, overuse of read zoom can actually reduce the image quality. Zoom function should be used after the correct depth is chosen.
- *Sector angle/field of view (FOV)*: The FOV can be altered/reduced when assessing smaller structures and using it improves visual acuity because extraneous tissue is removed from the image; image resolution is also improved. Having an extended FOV is excellent in musculoskeletal applications because it provides a panoramic view of the region of interest.
- *Harmonics*: Harmonics is a function that can help to improve the image quality in some patients, particularly those with a high body mass index (BMI), because it gives increased penetration without loss of detail, it reduces artefact such as reverberation, and reduces 'noise' and image clutter. Harmonics is usually included during equipment 'presets' but can be switched on and off by the operator.

Equipment and Technology

There are a wide variety of ultrasound machines available commercially, from wireless, cable-free hand-held systems to the larger machines seen in ultrasound departments. It is essential that the correct machine is available to practitioners based on the case mix to be scanned, the throughput of patients expected and the location. The decision on which machine to buy should always be made in consultation with all stakeholders, particularly those who will be using it. Factors to be taken into consideration are:

- Case mix and throughput of patients
- Location in which the machine is to be used
- Ergonomics
- Cost

ROOM REQUIREMENTS AND ANCILLARY EQUIPMENT

In 2014, a joint document produced by the Royal College of Radiologists (RCR) and Society and College of Radiographers (SCoR) set out the 'Standards for Provision of an Ultrasound Service'.[6] The document was intended to provide advice and guidance for both suppliers and commissioners of ultrasound services. As well as discussion on equipment, training and education, quality assurance and audit, governance and report writing, the document also discusses the minimum requirements for the working environment, as the environment in which the ultrasound equipment is used will have a profound effect on its efficacy.

Ultrasound scans should be undertaken in an appropriately sized and accessible lockable room with dimmable lighting (no natural light), air conditioning, a rise and fall examination couch, a privacy curtain or screen, a chair for the patient, an appropriate 'ergonomic' seat for the sonographer, a desk and computer with connectivity for image and report storage, a hand wash basin and adjacent toilet facilities. Obviously where ultrasound is used in PoCUS or a FAST scan is performed away from the 'ideal', this should be documented in the report as the quality of the scan could be compromised.

A supply of the relevant consumables for the case mix should be easily accessible; examples may be:

- Ultrasound gel, sterile and non-sterile
- Probe covers (including latex free)

- Couch roll
- Sterile and non-sterile gloves (including latex free)
- Sterile packs, needles etc. for biopsy or joint injections
- Contrast agents
- Appropriate waste disposable facilities (for general and contaminated waste)
- Infection control consumables – these will be different for different providers and depend on, amongst other things, equipment manufacturer's recommendations and local infection prevention and control policies

The type of 'cleaning' will be determined by equipment used and scans performed and can include sterilisation, or high- or low-level disinfection. It must be remembered that all equipment must be cleaned – including the couch, computer, key boards etc.

Where obstetric studies are undertaken, thermal imaging paper (for 'keepsake' images) must be stored appropriately because it is temperature-sensitive. There should also be a 'slave monitor' to enable the patient and those attending the scan with her to see the baby on screen without the practitioner having to adjust the ultrasound monitor and scan in awkward positions, which has been shown to contribute to work-related upper limb disorder (WRULD) in the sonographer population.[7]

IMAGING METHODS

Several different imaging methods or 'modes' are used in ultrasound imaging.

A-mode

Amplitude (A)-mode was the first type of ultrasound and is best described as a one-dimensional amplitude modulation scan. A-mode is still used in ophthalmic applications. The received echoes are plotted with the x axis representing depth and the y axis the intensity of the reflected wave.

B-mode

Brightness modulated (B)-mode ultrasound is two-dimensional (2D) and is the most commonly used application of ultrasound. 2D has generally been replaced by the term 2D imaging, the two dimensions being height and width and, depending on the position of the transducer, a cross-section of the body can be demonstrated in real time. Real time 2D imaging gives information such as size, volume, shape, wall outline, internal architecture of organs and masses, relationship to adjoining structures, movement of organs and presence of fluid.

M-mode (Fig. 29.3)

Motion (M)-mode is a variation in which rapidly generated pulses are imaged in succession: as interfaces move relative to the probe their velocities can be calculated. This mode is used in echocardiography for assessing valve motion and timing and in obstetrics is used to document the presence of fetal heart pulsations, particularly in early/embryonic stages when the use of Doppler is not recommended because of potential harm.

Doppler Mode

The Doppler principle is applied to evaluate venous and arterial systems, cardiology and perfusion within an organ of interest. There are four types of Doppler ultrasound techniques in common use:

- *Continuous wave (CW) Doppler*: The transducer has two crystals, one transmits the pulse at a known frequency whilst the other simultaneously receives the returning echoes and records their frequencies. The difference between the transmitted and received frequencies is

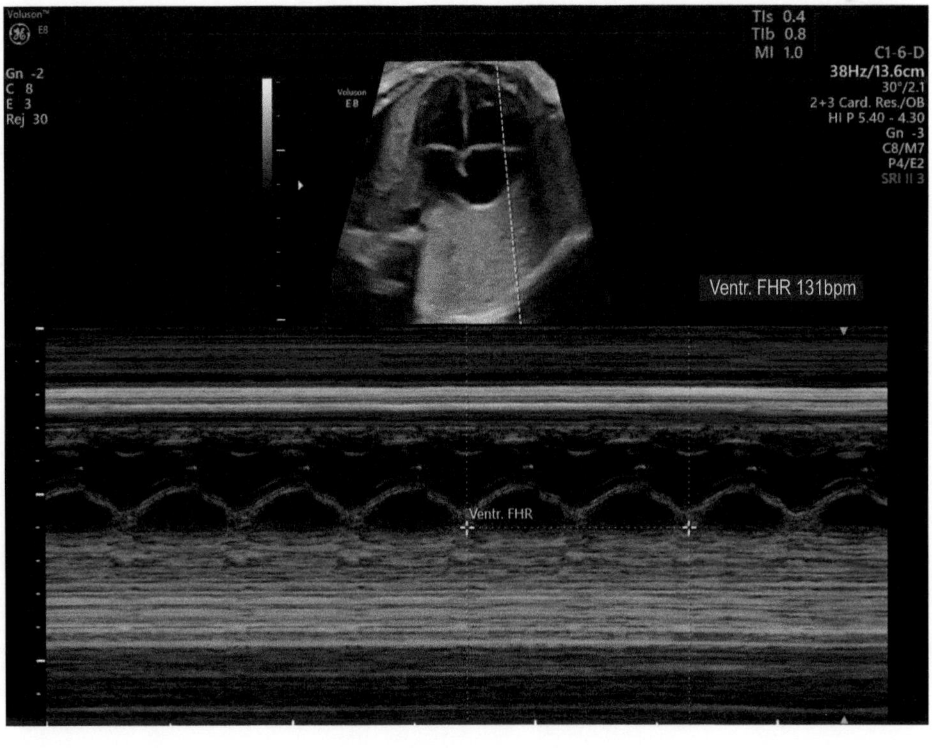

Fig. 29.3 Fetal heart with M-mode trace. (Used with permission of GE Healthcare. Voluson is a trademark of GE Healthcare.)

called the 'Doppler shift'. CW Doppler detects blood flow but does not give any other information such as depth of the vessel, or the direction and velocity of the flow.

- *Pulsed wave (PW) or spectral Doppler* (Fig. 29.4). PW Doppler allows the collection of signals from a specific area of the body. The operator uses 2D imaging to select the vessel to be assessed and a 'sample volume' is investigated.
- *Colour/Duplex Doppler*. Generally used when additional information is required, such as a pattern of flow within a conventional 2D image, e.g. perfusion of a specific organ, neovascularity, the direction of blood flow, or to highlight regions of interest such as jets and stenoses. The 2D image is used to identify the structure to be assessed and 'colour' is usually a push button control with the colour image superimposed on the 2D image.
- A colour box (sample volume) is placed over the region of interest, the resultant flow is colour coded and is calculated by positive Doppler shift (red) for flow towards the transducer and negative Doppler shift (blue) for flow away from the transducer. There may also be shades of orange and yellow, either where there is turbulent flow or the Doppler settings on the ultrasound equipment are not set correctly. Because the image produced is the result of both 2D and colour Doppler imaging, it is also known as duplex imaging.
- *Power Doppler*: Power Doppler maps the magnitude of the Doppler signal rather than the Doppler shift. Duplex imaging is used to superimpose a colour box onto the 2D image, the resultant colour image is in shades of yellow, orange and red, depending on the strength of the Doppler signal. This imaging mode is sensitive and therefore useful in detecting slow flow and flow through smaller vessels; however, unlike colour Doppler imaging there is no information on the direction of blood flow; and because of its sensitivity it is prone to motion artefact.

The use of Doppler ultrasound requires a good knowledge base as there are many things that can affect the quality and therefore have an impact on patient management. Doppler should never be performed without the relevant competencies.

Harmonic Mode (Fig. 29.5)

The physics behind harmonic imaging is complex; it involves the use of resonant properties of tissue to improve image quality by removing some of the artefacts. Instead of the transducer 'listening' for the returning pulse which has the same frequency as the transmitted wave, when the frequency is low (and therefore the penetrative ability of the wave is greater), the frequencies that can be detected by the 'broad bandwidth' transducer are multiples of the

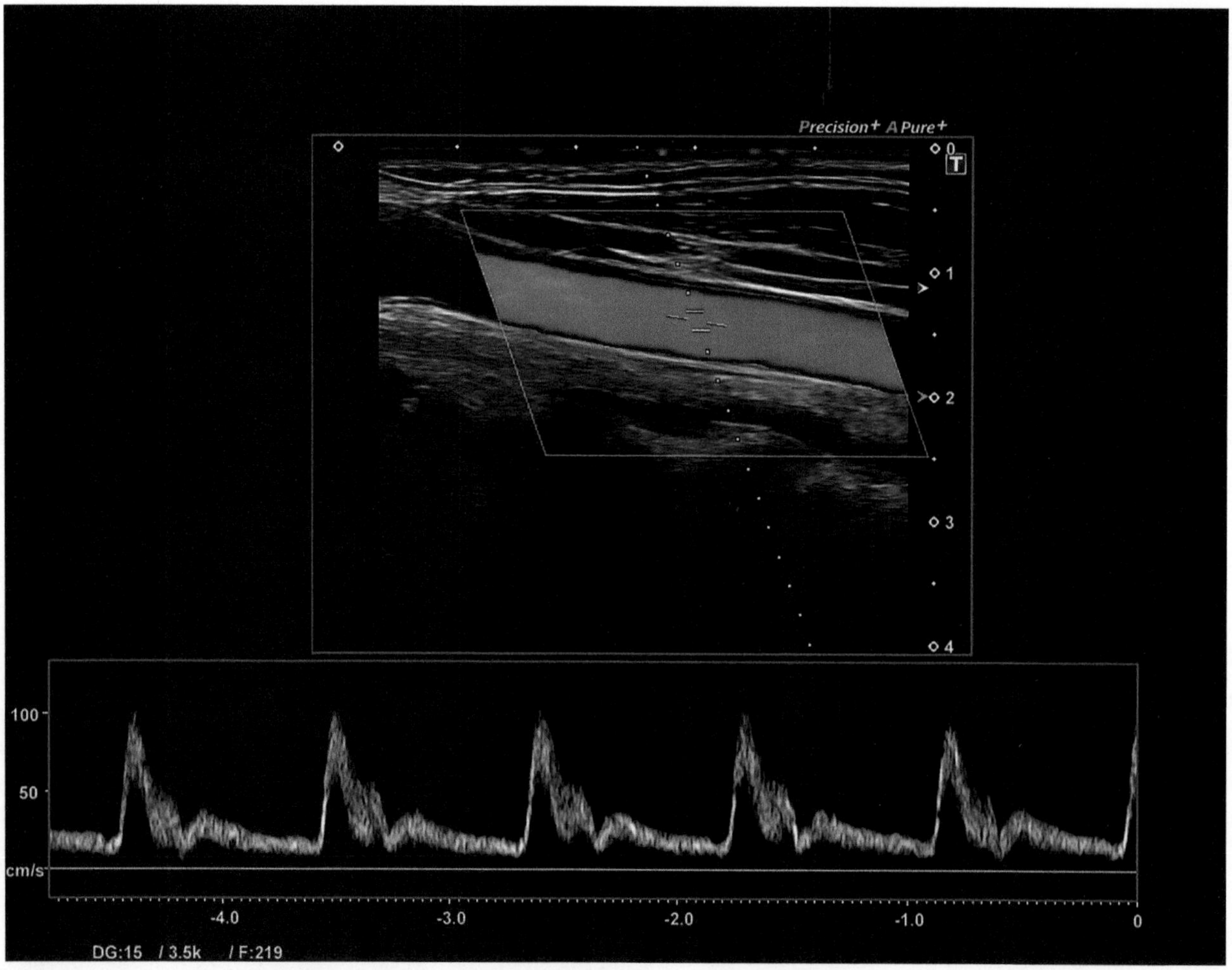

Fig. 29.4 Carotid with pulsed wave Doppler. (Reproduced with permission from Canon Medical Systems.)

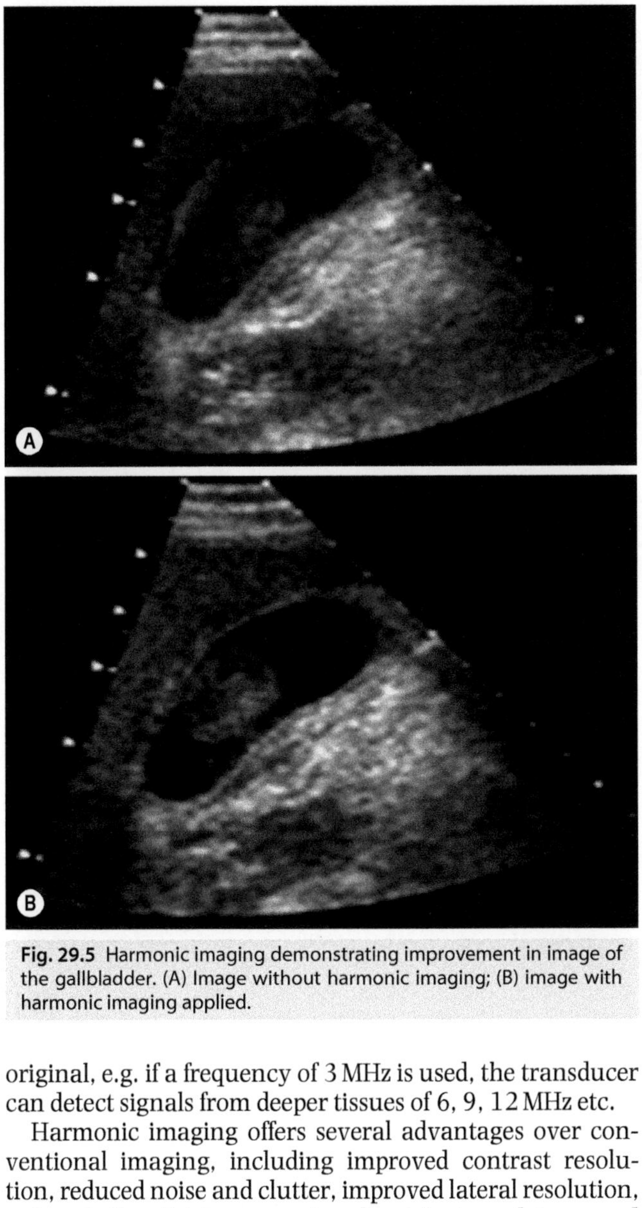

Fig. 29.5 Harmonic imaging demonstrating improvement in image of the gallbladder. (A) Image without harmonic imaging; (B) image with harmonic imaging applied.

original, e.g. if a frequency of 3 MHz is used, the transducer can detect signals from deeper tissues of 6, 9, 12 MHz etc.

Harmonic imaging offers several advantages over conventional imaging, including improved contrast resolution, reduced noise and clutter, improved lateral resolution, reduced slice thickness, reduced artefacts and improved signal-to-noise ratio. In general, harmonic imaging is useful when examining deeper structures and its use is recommended when scanning obese patients.[8]

Compound Imaging

In conventional imaging the tissue is insonated from one direction, but in compound imaging multiple beams from different angles are used to interrogate the tissue and a single 'composite' image is produced in real time.

Compound imaging improves image quality by reducing acoustic artefacts such as 'speckle' (caused by coherent wave interference), 'clutter' (which can result from side lobes and reverberations) and noise. Applications include imaging of the breast, peripheral blood vessels and musculoskeletal injuries.[9,10]

Extended Field of View (EFOV) (Fig. 29.6)

Most equipment manufacturers offer EFOV on their machines but will each have their own name for it. The advantage of EFOV is that it can produce spatially

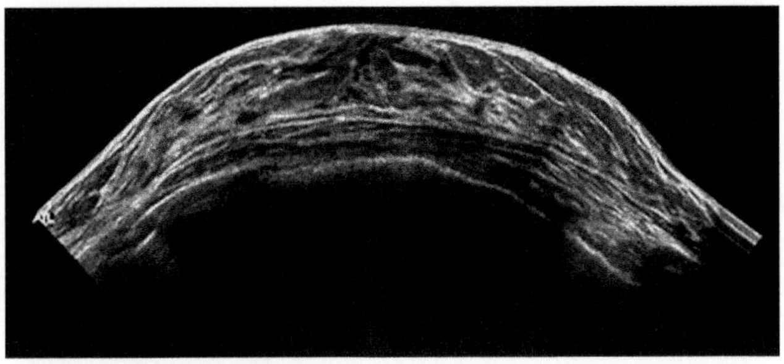

Fig. 29.6 EFOV – scan of breast. (Reproduced with permission from Philips Medical Systems.)

accurate images of larger organs or pathology in one single 'panoramic' image. The basic premise is that as the transducer moves across the skin surface, the computer within the machine recognises subtle differences between each successive frame and registers them, creating the image.

EFOV is especially useful for superficial organs such as the thyroid or breast, and for musculoskeletal imaging, where the entire length of a muscle and surrounding organs can be visualised. Because EFOV relies on the movement of the probe to generate the image, it is of no use in scanning anything with inherent movement, such as a fetus.[10]

Very High-Frequency Imaging and Intracavity Transducers

Miniature transducers offering very high-resolution imaging at frequencies ranging from 20 to 100 MHz can be placed within cavities to give high-resolution images of structures close to the cavity walls; examples of applications include transurethral, transoesophageal and intravascular scanning.[10]

Elastography

Elastography is an ultrasound technique for assessing the relative elastic properties of soft tissue.

Different tissue types have different elasticity (the ability of the tissue to resume its original shape or size after a force has been applied and then removed) and some disease processes/pathologies affect change in the elasticity of tissues. This change in elasticity can be detected non-invasively by using ultrasound elastography.

Elastography is commonly used to assess liver fibrosis, the presence of which causes the liver to be stiffer, i.e. less elastic. It is also commonly used in the differentiation of benign and malignant breast lesions and in assessment of the thyroid and prostate glands, and in renal, lymph node and some musculoskeletal applications.

There are two main types of elastography in practice:

- *Strain/compression elastography*: The first type of elastography to be introduced, this is a qualitative technique that provides information between the relative stiffness of one tissue compared to another by compressing tissue with the ultrasound transducer. Assessing the stiffness of a tissue to check for pathology has been done by doctors for centuries, e.g. palpating the abdomen for masses.
- *Shear wave elastography* (Fig. 29.7): Shear wave elastography (SWE) is a quantitative method providing an

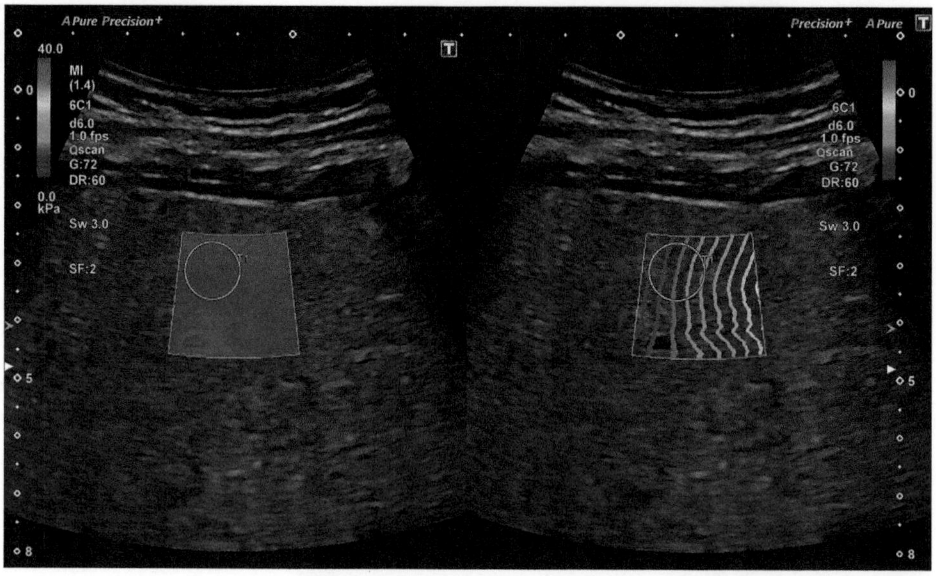

Fig. 29.7 Normal liver with shearwave. (Reproduced with permission from Canon Medical Systems.)

estimated value of predicted stiffness. This is used for differentiating between benign and malignant tumours. Low-frequency (100–500 Hz), low-amplitude shear waves (a transverse wave that occurs when tissue is subjected to a change in shape without a change in volume) are transmitted into tissue and the resultant vibration is detected using colour Doppler. When a discrete hard mass, such as a tumour, is present in a region of soft tissue, a decrease in the vibration amplitude will occur at its location. SWE is commonly used in the assessment of liver fibrosis, although different methods used by equipment manufacturers mean that results are often not transferable across different makes of machine.[10] The use of SWE frequently negates the need for liver biopsy and so is much better tolerated by the patient and also provides cost savings.

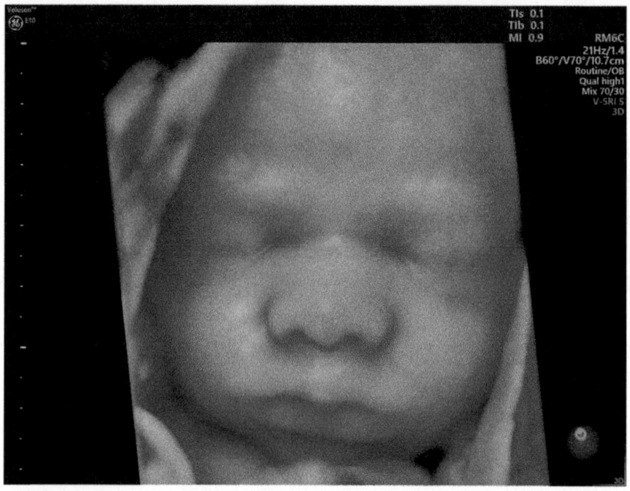

Fig. 29.8 3D fetal face at 31 weeks. (Used with permission of GE Healthcare. Voluson is a trademark of GE Healthcare.)

3D and 4D Ultrasound Imaging (Fig. 29.8)

The use of 3D ultrasound imaging is perhaps best known for its use in obstetrics for the provision of keepsake or 'souvenir' scans where parents can see images of their unborn baby in three dimensions. However, 3D ultrasound is an excellent adjunct to 2D ultrasound and is used in a number of applications, including gynaecology, obstetrics, breast, prostate and cardiology.

4D ultrasound is also known as 'real-time 3D ultrasound'. The basic concept is that the ultrasound equipment can acquire and display the 3D datasets with their multiplanar reformations and renderings in real time. However, 3D or 4D can only build on the 2D images, therefore the limitations and artefacts that affect 2D imaging, such as presence of gas and overlying structures, will also affect the quality of the 3D and 4D imaging.

3D probes are generally larger and heavier than 2D probes and as such there is a greater risk of the user suffering a work-related musculoskeletal injury. With this in mind, ultrasound equipment manufacturers work continuously to reduce this risk when developing their machines.

Contrast-Enhanced Ultrasound (CEUS) (Fig. 29.9)

The use of contrast media has enhanced the performance of some aspects of ultrasound imaging.

Ultrasound microbubble contrast agents are smaller than the mean diameter of a red blood cell, non-toxic, injectable intravenously, capable of crossing the pulmonary capillary bed after a peripheral injection, and stable enough to achieve enhancement for the duration of the examination.

CEUS is well known for use in liver disease,[11] but is now also used in other applications.[12,13]

The most common uses of liver CEUS are to characterise liver lesions, to detect metastases and to identify soft tissue damage in the cases of trauma. Non-liver applications include classification of renal cysts, sentinel node assessment for breast cancer patients and hysterosalpingo-contrast-sonography (HyCoSy) for tubal patency testing. Other applications include the spleen, gastrointestinal tract, prostate and scrotum.

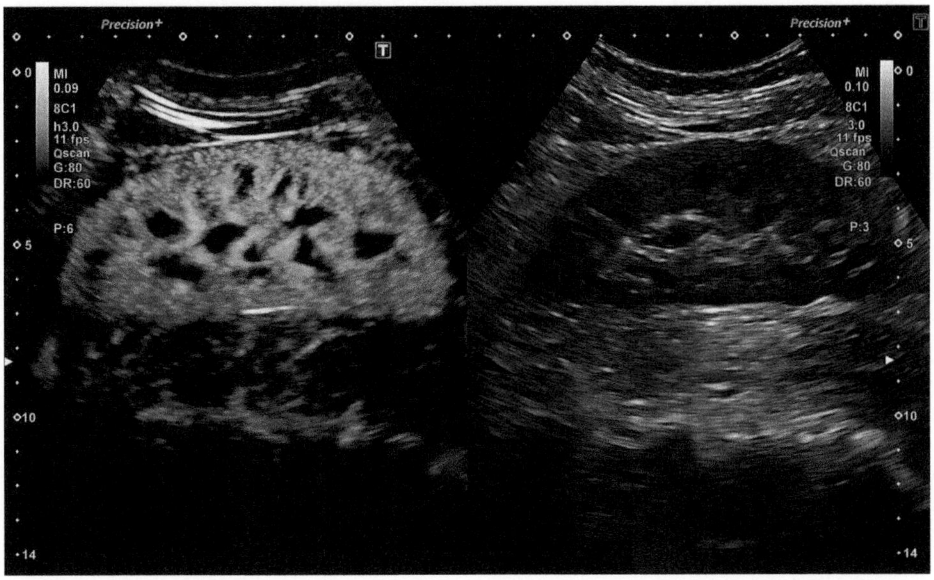

Fig. 29.9 **CEUS of the kidney.** (Reproduced with permission from Canon Medical Systems.)

Ultrasound Safety

Ultrasound is now accepted as being of considerable diagnostic value. There is no evidence that diagnostic ultrasound has produced any harm to patients in the time it has been in regular use in medical practice. However, the acoustic output of modern equipment is generally much greater than that of the early equipment and, in view of the continuing progress in equipment design and applications, outputs may be expected to continue to be subject to change. Also, investigations into the possibility of subtle or transient effects are still at an early stage. Consequently, diagnostic ultrasound can only be considered safe if used prudently.[11]

There are two groups to consider when discussing ultrasound safety – the patient and the operator.

PATIENT

Ultrasound has been used in medicine for decades and whilst there is no evidence that it has caused harm, it is important that users do their utmost to protect patients from any possible effects. More detail on ultrasound safety than is covered here can be found via BMUS.[14]

All machines display two safety indices during scanning: thermal and mechanical.

- *Thermal effect*: There can be a localised rise in tissue temperature due to the ultrasound energy being absorbed and converted into heat. This effect is displayed on the ultrasound monitor as a thermal index (TI); it is there to guide the operator of the potential for tissue heating. For example, a TI of 1 indicates a temperature rise of 1 °C. This is particularly important in obstetric scanning during development of the embryo and fetus. Temperature rises >1.5 °C may cause harm and the longer an embryo is exposed, the greater the risk of harm.
- *Mechanical (non-thermal) effect*: This can occur in the presence of very high ultrasound pressures, causing oscillation of microbubbles – cavitation, which can result in biological damage to tissue cells. The likelihood of cavitation occurring is related to the peak pressure and is referred to as the mechanical index (MI). Given that cavitation is the excitation of gas bubbles, the areas most at risk of this kind of damage are those where gas pockets occur, e.g. lung and bowel. The likelihood, however, is low if the MI is kept <0.3.[11] For all ultrasound imaging techniques, prudent use is advised.

The modes used during scanning have different inherent safety risks, for example, pulsed Doppler and colour Doppler imaging, with a narrow sample volume, carry a higher risk of thermal effects than a conventional 2D scanning examination, and the use of contrast agents can increase the potential for cavitation.

Infection Prevention and Control (IPC)

Hand hygiene before and after each patient contact is important in preventing the spread of disease, as is the correct sterilisation/disinfection of all equipment that comes into contact with either the patient or the operator. IPC is the responsibility of everyone; it is essential that all gel is removed from the probe and its cable after scanning a patient. It is good practice to let a patient see the cleaning of the probe and the use of hand gel before the start of the examination. Couch roll must be changed between patients and couches wiped down with appropriate clinical wipes. Departments will have local IPC policies that must be followed to reduce the risk to patients. There are a number of systems commercially available for the appropriate cleansing of equipment (particularly intracavity probes) and manufacturers provide details of which are recommended for their equipment.

Governance

Ultrasound scans should only be performed when there is a perceived benefit to the patient and should be undertaken by appropriately trained staff using equipment suitable for the case mix.

Reports should be written as soon after the examination as possible, by the person performing the scan, and support must be available for operators to seek advice where there are equivocal findings.

Staff should be aware of and supported in their role in safeguarding, and should undergo regular update, continuing professional development (CPD) and audit of practice. There should be processes in place to ensure equipment is regularly serviced and undergoes quality assurance testing. Policies should be reviewed regularly and always when there is new guidance published by the relevant bodies.

Consent

To ensure the patient is actively involved in their own care, they must be given information in a format they can understand so they can make informed decisions. Consent must be obtained prior to any scan, and for it to be valid the patient must be given information about the benefits and risks, limitations and how results will be imparted. If, for example, a pregnant woman does not wish to be told if a problem is identified with her baby during an ultrasound scan, she should be advised that any abnormalities will be documented and for this reason, she should consider declining the scan to be certain she will not inadvertently discover that an abnormality has been detected. Conversations had and decisions made must be documented in the patient notes.

OPERATOR

There are many factors that have the potential to cause harm to sonographers and there are numerous articles citing these, and advice from professional bodies and others.[6,7,15] Although the majority of papers and advice are centred on the physical impact of ultrasound scanning on sonographers, consideration must also be given to the mental well-being of staff. Delivering bad news can cause distress. Workload and expectations that do not give sufficient time to undertake a scan thoroughly can cause stress. Both the employer and the employee have a duty of care to reduce the risk of injury (mental and physical).

Employers must ensure that the working conditions are the best they can be, including such issues as environment, equipment, case load and type, workload and policies that support staff.

The rising levels of patient obesity are of increasing concern and there is advice available on management of the high BMI patient.[7,11]

Equipment manufacturers consider ergonomics in equipment design; additional ancillary equipment, e.g. saddle seats, should be made available. Employees have a duty of care to look after themselves and follow the guidance and advice issued to them in the workplace. Employees should report any concerns they have about their own health and safety and that of colleagues to enable the employer to respond as required.

Clinical Applications

Ultrasound is constantly evolving and parts of the body which even 15 years ago were difficult to assess, such as the bowel and joints, are now scanned routinely. The creation of 'specialist' training courses has enabled role extension in physiotherapy and midwifery, the advent of the AAA screening programme, FAST and PoCUS scanning and RCR guidelines on training for non-radiologist physicians have all contributed to the growth in the use of ultrasound.

SCANNING TECHNIQUE

All sonographers develop their own way of obtaining the information needed from a scan to enable interpretation and a clear and succinct report of findings to be written; it is essential that the method applied is systematic and thorough.

Prior to calling a patient into the room, it is incumbent on the sonographer to:

- Read the referral form so as to understand the reason for the scan and to determine if the patient has any needs, e.g. relating to language or mobility issues and to review previous images and reports.
- Confirm the patient's identity in accordance with protocol but should, as a minimum, include full name and date of birth. It is sensible to check this again when entering patient details on to the ultrasound system or before selecting the patient from the electronic work list.
- Introduce themselves and any colleagues in the room and the status of those present.
- Explain the scanning procedure to the patient in a way in which they can understand, including the fact that the patient may be required to hold their breath or to position themselves differently as the examination progresses.
- Explain the limitations, risks and benefits of the examination/procedure to the patient.
- Answer any questions the patient may have concerning the examination/procedure.
- Obtain valid informed consent from the patient, or their carer where necessary/appropriate, taking into account their capacity to understand.
- Ensure that the patient has understood any literature pertaining to the appointment which they may have been given and followed any instructions, e.g. fast or fill their bladder, but consider that it may be possible to undertake a satisfactory examination even if they have not followed the instructions.
- Allow the patient privacy to prepare themselves for the examination and be mindful of the possible need for a chaperone.
- Take a clinical history and not just rely on the information given on the referral form. Patients often wait some weeks from referral to appointment and any additional information regarding a change in or worsening or lessening of symptoms or results of blood tests for example can be useful.
- Communicate with the patient throughout the scan, even if only to confirm that they are comfortable or to advise how much longer the scan might take.
- Undertake the scan competently and thoroughly, being certain to address the clinical question and where necessary extend the scan according to local protocol.
- Allow the patient privacy to remove the gel and dress themselves.
- Explain to the patient the next step in their pathway, e.g. when and how they should get the results.

THE EXAMINATION

Often a negative, i.e. normal, ultrasound scan is as useful as a scan report detailing abnormal findings. This is because ultrasound is often the first form of imaging requested and as there are frequently multiple differential diagnoses for a patient's symptoms, the exclusion of pathology is very useful to the referrer and guides them towards other diagnoses/investigations.

No matter what the examination to be performed, the area must be exposed to allow access and consideration must be given to the patient's privacy and dignity and if they need to wear a hospital gown or simply be given sufficient paper roll to protect their garments, as ultrasound gel is always used.

The correct probe and equipment 'preset' is chosen and the sonographer optimises the image at the commencement and then throughout the scan to facilitate optimum visualisation.

Images archived are only a representation of the scan performed and are not proof absolute that organs have been examined in their entirety; they can, however, be used to determine if a scan has been undertaken with due care and attention. For audit purposes or in the event a claim is made that a practitioner has 'missed' pathology, a retrospective assessment of the images archived and, if necessary, multiple scans performed by the member of staff can demonstrate trends and patterns of scanning which can either work for or against the practitioner. When undertaking a review of a practitioner, things such as image quality, time taken to perform the scan, adherence to protocol, manipulation of machine controls, report written correlating with images archived re. findings and measurements, are all considered.

The following are examples of commonly requested ultrasound examinations and some common indications. Examinations, indications and pathology discussed are not exclusive and are meant as a guide only.

UPPER ABDOMEN

The patient is usually required to fast for 4—6 hours prior to the scan to facilitate visualisation of the gallbladder and to minimise bowel gas.

Organs are not routinely scanned in isolation. A referral stating '? gallstones' would not result in only the gallbladder being scanned, although some departments will have local rules where patients attend for repeat scans of a known disease process which allow for organ-specific scanning.

A typical upper abdominal scan will include assessment of the liver, gallbladder, bile ducts, pancreas, kidneys, spleen and the associated vasculature; abdominal aorta, IVC, para-aortic regions; and both hemidiaphragms. It is usual to turn the patient into decubitus and oblique positions and position the probe both sub- and intercostally to ensure full visualisation of the upper abdominal organs.

Common clinical indications include:

- RUQ (right upper quadrant) pain
- Abnormal blood test results, e.g. LFTs (liver function tests)
- Confirm/exclude gallstones/renal calculi/organomegaly
- Palpable upper abdominal mass
- Hypertension
- Weight loss
- General malaise
- Jaundice

All the organs should be assessed in long and transverse axis (as a minimum) and images evidencing this archived. An understanding of normal anatomy and variants as well as age-related changes should be understood.

Additional images should evidence pathology identified or suspected and the presence of any free fluid or masses.

Measurements are useful, particularly if an organ is out of the normal range.

Because ultrasound is in real time, it can only show what is happening at the time of the scan, it cannot predict what organs will look like in the future or how they looked in the past.

Liver (Fig. 29.10)

The size of the liver means that it must often be examined with the patient in different positions (e.g. supine, decubitus) and from a subcostal or intercostal approach to ensure the whole of the organ is visualised.

Assessment of the liver should include its shape, size, contour and ultrasound characteristics.

The liver parenchyma is normally homogeneous and of a similar reflectivity (isoechoic) to the renal cortex. The liver contour/outline should be smooth and this is often best confirmed using a high-frequency probe. The vasculature (portal venous, hepatic venous and arterial supply), ductal system and porta hepatis should all be assessed – the extent is determined by known or suspected pathology.

Focal lesions, benign and malignant, are usually readily demonstrated and whilst some have very distinctive characteristics and are easy to identify, others may need further imaging to determine their nature.

Many pathophysiological processes can lead to diffuse parenchymal liver diseases and the end-result of all chronic liver diseases (CLD) is healing by fibrosis and regeneration.[16]

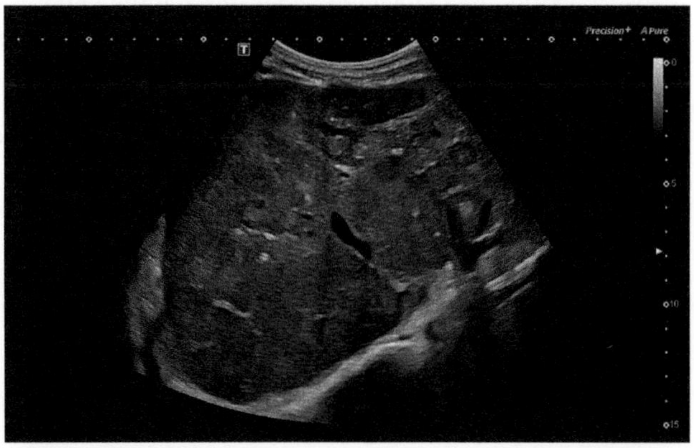

Fig. 29.10 Liver metastases. (Reproduced with permission from Canon Medical Systems.)

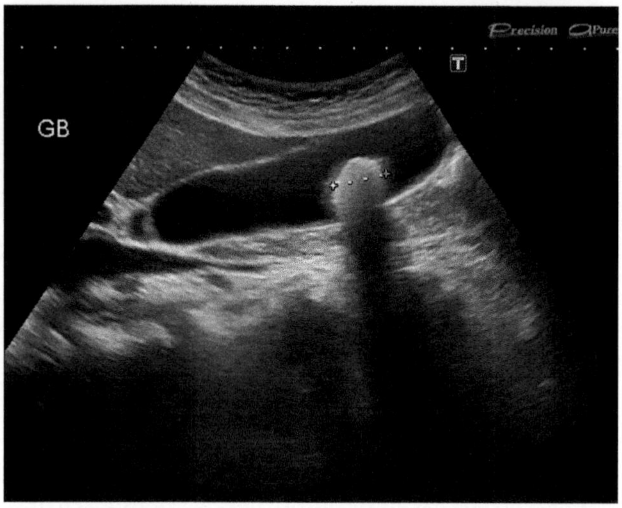

Fig. 29.11 Gallbladder demonstrating calculus.

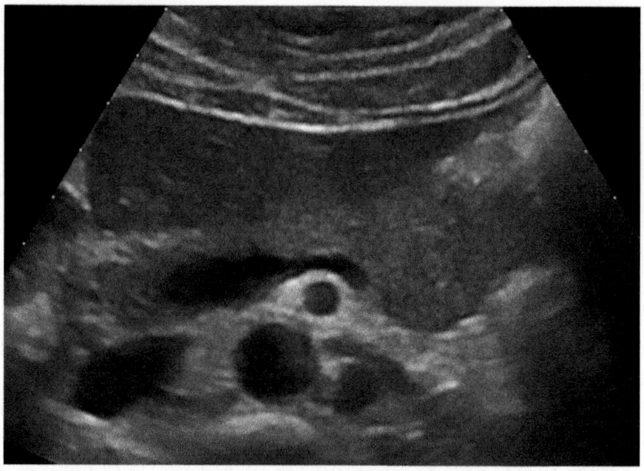

Fig. 29.12 Midline transverse pancreas with left lobe liver anteriorly, acting as a transonic window. (Reproduced with permission from JB Imaging.)

Ultrasound is good in detecting fatty change (hepatic steatosis) in the liver, the parenchyma becomes echobright when compared to the renal cortex, but it is non-specific and so CT, MR and elastography are widely used.

Gallbladder and Biliary Tree (Fig. 29.11)

The gallbladder usually lies under the right lobe of the liver. Its size and shape vary and the position of the fundus often varies with patient position and body habitus.

Because of the number of variants, it is important to assess the gallbladder with the patient in different positions, including erect – a good tip is to ask the patient to sit up at the end of the examination and have a look one last time at the gallbladder. If there are folds or a phrygian cap, or the neck has a 'J' shape, small stones can become apparent when the patient is moved into a different position.

Gallstones are one of the most common causes of upper abdominal pain and taking a clinical history is useful. On questioning, patients often report post prandial pain/sickness, lighter stools and darker urine and symptoms which are intermittent (the patient can be asymptomatic for months) and do not seem to follow a particular pattern.

It is important to assess the gallbladder wall thickness to determine if there is cholecystitis present as gallstones are often asymptomatic and may have nothing to do with the reason the patient attended. It can be useful to use the probe to gently press the gallbladder to see if the patient is tender, an indicator that you may have found the cause of the patient's pain. If there is tenderness on palpation this is known as a positive Murphy's sign.

There are three reasons why a gallbladder may not be seen:

- It is absent (either through surgical removal or, rarely, it is congenitally absent)
- The patient has not fasted and the gallbladder is contracted
- The gallbladder is diseased and contracted

The presence of dilated intra- and extrahepatic ducts suggests a diagnosis of surgical jaundice (caused by stones or tumours for example) as distinct from medical jaundice (caused by a form of liver disease) when the ducts appear essentially normal. The level of obstruction can often be clearly demonstrated by the level at which the ducts or gallbladder are seen to be normal. For example, a dilated common hepatic duct and intrahepatic ducts with a normal or small gallbladder and common bile duct would suggest a high obstruction of the cystic duct or above, while a fully dilated biliary system would indicate an obstruction at the lower end of the bile duct.

The common bile duct can be seen lying anteriorly to the portal vein and ideally should be followed to the pancreatic head, but the distal portion is often quite difficult to see owing to the gas-filled duodenum. The common duct should have a maximum diameter of 6 mm but this can vary with age and in post-cholecystectomy patients. The intrahepatic ducts should be checked – intrahepatic duct dilatation is always abnormal; likewise, duct wall thickening is abnormal.[17]

Pancreas (Fig. 29.12)

The pancreas can be notoriously difficult to see in its entirety on ultrasound and consequently early disease can be missed; i.e., there is a high false-negative rate. For this reason, CT and MR are the imaging modalities of choice where pancreatic disease is suspected.

In an abdominal ultrasound examination for vague symptoms such as epigastric pain, attempts should be made to visualise the whole pancreas, but if this is not possible then the report should reflect this. To report that 'the pancreas appears/is normal' when it has not been seen in its entirety (head/uncinate process, neck, body and tail) is misleading.

The pancreas is best visualised with the patient supine and the probe in the transverse position just below the xiphisternum, using the left lobe of the liver as a transonic 'window'. The pancreas must be examined in all planes, not just in its long axis.

In some cases asking the patient to drink water to fill the stomach so as to create an acoustic window in the gastric antrum through which the pancreatic tail can be visualised is helpful.

As well as the pancreas itself, the pancreatic duct and distal portion of the common bile duct and the associated vasculature (coeliac axis, superior mesenteric artery, portal veins and splenic and superior mesenteric veins) should be assessed.

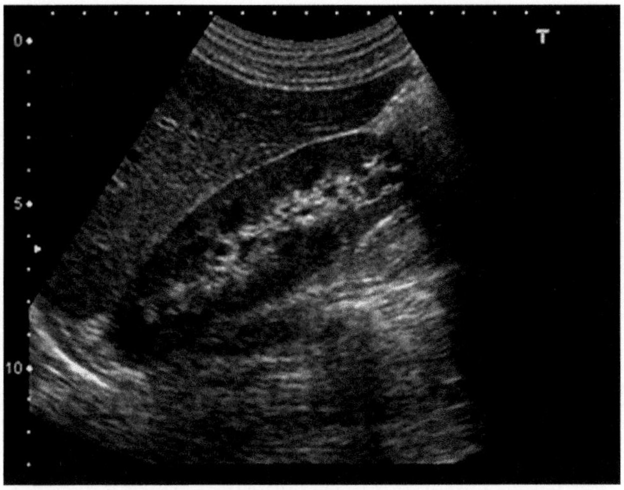

Fig. 29.13 Longitudinal view of right kidney. (Reproduced with permission from Toshiba Medical Systems Ltd.)

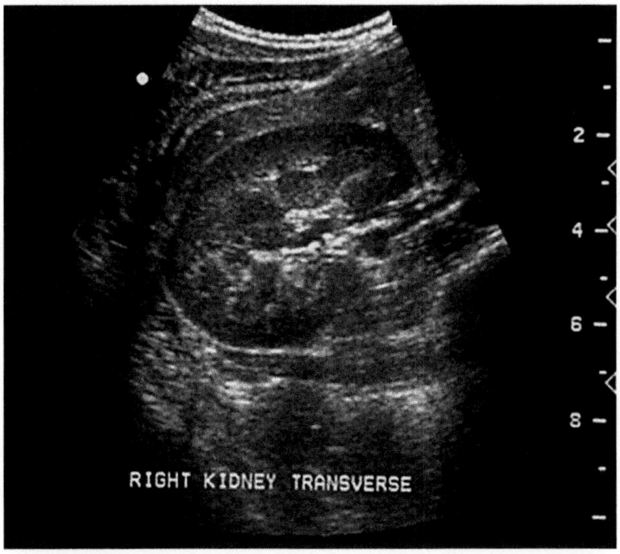

Fig. 29.14 Transverse view of right kidney. (Reproduced with permission from Philips Medical Systems.)

Spleen

Common indications for examination of the spleen are:

- Palpable mass LUQ (left upper quadrant)
- Abnormal blood results, e.g. white cell count, anaemia, low platelets
- Fatigue
- Trauma

The spleen is usually scanned as part of the whole upper abdominal examination. Ultrasound can be used to measure the size of the spleen but because there is such a wide variation of 'normal' (5–12 cm), it is important to know the local protocol for exactly how to measure it so that when monitoring disease processes the same parameters are used. It should measure about the same as the, assumed normal, left kidney.

If there is splenomegaly, the portal and hepatic veins should be assessed with Doppler (as well as the splenic vasculature).

In cases of trauma, ultrasound is invaluable for detecting haematoma; it can detect splenic lacerations and ruptures, and because of its portability is often the first imaging used (FAST). Contrast-enhanced CT is, however, the gold standard in splenic trauma imaging.

Solitary and multiple, benign and malignant lesions can be seen on ultrasound; Hodgkin's and non-Hodgkin's lymphoma are the commonest splenic malignancies.[18]

URINARY SYSTEM, INCLUDING PROSTATE GLAND (FIGS 29.13, 29.14)

Common indications for examination of the urinary tract as a whole are:

- Urinary tract infection (UTI)
- Haematuria
- Acute or chronic kidney injury – AKI (previously known as renal failure)
- Loin pain
- Family history of polycystic kidney disease
- Urinary retention/reduced urinary output
- Poor stream/dribbling/nocturia
- Frequency/urgency

The kidneys are included in an upper abdominal scan but if the urinary tract as a whole is to be assessed (i.e. if the patient presents with renal tract symptoms) then the patient will need a full bladder, although fluid loading should be avoided in the case of acute kidney injury and local protocol should be observed. The presence, location and size of the kidneys are easily determined on ultrasound and if they are not seen in their 'usual' place – posterior upper abdomen, right below the liver, left below the spleen – then the pelvis should be scanned as pelvic kidneys are a common finding.

Normal variants can be the cause of some symptoms, for example duplex or horseshoe kidneys can have a predisposition to UTI.

In cases of haematuria (microscopic or macroscopic), ultrasound can be part of a dedicated haematuria pathway or 'one stop' clinic with the patient also having a cystoscopy. In the case of unexplained macroscopic haematuria, a CT scan may also be performed and CT can be helpful in excluding abnormality where normal variants such as splenic hump or prominent columns of Bertin can sometimes mimic tumours.

Ultrasound is excellent in assessing the presence of hydronephrosis and can be useful in determining the cause; e.g. renal calculi or ureteric obstruction. The presence or absence of ureteric jets can also be easily demonstrated and can help with the diagnosis.

Renal cysts are very common and are usually incidental findings with the incidence increasing with age over the age of 50. Simple renal cysts are very different to polycystic kidney disease, which is a genetic condition with variable complications.

Ultrasound can clearly demonstrate the bladder wall (if the bladder is distended with urine), and any inherent pathology such as tumours (fixed irregular masses), calculi or foreign bodies. Ultrasound is useful in being able to measure the bladder wall thickness when distended and when empty, and can demonstrate any residual volume after micturition. Transitional cell carcinomas (the most common bladder tumour) can be detected along the posterior wall near the trigone but very small tumours may not be seen. Bladder diverticula and ureteroceles are easily detected by ultrasound.

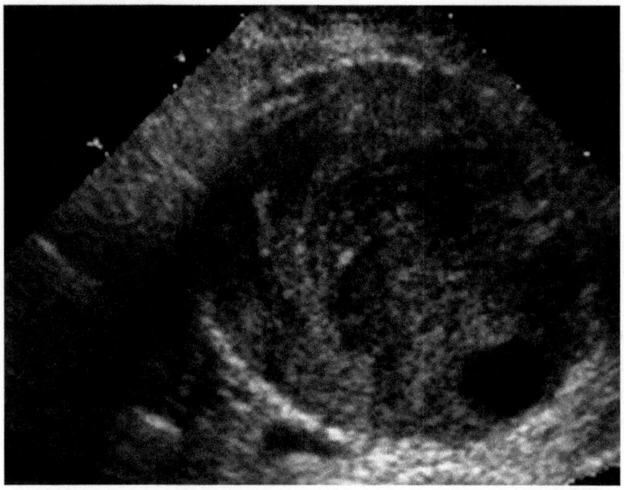

Fig. 29.15 Transverse section of abdominal aortic aneurysm (AAA).

Prostate enlargement, a common condition in older men, can be seen by scanning transabdominally. Scanning in this way will give an indication of the size of the prostate, its overall shape and reflectivity and whether calcification is present. The most common cause of prostate enlargement is due to benign prostatic hypertrophy (BPH).

Transrectal sonography of the prostate gives more detail and is used where biopsy is deemed necessary. Other imaging modalities, such as CT, MR, mpMR (multi-parametric MR) and nuclear medicine, are used in the TNM (Tumour, Node, Metastasis) staging of prostate cancer.

AORTA AND INFERIOR VENA CAVA (IVC) (FIG. 29.15)

Ultrasound is used to scan both the great vessels in the abdomen. The IVC is examined with ultrasound and colour Doppler in cases of newly found renal tumours and suspected IVC thrombosis.

In April 2009 the roll-out of a national screening programme in England (2012 in Scotland and Northern Ireland, 2013 in Wales) for abdominal aortic aneurysm (AAA) began, its aim being to reduce deaths from AAA by early detection. The programme invites all eligible men for screening by ultrasound in the year they turn 65, offering either treatment or monitoring, depending on the size of any aneurysm found.[19]

Once screened, men will be placed on a pathway based on the results of their scan:

- The aorta has a diameter of less than 3 cm: No aneurysm has been detected. The patient is informed of the result and will not require any further scans.
- The aorta has a diameter of between 3 and 4.4 cm: Patients with a small aneurysm do not need treatment but are invited to have follow-up scans at 12 months.
- The aorta has a diameter 4.5–5.5 cm: this is classed as a medium AAA and patients have a repeat scan every 3 months for monitoring purposes.
- The aorta has a diameter of 5.5 cm or above: The patient is referred to a vascular surgeon within 2 weeks to discuss treatment options.

AAA screening is undertaken by technicians who have undergone formal training in their role and who are supported and mentored by qualified sonographers and/or vascular technologists.

Abdominal aortic aneurysms are easily detected on ultrasound, and although there is a national screening programme it is still often detected outside of this, for example when a patient attends for an unrelated ultrasound scan.

ALIMENTARY CANAL

Ultrasound plays an integral part in the diagnosis and monitoring of conditions such as acute appendicitis, diverticulitis and inflammatory bowel diseases; and in the diagnosis of pyloric stenosis and intussusception in paediatrics.

An overall initial assessment of the bowel should be made using a curvilinear probe as abnormal bowel is easier to see on ultrasound than normal bowel. Masses, and dilated bowel loops with gas/faeces displaced are easy to detect. For detailed assessment of the bowel wall, linear array probes (high frequency) are required.

Where possible, the patient should be fasted for 6 hours to reduce bowel gas in the small intestine and scanning with the patient in the left decubitus position means that some bowel loops will be displaced allowing access to the appendix. The normal appendix can be difficult to see but if there is the suspicion of acute appendicitis and a normal appendix is not seen then a CT scan should be considered.

Thickening of the bowel wall is the most common feature identified on ultrasound.[11] Thickening of the wall can be due to a variety of reasons, e.g. oedema, tumour, inflammation; this can cause narrowing of the lumen and reduced or absent peristalsis.

Endoscopic ultrasound (EUS) is used in the detection of upper gastrointestinal malignancies, including in the oesophagus, stomach, gallbladder, extrahepatic bile ducts and pancreas and in the staging of oesophageal, gastric and pancreatic cancers. The procedure allows for biopsies to be taken to facilitate diagnosis.

LYMPH NODES

Lymph node enlargement can be demonstrated with ultrasound, depending on location and size of the nodes. Enlarged lymph nodes can often be seen in the upper abdomen, para-aortic region, neck and axilla. Enlarged lymph nodes are often the cause of a 'palpable lump', and taking a history from the patient is useful in these instances.

ADULT HEAD AND NECK (FIG. 29.16)

In many departments ultrasound assessment of the head and neck has evolved into a specialist role as, depending on the findings, the scan may extend beyond the region of interest and the whole neck be examined and biopsies undertaken. The main reasons for referral relate to the thyroid gland, lymph nodes and salivary glands.

Having a machine with EFOV capabilities is preferred when assessing the thyroid gland. Common indications are:

- abnormal TFTs (thyroid function tests)
- enlarged thyroid

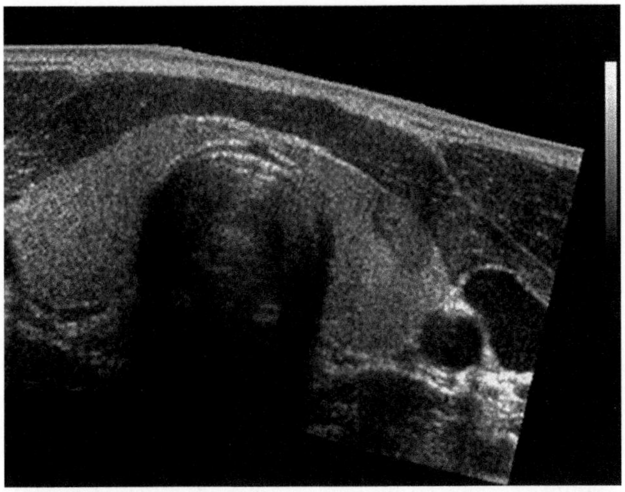

Fig. 29.16 Image of thyroid. (Reproduced with permission from Philips Medical Systems.)

- confirm/exclude multinodular goitre

In the UK, the British Thyroid Association has produced guidelines which support the classification of thyroid masses and it is important that the report describes the features of a lesion and into which category it falls.[20]

NEONATAL HEAD

The portability of ultrasound means that it can be used to scan an infant in a special care baby unit either in or out of an incubator. Using a high frequency probe, the most common approach is through the anterior fontanelle but the posterior fontanelle and mastoid suture can also be used, depending on the anatomy being examined. Consideration must always be given to the potential bio effects of ultrasound, in particular the heating effects at the brain/skull interface and the power should be set as low as possible.[11]

NEONATAL HIP

In the UK, when a newborn baby is suspected of having an unstable hip on clinical examination the baby should be scanned in the first 2 weeks following delivery. If there are known risk factors but the hips appear clinically stable, they should be scanned within 6 weeks.[21]

Each hip is scanned with the baby in a lateral position and the hip is moved and manipulated to assess the depth of acetabulum to determine the degree (if any) of subluxation or dislocation.

BREAST

The use of ultrasound in breast imaging is discussed in Chapter 25.

SUPERFICIAL ORGANS: 'SMALL PARTS'

High-frequency transducers in the region of 7–18 MHz are generally used for small parts imaging because there is, usually, no need for depth penetration.

Testes

Ultrasound is the main imaging modality for the investigation of the scrotum. As with all superficial structures, a linear-array high-frequency probe is required; however, in cases where there is a large scrotal mass, one or both testes may be displaced and it may be necessary to use a lower-frequency probe to find the testicle, which may have been displaced out of the FOV of the higher-frequency transducer. Both testes are assessed and compared; and the bilateral epididymal head, body and tail are scanned. A clinical history is important as previous vasectomy can cause thickening of the epididymis which is not pathological.

Common clinical indications are:

- Palpable lump/mass
- Pain
- Trauma
- Testicular/scrotal enlargement
- Varicoceles
- Infertility

Testicular masses are well seen if they are of a different reflectivity from the main body of the testis. Comparison with the unaffected side on the same image should always be made, because some tumours can infiltrate the whole testis and so there would be no difference in echotexture visible unless direct comparison was made with the contralateral side.

Depending on findings, the ultrasound scan will often require extending to the upper abdomen (testicular or epididymal masses), or the renal tract and aorta if varicoceles are found.[22]

The patient should always be asked to identify the lump to enable the sonographer to scan directly over the area indicated. This has twofold benefits; first, the patient knows that the sonographer has looked at the area of their concern, and second, to ensure that where the sonographer has identified a problem it directly relates to that with which the patient presented and is not an incidental finding.

Epididymal cysts are the most common cause of scrotal lumps in patients presenting for ultrasound, and the patient can be reassured that these are not of clinical significance.

Testicular torsion cannot always be excluded on ultrasound and as torsion is a clinical emergency (to preserve the viability of the testicle) it is often a clinical decision to take the patient for exploratory surgery.

When testicular microlithiasis is identified, the importance of regular review should be stressed to the patient because of the potential risk of malignancy.[23]

Ultrasound is used to confirm the presence of an undescended testis – usually identified in the inguinal canal, but which is important because of the increased risk of testicular cancer in such cases.

MUSCULOSKELETAL

The use of ultrasound in the diagnosis and treatment of musculoskeletal (MSK) problems has become commonplace because it allows a dynamic assessment and ease of comparison with the contralateral side.

Commonly undertaken MSK scans and clinical indications are:

- Shoulder: rotator cuff, pain, reduced range of movement
- Elbow: 'tennis' or 'golfer's' elbow, olecranon bursitis, pain or restricted movement
- Wrist and hand: swelling, synovitis, tendon tears
- Hip: effusion or bursitis
- Knee: bursitis, effusion, popliteal cyst
- Foot and ankle: Morton's neuroma, Achilles' tendon tear
- Patients with known or suspected rheumatoid arthritis

Soft tissue, palpable lumps are included in the MSK subspecialty training because of the multitude of benign and malignant masses which can occur. The most common palpable soft tissue mass demonstrated on ultrasound is a lipoma (often multiple), but taking a clinical history is important: for example, a lump increasing in size, painful or above a certain size when scanned (local protocol) can be an indication of malignancy and prompt referral is necessary. The examination should include an evaluation of the size of the mass and its location (relationship to fascia), the echotexture, e.g. if cystic, solid or mixed echogenicity, and the Doppler characteristics (using low flow settings).

VASCULAR

The majority of specialist and complex vascular ultrasound examinations are performed in dedicated vascular departments (often called vascular labs) although many general sonographers perform lower limb examinations to exclude deep vein thrombus (DVT) and carotid ultrasound examinations.

Lower Limb DVT Scans

There is a close relationship between DVT and a pulmonary embolus (PE) and if a patient has a DVT, or high clinical suspicion of one, then it is important that the patient receives appropriate care promptly.

The decision to scan is based on the clinical probability of the patient having a DVT, using Wells' Diagnostic Algorithm.[24] Points are accumulated based on specific risk factors. A score of 2 or more means they are high risk of DVT and 1 point or less means a DVT is unlikely.

One point is scored for each of the following:

- Active cancer (treatment ongoing or within the previous six months, or palliative)
- Paralysis, paresis or recent plaster immobilisation of the legs
- Recently bedridden for 3 days or more, or major surgery within the previous 12 weeks, requiring general or regional anaesthesia
- Localised tenderness along the distribution of the deep venous system (such as the back of the calf)
- Entire leg is swollen
- Calf swelling by more than 3 cm compared with the asymptomatic leg (measured 10 cm below the tibial tuberosity)
- Pitting oedema confined to the symptomatic leg
- Collateral superficial veins (non-varicose)
- Previously documented DVT
- Subtract 2 points if an alternative cause is considered at least as likely as DVT.

There is no national consensus on whether scanning the calf veins is necessary and individual departments make the decision based on local preference.

The scan starts in the groin of the affected leg with the common femoral vein (CFV) assessed using grey scale and colour Doppler. (If there is thrombus present in the groin an attempt should be made to visualise the iliac veins and IVC to try to determine the highest point of thrombus extension.) If no thrombus is present/suspected in the CFV at the level of the groin then compression can be utilised and the vein assessed by compression ± colour Doppler at regular intervals down to the level of the knee. The popliteal fossa should be assessed initially for any presence of a Baker's cyst or any other pathology.

Depending on protocol, the popliteal, posterior tibial and peroneal veins can be assessed and compression used if no clot is seen/suspected.

Carotid Artery Scans

Ultrasound is a safe and effective investigation in the initial diagnosis and staging of carotid artery disease. If the ultrasound findings are positive for atheroma and show evidence of stenoses the patient should be referred for further non-invasive imaging, e.g. CT or MR angiography prior to endarterectomy.

Duplex ultrasound provides both grey-scale images of the artery under investigation and Doppler to look at the actual flow. Carotid artery duplex scanning is part of the care pathway for patients who have had a stroke or transient ischaemic attack (TIA).

ECHOCARDIOGRAPHY

The majority of echocardiography examinations are performed by cardiac technicians/cardiac physiologists rather than generic sonographers.

Echocardiography is used to help detect:

- Endocarditis
- Cardiomyopathy
- Heart failure
- Damage caused by cardiac incident
- Congenital cardiac conditions

The majority of scans are performed 'transthoracic', although patients may also have transoesophageal, a stress (post exercise) echocardiogram, or contrast echocardiogram.

EMERGENCY FAST AND PoCUS SCANNING

Since 2010, the Royal College of Emergency Medicine (RCEM) included Point-of-Care Ultrasound (PoCUS) as a mandatory element for emergency medicine trainees.[25] Focused Assessment (or Abdominal) Sonography in Trauma (FAST) scanning can facilitate timely diagnosis in potentially life-threatening cases, such as patients who are haemodynamically unstable and have intra-abdominal haemorrhage, or to assess for pericardial effusion in cases of potential cardiac problems, enabling decisions around patient management to be made more promptly.

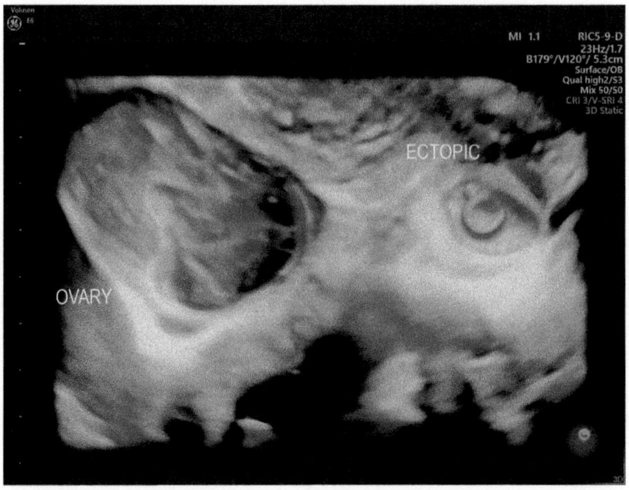

Fig. 29.17 **Ectopic pregnancy adjacent to the ovary. The yolk sac and fetal pole are clearly seen.** (Used with permission of GE Healthcare. Voluson is a trademark of GE Healthcare.)

FAST looks at four areas for the presence of free intraperitoneal fluid and cardiac tamponade:

- Right upper quadrant (Morison's pouch and right costophrenic recess)
- Left upper quadrant (spleno-renal recess and left costophrenic recess)
- Pericardial sac
- Pelvic cavity

There are other components in emergency medicine training – assessment of the abdominal aorta for aneurysm (AAA), focused echocardiography in life support (ELS) and ultrasound-guided vascular access (VA).[25]

Emergency Ultrasound in Obstetrics and Gynaecology (Fig. 29.17)

The RCEM include obstetric and gynaecology emergency ultrasound in their level 2 ultrasound training. The use of ultrasound is as a part of the overall examination of the patient and in conjunction with medical history, symptoms, blood tests, pregnancy tests, observations etc.

Gynaecology patients presenting to the Emergency Department usually do so with acute pelvic pain or vaginal bleeding.

In the case of a non-pregnant patient, acute pain can be the result of torsion (ovary, fibroid, ovarian cyst), tubo-ovarian abscess etc.

In the pregnant woman the role is primarily to exclude an ectopic pregnancy by the identification of intrauterine implantation or to identify an ectopic pregnancy. In later pregnancy, ultrasound can be used in the emergency situation following trauma, placental abruption or premature labour, for example.

Gynaecology

Gynaecological ultrasound is used in the assessment of the non-pregnant female reproductive organs, which are the uterus, cervix, vagina, ovaries, adnexae and rectouterine pouch. Other structures can also be visualised during a pelvic scan, such as the bowel, pelvic vessels and musculature, and the urinary bladder.

There are two main methods of assessing the female pelvic organs by ultrasound – transabdominal (TA) and transvaginal (TV) approach. The two approaches are adjuncts to each other and certainly in the diagnostic stage should be used together.

In a premenopausal woman, the ovaries and endometrium undergo cyclical changes and because of this it is important to take a clinical history from the woman so as to better understand during which stage of her cycle the ultrasound scan is being performed (and therefore what is 'normal'). Important things to note are:

- Menstrual status, i.e. prepubertal, premenopausal, menopausal
- Last menstrual period (LMP) if known
- Length of cycle if known
- Use of oral contraceptive, hormone replacement therapy (HRT), tamoxifen or any other medication that may affect cycle
- Previous pelvic or gynaecological surgery

Common clinical indications for ultrasound examination are:

- Abdominal distension
- Palpable pelvic mass
- Abnormal vaginal bleeding
- Pelvic pain
- Dyspareunia
- Amenorrhoea
- Dysfunctional menstrual bleeding
- Failure to conceive
- Postmenopausal bleeding
- Lost threads of an intrauterine contraceptive device
- Periods have not started at expected age

TECHNIQUE

Transabdominal (TA) Approach

TA approach allows a wide field of view. It is sensible to inform the patient prior to performing a TA scan that a TV scan may be needed before a diagnosis can be made; because often not everything can be seen on TA only. This gives the patient time to consider if she wishes to have a TV scan and by advising her beforehand of the possible need, removes any concerns she may have that you are doing the TV scan because you have 'seen something' on the TA scan.

The patient attends with a full bladder (to help to displace bowel, push the uterus out of the pelvis and to straighten the long axis of the uterus so that it lies perpendicular to the ultrasound beam), and the pelvic organs are assessed in sagittal and transverse planes. Images are archived, even if the bladder is empty and no anatomy can be seen, as this is evidence that an attempt was made to assess the pelvis in TA approach. Any large pathology will be seen even with an empty bladder, and measurements should be taken in TA approach as large pathologies are often out of the FOV of a TV scan. Where there is evidence of pathology, e.g. large fibroids which may compromise the kidneys and cause hydronephrosis for example, the examination can be easily extended when using the TA approach.

Transvaginal (TV) Approach

Ensuring that the patient understands the reason for a TV scan and what they can expect is essential in obtaining her consent. The patient should be offered a chaperone (who ideally should be present when the sonographer is explaining the rationale for proceeding to a TV scan and what will happen during the scan), and be afforded privacy in order to maintain her dignity before, during and after the examination. A TV scan may not be appropriate for some women, e.g. those who are virgo intacta or do not have capacity to consent.

A TV scan should always be offered to a patient where there is the possibility that performing it will improve visualisation and therefore the ability to write a useful report. TV scan is recommended in obese patients, where the uterus is retroverted, where pathology can be seen on TA and closer inspection is required, where the endometrium needs to be assessed, e.g. postmenopausal bleeding, or simply where organs cannot be seen.

Owing to the proximity of the organs to the transducer a higher frequency can be used, typically between 4 and 10 MHz. This gives an increased resolution, which is essential when evaluating endometrial thickness or assessing ovarian architecture.

UTERUS (FIG. 29.18)

The uterus can be assessed for its size, shape and outline as it undergoes normal physiological changes with age. Ultrasound is useful in diagnosing uterine congenital abnormalities, such as bicornuate uterus, didelphic (double uterus), unicornuate and septate uterus.

A common finding on ultrasound is fibroids (leiomyoma). Where fibroids are identified, the location, type (submucosal, intramural, subserosal or pedunculated), number and size, should be reported.

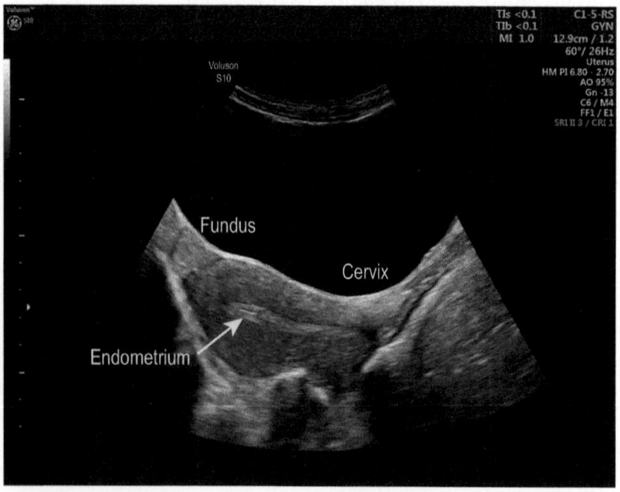

Fig. 29.18 Transabdominal long axis of uterus. (Used with permission of GE Healthcare. Voluson is a trademark of GE Healthcare.)

ENDOMETRIUM (FIG. 29.19)

The endometrium is best assessed on TV approach. Knowledge of the patient's menstrual history is particularly important in the presence of abnormal vaginal bleeding. In a menstruating woman the endometrial thickness and echo pattern vary according to the stage in the menstrual cycle. The upper limit of normal varies but if the endometrium is considered thickened, a repeat scan following menstruation should be arranged.

Vaginal bleeding in a postmenopausal woman can be a cause for concern, as there is a higher incidence of endometrial malignancy; however, in the majority of these women there will be a benign cause for the bleeding, such as hyperplasia or polyps. The upper limit of normal for a postmenopausal woman varies but is usually 4–5 mm. Local protocols will dictate the cut-off points for normal/abnormal and in the use of HRT or tamoxifen the upper limit is increased as these can induce endometrial hyperplasia. Generally in a postmenopausal woman, an endometrial thickness that is well defined and 5 mm or below is unlikely to be cancerous.[26,27]

However, as local protocols vary it is important that pathways are understood. Some departments will use 4 mm as the cut-off.[28]

OVARIES (FIG. 29.20)

The size and texture of the ovaries varies dramatically depending on the reproductive status of the patient. Immature follicles can be visualised in prepubescent ovaries; in a woman of reproductive age, follicles can be visualised as they mature; and in the postmenopausal patient the ovaries appear atrophied, with no evidence of follicular activity.

There are a range of pathologies that can affect the ovaries, for example: ovarian cysts, polycystic ovarian syndrome (PCOS) and ovarian torsion.

Ovarian Cysts

The management depends on the size and characteristics of the cyst and the menstrual status of the woman. These recommendations are a guide as protocols may vary locally.

- Premenopausal:
  - Simple and under 30 mm require no follow-up as these are almost certainly physiological

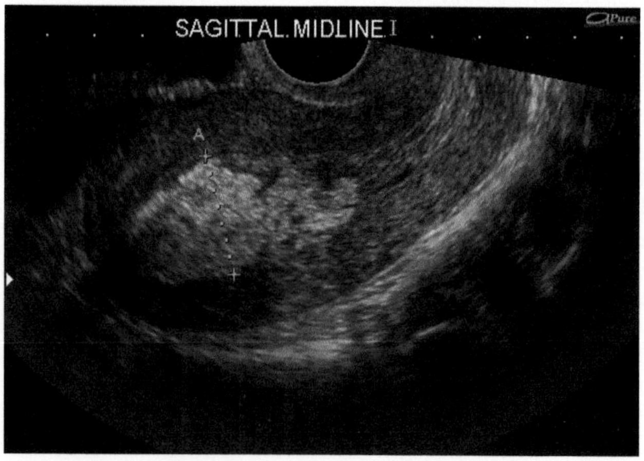

Fig. 29.19 Endometrial carcinoma.

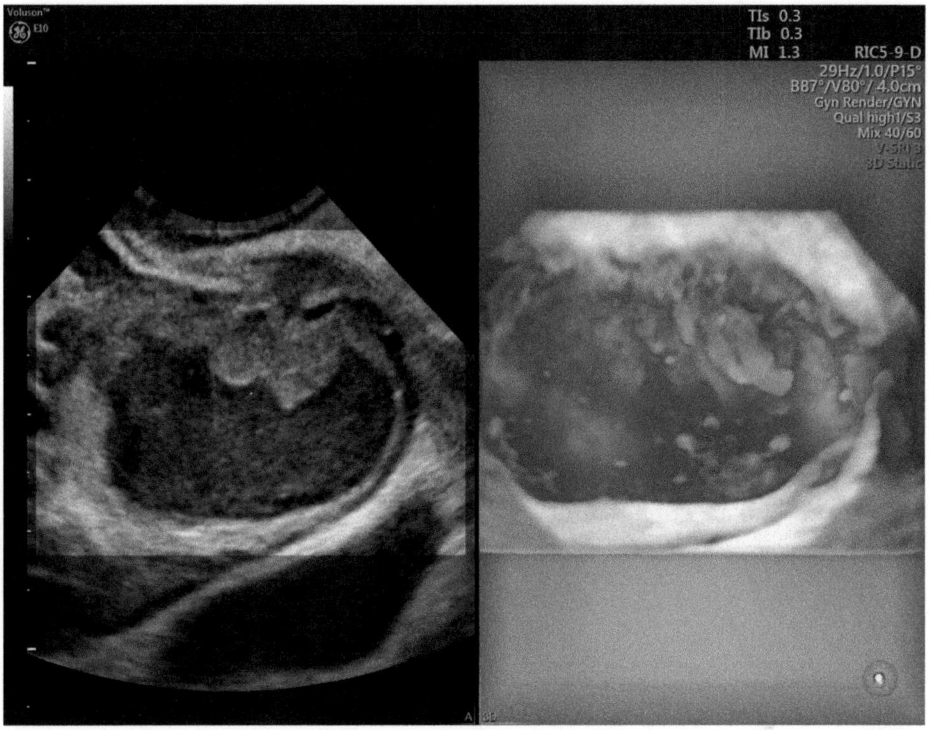

Fig. 29.20 Ovarian mass. 2D on the left, 3D render to the right. (Used with permission of GE Healthcare. Voluson is a trademark of GE Healthcare.)

  - Simple 30–49 mm require no follow-up as these are almost certainly benign
  - Simple 50–70 mm, follow-up scan in one year. If cyst is reduced in size, no further follow-up. If unchanged or larger, gynaecological referral suggested.
  - Simple and more than 70 mm, consider MR and/or gynaecological referral.

Non-simple ovarian masses such as dermoid tumours over 50 mm or a complex mass, e.g. indeterminate, solid, multilocular, or with thick vascular septa require gynaecological referral.[29]

- Postmenopausal:
  - Unilocular and under 50 mm: low risk of malignancy and as long as CA125 test is normal, 4–6 monthly ultrasound surveillance for one year is appropriate. If cyst is unchanged or smaller at the end of this time, the woman can be discharged, again assuming CA125 is normal.
  - Complex adnexal mass – with solid, multilocular appearance or focal thickening requires gynaecological referral.

Ultrasound findings in suspected ovarian cancers form part of the 'Risk of Malignancy Index',[30] alongside the menopausal status and CA125 results.

Infertility

Ultrasound is used to exclude the presence of pathology that may be the cause of infertility; for example, conditions that may prevent successful implantation such as fibroids or endometrial polyps or ovarian dysfunction such as PCOS.

Hysterosalpingo-contrast-sonography (HyCoSy) for tubal patency testing is used to help in confirming tubal patency and saline can be introduced into the endometrial cavity to outline any pathology, such as polyps, submucosal fibroids or adhesions.

During assisted fertility, ultrasound is primarily used to monitor the efficacy of administered drugs on the endometrium and ovaries and throughout the process of egg retrieval.

Ovarian hyperstimulation is a dangerous condition and the use of ultrasound to monitor the number and size of follicles will help to prevent this from occurring.

After successful conceptions/implantations, ultrasound is used to determine the number of gestational sacs and embryos and to exclude ectopic pregnancies.

Obstetrics

In the four countries of the United Kingdom, advice on the use of ultrasound screening in the routine care of obstetric patients is given by the National Screening Committee. In England, the Fetal Anomaly Screening Programme (FASP) sets the screening standards for obstetric ultrasound; with Scotland, Wales and Northern Ireland having similar programmes. There is literature available which details the detection rates and acceptable positive rates for the screening programme. The detail in this section relates to the standards set out by FASP in England.[31]

For both first and second trimester scans, two attempts must be made to obtain the necessary measurements and images. This can mean the woman is given a further appointment on another day or is rescanned later in the same day. Local protocol allows departments to choose what best suits them but in the case of the second trimester scan the second attempt must be by 23 weeks 0 days.

FASP guidelines do not give any advice or recommendations on any other obstetric ultrasound scans; e.g. those dealing with problems in early pregnancy or growth scans in the third trimester.

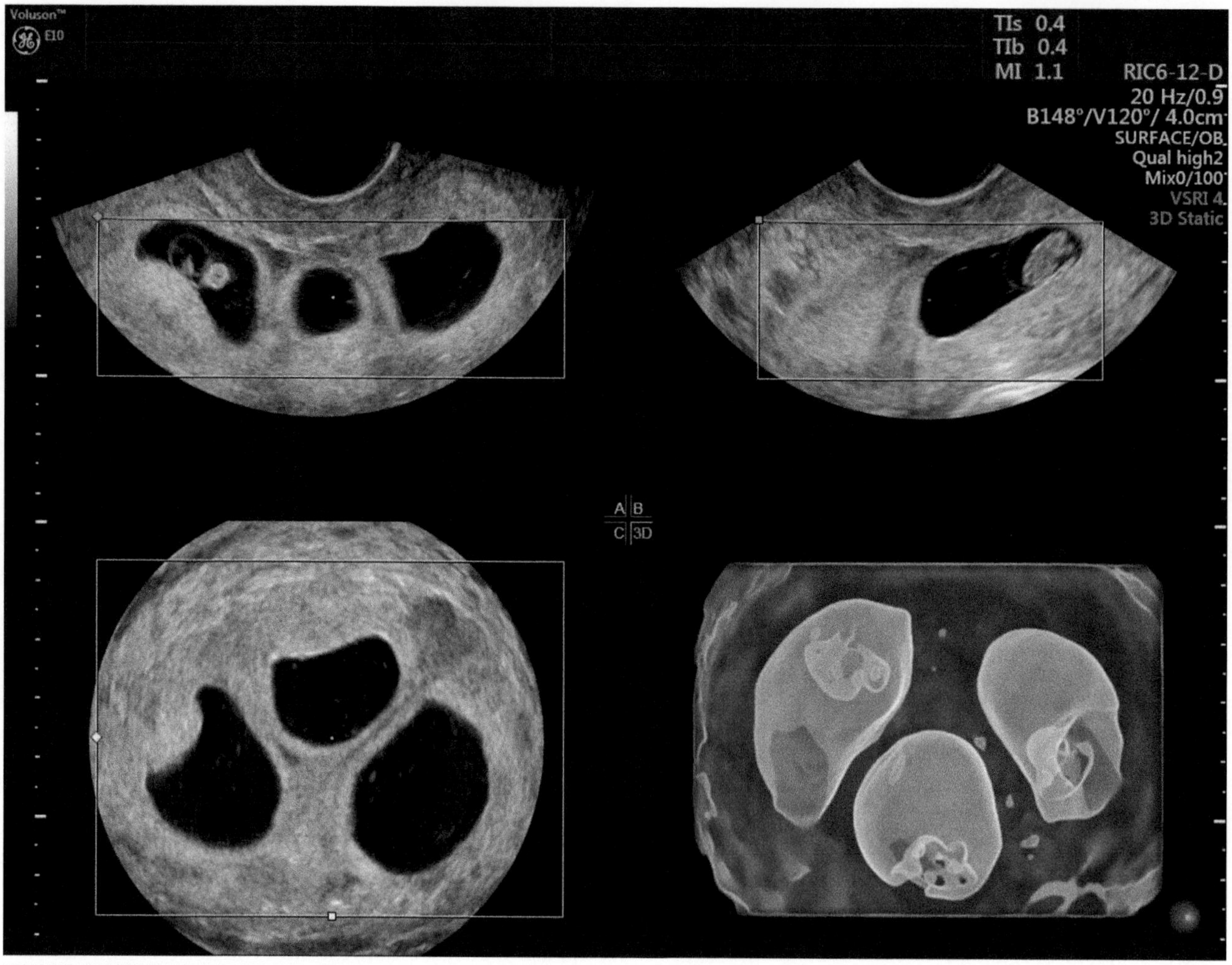

Fig. 29.21 Triplet pregnancy in 2D and 3D. (Used with permission of GE Healthcare. Voluson is a trademark of GE Healthcare.)

It is important to remember that women are offered ultrasound screening in pregnancy but that it is a choice and not compulsory. Some women may choose to have ultrasound scans but choose to not be screened for chromosomal or fetal structural abnormalities and the wishes of these women must be respected. Women must be given sufficient information about what can and cannot be detected and the limitations of ultrasound in a way they can understand to enable them to make an informed decision about their care. It is also important that women understand that a 'normal' scan is not a guarantee that their baby will not have other non-detectable conditions.

FIRST TRIMESTER

The main aims of a first trimester scan are:

- To exclude an ectopic pregnancy
- To confirm ongoing pregnancy, especially in the setting of vaginal bleeding and pain
- To date the pregnancy accurately by establishing gestational age and estimated date of delivery. Decidual reaction can be visible within the uterus as early as 4 weeks, with the presence of a gestation sac at 5 weeks. The gestation sac should be eccentrically placed, with the presence of a yolk sac and amnion within the sac. This observation can help distinguish between the pseudosac of an ectopic pregnancy or fluid collection in the cavity and a true gestation sac
- To determine the number of pregnancies (Fig. 29.21) and if multiple the amnionicity and chorionicity to ensure the patient is placed on the correct care pathway (monochorionic twins are at higher risk of fetal structural anomalies and of developing complications such as twin-to-twin transfusion syndrome and intrauterine growth restriction). Sonographic criteria used in the diagnosis of chorionicity are the Lambda sign, which is present when there is placental tissue between the amniotic membranes; the T sign, where there is no placental tissue between the amniotic membranes, suggesting that there is a single placenta; and the thickness of the inter-twin membrane
- To enable the patient to access screening services offered in a timely manner. Patients are offered screening for Down (trisomy 21), Edwards (trisomy 18) and Patau (trisomy 13) syndromes between 11 weeks +2 days to 14 weeks +1 day, so knowing the gestational age is essential to enable effective screening (if requested)
- To detect major structural anomalies that may be identified in early pregnancy, e.g. anencephaly.

Early Pregnancy Assessment (Fig. 29.22)

Prior to their scheduled first trimester ultrasound scan many women attend an early pregnancy unit because of

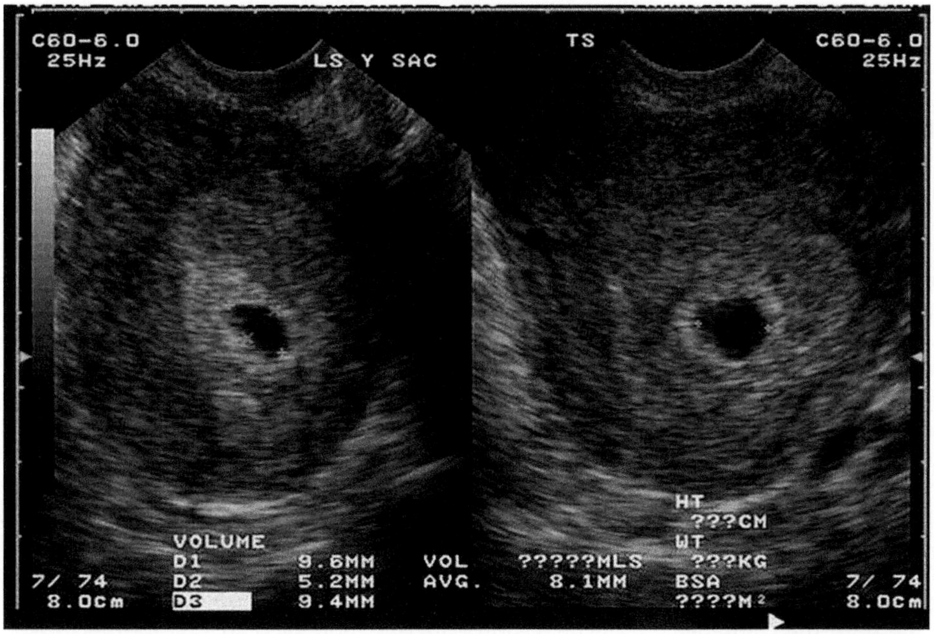

Fig. 29.22 Gestational sac measurements in three planes. (Reproduced with permission from Toshiba Medical Systems Ltd.)

pain or bleeding and ultrasound is used in the assessment of these women to ensure they do not have an ectopic pregnancy and to diagnose a failed or failing pregnancy.

A TV scan should always be performed if a pregnancy cannot be demonstrated in the uterine cavity and in cases where a failed pregnancy is suspected.

The visualisation of a gestation sac is the first sonographic sign of pregnancy. The spherical sac should be eccentrically placed in one layer of the decidua and will have an echogenic rim. The yolk sac is usually visible by the time the gestation sac diameter reaches 8 mm which equates to a pregnancy of around 5 weeks. The embryo is visible around 6 weeks and cardiac activity is usually seen at this time. An early pregnancy will be visible on TV scan earlier than on TA scan because of the closer proximity of the probe to the uterus.

The gestational sac is measured in three different planes and a mean sac diameter (MSD) calculated. MSD is not performed once a fetal pole/embryo is identified.

A failed pregnancy can be diagnosed where an embryo has a crown–rump length of 7 mm or more with no fetal heart pulsations seen. Where there is no visible embryo the empty gestation sac must have a MSD of greater than 25 mm to diagnose a failed pregnancy. If the MSD is less than 25 mm, conservative management is prudent and a repeat scan performed in 7 days.[32,33]

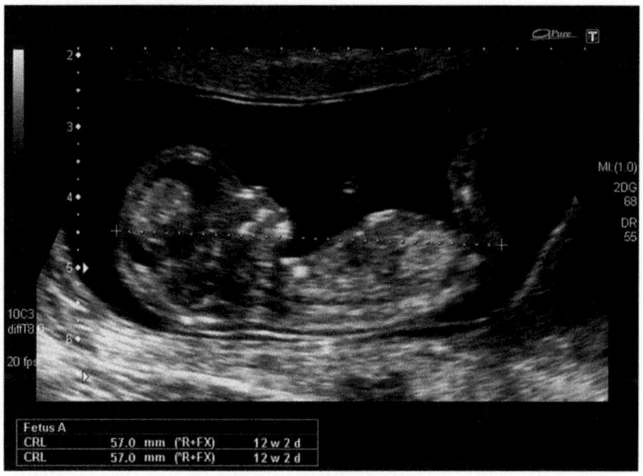

Fig. 29.23 CRL measurement.

Crown–Rump Length (CRL) (Fig. 29.23). Once an embryo is visible, the CRL can be used to determine gestational age to ensure future antenatal care is offered and undertaken in a timely manner. Care must be taken to ensure that the yolk sac is not included in the measurement as this will result in overestimation of the gestational age. A correctly measured CRL provides the most accurate estimation of a gestational age when performed in the latter part of the first trimester and the 'due date' or estimated date of delivery (EDD) determined at this time will be used throughout the pregnancy.

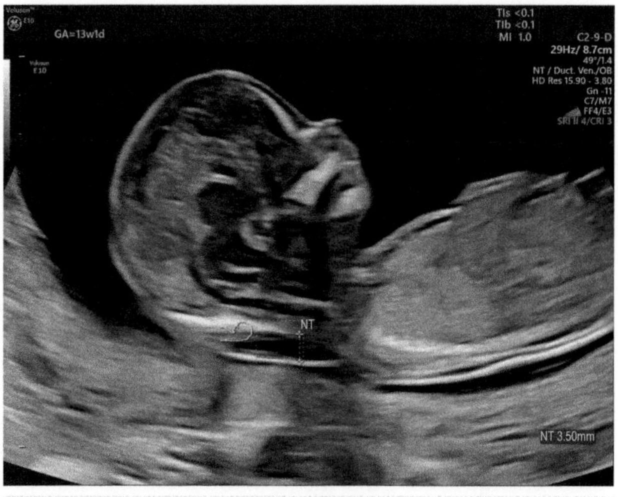

Fig. 29.24 First trimester: NT measurement. (Used with permission of GE Healthcare. Voluson is a trademark of GE Healthcare.)

Screening for Chromosomal Abnormalities (Fig. 29.24). In the first trimester, combined screening using maternal age, the nuchal translucency (NT) measurement and two biochemical markers (free beta hCG and PAPP-A), along with the gestational age determined by CRL (which must be between 45 mm and 84 mm), in order to determine the risk of a fetus having certain chromosomal abnormalities is offered to all eligible pregnant women.[31] If the fetus is at high risk, the woman is then offered invasive testing to confirm a diagnosis and enable decisions to be made about the pregnancy.

The FASP makes clear that women who wish to have screening for chromosomal abnormalities but who attend too late in their pregnancy to have the combined test in the first trimester must be offered serum screening in the second trimester.[31]

Second trimester serum screening is also known as the quadruple test and uses maternal age and four biochemical markers – AFP (alpha-fetoprotein), hCG (human chorionic gonadotropin), uE3 (unconjugated oestriol) and inhibin-A – and can be used 14 weeks +2 days until 20 weeks 0 days.

Although this combination of markers has a lower detection and a higher screen-positive rate than the combined test, it is the FASP recommended screening strategy in the second trimester.

In some areas, women who are found to be high risk following combined screening are offered Non-Invasive Pre-Natal Testing (NIPT) prior to invasive testing. NIPT is a blood test that detects placental DNA in the mother's blood and as placental DNA is, in most cases, the same as fetal DNA, sequencing and counting it means that any increase in T21, T18 and T13 can be detected. A woman can choose to have the combined screening or just part of it, she can also decline all screening and opt to have the first trimester scan only. It is important that the woman's informed decision is documented.

Complications in First Trimester

Gestational Trophoblastic Disease (GTD) (Hydatidiform Mole). Complete (no fetus present) and partial (presence of a coexisting fetus) hydatidiform mole are the most common forms of trophoblastic disease and although diagnosis of the condition is by histology they have typical appearances on ultrasound – the uterine cavity is filled with trophoblastic tissue with swollen villi presenting as cystic areas.

The diagnosis of GTD is important because women will need follow-up treatment and monitoring and in some cases may need chemotherapy.

Ectopic Pregnancy. An ectopic pregnancy is one that forms outside the endometrial cavity and is one of the causes of maternal death. Taking a clinical history is important in the care of a woman with a possible ectopic pregnancy as there are recognised predisposing factors such as a history of infertility. In vitro fertilisation (IVF), previous tubal surgery, e.g. sterilisation, previous sexually transmitted disease, history of previous caesarean section and a history of endometriosis all increase the risk of an ectopic pregnancy.

Symptoms of an ectopic pregnancy are often not recognised as such as they can be present in less serious conditions; examples are pain (usually unilateral), bleeding, or vaginal discharge.

All women are at risk of an ectopic pregnancy, and until the pregnancy is proven beyond doubt to be intrauterine, she has a pregnancy of unknown location (PUL), and should be presumed to have an ectopic and monitored/treated accordingly. It is possible to have an intrauterine and co-existing ectopic pregnancy, but this is rare. The commonest place for an ectopic pregnancy to implant is in the fallopian tube but they can also be ovarian, cervical, within a caesarean section scar and in the abdomen. It is essential to perform both a TA and a TV scan if there is any concern that a pregnancy cannot be confirmed to be intrauterine.

SECOND TRIMESTER (FIGS 29.25–29.30)

The FASP requires that the second trimester scan be performed between 18 weeks 0 days' and 20 weeks 6 days' gestation (assuming that the woman 'opts in' and presents for antenatal care early enough). Women can still have their scan if they present late but some conditions/abnormalities are harder to see as the pregnancy progresses.

The second trimester anomaly scan is performed to assess the fetus for the presence of 11 specific conditions and there is a base menu of images which must be archived.[31]

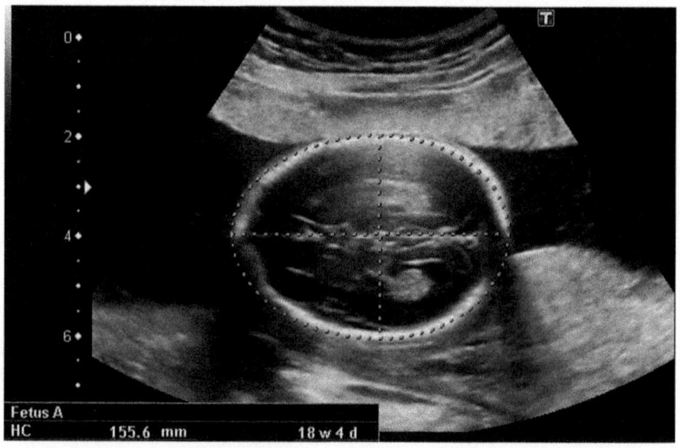

Fig. 29.25 HC measurement.

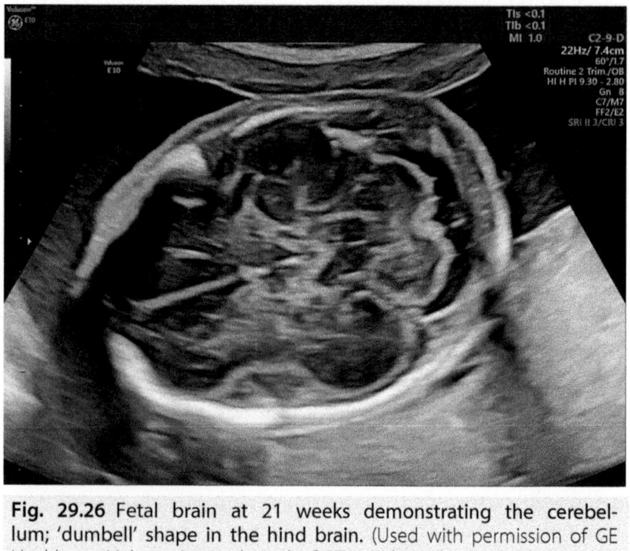

Fig. 29.26 Fetal brain at 21 weeks demonstrating the cerebellum; 'dumbell' shape in the hind brain. (Used with permission of GE Healthcare. Voluson is a trademark of GE Healthcare.)

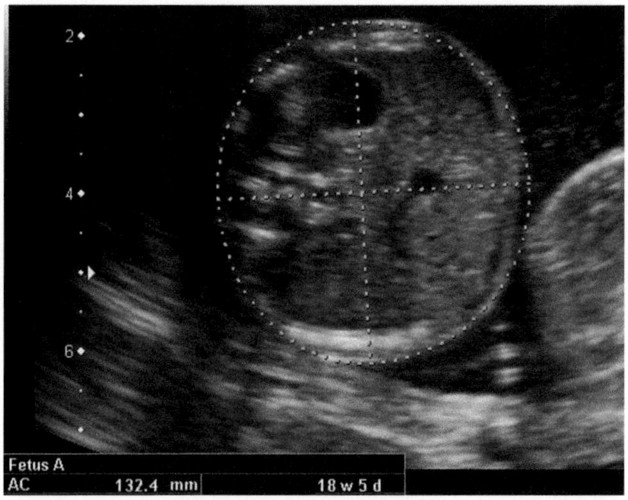

Fig. 29.27 AC measurement.

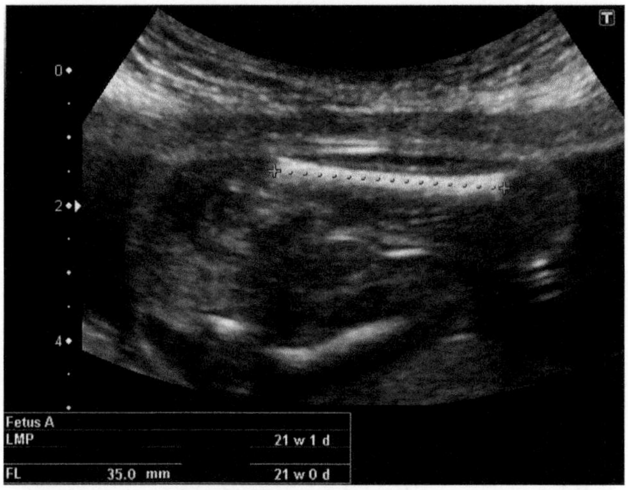

Fig. 29.28 FL measurement.

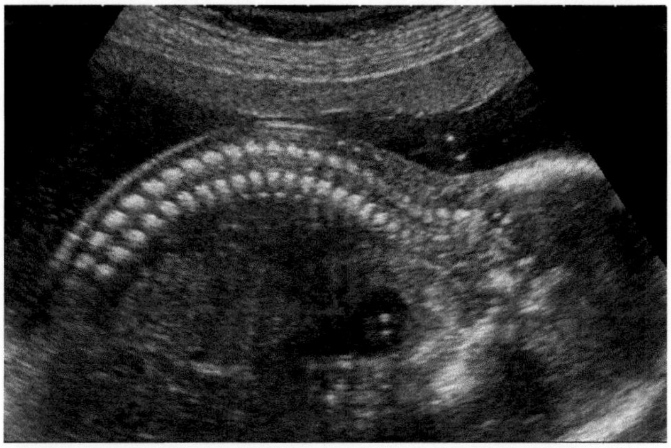

Fig. 29.29 Fetal spine in sagittal plane showing skin covering.

Specific Conditions

- Anencephaly
- Open spina bifida
- Cleft lip
- Diaphragmatic hernia
- Gastroschisis

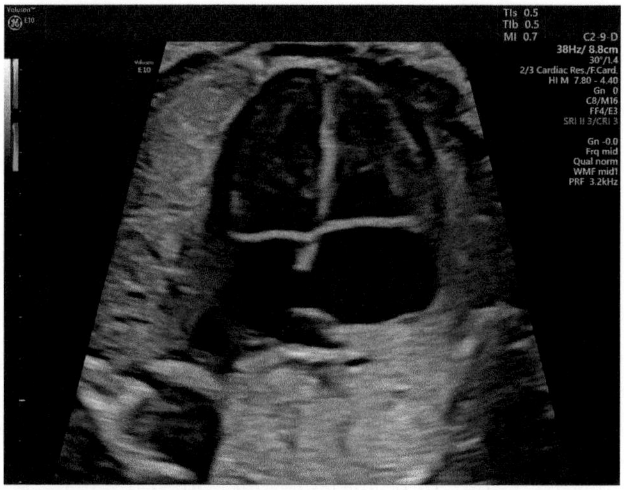

Fig. 29.30 Four-chamber fetal heart at 28 weeks. (Used with permission of GE Healthcare. Voluson is a trademark of GE Healthcare.)

- Exomphalos
- Serious cardiac abnormalities
- Bilateral renal agenesis
- Lethal skeletal dysplasia
- Edwards' syndrome (trisomy 13)
- Patau syndrome (trisomy 18)

Base Menu

The fetal anatomy to be examined and measured is:

1. Head circumference (HC) measurement and measurement of the atrium of the lateral ventricle
2. Suboccipitobregmatic view measurement of the transcerebellar diameter
3. Coronal view of lips with nasal tip
4. Abdominal circumference (AC) measurement
5. Femur length (FL) measurement
6. Sagittal view of spine including sacrum and skin covering

The fetal cardiac protocol requires the following images to be obtained:

1. Situs/laterality
2. Four-chamber: transverse section of the thorax including a complete rib and crux of the heart
3. Aorta/left ventricular outflow tract: this view shows the outflow tract of the left ventricle
4. Pulmonary/right ventricular outflow tract: this view shows the outflow tract of the right ventricle only; or the three-vessel view (3VV), which shows the outflow tract of the right ventricle, including the pulmonary artery
5. The three-vessel and trachea view (3VT): a transverse view of the fetal upper mediastinum; it depicts the main pulmonary artery in direct communication with the ductus arteriosus, the transverse aortic arch and the superior vena cava

As well as the requirements of the screening programme, the sonographer must also assess the placenta to ensure there is no placenta praevia (the placenta is close to or covering the internal os); consider the possibility of placenta accreta (the placenta tissue embeds deeply into the uterine wall and cannot be delivered resulting in sometimes catastrophic maternal bleeding); or vasa praevia (vessels from the fetus are adjacent to the cervix and can rupture causing bleeding that often results in fetal demise).

NICE guidelines suggest when to assess cervical length in women presenting at risk of pre-term birth:

If clinical assessment suggests that the woman is in suspected preterm labour and she is 30 weeks plus 0 days pregnant or more, consider transvaginal ultrasound measurement of cervical length as a diagnostic test to determine the likelihood of birth within 48 hours ... If cervical length is more than 15 mm, it is unlikely that the woman is in preterm labour. If cervical length is 15 mm or less, view the woman as being in preterm labour and offer treatment ...[34]

Interventional Ultrasound Guided Techniques

Invasive testing of this type carries with it a risk of miscarriage, infection, rhesus sensitisation and talipes (if performed before 15 weeks).

Amniocentesis. Usually undertaken during the second trimester after 15 weeks for fetal karyotyping and as well as Down, Edwards and Patau syndromes, can also detect cystic fibrosis, muscular dystrophy, sickle cell disease and thalassaemia. A transabdominal approach is used with the needle passing through the maternal abdominal wall into the amniotic sac and fluid withdrawn. Fetal cells are cultured enabling analysis to be carried out.

Chorionic Villus Sampling (CVS). CVS can be performed in the first trimester of pregnancy, usually between 11 and 14 weeks of gestation. In addition to the risks of amniocentesis, there is the possibility of insufficient tissue sample being obtained.

CVS is performed transabdominally or transcervically depending on the location of the placenta; under ultrasound guidance a sample of proliferating placental tissue is taken.

Fetal Blood Sampling. Cordocentesis or percutaneous umbilical blood sampling under ultrasound guidance is a means of obtaining fetal blood cells. It enables karyotyping/chromosome analysis as well as being used for the assessment and treatment of rhesus iso-immunisation. Intrauterine blood transfusions may be performed using this technique.

THIRD TRIMESTER

Scanning in the third trimester is not part of antenatal care for 'normal' singleton pregnancies.

Possible reasons for third trimester scans are:

- Fetal surveillance, for clinically small or large for dates gestations
- Poor obstetric history
- Multiple pregnancies: multiple pregnancies are at increased risk of complications
- Maternal conditions, such as hypertension and diabetes
- Reduced fetal movement
- To assess the placenta position where it has been previously thought to be low lying
- Suspicion of poly- or oligohydramnios
- Suspected fetal malpresentation

Future Developments

Artificial intelligence (AI) is likely to have a huge impact on ultrasound provision in the very near future.[35] It is already used in training simulation phantoms and data bases of ultrasound images are being collected which will be used to create algorithms to identify and grade images to be used in the audit of protocol-based examinations.

The use of ultrasound in radiotherapy is now recognised as a useful part of image-guided radiotherapy. Given the safety of ultrasound, its relative low cost and availability, its use in radiotherapy applications is likely to increase.

References

1. Royal College of Radiologists. *Ultrasound Training Recommendations for Medical and Surgical Specialties*. 3rd ed. London: RCR; 2017.
2. CASE. http://www.case-uk.org/course-directory/.
3. Edler I, Hertz C. The use of ultrasonic reflectoscope for the continuous recording of the movements of heart walls. *Clin Physiol Funct Imaging*. 2004;24:118–136.
4. Donald I, MacVicar J, Brown TG. Investigation of abdominal masses by pulsed ultrasound. *Lancet*. 1958;i:1188–1195.
5. Kasai C, et al. Real time 2 dimensional blood flow imaging using an autocorrelation technique. *IEEE TransSonics Ultrasonics*. 1985;32:458–464.
6. Royal College of Radiologists and Society and College of Radiographers. *Standards for Provision of an Ultrasound Service*. London: RCR; 2014.
7. Society and College of Radiographers. *Work Related Musculoskeletal Disorders (Sonographers)*. 3rd ed. London: SCoR; 2019.
8. Chiou S, Fox T. Comparing differential tissue harmonic imaging with tissue harmonic and fundamental gray scale imaging of the liver. *J Ultrasound Med*. 2007;26:1557–1563.
9. Lewin P. Quo vadis medical ultrasound? *Ultrasonics*. 2004;42:1–7.
10. Dogra V. *Advances in Ultrasound: An Issue of Ultrasound Clinics*. Vols. 4–3. Saunders; 2010.
11. Society and College of Radiographers and British Medical Ultrasound Society. *Guidelines for Professional Ultrasound Practice*. London: SCoR; 2019. Revision 4.
12. NICE (National Institute for Health and Care Excellence). *SonoVue (sulphur Hexafluoride Microbubbles) – Contrast Agent for Contrast-Enhanced Ultrasound Imaging of the Liver*. Diagnostics guidance [DG5]; 2012. https://www.nice.org.uk/Guidance/DG5.
13. Sidhu P, et al. The EFSUMB guidelines and recommendations on the clinical practice of contrast enhanced ultrasound (CEUS) in non-hepatic applications. *Ultraschall der Med*. 2018;39(2):2–44.
14. British Medical Ultrasound Society (BMUS). [Homepage] http://www.bmus.org.
15. Monnington S, et al. *Risk Management of Musculoskeletal Disorders in Sonography Work*. Cardiff: Health and Safety Executive; 2012.
16. Boll D, Merkle E. Diffuse liver disease: strategies for hepatic CT and MR imaging. *Radiographics*. 2009;29(6):1591–1614.
17. Penny SM. *Examination Review for Ultrasound: Abdomen & Obstetrics and Gynecology*. Philadelphia: Wolters Kluwer; 2018.
18. Walsh M, Manghat NE, Fox BM, et al. A pictorial review of splenic pathology at ultrasound: patterns of disease. *Ultrasound*. 2005;13(3):173–185.
19. Public Health England. *Service Specification 23: NHS Abdominal Aortic Aneurysm Screening Programme*. London: NHS; 2018.
20. Perros P, et al. *Guidelines for the Management of Thyroid Cancer*. 3rd ed. British Thyroid Association; 2014.
21. Public Health England. *Newborn and Infant Physical Examination Screening Programme Handbook*. London: PHE; 2020. https://www.gov.uk/government/publications/newborn-and-infant-physical-examination-programme-handbook/newborn-and-infant-physical-examination-screening-programme-handbook.
22. Mittal P, Little B, Harri PA, et al. Role of imaging in the evaluation of male infertility. *Radiographics*. 2017;37(3).
23. Richenberg J, Belfield J, Ramchandanai P, et al. Testicular microlithiasis imaging and followup: guidelines of the ESUR scrotal imaging subcommittee. *Eur Radiol*. 2015;25(2):323–330.
24. Wells P. Integrated strategies for the diagnosis of venous thromboembolism. *J Thromb Haemostasis*. 2007;5(1):41–50.

25. College of Emergency Medicine Ultrasound Subgroup. *Ultrasound Curriculum*. London: CEM; 2010.
26. Smith-Bindman R, Weiss E, Feldstein V. How thick is too thick? When endometrial thickness should prompt biopsy in postmenopausal women without vaginal bleeding. *Ultrasound Obstet Gynecol.* 2004;24(5):558–565.
27. Wolfman W, Leyland N, Heywood M, et al. Asymptomatic endometrial thickening. *J Obstet Gynaecol Canad.* 2010;32(10):990–999.
28. Sundar S, Balega J, Crosbie E, et al. *BGCS Uterine Cancer Guidelines: Recommendations for Practice*. British Gynaecological Cancer Society; 2017. https://www.bgcs.org.uk.
29. RCOG/BSGE. *Management of Suspected Ovarian Masses in Premenopausal Women.* Royal College of Obstetricians and Gynaecologists; 2011. [Green-top Guideline No. 62]. https://www.rcog.org.uk/en/guidelines-research-services/guidelines/gtg62/.
30. RCOG. *Ovarian Cysts in Postmenopausal Women.* Royal College of Obstetricians and Gynaecologists; 2016. [Green-top Guideline No. 34]. https://www.rcog.org.uk/en/guidelines-research-services/guidelines/gtg34/.
31. Public Health England. *NHS Fetal Anomaly Screening Programme Handbook*. London: PHE; 2018.
32. RCOG. *The Management of Early Pregnancy Loss.* Royal College of Obstetricians and Gynaecologists; 2011. [Green- top Guideline No. 25]. https://www.rcog.org.uk/en/guidelines-research-services/guidelines/gtg25/.
33. NICE (National Institute for Health and Care Excellence). *Ectopic and Miscarriage Diagnosis and Initial Management.* Clinical guideline [CG154]; 2012. https://www.nice.org.uk/guidance/cg154.
34. NICE (National Institute for Health and Care Excellence). *Pre-term Labour and Birth.* NICE guideline [NG25]; 2015. https://www.nice.org.uk/guidance/ng25.
35. Matthew J. Deep ultrasound: how artificial intelligence could impact sonography. In: *Intelligent Fetal Imaging & Diagnosis (IFIND) Project.* London: King's College; 2019.

30 Dual Energy X-ray Absorptiometry

KAREN KNAPP

Dual energy X-ray absorptiometry (DXA) is used for the prediction of fracture risk in the diagnosis of osteoporosis, and to monitor disease progression or therapeutic intervention. DXA is commonly considered to be the gold standard for the diagnosis of osteoporosis and is supported by the widest evidence-base and clinical utilisation.[1,2] Radiographs are an insensitive method to accurately quantify bone mineral density (BMD) changes and require a 30–50% loss of BMD before changes become apparent.[3] However, the quantification of BMD using DXA provides much greater sensitivity to bone changes. Imaging undertaken using DXA can also be used to identify vertebral fractures, and to identify thickening of the femoral cortex associated with incomplete atypical femoral fractures.[1,4]

Osteoporosis is defined as 'a progressive systemic skeletal disease characterised by low bone mass and microarchitectural deterioration of bone tissue, with a consequent increase in bone fragility and susceptibility to fracture'.[5] One in two women and one in five men over the age of 50 in the UK will fracture a bone, often as a result of osteoporosis.[6] Fragility fractures occur primarily, but not exclusively, at the distal radius, vertebrae and hip.[6] Worldwide, osteoporosis is estimated to affect 200 million women and causes more than 8.9 million fractures annually, resulting in an osteoporotic fracture every three seconds.[7,8]

Quality Assurance

The quality assurance requirements for DXA scanners are of utmost importance, with the best practice being to perform a quality assurance (QA) phantom scan daily. Daily QA scans should always be undertaken before scanning of patients begins for the day. This assures the scanner is operating within its recommended limits to ensure the accuracy of the results. Daily QA data must be plotted and assessed for sudden changes, or long-term slow drifts, as both can impact on the accurate measurement of BMD.[9] Shewart rules can provide a useful aid to clinical decision-making on the performance of a scanner, and offer a more robust statistical method for identifying scanner drifts than the subjective visualisation of plotted data.[10,11] Identifying slow drifts early is important, to prevent sudden catastrophic scanner failure with the associated cancellation of patient lists until the scanner is repaired. The identification of slow drift needs to lead to planned exploration and repair.

Scanners that fail QA must not be used for patient scanning until they are within the limits set by the manufacturers. For both QA and clinical scans the temperature in the scanning room should be within the limits specified by the manufacturer. This is of particular importance in mobile scanners, where larger temperature fluctuations might be expected in very cold or very warm weather. Records of QA must be kept, along with essential tests such as the emergency stop button check, which should be undertaken on a regular basis. Contingency plans should be included in standard operating procedures for decision-making regarding the operation and non-operation of the scanner.[12]

Multiple Scanner Departments

In a department with more than one scanner, it is best practice to ensure that patients are scanned on the same machine each time they return. However, this may not always be possible, especially when patients may have their first scan in the community on a mobile scanner, and might be seen in the hospital setting on other occasions. In this case a cross-calibration should be undertaken to investigate the comparability of the two scanners.[13] This can identify any systematic differences on the agreement of the scanners, providing essential information for the practitioner reporting the scan.

Referral Criteria for DXA

As for all medical imaging referrals, DXA scans must be appropriately justified and the radiation dose kept as low as reasonably practicable.[14] Referral criteria should align to national or international guidelines. In the UK there are guidelines from the National Institute for Health and Care Excellence (NICE), which has published evidence-based criteria for the assessment of those at risk of fragility fracture.[15]

Consider assessment of fracture risk:

- In all women aged 65 years and over and all men aged 75 years and over
- In women aged under 65 years and men aged under 75 years in the presence of risk factors. For example:
  - Previous fragility fracture
  - Current use or frequent recent use of oral or systemic glucocorticoids*
  - History of falls
  - Family history of hip fracture
  - Other causes of secondary osteoporosis
  - Low body mass index (BMI) (less than 18.5 kg/m^2)
  - Smoking
  - Alcohol intake of more than 14 units per week for men and women

*Glucocorticoid use for 3 or more months of a dose of prednisolone of 5 mg daily, or an equivalent dose of other glucocorticoids.

Other secondary risk factors for fracture include:

- Rheumatoid arthritis
- Premature menopause (<45years of age)
- Type 1 insulin-dependent diabetes
- Osteogenesis imperfecta in adults
- Untreated, longstanding hyperthyroidism
- Chronical malnutrition or malabsorption, coeliac disease
- Chronic liver disease
- Alcohol intake of 3 or more units daily[16]
- Cystic fibrosis[17]
- Hyperparathyroidism (primary or secondary)[18]

Bone loss is also seen in patients within these groups:

- Post-amputation[19]
- Following cardiovascular events[20]

In addition to glucocorticoids there are also multiple drugs known to affect bone metabolism, which provide appropriate justification for a DXA scan. These include:

- Over treatment with thyroxine
- Aromatase inhibitors[21]
- Androgen deprivation therapy[22]
- Anti-epileptic drugs
- Chemotherapy
- Anticonvulsants
- Selective serotonin reuptake inhibitors
- Proton pump inhibitors
- Anti-retroviral drugs
- Thiazodinediones[15,23]

This is not an exhaustive list and, as the evidence-base increases, more risk factors will be identified. It is important to also weigh up each referral outside of these criteria in conjunction with the current evidence-base and consideration of the pathophysiology of the disease, along with the potential impact on bone strength.

This chapter does not include referral criteria for a paediatric population; these should be scanned in specialist centres and interpreted by those with expertise in this population.[24,25]

Prior to referral for a DXA scan, an estimate of absolute fracture risk over 10 years is recommended. This can be undertaken using either FRAX[26] or QFracture.[27] Figure 30.1 shows an example of a fracture risk assessment using FRAX and Fig. 30.2 demonstrates the associated National Osteoporosis Guideline Group (NOGG) guidelines based on the fracture risk prediction.

It is recommended that DXA services do not routinely assess fracture risk in people aged under 50 years unless they have major risk factors (for example, current or frequent recent use of oral or systemic glucocorticoids, untreated premature menopause, or previous fragility fracture), because they are unlikely to be at high risk.[15]

Prior to the Scan

- The scan must be justified in accordance with local standard operating procedures by the practitioner.[14]
- It is important to have all the information required for the clinical interpretation of the scan. This means either the referral criteria must include all the clinical risk factors for osteoporosis and fragility fracture, or the patient has completed a questionnaire to collate this information. At a basic level, this can include the questions from either FRAX (Fig. 30.1) or QFracture,[16,27] along with a list of fractures a patient has sustained and a list of any drugs they are currently taking. Not all fractures are considered to be related to osteoporosis, such as metatarsal, phalangeal, and skull fractures.[28] It is important to also understand the level of trauma related to any fracture, so asking the patient to also detail how the fracture occurred is useful. An atraumatic or low trauma fracture is characterised as a fracture that has occurred from a fall from standing height, or less, and would not normally have resulted in a fracture in a healthy individual.[29]
- The patient should arrive in appropriate clothing for the scan or be changed into a gown. The recommended appropriate clothing should be detailed in the

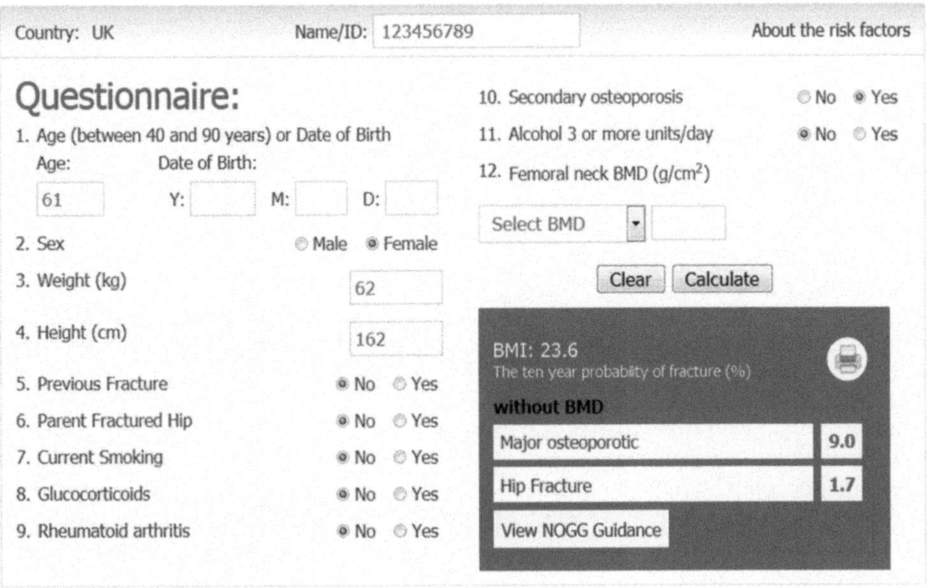

Fig. 30.1 Example of the FRAX Calculation Tool.

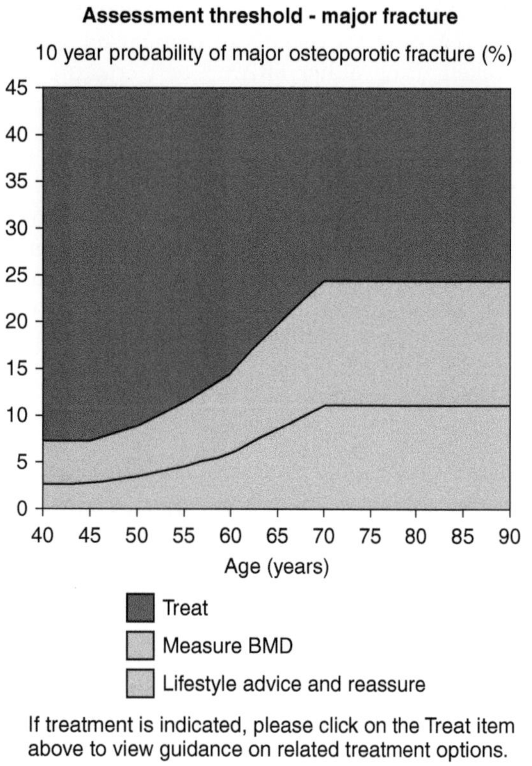

Fig. 30.2 National Osteoporosis Guideline Group modelling.

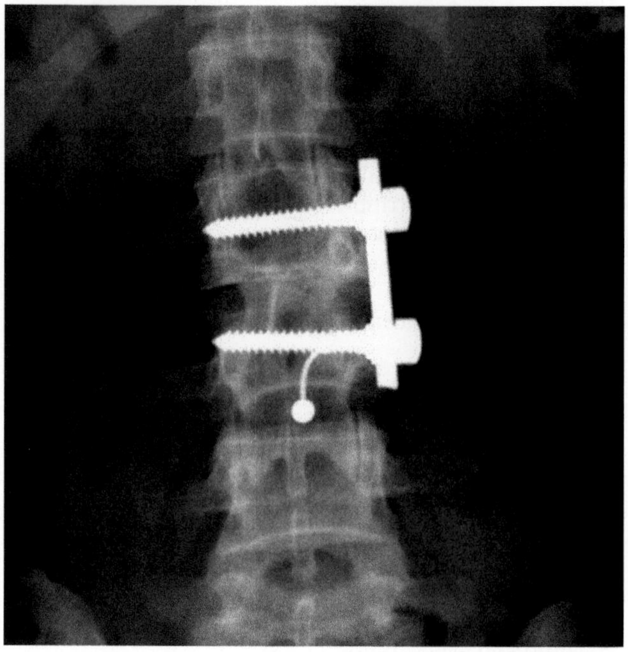

Fig. 30.3 Lumbar spine with metal work and a navel piercing.

appointment letter or an accompanying leaflet. DXA scans are sensitive to many artefacts and these include: buttons, items placed in pockets, piercings and tight waistbands (which can alter the measured BMD through compression of the surrounding soft tissue). Navel jewellery artefacts have been demonstrated to result in clinically significant errors in BMD measurement of the lower lumbar vertebrae,[30] while small metallic clothing clips can result in 'black hole' artefacts. These are not readily visualised, but have the potential to alter the BMD of a single vertebra.[31]

- If the patient is female and of child-bearing age, between the ages of 12 and 55 years (10 and 55 years in some departments), then pregnancy or the risk of pregnancy must be excluded in line with departmental protocol prior to the scan.[14]
- Previous imaging must be checked. A DXA scan should not have been conducted within the previous 2 years unless this is in line with departmental protocols, for example in patients on teriparatide, where rapid and large increases in BMD are seen. Artefacts can result from recent contrast investigations such as barium or water-soluble CT contrast studies of the gastrointestinal tract. Patients who have had a recent barium contrast examination should not be scanned for at least 2 weeks following the procedure, to prevent possible artefacts on the DXA scan due to slow bowel transit times or sequestration in diverticulae.[32] Patients who have had a recent iodine-based contrast examination should wait 1 week prior to undergoing DXA scan.[33] Patients who have undergone a recent technetium 99m (^{99m}Tc) bone scan or positron emission scan not be should be scanned until at least the following day.[34]
- Any previous surgery that might affect the scan result must also be identified. Hip replacements require scanning of the contralateral hip, while internal fixations in the spine (Fig. 30.3) require consideration as to whether they will yield a diagnostic scan. At least two vertebrae should be visible in order to make a diagnosis. The scan in Fig. 30.3 would yield a diagnostic scan since L1 and L4 are available. However, the navel ring should have been removed.
- It is also useful to know if the patient has suffered a recent lower limb fracture, since these can result in disuse osteopenia at the hip, which does recover over time, and it may be pertinent to scan the contralateral hip in these circumstances.[35]

Site Selection

The most appropriate sites for the diagnosis of osteoporosis using DXA are the hip (proximal femur) and lumbar spine. This is because these are clinically important fracture sites and thus have the strongest predictive power for fracture at those sites.[36]

The use of a single hip is sufficient and is statistically more appropriate for diagnosis in line with the reporting guidelines.[37] However, some departments will scan bilateral hips and this is also acceptable practice. Bilateral hips are recommended in patients who have experienced a recent lower limb fracture[35] and are also useful in amputees.

A scan of the forearm is not usually required, but may be of use in some circumstances. In particular, increased cortical bone at the ⅓ radius region of interest is useful in hyperparathyroidism where there is preferential cortical bone loss.[37] In some centres, a forearm scan may be undertaken in patients with bilateral hip replacements or where a lumbar spine measurement is impossible due to widespread degenerative disease or internal fixation.

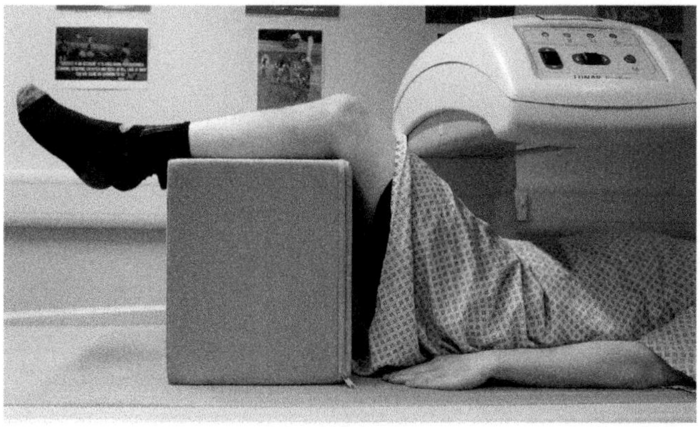

Fig. 30.4 Lumbar spine positioning – side view. (Courtesy Paul Quinn, University of Exeter.)

Fracture prediction can be further improved through identification of existing or previous vertebral fractures, a strong predictor of future fracture. DXA affords the ability to undertake imaging for vertebral fractures, while still maintaining a low radiation dose (0.002–0.5 mSv). In some patient groups, such as women over 70 and men over 80 with osteopenia,[38] vertebral fracture assessment (VFA) (performed using the DXA scanner) is an important addition to standard lumbar spine and proximal femur BMD measurements, and one that can help to optimise therapeutic interventions.[39] Furthermore, in some patients where use of standard DXA measurement sites is impossible due to fractures, surgical implants or other artefacts, the combination of VFA with clinical risk factors can provide a better assessment of fracture risk than clinical risk factors alone. These scans provide a lateral (and a posteroanterior (PA) if required) scan from L4 to T4. The International Osteoporosis Foundation and the International Society for Clinical Densitometry recommend VFA in patients with:

- T-score <−1.0 (see section on calculation and interpretation of BMD for explanation and further information on T-scores)
- Women ≥70 years old
- Men ≥80 years old
- Height loss >4 cm
- Self-reported, undocumented previous vertebral fracture
- Or height loss >2–4 cm with glucocorticoid therapy ≥5 mg prednisolone daily for ≥3 months[40]

LUMBAR SPINE POSITIONING

- Following appropriate patient preparation, the patient is positioned supine in the midline of the scanner bed with their legs raised on the positioning block (Fig. 30.4). It is important for this population to have plenty of pillows to make them comfortable. Some patients will have a significant kyphosis as a result of their vertebral fractures and their head must be adequately supported on pillows. This position is actually PA, since the X-ray tube is under the patient.
- Correct positioning is important and the patient should be straight and not rotated. The anterior superior iliac spines (ASISs) should be equidistant from the bed. The median sagittal plane (MSP) should be coincident with the long axis of the bed.

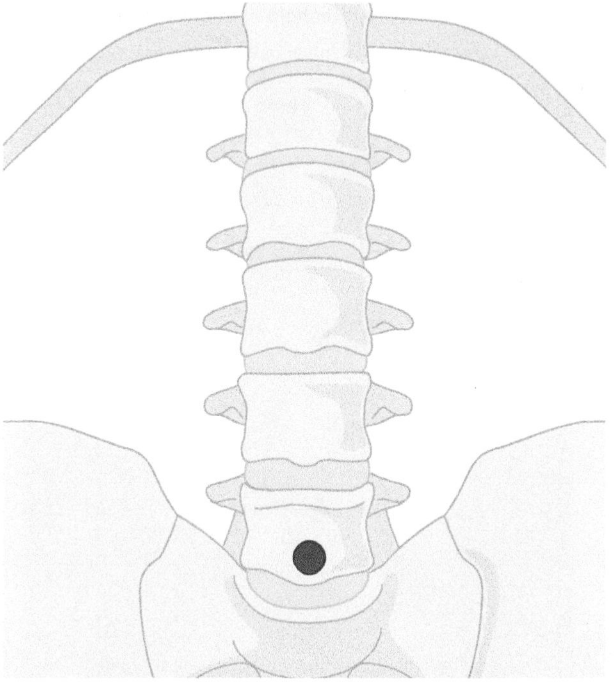

Fig. 30.5 Lumbar spine positioning – starting point.

- The laser cross should be positioned over the MSP, midway between the iliac crests and ASISs. The scan should start within the 5th lumbar vertebra (L5), or on a Hologic scanner may include the bottom of L5 (Fig. 30.5).
- The correct scan mode must be selected in line with the manufacturer's recommendations or departmental protocol. Most scanners will automatically default to the optimum scan mode based on the height and weight entered on the scanner. However, for some patients this may not be appropriate; it is important to check the tissue depth or weight and ensure the mode is appropriate.
- It is important to check the scan during acquisition and stop the scan early and re-position if needed, in order to ensure correct positioning and inclusion of region of interest.
- The scan should include half of L5 through to half of T12 (Fig. 30.6).
- It should be noted that anomalous vertebrae are present in 16–17% of the population. Of these atypical vertebrae 13% have rib anomalies, while the remainder result from lumbarisation of S1 or sacralisation of L5. Lumbarisation or sacralisation can result in the false impression of six or four lumbar vertebrae. It is important to identify the correct vertebrae for analysis on a DXA scan and the practitioner will statistically manage this most of the time if they use a system of counting from L5 upwards. As an example of vertebral variants, Fig. 30.7 demonstrates a partial sacralisation of L5 demonstrated on a DXA scan. Occasionally, a vertebral fracture assessment scan or other imaging may be available to assist in vertebral level identification, but this is not an indication to undertake further imaging. Before the patient gets off the table it is essential to check the scans on the analysis screen to ensure the acquisitions are appropriate, and that errors or artefacts have not been missed at the time of scanning. If artefacts are noted, it is essential to check

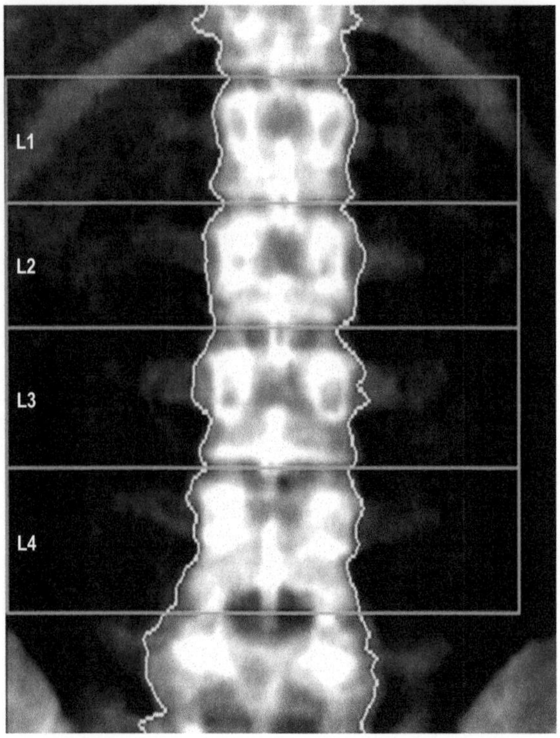

Fig. 30.6 Lumbar spine DXA.

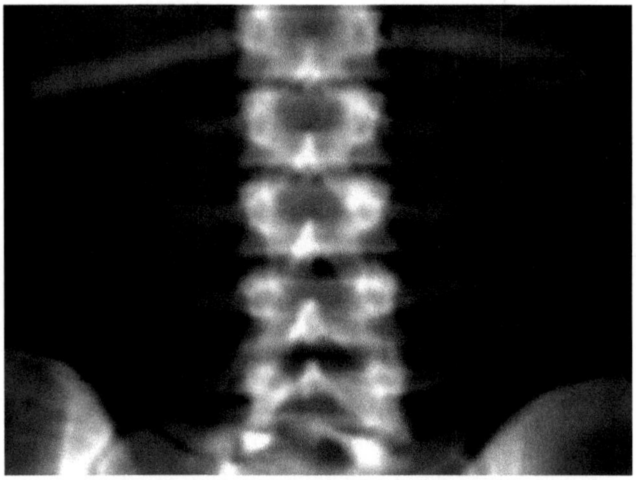

Fig. 30.7 Partial sacralisation of L5 demonstrated on a DXA scan.

whether they are internal or external to the patient. Not only can these artefacts impact on scan results, external artefacts may be mistaken for pathology on the low resolution scans.

HIP POSITIONING

- A hip positioning aid must always be used to help standardise positioning and assist the patient in holding the correct position for the duration of the scan. The patient lies supine on the table and the hip positioner is placed between their feet (Fig. 30.8).
- The hip to be scanned must be abducted by approximately 15° to separate the ischium from the lesser trochanter. The leg needs to be internally rotated by approximately 25° (Fig. 30.9). The foot should be in contact with the hip positioner and it is important to check the entire leg has been rotated and that it is not just the foot that has been internally rotated. The long axis of the femur should run parallel to the edge of the table.
- The laser cross hairs are placed 5 cm below the greater trochanter, in the midline of the femur, to start the scan (Fig. 30.10). There needs to be 3–5 cm on the scan before the ischium will be seen and the scan should finish 3–5 cm above the greater trochanter.
- It is important to check the scan during acquisition and stop the scan early and re-position if needed, in order to ensure correct positioning and inclusion of region of interest (Fig. 30.11).
- As previously discussed, bilateral hip scans are not essential. There is a high correlation between the two hips under normal circumstances (Fig. 30.12) but, for patients with amputations or with long-term disuse of a limb, it is may be advantageous to scan both hips because there is likely to be unilateral bone loss and increased fracture risk as a result. Figure 30.13 shows long-term bone loss in a patient with disuse osteopenia following a tibia and fibula fracture that resulted in an external fixator in situ for a period of 4 years.[41]

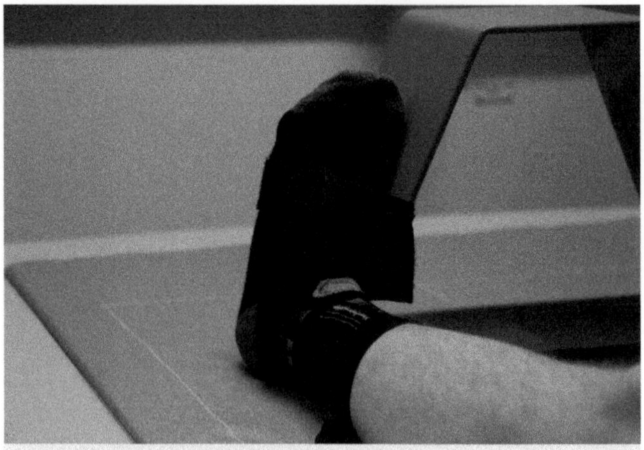

Fig. 30.8 DXA hip positioner. (Courtesy Paul Quinn, University of Exeter.)

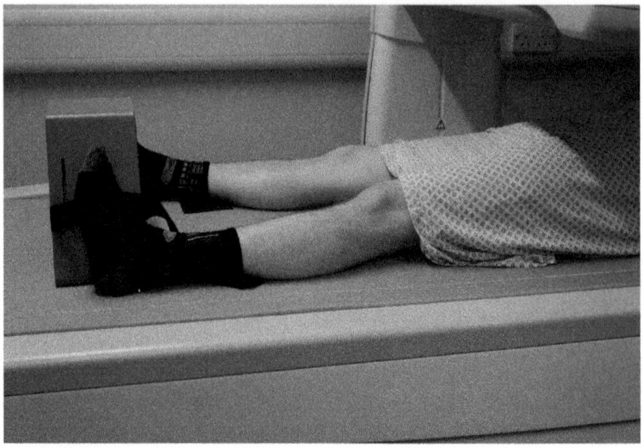

Fig. 30.9 Left hip positioning – leg position. (Courtesy Paul Quinn, University of Exeter.)

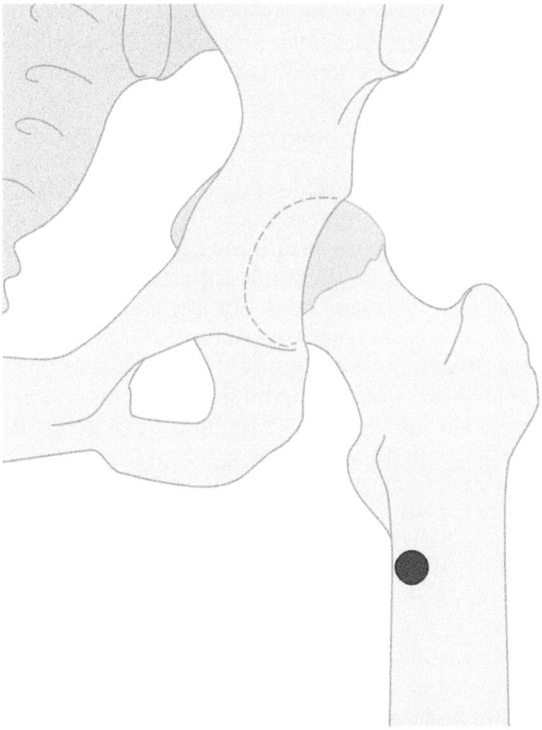

Fig. 30.10 Left hip positioning – with start point.

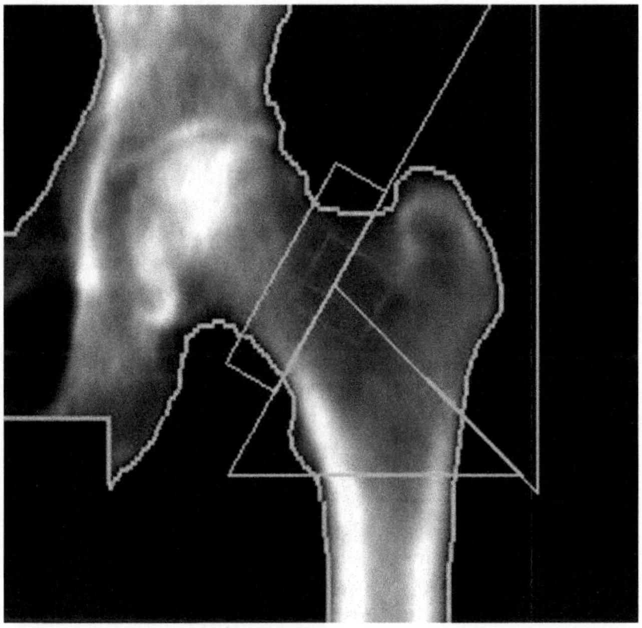

Fig. 30.11 DXA of the left hip.

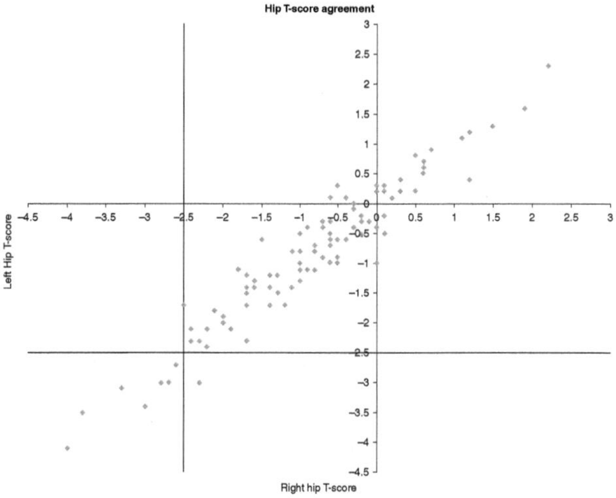

Fig. 30.12 Correlation between left and right hips.

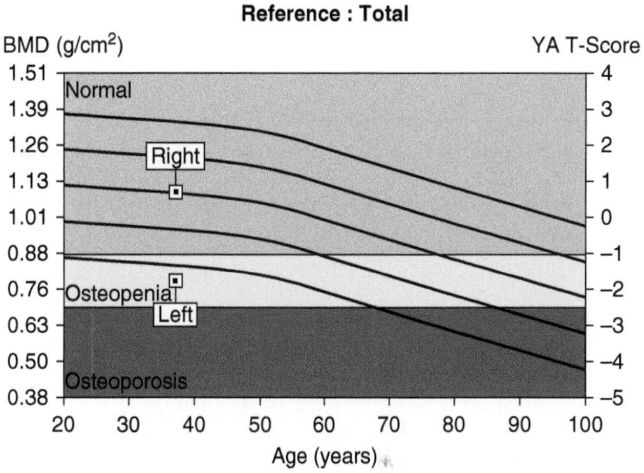

Fig. 30.13 Disuse osteopenia in the left hip.

FOREARM POSITIONING

- The patient sits with their non-dominant arm next to the DXA scanner. Their arm is measured using a tape measure from the olecranon process to the ulnar styloid process.
- The arm is positioned in the forearm positioning aid, in an anteroposterior (AP) position (remember that the X-ray tube is below the scanner bed in DXA) (Fig. 30.14), with the patient's fist lightly clenched.

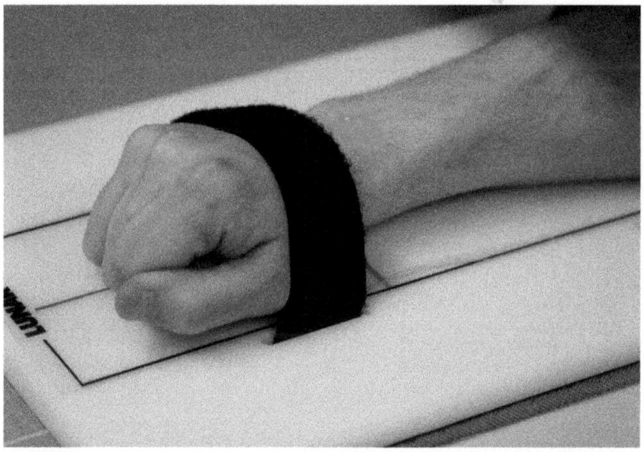

Fig. 30.14 Forearm positioning. (Courtesy Paul Quinn, University of Exeter.)

- The radial and ulnar styloid processes should be equidistant from the table. The scan is started in the midline between, and distal to, the radial and ulnar styloid processes. The forearm length is entered onto the computer system prior to analysis (Fig. 30.15).

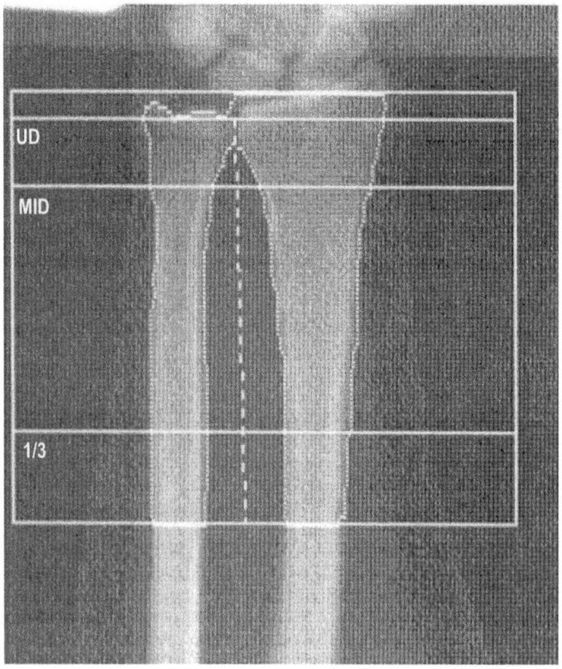

Fig. 30.15 Forearm DXA scan.

Vertebral Fracture Assessment (VFA)

VFA scans may be done as single energy or dual energy. Single-energy scans are the default mode for Hologic scanners and are faster, with a lower radiation dose. A focused dual energy scan is possible for any suspicious, but difficult to visualise areas. Dual energy scans are the mode available for the GE Lunar scanner and while these are slower and a slightly higher radiation dose, they afford better visualisation of the thoracic vertebrae.

Some scanners require a lateral decubitus position, while others will have a C-arm that will allow the patient to remain supine during the scan.

SUPINE POSITIONING FOR VFA

- Prior to positioning the patient, explain the positioning and the need for the patient to be as comfortable as possible to enable them to hold the position.
- The patient remains supine following their lumbar spine scan and positioned as for the PA (supine) lumbar spine. Ensure the patient is centred along the midline of the table and ask them to raise their arms above their head with their elbows bent. This is an intensely uncomfortable position for a patient with a recent vertebral fracture, so pads to rest their arms on or alternative positioning needs to be considered in line with their ability to hold the position. If raising their arms proves impossible, patients can have their arms folded across their chest.
- Correct positioning is important and the patient should be straight and not rotated. The ASISs should be equidistant from the bed. The MSP should be coincident with the long axis of the bed.
- The laser cross should be positioned over the MSP, midway between the iliac crests and ASISs. The scan should start within the 5th lumbar vertebra (L5) (Fig. 30.5).

LATERAL DECUBITUS POSITIONING FOR VFA

- The patient is positioned on their side with their back against the positioning aid. Ensure their back is positioned flat against the positioning aid and ensure their MSP is parallel to the table-top. The knees should be bent and the arms raised in front of their face. In patients with a recent vertebral fracture, correct positioning may be difficult but a position as close as possible to that required should be attempted. A pad between the knees can help to maintain a good lateral position, particularly in thinner patients. A pad may be required under the waist of the patient, again particularly for thin patients, to ensure the MSP remains parallel with the table throughout the spine. It is important that the patient is as comfortable as possible to hold this position for 3–4 minutes during the acquisition of the scan (Fig. 30.16).
- Position the laser cross hairs approximately 15 cm anterior (the distance will vary based on patient size) to the posterior processes of the spine and at a level midway between the ASIS and the iliac crest to start the scan in the middle of L5 (Fig. 30.17).

Total Body Scans

Total body scans are not routinely used in clinical practice in an adult population, but are a common research tool. However, they do form part of routine practice in paediatric scanning. Total body scans provide an assessment of body composition in addition to BMD and as such are of interest in populations where this may be of interest, for example in drug trials where body composition or fat distribution may be altered.

POSITIONING

The patient must be changed into a radiolucent gown for a total body scan since most clothing contains metal zips or buttons which will result in artefacts.

The patient is asked to lie supine on the table, within the line that runs around the edge of the table. MSP of their head and trunk should be perpendicular to the table-top (in a PA position) and there should be approximately 5 cm between the top of their head and the top line on the table. Legs are extended and slightly separated. Positioning of the patient's feet is often dictated by departmental protocol, but one method to aid patients to keep still and standardise positioning is to ask them to separate their legs slightly, with their toes touching together. A small band can be placed around the feet to help the patient hold the position (Fig. 30.18).

The patient's arms are extended and rested by their sides (but not touching the trunk) and their legs straight and slightly separated. If a patient is slim, their hands can be placed by their sides palm down on the table, or in a lateral

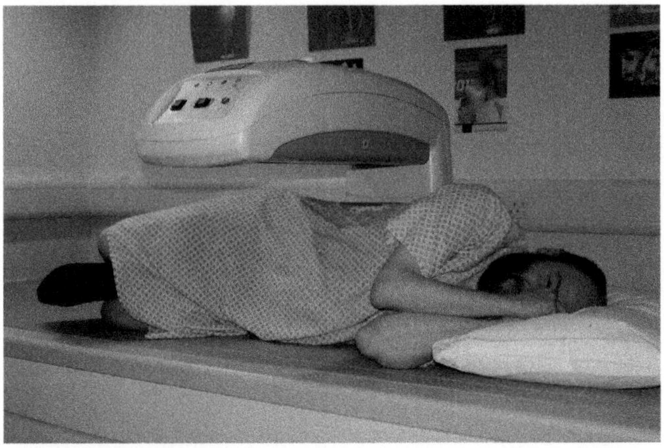

Fig. 30.16 VFA positioning – anterior view. (Courtesy Paul Quinn, University of Exeter.)

position if there is insufficient room for the former option (Fig. 30.19A,B).

CHECKING THE SCANS AND ARTEFACTS

Following the scan, all images must be checked in the analysis mode before the patient leaves. Scans must to be checked for artefacts and to ensure that they cover the correct anatomy, and that the positioning is acceptable.

Errors and artefacts which should be considered when interpreting a DXA scan can be broken down into two main areas: those that are avoidable and those that are unavoidable. Avoidable artefacts can be rectified by rescanning the patient or removing them from the scan during analysis. The decision regarding whether to rescan the patient must be made based on whether the scan analysis can sufficiently address the artefact. Unavoidable artefacts require careful scan analysis and interpretation or they may render the measurement uninterpretable.

Most artefacts result from patient-related factors. These may be in the form of clothing, prostheses, recent contrast or nuclear medicine investigations, other known or unknown pathologies and the positioning and size of the patient.

Artefacts commonly arise from clothing or items placed in pockets, piercings and occasionally patients failing to follow positioning instructions. Artefacts visible on the scan within one of the bone or soft-tissue regions of interest should have been checked with the patient at the time of the scan and removed if possible. Artefacts in the soft-tissue regions of interest (ROI) are equally as important as those within the bone itself, due to the use of both bone and soft-tissue ROIs in the calculation of BMD. Navel jewellery artefacts (see Fig. 30.3) have been demonstrated to result in clinically significant errors in the BMD measurement of the lower lumbar vertebrae,[30] while small metallic clothing clips can result in 'black hole' artefacts. These are not readily visualised, but have the potential to alter the measured BMD of a single vertebra[31] and therefore need to be excluded from the analysis if they cannot be removed.

Internal artefacts such as prostheses, drug pumps and lines cannot be removed, so the contralateral side should be scanned where possible, or vertebrae with overlying artefacts excluded from analysis as per the manufacturer's guidelines. It is recommended that a minimum of two

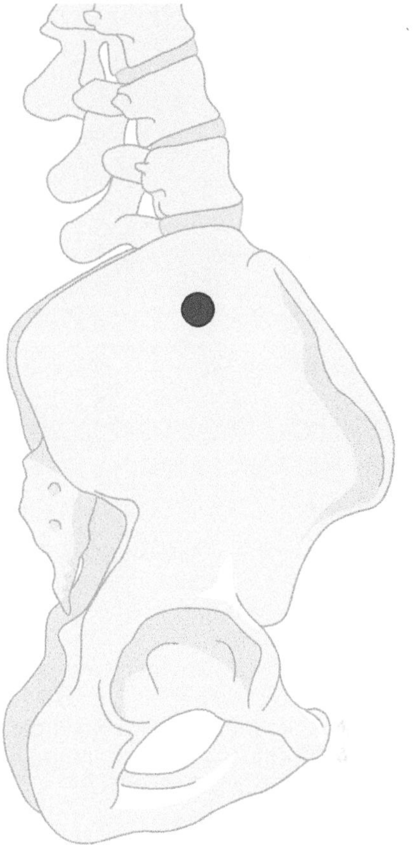

Fig. 30.17 VFA positioning – start point.

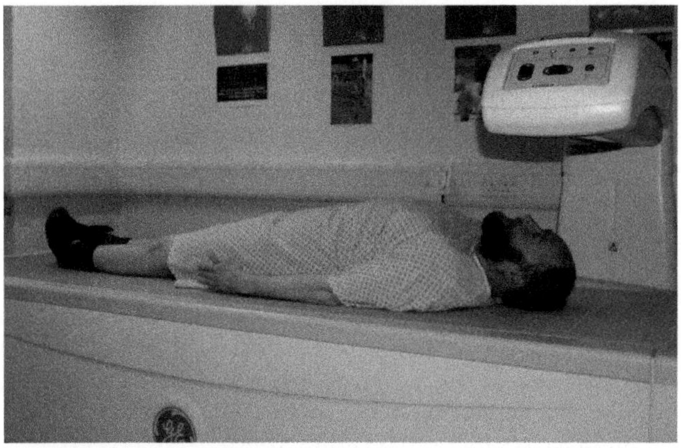

Fig. 30.18 Total body positioning. (Courtesy Paul Quinn, University of Exeter.)

vertebrae are used for the diagnosis of osteoporosis. Any fewer than this renders the scan too unreliable and a diagnosis should not be made on the basis of the result at a single vertebra.[42] Pathology within the soft tissue may result in artefacts that will not only affect the scan result, but may require highlighting in the DXA report if it is unknown. Figure 30.20 demonstrates a gallstone, while Fig. 30.21 demonstrates a calcified fibroid. While this will not impact on the BMD in this case, it is nonetheless worthy of note. It is possible that some artefacts may not be readily visualised

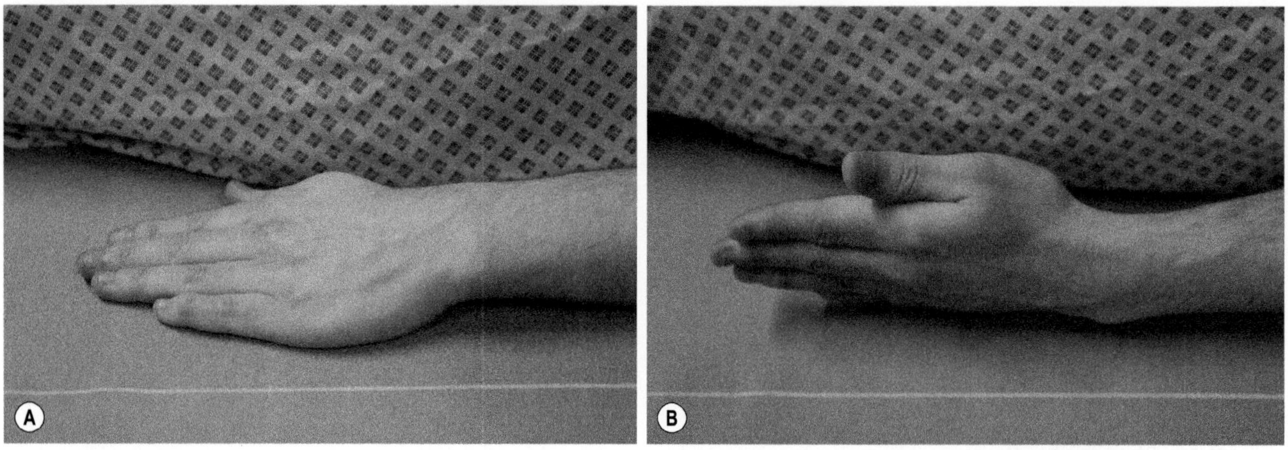

Fig. 30.19 (A,B) Hands in a palm down position and in a lateral position for total body positioning. (Courtesy Paul Quinn, University of Exeter.)

on the PA image, but are subsequently detected on VFA images. It is relatively common to note aortic calcification on the VFA image which may not be visualised on the PA image.

Poor positioning can lead to inaccurate results, difficulty identifying the correct vertebrae, insufficient soft tissue within the regions of interest for reliable measurement of BMD and up to 9% difference in the femoral neck BMD due to inaccurate positioning in hip scans.[43]

Image Analysis

LUMBAR SPINE

Analysis needs to be accurate and performed in line with the manufacturer's guidelines. Vertebral bodies must be correctly identified in the correct position, based on the manufacturer's guidelines. The edge detection of the bone needs to be correct; if this is inappropriately delineated, the scan should be classified as unreliable. Amendments of the edge detection by the operator are only recommended on GE Lunar scanners for obvious errors, but are not recommended by Hologic where manual amendment can cause inaccuracies in the measurement. Figure 30.22 demonstrates accurate edge detection and correct ROI placement in the spine. Not all spines are as easy; one of the biggest challenges in the ageing population is the presence of additional pathologies and normal variants of ageing. Osteoarthritis (OA) is the most prevalent form of arthritis[44] and common in an older population, meaning that a large proportion of patients scanned within an osteoporosis service will also have OA. The presence of OA will artificially elevate BMD, and vertebrae with obvious sclerotic focal defects and those with a greater than one T-score standard deviation (SD) increase should be excluded from the analysis.[42] Figure 30.23 demonstrates a spine with vertebrae excluded due to focal sclerotic defects and a T-score difference ≥1.0.

Normal variants within the spine are common[45] and can cause challenges for the correct identification of vertebrae, with some patients apparently presenting with four or six, instead of the usual five, lumbar vertebrae. Incorrectly identifying T12 as L1, for example, leads to reduced BMD being reported and therefore should be avoided[45] although, if other imaging is not available, the impact on diagnosis is minimal and other imaging is not warranted merely for confirmation. The use of VFA, where this is used in routine clinical practice, or historic imaging can assist with correct identification of vertebral levels.

HIP

Analysis is performed as instructed by the manufacturer's guidelines. The edge detection must be correctly identifying the bone. In patients with low bone mineral density, it is not uncommon for edge detection to miss part of the head of femur. It is important to address this error by using edge detection correction (point typing) so that it is clearly defined as bone, otherwise the femoral neck region of interest will be positioned too close to the femoral head and will give an inaccurate result. Figure 30.24 demonstrates a well-positioned and correctly analysed hip scan.

Beware of patients who have a fat panniculus that overlies the femoral neck area (Fig. 30.25). This can cause spurious results due to the inconsistencies in tissue thickness. In these patients, attempts should be made to retract the fat panniculus if at all possible. This can be done by asking the patient to move the panniculus out of the way and support it with their hand during the scan. However, this is not always successful and can be a difficult topic to broach with patients.

FOREARM

Analysis must be performed as instructed by the manufacturers. Generally, the forearm length is entered into the computer system and the region of interest (ROI) placed so that the upper border of the region of interest is located distally on the radius in accordance with the manufacturer's guidelines. If the positioning of the ROI is correct, there should be no need to change the size or position of the ultradistal, mid or 1/3 regions.

VERTEBRAL FRACTURE ASSESSMENT (VFA)

Most DXA scanners have morphometric software which can be used to identify vertebral fractures using the Genant scale.[46] However, visual assessment by those trained to interpret VFA scans is considered to be an accurate method

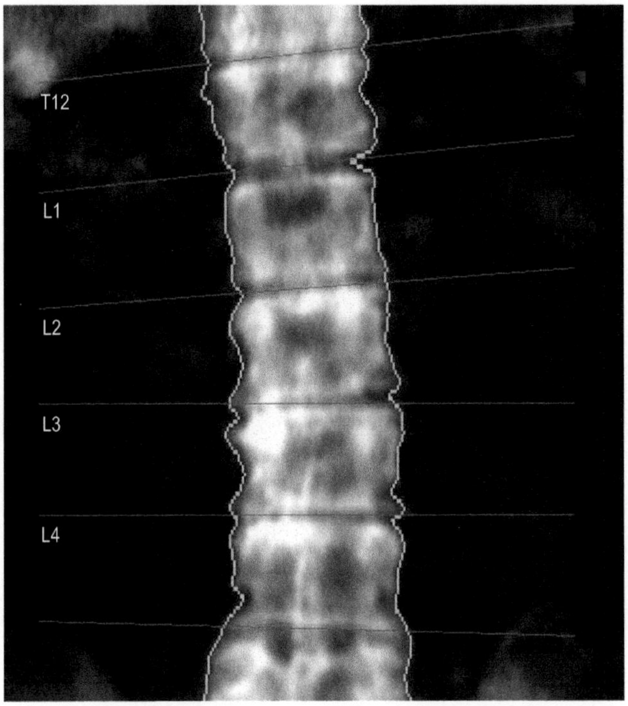

Fig. 30.20 Gallstone on a lumbar spine image.

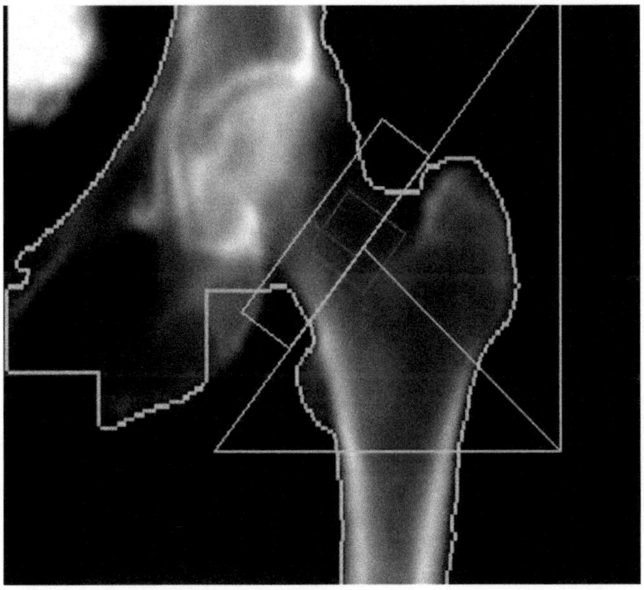

Fig. 30.21 Calcified fibroid on a left hip image.

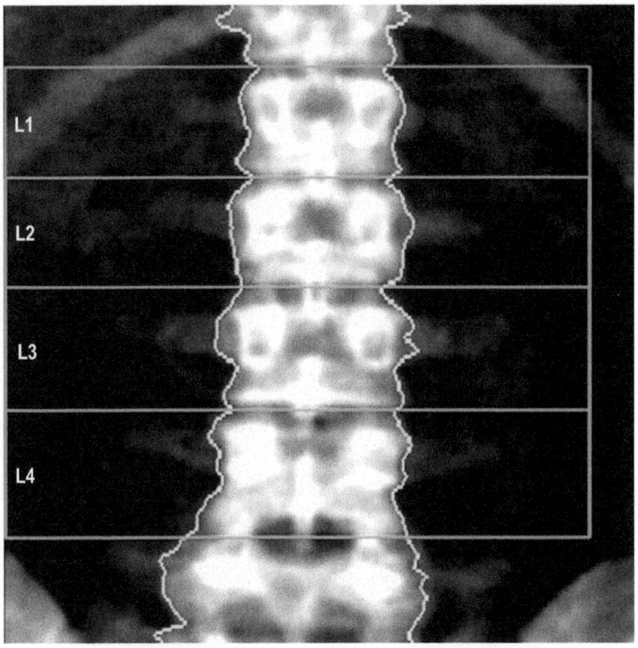

Fig. 30.22 Lumbar spine correct analysis.

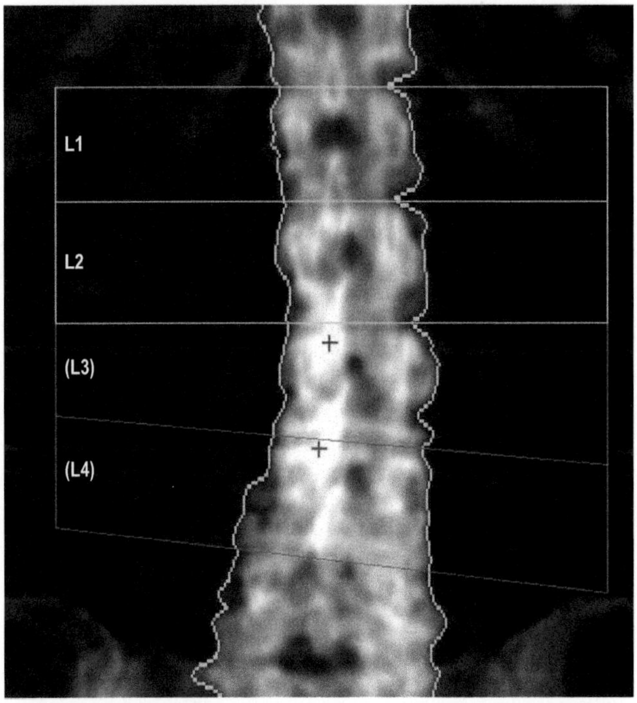

Fig. 30.23 Lumbar spine with vertebrae excluded resulting from degenerative changes.

and is used most frequently in clinical practice because it is faster.[47] Figure 30.26 demonstrates a T7 fracture on a VFA scan. Where a vertebral fracture is identified on the scan, projection radiographs are recommended to characterise the fracture and exclude any other underlying pathologies. Osteoporosis and other reasons for pathological fracture are not mutually exclusive and therefore other pathologies should be ruled out in patients where a new fracture is identified.[38,48] Furthermore, VFA has poor accuracy for detecting mild vertebral fractures[49,50] and further imaging may be required to confirm an equivocal fracture. Other congenital and developmental pathologies can mimic fractures, particularly with the poorer resolution on VFA compared to projection radiography.[51] Further imaging may be required to differentiate between non-fracture deformities such as Scheuermann's disease, degenerative changes, or to examine for another fracture-causing pathology such as Paget's disease of bone, or malignancy.[38] This follow-up imaging may include projection radiography, magnetic resonance imaging (MRI), computed tomography (CT), nuclear medicine or positron emission tomography CT (PET-CT) depending on the pathology suspected.[48]

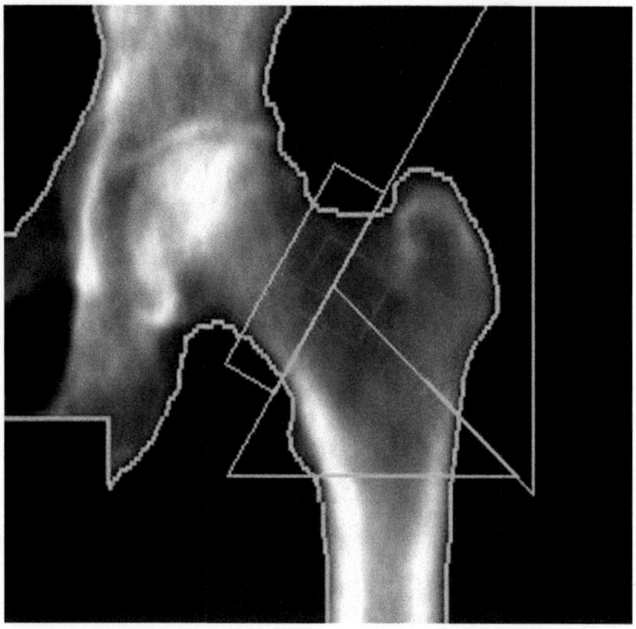

Fig. 30.24 Correctly analysed hip (GE Lunar scanner).

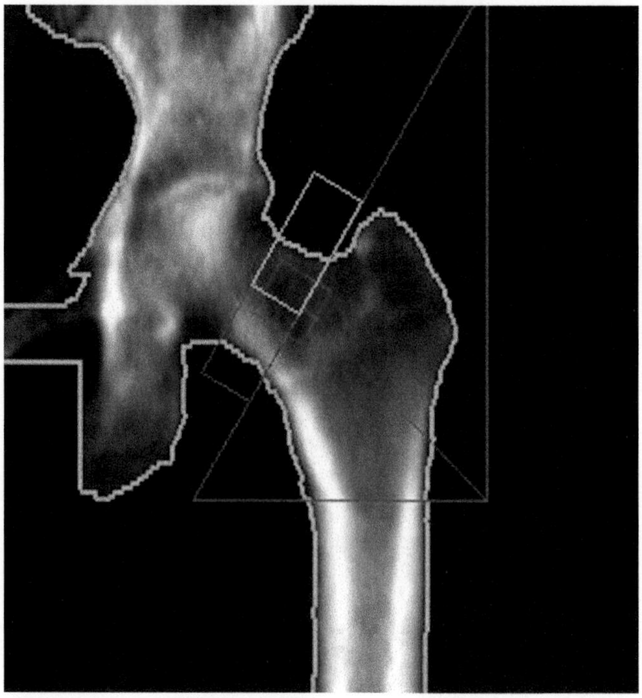

Fig. 30.25 A fat panniculus.

TOTAL BODY (TB)

Analysis must be undertaken as recommended by the manufacturer's guidelines. The ROIs for the TB scan include a number of lines that require correct positioning on the scan. In general, the horizontal line above the shoulders is placed just below the chin. The vertical lines at the shoulders are placed at the glenoid fossa. The vertical lines on either side of the spine are moved close to the spine and angled to match any curvature if required. The small horizontal line is placed at the level of T12–L1. The horizontal lines above the pelvis are placed just above the iliac crests and the angled lines below the pelvis are placed so they bisect both femoral necks. The vertical line between the legs is placed between the feet and the vertical lines lateral to both the legs are placed to include as much of the soft tissue as possible laterally, but without including the patient's fingers within the ROIs, as demonstrated in Fig. 30.27.

GENERAL CONSIDERATIONS

It must be remembered that BMD is an areal measurement and as such does not fully adjust for bone size in the way a 3D volumetric measurement would. This means that BMD will be underestimated in very small people who have small bones, while the opposite is true for tall people with bigger bones.

Care should be taken to note any significant changes in the patient's body habitus when evaluating sequential or follow-up scans, as obesity has been shown to increase precision errors.[52] Caution should also be taken in interpreting femur scans in obese patients with an overlying fat panniculus.[53] If an operator has asked the patient to retract this then it should be noted, and also retracted for subsequent examinations. Aortic calcification is frequently seen in ageing populations and this can also affect BMD results since it overlies the lumbar vertebrae. This can be difficult to identify on a PA lumbar spine DXA scan and might only be seen if the patient has vertebral fracture assessment (VFA), or on projection radiographs where it may be visualised anterior to the vertebral bodies.[54] Exclusion of vertebrae from the analysis may be appropriate if aortic calcification is limited to defined areas and is resulting in a greater than 1 T-score elevated discrepancy. Of particular note in an osteoporotic population are vertebral fractures, which may also elevate the BMD of the affected vertebrae. These can often show reduced vertebral height with dense sclerotic vertebrae and disproportionately high BMD. Again, these should be excluded from the analysis, with interpretation made from the remaining non-fractured vertebrae. If the patient is not known to have a vertebral fracture, but the image findings are suggestive of this, VFA may be useful if available. If not, the patient should be referred for further radiographic assessment to confirm the fracture and this may be performed at the time of assessment, or recommended in the report. Other diseases of note which will increase BMD either locally or systemically include Paget's disease of bone,[55] primary bone tumours and sclerotic bone metastases. A reason for variability in BMD across each individual vertebra is not always apparent. In a study of 2391 females the incidence of large T-score differences, greater than 1 standard deviation between vertebrae, was found to vary with age and body weight but was still common in a younger population; this shows that clinically significant T-score differences can occur in the absence of other pathology. This study demonstrated that there is likely to be a natural variance in some patients, which is not associated with any pathology; careful visual assessment of vertebrae must be made before any decision is reached to exclude a vertebra from the analysis.[56]

Occasionally, conditions other than osteoporosis can lead to low BMD and can cause confusion in the interpretation of DXA scans. This may be generalised, or may be focal. Examples of focal conditions leading to locally reduced BMD

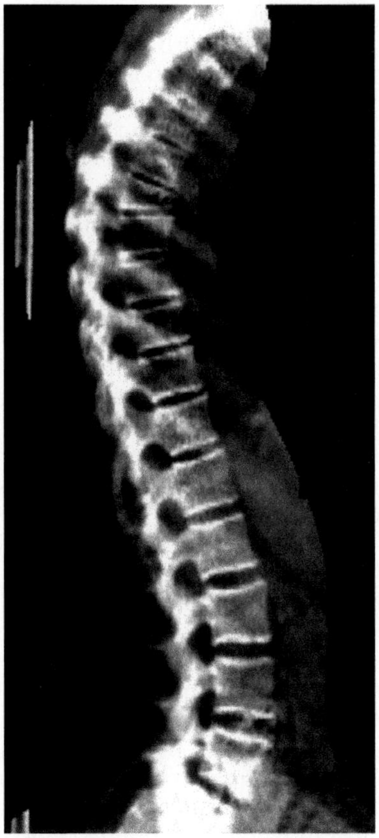

Fig. 30.26 A fracture of T7 identified on a VFA scan.

include previous spine surgery such as laminectomy or anatomical anomalies such as spina bifida occulta. These may not have been previously recognised in the patient. If T-score discrepancies are noted without any visual evidence of pathology in the vertebrae with higher BMD, it is important to consider whether the vertebrae with the low T-scores may be providing the spurious results. Lytic bone metastases may occur in breast cancer, so T-score discrepancies or unusual image appearances in patients known to have malignancy should be considered seriously for follow-up with further imaging.[57]

Calculation and Interpretation of Bone Mineral Density

Bone mineral density from a DXA scan is calculated using the following formula:

$$\text{Bone mineral density}(BMD) = \frac{\text{Bone mineral content}(BMC)}{\text{projected area of bone}}$$

The units used for BMD are in g/cm^2.

The spine regions of interest are combined to provide a single BMD measurement, usually from L1 to L4. This is done using the formula below:

$$BMD_{L1-L4} = \frac{BMC_{L1} + BMC_{L2} + BMC_{L3} + BMC_{L4}}{Area_{L1} + Area_{L2} + Area_{L3} + Area_{L4}}$$

A BMD value alone is of little value without an understanding of how it compares to a wider population. To do this, each

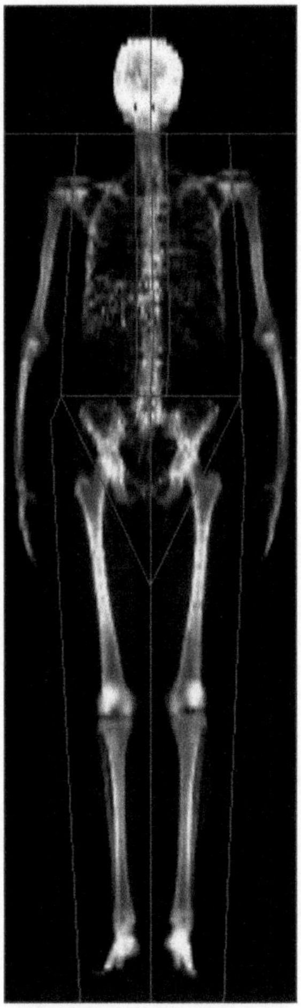

Fig. 30.27 A total body scan with appropriate analysis.

scanner contains reference data from a large population. The Royal Osteoporosis Society recommend the use of third National Health and Nutrition Examination Survey (NHANES III) reference data from the USA[58] for proximal femur DXA measurements, and DXA scanner manufacturers' UK reference data for the lumbar spine and forearm.[37]

The reference population is frequently described as the mean BMD and the population standard deviation matched for age, sex and race. Results are often displayed as a diagram against age, which shows the reference population ± 1 or 2 standard deviations. A patient's result may also be expressed numerically as a Z-score and T-score. This expresses how many standard deviations a person's BMD differs from the mean value for an age-, sex- and race-matched population or compared to a young population.

A T-score represents a comparison with a young population representing peak bone mass, while a Z-score provides an age-matched comparison.

A T-score is calculated using the following equation:

$$T-\text{score} = \frac{\text{Measured BMD} - \text{Young adult } \overline{x}}{\text{Young adult } \sigma}$$

Where $\overline{x}$ is the mean and σ is the standard deviation.

A Z-score is calculated using the following equation:

$$Z - score = \frac{Measured\ BMD\ -\ age\ matched\ \overline{x}}{Age\ matched\ \sigma}$$

Where $\overline{x}$ is the mean and σ is the standard deviation.

T-scores compare the result to the mean and standard deviation of a young adult population (20–40 years) regardless of the age of the patient, thus comparing the patient to the sex- and race-adjusted maximum BMD achieved in life. In 1994 WHO criteria were introduced as a guideline for the diagnosis of osteoporosis using spine, hip or forearm BMD. The WHO criteria advocated interpretation of spine, proximal femur and forearm BMD results using T-scores in the following four categories:

Normal: A BMD value of greater or equal to 1 SD below the young adult mean value (T >−1.0)

Osteopenia: A BMD value that lies between 1 and 2.5 SD below the young adult mean (T −1.0 to T −2.49)

Osteoporosis: A BMD value greater than or equal to 2.5 SD below the young adult mean value (T ≤−2.5)

Established osteoporosis: A BMD value greater than or equal to 2.5 SD below the young adult mean value (T ≤−2.5) in the presence of one or more fragility fractures.[4]

These criteria are still used today, but a more holistic approach should be considered, including the number of clinical risk factors. Considering both BMD and clinical risk factors increases the fracture prediction and thus can enable better targeting of therapeutic interventions.

T-scores are appropriate for postmenopausal women and they can also be used for men over the age of 50 years. However, they must never be used in children and should be avoided in younger adults, where Z-score should be used for interpretation instead. This is because peak bone mass is achieved approximately a decade after the cessation of linear bone growth, and it is thus inappropriate to compare someone who has not yet achieved peak bone mass to a population mean for peak bone mass.

Some scanners also provide the T-score and Z-score equivalents as a percentage. While these are not used clinically for diagnostic purposes, they are useful for explainin results to the patient.

Interpretation of DXA scans must be undertaken by appropriately qualified staff who have expertise in not only DXA, but in the pathophysiology of osteoporosis and metabolic bone diseases. It is important that the person providing the final clinical report understands the requirements for an appropriately positioned and analysed scan, and the impact of poor scanning technique on the result.

The presence of generalised low BMD on a DXA measurement, with or without fracture, may not be diagnostic of osteoporosis. Vitamin D deficiency is especially prevalent in some ethnic groups and among the elderly population in the UK, and therefore osteomalacia should be considered, particularly in those at risk of low vitamin D.[59] There may be other imaging findings in osteomalacia, which are not seen in osteoporosis. A Loosers zone, or pseudofracture, may be observed in association with reports of bone pain and muscle weakness[60] which are not typical symptoms of osteoporosis when a fracture is not present.[61] Milder variants of osteogenesis imperfecta may present in adults; this typically results in very low BMD and may be suspected from a characteristic fracture history in childhood. Multiple myeloma typically leads to focal lytic lesions but occasionally presents as generalised low BMD indistinguishable from osteoporosis.[62] Differential diagnosis requires appropriate work-up through blood analysis and appropriate imaging in any patient with unexplained low BMD.

Longitudinal Monitoring

Longitudinal monitoring of disease progression and the effects of therapeutic intervention makes up a proportion of the workload in many departments and, in addition to the considerations above, these scans should be considered in line with the expected clinical changes in BMD in light of the patient's history. Changes in BMD are generally slow and of similar magnitude annually to the error of the DXA measurement technique. A scan interval of at least 2 years is therefore usually required for the least significant change to be exceeded and to be confident that there has been a clear change in BMD.[52] This time may be reduced in some populations, such as individuals treated with anabolic agents when more rapid increases in BMD are seen. However, in some patients, in whom measurements are more variable, this interval may require extending. For example, in obese individuals the precision error is significantly greater than the 1% reported in the normal size population.[52,63] Furthermore, large changes in weight between scans can adversely impact on the reliability of DXA measurements, as demonstrated in patients who have undergone bariatric surgery.[64] Caution is advised on the interpretation of longitudinal measurements in patients being treated with strontium ranelate, due to its high atomic number which will artificially elevate measurements at all anatomical sites.[65,66] Quantifying changes in bone mass for this group of patients is not reliable, however increases in bone mass correlates directly to efficacy and may also indicate patient compliance with medication.

The Royal Osteoporosis Society (ROS) has published standards that provide best practice guidance for reporting DXA scans. The reporting requirements are not covered in this chapter because this is beyond the scope of this book. The reporting standards can be found on the website of the ROS.[37]

References

1. Blake GM, Fogelman I. The clinical role of dual energy X-ray absorptiometry. *Eur J Radiol.* 2009;71(3):406–414.
2. Kanis JA, McCloskey EV, Johansson H, et al. European guidance for the diagnosis and management of osteoporosis in postmenopausal women. *Osteoporos Int.* 2013;24(1):23–57.
3. Masud T, Mootoosamy I, McCloskey EV, et al. Assessment of osteopenia from spine radiographs using two different methods: the Chingford Study. *Br J Radiol.* 1996;69(821):451–456.
4. World Health Organization. *Assessment of Fracture Risk and its Application to Screening for Post-Menopausal Osteoporosis.* Geneva: WHO; 1994. Report of a WHO Study Group. (WHO Technical Report Series 843.).
5. Kanis JA, Delmas P, Burckhardt P, et al. Guidelines for diagnosis and management of osteoporosis. The European Foundation for osteoporosis and bone disease. *Osteoporos Int.* 1997;7(4):390–406.
6. van Staa TP, Dennison EM, Leufkens HG, et al. Epidemiology of fractures in England and Wales. *Bone.* 2001;29(6):517–522.
7. Kanis JA. *WHO technical report. Assessment of Osteoporosis at the Primary Health Care Level.* UK: WHO Scientific Group University of Sheffield; 2007:66.

8. Johnell O, Kanis J. An estimate of the worldwide prevalence and disability associated with osteoporotic fractures. *Osteoporos Int.* 2006;17(12):1726–1733.
9. Wells J, Ryan PJ. The long-term performance of DXA bone densitometers. *Br J Radiol.* 2000;73(871):737–739.
10. Lu Y, Mathur AK, Blunt BA, et al. Dual X-ray absorptiometry quality control: comparison of visual examination and process-control charts. *J Bone Miner Res.* 1996;11(5):626–637.
11. Koetsier A, van der Veer SN, Jager KJ, et al. Control charts in healthcare quality improvement. A systematic review on adherence to methodological criteria. *Methods Inf Med.* 2012;51(3):189–198.
12. Knapp KM, Griffin JGL, Blake GM. Dual energy x-ray absorptiometry: quality assurance and governance. *Osteoporos Rev.* 2014;22(1):1–6.
13. Griffin JGL, Knapp KM, Pearce G. Static and mobile DXA scanner invivo cross-calibration study. *Radiography.* 2013;19(1):7–10.
14. *The Ionising Radiation (Medical Exposure) Regulations.* UK Statutory Instrument 2017 No. 1322; 2017. https://www.legislation.gov.uk/uksi/2017/1322/contents/made.
15. NICE (National Institute for Health and Care Excellence). Osteoporosis: Assessing the Risk of Fragility Fracture. Clinical guideline [CG146]. https://www.nice.org.uk/guidance/cg146.
16. Kanis J, Johnell O, Odén A, et al. FRAX™ and the assessment of fracture probability in men and women from the UK. *Osteoporos Int.* 2008;19(4):385–397.
17. Anabtawi A, Le T, Putman M, Tangpricha V, et al. Cystic fibrosis bone disease: pathophysiology, assessment and prognostic implications. *J Cystic Fibrosis.* 2019;18(suppl 2):S48–S55.
18. Bilezikian JP, Brandi ML, Eastell R, et al. Guidelines for the management of asymptomatic primary hyperparathyroidism: summary statement from the Fourth International Workshop. *J Clin Endocrinol Metabol.* 2014;99(10):3561–3569.
19. Bemben DA, Sherk VD, Ertl WJJ, et al. Acute bone changes after lower limb amputation resulting from traumatic injury. *Osteoporos Int.* 2017;28(7):2177–2186.
20. Poole KE, Vedi S, Debiram I, et al. Bone structure and remodelling in stroke patients: early effects of zoledronate. *Bone.* 2009;44(4):629–633.
21. McCloskey E. Effects of third-generation aromatase inhibitors on bone. *Eur J Cancer.* 2006;42(8):1044–1051.
22. Daniell HW, Dunn SR, Ferguson DW, et al. Progressive osteoporosis during androgen deprivation therapy for prostate cancer. *J Urol.* 2000;163(1):181–186.
23. Vestergaard P. Drugs causing bone loss. In: Barrett JE, ed. *Handbook of Experimental Pharmacology.* Cham: Springer; 2019.
24. Crabtree NJ, Arabi A, Bachrach LK, et al. Dual-energy X-ray absorptiometry interpretation and reporting in children and adolescents: the revised 2013 ISCD Pediatric Official Positions. *J Clin Densitom.* 2014;17(2):225–242.
25. Shuhart CR, Yeap SS, Anderson PA, et al. Executive summary of the 2019 ISCD position development Conference on monitoring treatment, DXA cross-calibration and least significant change, spinal Cord injury, Peri-prosthetic and Orthopedic bone health, Transgender medicine, and Pediatrics. *J Clin Densitom.* 2019;22(4):453–471.
26. Hillier TA, Cauley JA, Rizzo JH, et al. WHO absolute fracture risk models (FRAX): do clinical risk factors improve fracture prediction in older women without osteoporosis? *J Bone Miner Res.* 2011;26(8):1774–1782.
27. Hippisley-Cox J, Coupland C. Derivation and validation of updated QFracture algorithm to predict risk of osteoporotic fracture in primary care in the United Kingdom: prospective open cohort study. *BMJ (Clin Res).* 2012;344:e3427.
28. Warriner AH, Patkar NM, Curtis JR, et al. Which fractures are most attributable to osteoporosis? *J Clin Epidemiol.* 2011;64(1):46–53.
29. Morrison A, Fan T, Sen SS, et al. Epidemiology of falls and osteoporotic fractures: a systematic review. *ClinicoEconom Outcomes Res CEOR.* 2013;5:9.
30. Ott SM, Ichikawa LE, LaCroix AZ, et al. Navel jewelry artifacts and intravertebral variation in spine bone densitometry in adolescents and young women. *J Clin Densitom.* 2009;12(1):84–88.
31. Morgan SL, Lopez-Ben R, Nunnally N, et al. 'Black hole artifacts'– new potential pitfall for DXA accuracy? *J Clin Densitom.* 2008;11(2):266–275.
32. Xu HM, Han JG, Na Y, et al. Colonic transit time in patient with slow-transit constipation: comparison of radiopaque markers and barium suspension method. *Eur J Radiol.* 2011;79(2):211–213.
33. Sala A, Webber C, Halton J, et al. Effect of diagnostic radioisotopes and radiographic contrast media on measurements of lumbar spine bone mineral density and body composition by dual-energy x-ray absorptiometry. *J Clin Densitom.* 2006;9(1):91–96.
34. Blake GM. The effect of radiopharmaceutical administration on dual-energy X-ray absorptiometry scans. *J Clin Densitom.* 2013;16(3):257–258.
35. Hopkins SJ, Toms AD, Brown M, et al. Disuse osteopenia following leg fracture in postmenopausal women: implications for HIP fracture risk and fracture liaison services. *Radiography (Lond).* 2018;24(2):151–158.
36. Marshall D, Johnell O, Wedel H. Meta-analysis of how well measures of bone mineral density predict occurrence of osteoporotic fractures. *BMJ (Clin Res).* 1996;312(7041):1254–1259.
37. Peel N, Griffith J. *Reporting Dual Energy X-ray Absorptiometry Scans in Adult Fracture Risk Assessment: Standards for Quality.* London: Royal Osteoporosis Society; 2019. Available at: https://theros.org.uk/clinical-publications-and-resources/.
38. Schousboe JT, Vokes T, Broy SB, et al. Dual-energy X-ray absorptiometry technical issues: the 2007 ISCD Official Positions. *J Clin Densitom.* 2008;11(1):92–108.
39. Kuet KP, Charlesworth D, Peel NFA. Vertebral fracture assessment scans enhance targeting of investigations and treatment within a fracture risk assessment pathway. *Osteoporos Int.* 2013;24(3):1007–1014.
40. Lewiecki EM, Gordon CM, Baim S, et al. International Society for clinical densitometry 2007 adult and Pediatric Official positions. *Bone.* 2008;43(6):1115–1121.
41. Knapp KMRA, Welsman JR, MacLeod KM. Prolonged unilateral disuse osteopenia 14 years post external fixator removal: a case history and critical review. *Case Reports in Medicine.* 2010. https://doi.org/10.1155/2010/629020. (2010:629020).
42. *ISCD. Official Positions – Adult Positions.* International Society for Clinical Densitometry; 2007. https://iscd.org/learn/official-positions/adult-positions/.
43. Palmer RM. *An Evaluation of the Limitations for the Technique of Dual Energy Absorptiometry in the Measurement of Bone Disease.* The University of Glamorgan; 1996.
44. CYJ W, Conaghan PG. New horizons in osteoarthritis. *Age Ageing.* 2013;42(3):272–278.
45. Peel NFA, Johnson A, Barrington NA, et al. Impact of anomalous vertebral segmentation on measurements of bone-mineral density. *J Bone Miner Res.* 1993;8(6):719–723.
46. Genant HK, Jergas M, Palermo L, et al. Comparison of semiquantitative visual and quantitative morphometric assessment of prevalent and incident vertebral fractures in osteoporosis. The Study of Osteoporotic Fractures Research Group. *J Bone Miner Res.* 1996;11(7):984–996.
47. Rea JA, Steiger P, Blake GM, et al. Optimizing data acquisition and analysis of morphometric X-ray absorptiometry. *Osteoporos Int.* 1998;8(2):177–183.
48. Aggarwal A, Salunke P, Shekhar BR, et al. The role of magnetic resonance imaging and positron emission tomography-computed tomography combined in differentiating benign from malignant lesions contributing to vertebral compression fractures. *Surg Neurol Int.* 2013;4(suppl 5):S323–S326.
49. Rea JA, Chen MB, Li J, et al. Morphometric X-ray absorptiometry and morphometric radiography of the spine: a comparison of prevalent vertebral deformity identification. *J Bone Miner Res.* 2000;15(3):564–574.
50. Jiang G, Eastell R, Barrington NA, et al. Comparison of methods for the visual identification of prevalent vertebral fracture in osteoporosis. *Osteoporos Int.* 2004;15(11):887–896.
51. Rea JA, Li J, Blake GM, Steiger P, et al. Visual assessment of vertebral deformity by X-ray absorptiometry: a highly predictive method to exclude vertebral deformity. *Osteoporos Int.* 2000;11(8):660–668.
52. Knapp KM, Welsman JR, Hopkins SJ, et al. Obesity increases precision errors in dual-energy x-ray absorptiometry measurements. *J Clin Densitom.* 2012;15(3):315–319.
53. Binkley N, Krueger D, Vallarta-Ast N. An overlying femur bone fat panniculus affects mass measurement. *J Clin Densitom.* 2003;6(3):199–204.
54. Cecelja M, Frost ML, Spector TD, et al. Abdominal aortic calcification detection using dual-energy X-ray absorptiometry: validation study in healthy women compared to computed tomography. *Calcif Tissue Int.* 2013;92(6):495–500.
55. Ralston SH, Langston AL, Reid IR. Pathogenesis and management of Paget's disease of bone. *Lancet.* 2008;372(9633):155–163.

56. Blake GM Noon E, Spector TD, et al. Intervertebral T-score differences in younger and older women. *J Clin Densitom.* 2013;16(3):329–335.
57. Quattrocchi CC, Piciucchi S, Sammarra M, et al. Bone metastases in breast cancer: higher prevalence of osteosclerotic lesions. *Radiol Med.* 2007;112(7):1049–1059.
58. Looker AC, Orwoll ES, Johnston JR, et al. Prevalence of low femoral bone density in older US adults from NHANES III. *J Bone Miner Res.* 1997;12(11):1761–1768.
59. Mavroeidi A, Aucott L, Black AJ, et al. Seasonal variation in 25(OH) D at Aberdeen (57 degrees N) and bone health indicators – could holidays in the sun and cod liver oil supplements alleviate deficiency? *PloS One.* 2013;8(1). e53381.
60. Reginato AJ, Falasca GF, Pappu R, et al. Musculoskeletal manifestations of osteomalacia: report of 26 cases and literature review. *Semin Arthritis Rheum.* 1999;28(5):287–304.
61. Zhao Y, Liu Y, Zheng Y. Osteoporosis and related factors in older females with skeletal pain or numbness: a retrospective study in East China. *J Int Med Res.* 2013;41(3):859–866.
62. Roux S, Bergot C, Fermand JP, et al. Evaluation of bone mineral density and fat-lean distribution in patients with multiple myeloma in sustained remission. *J Bone Miner Res.* 2003;18(2):231–236.
63. Rajamanohara R, Robinson J, Rymer J, et al. The effect of weight and weight change on the long-term precision of spine and hip DXA measurements. *Osteoporos Int.* 2011;22(5):1503–1512.
64. Yu EW, Bouxsein M, Roy AE, et al. Bone loss after bariatric surgery: discordant results between DXA and QCT bone density. *J Bone Miner Res.* 2014;29(3):542–550.
65. Fogelman I, Blake GM. Strontium does accumulate in bone. *Osteoporos Int.* 2012;23(3):1187.
66. Liao J, Blake GM, McGregor AH, et al. The effect of bone strontium on BMD is different for different manufacturers' DXA systems. *Bone.* 2010;47(5):882–887.

Glossary of Radiographic Terms

Abduction: Refers to limbs or digits, when they are moved away from the median sagittal plane or trunk. An abducted thumb is moved away from the rest of the hand.
Adduction: Refers to limbs or digits, when they are brought towards the median sagittal plane or trunk. An adducted thumb is moved towards the rest of the hand.
Anatomical position: The trunk and limbs are extended fully, with the arms slightly abducted at the side. The palms of the hands face forwards. The front of the patient faces forwards.
Anterior: The front of the patient, or body part, when the patient is in the anatomical position.
Anterior oblique: An oblique position, when the anterior aspect of the patient is nearest the image receptor *or* a posteroanterior position with an oblique angle applied in a lateral or medial direction.
Anteroposterior: A position where the anterior aspect of the patient faces the X-ray tube, and the central ray passes through this aspect and exits through the posterior aspect.
Anthropological baseline: Baseline used in radiography of the head, dental radiography and CT (see Chs 11 and 14). Also known as the Frankfurt/ Frankfort plane.

Bucky: Antiscatter device.

Caudal: Relating to the lower part of the body, or feet. Used mainly in conjunction with beam angulation, meaning to direct the beam towards the feet.
Coronal plane: An imaginary line that divides the front and back of the head and trunk vertically. It is perpendicular to the median sagittal plane.
Cranial: Relating to the head. Used mainly in conjunction with beam angulation, meaning to direct the beam towards the head.
Craniocaudal: Mammographic term used when the breast is placed with its inferior aspect on the image receptor and the X-ray beam directed vertically to enter the breast on its uppermost surface, exiting inferiorly.

Decubitus: The patient is in a horizontal position. Used in conjunction with a qualifying term to indicate which aspect of the body is nearest the image receptor, as in 'lateral decubitus', 'prone decubitus'.
Dorsal: The back of the patient or body part; sometimes used instead of 'posterior'.
Dorsiflexion: Flexion of the hand at the wrist when the dorsum of the hand moves in a posterior direction, or flexion of the foot at the ankle when the dorsal aspect of the foot moves towards the ankle.
Dorsipalmar: The hand is placed with its palmar aspect on the image receptor.
Dorsiplantar: The foot is placed with its sole on the image receptor.
Dorsum: The back of the hand or the top of the foot.

Erect: The patient is standing or sitting, with the median sagittal and coronal planes vertical.
Eversion: Lateral flexion at the ankle joint, where the plantar aspect of the foot moves in a lateral direction. Excessive forced eversion can cause injury in the ankle or other joints.
Extension: Typically, effecting 'opening' or straightening of a joint. For example, the extended elbow will place the arm in a position where the forearm and humerus continue in the same plane. Lumbar or thoracic spine: the patient usually bends backwards. Cervical spine: the head is tipped backwards to lift the chin. Foot: the foot is moved at the ankle so that the toes point downwards or posteriorly (although this is usually referred to as plantar flexion).
External: On the outside/towards the outside/away from the median sagittal plane. Usually used in conjunction with describing rotation of a limb, when the big toes or thumbs are turned outwards, away from the trunk or median sagittal plane.
External auditory meatus: Surface marking used in radiography of the head (see Ch. 11).
External occipital protuberance: Surface marking used in radiography of the head (see Ch. 11).

Flexion: Typically, effecting 'closing' of a joint such as bending the knee or elbow. Can be described in conjunction with description of the direction of flexion, such as lateral/dorsal/palmar flexion for other body parts, such as the hands and feet. Lumbar or thoracic spine: the patient usually bends forwards but lateral flexion may also be described. Cervical spine: the head is bent forwards to tuck the chin down.
Focus film distance: When film is used, distance from the focal spot to the image receptor (known as source image distance in some countries).
Focus object distance: Distance from the focal spot to the body part (known as source object distance in some countries).
Focus receptor distance: Distance from the focal spot to the body part (known as source image distance in some countries).
Frankfurt/Frankfort plane: (see Anthropological baseline).
Fronto-occipital: Refers to positioning of the head, when the X-ray beam enters the frontal aspect and exits via the occiput.

Glabella: Surface marking used in radiography of the head (see Ch. 11).
Grid: Antiscatter device.

Image receptor: A plate, upon which X-radiation impinges and creates a latent image. Can be a film which is placed in a cassette, or a radiosensitive structure which converts the image digitally for reproduction on a display screen (see Ch. 1).

Inferior: Below or underneath.
Inferosuperior: A position where the inferior aspect of the body part is nearest the X-ray tube and the central ray passes through this aspect, exiting through the superior aspect. Mainly used in examination of limbs and the shoulder girdle.
Internal: On the inside/towards the inside/towards the median sagittal plane. Often used in conjunction with describing rotation of a limb, when the big toes or thumbs are turned inwards, towards the trunk or median sagittal plane.
Inversion: Medial flexion of the ankle joint, where the plantar aspect of the foot moves in a medial direction. Excessive forced inversion can cause injury in the ankle or other joints.

Lateral: The outermost side of the trunk or body part, furthest from the median sagittal plane. Can be used in description of rotation of limbs (see Rotation). Also a radiographic position/projection where one side of the trunk or body part faces the X-ray tube and the opposite side faces the IR.
Lateral oblique: Initially a lateral position, the body part is rotated towards the image receptor *or* the lateral patient position is maintained but a tube angle is employed.
Lateromedial: A position where the lateral aspect of the body part faces the X-ray tube and the central ray passes through this aspect, exiting via the medial aspect. Mainly used in mammography but can be used in some limb radiography to describe beam direction.
Left anterior oblique: An oblique position, when the anterior aspect of the left side lies nearer the image receptor than the right side.
Left posterior oblique: An oblique position, when the posterior aspect of the left side lies nearer the image receptor than the right side.
Lordosis/lordotic: The patient is leaning back.

Medial: Towards or nearest the median sagittal plane. Can be used in description of rotation of limbs (see Rotation).
Median sagittal plane: An imaginary line that divides the left and right sides of the head and trunk vertically, in the midline.
Mediolateral: A position where the medial aspect of the body part faces the X-ray tube and the central ray passes through this aspect, exiting via the lateral aspect. Mainly used in mammography but can be used in some limb radiography to describe beam direction.

Nasion: Surface marking used in radiography of the head (see Ch. 11).

Object film distance: When film is used, distance from the body part to the image receptor (known as object image distance in some countries).
Object receptor distance: Distance from the body part to the image receptor (known as object image distance in some countries).
Oblique: The body part position lies between the lateral and anteroposterior or posteroanterior positions. For hands and feet, the palm or sole is raised from the image receptor along the medial or lateral aspect.
Occipitofrontal: Refers to positioning of the head, when the X-ray beam enters the occipital aspect and exits via the forehead (frontal bone).
Occipitomental: Refers to positioning of the head, when the X-ray beam enters the occipital aspect and exits via the chin.
Orbitomeatal baseline: Baseline used for skull radiography (see Ch. 11).

Palmar: Relating to the palm of the hand.
Plantar: Relating to the sole of the foot.
Plantar flexion: Flexion of the foot at the ankle when the dorsal aspect of the foot moves away from the ankle.
Posterior: The back of the patient or body part, when the patient is in the anatomical position.
Posterior oblique: An oblique position, when the posterior aspect of the patient is nearest the image receptor *or* an anteroposterior position with an oblique angle applied in a lateral or medial direction.
Posteroanterior: A position where the posterior aspect of the patient faces the X-ray tube and the central ray passes through this aspect and exits through the anterior aspect.
Pronation: Used when referring to the position of the hand when it is placed palm down.
Prone: The patient is lying horizontally face down.

Right anterior oblique: An oblique position, when the anterior aspect of the right side lies nearer the image receptor than the left side.
Right posterior oblique: An oblique position, when the posterior aspect of the right side lies nearer the image receptor than the left side.
Rotation: Turning the trunk or head laterally in relationship to the median sagittal plane. External or lateral rotation: turning a limb when the hallux or thumb is turned outwards, away from the trunk or median sagittal plane. Internal or medial rotation: when the hallux or thumb is turned inwards, towards the trunk or median sagittal plane.

Semi-prone: One side of the patient is partly raised from the prone position, as in the anterior oblique position.
Semi-recumbent: The patient is leaning back, between the erect and supine positions.
Submentovertical: A position of the head where the beam enters below the chin and exits via the top of the skull (vertex).
Superior: Above or uppermost.
Superoinferior: A position where the superior aspect of the body part is nearest the X-ray tube and the central ray passes through this aspect, exiting through the inferior aspect. Mainly used in examination of limbs.
Supine: The patient is lying horizontally on their back.

Tilt: Tipping the trunk or head away from the median sagittal plane, anteriorly, posteriorly or laterally.

Index

Page numbers followed by "f" indicate figures, "t" indicate tables, and "b" indicate boxes.

Notes

All entries refer to plain X-radiography, unless another method has been indicated.

vs. indicates a comparison.

To save space in the index, the following abbreviations have been used:

AO – anterior oblique
AP – anteroposterior
CR – computed radiography
CT – computed tomography
DP – dorsiplantar or dorsipalmar
DPO – dorsiplantar or dorsipalmar oblique
DR – digital radiography
DXA – dual energy X-ray absorptiometry
FO – fronto-occipital
IVU – intravenous urography
LAO – left anterior oblique
LPO – left posterior oblique
MRI – magnetic resonance imaging
OF – occipitofrontal
OM – occipitomental
PA – posteroanterior
RNI – radionuclide imaging
RAO – right anterior oblique
RPO – right posterior oblique
SMV – submentovertical

A

D

I

J

K

L

U

V

W

X

Y

Z